AF837682

Forensic Histopathology

Reinhard B. Dettmeyer

Forensic Histopathology

Fundamentals and Perspectives

Second Edition

Springer

Reinhard B. Dettmeyer
University Hospital Giessen Institute of Forensic Medicine
Giessen
Germany

ISBN 978-3-030-08595-7 ISBN 978-3-319-77997-3 (eBook)
https://doi.org/10.1007/978-3-319-77997-3

Softcover re-print of the Hardcover 2nd edition 2018

Printed on acid-free paper

This Springer imprint is published by the registered company Springer International Publishing AG part of Springer Nature.
The registered company address is: Gewerbestrasse 11, 6330 Cham, Switzerland

Foreword to the Second Edition

In the first edition of his book, *Forensic Histopathology—Fundamentals and Perspectives*, Reinhard Dettmeyer expanded and deepened, very convincingly, the relevance of histomorphological investigation and diagnostics in forensic medicine. In this extended and revised second edition, he succeeds in creating a working basis, as well as a handbook, for the entire field of medical scientific forensics. It highlights the ever growing importance of expert histomorphological evidence. One can anticipate the beneficial outcome that expert opinions on fatalities that do not draw on histology will become a thing of the past. This is particularly apparent in the important border area of natural and unnatural damage, where pathology and forensics are closely linked and interrelated.

As such, this work by Reinhard Dettmeyer represents a real step forward in establishing the truth by forensic methods and, looking back at his own "histological past," it is a source of pleasure and satisfaction for the author of this foreword.

Hamburg, Germany
Spring 2018

Werner Janssen

Preface to the Second Edition

It is beyond dispute that cytology plays an important role in trace analysis, as does histopathology in cause-of-death determination; both also play an important role in the preparation of expert opinions on cause-of-death determination on behalf of the authorities and private individuals. This applies not only in general pathology but also in forensic medicine. The good acceptance of the first edition of *Forensic Histopathology—Fundamentals and Perspectives*, published in 2011, led to much predominantly positive feedback.

Compared with the first edition, this second edition largely closes gaps in the spectrum of frequent and classic histopathological findings relevant to cause of death, as well as rarer but nevertheless relevant findings. This covers, for instance, fatal amniotic fluid embolism, heroin-related anthrax infection, and ecstasy-induced malignant hyperthermia with rhabdomyolysis, as well as surprising and also rare findings such as sickle-cell anemia, ochronosis, and fatal hemorrhage in Osler-Weber-Rendu disease.

Data provided in tabular form on the histological determination of the age of findings have been supplemented; some new tables have been included, e.g., on the determination of fetal and neonatal age using lung histology; and a number of histological findings in iatrogenic injury have been added.

Additional comments can now be found on quality assurance and interpretation in the microscopic analysis of tissue sections, as well as remarks on investigations deemed important by the author in terms of their further scientific consideration. Although this revised second edition takes most histopathological findings encountered in daily routine into consideration, gaps will always remain; naturally, the reader continues to be referred to the relevant literature for a more in-depth analysis of specific questions.

The author has endeavored to incorporate the most recent literature (up to November 2017) relating to forensic histopathology in the reference lists of each chapter.

This second edition raises the hope that some of the feedback may lead to the pursuit of current issues within the framework of scientific and, in particular, immunohistochemical studies, while taking into consideration the necessary scientific standards in the technical application of stains and the interpretation of microscopic findings. Once again, the author welcomes feedback and suggestions of any kind.

Sincere thanks go to the "father" of forensic histology and forensic histopathology in Germany, Professor Dr. Werner Janssen, Director Emeritus of the Institute for Forensic Medicine at the University of Hamburg, for his willingness to also write a foreword to this second edition.

Some of the images contained in this work were created by the author at the University of Bonn's Forensic Medicine Department.

Giessen, Germany Reinhard B. Dettmeyer
Spring 2018

Acknowledgments

For their valuable support in the preparation of this second edition by permitting the use of images, my gratitude goes to Dr. med. S. Afram (Gronau, Germany), Dr. med. R. Amberg (Freiburg, Germany), Dr. med. C.G. Birngruber (Gießen, Germany), Dr. med. B. Busch† (Gießen, Germany), Dr. med. D. Farkäs (Kosice, Slovakia), Dr. med. I. Gerling (Kiel/Lübeck, Germany), Dr. med. C. Haag (Solingen, Germany), Prof. Dr. R. Kandolf† (Tübingen, Germany), Dr. med. J. Lang (Gießen, Germany), Dr. med. G. Lasczkowski (Gießen, Germany), Prof. Dr. J. Preuss-Wössner (Kiel/Lübeck, Germany), Dr. Dr. med. F. Ramsthaler (Homburg, Germany), Prof. Dr. med. M. Riße (Gießen, Germany), Prof. Dr. med. M. Schlamann (Gießen, Germany), Dr. K. Varchmin-Schultheiß (Münster, Germany), Prof. Dr. med. M. A. Verhoff (Frankfurt, Germany), Prof. em. Dr. med. G. Weiler (Gießen, Germany), and Dr. rer. nat. H. Wollersen (Gießen, Germany).

Again, I would like to thank our medical assistant, N. Weil, for the excellent conventional histological and immunohistochemical staining of numerous tissue sections, as well as M. Witte and I. Martytschan for the technical processing of the many images used in this book. Finally, my thanks go again to the translator, C. Schaefer (Heidelberg), for her work on the translation of the manuscript.

Contents

Abbreviations

α7-nAChR	α7-nicotinic acetylcholine receptor
β-APP	β-Amyloid precursor protein
ABC	Avidin–biotin complex
ACTH	Adrenocorticotropic hormone
AEC	Amino ethyl carbazole
AHA	American Heart Association
AIDS	Acquired immune deficiency Syndrome
AIS	Amniotic infection syndrome
AMH	Anti-Mullerian hormone
APAAP	Alkaline-phospatase-anti-alkaline-phosphatase
AQP5	Aquaporin-5
ARDS	Adults respiratory distress syndrome
ARVCM	Arrhythmogenic right-ventricular cardiomyopathy
ASS	Acetylsalicylic acid
AV	Adenovirus
AV node	Atrioventricular node
AVM	Arteriovenous malformation
AVN	Atrioventricular node
BALT	Bronchus-associated lymphoid tissue
BCG	Bacillus Calmette-Guérin
bFGf	Basic Fibroblast growth factor
BPD	Bronchopulmonary dysplasia
$C5b\text{-}9_{(m)}$	Monoclonal complement factor $C5b\text{-}9_{(m)}$; terminal complement complex
CAB	Chromotrope aniline blue
CAR	Coxsackie-adenovirus receptor
CBN	Contraction band necrosis
CCl_4	Tetrachloride carbon
CCR2	Chemokine receptor2 (CD192)
CCS	Cardiac conduction system
CD	Cluster of differentiation
CDC	Centers for disease control
cDNA	Complementary DNA
CK	Creatine kinase
CLSM	Confocal laser scanning microscopy
CMV	Cytomegalovirus
CNS	Central nervous system

CO	Carbon monoxide
CO-Hb	Carboxyhemoglobin
CPM	Central pontine myelinolysis
CSF	Colony stimulating factor
CSS	Churg-Strauss syndrome
CTE	Chronic traumatic encephalopathy
CVB	Coxsackie virus type B
CX3CR1	Fractalkine receptors, which mediate both leukocyte migration and adhesion
DAB	Diaminobenzidine
DAI	Diffuse axonal injury
DAO	Diaminoxidase determination
DCM	Dilative cardiomyopathy
DCMi	Dilative cardiomyopathy, inflammatory type
DIC	Disseminated intravascular coagulation
DIHS	Drug-induced hypersensitivity syndrome
DNA	Desoxyribonucleic acid
DRESS	Drug rash with eosinophilia and systemic symptoms
dUTP	Deoxyuridine triphosphate
E-605	Parathion
EBV	Epstein-Barr virus
ECG	Electrocardiogram
ECP	Eosinophil cationic protein
EDS	Ehlers-Danlos syndrome
EDX	Energy dispersive microanalysis
ELAM	Endothelial leukocyte adhesion molecule
EMB	Endomyocardial biopsy
EPC	Endothelial progenitor cells
Epo	Erythropoietin
ERCP	Endoscopic retrograde cholangiopancreaticography
ESRD	End stage renal disease
EV	Enterovirus
EvG	Elastica van Gieson
FFP3	Filtering face piece
Figs	Figures
FISH	Fluorescence in situ hybridisation
FMD	Fibromuscular dysplasia
FNH	Focal nodular hyperplasia
FSGS	Focal segmental glomerulosclerosis
FSH	Follicle-stimulating hormone
FWD	Fresh water drowning
GA1	Glutaric aciduria type 1
gcl	Ganglion cell layer
GFAP	Glial fibrillary acidic protein
GH	Growth hormone
GPA	Glycophorin A
H&E	Hematoxylin and eosin
HBA1c	Glycated hemoglobin A1c

HBcAG	Hepatitis B core antigen
HBFP	Hematoxylin basic fuchsin picric acid
HBsAG	Hepatitis B surface antigen
HBV	Hepatitis B virus
HCM	Hypertrophic cardiomyopathy
HCV	Hepatitis C virus
HELLP	Hemolysis, elevated liver enzymes, low platet count
hfp	High power field
HHSV	Human herpes simplex virus
HHT	Hereditary hemorrhagic telangiectasia
HIF-1-α	Hypoxia inducible factor 1-α
HIV	Human immunodeficiency virus
HIVAN	HIV-associated nephropathies
HLA	Human leukocyte antigen
HMD	Hyaline membrane disease
HPS	Hemophagocytic syndrome
HPV	Human papilloma virus
HRV	Human rhinovirus
hsp	Heat shock protein
HSPG	Heparan sulphate proteoglycans
HVR	Hypervariable region
ICAM	Intracellular adhesion molecule
IHE	Ischemic heart disease
IHSS	Idiopathic hypertrophic subaortic stenosis
IL	Interleukine
inl	Inner nuclear layer
ipl	Inner plexiform layer
ISH	In situ hybridisation
LAB	Labeled avidin biotin
LALT	Larynx-associated lymphoid tissue
LCA	Leukocyte common antigen/left coronary artery
LE	Lupus erythematodes
LFB	Luxol fast blue
LH	Luteinizing hormone
LSAB	Labeled streptavidin biotin
LV	Left ventricle
LVNC	Left ventricular non-compaction cardiomyopathy
MALT	Mucosa-associated lymphoid tissue
MBP	Major basic protein
MCAD	Medium-chain acyl-coA dehydrogenase deficiency
MDMA	Methylenedioxymethamphetamine
MFD	Myo fibrillary degeneration
MGG	May-Grünwald-Giemsa stain
MHC	Major histocompatibility complex
MIB	Marker of cell proliferation
MLNS	Mucocutaneous lymph node syndrome
MMP	Metalloproteinases
MPGN	Membrane-proliferative glomerulonephritis

MPO	Myeloperoxidase
MRP	Mucin carbohydrate
MRSA	Methicillin-resistant Staphylococcus aureus
MTX	Methotrexate
NAHI	Non-accidental head injury
NAI	Non-accidental injury
NAME	National Association of Medical Examiners
NASD	Naphthol AS-D chloracetate esterase stain
NCBI	National Center for Biotechnology Information
NCCM	Non-compaction cardiomyopathy
nfl	Nerve fiber layer
NFP	Neuro filament protein
NMS	Neuroleptic malignant syndrome
NP57	Neutrophil elastase
NSAI	Non-steroidal anti-inflammatory agents
NSAR	Non-steroidal antirheumatics
NSE	Neuroendocrine specific enolase
OHSS	Ovarian hyperstimulation syndrome
onl	Outer nuclear layer
opl	Outer plexiform layer
OPSI	Overwhelming postsplenectomy infection
PAS	Periodic acid-Schiff reaction
PBS	Phosphate buffered saline
pc	Photoreceptors
PCAM	Platelet endothelial cell adhesion molecule
PCR	Polymerase chain reaction
PDS	Pokkuri death syndrome
PECAM	Platelet endothelial cell adhesion molecule
PGM-1	Phosphoglucomutase
PNEC	Pulmonary neuroendocrine cells
PPD	Paraphenylenediamine
PRL	Prolactin
PTAH	Phosphotungstic acid-hematoxylin
PVB19	Parvovirus B19
REM	Raster electron microscope
RNA	Ribonucleic acid
SAH	Subarachnoid hemorrhage
SBS	Shaken baby syndrome
SCD	Sudden cardiac death
SDH	Subdural hemorrhage
SEM	Scanning electron microscope
SES	Silicone embolism syndrome
SICM	Stress induced cardiomyopathy
SID	Sudden infant death
SIDS	Sudden infant death syndrome
SIRS	Systemic inflammatory response syndrome
SIRT	Selective internal radiotherapy
SMC-actin	Smooth muscle cell-actin

ssDNA	Single-stranded DNA
STN	Sialyl-Tn
STR	Short tandem repeats
SUDEP	Sudden unexpected death in epilepsy
SWD	Salt water drowning
TBI	Traumatic brain injury
TCA	Tooth cementum annulation
TdT	Terminal deoxynucleotidyl transferase
TEP	Total endoprosthesis
TGF-β	Transforming growth factor-β
TH	Tyrosine hydroxylase
TNF-α	Tumor necrosis factor-α
TSH	Thyroid-stimulating hormone
TTR	Transthyretin
TUNEL	Tdt-mediated dUTP-biotin neck labeling
TURP	Transurethral resection of the prostate
VCAM	Vascular cell adhesion molecule
VEGF	Vascular endothelial growth factor
vitr	Vitreous
VLA	Very late antigen
VMAT2	Vesicular monoamine transporter 2
VP	Viral protein
WBS	Williams-Beuren syndrome
WFS	Waterhouse-Friderichsen syndrome
WHO	World Health Organization
XIST ISH	X-inactive specific transcript RNA in-situ hybridization
ZnCP-I	Zinc coproporphyrin-I

1 Introduction

The importance of morphological investigations in the administration of justice was highlighted over two decades ago (Janssen 1988), as was the necessity for rules governing the performance of medicolegal autopsies, for which guidelines have since been set out (Brinkmann 1999). The purpose of a medicolegal autopsy is to identify and classify unnatural deaths and to establish facts for further inferences. In recent decades, in most parts of Europe, public prosecutors have increased the threshold for having a medicolegal autopsy performed, and autopsy rates have decreased. But a medicolegal autopsy might not only be essential for the recognition and correct investigation of a crime, it can also identify, e.g., a genetic disorder, and thus help affected relatives (Klintschar et al. 2009).

The forensic community has been unable to agree to date on the need to perform histological examination at forensic autopsy. Some authors want microscopic examination only to be used as needed but not as a matter of routine (Molina et al. 2007). Others conclude that there is a considerable discrepancy rate between macroscopic and microscopic findings in forensic autopsy. Histology is an important feature regarding autopsy quality and is essential to confirm, refine, or refute macroscopic findings (Madadin et al. 2017; de la Grandmaison et al. 2010). However, the usefulness of systematic histological examination was demonstrated in a recently published prospective study carried out on 428 autopsy cases (de la Grandmaison et al. 2010):

- A mechanism of death not shown by gross anatomic findings was discovered by histology in about 40% of cases.
- The cause of death was established by histology alone in 8.4% of cases.
- Microscopic findings affected the manner of death in 13% of cases.
- Histology provided additional information on prior medical condition of the deceased in approximately 49% of cases.
- Traumatic lesions were better documented by histology in approximately 22% of cases.

There is no doubt that systematic standard histology for the main organs should be used in routine forensic autopsies (de la Grandmaison et al. 2010). In addition, histological investigations may be necessary in cases of multiple interchanging of tissue samples (Banaschak et al. 2000). Needless to say, there are numerous other histological, immunohistochemical, and cytologic questions. Many diseases can explain sudden unexpected death, including specific syndromes with interesting microscopic findings. Histological findings in a number of syndromes will be presented and discussed here. However, for more detailed information on the multitude of syndromes and rare infections, the reader is referred to the specialist literature, e.g.:

- Williams syndrome or Williams–Beuren syndrome (WBS), which can cause sudden death in children and young adults in particular

R. B. Dettmeyer, *Forensic Histopathology*, https://doi.org/10.1007/978-3-319-77997-3_1

(Wessel et al. 2004; Krous et al. 2008; Suárez-Mier and Morentin 1999; Bird et al. 1996), especially in association with anesthetics (Gupta et al. 2010).
- Prader–Willi syndrome, first described in 1956, which can lead to sudden death particularly in childhood (Pomara et al. 2005).
- Lethal leptospirosis (Morbus Weil). Leptospirosis is an infectious disease caused by pathogenic bacteria of the genus *Leptospira*. Only 5–10% of patients with leptospirosis present with the icteric form, often complicated by multiorgan involvement such as meningitis, acute renal failure, myocarditis, and pulmonary symptoms (alveolar hemorrhage and acute respiratory distress syndrome) (Luchini et al. 2008).

Forensic autopsies often include histological analysis; however, this is not always the case. The standards for the practice of forensic pathology were proposed by the Forensic Pathology Committee of the College of American Pathologists. According to this proposal, the extent of histological examination of autopsy tissues is at the discretion of the pathologist (Randall et al. 1998). The Forensic Autopsy Performance Standards of the National Association of Medical Examiners (NAME) requires histological examination in cases with no gross anatomic cause of death unless remains are skeletonized (NAME 2006).

Although there are studies on the value of histological examination (Molina et al. 2007; Langlois 2006; Bernardi et al. 2005; Roulson et al. 2005; Zaitoun and Fernandez 1998), the usefulness of systematic histology in forensic autopsies should be determined irrespective of cause and manner of death (de la Grandmaison et al. 2010). Naturally, autopsy samples must be sufficient in quantity and quality. In the future, autopsy protocols and guidelines should include conventional histology and – where necessary – immunohistological techniques.

Autopsy investigations in forensic medicine raise numerous diagnostic questions, much like those seen in general pathology. Even evidence of a natural death can be of forensic significance, e.g., in the context of exculpating a suspect. Moreover, it provides relatives with an explanation for the often sudden and unexpected death of a person.

Thus, it is of little surprise that histomorphological diagnosis is to a great extent identical to diagnosis in both general and specialized pathology. Nevertheless, there are numerous specific forensic questions and histopathological findings which are more often, or exclusively, significant in forensic medicine. In addition to the special questions faced in forensic practice, the fact that frequently autolytic or markedly putrefied tissue requires investigation presents particular challenges in terms of diagnosis.

The Value of Forensic Histopathology Currently in European forensic medicine, histological organ and tissue investigations are carried out or ordered by the authorities (Ferrara et al. 2010) in only around 50% of all autopsies; enzyme and immunohistochemical methods are used even less frequently, while in situ hybridization, molecular pathological investigations, and electron microscopic diagnosis are less common again. In such situations, it is essential to emphasize the usefulness of conventional histological microscopy in the first instance, in the hope that it also underpins advanced diagnosis with the other methods. After all, there are numerous diseases which can only be diagnosed by means of microscopic investigations, including not only viral myocarditis but also extremely rare diseases, e.g., Williams–Campbell syndrome as a cause of death in neonates (Bohnert et al. 2003), and other relatively rare diseases that are attracting general scientific interest in terms of investigation and research. It is precisely such unusual and sudden fatalities due to rare causes that need to be investigated and elucidated by forensic pathologists (e.g., Ondruschka et al. 2016; Tong et al. 2016; Dean et al. 2014; Duan et al. 2013; Roll et al. 2009). Thus it is surprising that the discussion on the value of histological investigations continues (Byard and Winskog 2012; Cordner 2012; Davis 2012; Hunsaker 2012; Lau 2012; Pollanen 2012; Fronczek et al. 2014; de Giorgio and Vetrugo 2014). In contrast to this, studies,

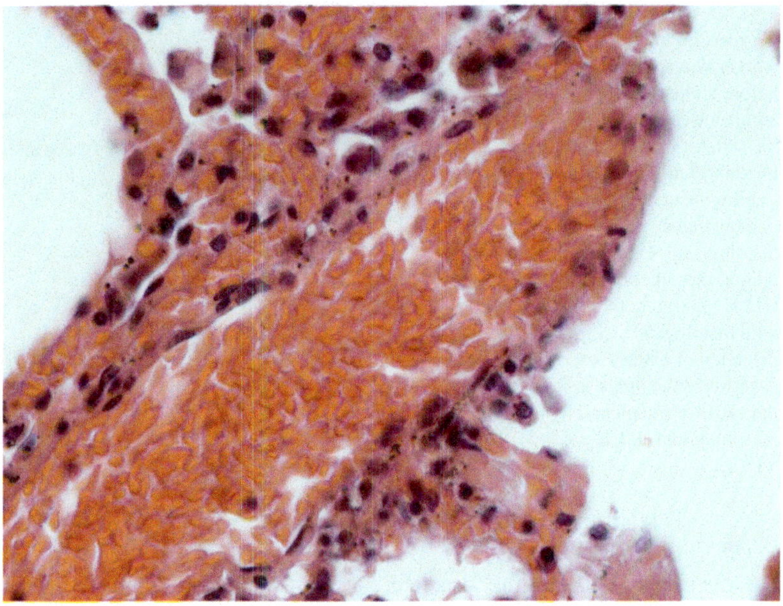

Fig. 1.1 Lung tissue showing acute blood congestion and sickle-shaped red blood cells in sickle cell anemia (H&E ×400)

overview articles, and a glance in the specialist publications on forensic medicine give examples of the benefits of forensic histopathology, even for the detection of diseases such as sickle cell anemia, which affects around 300 million people worldwide (Fig. 1.1; Podduturi and Guileyardo 2015). Moreover, numerous publications in specialist forensic medical journals demonstrate the benefits of histology in many – although by no means all – cases (de la Grandmaison et al. 2010; Dettmeyer et al. 2013; Dettmeyer 2014; Dettmeyer 2016).

Traditionally, forensic histopathology is an integral part of diagnostics not only to establish causes of death but also to answer a multitude of other legally relevant questions:

- Histomorphological chronology of a disease
- Postmortem histological findings as evidence of an intravital event, i.e., evidence of vital status
- Histomorphological determination of age, e.g., of a myocardial infarct, an injury, or a skin wound
- Classification of microscopic findings in the context of patient history, postmortem biochemical and chemico-toxic findings, as well as results of criminological investigations (e.g., into long-term i.v. drug abuse, condition following recurrent trauma in cases of ultimately lethal child abuse, deep vein thrombosis following lower leg fractures caused by traffic accidents, powder-burn particles at the site of bullet entry, determining the age of craniocerebral trauma, etc.)
- Microscopic identification of tissue fragments and cells for advanced trace analysis
- Microscopic detection of textile fibers carried into the bullet track in order to differentiate between shot entry and shot exit localization
- Histocytological detection of cells, e.g., spermatozoa following sexual offenses, or for molecular genetic analysis
- Histomorphological diagnosis to clarify lethal outcomes in occupational diseases, e.g., lethal asbestos-related pleural mesothelioma (Woitowitz et al. 1986; Churg 1982) (Fig. 1.2).

Conventional histology, including standard staining methods, has formed the basis of microscopic diagnosis for decades. Based on routine histology – and depending on the questions requiring clarification – enzyme histochemical and immunohistochemical methods for the detection of fine tissue structures or specific antigens

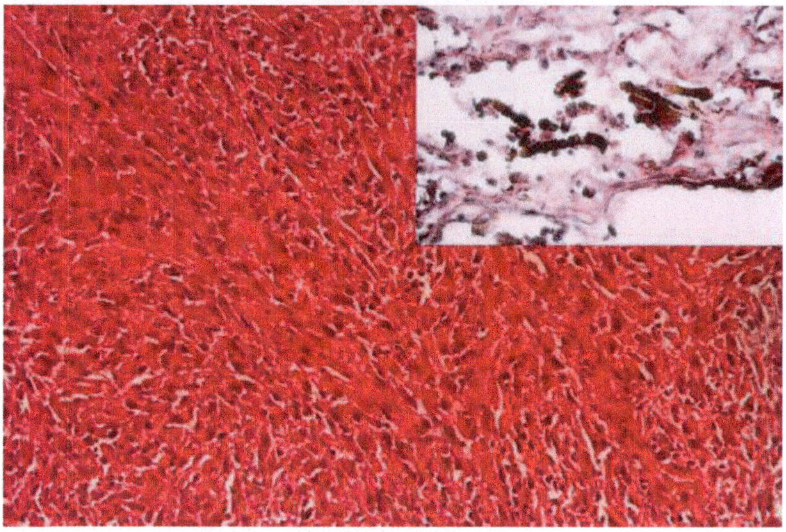

Fig. 1.2 The body of a 57-year-old metal worker was suspended before cremation. The autopsy was ordered by the statutory accident insurance/employer's liability insurance and demonstrated histologically extensive pleural mesothelioma (H&E ×200) together with histological detection of extensive asbestos in the lungs as the cause of the pleural mesothelioma (H&E ×400)

are considered. In routine practice, decisions need to be made regarding which methods will lead to both scientifically and legally relevant insights. Thus, a good knowledge of histology and immunohistochemistry is essential when writing expert opinions on causality and advising judicial bodies (police, public prosecutors, courts) or insurance institutions (private life or accident insurers, employer's liability insurance associations acting as accident insurers), in terms of which diagnostic measures are required following autopsy.

However, not all conventional histological or immunohistochemical investigations are essential; fine tissue diagnosis often yields precisely the additional information or indications which, in the context of individual cases, may enable a sufficiently plausible expert opinion to satisfy the strict standards of proof in criminal law or make a crucial contribution when convincing a court of law.

The focus in forensic medical practice is not, in the first instance, on answering questions in terms of correlating autopsy findings with a clinically documented disease course or particular aspects of tumor pathology. The primary goal in forensic practice is to either prove or exclude effects on the human body, whereby general processes (e.g., postmortem autolysis, putrefaction, decomposition) and final reactions of the organism (e.g., micromorphological signs of shock of varying causes, final chyme aspiration) need to be differentiated from specific, forensically relevant damage: effects of trauma, gunshot wounds, effects of heat (scalds and burns) and cold (death due to hypothermia, freeze), death due to strangulation, choking, drowning, and/or micromorphologically detectable (lethal) acute or chronic intoxication or indications thereof.

In addition, there is a wide spectrum of histologically and immunohistochemically diagnosable causes of sudden unexpected death from natural causes; infections in particular should be mentioned in this context, whereby in forensic medical practice rare infections are seen even in Germany, such as malaria, mumps, or bacterial and viral meningoencephalitis which remained undiagnosed in life.

The broadness of the diagnostic spectrum combined with the diagnostic questions faced in each individual case prevents a comprehensive – or even conclusive – picture of histological, enzymatic, and immunohistochemical diagnosis. Therefore, any description of histomorphological diagnosis in forensic medicine can and should relate to basic principles, deal with classical findings, and highlight options for further microscopic diagnosis which may yield additional information in some cases. A higher rate of autopsy tissue samples used in histological work-up is always associated with a higher yield of information.

Thus, in terms of tissue sampling for diagnosis, it is necessary at the outset to establish whether:

- Samples were chosen appropriately at the time of autopsy in terms of localization.
- The fixative chosen is appropriate for the diagnostic question.
- Fixation time still permits promising diagnosis.
- Tissue samples chosen for microscopic investigations are sufficiently representative.
- Tissue sections are technically sound.
- Avoidable artifacts are precluded when producing the tissue section.
- In staining, faultless representation of the structures to be analyzed is possible.

Needless to say, a sufficiently powerful microscope should be available, as well as the opportunity to consult with colleagues.

Although tissue samples in paraffin blocks and prepared tissue sections are associated with automatic documentation and storage of findings, extending the case-related documentation by printed or digitally stored findings should be considered. In particular, the stability of staining methods, primarily immunohistochemical staining, can be limited, such that the possibility of making later findings (after several years) is excluded.

Experience with Microscopy Only lay people are under the impression that, following staining, a look into the microscope is sufficient to observe findings and directly reach a diagnosis.

In actual fact, it is true to say:

The investigator can only correctly interpret those microscopic findings which he/she knows and recognizes.

In the absence of microscopy experience, misjudgments even in the evaluation of staining quality are unavoidable, leading necessarily to incorrect diagnosis. Although microscopic findings are frequently available, they are wrongly classified due to a lack of experience in microscopy. Significant interobserver variations can be explained, at least in part, in this way.

For these reasons, reciprocal checking and discussion at the microscope is all the more important in routine diagnostics, much as it is in microscopic investigations in the context of scientific studies. Inexperienced doctoral students generally need to be thoroughly familiarized with the problems of microscopic diagnosis. This applies not only to evaluating whether staining has been successful but also to recognizing pathological findings.

In forensic medicine in particular, primarily autoptic cell and tissue samples are investigated, ranging from cells and tissues which have undergone mildly autolytic changes to samples demonstrating marked autolysis, putrefaction, proliferation, as well as colonization by microbiological organisms. Thus, it should come as no surprise that cell and tissue structures which are clearly and ideally represented using staining techniques are not always encountered in microscopic findings:

The microscopic diagnosis of autolytic and putrefied cells and tissue requires a particularly high level of experience in microscopy.

In addition to the information on the most important standard staining methods and most useful immunohistochemical techniques, typical errors and artifacts arising during the preparation and evaluation of tissue samples are discussed, as well as the need to correctly select and evaluate structures intended for microanatomic analysis (Chap. 2).

Immunohistochemistry Current developments in immunohistochemical diagnosis for forensic purposes need to be considered. However, findings obtained under experimental conditions in immunohistochemical diagnosis and found under optimal technical and methodical conditions often cannot be reliably reproduced in routine forensic medical practice. This applies, for example, to the immunohistochemical determination of injury age.

Conventional histology remains the basis for determining the age of post-traumatic findings. At the same time, while forensic institutes and forensic physicians have at best laboratory equipment for conventional histological staining at their disposal, this is generally not true for special enzymatic histochemical or immunohistochemical diagnostic equipment. For this reason, the focus of information here will remain on conventional histological diagnosis while providing examples of and recommendations for further diagnostic options.

Recommendations on performing histological or immunohistochemical investigations include the following points (de la Grandmaison et al. 2010):

- Injuries found at autopsy should be sampled for histological study.
- In sudden cardiac death, early diagnosis of acute myocardial ischemia by immunohistochemistry should include myoglobin, desmin, cardiac troponin I, and the C5b-$9_{(m)}$ complex (Dettmeyer 2009, Campobasso et al. 2008).
- In closed head trauma, diffuse axonal injury (DAI) can be detected using β-amyloid precursor protein expression (Sheriff et al. 1994).
- For age estimation of skin wounds, immunohistochemical markers such as collagens, fibronectin, adhesion molecules, inflammatory cytokines, and chemokines may be helpful (Cecchi 2010; Kondo 2007).

Thus, this book aims to outline the basic principles and highlight the possibilities of diagnostics. It should be an aid in the decision-making process regarding type and extent of histological and immunohistochemical diagnosis, from sample selection to microscopic diagnosis. Furthermore, basic scientific studies are required on the value of individual diagnostic techniques in histology and in particular immunohistochemistry, including the application of new immunohistochemical markers in forensic investigations, e.g., basic fibroblast growth factor (bFGF) (Wang et al. 2009), P-selection (Nogami et al. 2000), or hypoxia-inducible factor-1α (HIF-1α) (Zhu et al. 2008).

In addition, it should be mentioned that advances in molecular biology have provided a procedure to investigate genetic bases of diseases that might be present with sudden death – so-called molecular pathology (Maeda et al. 2010).

Organization The organization chosen for this book is intended to cover the spectrum of frequent questions and classical findings encountered at autopsy with strong emphasis on general and specialized pathology while avoiding detailed repetition of self-evident findings. At numerous points in the text, the reader is referred to the relevant literature not only on forensic pathology and neuropathology. In addition to the effects of various types of violent trauma (Chap. 3), forensic pathology covers toxin- and drug-related histopathological findings, including the effects of alcohol (Chaps. 4, 5, and 6). Electricity, heat, and cold as causes of death require particular attention (Chaps. 7 and 8). In addition, cardiac causes of death are of particular interest in forensic pathology, whether resulting from embolisms (Chap. 9) or directly from cardiac or cardiovascular diseases (Chap. 13). Specific vascular and metabolic diseases can explain sudden death and therefore warrant particular attention in forensic pathology (Chap. 14). The histopathologically verifiable estimation of injury and skin wound age is of great forensic interest (Chap. 10), likewise the relevance of aspiration and inhalation of foreign substances to the time of death (Chap. 11) and the histological possibilities of diagnosing identity and evaluating osteological findings (Chap. 12). Primary and secondary infections by bacteria, viruses, and fungi, as well as septic processes, are very important in forensic autopsy and subsequent microscopy investigations (Chap. 15), while histopathological findings in endocrine organs are less frequently revealed as causes of death (Chap. 16). Autopsy in stillbirths, infants, and children are consistently required to identify not only a possible involvement of trauma in the cause of death but also any preexisting disease: the spectrum ranges from pathological lesions in the placenta and amniotic fluid infection as causes of intrauterine death to the phenomenon of sudden infant death syndrome (SIDS) and rare diseases – some undiagnosed prior to autopsy – which cannot be exhaustively investigated here, thus necessitating a focus on the most significant and frequently observed findings in such cases (Chap. 17). Trace analysis requires cytological diagnosis of biological materials on, e.g., textiles, objects, or smear samples to identify spermatozoa following sexual offenses (Chap. 18). A particular challenge faced almost exclusively in forensic medicine is the macroscopic and microscopic investigation of corpses following long postmortem intervals or exhumation, making a discussion of the possibilities offered by microscopy diagnosis an important contribution to the book (Chap. 19). As for the broad field of forensic neuropathology, however, only a limited number of frequent and particularly significant findings encountered in routine forensic medicine will be discussed (Chap. 20); the reader is referred to the relevant specialist literature for more detailed information.

References In view of the wealth of publications, a selection of references which would serve as a starting point for further research is needed to be made. Although conventional histological staining forms the essential and indispensible basis of diagnosis, care was taken to include recent scientific studies in the selection of references. This is intended to support the value of further histological and immunohistochemical investigations and to encourage case management, where diagnostic information gained from microscopy is indispensible. Primarily, publications in specialist forensics journals have been taken into account.

1.1 Microscopic Examinations and Medical Malpractice Cases

Forensic pathologists are often confronted with iatrogenic findings or undesired and unavoidable side effects of medical interventions, e.g., a lethal course in ovarian hyperstimulation syndrome (OHSS). OHSS is an iatrogenic disorder arising subsequent to ovulation induction or ovarian hyperstimulation for assisted reproduction techniques, which can lead to, e.g., adult respiratory distress syndrome (ARDS) as a cause of death (Fineschi et al. 2006). Uncommon histological findings at autopsy due to intramuscular administration of extended release drugs have also been observed (Hecht and Lamprecht 2010).

Contrary to public perception, autopsy investigations – depending on the country in question – are increasingly concerned with the clarification of medical malpractice cases. According to own (broad and varied) experience, histological investigations can form a vital basis for forensic expert opinions in cases of medical malpractice (Dettmeyer and Preuß 2009; Dettmeyer et al. 1998, 2004, 2005, 2006; Dettmeyer and Madea 1999), e.g., in cases of lethal infection resulting from nursing errors involving decubitus ulcers and purulent osteomyelitis (Türk et al. 2003, Tsokos et al. 2000).

Therefore, by way of illustration, case studies in which microscopic diagnosis played a decisive role in clarifying clinically unexplained disease courses and managing medical malpractice cases will be presented.

Case 1
Lethal hemorrhage 7 days after tonsillectomy in a 12-year-old boy. A suppurative, abscessed arterial vascular wall in the tonsillar bed could be identified as the origin of hemorrhage, thus explaining the acuteness of death (Fig. 1.3).

Case 2
A sprightly 82-year-old female patient collapsed in front of an X-ray screen during a chest radiograph, fell, and suffered head injury. Immediate resuscitation efforts were unsuccessful. Relatives alleged that the patient should have been supported by a personnel during the X-ray examination and that she had died as a result of her fall. No cause of death could be identified macroscopically at autopsy. Histologically, however, massive cardiovascular amyloidosis with amyloid plaques in the myocardium was found to be the cause of sudden cardiac death (Fig. 1.4).

Case 3
A case of death on the operating table during bronchoscopy and biopsy of a small pulmonary nodule, which lead to continuous hemorrhage. The 54-year-old patient aspirated blood and asphyxiated (so-called hemorrhagic emphysema). Histology showed the pulmonary nodule to be a metastasis of a well-vascularized clear-cell renal

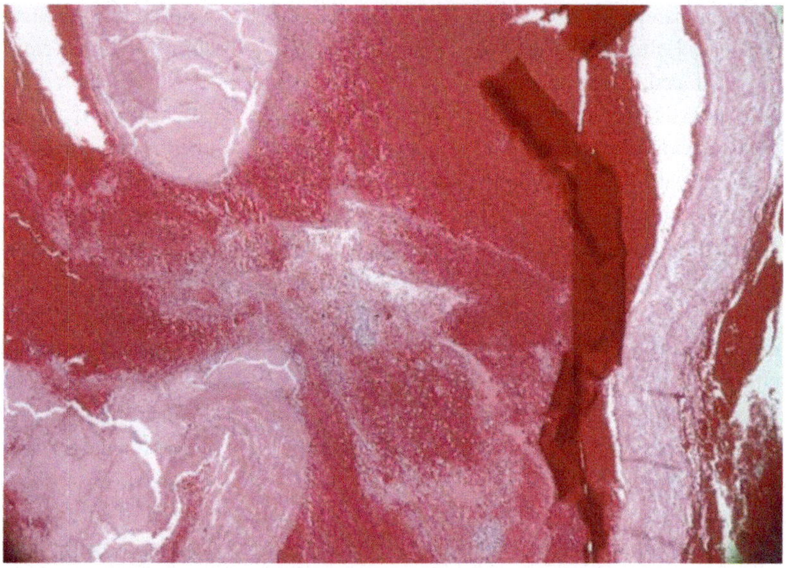

Fig. 1.3 A medical malpractice case: lethal hemorrhage 7 days following tonsillectomy in a 12-year-old boy with circumscribed suppurative melting of an arterial vascular wall in the tonsillar bed proven histologically (H&E ×40)

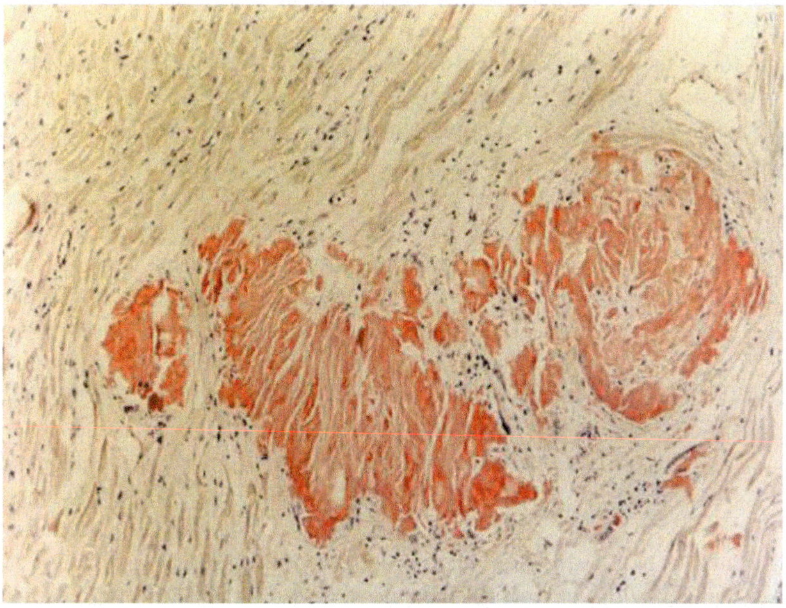

Fig. 1.4 Histologically, extensive cardiovascular amyloidosis with multiple amyloid plaques in the myocardium was seen with Congo red staining, as well as surrounding interstitial fibrosis in restrictive cardiomyopathy (×200)

carcinoma (Fig. 1.5). The patient had been made aware of the risk of hemorrhage prior to bronchoscopy.

Case 4

A 73-year-old woman with a fresh femoral neck fracture suffered acute asystole in the Palacos phase during total endoprosthesis. The decedent's relatives maintained that an error had been made during surgery. No cause of death could be found macroscopically. Histologically, a massive fat and bone marrow embolism in lung tissue was identified as the cause of death; a bone marrow embolism was also found in the myocardium (Fig. 1.6).

Case 5

As a rare complication during and after transurethral resection of the prostate (TURP), large quantities of irrigation fluid can be absorbed through periprostatic venous sinuses into the vascular compartment, causing cardiovascular

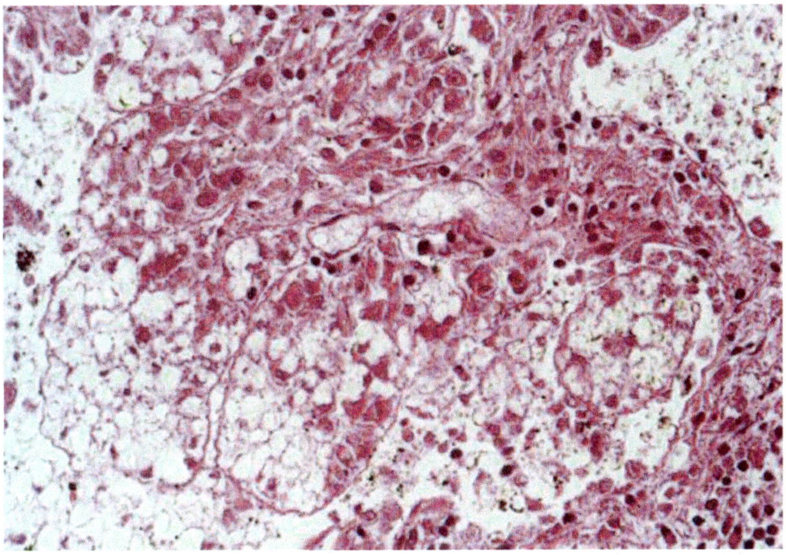

Fig. 1.5 Lethal aspiration of blood following bronchoscopic biopsy from a small node in the lung area suspicious for tumor involvement. Metastasis of a partially clear-cell, well-vascularized renal cell carcinoma was proven histologically (H&E ×400)

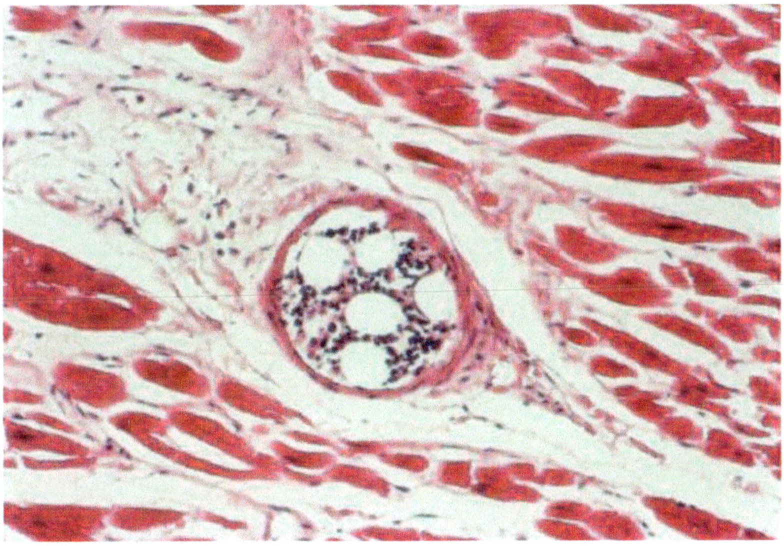

Fig. 1.6 Histologically proven intramyocardial bone marrow embolism, according to clinical information, acute intraoperative asystole occurred in the Palacos phase during femoral head endoprosthesis (H&E ×200)

and central nervous symptoms. The present case involved precisely this type of irrigation fluid absorption through the venous vascular system causing "fluid lung" (also known as TUR syndrome). The patient experienced a phase of hypoxia and died shortly thereafter. The relatives assumed that the patient had been insufficiently monitored during surgery. Histologically, massively fibrosed and calcified veins of the prostatic plexus were seen with barely collapsible tubular lumens, thereby favoring irrigation fluid absorption (Fig. 1.7) (Dettmeyer et al. 1999; Goel et al. 1992).

Case 6

The patient developed severe lethal sepsis within 24 h after liposuction. Histologically, extensive phlegmonous-suppurative panniculitis was found in the area around a puncture site (Fig. 1.8), while signs of shock were seen at autopsy. Fat embolism should also be considered in cases of sudden unexpected death following liposuction (Platt et al. 2002; Schmidt et al. 2001, 2002).

Case 7

Cytostatic drugs can have severe side effects, leading in particular to liver changes. In rare

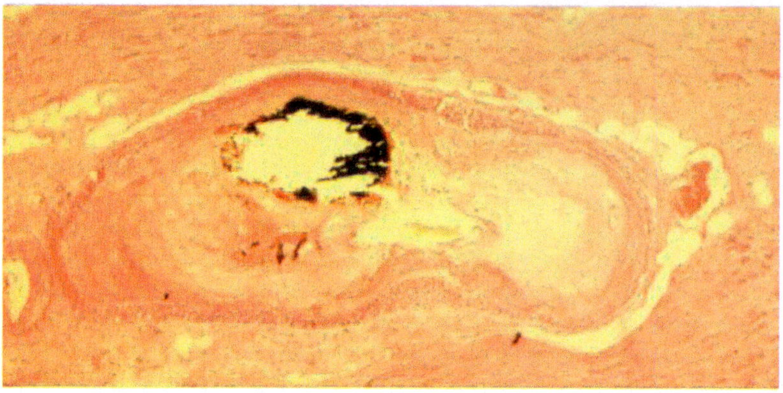

Fig. 1.7 "Fluid lung" resulting from absorption of irrigation fluid through surgically opened veins with calcified walls of the prostatic venous plexus during prostate surgery – TUR syndrome. Largely sclerotized periprostatic vessels (phlebosclerosis) with wall calcification and a narrow residual lumen (H&E ×100)

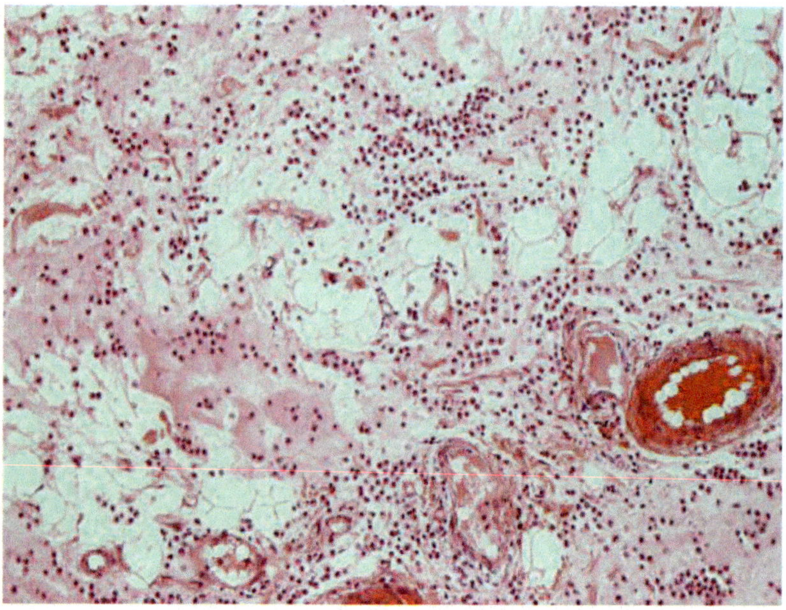

Fig. 1.8 Extensive phlegmonous-suppurative panniculitis in subcutaneous abdominal fatty tissue following liposuction and subsequent lethal sepsis (H&E ×100)

cases, cytostatic drug administration can lead to death. Dosage errors and inappropriate methods of administration are relevant in medical malpractice cases. Following inadvertent intrathecal injection of the cytostatic drug vincristine in a patient with acute lymphatic leukemia, the patient died. Extensive necrosis of spinal cord nerve tissue was seen histologically (Dettmeyer et al. 2001) (Fig. 1.9).

Although further findings following treatment errors have been described, not all can be mentioned here. There are only scant reports in the literature on accidental intravenous injection of enteral feeds leading to death, which is indeed an extremely rare complication (Fechner et al. 2002; Stellato et al. 1984; Casewell and Philpott-Howard 1983). In such cases, foreign materials can be found histologically in the pulmonary

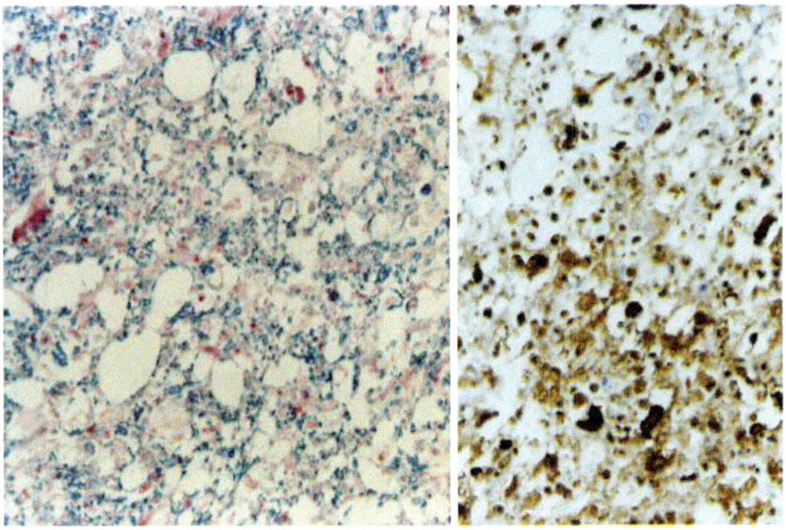

Fig. 1.9 Histomorphological finding in spinal cord tissue following inadvertent intrathecal administration of vincristine in a patient with acute lymphatic leukemia: degeneration of myelin and axons accompanied by a pseudocystic transformation (Luxol fast blue ×200) and immunohistochemical demonstration of neurofilament aggregates (×200)

arteries up to the peripheral branches and in small bronchial arteries and veins, as well as in renal, hepatic, and pancreatic arteries. This foreign material is also visible using polarized light.

1.2 Tissue Damage Due to Iatrogenic Interventions

Adverse side effects or damage can be caused in the context of medical or nursing measures without these necessarily representing errors in care or treatment. The spectrum ranges from vocal cord hemorrhage due to intubation (see Fig. 3.29), bleeding, infections, and resuscitation-related fractures to rare, undetected fatal side effects.

1.2.1 Silicone Implant Leakage

As a general rule, implanted foreign material, e.g., silicone breast implants, can leak into surrounding soft tissue (Fig. 1.10). This can cause considerable fibrosis in the area of the leaked silicone particles. This does not necessarily lead to the embolic spread of silicone particles, as reported for silicone oil, i.e., silicone embolism syndrome (SES) (see Chap. 9, Sect. 9.2.5).

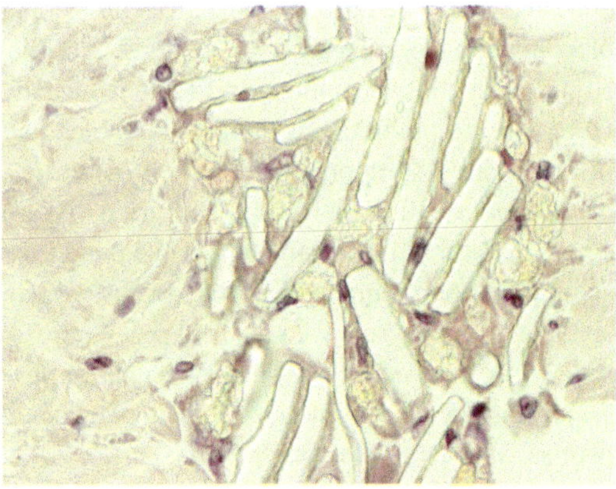

Fig. 1.10 Silicone deposited in the fiber capsule of a ruptured silicone breast implant (H&E ×400)

1.2.2 Iatrogenic Fistulas

In rare cases, tracheoesophageal or tracheo-aortic fistulas can develop at the lower edge of a

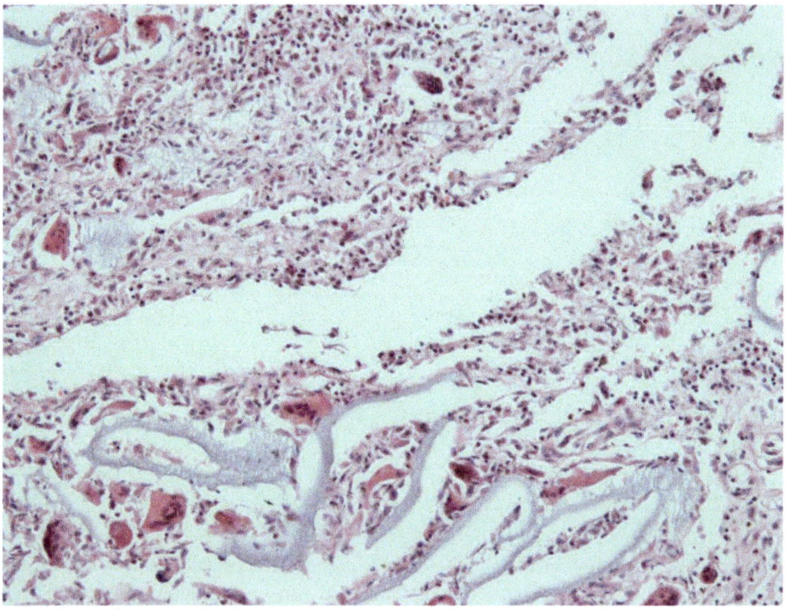

Fig. 1.11 Nonspecific, chronic, granulating, foreign body-reactive, and fistulating inflammation from the lower edge of a tracheal tube to the wall of the aortic arch in the form of a tracheal-aortic fistula with acute fatal hemorrhage in the upper and lower airways, blood aspiration, and hemorrhagic emphysema (H&E ×100)

respiration tube after it has been in place for several weeks; in the case of the latter, acute fatal bleeding into the upper airways occurs (Fig. 1.11). However, malignant tumors and their metastatic spread are a more frequent cause of fatal bleeding in the upper respiratory tract, with erosion of a blood vessel and acute blood aspiration (Byard 2014). As part of this, aspiration-related and final acute pulmonary emphysema may occur, which, similar to emphysema aquosum (see Chap. 3, Fig. 3.14), is referred to as hemorrhagic emphysema. Iatrogenically induced aorto-esophageal fistulas and fatal bleeding (Chan et al. 2017; Farkaš et al. 2015; Hadžisejdić et al. 2012), a ruptured aortic aneurysm in the esophageal lumen (Ambepitiya et al. 2010), and an aorto-duodenal fistula (Williams et al. 2015) and a fatal broncho-vascular fistula after lobectomy (Hinderberger et al. 2017) have also been described.

1.2.3 Decubitus Ulcers

Decubitus ulcers at various sites are relatively common. Ulcers of this kind may be present for long periods of time in bedridden, multimorbid patients (arterio-/arteriolosclerosis, diabetes, post-chemotherapy status, consumptive disorders, etc.) without the ulcers having any relevance in terms of cause of death.

However, large ulcers in particular, e.g., sacral ulcers, can prompt nursing malpractice claims, and, in some cases, it is necessary to investigate whether there is a causal link between a large decubitus ulcer and death. Histologically, one sees necrosis of the skin and subcutaneous soft tissue accompanied by a chronic inflammatory reaction that is often clearly demarcated deeper down: fibrin layers, leukocytes including granulocytes, and an adjacent dense lymphomonocytic infiltrate in a fibrotic granulation tissue with occasional branched capillary blood vessels (Fig. 1.12). Macrophages and siderophages are also found. Microbial colonization – primarily by cocci and bacilli and rarely fungi – is usually seen in the form of basophilic bacterial colonies only on the surface of the ulcer. This type of histological finding is usually irrelevant in terms of the cause of death if the patient showed no signs of fever or sepsis prior to death. If, however, the patient was septic, one should consider the possibility of the ulcer as an entry port for bacteria. In this case, it is advisable from a histological perspective to analyze phlegmonous/purulent or supperative inflammation of tissue beneath and adjacent to the ulcer in combination with the

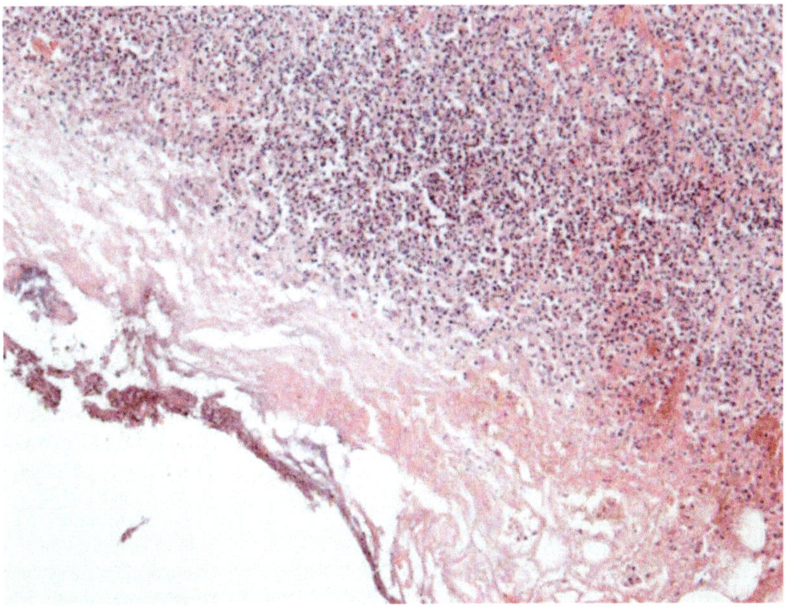

Fig. 1.12 Sacral decubitus ulcer with a necrotic zone on the surface and fibrinopurulent plaque at the level of subcutaneous fat tissue, transitioning to a deeper granulation tissue infiltrated by inflammatory cells (H&E ×100)

microbiological detection of bacteria in swabs from the ulcer and in a blood sample distant to the ulcer. In the case of extremely deep ulcers, the inflammatory process may reach the bone or bone marrow, producing histologically detectable osteomyelitis.

Immunohistochemical analysis addresses questions of wound healing in decubitus ulcers and, in particular, the expression of leukocyte and endothelial adhesion molecules (P-, E-selectin, VCAM-1, LFA-1, and VLA-4) from different areas of an ulcer (Fattouh et al. 2015).

References

Ambepitiya SGH, Michiue T, Bessho Y, Kamikodai Y, Ishikawa T, Maeda H (2010) An unusual presentation of thoracic aortic aneurysm rupturing into the esophagus: an autopsy case report. Forensic Sci Med Pathol 6:121–126

Banaschak S, Du Chesne A, Brinkmann B (2000) Multiple interchanging of tissue samples in cases of breast cancer. Forensic Sci Int 113:3–7

Bernardi FDC, Saldiva PHN, Mauad T (2005) Histological examination has a major impact on macroscopic necropsy diagnoses. J Clin Pathol 58:1261–1264

Bird LM, Billmann GF, Lacro RV, Spicer RL, Jariwala LK, Hoyme HE, Zamora-Salinas R, Morris C, Viskochil D, Frikke MJ, Jones MC (1996) Sudden death in Williams syndrome: report of ten cases. J Pediatr 129:926–931

Bohnert M, Thierauf A, Große Perdekamp M, Böhm N (2003) Das Williams-Campbell-Syndrome—eine seltene Todesursache bei Neugeborenen. 19th spring meeting—Southern Region. German Society of Forensic Medicine, Heidelberg, Germany, 26–27 Feb 2003

Brinkmann B (1999) Harmonisation of medico-legal autopsy rules. Int J Legal Med 113:1–14

Byard RW, Winskog C (2012) Histology in forensic practice: required or redundant? Forensic Sci Med Pathol 8:56–57

Byard RW (2014) Endobronchial/tracheal metastasis and sudden death. J Forensic Sci 59:1139–1141

Campobasso CP, Dell'Erba AS, Addante A, Zotti F, Marzullo A, Colona MF (2008) Sudden cardiac death and myocardial ischemia indicators. A comparative study of four immunohistochemical markers. Am J Forensic Med Pathol 29:154–161

Casewell MW, Philpott-Howard J (1983) Septicaemia from inadvertent intravenous administration of enteral feeds. J Hosp Infect 4:403–405

Cecchi R (2010) Estimating wound age: looking into the future. Int J Legal Med 124:523–536

Chan D, O'Donnell C, Parsons S (2017) Sudden cardiac death from aortoesophageal fistula: an autopsy case report of a rare complication of thoracic aortic aneurysm. Forensic Sci Med Pathol 13(4):504–507

Churg A (1982) Fiber counting and analysis in the diagnosis of asbestos-related disease. Hum Pathol 13:381–392

Cordner S (2012) Histology in forensic practice. Forensic Sci Med Pathol 8:71–72

de la Grandmaison GL, Charlier P, Durigon M (2010) Usefulness of systematic histological examination in routine forensic autopsy. J Forensic Sci 55:85–88
de Giorgio F, Vetrugo G (2014) Is histological examination always necessary to determine a cause of death? Of course it is! Forensic Sci Med Pathol 10:477–478
Davis GJ (2012) Histology in forensic practice. Forensic Sci Med Pathol 8:60–61
Dettmeyer R (2009) Unterlassene Aufklärung eines akuten Myokardinfarktes als Vergehen der fahrlässigen Tötung gemäß § 222 StGB. Anmerkung zum Urteil des AG Potsdam v. 12.03.2007—84 Ds 486 Js 6255/05. In: Dettmeyer R (ed) Rechtsreport, Rechtsmedizin, vol 19, pp 106–108
Dean DE, Jamison JM, Lane JL (2014) Spontaneous rupture of the gall bladder: an unusual forensic diagnosis. J Forensic Sci 59:1142–1145
Dettmeyer R, Verhoff MA, Schütz H (2013) Forensic medicine: fundamentals and perspectives. Springer, Heidelberg Dordrecht London New York
Dettmeyer R (2014) The role of histopathology in forensic practice: an overview. Forensic Sci Med Pathol 10:401–412
Dettmeyer R (2016) Histopathology. In: Payne-James J, Byard RW (eds) Encyclopedia of forensic and legal medicine, vol 3, 2nd edn, pp 35–46
Dettmeyer R, Madea B (1999) Rechtsmedizinische Gutachten in arztstrafrechtlichen Ermittlungsverfahren. Medizinrecht 17:533–539
Dettmeyer R, Preuß J (2009) Medical malpractice charges in Germany—a survey. Legal Med 11:S132–S134
Dettmeyer R, Schmidt P, Grellner W, Madea B (1998) Postoperative urämische Epikarditis und Pneumonitis nach irrtümlicher Nephrektomie wegen eines Angiomyolipoms. Urologe [B] 38:370–373
Dettmeyer R, Schmidt P, Grellner W, Madea B (1999) Lethal transurethral resection syndrome (TUR-syndrome)—morphological and medicolegal aspects. Rechtsmedizin 10:39–42
Dettmeyer R, Drieverf F, Becker A, Wiestler OD, Madea B (2001) Fatal myeloencephalopathy due to accidental intrathecal vincristine administration: a report of two cases. Forensic Sci Int 122:60–64
Dettmeyer R, Preuß J, Madea B (2004) Malpractice—role of the forensic pathologist in Germany. Forensic Sci Int 144:265–267
Dettmeyer R, Egl M, Madea B (2005) Medical malpractice charges in Germany—role of the forensic pathologist in the preliminary criminal proceeding. J Forensic Sci 50:423–427
Dettmeyer R, Preuss J, Madea B (2006) Behandlungsfehlervorwürfe nach Koronarangiographien. In: Kauert G, Mebs D, Schmidt P (eds) Kausalität—rechtsmedizinische, naturwissenschaftliche und juristische Beiträge. Festschrift für H-J, Bratzke, pp 67–76
Duan Y, Liu L, Liu Y, Sunnassee A, Liu Q (2013) Sudden death due to lupus-induced pancarditis diagnosed after necropsy: a case report. Forensic Sci Int 232:e9–e11
Farkaš D, Špak L, Švajdler M, Iannaccone SF, Sihotsky V, Katuchová J, Ginelliová A (2015) Traumatic pseudoaneurysm of descendent thoracic aorta solved by aortal stent graft repair followed by development of fatal aortoesophageal fistula. Soud Lek 60:46–50
Fattouh M, Buschmann CT, Thamm OC, Sperhake JP, Püschel K, Tsokos M (2015) Pressure ulcers and wound healing. Immunohistochemical analysis of leucocyte and endothelial adhesion molecules. Rechtsmedizin 25:299–308
Fechner G, Du Chesne A, Ortmann C, Brinkmann B (2002) Death due to intravenous application of enteral feed. Int J Legal Med 116:354–356
Ferrara SD, Bajanowski T, Cecchi R, Snenghi R, Case C, Viel G (2010) Bio-medical guidelines and protocols: survey and future perspectives in Europe. Int J Legal Med 124:345–350
Fineschi V, Neri M, Di Donato S, Pomara C, Riezzo I, Turillazi E (2006) An immunohistochemical study in a fatality due to ovarian hyperstimulation syndrome. Int J Legal Med 120:293–299
Fronczek J, Hollingbury F, Biggs M, Rutty G (2014) The role of histology in forensic autopsies: is histological examination always necessary to determine a cause of death? Forensic Sci Med Pathol 10:39–43
Goel CM, Badenoch DF, Fowler CG, Blandy JP (1992) Transurethral resection syndrome. Eur Urol 21:15–17
Gupta P, Tobias JD, Goyal S, Miller MD, Melendez E, Noviski N, De Moor MM, Mehta V (2010) Sudden cardiac death under anesthesia in pediatric patient with Williams syndrome: a case report and review of literature. Ann Card Anaesth 13:44–48
Hadžisejdić I, Mustać E, Krstulja M, Franjić N, Štimac D (2012) Thoracic aortic aneurysm rupture into the esophagus. Forensic Sci Med Pathol 8:327–329
Hecht L, Lamprecht A (2010) Intramuscular administration of extended release drugs. Uncommon histological finding at autopsy. Rechtsmedizin 20:510–514
Hinderberger P, Fliss B, Thali MJ, Schweitzer W (2017) Fatal bronchovascular fistula after lobectomy visualized through postmortem computed tomography angiography: a case report. Forensic Sci Med Pathol 13:234–239
Hunsaker JC (2012) Histology in forensic practice. Forensic Sci Med Pathol 8:66–68
Janssen W (1988) Morphologische Untersuchungen in der Rechtspflege—Anspruch und Wirklichkeit. Z Rechtsmed 100:5–17
Klintschar M, Bilkenroth U, Arslan-Kirchner M, Schmidke J, Stiller D (2009) Marfan syndrome: clinical consequences resulting from medicolegal autopsy of a case of sudden death due to aortic rupture. Int J Legal Med 123:55–58
Kondo T (2007) Timing of skin wounds. Legal Med 9:109–114
Krous HF, Wahl C, Chadwick AE (2008) Sudden unexpected death in a toddler with Williams syndrome. Forensic Sci Med Pathol 4:240–250
Langlois NF (2006) The use of histology in 638 coronial post-mortem examinations of adults: an audit. Med Sci Law 46:310–320

Lau G (2012) Histology in forensic practice. Forensic Sci Med Pathol 8:58–59

Luchini D, Meacci F, Oggioni MR, Morabito G, D'Amato V, Gabbrielli M, Pozzi G (2008) Molecular detection of Leptospira interrogans in human tissues and environmental samples in a lethal case of leptospirosis. Int J Legal Med 122:229–233

Madadin M, Molah R, Cordner S (2017) Autopsy histopathology where the prosector is not a histopathologist: a proposal. Forensic Sci Med Pathol 13:383–387

Maeda H, Zhu B, Ishikawa T, Michiue T (2010) Forensic molecular pathology of violent deaths. Forensic Sci Int 203:83–92

Molina DK, Wood LE, Frost RE (2007) Is routine histopathologic examination beneficial in all medicolegal autopsies? Am J Forensic Med Pathol 28:1–3

National Association of Medical Examiners (2006) Forensic autopsy performance standards. Am J Forensic Med Pathol 27:200–225

Nogami M, Takatsu A, Endo N, Ishiyama I (2000) Immunohistochemical localization of P-selectin in the glomeruli from forensic autopsies. Legal Med 2:21–25

Ondruschka B, Habeck JO, Hädrich C, Dreßler J, Bayer R (2016) Rare cause of natural death in forensic setting: hemophagocytic syndrome. Int J Legal Med 130:777–781

Platt MS, Kohler LJ, Ruiz R, Cohle SD, Ravichandran P (2002) Deaths associated with liposuction: case reports and review of the literature. J Forensic Sci 47:205–207

Podduturi V, Guileyardo JM (2015) Sickle cell trait as a contributory cause of death in natural disease. J Forensic Sci 60:807–811

Pomara C, D'Errico S, Riezzo I, de Cillis GP, Fineschi V (2005) Sudden cardiac death in a child affected by Prader-Willi syndrome. Int J Legal Med 119:153–157

Pollanen MS (2012) Histology in forensic practice. Forensic Sci Med Pathol 8:69–70

Randall BB, Fierro MF, Froede RS (1998) Practice guidelines for forensic pathology. Arch Pathol Lab Med 122:1056–1064

Roll P, Beham A, Beham-Schmid C (2009) Post-mortem histopathological investigation of the bone marrow in forensic medicine: an important issue for both the forensic and clinical pathologist. Forensic Sci Int 186:e17–e20

Roulson J, Benbow EW, Hasleton PS (2005) Discrepancies between clinical and autopsy diagnosis and the value of post mortem histology: a meta-analysis and review. Histopathology 47:551–559

Schmidt P, Dettmeyer R, Madea B (2001) Septisch-toxischer Schock nach Liposuktion. Rechtsmedizin 11:275–279

Schmidt P, Dettmeyer R, Madea B (2002) Commentary on: Platt MS, Kohler LJ, Ruiz R, Cohle SD, Ravichandran P. Deaths associated with liposuction: case reports and review of the literature. J Forensic Sci 47:205–207

Sheriff FE, Bridges LR, Sivaloganathan S (1994) Early detection of axonal injury after human head trauma using immunocytochemistry for beta-amyloid precursor protein. Acta Neuropathol 87:55–62

Stellato TA, Danziger LH, Nearman HS, Creger RJ (1984) Inadvertent intravenous administration of enteral diet. J Parenter Enteral Nur 13:453–455

Suárez-Mier MP, Morentin B (1999) Supravalvular aortic stenosis. Williams syndrome and sudden death. A case report. Forensic Sci Int 106:45–53

Tong F, Liang Y, Zhang L, Li W, Chen P, Duan Y, Zhou Y (2016) Fatal liver cyst rupture in polycystic liver disease complicated with autosomal dominant polycystic kidney disease: a case report. Forensic Sci Int 262:e5–e8

Tsokos M, Delling G, Lockemann U, Heinemann A, Püschel K (2000) Incidence and extent of osteomyelitis in advanced grade pressure sores—a histomorphological analysis following non-decalcified preparation of the Os sacrum. Rechtsmedizin 10:56–60

Türk EE, Tsokos M, Delling G (2003) Autopsy-based assessment of extent and type of osteomyelitis in advanced-grade sacral decubitus ulcers: a histopathologic study. Arch Pathol Lab Med 127:1599–1602

Wang Q, Ishikawa T, Quan L, Zhao D, Li DR, Michiue T, Chen JH, Zhu BL, Maeda H (2009) Immunohistochemical distribution of basic fibroblast growth factor (bFGF) in medicolegal autopsy. Legal Med 11:S161–S164

Wessel A, Gravenhorst V, Buchhorn R, Gosch A, Partsch CJ, Pankau R (2004) Risk of sudden death in the Williams-Beuren syndrome. Am J Med Genet A 127A:234–237

Williams AS, Little DL, Herath J (2015) Sudden unexpected death as a result of primary aortoduodenal fistula identified with postmortem computed tomography. Forensic Sci Med Pathol 11:596–600

Woitowitz HJ, Manke J, Breit S, Brückel B, Rödelsperger K (1986) Asbest- und sonstige Mineralfasern in der menschlichen Lunge. Pathologe 7:248–257

Zaitoun AM, Fernandez C (1998) The value of histological examination in the audit of hospital autopsies: a quantitative approach. Pathology 30:100–104

Zhu BL, Tanaka S, Ishikawa T, Zhao D, Li DR, Michiue T, Quan L, Maeda H (2008) Forensic pathological investigation of myocardial hypoxia-inducible factor-1alpha, erythropoietin and vascular endothelial growth factor in cardiac death. Legal Med 10:11–19

Staining Techniques and Microscopy

2

While conventional histological staining methods have been established for decades, some for more than a century, immunohistochemical techniques are not yet routinely used in forensic diagnostics. They are used, however, when specific problems occur. In such cases, depending on the problem, routine diagnostics may be supplemented with specific microscopic techniques, including electron microscopy, laser scanner microscopy, and laser microdissection techniques, in order to isolate single cells or cell groups. For important routine diagnostics, established standard histological staining methods are discussed here. Basic information on immunohistochemical techniques and on the best-practice use of immunohistochemical and other methods are mentioned only briefly and therefore do not substitute reference to the specialist literature. It is important to point out, however, that toxicological investigations can essentially be performed on formalin-fixed tissue as well as on paraffin-embedded tissue. In individual cases, one should consider carrying out a toxicological analysis of the formalin solution in which the tissue has been fixed (Nikolaou et al. 2013). Otherwise, determination of both fetus' and mother's blood type by immunohistochemistry from an autopsy case immersed in formalin for over 50 years is reported (Uno et al. 2016).

Immunohistochemical staining techniques, in particular the ABC method, the APAAP method, and the TUNEL technique, are used to label defined antigens with monoclonal and polyclonal antibodies. Commercially produced antibodies mostly originate from mice, less frequently from rabbits.

In these cases, a number of methodological and technical nuances must be considered in order to gain usable results. The degree of autolysis or putrefaction, the selection of fixation medium, fixation duration, incubation period, and concentration of the selected antibodies can be crucial. Different methods of antigen unmasking are significant in a number of immunohistochemical stainings.

The following chapter gives a general overview of staining and microscopy, highlighting the most important aspects, including potential sources of error and the recognition of typical mistakes and artifacts. For more detailed information, please refer to the relevant works on histological and immunohistochemical techniques.

2.1 Conventional Histological Staining

Conventional histological staining methods, including stain selection for specific situations, have long been established. Descriptions of the most frequently used staining methods should be sufficient for day-to-day practice (Table 2.1). Longer fixation in formaldehyde or in higher concentrations of formaldehyde can lead to sediments of formalin pigment. If the assessment of tissue sections will be affected by such sediments, pretreatment should be considered

R. B. Dettmeyer, *Forensic Histopathology*, https://doi.org/10.1007/978-3-319-77997-3_2

Table 2.1 Frequently used conventional histological staining methods (selection) and sample questions that arise in forensic practice

Staining	Presented structures	Examples from forensic practice
Alcian blue	Detection of acid mucopolysaccharides	Mucoid lakes, for example, in cases of idiopathic cystic Erdheim–Gsell medial necrosis and dissected aortic aneurysm
Azan staining (azo carmine and aniline blue)	Connective tissue staining (red): azo carmine stains cell nuclei, erythrocytes, fibrin, fibrinoid, acidophilic cytoplasm, epithelial hyaline Aniline blue (blue): collagen fibers, fibrous hyaline, basophil cytoplasm, mucus	Differentiates basophilic and chromophobe cells in the hypophysis; loss of detectability, for example, in the case of Sheehan syndrome
Best's carmine stain	Classified as a glycogen stain but is not specific; also stains mucus, fibrin, gastric glands, and mast cell granules	Glycogen detection in kidney distal tubular cells in the case of hyperglycemia (Armanni–Ebstein cells)
Elastin staining according to Weigert	Stains elastic fibers violet–black	For example, elastic fibers in the aortic media
Elastica van Gieson (EvG)	Combined staining of collagen fibers (red) and elastic fibers according to Weigert (black and brown); cytoplasm, musculature, amyloid, fibrin, and fibrinoid (yellow)	Fibrotic zones in the myocardium, fibrosis in other organs, liver cirrhosis, cystic medial necrosis
Iron stain (Prussian blue reaction)	Stains trivalent iron, in particular hemosiderin; detection of iron deposits	Siderosis of the lung, posttraumatically deposited siderophages, e.g., for wound age determination
Fibrin staining according to Weigert	Blue: fibrin and bacteria Red: cell nuclei; is not considered a specific fibrin stain	Detection of microfibrin in the placenta, hyaline membrane in the lung post shock event
Gomori's stain	Argyrophilic reticular fibers (silver)	Glomerular basal membranes in the case of a membrane-proliferative glomerulonephritis type I (MPGN)—the so-called tram tracks; reticular fiber network in the case of hepatic peliosis
Grocott stain	Ideal fungal stain: fungal conidia, fungal fibers stain black	Fungal infection
Hematoxylin–eosin (H&E) staining	Acidophilic cytoplasm is red, basophil nuclei are blue, erythrocytes are red	Routine staining
Congo red stain	Amyloid stain	Amyloidoses of any type, in particular cardiovascular
Kossa stain	Calcified bone tissue stains black in a non-calcified specimen	Sediments in renal tubules and vascular walls following ethylene glycol intoxication
Staining according to Lie et al. (1971)	Fresh myocardial ischemia in the absence (as yet) of demarcation of the infarction (so-called fuchsinorrhagia of the myocardium)	Fresh myocardial infarction or acute myocardial ischemia in stenosing coronary sclerosis
Luxol fast blue (LFB)	Evidence of myelin and phospholipids	Myelin sheath staining
Mallory's stain	Trichrome stain; collagen and reticular connective tissue is light blue, nuclei are red, smooth musculature is violet, striated musculature orange-red, mucus is blue	Connective tissue stain, for example, in the case of liver cirrhosis
Masson–Goldner stain	Red-orange: parenchyma and fibrin Green: mesenchyme Black: cell nuclei	Hyaline fibrin thrombi in the case of shock

Table 2.1 (continued)

Staining	Presented structures	Examples from forensic practice
May-Grünwald–Giemsa stain (MGG)	Nuclei are purple-red, nucleoli are blue, cytoplasm is light blue-gray to red-violet, erythrocytes are pink to orange (except in the case of alkaline pH where they are green-blue)	Hematopoietic marrow, differentiation of cells of the myeloid and lymphatic line; eosinophil granula is red
Methylene blue	Nuclei are sharp blue, plasma cells are deep blue, erythrocytes are greenish	Suitable to detect agents, e.g., helicobacter pylori
Naphthol AS-D chloroacetate esterase stain (Moloney et al. 1960) (enzyme-histochemical stain; abbreviated to ASD)	Neutrophil myeloid cells with all preliminary stages stain wine red	Mostly selective detection of neutrophil granulocytes in purulent inflammation of all kinds (phlegmons, abscesses)
Nissl stain	Detects cell nuclei and tigroid bodies in nerve cells; cell nuclei and Nissl substance violet, nerve cells light blue, the rest is colorless	Detection of nervous tissue
Osmium stain	Lipid vacuoles in the cytoplasm	Hepatic steatosis
Pagoda red stain	Splenic eosinophilia and accumulations of mast cells	Acute anaphylactic shock
Orcein stain	Detection of elastic fibers, used to identify the Australia HBsAG	Hepatocellular single cell necrosis in the case of active hepatitis B—detection of hepatitis B surface antigen; result should be checked immunohistochemically
Papanicolaou stain	Cells are blue to black, nucleoli are black to red, cytoplasm is blue-green (cyanophil) to pink-red (eosinophil); erythrocytes are bright red	Standard stain for vaginal wet mount
PAS (periodic acid–Schiff's reagent)	Stains carbohydrates, in particular glycogen, purple-red (magenta) and epithelial mucin	Glycogen positive Armanni–Ebstein cells in the renal tubules in the case of diabetic coma
Periodic acid—silver	Stains basal membranes, Alzheimer's plaques, and fungi black	Detection of basal membranes, for example, in the kidney
Picrosirius red	Decalcified bone tissue; visualization of collagen tissue	Determination of human specificity of bone tissue, bone age determination at the time of death (see Chap. 10)
PTAH	Phosphotungstic acid–hematoxylin according to Mallory	Used to differentiate between smooth and striated muscle fibers, detects fibrin; suitable in the case of muscle damage, also in the myocardium
Prussian blue	Blue: hemosiderin, Fe III	Siderosis of the lung, hemosiderin macrophages full of pigments
Reticulin stain	Silvering of fine (pre-) collagen reticulin fibers	Basal membranes, newly formed fibers
Sudan III	Fat stain; lipids stain yellowish-red; Sudan IV stains more orange-red	Fat embolisms, fatty liver
Toluidine blue	Detects striation of muscle fibers and metachromatic substances	Striated muscle tissue, mast cell granules
Silvering	Black: reticular fibers, nervous fibers Brown: collagen fibers	Hepatic peliosis, glomeruli
Ziehl–Neelsen stain	Acid-resistant rods, mycobacteria (also lepra bacteria) stain bright red	In particular tuberculosis; microscopy ×1000, oil immersion

There are numerous other simple and combined staining methods that are described in the relevant literature

(Kardasewitsch reaction; Kardasewitsch 1952). Depending on which tissue is to be investigated, the fixation technique can influence the microscopic image. Thus, for example, the influence of fixation on the development of pulmonary alveoli has been investigated (Hausmann et al. 2004). It is important to bear in mind that all stains can on occasion, and particularly in the case of specimens taken at autopsy, yield false-positive or false-negative results. For example, staining according to Lie et al. (1971) with fuchsinorrhagia in the case of extremely fresh myocardial necrosis is considered to be relatively reliable, although inexplicable false-positive findings were also reported at that time (Frick 1981). A handful of less well-known stains are supposed to be helpful for certain investigations. For example, pagoda red stain is recommended in acute anaphylactic shock to detect splenic eosinophilia, combined with a local accumulation of mast cells, the presence of which can be immunohistochemically investigated using CD117 (Trani et al. 2008). In addition to Sudan III staining to visualize lipid vacuoles, osmium staining also makes lipid vacuoles appear blackish-brown if the incubation time is adhered to (Fig. 2.1).

In some cases, alternative fixing solutions are used: Bouin's solution, Zamboni solution, "NoTox" (Meyer et al. 1996), pure alcohol, etc. In cases where an electron microscopic investigation is needed, glutaraldehyde is typically chosen as a fixative (3% solution for 24 h at 4 °C, followed by phosphate buffer solution; additional fixation in 1% osmium acid, embedded in Epon).

It should be noted that fixative selection and duration can have a direct bearing on potential molecular genetic investigations (Kuhn and Krugmann 1995). Such investigations can be difficult or even impossible, and special pretreatment methods are sometimes suggested (Ananian et al. 2010; Fracasso et al. 2009; Wiegand et al. 1996; Kok and Boon 1992; Kwok and Higuchi 1989; Ben-Ezra et al. 1991; Holgate et al. 1986).

Immunohistochemical evidence can be found in formalin-fixed tissue, depending on the antigen, as is the case for viral antigens (Lozinski et al. 1994), but also in other molecular genetic investigations (Miething et al. 2006). Antigen-conserving methods are also discussed in order to overcome antigen loss or difficult detectability due to autolysis (Pelstring et al. 1991). Microwave pretreatment can accelerate fixation with formaldehyde (Login et al. 1987). In addition to conventional histology, which has long been common practice, immunohistochemical techniques have also found their way into forensic diagnostics (Bratzke and Schröter 1995).

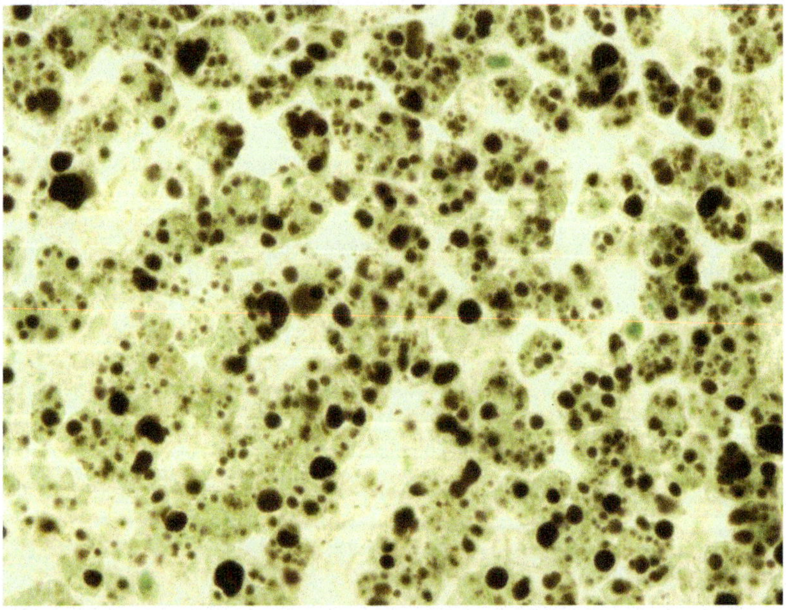

Fig. 2.1 Osmium stain to visualize lipid vacuoles in hepatocytes in hepatic steatosis (×400)

2.1.1 Background Staining and Artifacts in Conventional Staining Methods

In order to assess the quality of a tissue section, impurities and disturbing artifacts should be defined:

- Displaced tissue not belonging on the microscope slide (e.g., displaced splenic tissue, which can simulate a lymphocytic inflammatory infiltrate) (Fig. 2.2 and 2.3)
- Excessive formalin pigment
- Overstaining due to a coloring agent in the case of dye combinations
- Slice artifact with partly missing or torn tissue (Fig. 2.4 and 2.5)

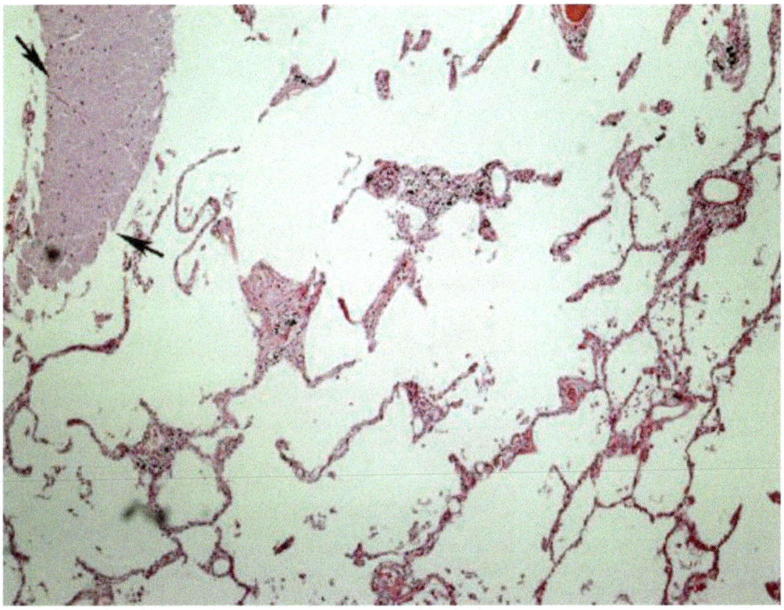

Fig. 2.2 Displaced brain tissue (*arrows*) in a pulmonary tissue section due to careless work (H&E ×40)

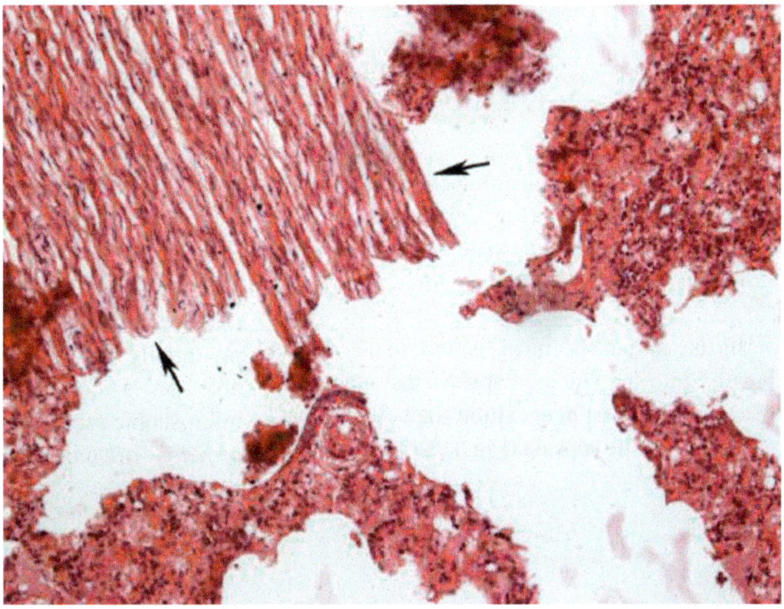

Fig. 2.3 Displaced portions of heart muscle tissue (*arrows*) in a pulmonary tissue section due to careless work (H&E ×40)

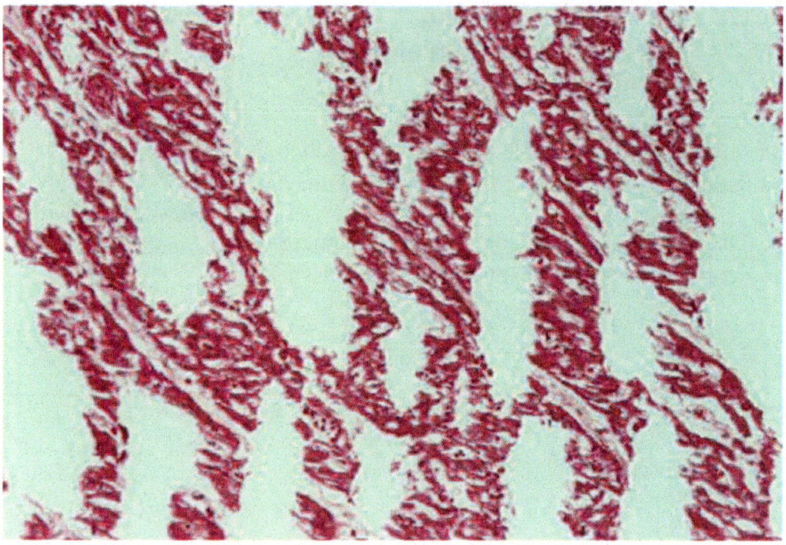

Fig. 2.4 Rough-slice artifact with tears in the tissue due to a blunt blade (H&E ×40)

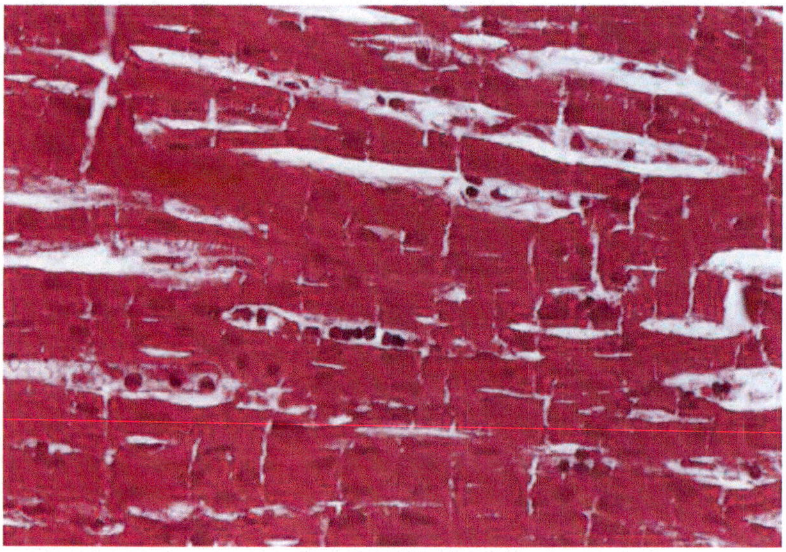

Fig. 2.5 Tear artifacts in the heart muscle tissue caused by a blunt blade and imprecise cutting (H&E ×400)

- Wave formation in histological sections with insufficient staining (Fig. 2.6)
- Artificially modified tissue due to incorrect treatment (Fig. 2.7)

If the tissue specimen is too thick and is pressed into the storage capsule, the superficial sections taken first may exhibit the hole-like pattern of the tissue capsule (Fig. 2.8).

2.2 Immunohistochemical Techniques

The ability to produce monoclonal antibodies (Köhler and Milstein 1975) resulted in numerous highly specific antibodies becoming available on a commercial basis. This enables microscopic representation of specific antigenic proteins or molecules in a section or cell

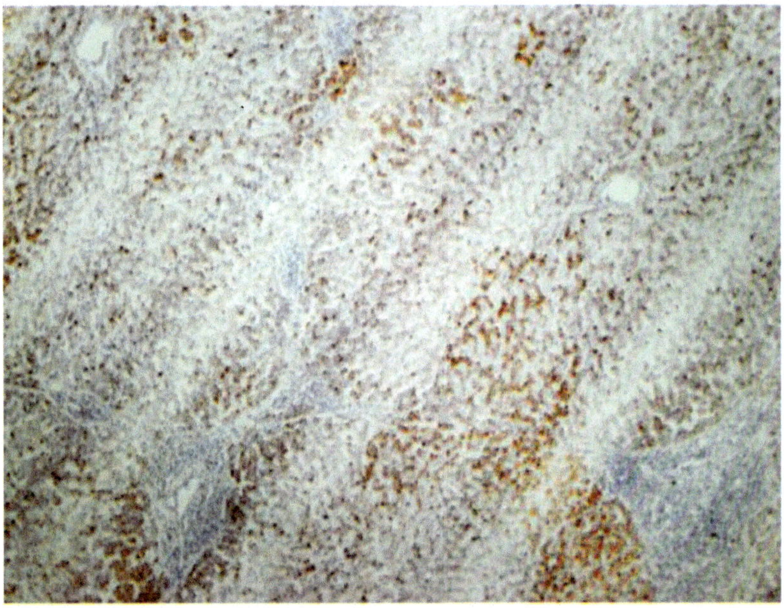

Fig. 2.6 Wave-like formation of a tissue section with insufficient lipid staining (Sudan III ×100)

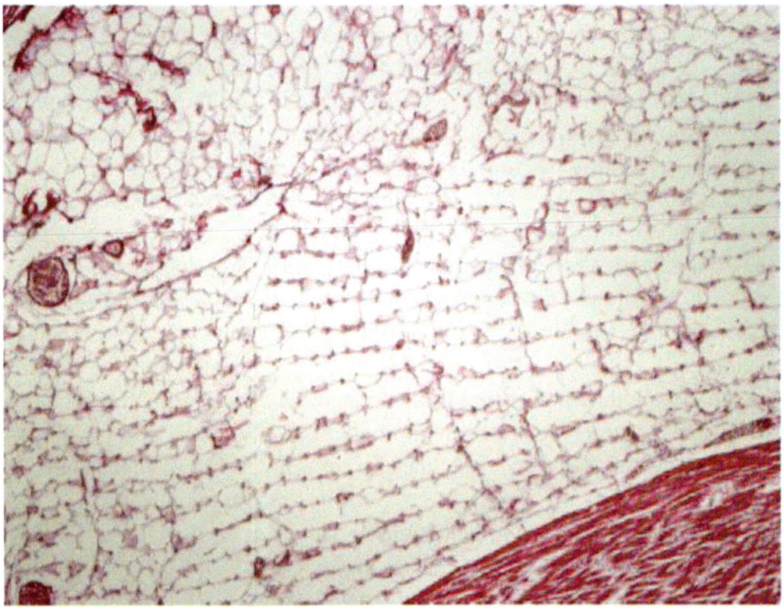

Fig. 2.7 Incision-related row formation of subepicardial adipose tissue with altered lipocytes (H&E ×40)

specimen (immunohistochemistry, immunocytochemistry). The range of immunohistochemically displayed cell and tissue proteins includes, e.g., collagens, basal membrane components, hormones, cytoskeleton proteins, glycoproteins of cell membranes, viral and bacterial antigens, cytokines, and complement factors.

Unlike conventional histological staining methods, immunohistochemical techniques are based on antigen–antibody bindings, which can be affected by inappropriate fixative selection and duration. Microwave-based fixation of tissue in formaldehyde may also have negative consequences (Login et al. 1987).

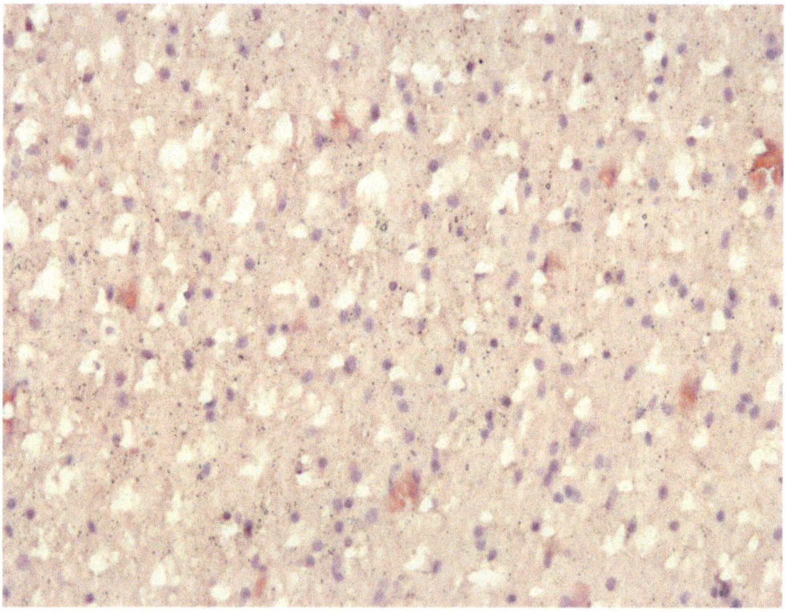

Fig. 2.8 Hole-like pattern of the tissue capsule in a brain tissue section after pressing an overly thick tissue specimen into the capsule (HE ×200)

Fixative selection must be considered individually for each antigen and each antibody. Manufacturers state, however, whether an antibody—following formaldehyde fixation –can be used on a paraffin section or not (Noll and Schaub-Kuhnen 2000).

In practice, formaldehyde has been acknowledged as a fixative for conventional routine staining methods for decades and can also be used for fixation in certain immunohistochemical techniques.

The compatibility of different concentrations of these solutions with specific immunohistochemical techniques has only been partially investigated.

Note: The current recommendation for immunohistochemical techniques is a maximum of 4% neutral buffered formaldehyde solution and for some antibodies a maximum fixation time of 48 h.

Tissue can then be dehydrated with various concentrations of alcohol in ascending order and can be embedded in paraffin according to Peterfi's methyl-benzoate method. Finally, 3–5 μm slices are prepared as unstained sections.

With longer fixation times, proteins are cross-linked more intensely due to the fixative, so that the antigen-binding sites are masked and the added primary antibodies cannot dock (Mason and O'Leary 1991), resulting in false-negative findings. To avoid this, various methods of antigen unmasking can be used, e.g., enzyme autodigestion or steeping in citrate solution. The antigen reactivity of proteins cross-linked due to fixation can be rebuilt (antigen retrieval).

Note: Temperatures of >60 °C cause a denaturation of the proteins or antigens and thus can also result in false-negative results. A temperature of approximately 58 °C is recommended, which must be considered when mounting tissue sections on microscope glass slides in a water bath.

Polyclonal and monoclonal antibodies are distinguished:

- Polyclonal antibodies bind to different parts of a macromolecular antigen.
- Monoclonal antibodies recognize only a single epitope of an antigen.

The binding of antigen and antibody (the antigen–antibody precipitate) in the tissue section must be made visible in further steps. For this purpose, an enzyme-labeled detection system is used: a secondary antibody (bridge antibody) reacts with the primary antibody, which is already specifically bound in the tissue. This leads to a local enrichment of attached enzymes. After adding a substrate solution, these enzymes become active and lead to a dye formation, which is also reflected locally. Horseradish peroxidase and alkaline phosphatase have proven successful as enzymes for this purpose. As a rule, one of these two enzymes is typically used with different coloring agents (chromogens). Even if few specific antigen quantities are visualized in this way, counterstaining of the cell nuclei is done with hemalaun (hematoxylin), so that a microscopic orientation is possible in the tissue section.

In order to label defined antigens, two methods have been established, which can vary in individual cases: the ABC method and the APAAP method. Depending on the enzyme, substrate, and chromogen used, a different color marking is made (Table 2.2). The various immunohistochemical methods have in part been compared and tested (Sabattini et al. 1998).

In many cases, better results are achieved when tissue sections are pretreated for antigen unmasking.

2.2.1 Methods of Antigen Demasking

Even if only a few antigens are detected immunohistochemically, a loss of antigenic reactivity is expected due to the use of fixative, fixation duration, and paraffin embedding (excessively high temperatures). Additionally, tissue extracted during autopsy can be autolytically modified at extraction (see Chap. 19). It still applies that a particular procedure must be determined for every antigen to be detected immunohistochemically and for every antibody (fixative choice, fixation duration, temperature, incubation period, etc.). Not all commercially available antibodies can be used on a paraffin section; some can only be used after appropriate pretreatment (Imam 1995), one reason being the strong cross-linking of proteins due to formaldehyde (Mason and O'Leary 1991). In this context, different methods have proven helpful to retrieve antigenic reactivity, i.e., to break up the proteins cross-linked due to fixation (antigen retrieval) (Table 2.3). Some

Table 2.2 Chromogen-dependent color marking in immunohistochemistry or immunocytochemistry

Enzyme	Substrate	Chromogen	Color
Peroxidase	Hydrogen peroxide (H_2O_2)	1. DAB = diaminobenzidine	Brown (when adding nickel sulfate black)
		2. AEC = amino ethyl-carbazole	Red-brown
Alkaline phosphatase	Naphthol phosphate	1. Fast red	Red
		2. Fast blue	Blue
		3. New fuchsine	Red

Table 2.3 Methods of antigen unmasking (antigen retrieval) in order to allow immunohistochemical staining on paraffin-embedded tissue (selection)[a]

Method	Approach
Proteolytic autodigestion (trypsin, pronase, pepsin, etc.)	Incubate tissue section with the enzyme. Note: an extremely intensive autodigestion can lead to undesired destruction of tissue structure
Cooking in citrate buffer	Cook tissue sections briefly in citrate buffer in the microwave; varying concentrations and cooking times apply (Brown and Chirala 1995; Cuevas et al. 1994; Gown et al. 1993; Leong 1996)
Cooking in aluminum chloride	Less-known method: the tissue sections are cooked in aluminum chloride in the microwave; varying concentrations and cooking times appl.
Wet-autoclaving	Influence of wet heat, e.g., 120 °C with citrate buffer pH 6.0 (Bankfalvi et al. 1994a, b; Dreßler et al. 1998); relatively simple handling, special microscope slides may be necessary to prevent detachment of the tissue section
Cooking in urea solution	Cook tissue sections in urea solution of various concentrations (Shi et al. 1994, 1995, 1997)

[a]Compare Williamson et al. (1998), Pileri et al. (1997), Werner et al. (1996), von Wasielewski et al. (1994), Dokhan et al. (1993), Leong and Milios (1993), and Shi et al. (1991)

antigens cannot be detected immunohistochemically without antigen retrieval (Merz et al. 1995a, b). The demand for better standardization, including methods of antigen unmasking, seems to be reaching its limit due to the fact that every tissue type is different, the duration before taking a tissue sample varies (at autopsy), and the duration of formalin fixation and paraffin embedding also varies considerably (Taylor et al. 1996). On the other hand, immunohistochemical visualization should be possible even with only a small number of antigens and when it is useful to strengthen their signal.

2.2.2 ABC Method

Immunohistochemical staining according to the avidin–biotin complex (ABC) method is done according to the procedure of Hsu et al. (1981a, b) (Table 2.4). This procedure has more recently been modified to the LAB or LSAB method (labeled avidin/streptavidin biotin, secondary antibodies with covalently linked biotin and enzyme-marked avidin or streptavidin). When using this method, the unconjugated primary antibody initially binds to the appropriate antigen. The avidin–biotin–peroxidase complex then binds to the biotin on the secondary antibody. The added chromogen reacts with the enzyme and is deposited where the antigen is located. Contrasting cell structures are presented through counterstaining with hemalaun. In doing so, antigens which are localized, e.g., at the cell surface, can be specifically identified (cell adhesion molecules). Color intensity may vary depending on the number of antigens.

2.2.3 APAAP Method

The APAAP immunohistochemical staining method is performed according to the method described by Cordell et al. (1984) (Table 2.5).

Withdrawal trials represent an important check made in immunohistochemical staining. The protocol for immunohistochemical staining is carried out completely; however, the primary antibody is left out in a withdrawal trial, and the secondary antibody is left out in a second withdrawal trial. In both cases, a color marking should be missing in the microscopic examination.

Table 2.4 Procedure when using the ABC method according to Hsu et al. (1981a, b)

Method	Procedure
Preparation of tissue sections	Mount 3–5 μm thin slices onto special microscope slides in order to prevent a detachment of tissue sections; water bath of maximum 58 °C
Deparaffining	Put tissue section into xylol (2 × 10 min), then 3 min into 100% alcohol
Blockage of endogenous peroxidase activity	0.5% hydrogen peroxide solution (H_2O_2)/methanol solution in order to block endogenous peroxidase, then 3 min into 100% alcohol
Rehydration	Rehydrate with various concentrations of alcohol in descending order, then washing in distilled water
Antigen unmasking	Optional: pretreatment with various methods, e.g., enzymatic autodigestion with pronase, pepsin, and trypsin or cooking in citrate solution or aluminum chloride solution, autoclaving; then washing in PBS buffer (10–20 min), incubate with normal serum (approximately 15–20 min)
Primary antibodies	Incubate with the desired polyclonal or monoclonal primary antibody (e.g., from mouse); incubation period varies depending on the primary antibody; then wash with PBS buffer for approximately 5 min, may be mixed with Brij solution (4–1000 mL of PBS buffer)
Secondary antibodies (bridge antibodies)	Incubate the tissue section with a biotinylated secondary antibody (incubation period varies); then wash in PBS buffer or Brij solution (approximately 5 min)
ABC reagent	Incubate with ABC reagent (duration varies)
Substrate solution	Add the substrate solution with the coloring agent consisting of: 30 mg AEC (3-amino-9-ethyl-carbazole) dissolved in 12 mL dimethyl sulfoxide, adding 200 mL 0.1 M sodium acetate buffer (pH 5.2) and 10 μL of 30% hydrogen peroxide (H_2O_2)—incubation period varies
Rinse	Rinse for 10 min with running tap water
Counterstaining and covering	Counterstain with hemalaun (stains cell nuclei blue) and fix cover slips with glycerol gelatin

Table 2.5 Procedure when using the APAAP method according to Cordell et al. (1984)

Method	Procedure
Preparation of tissue sections	Mount 3–5 μm thin slices onto special microscope slides in order to prevent detachment of the tissue section; water bath of maximum of 58 °C
Deparaffining	Put tissue section into xylol (2 × 10 min), then into 100% alcohol for 3 min
Blockage of endogenous peroxidase activity	0.5% hydrogen peroxide solution (H_2O_2)/methanol solution in order to block endogenous peroxidase, then into 100% alcohol for 3 min
Rehydration	Rehydrate with different concentrations of alcohol in descending order, then wash in distilled water
Antigen unmasking	Optional: pretreatment with various methods, e.g., enzymatic autodigestion with pronase, pepsin, and trypsin or cooking in citrate solution or aluminum chloride solution, autoclaving; then wash in PBS buffer (10–20 min), incubate with normal serum (approximately 15–20 min)
Primary antibodies	Incubation with the desired polyclonal or monoclonal primary antibody (e.g., from mouse); incubation period varies depending on the primary antibody; then wash with PBS buffer (or Tris buffer) for approximately 5 min
Secondary antibodies (bridge antibodies)	Incubation of the tissue section with a biotinylated secondary antibody (incubation period varies); then wash again in PBS buffer (approximately 5 min)
APAAP complex	Incubation with the APAAP complex at room temperature (incubation period varies)
Wash	Wash in Tris buffer (5 min)
APAAP complex	Optional: repeat incubation with the APAAP complex at room temperature (incubation period varies)
Substrate solution	Add the substrate solution with the coloring agent consisting of: 2 mg naphthol AS-MX phosphate dissolved in 0.2 mL dimethylformamide with 9.8 mL, 0.1 mL Tris buffer, 10 mL levamisole; add and filtrate 10 mg fast red TR salt prior to use
Wash	Wash in Tris buffer (5 min)
Counterstaining and covering	Counterstain with hemalaun (approximately 20 s, stains cell nuclei blue), annealing in H_2O, fix cover slips with glycerol gelatin

2.2.4 Background Staining and Artifacts in Immunohistochemical Staining

Undesirable changes to the tissue section may occur when conventional histological staining is used, as well as certain immunohistochemical techniques (see above). Artifacts in the histological section are predominantly caused by unprofessional work, incorrect fixation and embedding (e.g., tears), improper tissue cutting or mounting of the tissue section, or during staining (e.g., lighter or darker spots, etc.).

The abovementioned technical errors while preparing tissue sections are also possible when preparing tissue sections for immunohistochemical techniques. However, in immunohistochemistry, attention should be paid to other changes or artifacts, especially in the area of unspecified, marginal background stains or undesired dye deposits (Fig. 2.9). For this reason, positive and negative controls should be conducted parallel to examination of the compound. Nevertheless, an inexperienced examiner may confuse artifacts with a positive stain (Fig. 2.10). Excessively thick tissue sections or folded tissue sections may result in an accumulation of reagents with a false-positive reaction. During immunohistochemical representation of amorphous necrotic areas or those with cell detritus, nonspecific staining occurs regularly. This is also the case for strongly hemorrhagic imbibed compounds. If the desired antigen is also found in the serum following insufficient rinsing, partially intensive background stains will result.

The standardized blockade of endogenous peroxidase activity and preceding incubation with normal serum will help avoid contamination and artifacts. Nonspecific binding of primary and secondary antibodies to tissue structures, which may lead to false-positive results, should be avoided by increased diluting of the antibodies, which should be done in a separate procedure for each individual antibody.

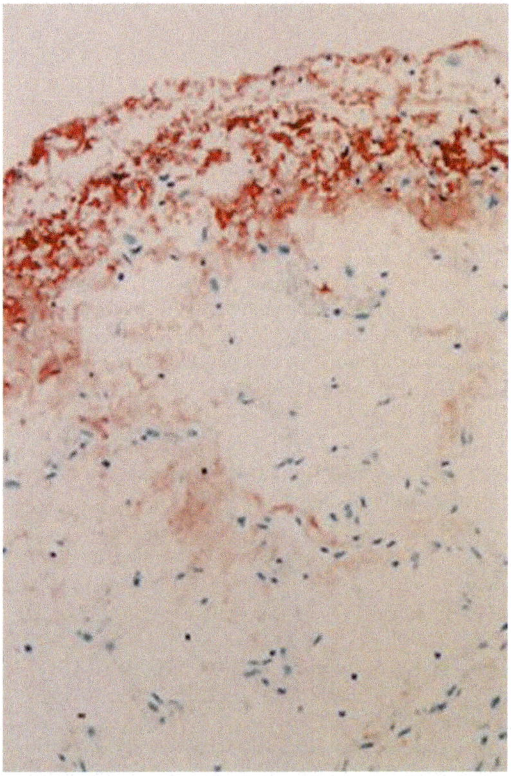

Fig. 2.9 Nonspecific stain deposit at the margin of the tissue section—ABC method (×100)

In forensic medicine, the dilutions prescribed by the manufacturer can be utilized initially, but, often, variations are needed for the distinct autolytic tissue to be examined.

In addition, a specificity control must be made even if immunohistochemical staining occurs on the anticipated structures microscopically. Here, positive and negative controls are critical; tissue sections containing the antigen to be detected should be stained parallel to the withdrawal trials. Specific tissue probes may be used for positive controls, e.g., tonsil tissue to detect lymphatic cells or epidermis to show cytokeratin. For the representation of individual cells, a control of identical tissue should be used, e.g., when qualifying and quantifying leukocytes in the renal glomeruli or in the myocardial interstitium. Nonspecific stain deposits may be mistaken for a positive reaction during a superficial observation (Fig. 2.11), a mistake that can be clarified by using magnification while making the observation (Fig. 2.12). For qualification and quantification purposes of defined cell types, control and observation under high magnification (×400) are essential.

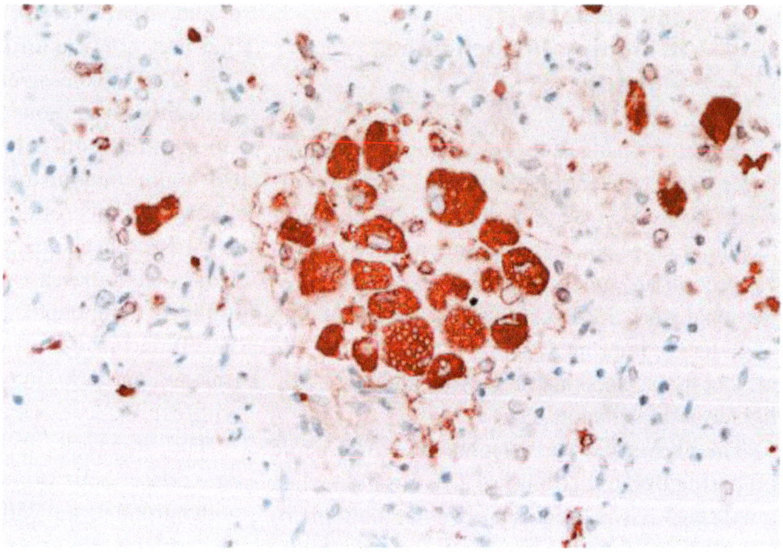

Fig. 2.10 Nonspecific false-positive staining of obviously intravascular, agglutinated structures with an antibody for macrophages (CD68 ×200)

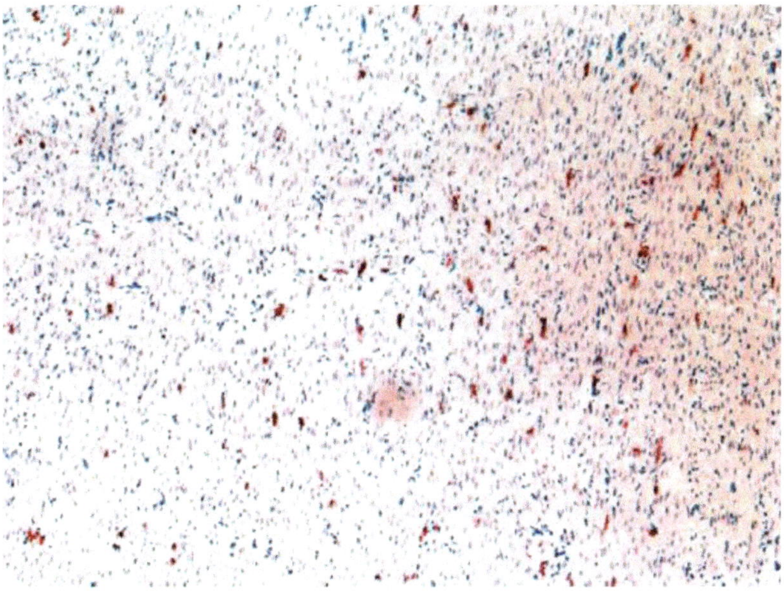

Fig. 2.11 False-positive detection of intramyocardial CD45R0-positive T-lymphocytes with minimal enlargement (×100)

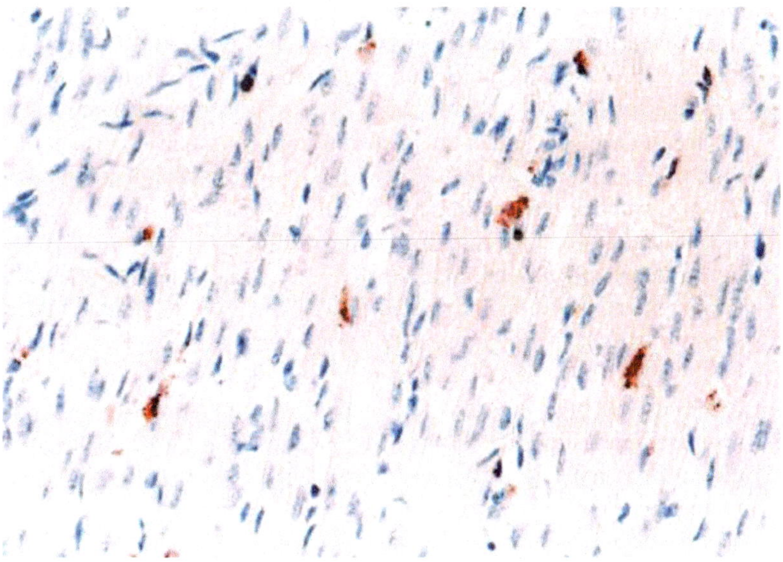

Fig. 2.12 Identical compound, as in Fig. 2.11, with significant enlargement: despite stain deposit, no representation of cellular structures, unspecified stain deposit, no display of CD45R0-positive T-lymphocytes (×400)

In immunohistochemistry, background staining can have different causes (Feiden 1995).

- It can be frequently caused by blocking of endogenous peroxidase activity; for this reason, H_2O_2 block (or alternatively use of the APAAP method), as well as incubation with normal serum, is part of the standard protocol for immunohistochemical staining.
- When antibodies show nonspecific binding, the most effective way to counteract this is by significantly diluting the antibodies. This process must be repeated individually for each antibody. In general, the manufacturer's dilution ratio is valid.

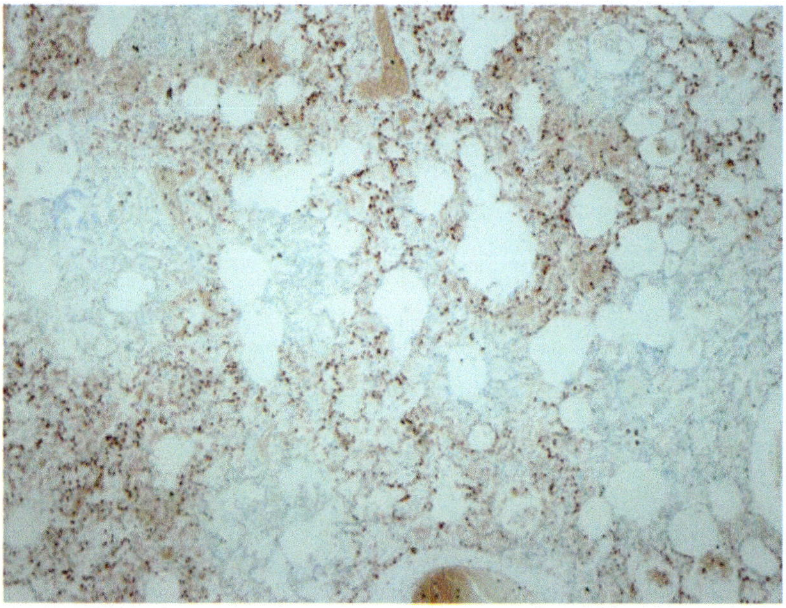

Fig. 2.13 Irregular distribution of the antibody in immunohistochemical staining with leukocyte common antigen (LCA) and the resultant gaps in the specimen (×40)

- Increased activity of alkaline phosphatase can be counteracted by adding levamisole to the substrate solution.
- Drying of the compound or complete deparaffinization should be avoided.
- When disruptive electrostatic binding forces are present, the ion concentrations in the dilution buffer should be increased.
- When antigen diffusion is followed by a false negative or an increasingly weak reaction, tissue or cell fixation must be examined.
- In the case of polyclonal antibodies and cross-reactivity of the antibody, one should consider absorption; changing to a monoclonal antibody is better.
- Tissue necrosis and advanced autolysis may lead to immunohistochemical staining which should not be regarded as specific.

It should be taken into consideration that interpretation of immunohistochemical stains presumes that the results of conventional histological stains are known. Immunohistochemical findings that do not fit within this context should be examined critically; in the case of ambiguity, findings should be limited to histological routine staining. Erroneous evaluations may occur when a finding is based on only one immunohistochemical stain. A spectrum of several antibodies should be used. Another artifact in immunohistochemical staining worthy of mention is the gaps in tissue section visualization that are occasionally caused by irregular distribution of the antibody (Fig. 2.13).

2.3 Selection of Antigens and Antibodies

The selection of antigens to be detected or the antibodies to be used depends on the questions being asked. Thus, in the case of a newborn found dead, aspirated epidermal cells floating in the amniotic fluid of the fetus may be immunohistochemically shown under the microscope with an antibody against cytokeratin, proving amniotic fluid aspiration (see Chap. 11). A spectrum of immunohistochemical markers (antibodies) is recommended as ischemia markers for the myocardium to prove acute death following stenosing coronary sclerosis (clinical, acute lethal coronary insufficiency) (see Chap. 13) as well as to determine the age of injuries or skin lesions (see Chap. 10). The recommendation to use a spectrum of immunohistochemical markers is also valid when determining the age of brain or myocardial infarcts.

Numerous functionally relevant surface molecules of immunocompetent cells previously discovered have been given multiple descriptions. For simplification, CD nomenclature was introduced (CD, cluster of differentiation). The molecules are named with a prefix, "CD," and they are assigned a number. The basis for assigning a CD number to a surface molecule is the availability of monoclonal antibodies that clearly define the respective surface molecule.

After an antibody has been selected, the manufacturer's specifications for the antibody must be verified, especially in terms of whether the antibody is only to be used for a frozen section or also for a paraffin section and thus whether it is "paraffin-compatible." The term paraffin-compatible may be misunderstood since formaldehyde, which is the most frequently selected fixative, can hinder immunohistochemical detection of antigens. Formaldehyde results in a relatively intensive interlacing of proteins such that—initially also according to manufacturer's specifications—a procedure for antigen unmasking may be needed (see above). If sufficient reproducibility of antigen detection is ultimately achieved, modification of the antigen demasking pretreatment may be established in one's own laboratory; different methods, solutions, and incubation times (microwave pretreatment, damp autoclave treatment, etc., see also above) are possible.

There is a differentiation between antigens of the extracellular matrix and membrane-bound antigens, e.g., of the cell or basal membranes. For example, it is feasible to select the immunohistochemically detectable basal membrane components collagen IV and laminin as representative intact basal membrane antigens. Fibronectin and complement C5b-$9_{(m)}$ antibodies are indicated to prove prior myocardial necrosis in the myocardium. However, in each case, the goal of immunohistochemical techniques is to gain knowledge in addition to conventional histological staining. Thus, in conventional myocarditis diagnosis according to the Dallas criteria, significant diagnostic insecurity exists due to interobserver variability. Immunohistochemical qualification and quantification of interstitial inflammatory cells leads to the confirmation of a high quota of inflammatory cardiac myopathies (chronic myocarditises) with dilative cardiomyopathies (see Chap. 13).

Immunohistochemical examination of injuries, in particular skin and soft tissue lesions, may lead to an approximate age determination of the lesion, which is helpful and may be significant in criminal investigations. However, in many cases, caution should be taken when basing conclusions solely on immunohistochemical findings, even if this may be possible for an individual case. Table 2.6 contains a list of current antibodies with reference to forensic medical problems.

Table 2.6 List of selected immunohistochemical primary antibodies (according to bibliographical references)[a] frequently used in forensic medicine

Antibodies	Destination structure/localization	Problem
Adhesion molecule, e.g., ICAM-1, VCAM-1	Surface membranes, especially on endothelial cells for cell–cell interaction	Activation of leukocyte invasion with inflammatory processes
Anti-C5b-$9_{(m)}$ complement	Complement factor C5b-9	Early necrosis marker, e.g., with myocardial infarct
Anti-fibrinogen	Fibrinogen	Early necrosis marker, e.g., with myocardial infarct
Anti-fibronectin	Fibronectin	Early myocardial necrosis
Anti-IgG	Immunoglobulin type IgG	Immunoglobulin deposit in glomerulus loops with heroin-associated nephropathy
Anti-IgM	Immunoglobulin type IgM	Immunoglobulin deposit in glomerulus loops with heroin-associated nephropathy
Anti-myoglobin	Myocardial and skeletal muscle cells	Myoglobin-containing protein cylinder with rhabdomyolysis
CD3	T-lymphocytes	Viral infections
CD68	Macrophages	Cellular histiocytic reaction when determining age of lesion

(continued)

Table 2.6 (continued)

Antibodies	Destination structure/localization	Problem
CD45R0	Activated T-lymphocytes	Viral infections
Chromogranin A	Enterochromaffin-like cells, neuroendocrine tumors	Pheochromocytoma
Collagens	Basal membrane component	Intact basal membranes
Cytokeratin	Epithelial cells, among others keratinizing squamous epithelial cells	Amniotic fluid embolism in pregnant women or amniotic fluid aspiration in newborns
Cytokines—generic term for peptide mediators with biological effect on cells, especially interleukins, interferons, chemokines, TNF-α, TGF-ß, colony-stimulating factors (CSFs)	In part many somatic cells, among others vascular endothelial cells, different types of leukocytes, including T-lymphocytes, monocytes, macrophages, T-helper cells, stroma cells, etc.	For example: emphasized expression in inflammatory processes, activation factors for natural killer cells, etc.; thus, TNF-α is produced by monocytes/macrophages in particular
Cytomegalovirus (CMV)	Infected cells	CMV sialadenitis in particular with SIDS, CMV pneumonia
Desmin	Smoothly and horizontally striped muscle cells, myocardial structure protein (Paulin and Li 2004)	Absent in the case of myocardial necrosis
Heat shock proteins (HSP)	Different proteins which help other proteins maintain their secondary structure; this means protecting cellular proteins from denaturation (Javid et al. 2007; Hasday and Singh 2000)	Increased expression following cellular stress caused by heat, radiation, toxins, etc.
Laminin	Basal membrane component	Intact basal membranes
LCA (CD45)	Pan-leukocyte marker (leukocyte common antigen)	Inflammatory processes
MHC molecules (major histocompatibility complex = MHC)	MHC molecules function in different cells as binding and presentation molecules for intracytoplasmic and endocytic antigens	More emphasized expression of certain MHC molecules with, e.g., viral infections
Myosin	Cells of the skeletal musculature	Rhabdomyolysis; myosin cylinder in renal tubules
PCAM-1 = platelet endothelial cell adhesion molecule (CD31)	Endothelial cells, thrombocytes, monocytes, neutrophil granulocytes	On endothelial cells involved in leukocyte transmigration
Selectins (E-, P-, and L-selectin)	E-selectin in plasma membranes of endothelial cells, P-selectin in endothelial cells and thrombocytes; L-selectin is made by all leukocytes: surface molecules to organize leukocyte invasion: rolling, trapping, diapedesis	Proinflammatory marker, in inflammatory processes
Tenascins	Extracellular matrix glycoproteins (Chiquet-Ehrisman and Chiquet 2003)	Repair processes surrounding healing lesions, including myocardial necrosis
Troponin I	Myocardial structure protein which builds the contractile part of the muscle cell with myosin and actin	Absent in the case of myocardial necrosis
Tyrosine kinase KIT (CD117)	For instance, surface molecules on mast cells	Mast cells can also be visualized following expression of tryptase (degranulated mast cells)
Vimentin	Intermediate filament of mesenchyme cells (e.g., fibroblasts, endothelial cells, smooth muscle cells)	Wound healing in skin lesions

[a]There are numerous other antibodies which have not been checked for suitability in connection with forensics but which are used in individual forensic studies for defined problems

However, the number of available antibodies is so high that only selected antibodies can be listed. In the area of neurotraumatology, antibodies are used against glial and neuronal cells, as well as to determine the age of brain injuries (please see the specialized literature for general and forensic neuropathology).

The following antibodies or markers have been intermittently available for the group of infectious agents: *Chlamydia pneumoniae* (Dettmeyer et al. 2006), *Cytomegalovirus* (Dettmeyer et al. 2007), *Cryptococcus neoformans*, Epstein–Barr virus (EBV), *Helicobacter pylori*, hepatitis antigens HBs and HBc, HIV (p. 24), herpes simplex, human papilloma virus (HPV), Pneumocystis carinii, and Toxoplasma gondii.

The following is valid for the evaluation of immunohistochemical stains:

1. Methodical errors and artifacts must be excluded. Both positive and negative controls must yield expected results. An "internal positive control" is conceivable [e.g., thrombocytes and megakaryocytes show constitutive expression of P-selectin (Ortmann and Brinkmann 1997)].
2. When cellular antigens are specifically detected, this results in a stained cell (e.g., leukocytes, T-lymphocytes, B-lymphocytes, macrophages, etc.); at low cell counts, quantification may be done by counting cells per visual field (high power field, ×400) or per surface (mm^2).
3. Cell-bound antigens may also show different intensities of expression, which correlate with color intensity. A graduation of the extent of expression is possible.
4. In the case of non-cell-bound antigens, which can be found in the intra- and extra-cellular matrix, a graduation of color intensity is normal, for example, to evaluate the expression of MHC class I and II molecules. The following graduation is used:
   0 = no staining
   + = minimal
   ++ = moderate
   +++ = intense
   ++++ = extreme

Such a semiquantitative analysis of the staining results can be found in published forensic medicine studies and may be included in statistical analysis (Dettmeyer et al. 2004a, b; Ortmann and Brinkmann 1997; Nwariaku et al. 1995). Microscopic evaluation of the compounds should be carried out in a timely manner, since—also according to own experience—depending on the antibody selected and storage of the tissue section, a reduction in color intensity can be possible after only a few months, which directly affects the quantification of immunohistochemical findings (Dettmeyer et al. 2009a, b, c).

2.4 Special Examination Techniques

A number of special examination techniques are used in forensic medicine, mainly in the context of scientific studies, including TUNEL assay, in situ hybridization, confocal laser scanning microscopy, electron microscopy, and laser microdissection.

2.4.1 TUNEL Assay

The TUNEL assay (TdT-mediated dUTP-biotin nick end labeling) is used to detect cell nuclei in apoptotic cells. "TdT" describes an enzyme, "terminal deoxynucleotidyl transferase," which is needed for an intermediate step. The enzyme TdT causes marked nucleotides to be added to the hydroxyl groups (3′-OH groups) released on the fragmented DNA string when apoptosis occurs. These hydroxyl groups can be made visible with the help of fluorescence microscopy. The method was first described in 1992 (Gavrieli et al. 1992). Critics find fault with the fact that reliable differentiation between apoptotic and necrotic cells is not possible (Grasl-Kaup et al. 1995). Improvements to the method have since been reported (Labat-Moleur et al. 1998). Currently, the TUNEL assay is not relevant for routine forensic medicine diagnostics, but it is used within the scope of scientific studies. Tumor tissue may be used as a positive control, since it contains many apoptotic cells, e.g., a malignant lymphoma (Fig. 2.14).

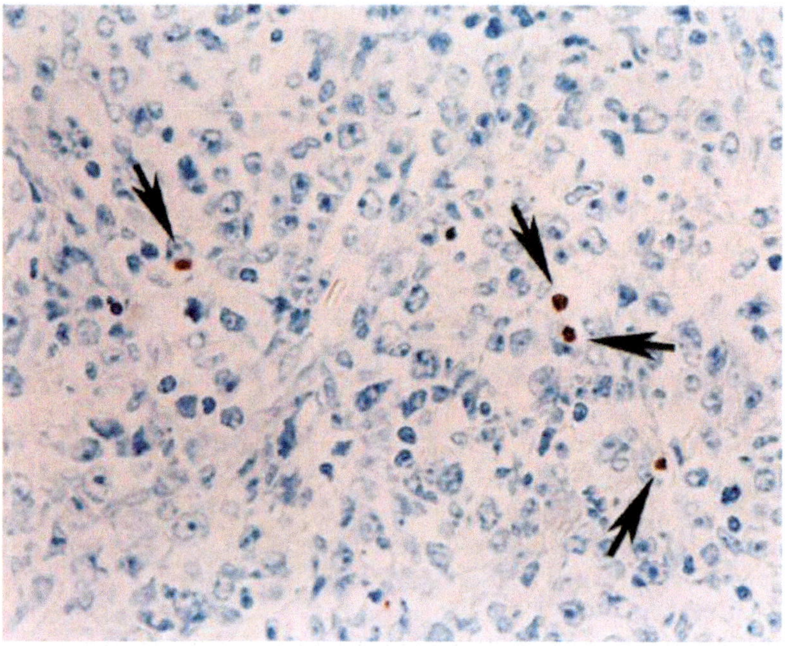

Fig. 2.14 TUNEL assay with detection of individual apoptotic cells (*arrows*) in a malignant lymphoma as a control specimen (×200)

A handful of publications present apoptosis which, given that single cells are affected, is easily recognized at 400× magnification. Studies that show (purportedly) positive apoptosis reactions using the TUNEL technique, but fail to present their findings at higher magnification, are to be viewed with skepticism.

The first thing that needs to be verified is whether apoptosis is to be expected in the first place and how one should interpret positive or negative findings. Tissue identical to the organ in question and which has also been obtained at autopsy needs to be selected as a positive control. The problem can be elucidated using the example of viral myocarditis and the hypothesis that, without apoptotic cardiomyocytes, there would be no viral myocarditis. This hypothesis ignores three aspects.

Firstly, postmortem autolytic processes can prevent positive detection of apoptosis; secondly, viruses (particularly enteroviruses), as the most frequent cause of myocarditis, can have anti-apoptotic effects; and thirdly, apoptosis in the early phase of myocarditis, which can last days, has not (yet) been detected (see Chaps. 13 and 17 for more details).

The literature states the following in this regard: "Other authors could only present a positive result in TUNEL staining in cases autopsied within 20 h of death and where the time lapse between onset and death was within 2 h" (Nakatone et al. 2002). To simply purport a "short" postmortem interval in a publication against this backdrop, despite it being generally known that an autopsy can rarely be carried out within 20 h, raises doubt about the accuracy of the diagnosis. If the chronology of the disease also undermines the assumption that positive apoptosis detection is to be expected, then one's own interpretation of a supposedly positive or negative microscopy finding should be viewed with particular skepticism. Thus, it is incorrect to infer that: "A causal link between myocarditis and cases of sudden child death cannot be assumed on the basis of this investigation." For the purposes of comparison, if myocardial infarction is no longer microscopically identifiable due to putrefaction, it would be wrong to conclude that, due to the putrefaction-related failure to detect myocardial infarction, there was no myocardial infarction. A certain skepticism regarding the reliability of the TUNEL technique is formulated in the literature: "It is not certain that they represent true apoptosis induced by ischemia" (Edston et al. 2002) and "…we think that its use may be insufficient due to its low specificity" (Erel et al. 2014).

2.4.2 In Situ Hybridization

In situ hybridization is a molecular biological method used to detect nucleic acids, RNA or DNA in tissue, single cells, or metaphase chromosomes. To this end, an artificial nucleic acid probe is used. The probe hybridizes (binds) to the nucleic acid of interest with the help of base pairing. The description "in situ" means that the analysis occurs directly in the cell or tissue and not in a test tube. The probes involved are generally DNA probes that are more stable than RNA probes. Marking of the probe can be done directly with haptens (e.g., digoxigenin, biotin, or 2,4-dinitrophenol) or with fluorescing molecules (fluorescence in situ hybridization, FISH). Hybridization may take from 1 h to several days depending on the probe material and destination sequence. Probe molecules which are not specifically bound are washed out. The method used depends on the problem, e.g., proving cytomegaloviruses in the parotid gland in cases of assumed sudden infant death (Fig. 2.15). In principle, in situ PCR and PCR in situ hybridization are also possible in paraffin-embedded tissue (Schiller et al. 1998).

2.4.3 Confocal Laser Scanning Microscopy

Confocal laser scanning microscopy (CLSM) uses two channels, e.g., laser line 1 (argon ion 488 nm) and laser line 2 (krypton 568 nm) and allows detection of two fluorescent signals (double markers) from the same specimen scanned simultaneously and digitally converted into an image. This technique of microscopic imaging has transformed the field of biology and forensic histopathology in particular (Wyss and Lasczkowski 2008; Turillazzi et al. 2007; Lucitti and Dickinson 2006). By allowing greater resolution, optical sectioning of the sample and three-dimensional reconstruction, CLSM has found a wide field of application (e.g., sudden cardiac death, neonatal hypoxic–ischemic lesions, electrical, and explosion injuries). For example, CLSM was used to investigate the vitality and age of conjunctival petechiae by investigating the expression of the endothelial adhesion molecule P-selectin (Wyss and Lasczkowski 2008; Fig. 2.16).

2.4.4 Electron Microscopy

The development of electron microscopy has opened new horizons for medical and physical

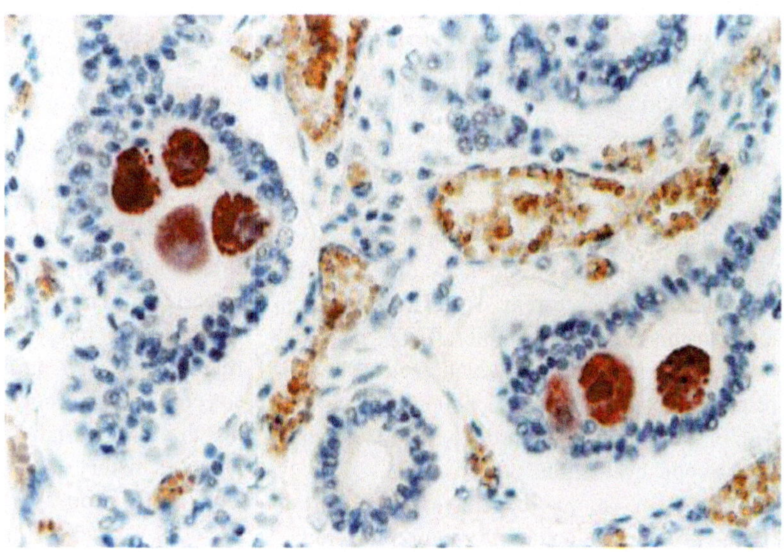

Fig. 2.15 Detection of cytomegaloviruses using in situ hybridization in glandular epithelial cells of the parotid gland (×200)

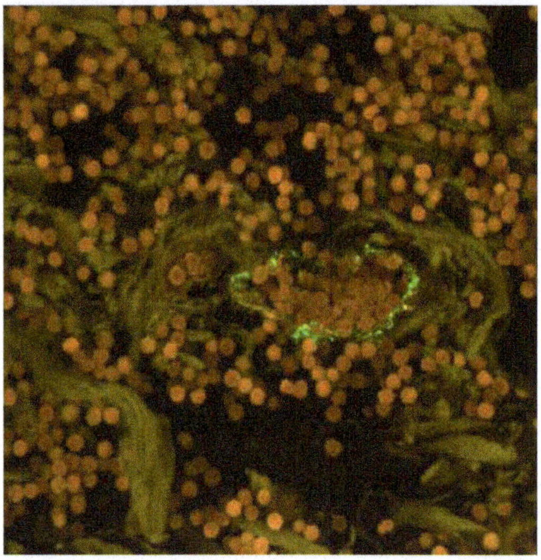

Fig. 2.16 Confocal laser scanning microscopy to investigate the vitality and age of conjunctival petechiae by investigating the expression of the endothelial molecule P-selectin (image courtesy of Dr. Lasczkowski, Gießen, Germany)

research (Biro et al. 2010). The interior of an object, or its surface, can be displayed with the help of an electron microscope. While the optical microscope only reaches a resolution of approximately 200 nm, the current resolution of the electron microscope is approximately 0.1 nm. There are different types of electron microscope. When creating a picture, the raster electron microscope (REM) (scanning electron microscope) is differentiated from the still-life microscope. In view of the geometry of the arrangement, scanning transmission electron microscopy is considered to be a technical variation of still-life microscopy.

With the scanning electron microscope (SEM), a thick electron ray is guided over the object. During this process, emitted or backscattered electrons, including other signals, are synchronously detected; the intensity of the pixel is determined by the current. When working with the transmission electron microscope, electrons travel through the object, which need to be correspondingly thin. The object should be embedded in the fixative glutaraldehyde for electron microscopic evaluation.

SEM with energy dispersive microanalysis (EDX) provides valuable information in forensic medicine about the morphology of injuries and injury implements. The use of SEM is not limited by autolysis to the same degree as transmission electron microscopy, for example. SEM can be used for the study of various types of wounds and particularly for the study of bullet wounds (Havel 2003; Havel and Zelenka 2003; Kage et al. 2001; Torre et al. 2002; Fechner et al. 1990; Brinkmann et al. 1984). Also, other authors concluded that SEM, together with EDX, can provide explicit information in bullet wound investigations (Cardinetti et al. 2004) and can be useful for diagnosis in cases of electrocution (Kinoshita et al. 2004).

Electron microscopy plays an important role in forensic medicine for the detection of metallic particles, but otherwise it is used foremost within the scope of scientific studies. In certain cases, SEM together with EDX enables the determination of projectile parameters in firearm wounds, as well as an approximate determination of firearm distance (Biro et al. 2010; Dubrovin and Dubrovina 2003).

2.4.5 Laser Microdissection

Laser microdissection is a technique to isolate certain cells from microscopically analyzed smears, tissues, and/or organs. The tissue or single cells are cut open with a laser without damaging their morphology. This technique is used to collect cells for specific DNA or RNA analyses, e.g., sperm following a sexual offense (Vandewoestyne et al. 2009; Seidl et al. 2005).

2.5 Tissue Sample Selection

Information on previous history can be relevant as early on as at the sample selection stage, since one can either pay special attention to a particular finding (e.g., myocardial infarction, liver cirrhosis, etc.) or one is able to demonstrate that a finding that was actually expected according to the previous history is in fact not present (e.g., exclusion of amyloidosis, a particular tumor, meningitis, etc.). A lack of microscopy experience can already result in misinterpretations during the assessment of staining quality, and misdiagnoses necessarily ensue. It is not uncommon for microscopic findings to be present but to be overlooked or incorrectly classified due to a lack of microscopy experience. This partially explains interobserver variability.

With some organs, one can proceed on the basis of the "pars pro toto" principle: viral hepatitis often affects the entire organ and can generally be detected or excluded with two samples (left and right hepatic lobes); the same usually applies in, e.g., hepatic steatosis, liver fibrosis/cirrhosis, acute glomerulonephritis, severe ascending cholangitis, and fibroadenia of the spleen.

Other diseases require several samples to be taken in order to reliably diagnose certain disorders, e.g., adrenocortical hyperplasia, lipoid loss in adrenocortical cells, nonspecific thyroiditis, generally acute congestive hyperemia, and edema.

In the case of special diagnoses, tissue samples need to be taken from defined sites, not least for the purposes of adequate documentation: e.g., from the margins of the infarction or the center of the infarction or lesion in the case of macroscopically visible fresh myocardial infarction, tumors, cerebral infarction, splenic infarction, and other focal findings [e.g., focal nodular hyperplasia (FNH), focal tuberculous lesions, etc.).

The problem of the representativeness of selected samples is more relevant in forensic practice, e.g., in lung tissue, the myocardium, and wound age determination. Lung tissue—more so in adults of advancing age than in infants and children—exhibits areas of varying perfusion and ventilation associated with aging processes and possibly with previous inflammatory episodes (emphysema, increasing interstitial fibrosis, etc.). Cardiac findings (e.g., coronary sclerosis, coronary thrombosis, interstitial myocardial fibrosis, disorders of cardiac fiber structure in cardiomyopathies, myocarditis, fibromuscular dysplasia of the AV node artery, sinus node fibrosis, acute and chronic hypoxic–ischemic myocardial damage, cardiovascular amyloidosis, etc.) may occur only focally and (partially) escape detection if only a small number of samples are used for microscopy investigations.

2.6 Interpreting Histological and Immunohistochemical Staining

The microscopic analysis of even a large number of samples may prove unhelpful in the absence of basic pathophysiological knowledge. The following example illustrates this well:

Example: Histopathological Classification of Pulmonary Edema

If the body is in a supine position, reddish-brown discoloration is often macroscopically visible on the dorsal parts of the lung, and more fluid is found in these areas (internal livor mortis). Histologically, lung tissue of this kind exhibits (hemorrhagic) pulmonary edema depending on postmortem interval, while, in contrast, the ventral parts of the lung are more likely to show empty pulmonary alveoli and no pulmonary edema. This example illustrates how microscopic-histopathological grading of the extent of pulmonary edema is unhelpful. The lung weight measured at autopsy, on the other hand, is significantly more reliable for the diagnosis of "pulmonary edema." Whoever classifies microscopically unequivocal pulmonary edema in H&E staining as, e.g., grade 3 pulmonary edema, needs to explain what grade 1 and 2 pulmonary edema looks like under the microscope and what level of reliability should be conferred to such a grading.

In addition to also taking macroscopic findings and postmortem interval into consideration in the interpretation of histological findings, it may be that a diagnosis can only be established, depending on the diagnostic question, if a sufficient number of samples and tissue sections are analyzed. An example to illustrate this point would be:

Example: A Sufficient Number of Myocardial Specimens in Suspected Viral Myocarditis

Macroscopically abnormal findings in the heart should be removed for microscopic analysis. If this type of finding is absent and cardiomyopathy or myocarditis, for instance, needs to be ruled out, numerous myocardial specimens, which possibly need to be analyzed in serial sections using special stains, are required for the purely focal detection of these two diseases. The removal of eight myocardial samples from a defined site is recommended in infants; according to more recent literature, nine myocardial samples and six samples frozen for molecular genetic diagnosis to detect the viral genome are recommended (Gaaloul et al. 2016). This number of myocardial samples enables a representative overview at an infant-heart weight of around 25–30 g. However, eight samples do not permit comparable representativeness in larger adult hearts (350–450 g); nevertheless, the methodology proposed for infant hearts is sometimes extrapolated indiscriminately to adult hearts for the diagnosis of myocarditis.

Even in the case of a sufficient number of samples and correct immunohistochemical staining, a meaningful interpretation of microscopic findings is only possible if the examiner possesses the relevant basic knowledge of histology. This is also well illustrated by an example (that should not be followed).

Example: Grading the Number of Alveolar Macrophages in Pulmonary Tissue

The macrophage marker CD68 identifies the abundant local alveolar macrophages physiologically present in pulmonary tissue (Fig. 2.17). These alveolar macrophages are often found postmortem, artificially desquamated and accumulated, e.g., in atelectatic areas (Fig. 2.18). Thus, quantifying CD68-positive macrophages in pulmonary tissue taken at autopsy by counting per high power field (hpf) or mm^2 is wholly unsuited to the visualization of pulmonary inflammation, since the preexisting macrophages are always included in the count or cannot be differentiated. Therefore, the introduction of a grading system for inflammatory processes according to the number of CD68-positive macrophages per hpf or mm^2 is wholly meaningless, even though this diagnostically pointless procedure is occasionally practiced. The authors of studies such as these are subsequently unable to explain how they differentiated from preexisting (alveolar) macrophages in the count and how they propose to exclude postmortem autolytic distortions.

2.7 Selecting a Suitable Positive Control

Particularly in the case of tissue samples taken at autopsy, it is important to establish whether the epitopes to be visualized immunohistochemically are still present, i.e., are sufficiently resistant to autolysis. There are only scant

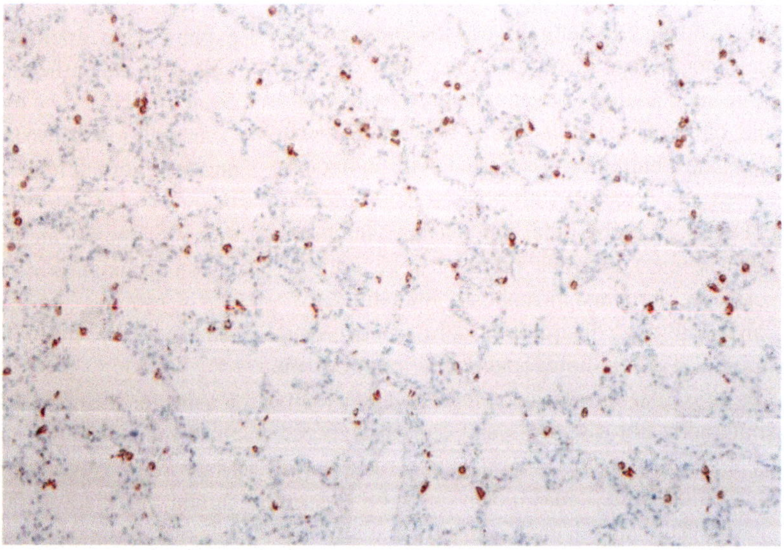

Fig. 2.17 Normal finding with evidence of preexisting local CD68-positive alveolar macrophages in pulmonary tissue (×100)

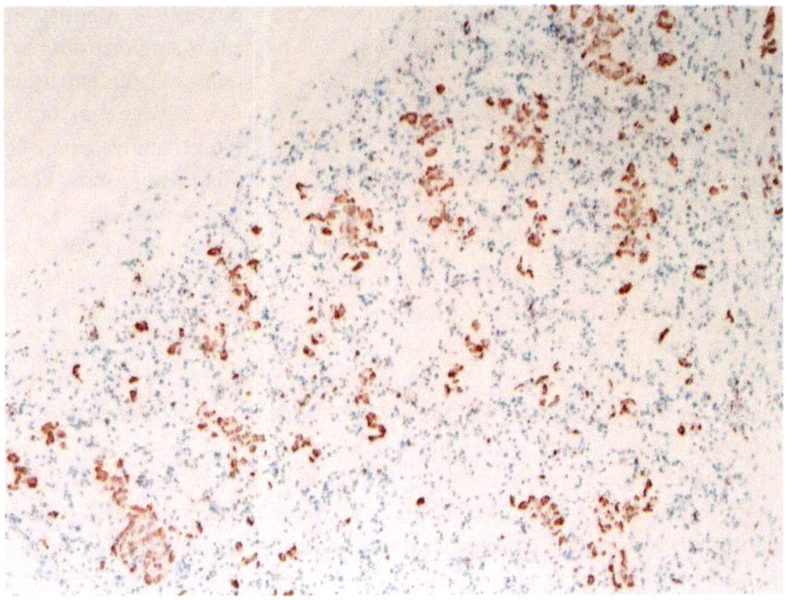

Fig. 2.18 Subpleural atelectasis with an accumulation of preexisting CD68-positive alveolar macrophages in pulmonary tissue; comparable areas of macrophage accumulation are also found in central sections of pulmonary tissue (CD68 ×100)

qualitatively good, systematic investigations on the ability of molecules detectable immunohistochemically to resist autolysis or putrefaction; experience has nonetheless been garnered (see Chap. 19). For example, cell-bound antigens are considered to be more stable on the whole compared with non-cell-bound molecules (with exceptions, naturally). This applies, for example, to the frequently used immunohistochemical markers LCA, CD68, CD45, CD3, as well as many more; according to own experience, the necrosis marker $C5b9_{(m)}$ is also relatively resistant to autolysis and can be successfully used to detect myocardial infarction for instance (see Chap. 13). In any event, one should carry out a positive control on tissue that has also been taken at autopsy. If diagnostic work is restricted to a semiquantitative estimation of the expression of certain immunohistochemical markers, a relevant positive control in which the antigens to be identified are present in abundance is adequate. For example, if leukocytes or lymphocytes are to be measured only semiquantitatively and graded according to a normal, low, moderate, or high number of cells detectable in tissue (0, +, ++, +++), then tonsil tissue or a lymph node taken at autopsy can be used as a positive control. However, a positive control of this sort is not adequate if the objective is to identify individual cell types or individual cells in tissue in order to count them.

2.8 Immunohistochemical Qualification and Quantification of Individual Cell Types

Even if individual cells are to be identified (qualified) and counted (quantified), e.g., as cell count per hpf (×400) or per mm^2, it is once again necessary to select an organ-identical positive control taken at autopsy.

The best known analysis in this context is the qualification and quantification of interstitial leukocytes in the myocardium in the case of (suspected) myocarditis. However, even if the immunohistochemical identification of leukocytes, lymphocytes, and macrophages appears to have been successful and error-free in the positive control, it is essential to check whether all cells in each individual specimen were in fact detected on staining, a task barely feasible without microscopy experience. Added to this is the fact that a high rate of insufficient staining occurs when performing immunohistochemical stains "by hand" with wet chambers. This problem can also be illustrated using an example.

Example: Macrophage Detection in the Infant Myocardium
Cases where patently unsuccessful stains are not recognized as such lead to, e.g., statements according to which no CD68-positive macrophages were detectable in over 90% of cases of infant myocardia investigated. This was asserted for the first time, as yet, by a working group, apparently without registering that, as a result and as far as it would appear, they were the first to (purportedly) detect macrophage-free infant myocardium in a large collective. If results such as these, based on patently erroneous stains, are published as normal values for instance, and if other working groups let themselves be guided by these results, it is possible that misinterpretations will ensue. A case in point would be the hasty assumption of an inflammatory process in the myocardium on the basis of successful immunohistochemical visualization of macrophages, since the infant myocardium is, in general, supposedly macrophage-free. Cases of relatively macrophage-rich myocarditis are known.

Immunohistochemical diagnostics have led to advances particularly in the diagnosis of viral myocarditis, as evidenced by numerous publications (see Chaps. 13 and 17). Should these advances be ignored, it is possible that an author will end up supporting wholly contradictory findings.

An example here would be a statement made in 2005: "Modern immunohistochemical techniques provide a powerful tool to prove lethal myocarditis in cases devoid of traditional histological findings according to the Dallas criteria," compared with a 2015 statement by the same author: "At in least infants, the diagnosis of myocarditis from autopsy tissues still requires application of the Dallas criteria. Immunohistochemical methods cannot replace the conventional diagnosis of myocarditis."

The publication of conflicting results by an author may subsequently continue. For example, "Using immunohistochemical methods with qualification and quantification of interstitial leucocytes, PCR and Rt-PCR methods for identifying virus genome within the myocardium, it is possible to identify in about one third of SIDS cases a myocarditis as cause of death," compared with a statement by the same author, "A causal link between myocarditis and cases of sudden infant death cannot be assumed on the basis of this investigation." Poor methodological mastery and a disinclination toward self-critical review within a working group can result in other investigators being gravely misled.

2.9 Histopathological Studies: Findings and Comparability

Prior to conducting a study or bringing out a subject-related publication, the relevant literature should be consulted in order gain an awareness of the current state of research. Against this backdrop, the following statement is somewhat surprising: "Myocarditis was relatively rarely identified in SIDS collectives in older studies, whereas newer investigations report a higher incidence, some as high as 20%." Although there are indeed older and newer studies reporting a high incidence of myocarditis, the authors of the above statement have chosen not to elaborate on what "older" and what "newer" investigations are but arrive nevertheless at the following conclusion: "Thus, overall, there is no evidence to suggest that myocarditis represents a pathomechanism that contributes in any significant way to death in fatalities considered to be SIDS." This statement is valid if one deems an incidence of, e.g., 20% to not be an "important pathomechanism."

When evaluating and comparing studies, it is important to verify whether comparable samples were indeed investigated using comparable methods. For example, a prospective study using immunohistochemical markers and molecular genetic virus detection on samples taken from a defined site in the infant myocardium and fixed for a maximum of 48 h in neutral phosphate-buffered formalin yielded the result that lethal viral myocarditis could be a plausible cause of death in some cases of purported SIDS (Dettmeyer et al. 2004a, b; Dettmeyer 2016). A second study confirmed this result (Dettmeyer et al. 2009a, b, c). A third, albeit retrospective, study, whose authors provided no details on the number of specimens investigated per case or for how long (or in which fixative) the specimens were kept, arrived at the conclusion that myocarditis played no relevant role in SIDS (Krous et al. 2009), a statement which drew critical comment (Dettmeyer et al. 2009a, b, c). The differing methodology backs up both studies, since the methodology could also have worked retrospectively to an extent. However, formulating the following without providing more details "For instance a study on viral infection of the myocardium in SIDS cases claimed that nearly in 30% of cases viral genome was detected in the myocardium, a finding that could not be confirmed in succeeding studies" is incorrect on two levels. Firstly, this relates to merely one follow-up histopathological and molecular genetic study, not "studies" (plural), and secondly, the crucial methodological differences in the first two studies compared with the third were simply not mentioned. This is despite the fact that the statement "nearly in 30%" likely refers to a publication that was unfortunately not specified in the publication but which can nevertheless be found and which states that: "… it is possible to identify in about one third of SIDS cases a myocarditis as cause of death." More recent studies support the reasonable suspicion of fatal myocarditis in a portion of SIDS victims (Gaaloul et al. 2016; see Chap. 17).

The list of methodologically unhelpful investigations, incorrect diagnoses, and conflicting statements encountered also in forensic histopathology goes on. Table 2.7 provides a non-exhaustive overview of possible errors in and misinterpretations of histological, histopathological, and immunohistochemical findings.

Table 2.7 Some examples of errors in or questionable interpretations of histological, histopathological, and/or immunohistochemical findings

Example	Invalid interpretation/comment
Immunohistochemical CD68-positive macrophage count in lung tissue to diagnose inflammation	The CD68 antibody detects physiologically present alveolar macrophages; postmortem autolytic processes cause a buildup of these macrophages; a CD68-positive cell count does not permit any conclusions to be drawn on the possible presence of pneumonia
Grading the number of CD68-positive macrophages counted in lung tissue	For the abovementioned reasons, the distribution of macrophages in lung tissue is severely affected by postmortem autolytic processes; as such, there is absolutely no basis for a grading, e.g., according to grades 1, 2, or 3 as part of the supposed diagnosis of inflammation in lung tissue
Histological detection of pulmonary edema	The detection of local edema in pulmonary tissue has in itself no validity, since pulmonary edema can ultimately develop at any site in lung tissue
Histological classification of pulmonary edema	Grading the extent of pulmonary edema on the basis of histological findings is not beneficial. The severity of pulmonary edema is more reliably established from the weight of the lungs
Immunohistochemical qualification and quantification of interstitial macrophages in the infant myocardium	The non-critical acceptance of negative immunohistochemical findings as a result of poor mastery of the staining method—and despite basic medical knowledge and the relevant literature suggesting that, e.g., it is not possible to have macrophage-free infant myocardium in numerous cases—leads to invalid results. Publishing false-negative findings as normal findings can result in considerable confusion
Postmortem interval as an influencing factor	If no one has hitherto detected an apoptosis-positive reaction, e.g., in myocardial tissue taken at autopsy at a postmortem interval of over 20 h, then some apoptosis-negative results at longer postmortem intervals have no validity whatsoever
Publishing meaningless and trivial findings	Age-appropriate findings, or even histopathological findings that are relatively pronounced for the given age, need to be classified in a meaningful context; otherwise, they are completely devoid of meaning and validity. Banal endothelial coronary sclerosis generally has no reconstructive or pathophysiological validity whatsoever

(continued)

Table 2.7 (continued)

Example	Invalid interpretation/comment
Invalid comparison of studies	To argue, one study does not confirm the findings of another study when the findings came from studies with widely differing methodologies (e.g., retrospective rather than prospective; differing fixatives, fixation times, and number of specimens), while at the same time not mentioning these methodological differences is not to be taken seriously and conveys a false impression
Invalid extrapolation of a method	Eight myocardial specimens from an infant heart weighing 25 g are able to yield overall histologically representative findings in terms of the diagnosis of myocarditis, not however from an adult heart weighing 350–450 g. The indiscriminate extrapolation of specimen number to adult hearts and the unclear results that can be expected from this is not a reason to reject the method in infant hearts
Invalid inference about a functional process based on morphological findings	Example: hepatic steatosis can be "starting" or "abating"; neither stage can be inferred from histopathological findings
Lymphocytic infiltrates with germinal center formation in thyroid tissue	The detection of lymphocytic infiltrates with germinal center formation in interstitial thyroid tissue does not on its own justify the diagnosis of Hashimoto's goiter

References

Ananian V, Tozzo P, Ponzano E, Nitti D, Rodriguez D, Caenazzo L (2010) Tumoural specimens for forensic purposes: comparison of genetic alterations in frozen and formalin-fixed paraffin-embedded tissues. Int J Legal Med 125(3):327–332

Bankfalvi A, Navabi H, Bier B, Böcker W, Jasani B, Schmid W (1994a) Wet autoclave pretreatment for antigen retrieval in diagnostic immunohistochemistry. J Pathol 174:223–228

Bankfalvi A, Riehemann K, Öfner D, Checci R, Morgan JM, Piffko J, Böcker W, Jasani B, Schmid KW (1994b) Feuchtes Autoklavieren. Pathologe 15:345–349

Ben-Ezra J, Johnson DA, Rossi J (1991) Effect of fixation on the amplification of nucleic acids from paraffin-embedded material by the polymerase chain reaction. J Histochem Cytochem 39:351–354

Biro C, Kovac P, Palkovic M, El-Hassoun O, Caplovicova M, Novotny J, Jakubovsky J (2010) Potentialities of scanning electron microscopy and EDX analysis in bullet wounds. Rom J Leg Med 18:225–230

Bratzke H, Schröter A (1995) Immunhistochemie in der Rechtsmedizin. Hänsel-Hohenhausen, Egelsbach

Brinkmann B, Fechner G, Püschel K (1984) Identification of mechanical asphyxiation in cases of attempted masking of the homicide. Forensic Sci Int 26:235–245

Brown RW, Chirala R (1995) Utility of microwave-citrate antigen retrieval in diagnostic immunohistochemistry. Mod Pathol 8:515–520

Cardinetti B, Ciampini C, D'Onofrio C, Orlando G, Gravina L, Ferrari F, Di Tullio D, Torresi L (2004) X-ray mapping technique: a preliminary study in discriminating gunshot residue particles from aggregates of environmental occupational origin. Forensic Sci Int 143:1–19

Chiquet-Ehrisman R, Chiquet M (2003) Tenascins: regulation and putative functions during pathological stress. J Pathol 200:488–499

Cordell JL, Falini B, Erber WN, Ghosh AK, Abdulaziz Z, McDonald S, Pulford AF, Stein H, Mason DY (1984) Immunoenzymatic labeling of monoclonal antibodies using immuno complexes of alkaline phosphatase and monoclonal anti-alkaline phosphatase (APAAP-complex). J Histochem Cytochem 32:219–229

Cuevas EC, Bateman AC, Wilkins BS, Johnson PA, Williams JH, Lee AHS, Jones DB, Wright DH (1994) Microwave antigen retrieval in immunocytochemistry: a study of 80 antibodies. J Clin Pathol 47:448–452

Dettmeyer R (2016) Postmortem diagnostics of a (post-) viral myocarditis in putative sudden infant death syndrome. Case report for avoidance of errors in the diagnostics. Rechtsmedizin 26:514–519

Dettmeyer R, Baasner A, Schlamann M, Padosch SA, Haag C, Kandolf R, Madea B (2004a) Role of virus-induced myocardial affections in sudden infant death syndrome (SIDS): a prospective post-mortem study. Pediatr Res 55:947–952

Dettmeyer R, Baasner A, Schlamann M, Padosch SA, Haag C, Kandolf R, Madea B (2004b) Role of virus-induced myocardial affections in sudden infant death syndrome: a prospective postmortem study. Pediatr Res 55:1–5

Dettmeyer R, Stiel M, Madea B (2006) Heat shock protein 60 (cHSP60) as a marker for chronic infection with *Chlamydia pneumoniae* in atherosclerosis—investigation of atherosclerotic coronary arteries by immunocytochemistry. Forensic Sci Med Pathol 2:173–178

Dettmeyer R, Sperhake JP, Müller J, Madea B (2007) Cytomegalovirus-induced pneumonia and myocarditis in 3 cases of suspected sudden infant death syndrome (SIDS): diagnosis by immunohistochemical techniques, in-situ-hybridisation and molecular pathologic investigations. Forensic Sci Int 174:229–233

Dettmeyer R, Baasner A, Haag C, Bruch S, Schlamann M (2009a) Immunohistochemical and molecular pathological diagnosis of myocarditis in cases of suspected sudden infant death syndrome (SIDS)—a multicenter study. Legal Med 11:S124–S127

Dettmeyer R, Bruch S, Haag C (2009b) Letter to the editor on “myocardial inflammation, cellular death, and viral detection in sudden infant death caused by SIDS, suffocation, or myocarditis”. Pediatr Res 66:714

Dettmeyer R, Friedrich K, Schmidt P, Madea B (2009c) Heroin-associated myocardial damages—conventional and immunohistochemical investigations. Forensic Sci Int 187:42–46

Dokhan DB, Kovatich AJ, Miettinen M (1993) Nonenzymatic antigen retrieval in immunohistochemistry—comparison between different antigen retrieval modalities and proteolytic digestion. Appl Immunohistochem 1:149–155

Dreßler J, Bachmann L, Koch R, Müller E (1998) The detection of P-selectin in paraffin embedded sections by wet autoclave technique. J Cell Pathol 3:139–143

Dubrovin IA, Dubrovina IA (2003) The influence of a shot distance on a profile of a wound canal in flat bones. Sud Med Ekspert 46:11–13

Edston E, Gröntoft L, Johnsson J (2002) TUNEL: a useful screening method in sudden cardiac death. Int J Legal Med 116:22–26

Erel O, Gun B, Tataroğlu C, Dirlik M (2014) Evaluation of apoptosis in myocardial injury in cases of medico-legal death. Rom J Leg Med 22:267–274

Fechner G, Petkovits T, Brinkmann B (1990) Ultrastructural pathology of mechanical skeletal muscle damage. Z Rechtsmed 103:291–299

Feiden W (1995) Einführung in die Immunhistochemie. In: Bratzke H, Schröter A (eds) Immunhistochemie in der Rechtsmedizin. Hänsel-Hohenhausen, Egelsbach, pp 7–13

Fracasso T, Heinrich M, Hohoff C, Brinkmann B, Pfeiffer H (2009) Ultrasound-accelerated formalin fixation improves the preservation of nucleic acids extraction in histological sections. Int J Legal Med 123:521–525

Frick R (1981) Stenosierende Koronarsklerose und Färbung des Myokards nach Lie et al. 1971 (Fuchsinorrhagie). Pathologe 2:246–254

Gaaloul I, Riabi S, Evans M, Hunter T, Huber S, Aouni M (2016) Postmortem diagnosis of infectious heart diseases: a mystifying cause of sudden infant death. Forensic Sci Int 262:166–172

Gavrieli Y et al (1992) Identification of programmed cell death in situ via specific labeling of nuclear DNA fragmentation. J Cell Biol 119:493–501

Gown AM, de Wever N, Battifora H (1993) Microwave-based antigenic unmasking—a revolutionary new technique for routine immunohistochemistry. Appl Immunohistochem 1:256–266

Grasl-Kaup B et al (1995) In situ detection of fragmented DNA (TUNEL-assay) fails to discriminate among apoptosis, necrosis, and autolytic cell death: a cautionary note. Hepatology 21:1465–1468

Hasday JD, Sing IS (2000) Fever and the heat shock response: distinct, partially overlapping processes. Cell Stress Chaperones 5:471–480

Hausmann R, Bock H, Biermann T, Betz P (2004) Influence of lung fixation technique on the state of alveolar expansion—a histomorphometrical study. Legal Med 6:61–65

Havel J (2003) Energy-dispersive X-ray fluorescence spectrometry—a forensic chemistry method for determination of shooting distance. Soud Lek 48:57–60

Havel J, Zelenka K (2003) Energy dispersive x-ray fluorescence spectrometry—a forensic chemistry method for detection of bullet metal residue in gunshot wounds. Soud Lek 48:22–27

Holgate CS, Jackson P, Pollard K, Lunny D, Bird CC (1986) Effect of fixation on T and B lymphocyte surface membrane antigen demonstration in paraffin processed tissue. J Pathol 149:293–300

Hsu SM, Raine L, Fanger H (1981a) Use of avidin-biotin-peroxidase complex (ABC) in immunoperoxidase techniques: a comparison between ABC and unlabeled antibody (PAP) procedures. J Histochem Cytochem 29:577–580

Hsu SM, Raine L, Fanger H (1981b) A comparative study of the peroxidase-antiperoxidase method and an avidin-biotin-complex method for studying polypeptide hormones with radioimmunoassay antibodies. Am J Clin Pathol 75:734–739

Imam SA (1995) Comparison of two microwave based antigen-retrieval solutions in unmasking epitopes in formalin-fixed tissue for immunostaining. Anticancer Res 15:1153–1158

Javid B et al (2007) Structure and function: heat shock proteins and adaptive immunity. J Immunol 179:2035–2040

Kage S, Kudo K, Kaizoji A, Ryumoto J, Ikeda H, Ikeda N (2001) A simple method for detection of gunshot residue particles from hands, hair, face, and clothing using scanning electron microscopy/wavelength dispersive X-ray (SEM/WDX). J Forensic Sci 46:830–834

Kardasewitsch B (1952) Eine Methode zur Beseitigung der Formalinsedimente (Paraform) aus mikroskopischen Praeparaten. Z Wiss Mikrosk 42:322–324

Kinoshita H, Nishiguchi M, Ouchi H, Minami T, Kubota A, Utsumi T, Sakamoto N, Kashiwagi N, Shinomiya K, Tsuboi H, Hishida S (2004) The application of a variable-pressure scanning electron microscope with energy dispersive X-ray microanalyser to the diagnosis of electrocution: a case report. Legal Med 6:55–60

Köhler G, Milstein C (1975) Continuous cultures of fused cells secreting antibodies of predefined specificity. Nature 256:495–497

Kok LP, Boon ME (1992) Microwave cookbook for microscopists. Art and science of visualization, 3rd edn. Coulomb Press, Leiden

Krous HF, Ferandos C, Masoumi H, Arnold J, Haas EA, Stanley C, Crossfeld PD (2009) Myocardial inflammation, cellular death, and viral detection in sudden infant death, caused by SIDS, suffocation or myocarditis. Pediatr Res 66:17–21

Kuhn H, Krugmann J (1995) Einfluß von Formalinfixierung und Fixationsdauer auf die DNA-Amplifizierung von verschiedenen Paraffineingebetteten Geweben. Verh Dtsch Ges Pathol 79:600

Kwok S, Higuchi R (1989) Avoiding false positives with PCR. Nature 339:237–238

Labat-Moleur F et al (1998) TUNEL apoptotic cell detection in tissue sections: critical evaluation and improvement. J Histochem Cytochem 46:327–334

Leong ASY (1996) Microwaves in diagnostic immunohistochemistry. Eur J Morphol 34:381–383

Leong ASY, Milios J (1993) An assessment of the efficacy of the microwave antigen-retrieval procedure on a range of tissue antigens. Appl Immunohistochem 1:267–274

Lie JT, Holley KE, Kampa WR, Titus LL (1971) New histochemical method for morphologic diagnosis of early stages of myocardial ischemia. Mayo Clin Proc 46:319–327

Login GR, Schnitt SJ, Dvorak AM (1987) Methods in laboratory investigation—rapid microwave fixation of human tissues for light microscopic immunoperoxidase identification of diagnostically useful antigens. Lab Investig 57:585–591

Lozinski GM, Davis GG, Krous HF, Billmann GF, Shimizu H, Burns JC (1994) Adenovirus myocarditis: retrospective diagnosis by gene amplification from formalin-fixed, paraffin-embedded tissues. Hum Pathol 25:831–834

Lucitti JL, Dickinson ME (2006) Moving toward the light: using new technology to answer old questions. Pediatr Res 60:1–5

Mason JT, O'Leary TJ (1991) Effects of formaldehyde fixation on protein secondary structure: a calorimetric and infrared spectroscopic investigation. J Histochem Cytochem 39:225–229

Merz H, Malisius R, Mannweiler S, Zhou R, Hartmann W, Orscheschek K, Moubayed P, Feller AC (1995a) ImmunoMax—a maximized immunohistochemical method for the retrieval and enhancement of hidden antigens. Lab Investig 73:149–156

Merz H, Malisius R, Mannweiler S, Zhou R, Hartmann W, Orscheschek K, Moubayed P, Feller AC (1995b) Methods in laboratory investigation ImmunoMax. Lab Investig 73:149–156

Meyer R, Niedobitek F, Wenzelides K (1996) Erfahrungen mit der Formalinersatzlösung NoTox. Pathologe 17:130–132

Miething F, Hering S, Hanschke B, Dressler J (2006) Effect of fixation to the degradation of nuclear and mitochondrial DNA in different tissues. J Histochem Cytochem 54:371–374

Moloney WC, McPherson K, Fliegelman L (1960) Esterase activity in leucocytes demonstrated by the napthol-ASD-chloracetate substrate. J Histochem Cytochem 8:200

Nakatone M, Matoba R, Ogura Y, Tun Z, Iwasa M, Maeno Y, Koyama H, Nakamura Y, Inoue H (2002) Detection of cardiomyocyte apoptosis in forensic autopsy cases. Int J Legal Med 116:17–21

Nikolaou P, Papoutsis I, Dona A, Spiliopoulou C, Athanaselis S (2013) Toxicological analysis of formalin-fixed or embalmed tissues: a review. Forensic Sci Int 233:312–319

Noll S, Schaub-Kuhnen S (2000) In: Höfler H, Müller KM (eds) Praxis der Immunhistochemie. Urban and Fischer, München

Nwariaku FE, Mileski WJ, Lightfoot E, Sikes PJ, Lipsky PE (1995) Alterations in leukocyte adhesion molecule expression after burn injury. J Trauma 39:285–288

Ortmann C, Brinkmann B (1997) The expression of P-selectin in inflammatory and non-inflammatory lung tissue. Int J Legal Med 110:15–158

Paulin D, Li Z (2004) Desmin: a major intermediate filament protein essential for the structural integrity and function of muscle. Exp Cell Res 301:1–7

Pelstring RJ, Allred DC, Esther RJ, Lampkin SR, Banks PM (1991) Differential antigen preservation during tissue autolysis. Hum Pathol 22:237–241

Pileri SA, Roncador G, Ceccarelli C, Piccioli M, Briskomatis A, Sabattini E, Ascani S, Santini D, Piccaluga PP, Leone O, Damiani S, Ercolessi C, Sandri F, Pieri F, Leoncini L, Falini B (1997) Antigen retrieval techniques in immunohistochemistry: comparison of different methods. J Pathol 183:116–123

Sabattini E, Bisgard K, Ascani S, Poggi S, Piccioli M, Ceccarelli C, Pieri F, Fraternali-Orcioni G, Pileri SA (1998) The ENVision system: a new immunohistochemical method for diagnosis and research: critical comparison with the APAAP, ChemMate, CSA, LABC and SABC techniques. J Clin Pathol 51:506–511

Schiller PI, Puchta U, Ogilvie AJL, Graf A, Kind P, Sander CA (1998) In-situ-PCR und PCR-in-situ-Hybridisierung am Paraffingewebe. Pathologe 19:313–317

Seidl S, Burmeister R, Hausmann R, Betz P, Lederer T (2005) Contact-free isolation of sperm and epithelial cells by laser microdissection and pressure catapulting. Forensic Sci Med Pathol 1:153–157

Shi SR, Key ME, Kalra KL (1991) Antigen retrieval in formalin-fixed, paraffin-embedded tissues: an enhancement method for immunohistochemical staining based on microwave oven heating of tissue sections. J Histochem Cytochem 39:741–748

Shi SR, Chaiwun B, Young L, Imam A, Cote RJ, Taylor CR (1994) Antigen retrieval using pH 3.5 glycine-HCI buffer or urea solution for immunohistochemical localization of Ki-67. Biotech Histochem 69:213–215

Shi SR, Imam A, Young L, Cote RJ, Taylor CR (1995) Antigen retrieval immunohistochemistry under the influence of pH using monoclonal antibodies. J Histochem Cytochem 43:193–201

Shi SR, Cote RJ, Taylor CR (1997) Antigen retrieval immunohistochemistry: past, present, and future. J Histochem Cytochem 45:327–343

Taylor CR, Shi SR, Cote RJ (1996) Antigen retrieval for immunohistochemistry. Status and need for greater standardization. Appl Immunohistochem 4:144–166

Torre C, Mattutino G, Vasino V, Robino C (2002) Brake linings: a source of non-GSR particles containing lead, barium, and antimony. J Forensic Sci 47:494–504

Trani N, Bonetti LR, Gualandri G, Barbolini G (2008) Immediate anaphylactic death following antibiotics injection: splenic eosinophilia easily revealed by pagoda red stain. Forensic Sci Int 181:21–25

Turillazzi E, Karch SB, Neri M, Pomara C, Riezzo I, Fineschi V (2007) Confocal laser scanning microscopy. Using new technology to answer old questions in forensic investigations. Int J Legal Med 122:173–177

Uno AT, Morita S, Furukawa S, Nishi K, Hitosugi M (2016) Determination of both fetus'and mother's blood type from an autopsy case immersed in formalin for over 50 years. J Forensic Sci 61:1131–1134

Vandewoestyne M, van Hoofstat D, van Nieuwerburgh F, Deforce D (2009) Automatic detection of spermatozoa for laser capture microdissection. Int J Legal Med 123:169–175

von Wasielewski R, Werner M, Nolte M, Wilkens L, Georgii A (1994) Effects of antigen retrieval by microwave heating in formalin-fixed tissue sections on a broad panel of antibodies. Histochemistry 102:165–172

Werner M, Wasieleweski VR, Komminoth P (1996) Antigen retrieval, signal amplification and intensification in immunohistochemistry. Histochem Cell Biol 105:253–260

Wiegand P, Domhöver J, Brinkmann B (1996) DNA-degradation in formalin-fixiertem Gewebe. Pathologe 17:451–454

Williamson SLH, Steward M, Milton I, Parr A, Piggott NH, Krajewski AS, Angus B, Horne CW (1998) Technical advance—new monoclonal antibodies to the T cell antigens CD4 and CD8—production and characterization in formalin-fixed paraffin-embedded tissue. Am J Pathol 152:1421–1426

Wyss A, Lasczkowski G (2008) Vitality and age of conjunctival petechiae: the expression of P-selectin. Forensic Sci Int 178:30–33

3 Histopathology of Selected Trauma

The task of forensic traumatology and histopathological diagnosis is to:

- Prove an inflicted injury as such
- Establish whether the trauma was inflicted while alive (intravital) or following death (postmortem)
- Establish whether, in the case of intravital trauma, the age of the injury can be determined and thus also whether survival time following injury infliction can be determined (Chap. 10)
- Establish whether trauma-related injuries correspond with an alleged crime
- Establish whether histopathological findings in individual cases are sufficiently specific to either prove or exclude a particular event or alleged crime

These requirements apply to injuries resulting from blunt or sharp trauma, e.g., hematoma with tissue necrosis, to blunt chest trauma with cardiac contusion, and craniocerebral trauma with cerebral contusion (see Chap. 20). In addition, other injuries to internal organs and polytrauma with multiple injuries, including fractures, need to be considered. The multitude of possible and described histopathological findings cannot be described and referred to in full here. However, of particular note is the importance of histological pulmonary findings in polytrauma patients whom an increasing incidence of fat and bone marrow embolisms is seen according to survival time, while findings corresponding to shock (leukocyte sequestration, leukocyte sticking) are seen at shorter trauma survival times (1.5–3.5 h). Megakaryocyte embolism is more likely to be seen in cases of late death with occasionally large numbers of immature myeloid cells in the pulmonary capillary system or in the medullary vasa recta in "shock kidney" (Pedal and König 1983).

Skin wounds, which provide orientation in terms of wound healing phases with re-epidermalization of the surface, will receive particular attention (see Chap. 10). Death from drowning can also be considered an effect of external trauma in a wider sense.

Findings following trauma or a known act of violence can be proven histologically as well as immunohistochemically (Wang et al. 2012). Many of these findings can be found in the literature including rare cases, e.g., traumatic infarction following stab wound of the heart (Kampmann and Bode 1982). However, these findings often relate to wholly nonspecific lesions such as acute congestion, circumscribed emphysema-like areas in lung tissue, cardiomyocyte contraction bands, or even vacuolization in hepatocyte cytoplasm. Although these and many other findings can be the result of the given trauma or known impact, conversely they are in no way pathognomonic and do not enable a conclusion regarding trauma type to be drawn. The same applies to signs of intravascular leukocytosis following non-immediate fatal traumatic death (craniocerebral injury, hemorrhage,

R. B. Dettmeyer, *Forensic Histopathology*, https://doi.org/10.1007/978-3-319-77997-3_3

protracted asphyxiation, anesthetic intoxication) (Schulz 1968). Additionally, there are stress proteins including ubiquitin which rapidly respond to various types of stress. Changes in these reactants have been studied by immunohistochemical and biochemical methods in fire fatalities, brain injury, hypoxia, hyperthermia, and hypothermia (Ishikawa et al. 2007).

3.1 Hemorrhage, Necrosis, and Skeletal Muscle Trauma

Typical effects of blunt trauma to the body at the site of trauma impact include local destruction of cells in tissue and smaller capillary or even larger blood vessels, with subsequent acute hemorrhage in the affected tissue. Injury to the tissue itself should be differentiated from trauma-related hemorrhage within the tissue. In this context, fat, muscle, bone, and nerve tissue can be injured. Particular attention should also be given to internal organ injury, i.e., organ-specific tissue. Surgery-related, i.e., iatrogenic, hemorrhage can also occur.

3.1.1 Hemorrhage

Although hemorrhage can be detected macroscopically, it is occasionally only visible microscopically. Examples include:

- Intra- and subcutaneous hemorrhage, e.g., following blunt trauma from blows and falls
- Hemorrhage in subcutaneous soft tissue and musculature following (compression) trauma, e.g., to the throat (hanging, choking, strangulation)
- Contusion hemorrhage in internal organs (e.g., cardiac, cerebral, and pulmonary contusion, as well as subcapsular hemorrhage beneath the liver and/or splenic capsule with later rupture of the organ capsule)
- Fall- and blow-related hemorrhage in combination with fractures
- Hemorrhage related to specific trauma (e.g., following "décollement")
- Other trauma-related types of hemorrhage, e.g., following sharp or piercing trauma to the body (stab wounds, cuts, etc.)
- Injection-related hemorrhage
- Hemorrhage in a resuscitation setting
- Macro- and microhemorrhage due to pressure increases (e.g., Perthes pressure congestion)
- Hemorrhage due to natural causes, including alcohol-related esophageal variceal hemorrhage, Mallory-Weiss syndrome, or ulcer hemorrhage (duodenal, ventricular), including ulcer hemorrhage arising from (generally) a single ulcer following submucosal artery erosion (Dieulafoy's lesion) (Hosemann 1983; Donaldson and Hamlin 1950); tumor-related acute fatal hemorrhage is also not rare
- Retropharyngeal hemorrhage of varying etiology with obstruction of the upper respiratory tract and death by asphyxiation
- Postoperative hemorrhage
- Iatrogenic hemorrhage of different causes, e.g., due to endoscopy (Ginellivá et al. 2016)
- Hemorrhage in the context of incarcerated or twisted intestinal segments in acute circulatory disorders, particularly in hernias and due to adhesions in the abdominal cavity

Posttraumatic local hemorrhage is frequently a histopathological correlation. This type of hemorrhage is more pronounced when located adjacent to bony structures, e.g., subcutaneous hemorrhage in soft tissue of the extensor surface of the lower arm in the context of a "self-defense injury" (Fig. 3.1).

In general, considerable gross blunt force trauma is needed to cause contusion hemorrhage. In such cases, diffuse, unclearly demarcated bleeding into, e.g., the subepicardial fatty tissue (Fig. 3.2) and the myocardium in the case of cardiac contusion or extensive hemorrhage in the pulmonary interstitium and pulmonary alveoli in the case of pulmonary contusion (Fig. 3.3) is seen.

Focal contusion in cerebral tissue presents predominantly in a coup-contrecoup localization, initially as fresh intracerebral hemorrhage, partially striated and, depending on trauma intensity, restricted to the cerebral cortex (Chap. 20).

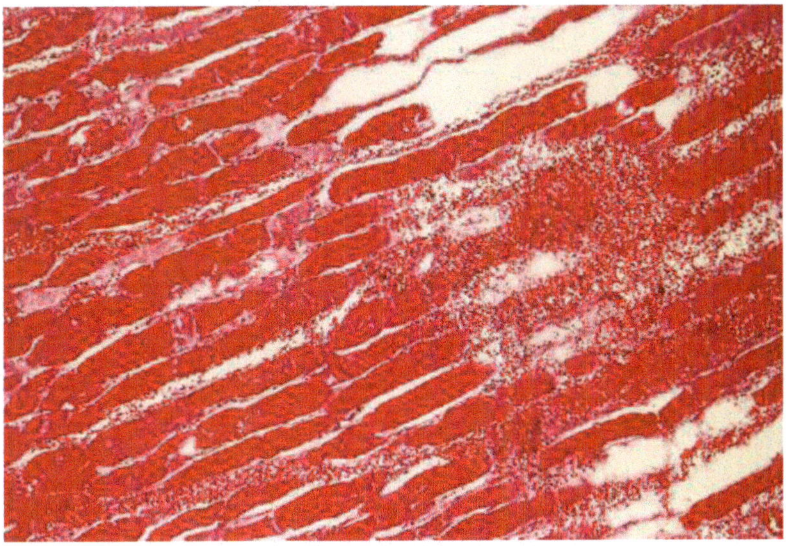

Fig. 3.1 Fresh hemorrhage in subcutaneous musculature tissue of the extensor surface of the right arm (self-defense injury) following blunt trauma caused by a blow with a stick (H&E ×200)

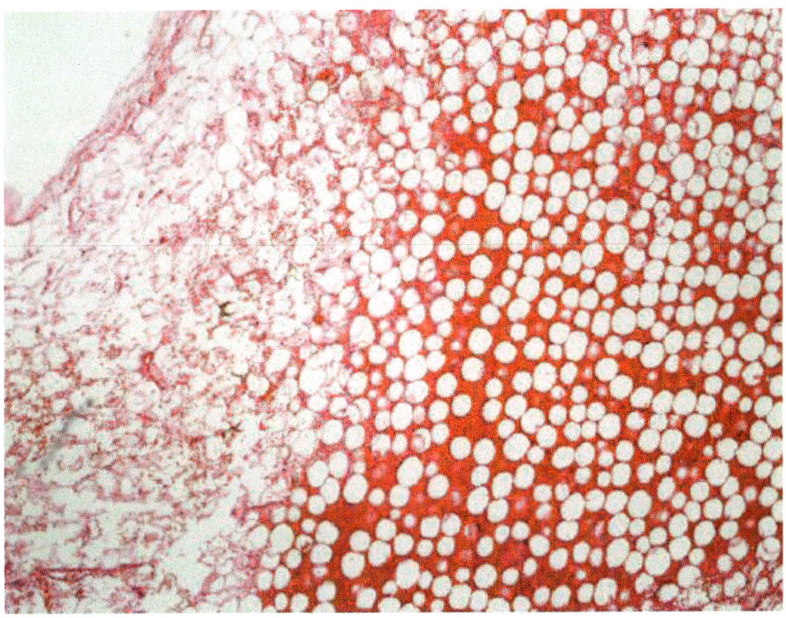

Fig. 3.2 Subepicardial hemorrhage following blunt chest trauma and cardiac contusion (H&E ×40)

In cases where hemorrhage is survived, wound healing begins with resorption and increased organization of the hemorrhage. In larger hemorrhages and hemorrhage cavities, wound healing begins in peripheral areas, which should therefore be resected in a targeted fashion for microscopic investigation. Depending on the suspected course of events, attention should be paid to hemorrhage in particular areas. In the case of anal penetration, careful work-up of the anorectal region at the level of the dentate line may be necessary for the detection of hemorrhage (Fig. 3.4).

During wound infliction, foreign bodies may enter the wound and occasionally be detectable microscopically (Fig. 3.5). In such cases, wound age is once again of importance. In addition to signs of infection and organization of hemorrhage, attention should also be paid to foreign-body giant

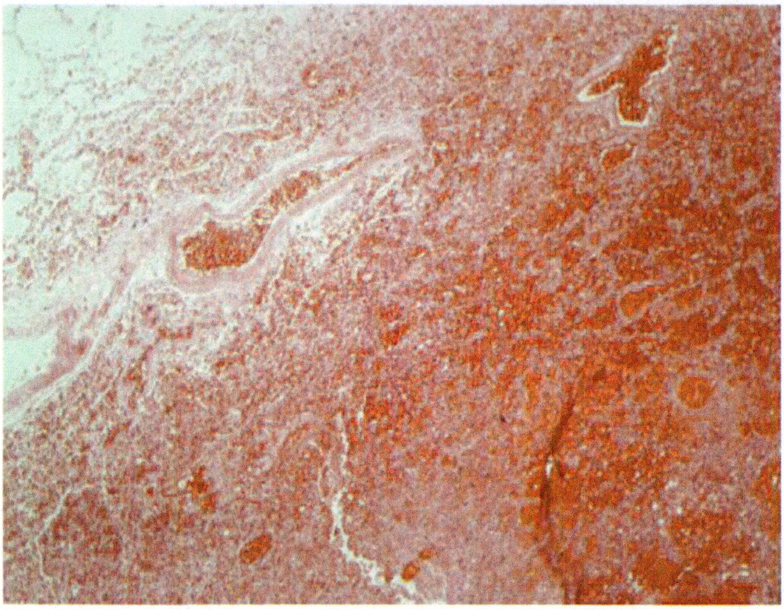

Fig. 3.3 Extensive intrapulmonary hemorrhage in a case of pulmonary contusion (H&E ×40)

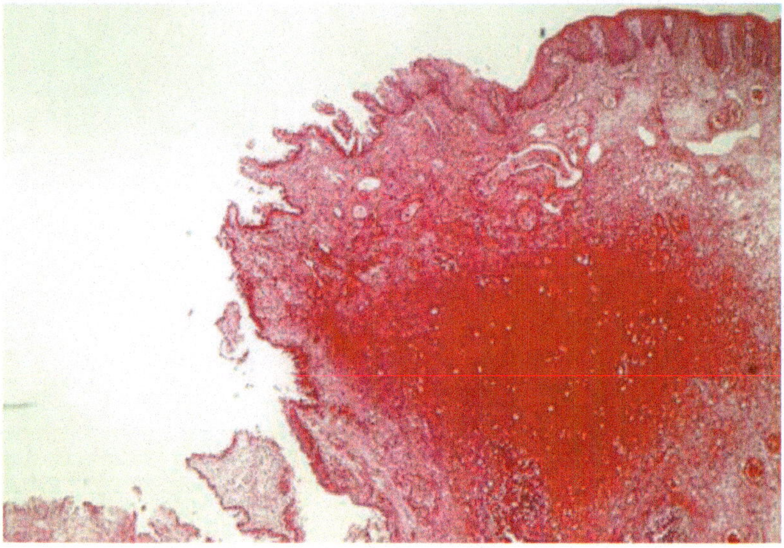

Fig. 3.4 Localized hemorrhage at the level of the dentate line following anal penetration (rape) (survival time, 4–6 h) (H&E ×40)

cells as well as to hemosiderin-loaded macrophages resulting from resorption of ferrous hemoglobin in erythrocytes.

In the case of soiled crime instruments, microscopic remnants of dirt or broken-off particles from the surface of the instrument may enter the wound – in the case of glass instruments, possibly also tiny glass splinters.

Retropharyngeal Hematoma Extensive hemorrhage in the retropharyngeal soft tissue can lead to obstruction of the upper respiratory tract, although final inspiratory stridor and intubation complications have been reported. Histologically, fresh hemorrhage can be seen, as can small tissue necrosis focally, which may also be the result of intensive resuscitation measures. Trauma and surgical interventions are mentioned as the main causes here, while blood coagulation disorders and anticoagulation therapy are favoring factors (Bapat et al. 2002; Sandooram et al. 2000; Tsai and Huang 1999; Chin et al. 1998; Mazzon et al.

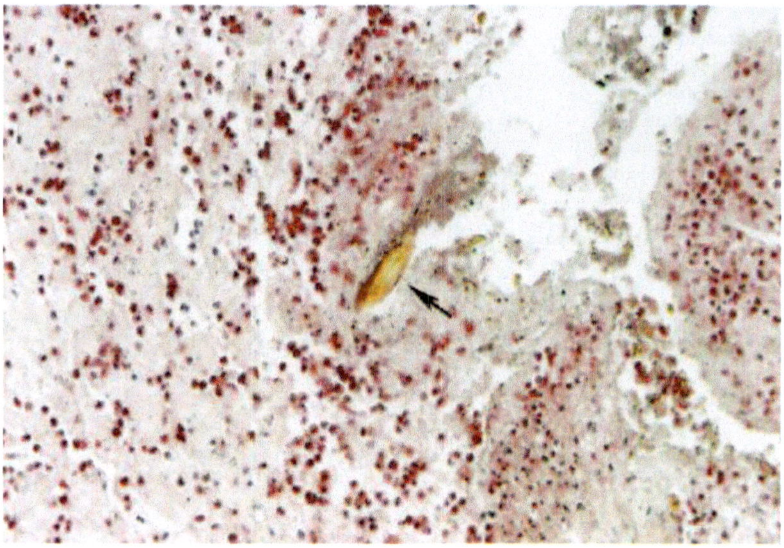

Fig. 3.5 Same case as in Fig. 3.4: microscopic wood splinter found in the rectal mucosa following anal penetration with the handle of a wooden brush (survival time, 4–6 h) (H&E ×200)

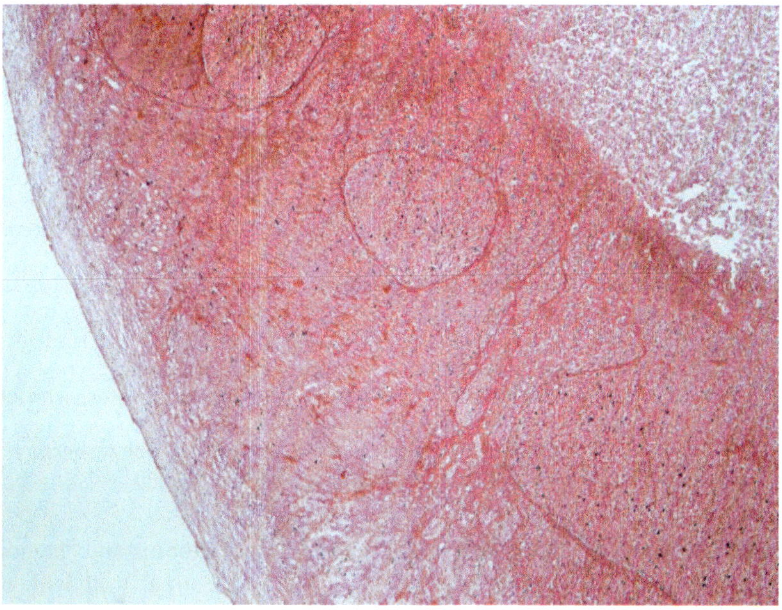

Fig. 3.6 Hemorrhage beneath the splenic capsule following blunt upper abdominal trauma (H&E ×40)

1998; Cox 1998; O'Donnell et al. 1997; Hughes et al. 1972).

Subcapsular Hemorrhage In addition to hemorrhage in the adipose capsule of the kidneys, trauma-related hemorrhage beneath the liver or splenic capsule can occur following blunt abdominal trauma; this may cause subsequent rupture in a time-delayed manner following trauma and cause fatal abdominal hemorrhage (Figs. 3.6 and 3.7). Determining the age of subcapsular hemorrhage may be relevant in some cases (Riezzo et al. 2014).

Incarcerated Intestinal Segment It is occasionally important to establish the age of incarceration in claims of medical malpractice relating to the late diagnosis of an incarcerated intestinal segment. One does not always see ischemic necrosis of, e.g., the incarcerated intestinal segment in a hernia, but sometimes, instead, hemorrhagic infarction with varying histological

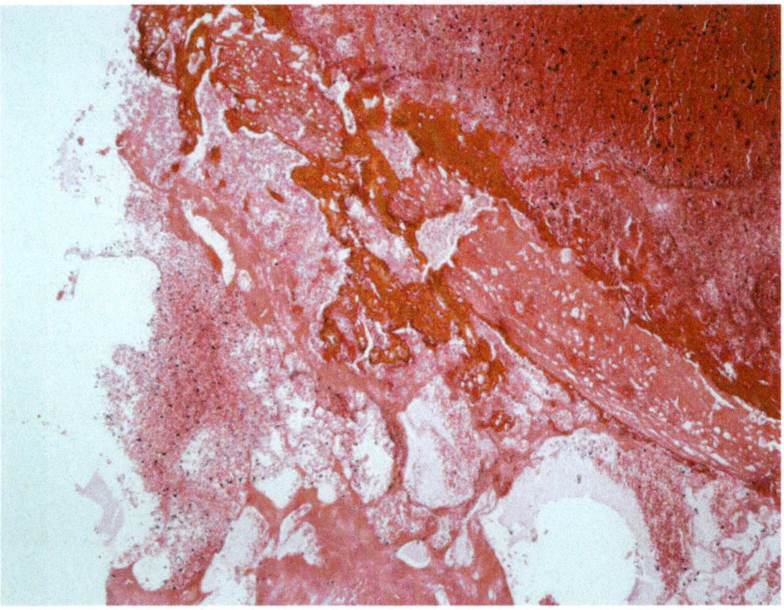

Fig. 3.7 Freshly ruptured subcapsular hemorrhage beneath the splenic capsule following blunt upper abdominal trauma with coagulated blood and fibrin strands (H&E ×40)

Table 3.1 Histological findings in incarcerated intestinal segment, roughly correlated with the duration of incarceration

Age	Histological finding
Acute	Acute blood congestion and erythrocyte extravasation in the intestinal mucosa
Subacute	Acute blood congestion and extensive bleeding into the mucosa of the intestinal wall, as well as in the submucosa and down to the serosa of the visceral peritoneum with edema in the entire intestinal wall (Fig. 3.8)
No longer fresh	Leukocyte invasion of the mucosa, focal invasion of the intestinal wall, and microfocal necrosis
Of longer duration	Intensive leukocyte penetration of the intestinal wall involving numerous segmented neutrophil granulocytes, microfibrin deposits on the serosa of the visceral peritoneum, overall consistent with so-called purulent transmigration peritonitis (rupture of the intestinal wall possible)
Older	Large areas of necrosis in the intestinal wall with significant risk of intestinal wall rupture and accompanying fibrinous purulent peritonitis

findings depending on the duration of incarceration (Table 3.1).

Specifying more precise times for histological findings in the course of intestinal incarceration poses difficulties, since there can often have been phases of brief recovery or improvement of the circulatory status on the one hand, while on the other, and as far as is known, there are no systematic studies that include a correlation of histological findings with the clinical course of intestinal segment incarceration. At autopsy, one most commonly sees a segmental, partially discrete fibrinous peritonitis and "hemorrhagic infarction" of the intestinal wall with more or less pronounced leukocyte infiltration involving segmented granulocytes.

In the findings already visualizable macroscopically in segmental hemorrhagic infarction of an intestinal segment (usually a small intestine segment), one also sees hemorrhages, focal necrosis, and a marked leukocytic inflammatory reaction as a result of torsion of the associated mesenteric adipose tissue (Fig. 3.9).

Tumor-Related Bleeding Acute bleeding due to tumor-related infiltration of vessel walls with bleeding inward or outward is known in almost all malignancies. In some cases, even primary benign tumors can trigger unexpected fatal bleeding. In such cases, histologically definable special forms of above all solely histologically benign tumors may have developed. Von Recklinghausen's type 1 neurofibromatosis is an example in point. Here, numerous, frequently subcutaneous neurofibromas develop. These neurofibromas can sometimes trigger bleeding as a result of infiltration of the vessel walls of larger arteries or veins (Liang et al. 2016; Kettner et al. 2007; Hines et al. 2002; Greene et al. 1974). In addition to identifying tumor tissue at the level of the source of bleeding, histological analysis in such cases should also include the identification of tumor-related destruction of vessel walls, e.g., by demonstrating damaged

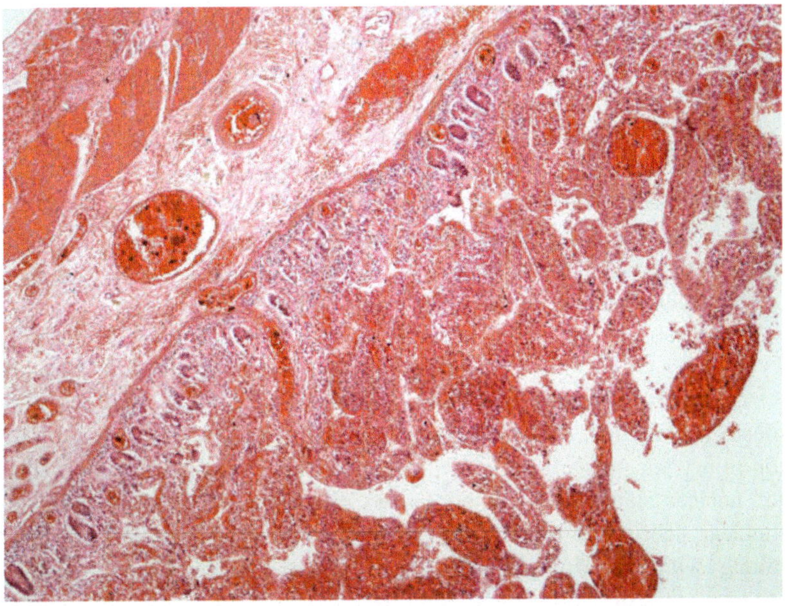

Fig. 3.8 Subacute hemorrhagic infarction (circulatory disorder) of a segment of the small intestine with extensive hemorrhages in the mucosa and focal hemorrhages in the deeper parts of the intestinal wall (H&E ×40)

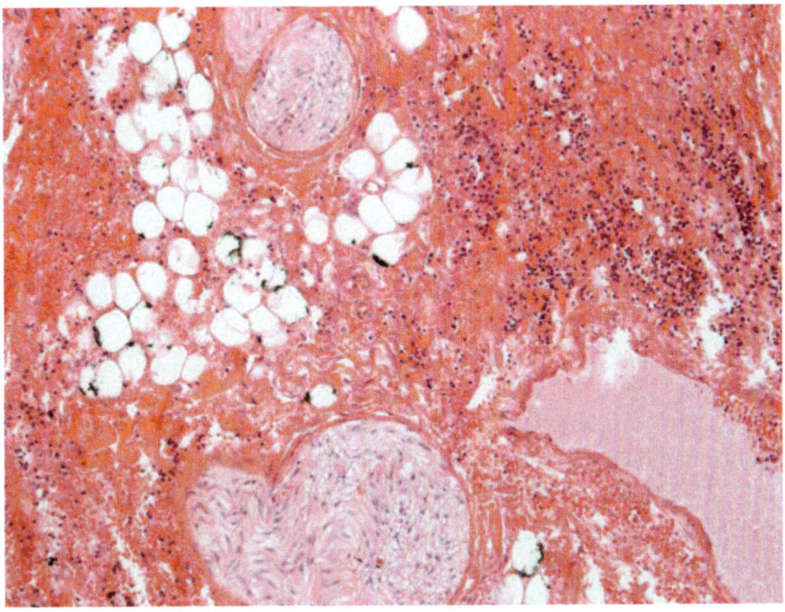

Fig. 3.9 Twisted segment of the mesenteric root with acute blood congestion, edema, hemorrhages, small necroses, and a leukocyte reaction here in the setting of segmental hemorrhagic infarction of a segment of the small intestine (H&E ×100)

structures in the internal lamina, as well as damaged or ruptured elastic fibers in the arterial wall, visualizable using the Elastica van Gieson stain.

3.1.2 Necrosis

Intravital trauma-related tissue necrosis is often accompanied by hemorrhage. In addition, however, there is destroyed tissue to which the organism can react with:

- Resorption – the most frequent case
- Demarcation and rejection without extensive cellular resorption, as can be the case in short-term, localized effects of extreme heat applied to a small area, e.g., third-degree heat injury with so-called active necrosis
- Resisting attack from cell destruction products

In the case of resorption, necrotic tissue with destroyed and lost tissue structures, depending on injury age, as well as tamped nuclei or loss of nuclear stainability can be seen. Cell and nuclear debris can be detected histologically, along with a peripheral increase of macrophages, invading fibrocytes, fibroblasts, lymphocytes, and granulocytes; later, granulation tissue with capillary blood vessels forms. Hemosiderin-loaded macrophages can often be seen from the third day: in the case of fatty tissue, lipophages are seen and in hemorrhage, erythrophages. Comparable systematic investigations to determine injury age, as in skin wounds (Chap. 10), are not available for tissue-only wounds, with the exception of cerebral tissue injury (Chap. 20), myocardial infarction (Chap. 13), and posttraumatic injury to the skeletal musculature (see Sect. 3.1.3) following fractures (Chap. 10). In the case of high numbers of proteins and cell destruction products related to trauma, the histological picture is that of “crush kidney” (Ishikawa et al. 2007; Abe et al. 2001; Heintz 1961).

3.1.3 Skeletal Muscle Trauma

The skeletal musculature is frequently affected by trauma to the body. Extensive investigations into vitality in muscle injury using phosphoric and tungstic acid staining date back to the 1980s (Sigrist 1986, 1987).

Thereafter, the following signs were considered as intravital reactions following muscle trauma:

- Evidence of destruction of skeletal muscle fiber integrity including funnel-shaped demarcation of areas of fiber rupture
- Loss of cross-striation in skeletal muscle fibers
- The appearance of longitudinal fibrillar structures
- Segmental and discoid decay of skeletal muscle fibers

In forensic medical practice, evidence of local hemorrhage remains an indication of vitality if it exceeds a critical extent. In addition, attention should be paid when using greater magnifications in light microscopy to whether the continuity and integrity of the skeletal muscle fibers can be visualized or whether invaginations already detectable using staining occur (Fig. 3.10). Difficulties may be encountered in the differentiation between intravital and postmortem changes in the case of contraction band detection (Ojala and Lempinen 1968). However, there are no grounds to doubt vitality on detection of a cellular reaction and distinct tearing of individual skeletal muscle fibers (Oehmichen et al. 1986) (Fig. 3.11).

Uncertainty remains, however, in the differentiation of intravital injuries from postmortem changes. Samples of skeletal muscle where mechanical or electrical stimulation had been carried out up to 8 h postmortem (hpm) were examined for structural changes to the fibers by light microscopy. A comparison with control muscle samples taken contralaterally from the same corpse showed that the findings interpreted as being of intravital origin, e.g., destruction of

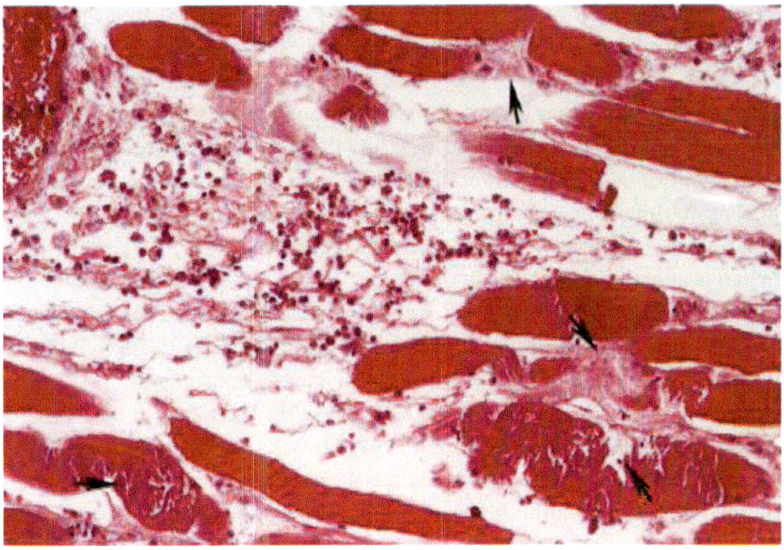

Fig. 3.10 Slightly older trauma to the skeletal musculature including a cellular reaction and tearing of muscle fibers (*arrows*) (H&E ×200)

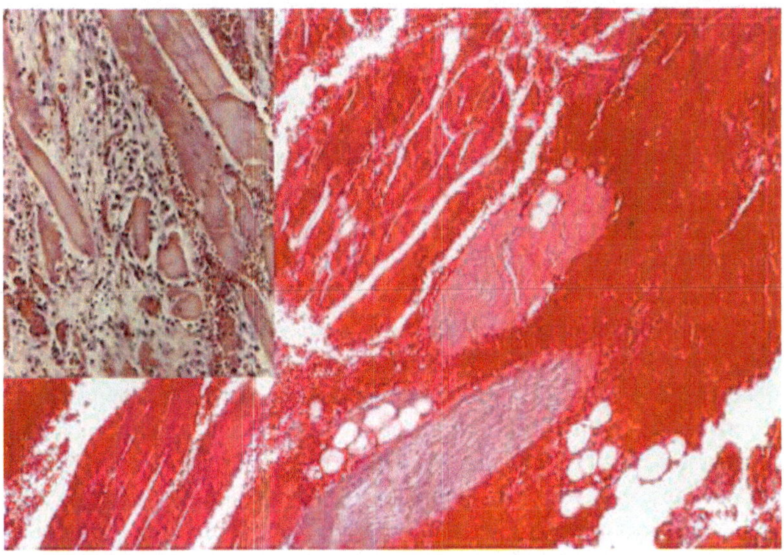

Fig. 3.11 Fatal compression trauma to the neck (massive strangulation) with strong resistance on the part of the victim: extensive hemorrhage in the neck musculature, single muscle fiber necrosis (HE ×100), and "opaque" muscle fibers (H&E ×200)

fiber integrity, invagination, and contraction bands, could also be due to postmortem alterations (Henssge et al. 2002). It is also unclear whether the positive identification of intravital injury is of any value or whether a negative finding reliably excludes intravital trauma. Up until the investigations carried out by Fechner et al. 1990, 1991 and Fechner 1995, it was unclear when exactly the earliest appearance of intravital findings could be expected with regard to injury age determination.

Sigrist's findings (1986, 1987) could initially be confirmed by subsequent investigations using paraffin sections and semi-thin sections (Fechner et al. 1990, 1991). In addition, contraction bands and large cystic changes supported intravital infliction of injury. Disintegration of the fiber structure, including longitudinal fibrillar structures, should be detectable after 30 min, although only reliably so at stronger, e.g., 1100-fold magnification. Immediately following trauma, electron microscopic findings are detectable, alternating between hypercontraction bands and rupture zones (Fechner 1995, Fechner et al. 1990, 1991).

Staining of the structural proteins actin, myosin, and desmin, as well as the functional protein myoglobin, enables immunohistochemical differentiation between intravital and postmortem muscle trauma. The shift from positive and negative reactions or from depletion and accumulation in intravitally injured skeletal muscle fibers is particularly noteworthy here, while detection is homogeneous in postmortem muscle trauma (Fechner 1995; Fechner et al. 1990, 1993). In the case of intravital trauma to skeletal muscle, depletion of all proteins investigated (actin, myosin, desmin, myoglobin) has been reported. These antigens may also be detected in the otherwise empty muscle fiber tubules, the areas of discoid decay in muscle fibers, as well as outside the fibers (Fechner et al. 1991). Depletion begins within minutes of trauma, myoglobin being the earliest. The proteins mentioned could be reliably detected up to 72 h postmortem. Thus, the light microscopic detection of muscle protein depletion can be a valuable aid in the determination of intravital muscle fiber changes.

In immunohistochemical staining of molecules not found in uninjured skeletal muscle, fibers, fibrinogen, and fibrin are particularly noteworthy as the end product of coagulation. These proteins are usually found in intravitally injured skeletal muscle in otherwise empty muscle fiber tubules and spaces between myofibrils, as well as in areas of fiber rupture. The detection of complement factor $C5b\text{-}9_{(m)}$ as a necrosis marker was possible on human skeletal muscle fiber, gradually increasing from an injury age of 1 h. $C5b\text{-}9_{(m)}$ is not detectable in skeletal muscle lesions inflicted postmortem (Fechner 1995). According to Fechner's investigations, immunohistochemical detection of fibrin, fibrinogen, fibronectin, and complement factor $C5b\text{-}9_{(m)}$, as well as an accumulation of myoglobin, is only possible in skeletal muscle injury inflicted during life; depletion alone, without an accumulation of actin, myosin, desmin, and myoglobin, can apparently also occur in lesions incurred postmortem.

Therefore, following muscle trauma, a depletion and accumulation of muscle-specific (actin, myosin, desmin, myoglobin) and non-muscle-specific proteins (fibrin, fibrinogen, fibronectin) can be seen within hours. From a posttraumatic interval of approximately 1 h, necrosis factor $C5b\text{-}9_{(m)}$ can be increasingly detected (Fechner et al. 1991, 1993; Fechner 1995). Further histological and immunohistochemical investigations point to the relevance of "opaque fibers" as evidence of intravital trauma or compression of the musculature: opaque fibers were swollen and rounded in transverse section and showed loss of cross striations. They also stained deep pink with H&E, blue-green, and sometimes red in modified Gomori trichrome and showed a negative reaction for myoglobin immunohistochemically, while fibronectin was localized around the muscle fibers. These findings were not observed in the cervical muscles without the effects of compression (Tabata 1998). Other studies have investigated skeletal muscle damage for the time-dependent expression of markers such as α7 nicotinic acetylcholine receptor (α7 nAChR)–however, only in animal models (Fan et al. 2014).

3.2 Neck Trauma

In the case of neck trauma, in particular strangulation, hanging, and choking, findings relating to local injury may be of interest. Earlier investigations concentrated on the histology of strangulation (Brinkmann and Püschel 1981; Brinkmann 1978). In addition to findings relating to skin injury, changes to the carotid body should be considered, particularly in the case of violent strangulation. In cases where there is known or suspected localized trauma, microscopic investigations can show tissue injury in the affected area (Maxeiner 1983, 1985). This also applies to intra- and subcutaneous hemorrhage and bleeding, e.g., in the neck musculature or other sites exposed to trauma. In some cases, necrosis and compression of muscle tissue may be detectable (Sigrist and Germann 1989; Sigrist 1986, 1987). However, a differential diagnostic distinction from nontraumatic posterior cricoarytenoid muscle hemorrhage is necessary

(Weiler and Risse 1988; Maxeiner 1987a; Paparo and Siegel 1976).

Thus, in many cases of compression trauma to the neck, discrete, although occasionally also marked, microscopically detectable findings can be made including erythrocyte extravasates, hemorrhage, damage to the skeletal musculature of the neck, and – depending on survival time – cellular reactions: leukocytes and early leukocyte migration, with the help of which at least vitality at the time of trauma to the neck, can be proven (Maxeiner 1987b, 1996; Chap. 10). In the absence of a cellular reaction, segmental and discoid decay of muscle cells with loss of cross-striation and newly formed pathological longitudinal striations point to intravital trauma (see Figs. 3.12 and 3.13) (Sigrist and Germann 1989). Phosphoric and tungstic acid or PTAH staining is recommended for detection.

Histological appearances of fractured superior horns of the thyroid cartilage and the surrounding

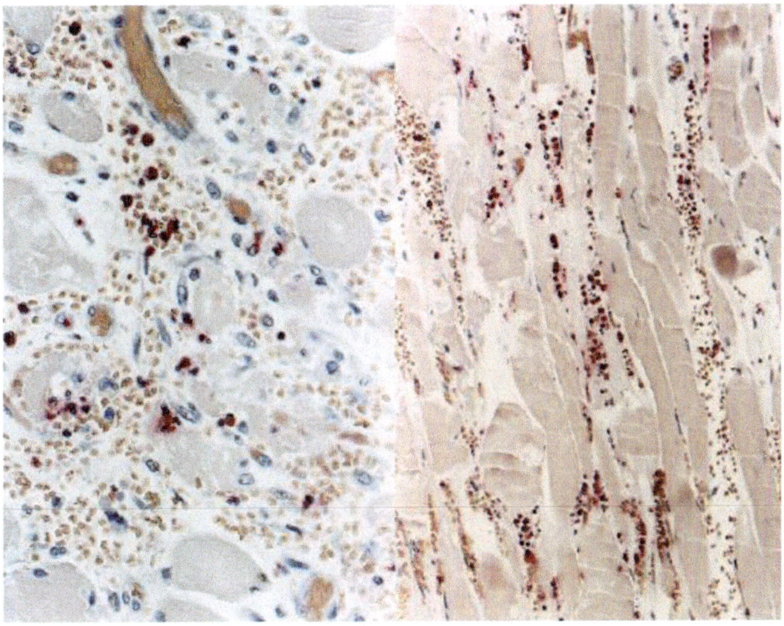

Fig. 3.12 Fatal compression trauma to the neck with hemorrhages (H&E ×200) and ASD-positive granulocytes (×400)

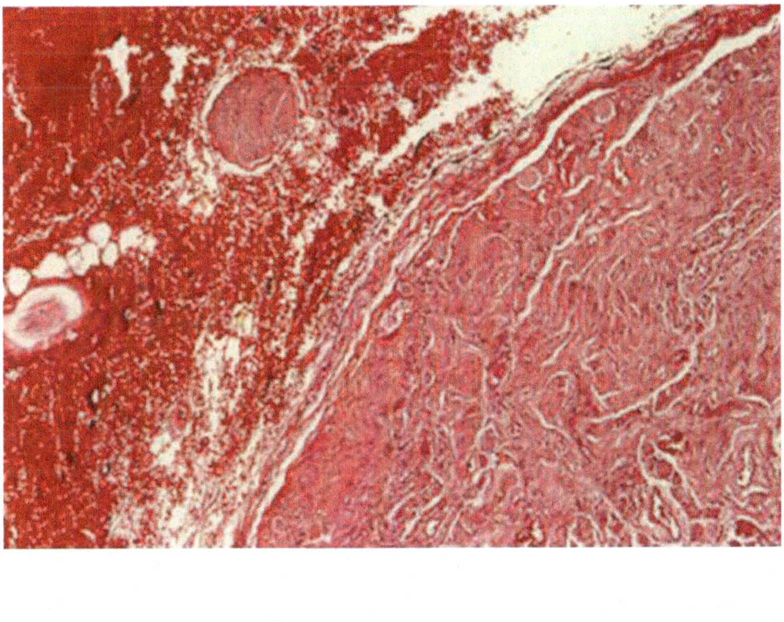

Fig. 3.13 Carotid body with pericapsular hemorrhage following violent compression trauma to the neck (H&E ×40)

tissues have been described. Many histological findings, including hemorrhage and fractures, had not been evident at gross examination. Therefore, some authors conclude that histological examinations of superior horns may not only uncover macroscopically overlooked injuries but may also facilitate the clarification of an injury's vital origin (Rajs and Thiblin 2000).

In some cases of compression trauma to the neck, damage to the carotid body should be considered. This is particularly true in cases where intravital hemorrhage can be detected in the pericapsular or subcapsular regions of the carotid body (Fig. 3.13) or even in the region of afferent and efferent nerve fibers (Fig. 3.14). Recent studies indicate that myocardial hypertrophy is associated with carotid body hyperplasia (Sivridis et al. 2011; see also Smith et al. 1982; Heath et al. 1970).

Lymphangiectasia may occur within the carotid body, possibly as the result of massive congestion due to neck compression (Fig. 3.15). In cases of a histological or immunohistochemical indication of damage to the carotid body,

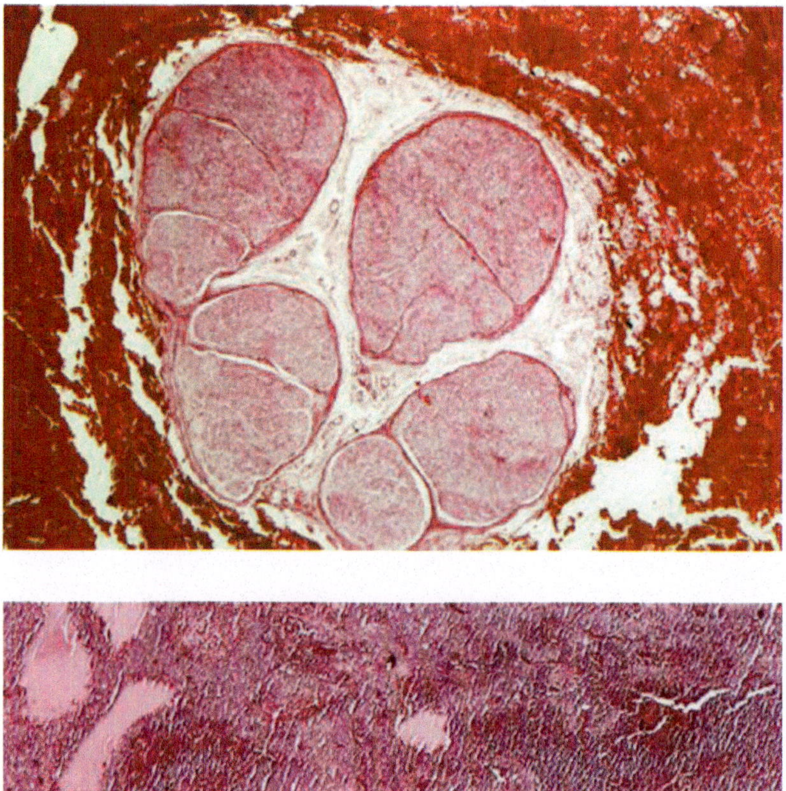

Fig. 3.14 Afferent and efferent nerve fibers of the carotid body surrounded by hemorrhage following lethal strangulation (H&E ×100)

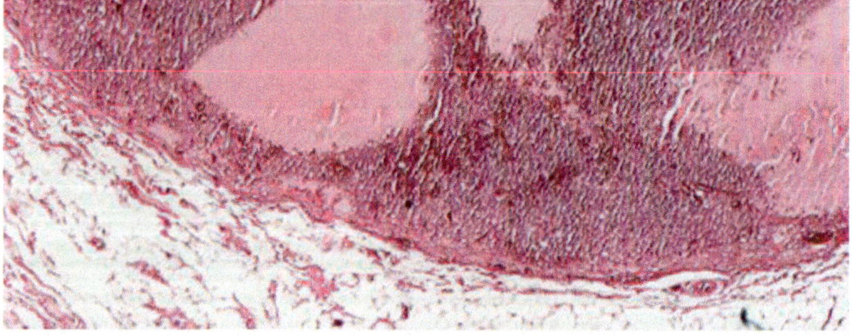

Fig. 3.15 Lymphangiectasis detectable within the carotid body following compression trauma to the neck (H&E ×40)

lethal carotid sinus reflex, although very rare, should be taken into consideration in the differential diagnosis, depending on the crime (Dettmeyer et al. 2004; Anscombe and Knight 1996; Kubo et al. 1994; Sigrist et al. 1989; Schollmeyer 1961; Camps and Hunt 1959).

Despite the absence of direct trauma due to blunt impacts, fatal rhabdomyolysis with myoglobinuric renal failure (see Chap. 4) can occur by positional torture in a stress position as in cases of reverse hanging, also known as Palestinian hanging. This is a form of positional torture where the victim is suspended for a prolonged period of time by the wrists, after the wrists were bound at the back (Pollanen 2016).

3.3 Cardiac Concussion and Cardiac Contusion

With regard to the cardiac muscle, a conceptual distinction is made between cardiac "contusion" and cardiac "concussion." In the case of cardiac contusion (as in, e.g., cerebral contusion) and in addition to hemorrhage, damage to the cardiac muscle fibers is frequently detected macroscopically, while microscopic detection is always reliable following blunt trauma (Staak 1968). The detection of troponins may also be helpful (Peter et al. 2006). Coronary artery involvement is possible, as is traumatic rupture of the ventricle wall following chest trauma (Chen et al. 2015; Barbesier et al. 2015; Dobiáš et al. 2013; Schwaiblmair and Höfling 1997; Goffin and Heyndrickx 1974; Sevitt 1973) and as are changes in the cardiac conduction system (Zhu et al. 1999). Histologically, lesions of myocardial contusions can be identified at subepicardial, myocardial, or subendocardial layers as interstitial hemorrhage, disruption, or coagulative necrosis as well as contraction band necrosis of the muscle fibers (Guan et al. 2007).

In the case of cardiac concussion, there are no macroscopic findings at autopsy (as in cerebral concussion) for which a macroscopic morphological correlation is as yet known.

There are series of reports on cardiac concussion, including fatal and nonfatal cases (Maron et al. 1995, 1997; Kaplan et al. 1993; Viano et al. 1992; Abrunzo 1991; Karofsky 1990; Tenzer 1985; Frazier and Mirchandani 1984; Green et al. 1980; Froede et al. 1979; Dickman et al. 1978; Parmley et al. 1958). Immunohistochemical investigations using canine models and a control group led to pathological findings following cardiac concussion (Guan et al. 1999). At autopsy of the animals, however, neither macroscopically nor conventional histologically detectable myocardial lesions could be seen. However, immunohistochemically, focal patchy loss of myocardial myoglobin, creatine kinase BB, and creatine kinase MM was identified with scattered deposition of these substances between myocardial fibers elsewhere. Such changes as relaxed myofibrils with widened I band, contracted myofibrils, and broken cristae of the mitochondria were observed in the myocardial ultrastructure. In addition, lanthanum particles deposited within mitochondria with blurred mitochondrial cristae, which were identified at the subepicardial layer of the right ventricle postimpact, were observed (Guan et al. 1999). Nevertheless, these findings cannot be regarded as morphologically specific or absolute ones in cardiac concussion.

It is established, however, that there may be a morphological, immunohistochemically detectable correlation in the case of cardiac concussion. Some morphological changes may be detected if detailed examinations are conducted with more sophisticated or sensitive techniques in cases of instantaneous death from cardiac concussion.

In the case of cardiac contusion and other direct trauma to the cardiac musculature, comparisons between intravital injury and postmortem injury showed that wound reactions in intravital injury are significantly more detectable than in postmortem injuries. Intrasarcolemmal accumulation of fibrinogen and fibronectin has been observed, while the formation of contraction bands is more pronounced than in postmortem wounds. The whole pattern of pathological changes is described as much more variegated and pronounced (Ortmann et al. 2001). To determine whether injury to the cardiac muscle is intravital or not, a spectrum of immunohistochemical markers are recommended: troponin C, fibronectin, or fibrinogen and C5b-$9_{(m)}$ (Ortmann et al. 2001), as well as conventional histological methods (H&E, Elastica van Gieson, Luxol fast blue, etc.).

3.4 Drowning: Water-Submerged Victims

Diagnosing death by drowning can occasionally be challenging (Piette and de Letter 2006), including the interpretation of periorbital and conjunctival petechiae which may be present (Somers et al. 2008). Detectable findings may vary depending on the depth at which the airways were covered by fluid (Toklu et al. 2006). Histological investigations on drowning victims are performed to:

- Determine postmortem interval
- Establish whether injuries were incurred intravitally
- Confirm suspicion of death by drowning (determine cause of death)
- Assist in determining the drowning medium where necessary
- Establish an alternative cause of death

Despite numerous studies, the value of histological investigations into deaths by drowning is to be viewed with caution. The investigation of drowning-related findings focuses on the lungs and skin (An et al. 2011 Brinkmann et al. 1983a, b, 1997; Brinkmann and Butenuth 1982; Janssen 1977; Heinen and Dotzauer 1973; Kunz 1960; Goldbach and Hinüber 1956; Schleyer 1951; Dierkes 1938; Ökrös 1938; Wachholz 1907). Additionally, histological investigations of injuries and hemorrhage, particular on the neck and chest wall musculature, can be carried out. Paltauf's spots which cannot be unequivocally evaluated macroscopically in the case of death by drowning can be confirmed histologically by detecting erythrocyte extravasates. The possibility of impairment to histological findings as a result of changes caused by putrefaction should always be borne in mind. Histological findings on drowning victims should be analyzed in particular detail.

3.4.1 Determining the Postmortem Interval in Water-Submerged Corpses

While macroscopic criteria for determining the postmortem interval in water are available (Reh 1970), investigations on the epidermis and subepidermal soft tissue (corium, subcutaneous fatty tissue) were carried out to histologically determine postmortem interval in water (Table 3.2).

Table 3.2 Histological criteria for the epidermis, subepidermal tissue, and lung to determine postmortem interval and vital status as described in the older literature

Histological findings	Presumed postmortem interval
General histological changes to the epidermis	No definite correlation
Evidence of large particles of water components (algae, plant components) in the peripheral branches of the bronchial tree and the alveoli in cases of submersion in a water depth of 3 m	Indicates intravital drowning in the case of a postmortem interval of less than 1 day (Janssen 1977)
Good elastic fiber staining in the subepidermal corium of plantar skin	Maximum 1 week (Dierkes 1938)
Evidence of pigment-producing bacterial colonies (rare finding)	At least 1–2 weeks (Berg 1975)
Moderate stainability of elastic fibers in the corium of plantar skin; wrinkling of the epidermis without detachment from the superficial corium	Approximately 2–3 weeks (Dierkes 1938)
Early adipocere formation at the cutis–subcutis border	At least 3–4 weeks (Janssen 1977)
Poor or lacking stainability of elastic fibers in the corium of plantar skin	4 weeks, possibly longer (Dierkes 1938)
Complete loss of stainability of elastic fibers in abdominal and back skin	3–10 weeks (Ökrös 1938)
Preserved elastic fibers in lung tissue	Less than 2 months (Kunz 1960)
Evidence of struvite crystals in sea-water corpses	9 months and longer (Cherkavsky and Stukochenko 1965)

Determining stainability of elastic fibers apparently also depends on the fixative, the stain (e.g., according to Weichert), and the age of the deceased. Thus, elastic fibers may be better detected in children using unfixed sections (Goldbach and Hinüber 1956)

Epidermis Cases where corpses remain in water result in so-called washerwoman's skin: wrinkling and grayish-white discoloration of skin areas without sebaceous glands, i.e., nipple-areola complex, palms of the hands, and soles of the feet. The following histological signs of water absorption are observed:

- Swelling of the epidermal keratinizing squamous epithelium
- Detachment of the horny layer
- Fraying of the keratin lamellae
- Vacuoles appear in the epithelial cells of the (basal) germinative layer
- Gradually, although with no exact chronological correlation, cell and nuclear borders disappear, as do the keratohyaline granules
- With increasing wrinkling, the epidermis detaches from the subepidermal corium

Elastic Fibers in Subepidermal Soft Tissue (Corium) Parallel to the development of macroscopically visible washerwoman's skin, tissue swelling and detachment are found in the corium. The usually thickly layered elastic fibers are particularly affected. However, no consistent picture can be taken from the literature: in cases where fibers stain well, a postmortem interval of maximum 1 week is likely (Dierkes 1938); a postmortem interval of less than 2 months is assumed in the case of good detectability in the lungs. Thus, histological investigations to determine the postmortem interval in water can only be of secondary importance. Given the strong variations in water type, temperature, movement, and pollution, as well as variations in victim age and epidermal thickness, histological investigations of the epidermis are unable to make a decisive contribution in determining the postmortem interval in water.

Other histological findings in corpses submerged in water as described in the literature include occasional "calcium soap" nodules, particularly on hepatic veins and the endocardium, while similar nodular formations occur on the skin (Janssen 1977). In the case of long-term submersion in sea water, struvite crystals may be found (Cherkavsky and Stukochenko 1965), indicating a postmortem interval of 9 months or longer. Adipocere formation at the cutis–subcutis border is also found in corpses submerged in water, although this can equally occur outside water. Even after histological analysis, the finding of adipocere formation in relation to determining the postmortem interval is to be viewed with caution, although it should be included in the overall evaluation (see Chap. 19). This also applies to the detection of pigment-forming bacterial colonies (*B. prodigiosum*, *B. Violaceum*), which are found only rarely and can be seen after 1–2 weeks at the earliest in the cutis of corpses submerged in water (Berg 1975). Janssen quite rightly points out that pigment-forming bacterial colonies with a patterned arrangement together with skin appendages can lead to erroneous identification as a tattoo (Janssen 1977).

Also true of corpses submerged in water is that, depending on survival time, existing injuries can very well be investigated successfully for a possible intravital origin; to this end, histological investigation of tissue from the marginal area of the injury is necessary. The same applies to determining preexisting disease, since internal organs can remain relatively well-preserved even after several months of submersion in water.

3.4.2 Histology of the Drowned Lung

In the case of drowning, the drowning medium is aspirated, most commonly water (fresh- or saltwater; Chap. 11), in some cases together with corresponding constituents, e.g., bath salts (Mukaida et al. 1998; Reh 1970, Holden and Crosfill 1955). From a pathophysiological perspective, death by drowning is classified as asphyxiation; however, it has some particular features.

In the case of freshwater drowning, algae (diatoms) present in the water are aspirated and can be subsequently detected not only in the lungs but also in internal organs as a result of hematogenous spread. At the same time, final strong respiratory efforts lead to the overinflation of

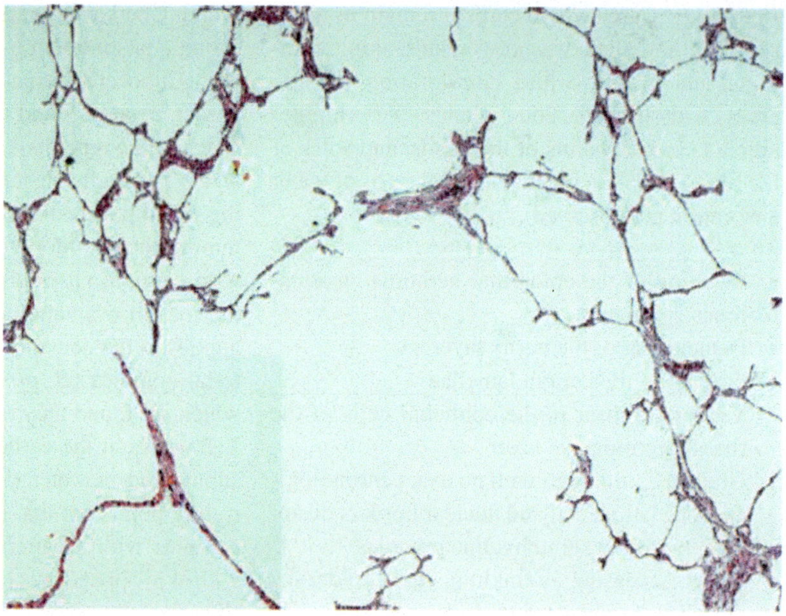

Fig. 3.16 Histological correlation of emphysema aquosum in a case of death by drowning: extremely narrow to flattened interalveolar septa, occasionally stump-like at the margin of blister cavities (H&E ×40)

lung tissue (emphysema aquosum), which is more pronounced in the peripheral region. This results in the rupture of narrow interalveolar septa, which coalesce to small blister cavities. The pulmonary alveoli are acutely dilated, while the septal capillaries are compressed and contain scant erythrocytes (Fig. 3.16) (Lunetta et al. 2004).

Emphysema aquosum in "drowned lung" shows histological findings including changes to lung architecture (Brinkmann et al. 1983a, b; Brinkmann 1978), although activation of type II pneumocytes and a marked increase in alveolar macrophages may also be observed, as well as increased phagocytic activity (Püschel et al. 1983; Brinkmann and Butenuth 1982). In the setting of basal membrane rupture in the alveolar septa, alveolar macrophages reached the blood circulation and could be detected in cardiac blood in a case of death by drowning (Reiter 1984). In this context, so-called smoker cells are washed from the pulmonary alveoli into the cardiac blood. There is general agreement that significant volumes of water reach the alveolar spaces and, following rupture of capillary walls, the blood circulation in the case of death by drowning. The histological finding of pulmonary acini with alternating normal blood levels and extensive anemia, so-called pulmonary dysemia, has also been described in cases of death by drowning.

The following pathological-anatomic criteria or means of microscopic investigation in lung tissue in the case of death by drowning warrant mention:

- Determining emphysema aquosum
- Detecting damage to the alveolar–capillary membrane
- Determining so-called pulmonary dysemia
- Alveolar macrophage count (Betz et al. 1993a)
- Detecting pigmented pulmonary macrophages in association with dust particles and crystals in left heart blood (Karkola and Neittaanmaki 1981)
- Histochemical typing of myelomonocytes in lung tissue (Brinkmann et al. 1997)
- Determining pulmonary surfactant
- Scanning electron microscopic investigation of lung tissue

The intensity of emphysema aquosum should correspond to the duration of the drowning process; however, only scant morphometric investigations are available in which the extent of emphysema aquosum has been determined (Kohlhase and Maxeiner 2003; Fornes et al.

1998). Acute pulmonary emphysema has also been described in cases of mechanical asphyxia such as ligature or manual strangulation, rarely in cases of (incomplete) hanging. The mean alveolar space can be measured by image analysis software, demonstrating acute pulmonary emphysema also in cases of incomplete hanging as vital sign (Castiglioni et al. 2016). Similarly, only individual investigators refer to the detection of smoker cells in left heart blood in the case of drowning (Reiter 1984), while others concentrate on the role of alveolar macrophages (Betz et al. 1992, 1993a, b) or have undertaken ultrastructural or electron microscopic investigations (Torre and Varetto 1985; Püschel et al. 1983; Böhm 1973; Schneider 1972).

Other causes of emphysema which could predate submersion in water should always be considered in the differential diagnosis, e.g., chronic obstructive pulmonary disease (COPD), chronic asthma, preexisting mucoviscidosis, exogenous respiratory impairment (suffocation with a soft object), aspiration (e.g., of blood as in hemorrhagic emphysema), or cardiopulmonary resuscitation.

In addition to tears in the alveolar membrane, aspirated foreign-body particles can occasionally be seen microscopically in the lumen of peripheral branches of the bronchial tree. This finding may be an indication of intravital drowning in the case of a postmortem interval of less than 1 day and a water depth of less than 3 m (Janssen 1977). Diatoms are not detected using staining and, as colorless particles, can only be defined by an experienced investigator using microscopic methods at strong magnifications. Since the lungs represent a very large organ – increasingly so with advancing age – with varying ventilation and perfusion ratios, the histological correlation of macroscopically diagnosed drowned lung can only be determined in lung tissue taken from appropriate, representative regions, when the patient history is taken into account in the interpretation of findings (e.g., intensive cardiopulmonary resuscitation measures following the onset of rigor mortis in chest muscles), and on comparison with macroscopic findings.

Taking two lung samples from each pulmonary lobe (one central, one peripheral) is recommended. H&E, Gomori staining, and frozen sections using Sudan III (fat staining) are recommended as routine staining methods (Janssen 1977). Findings similar to those in drowned lung can result simply from the hydrostatic pressure caused by submersion in a water depth of 4 m or more (Janssen 1977). Histological criteria for death by drowning, including detection of a reticular fiber structure in lung tissue considered to be specific (Reh 1970), could not be confirmed in later investigations (Heinen and Dotzauer 1973).

Freshwater and Saltwater Drowning While so-called dry lung with emphysema aquosum can be seen in the case of freshwater drowning, lung edema as a result of osmotic processes is seen in saltwater drowning. "Near drowning" describes cases where a previously submerged person dies within at least 24 h of being rescued. Pathophysiological mechanisms, symptoms, and histological findings in cases of freshwater drowning, saltwater drowning, and near drowning are listed in Table 3.3. Restricting histological investigations to the lung in cases of death by drowning is advised against; in particular, heart, liver, kidney, and brain tissue should be analyzed for signs of acute hypoxia or asphyxiation. Hemorrhage possibly present in the neck musculature or chest wall should be investigated for signs of intravital origin. The significance of hemolytic staining of the aorta is unclear; however, it appears to be associated with freshwater drowning (Byard et al. 2006a, b).

To differentiate between freshwater drowning and saltwater drowning, investigations of intrarenal aquaporin-2 expression as a valuable marker have been suggested (An et al. 2010). Additionally, intracerebral aquaporin-4 expression was found to be significantly lower in saltwater drowning than in a control group (An et al. 2010). Other authors have shown in animal experiments that the analysis of aquaporin-5 expression could be forensically useful for differentiation between freshwater drowning and saltwater drowning or

Table 3.3 Pathophysiological mechanisms, symptoms, and histologic findings in freshwater drowning, saltwater drowning, and "near drowning"

Freshwater	Salt water	Near drowning
Hypotonic	Hypertonic	–
Large volumes of water quickly pass through the alveoli	Plasma is osmotically drawn into pulmonary alveoli	–
Increase of blood volume	Decrease of blood volume	–
Hemolysis with potassium release	Hemoconcentration	–
Denaturation of pulmonary surfactant	Dilution of pulmonary surfactant	Pneumonitis, fever, sepsis
Emphysema aquosum ("dry lung")	Pulmonary edema	Pulmonary edema
Expansion, thinning, and occasionally tearing of alveolar septa; ruptured elastic fibers (EvG staining)	–	Hemoglobinuria
Rupture of capillary walls with hemorrhage (Paltauf's spots) – extravascular detection of erythrocytes	–	Signs of cerebral hypoxia: amnesia, convulsions, confusion, coma
Possibly aspirated foreign bodies in water, rarely aspiration of chyme	Rarely aspiration of chyme	Sudden development of cerebral edema

In the case of longer postmortem intervals, autolysis and putrefaction may alter findings to the extent that drowning by death is no longer morphologically detectable. In some cases, staining of alveolar reticular fiber structures to detect alveolar expansion may be helpful

between freshwater drowning and postmortem immersion (Hayashi et al. 2009).

Hemorrhage in the neck and nape muscles is occasionally found at autopsy investigations into cases of death by drowning. These hemorrhages and histological muscle alterations are attributed to agonal convulsions, hypercontraction, and overexertion of the affected muscle groups. As long as no cutaneous or subcutaneous hematomas above the hemorrhages can be found, these autopsy findings – with special reference to histology – can serve as an additional criterion to differentiate drowning from other causes of death (Püschel et al. 1999; Carter et al. 1998).

A number of immunohistochemical and electron microscopic investigations relate to pulmonary surfactant (Zhu et al. 2000a, b, 2001, 2002; Lorente et al. 1990), findings in the spleen (Haffner et al. 1994), and the pulmonary structure (Torre and Varetto 1985; Torre et al. 1983). Morphometric investigations into the relevance of alveolar macrophages in drowning diagnosis included determination of the areal density of the pulmonary interstitium and alveolar macrophages. In this context, the values in lung samples taken from drowning victims were significantly lower than in the control group and lower than in severe emphysema.

Near Drowning and Mycotic Infection Fungal infections can be a rare late effect in near drowning with aspiration of water (Ortmann et al. 2010; Buzina et al. 2006; Fisher et al. 1982), in particular involving cerebral infection (Wilichowski et al. 1996; Rüchel and Wilichowski 1995; Dworzack et al. 1989; Fisher et al. 1982) with *Pseudallescheria boydii* or *Scedosporium apiospermum* (Katragkou et al. 2007). Mycotic encephalitis and intracerebral abscesses following initial survival of near drowning have been reported. After death, *Pseudallescheria boydii* can be easily cultured from heart blood and affected tissue. Using conventional histologic staining, hyphae with conidiophores and conidia can be detected with the Grocott–Gomori methenamine silver stain.

3.4.3 Detection of Diatoms in Death by Drowning

The diagnosis of death by drowning can be very difficult. It must be proven that covering of the airways by fluid has occurred by active aspiration of the drowning medium. The comparative identification which combines a qualitative and quantitative investigation of diatoms from tissues of the corpse with that of the drowning medium is a specific detection procedure. Positive results allow the diagnosis of typical drowning (Kakizaki and Yukawa 2015; Farrugia and Ludes 2010; Takeichi and Kitamura 2009; Hendey 1973). A prerequisite of this is that the water in which the individual drowned contains sufficient diatoms. The growth of diatoms in water largely depends on weather conditions and/or the season and the associated fluctuations in water temperature. Colonization by diatoms may be reduced to a minimum during the cold winter months. As a result, there are no, or only scant, diatoms present to enter the body during drowning. However, in typical drownings in waters sufficiently colonized by diatoms, one finds abundant diatoms in pulmonary tissue; the number of diatoms in other organs is also increased. In principle, however, diatoms are also present in small numbers in living individuals, as well as in deceased individuals that did not die due to drowning. For this reason, it is crucial to perform a quantitative differentiation of the diatom content in individual organs while taking threshold values into account.

Diatoms are eukaryotic unicellular or colonial algae, which are ubiquitous in water, air, and soil. Numerous publications on investigation methods are available (Lunetta and Modell 2005; Hurlimann et al. 2000; Sidari et al. 1999; Lunetta et al. 1998; Pollanen 1998; Auer and Mottonen 1991; Fukui et al. 1980; Peabody 1980; Udermann and Schuhmann 1975; Spitz and Schneider 1964; Otto 1961; Thomas et al. 1961; Weinig and Pfanz 1951; Buhtz and Burkhardt 1938). In cases where a diatom-containing drowning medium is aspirated, some diatoms may reach the blood circulation via the airways following pre-final rupture of pulmonary capillaries and spread through the organism. Small diatoms (e.g., *Melosira, Synedra, Cyclotella, Stephanodiscus, Navicula, Nitzschia, Amphipleura, Fragilaria*) cross from the pulmonary alveoli into the blood circulation, thereby reaching organs such as the brain, kidneys, liver, and bone marrow. However, in principle, diatoms may also be detected in the organs of non-drowning victims, since they can also be found in pulmonary dust (Otto 1961). By virtue of their robust resistance to putrefaction, acids, and heat, diatoms can essentially be detected even in adipocerous or markedly putrefied bodies. Diatoms found on clothing can be used to determine contact with surface water or a specific water source (Uitdehaag et al. 2010).

Diatoms have a silicate cell wall (frustule) and shell-like ornamentation. Distinction is made between pennate and centric diatoms: the latter have a radially symmetric pattern, while centric diatoms, a bilaterally symmetric pattern. Morphologically, these filigree structures vary widely, including tiny thorns and warts, spines, ribs, punctations, lineolations, and striations. Taxonomically, the identification of diatoms is carried out using light microscopy. The use of electron microscopy investigations to identify diatoms in tissue removed at autopsy has been suggested in the literature. However, a scanning electron microscope is not necessary for routine applications.

As a basic principle, diatoms found in the liver, kidneys, or bone marrow point to death by drowning as the cause of death. However, the diagnosis of death by drowning requires 20 diatoms/100 μL of sediment taken from 10 g of lung tissue and 5 diatoms/100 μL of sediment taken from 10 g of tissue from at least one other organ. Using these reference values, false-positive findings can be avoided, assuming that sources of contamination have been excluded and that the diatoms have been accurately identified. Those diatoms reaching inhalation pathways via the alveolar–capillary membrane or, following oral ingestion, the major circulation via the digestive tract mucosa are generally <10 μm, i.e., centric diatoms. These diatoms can usually be detected in only small numbers. A qualitative evaluation and comparison of diatoms found in tissue of the victim and those found in the drowning medium or water is required. In principle, diatoms can also penetrate to the peripheral bronchials via the upper respiratory tract postmortem. In particular, in cases of submersion at depths of over 2 m and a postmortem interval of at least 5–6 h, the possibility of postmortem penetration of diatoms should be considered.

Morphologically, diatoms can be roughly classified into centric, i.e., circular to elliptical, and pennate, i.e., linear to lanceolate (Fig. 3.17).

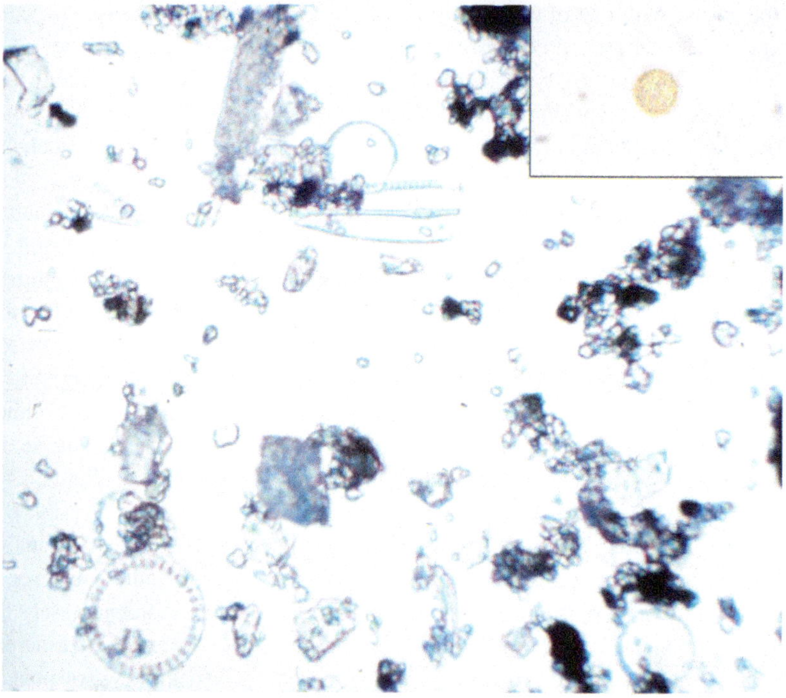

Fig. 3.17 Various forms of diatoms

3.5 Injury by Firearms and Explosives

Injury by firearms, guns, and explosives is characterized by significant local tissue destruction, including hemorrhage and necrosis. In the case of close-range gunshot injuries producing temporary cavities, microscopically fine powder-burn particles are frequently found at the level of bullet entry (Fig. 3.18), which can be traced along the bullet track (Fig. 3.19). Even at the level of bullet exit, powder-burn particles can be found microscopically in individual cases, albeit in lower concentrations. Furthermore, textile fiber displaced into the bullet track can be detected using microscopy. Attempts have been made to determine firing distance by analyzing residues (Neri et al. 2007). Additionally, scanning electron microscopy (SEM) with energy dispersive X-ray (EDX) microanalysis can provide valuable information about the morphology of injuries and injury implements. Meanwhile, the possibilities offered by the use of SEM together with EDX to evaluate the interaction of a bullet passing through human tissue have been confirmed (Biro et al. 2010).

Blast injuries. In addition to gunshot injuries, blast injuries have also been attracting increased attention in recent years (Neri et al. 2007; Stiel et al. 2006; Ladham et al. 2005; Shields et al. 2003; Tsokos et al. 2003; Rothschild and Maxeiner 2000; Varga and Csabai 1992; Laposata 1985).

Histological and immunohistochemical findings may include (Turillazzi et al. 2010):

- Lung sections with alveolar ruptures, thinning of alveolar septae, and enlargement of alveolar spaces (Fig. 3.20)
- Subpleural and intra-alveolar hemorrhage
- Soot aspiration in smaller bronchi
- Apparently empty spaces ("air bubbles") of various sizes in both pulmonary and renal microvasculature, surrounded by leukocytes and platelets
- Nuclear elongation may be found in residual fragments of the tracheal epithelium
- Diffuse hemorrhage in the liver and spleen

Signs of human blast lung injury include diffuse alveolar overdistension and circumscribed interstitial hemorrhage showing a cuff-like pattern around pulmonary vessels. In addition, venous air embolism, bone marrow embolism, and pulmonary

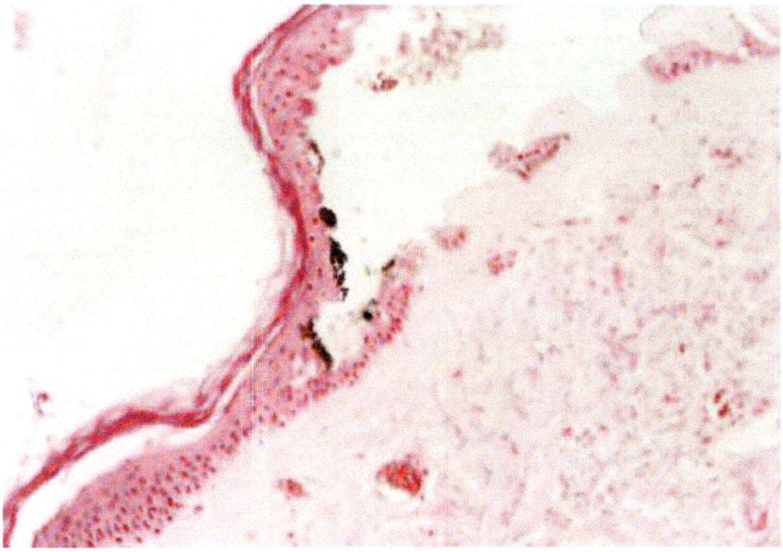

Fig. 3.18 Powder-burn particles detected in soft tissue at the point of bullet entry causing subepidermal undermining (H&E ×100)

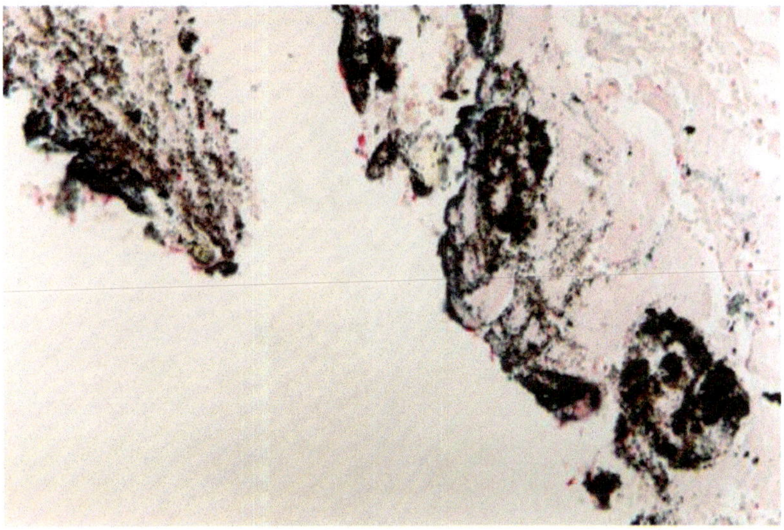

Fig. 3.19 Penetrating craniocerebral shot wound with traces of powder burn at the edge of the intracerebral bullet track (Prussian blue ×200)

fat embolism are possible (Tsokos et al. 2003). "Air bubbles" may present with peripheral platelet aggregates and an adsorbed fibrinogen layer to the interface (Turillazzi et al. 2010).

Simultaneously, multiple explosion splinters penetrate through clothing into the skin or body; correspondingly, a partially lacerated epidermis with encrusted black particles can be observed microscopically (Fig. 3.21).

Post-explosion residues from pyrotechnic compositions or explosives generated during an explosion can be examined by SEM/EDX. Results from various studies suggest that there might be a difference in morphology and composition of pyrotechnic residues formed at different levels of confinement. Moreover, it has been suggested that more experiments and improved sampling methods are necessary to determine which variables have the most pronounced effect on shape, size, and composition of pyrotechnic residues (Vermeij et al. 2009).

Neuropathological findings were described in a case with retained lead shot pellets in the brain of a man who survived 2 months. At the sites of lead shot retention, a local reaction developed, and many macrophages surrounding a focus of lead shot retention, as well as mild signs of diffuse axonal damage, were found throughout the brain (Malandrini et al. 2001).

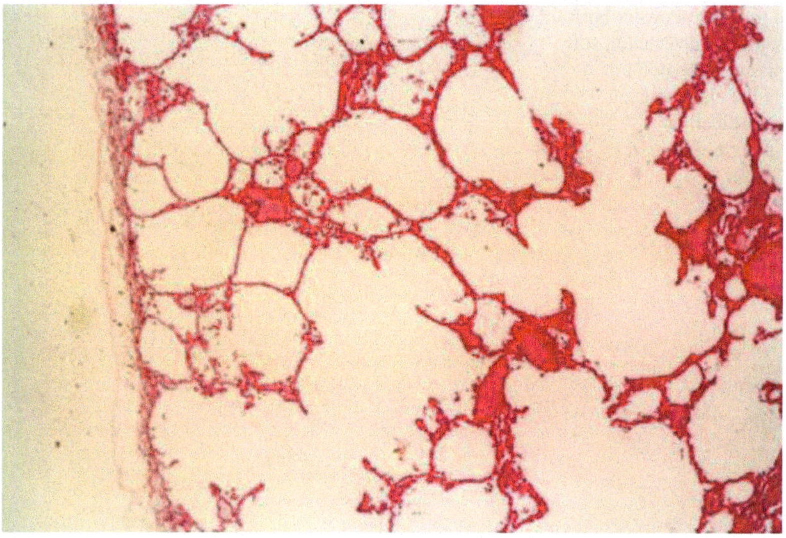

Fig. 3.20 Ruptured peripheral pulmonary alveoli with stump-like, preserved interalveolar septa in a blast victim; this finding, however, is insufficiently characteristic (H&E ×40)

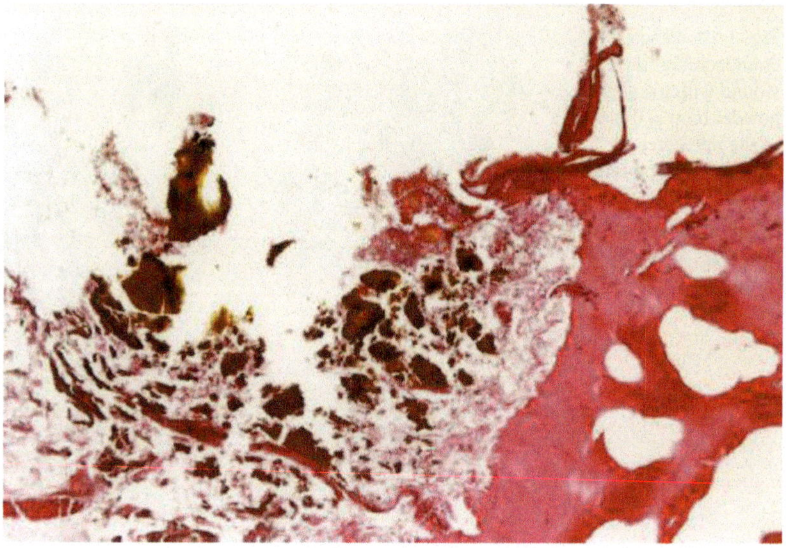

Fig. 3.21 Partially destroyed epidermis in a blast injury with multiple encrusted explosion splinters and particles (H&E ×100)

3.6 Stab Wounds and Hemorrhage

In addition to histological analysis of local findings in stab wounds, the possible existence of an embolism requires clarification, in particular an air embolism in the case of stab wounds to the throat.

3.6.1 Stab Wounds

In the case of stabs wounds sustained intravitally, external hemorrhage from the wound site may ensue, whereby particles adhering to the penetrating object or knife can be washed out. As long as hemorrhage persists or recurs, hemorrhage-related spread of early wound healing reactions in the organism should be considered (e.g., cells, fibrin threads; Figs. 3.22 and 3.23). The wound track created by a sharp instrument, usually a knife or scissors, is regularly surrounded by hemorrhage to the end of the wound track (Fig. 3.24).

If the penetrating object is soiled, particles may remain in the wound track and be histopathologically detectable (Fig. 3.25). In rare cases,

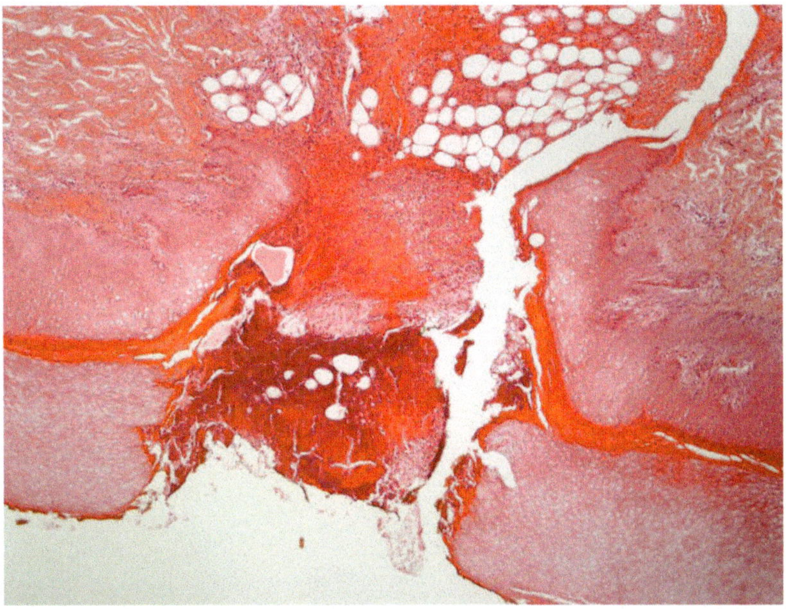

Fig. 3.22 Fresh knife stab wound on the skin (H&E ×40)

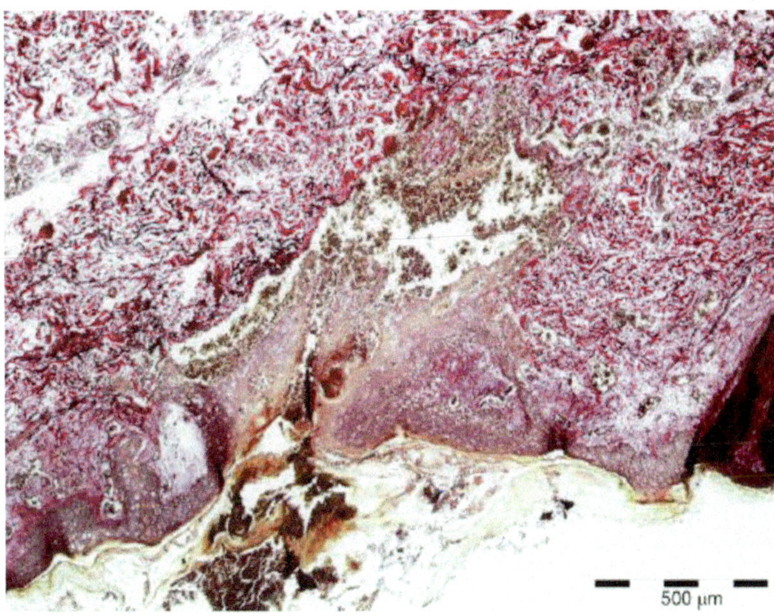

Fig. 3.23 Stab wound from a knife and wound track running through the epidermis with surrounding hemorrhage (H&E ×40)

embolic spread of a cartilage particle to the lungs following repeated deep stab wounds to the throat, jugular vein incision, and additional air embolism is possible (Fig. 3.26).

If a victim briefly survives a knife stab, one is able to see early signs of a phagocytic reaction along the wound track, in particular leukocyte invasion in areas of necrotic tissue (Fig. 3.27).

3.6.2 Fatal Hemorrhage with Subendocardial Hemorrhage

In forensic medical practice, cases of death by hemorrhage with hemorrhagic-hypovolemic shock are seen following violent crime involving serious injury. In cases with an acute course, mild vascular congestion can be seen

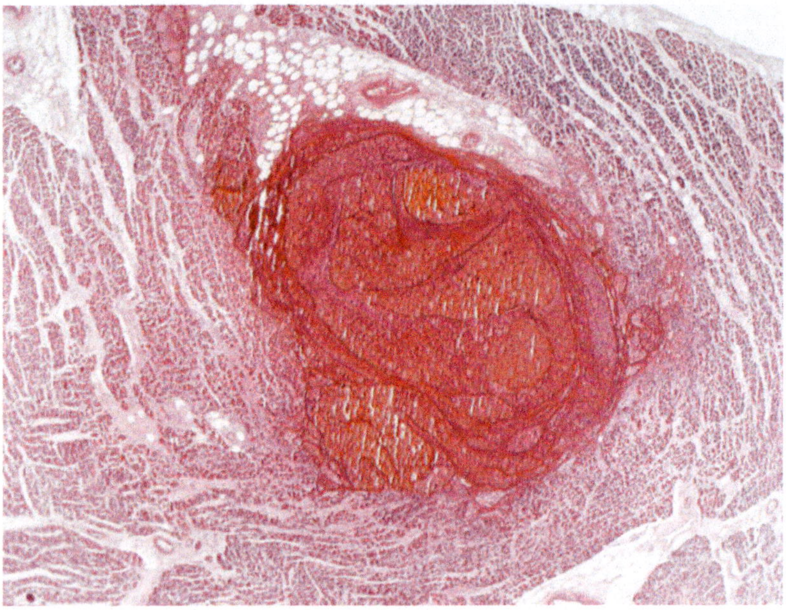

Fig. 3.24 The end of a wound track in the cardiac muscles surrounded by hemorrhage (H&E ×100)

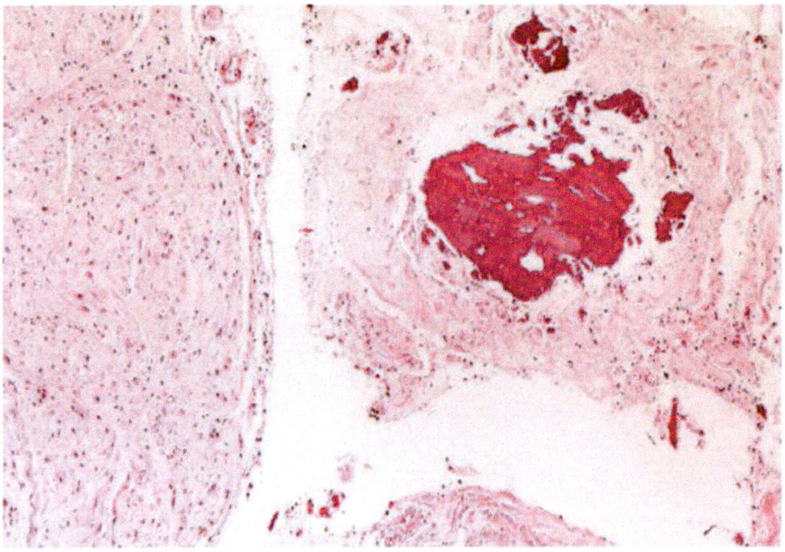

Fig. 3.25 Wound track of a knife stab wound through to the spinal cord ganglion with spread of microscopic bone particles (H&E ×100)

histologically, corresponding to the macroscopic finding of markedly pale internal organs following circulatory centralization, with, however, a pronounced renal corticomedullary junction and hyperemic capillaries in the medulla. In cases of protracted hemorrhage, capillary hyperemia in the glomeruli is apparent, in addition to marked hyperemia in the medullary region of the kidneys (Adebahr and Weiler 1976). At the same time, subendocardial hemorrhage is frequently seen in the case of significant blood loss (Fig. 3.28); this finding is considered to be an indication of both an intravital event and hypoxia (Weinke et al. 2000).

Subendocardial hemorrhage may occur following cardiac injuries and resuscitation, as well

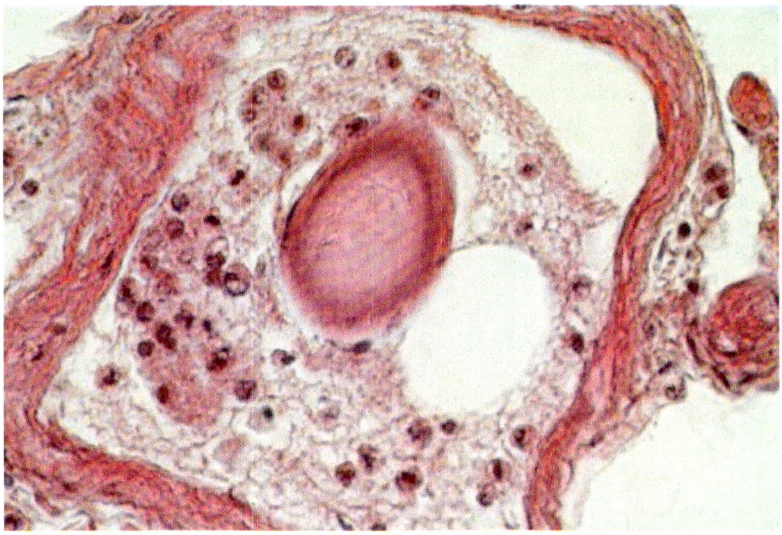

Fig. 3.26 Embolic spread of a cartilage particle to the lungs following repeated deep stab wounds to the throat, jugular vein incision, and additional air embolism (H&E ×400)

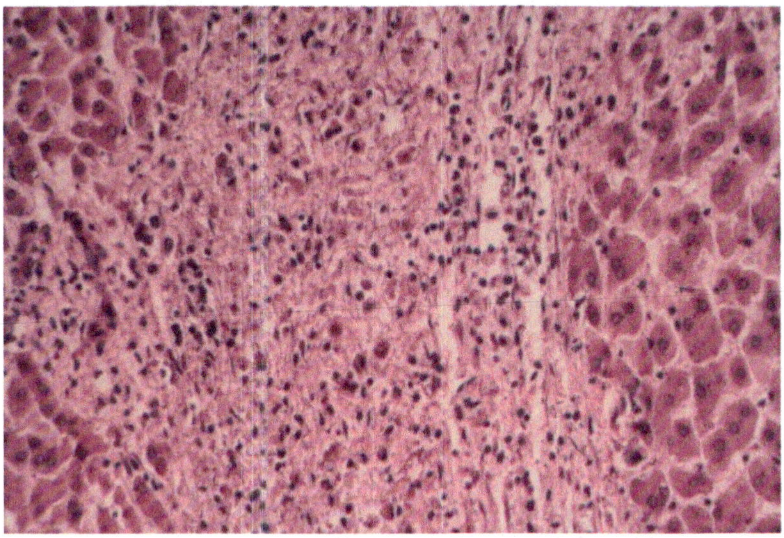

Fig. 3.27 A stab wound to the liver that was briefly survived, showing leukocyte invasion of necrotic areas of the adjacent liver tissue (H&E ×200)

as secondary to noncardiac injuries (Seidl 2005) such as:

- Head injuries
- Infectious diseases leading to shock
- Hemorrhagic diathesis, partly due to intoxication or disseminated intravascular coagulation
- Abdominal trauma
- Asthma
- Hemorrhagic-hypovolemic shock
- Intoxication (digitalis, cocaine)

Therefore, hemorrhage beneath the endocardium, predominantly found in the ventricle of the left heart, is seen in many forensic autopsy cases (Harruff 1993; Keil et al. 1991; Rajs 1977), e.g., in combination with intracranial lesions (Smith 1954), in cases of shock (Sheehan 1940), and as result of direct mechanical trauma (Chiu et al. 1972). Subendocardial hemorrhage can be accompanied by necrosis (Chiu et al. 1972). It is also described in cases of severe abdominal trauma (Caesar 1999). There is speculation that

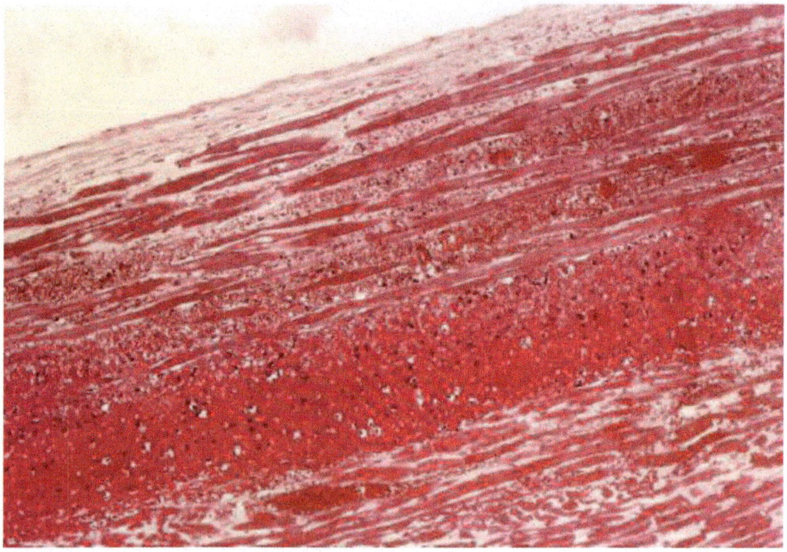

Fig. 3.28 Streaky subendocardial hemorrhage following death due to hemorrhage in hemorrhagic-hypovolemic shock following stab wounds to the upper abdomen with approximately 1400 mL blood in the abdominal cavity (H&E ×100)

subendocardial hemorrhage with necrosis in the case of cerebral processes is the result of increased catecholamine release (Caesar 1999). Of course, there are frequent cases of hemorrhage due to natural causes seen in forensic medical practice, e.g., ruptured aortic aneurysm or spontaneous peripheral varicose vein rupture (Doberentz et al. 2010). The infiltration of "primed" polymorphonuclear neutrophils into multiple organs has been reported in cases of traumatic or hemorrhagic shock. The results of a recently published study indicate that a massive MPO-positive neutrophil infiltration occurred in the lung and liver of elderly physical abuse victims and that the number of infiltrating neutrophils in these abuse cases was increased significantly compared with that in control groups. The endothelial expression of P-selectin and the number of IL-8-positive cells are also reported to be significantly increased in the lung and liver of abuse cases (Hayashi et al. 2010).

3.7 Asphyxiation

Asphyxiation can present challenging questions in terms of expert opinions, in particular in cases of homicidal asphyxiation with soft objects (Keil and Berzlanovich 2010; Banaschak et al. 2003; Hadley and Fowler 2003; Zhu et al. 2003; Ito and Kimura 1990; Robbins et al. 1988). In such cases, there are as a rule no – or only uncharacteristic – morphological findings. Forensic pathologists are often asked to provide evidence of asphyxia death in the trial, and a histological marker would be of great help. Potential markers of mechanical asphyxia were investigated using samples from the lung, e.g., P-selectin, E-selectin, or HIF1-α (Cecchi et al. 2014). Histological examinations are required in all cases to exclude any relevant acute disease. Death due to toxicological effects must also be excluded. Differentiating asphyxia-related or hypoxic tissue and organ damage from autolytic changes is not always possible.

Conjunctival petechiae The occurrence of petechial hemorrhage in the conjunctiva can be observed in cases of external suffocation, as well as in deaths due to other unnatural causes (e.g., electrocution, craniocerebral trauma, intoxication) or natural [e.g., cardiac, central nervous system (CNS), infectious] causes. They may also occur in the presence of altered intrathoracic or intra-abdominal pressure resulting in inflow congestion and increased pressure to veins and capillaries of the head and neck region (e.g., epileptic fit, asthma attack, sneezing, coughing, vomiting, giving birth, Valsalva). Using a confocal laser scanning microscope (CLSM), an attempt was made to verify whether conjunctival petechiae had been caused by diapedesis or by rhexis hemorrhage (Lasczkowski et al. 2005).

Histology of the Lung Particular importance is accorded to the investigation of lung tissue in the case of death by asphyxia (Strunk et al. 2010; Schmeling et al. 2009; Betz et al. 1993a, b; Brinkmann et al. 1984). However, varying ventilation and perfusion parameters are found in the lung with advancing age, in addition to which the effects of external factors mediated via aspirated air can be seen, e.g., the development of smoker macrophages. In the case of asphyxiation with a soft object, such as a pillow, microscopic investigation of the tracheal and bronchial lavage should be considered (Chap. 11). Hypercapnic and hypoxic conditions may affect the development of hemoglobin subtypes as well as extramedullary hematopoiesis (Kouno et al. 2000).

While histological findings in lung tissue have been described in cases of death by asphyxiation, as in death by strangulation, their specificity should be evaluated with caution. These findings include alveolar overdistension accompanied by alveolar rupture, intra-alveolar hemorrhage with alveolar edema, alveolar–capillary congestion, and swelling of pneumocytes (Byard and Tsokos 2005). Dystelectasis, collar-like periductal hemorrhage and lymphangiectasia, increased microthrombi, and endothelium alternations can be added to this picture (Brinkmann 1981).

The overall microscopic picture is decisive for the correlation of histological findings in the lung with a diagnosis of asphyxiation with a soft object: acute congestive hyperemia with focal hemorrhage immediately adjacent to overextended pulmonary alveoli, defined as "hemorrhagic-dysoric syndrome" (Brinkmann et al. 1984). The histological finding of "hemorrhagic-dysoric syndrome" has been partially confirmed in individual cases (Bohnert et al. 2004; Banaschak et al. 2003). Resuscitation as the cause of histological findings, e.g., intensive ventilation following the onset of rigor mortis, should be considered in the differential diagnosis. Findings in both the lung and the petechiae can have other causes and are not specific for asphyxiation.

A further important indication of asphyxiation is petechial hemorrhage. This is seen in vascular congestion following the rupture of capillaries or very small peripheral blood vessels, in particular in the eyelids and conjunctiva (see above), in the mucosa of the oral vestibule, and over the entire facial skin area in severe cases of compression trauma to the neck. Petechiae may also be found beneath the lung membrane and other serous membranes (subepicardial, subperitoneal).

Earlier histological investigations described increased numbers of alveolar macrophages and giant cells in the lung tissue of healthy persons who had died of protracted oxygen deficiency. The duration of asphyxiation was given as 15–60 min and causes of death as chest compression, throttling, and smothering (Janssen 1963, 1977). Janssen concluded that the proliferation of alveolar cells was stimulated by lack of oxygen, while pulmonary giant cells in healthy persons point to death by slow asphyxia. Other investigators demonstrated that numerous alveolar macrophages and pulmonary giant cells also appear in controls (Betz et al. 1993a, b, 1994). Immunohistochemically, strong positive reactions can be observed with the general macrophage marker PG-M1 (CD68). This antibody detects the CD68 antigen which is expressed as an intracytoplasmic molecule and absent from granulocytes and their precursor cells. Using this and other antibodies (LN-4, 27 E 10, 25 F 9, AMH 152, MIB 1 = Ki 67), the results of a further study were in concordance with the data of Betz et al. (Grellner and Madea 1996). In addition, animal tests with rats and guinea pigs killed by prolonged hypoxia varying from 30 min to 12 h provided similar histological pulmonary changes, with the occurrence of swollen and mobilized alveolar cells resulting in the formation of polynuclear giant cells (Janssen and Bärtschi 1964).

3.8 Differentiation Between SIDS and Asphyxiation

Sudden infant death syndrome (SIDS) is defined as the sudden death of an infant that is unexpected from the patient history and for which thorough postmortem examination is unable to reveal the cause of death (see Chap. 17). SIDS is therefore a diagnosis of exclusion. A differentiation between SIDS and death by asphyxiation, in particular due to smothering, can be very challenging, especially in cases where external findings such as scratches or abrasions to the skin of the nose, mouth, and neck, or bruises and tears of the mucous membranes of gums and lips are absent (Scheers et al. 1998).

Petechial hemorrhage of the conjunctivae and eyelids strongly indicate asphyxiation but can also be observed in other conditions, in particular following cardiopulmonary resuscitation (Adebahr 1981). With regard to a possible differentiation between SIDS and asphyxiation, it is of interest that most authors found no petechiae in SIDS except in cases showing vomit aspiration (Betz et al. 1998). Similar to the appearance of conjunctival petechiae, acute pulmonary emphysema is a frequent but also nonspecific finding in asphyxiation. Even though the lungs of suspected cases of SIDS tend to fill the pleural cavities (Valdes-Dapena 1982), dystelectasis of the lung is a more common finding. However, it seems to be reasonable to conclude that the simultaneous appearance of conjunctival petechiae and acute pulmonary emphysema strongly indicates death by asphyxiation (Betz et al. 1998). In the past, several cases have been described in which an infant or several siblings under 1 year of age were intentionally smothered, usually with fatal outcomes. Of special note in this regard is a 1972 description of multiple cases of SIDS in a single family. In 1994, however, it was proved that the case actually involved multiple infanticides by the children's mother (Pinholster 1994). Had the cause of death been correctly diagnosed as infanticide and not as SIDS in the first child, the death of the other children could have been prevented (Oehmichen et al. 2000).

Petechiae of the skin can result from smothering (Bohnert et al. 2004). But even if forensic findings are based on autopsies conducted according to the International Standardized Autopsy Protocol for Sudden Unexpected Infant Death, including complete histological, neuropathological, and toxicological investigations (Krous 1995), it may be impossible to verify smothering as the real cause of death (Oehmichen et al. 2000). In such cases, histological investigations alone can help to clarify the intensity of pulmonary emphysema and whether there is vomit aspiration into the small bronchi and bronchioli as an alternative explanation for petechiae of the skin.

3.9 Some Histopathologic Changes due to Cardiopulmonary Resuscitation

Of the spectrum of numerous injuries possibly resulting from cardiopulmonary resuscitation, only a few will be mentioned here, relating mainly to cardiac findings. Cardiac changes due to cardiopulmonary resuscitation (Bajanowski et al. 2003; Matsuda et al. 1997; Karch and Billingham 1984; Adebar 1966) are well known in the literature and may include:

- Myocardial hemorrhage
- Subepicardial hemorrhage
- Subjacent contraction bands
- Disruption of intercalated discs
- Hypereosinophilia on the epicardial surface or just below
- Coagulative necrosis without inflammatory infiltrates

Other findings resulting from cardiopulmonary measures can frequently be detected macroscopically at autopsy (serial rib fractures, ruptured liver and spleen, hemorrhage following puncture, etc.). In the case of patients intubated intravitally, striated hemorrhage in the subepithelial tissue of the larynx may be seen microscopically at the level of the vocal cords (Fig. 3.29). Intensive cardiopulmonary resuscitation may produce the histological picture of emphysema aquosum or a more or less intensive interstitial emphysema accompanied by septal ruptures (Saternus 1987).

In cases where prolonged high-pressure ventilation and administration of high-concentration oxygen are necessary, the histological picture of respirator lung may develop, characterized in the first exudative phase by capillary congestion, by intra-alveolar edema, by hyaline membranes, and in most cases by concomitant inflammatory alterations. In the subsequent irreversible phase, fibrous organization processes dominate and

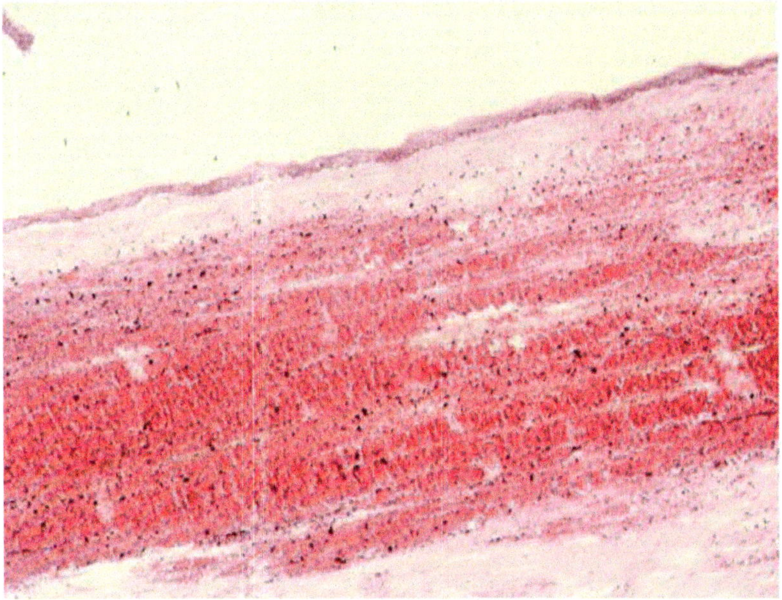

Fig. 3.29 Striated fresh subepithelial hemorrhage beneath nonkeratinized squamous epithelium of the vocal cords following intravital intubation (H&E ×100)

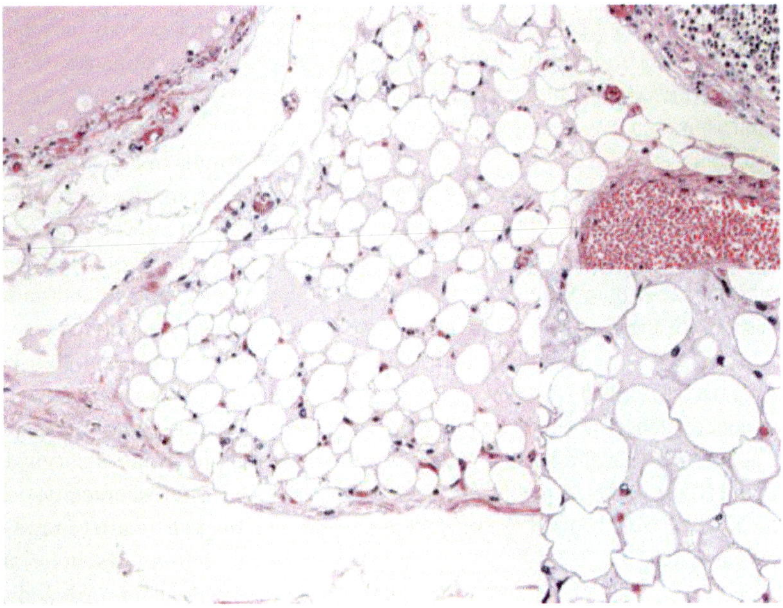

Fig. 3.30 Gelatinoid atrophy in fat tissue due to hunger strike (77 days) (H&E ×100; H&E ×400)

show a variable tendency toward pulmonary fibrosis (Ritter et al. 1985).

3.10 Death by Starvation/ Dehydration

The main focus of attention in cases of death by starvation and dehydration is on macroscopic findings (Riße et al. 2010). Cases sometimes involve hunger strikers (Altun et al. 2004; Beyon 1996) or fatalities in the setting of anorexia nervosa (Hewitt et al. 2001). Besides microvacuolar steatosis of hepatocytes, thymic involution has also been described histologically (Nishio et al. 2000; Tanegashima et al. 1999). However, there are histological findings which correlate with macroscopy and patient history: subcutaneous fatty tissue with gelatinoid atrophy (Fig. 3.30), in extreme cases even subepicardial fatty tissue is strongly rarefied,

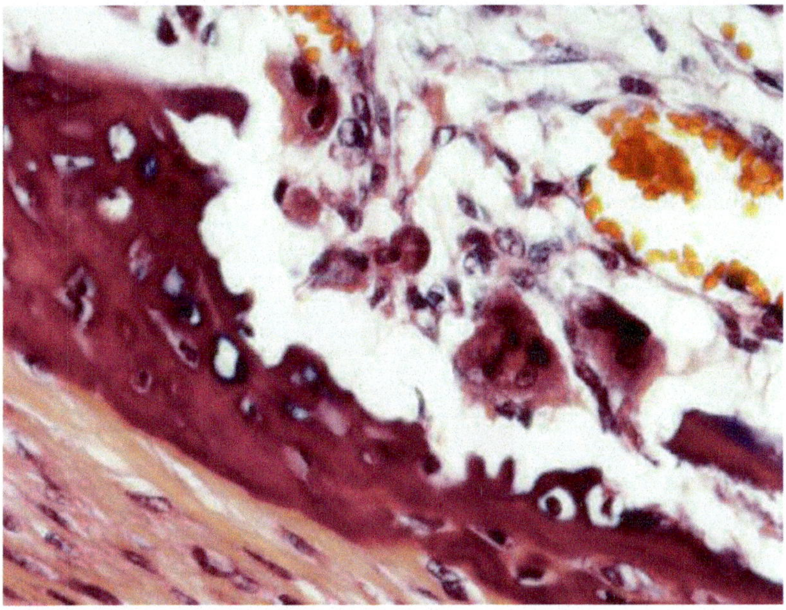

Fig. 3.31 Lacunar bone resorption with polynuclear osteoclasts in a case of death due to starvation (H&E ×400)

hepatocyte vacuolization may be observed in the liver, and endocrine organs have undergone degeneration (Piercecchi-Marti et al. 2006). Although a final aspiration may occasionally be seen, infection (bronchial pneumonia, urogenital infection, etc.) should also be considered as a possible direct cause of death (Edler et al. 2008; Fieguth et al. 2000; Püschel et al. 1987). Bone tissue demonstrates increased resorption lacunae and osteoclasts in the case of advanced rickets (Fig. 3.31), while frontal lobe atrophy as well as acute renal tubular necrosis have been described (Altun et al. 2004). In the case of concomitant child abuse involving abuse-related fractures, periosteal reactions in long bones can be found (Blum and Hausmann 2009), as well as fractures which may be used for fracture age determination (Chap. 10).

3.11 Traumatic Injury to the Kidneys, Liver, and Pancreas

In cases of upper abdominal contusion and/or penetrating injury to the abdomen and flanks, the kidneys, liver, and pancreas may be involved. Subcapsular as well as intraparenchymal hemorrhage may be seen in the liver; atraumatic hepatic hemorrhage is rare but may occur in, e.g., fatty liver hepatitis and hepatic peliosis.

Compression of the pancreas may result in localized necrosis and hemorrhage, contusion results in hematoma formation, while larger tears lead to involvement of the gland's excretory ducts. Subcapsular rupture may occur in pancreatic tissue, including incomplete rupture (pancreas capsule and pancreas parenchyma with an intact pancreatic duct) or complete rupture (complete pancreatic transection). Hemorrhage, internal pancreatic fistulas, abscesses, pseudocysts, as well as chronic fibrosing pancreatitis may ensue in the event of survival.

Microscopically, posttraumatic chronic fibrosing pancreatitis shows duct ectasia with secretion retention (dyschylia) and basophilic deposits of microcalcium, in addition to an increase in collagen fibers and a generally loose lymphocytic inflammatory infiltrate. Post-interventional pancreatitis following endoscopic retrograde cholangiopancreatography (ERCP) represents the most serious example of iatrogenic pancreatitis.

Although direct trauma to the kidneys can generally be diagnosed macroscopically, some investigations have focused on immunohistochemical findings, e.g., the expression of P-selectin in renal glomeruli following trauma.

P-selectin is a cell adhesion glycoprotein stored in Weibel-Palade bodies of vascular endothelial cells and in platelet α-granules and is an important regulator of the first phase of leukocyte–endothelium interaction (Nogami et al. 2000).

Although traumatic tissue or organ injury can heal, posttraumatic scarring often forms and may remain detectable for life. Histologically, scar tissue presents as collagenous or rough fibrous connective tissue, such that large areas of cord-like or extensive fibrosis in the abdominal region should arouse the suspicion of previous (possibly very old) trauma (Dye et al. 2008), which may even have taken place in childhood (Byard and Heath 2010).

In the context of chronic physical child abuse, hemosiderin deposits were found to be significantly more abundant in the lungs and liver of chronic abuse victims. In lung specimens, hemosiderin deposits were found in alveolar macrophages, which were diffuse in the lung parenchyma. In the liver, diffuse hemosiderin deposits could be seen in Kupffer stellate cells and hepatocytes (Dorandeu et al. 1999).

References

Abe M, Saitoh H, Sato Y, Hamaguchi K, Kiuchi M (2001) Immunohistochemical study of the kidneys after severe muscular injury. Int J Legal Med 114:232–236

Abrunzo TJ (1991) Commotio cordis: the single, most common cause of traumatic death in youth baseball. AJDC 145:1279–1282

Adebahr G (1981) Value of cyanosis and petechiae in strangulation and concurrent severe anemia. Z Rechtsmed 86:123–128

Adebahr G, Weiler G (1976) Blutverteilungsmuster in der Niere bei Tod durch Verbluten. Forensic Sci 7:179

Adebar G (1966) Histologische Befunde am Herzmuskel bei Wiederbelebungsversuchen. Dtsch Z Ges Gerichtl Med 57:205

Altun G, Akansu B, Altun BU, Azmak D, Yilmaz A (2004) Deaths due to hunger strike: post-mortem findings. Forensic Sci Int 146:35–38

An JL, Ishida Y, Kimura A, Kondo T (2010) Forensic application of intrarenal aquaporin-2 expression for differential diagnosis between freshwater and saltwater drowning. Int J Legal Med 124:99–104

An LJ, Ishida Y, Kimura A, Kondo T (2011) Immunohistochemical examination of intracerebral aquaporin-4 expression and its application for differential diagnosis between freshwater and saltwater drowning. Int J Legal Med 125:59–65

Anscombe AM, Knight BH (1996) Delayed death after pressure on the neck: possible causal mechanisms and implications for mode death in manual strangulation discussed. Forensic Sci Int 78:193–197

Auer A, Mottonen M (1991) Qualitative diatom analysis as a tool to diagnose drowning. Am J Forensic Med Pathol 12:213–218

Bajanowski T, Ortmann C, Teige K, Wedekind H, Zack F, Röse I, Brinkmann B (2003) Pathological changes of the heart in sudden infant death. Int J Legal Med 117:193–203

Banaschak S, Schmidt P, Madea B (2003) Smothering of children older than 1 year of age—diagnostic significance of morphological findings. Forensic Sci Int 134:163–168

Bapat VN, Brown K, Nakas A, Shabbo F (2002) Retropharyngeal hematoma—a rare complication of anticoagulant therapy. Eur J Cardiothorac Surg 21:117–118

Barbesier M, Boval C, Desfeux J, Lebreton C, Léonetti G, Piercecchi-Marti MD (2015) Acute fatal coronary artery dissection following exercise-related blunt chest trauma. J Forensic Sci 60:233–235

Berg S (1975) Leichenzersetzung und Leichenzerstörung. In: Mueller B (ed) Gerichtliche Medizin. Springer, Berlin, Heidelberg, New York, p 62

Betz P, Wilske J, Nerlich A, Tübel J, Peschel O, Penning R, Eisenmenger W (1992) Die Bedeutung der Alveolarmakrophagen für die Ertrinkungsdiagnosik—eine morphometrische Studie. Rechtsmedizin 2:143–147

Betz P, Nerlich A, Penning R, Eisenmenger W (1993a) Alveolar macrophages and the diagnoses of drowning. Forensic Sci Int 62:217–224

Betz P, Nerlin G, Penning R, Eisenmenger W (1993b) Pulmonary giant cells and their significance for the diagnosis of asphyxiation. Int J Legal Med 106:156–159

Betz P, Beier G, Eisenmenger W (1994) Pulmonary giant cells and traumatic asphyxia. Int J Legal Med 106:258–261

Betz P, Hausmann R, Eisenmenger W (1998) A contribution to a possible differentiation between SIDS and asphyxiation. Forensic Sci Int 91:147–152

Beyon J (1996) Hunger strike in Turkish prisons. Lancet 348:737

Biro C, Kovac P, Palkovic M, El-Hassoun O, Caplovicova M, Novotny J, Jakubovsky J (2010) Potentialities of scanning electron microscopy and EDX analysis in bullet wounds. Rom J Leg Med 18:225–230

Blum S, Hausmann R (2009) Periostreaktionen an langen Röhrenknochen im Kindesalter. Differentialdiagnose "battered child syndrome". Rechtsmedizin 19:228–230

Böhm E (1973) Rasterelektronenmikroskopische Untersuchungen an Lungenalveolen—Demonstration am Beispiel der Ertrinkungslunge. Beitr Gerichtl Med 30:24–29

Bohnert M, Grosse Perdekamp M, Pollak S (2004) Three subsequent infanticides covered up as SIDS. Int J Legal Med 119:31–34

Brinkmann B (1978) Vitale Reaktionen in der Lungenstrombahn bei Tod durch Strangulation. Z Rechtsmed 81:133–146

Brinkmann B (1981) Morphologie und Pathophysiologie des akuten Strangulations-Todes. Pathologe 2:122

Brinkmann B, Butenuth W (1982) Histology and ultrastructural pathology of the lung in experimental drowning. Beitr Gerichtl Med 40:95–98

Brinkmann B, Püschel K (1981) Die Lunge als Erfolgsorgan der Strangulationsagonie. Z Rechtsmed 86:175–194

Brinkmann B, Fechner G, Püschel K (1983a) Zur Lungenhistologie bei experimentellem Ertrinken. Z Rechtsmed 89:267–277

Brinkmann B, Fechner G, Püschel K (1983b) Zur Ultrastrukturpathologie des Alveolarapparates beim experimentellen Ertrinken. Z Rechtsmed 91:47–60

Brinkmann B, Fechner G, Püschel K (1984) Identification of mechanical asphyxiation in cases of attempted masking of the homicide. Forensic Sci Int 26:235–245

Brinkmann B, Hernandez MA, Karger B, Ortmann C (1997) Pulmonary myelomonocyte subtypes in drowning and other causes of death. Int J Legal Med 110:295–298

Buhtz G, Burkhardt W (1938) Die Feststellung des Ertränkungsortes aus dem Diatomeenbefund der Lungen. Dtsch Z Ges Gerichtl Med 29:469

Buzina W, Feierl G, Haas D, Reinthaler FF, Holl A, Kleinert R, Reichenpfader B, Roll P, Marth E (2006) Lethal brain abscess due to the fungus *Scedosporium apiospermum* (teleomorph *Pseudallescheria boydii*) after a near drowning incident: case report and review of the literature. Med Mycol 44:473–477

Byard RW, Heath K (2010) Mesenteric fibrosis—a histologic marker of previous blunt abdominal trauma in early childhood. Int J Legal Med 124:71–73

Byard RW, Tsokos M (2005) Infant and early childhood asphyxial deaths. In: Tsokos M (ed) Forensic pathology reviews, vol 2. Humana, Totowa, pp 101–124

Byard RW, Gains G, Simpson E, Eitzen D, Tsokos M (2006a) Drowning, haemodilution, haemolysis and staining of the intima of the aortic root—preliminary observations. J Clin Forensic Med 13:121–124

Byard RW, Gains G, Tsokos M (2006b) Haemolytic staining of the intima of the aortic root—a useful pathological marker of freshwater drowning? J Clin Forensic Med 13:125–128

Caesar R (1999) Subendokardiale Blutungen. In: Remmele W (ed) Pathologie, vol 1. Springer, Berlin, Heidelberg, New York, p 243

Camps FE, Hunt AC (1959) Pressure on the neck. J Forensic Med 6:116–135

Carter N, Ali F, Green MA (1998) Problems in the interpretation of hemorrhage into neck musculature in cases of drowning. Int J Legal Med 112:101–106

Castiglioni C, Baumann P, Fracasso T (2016) Acute pulmonary emphysema in death by hanging: a morphometric digital study. Int J Legal Med 130:1281–1285

Cecchi R, Sestili C, Prosperini G, Cecchetto G, Vicini E, Viel G, Muciaccia B (2014) Markers of mechanical asphyxia: immunohistochemical study on autoptic lung tissues. Int J Legal Med 128:117–125

Chen X, Zhang J, Deng Z, Hou Y (2015) A case of isolated ventricular septal rupture caused by blunt chest trauma. Rom J Leg Med 23:243–246

Cherkavsky NB, Stukochenko AG (1965) The findings of struvite crystals in serous cavities of sea water corpses. Subebnomed eksp (Mosk) 8, Nr. 1, 18; Ref. Dtsch Z Ger Med 59:129 (1967)

Chin KW, Sercarz JA, Wang MB, Andrews R (1998) Spontaneous cervical hemorrhage with near-complete airway obstruction. Head Neck 20:350–353

Chiu CJ, Mesereau WA, Scott HJ (1972) Subendocardial hemorrhagic necrosis. The role of direct mechanical trauma on the endocardium. J Thorac Cardiovasc Surg 64:66–75

Cox RG (1998) Retropharyngeal haematoma leading to airway obstruction in a child with closed head trauma. Paediatr Anaesth 8:353–356

Dettmeyer R, Graß H, Diefenbach C, Madea B (2004) Letales Karotissinussyndrom. Z Rechtsmed 14:117–121

Dickman GL, Hassan A, Luckstead EF (1978) Ventricular fibrillation following a baseball injury. Phys Sportsmed 6:85–86

Dierkes K (1938) Über die Histologie der Waschhaut. Dtsch Z Ges Gerichtl Med 30:262

Dobiáš M, Hejna P, Al Mawiri A (2013) Coronary artery dissection: a fatal complication following blut chest trauma. Forensic Sci Med Pathol 9:454–457

Doberentz E, Hagemeier L, Veit C, Madea B (2010) Unattended fatal hemorrhage due to spontaneous peripheral varicose vein rupture—two case reports. Forensic Sci Int 206(1–3):e12–e16

Donaldson GA, Hamlin E (1950) Massive hematemesis resulting from rupture of a gastric-artery aneurysm. N Engl J Med 243:369–373

Dorandeu A, Perie G, Jouan H, Leroy B, Gray F, Durigon M (1999) Histological demonstration of haemosiderin deposits in lungs and liver from victims of chronic physical child abuse. Int J Legal Med 112:280–286

Dworzack DL, Clark RB, Borkowski WJ Jr, Smith DL, Dykstra M, Pugsley MP, Horowitz EA, Connolly TL, McKinney DL, Hostetler MK, Fitzgibbons JF, Galant M (1989) Pseudallescheria boydii brain abscess: association with near-drowning and efficacy of high-dose, prolonged miconazole therapy in patients with multiple abscesses. Medicine 68:218–224

Dye DW, Peretti FJ, Kokes CP (2008) Histologic evidence of repetitive blunt force abdominal trauma in four pediatric fatalities. J Forensic Sci 53:1430–1433

Edler C, Schulz F, Tsokos M, Püschel K (2008) Forensische Pädopathologie: Tödliche Vernachlässigung. Prakt Paediatr 14:406–410

Fan YY, Zhang ST, Yu LS, Ye GH, Lin KZ, Wu SZ, Dong MW, Han JG, Feng XP, Li XB (2014) The time-dependent expression of α7nAChr during skeletal muscle wound healing rats. Int J Legal Med 128:779–786

Farrugia A, Ludes B (2010) Diatom detection and identification. Significance for the diagnosis of death by drowning. Rechtsmed 20:49–58

Fechner G (1995) Immunhistochemische Untersuchungen bei Muskeltraumen. In: Bratzke H, Schröter A (eds) Immunhistochemie in der Rechtsmedizin. Hänsel-Hohenhausen, Egelsbach, Frankfurt, Washington DC, pp 22–36

Fechner G, Petkovits T, Brinkmann B (1990) Zur Ultrastruktur-Pathologie mechanischer Skelettmuskelschädigungen. Z Rechtsmed 103:291–299

Fechner G, Hauser R, Sepulchre MA, Brinkmann B (1991) Immunohistochemical investigations to demonstrate vital direct traumatic damage of skeletal muscle. Int J Legal Med 104:215–219

Fechner G, Hernandez M, Bajanowski T, Sepulchre MA, Brinkmann B (1993) Immunohistochemical alteration after muscle trauma. Int J Legal Med 105:203–207

Fieguth A, Günther D, Kleemann WJ (2000) Tödliche Kindesvernachlässigungen infolge Mangelernährung. In: 9th spring meeting of the German Society of Forensic Medicine, Leipzig, 4–5 May 2000

Fisher JF, Shadomy S, Teabeaut R, Woodward J, Michaels GE, Newman MA, White E, Cook P, Seagraves A, Yaghmai F, Rissing JP (1982) Near drowning complicated by brain abscess due to *Petriellidium boydii*. Arch Neurol 39:511–513

Fornes P, Pepin G, Heudes D, Lecomte D (1998) Diagnosis of drowning by combined computer-assisted histomorphometry of lungs with blood strontium determination. J Forensic Sci 43:772–776

Frazier M, Mirchandani H (1984) Commotio cordis—revisited. Am J Forensic Med Pathol 5:181–184

Froede RC, Lindsey D, Steinbronn K (1979) Sudden unexpected death from cardiac concussion (commotio cordis) with unusual complications. J Forensic Sci 24:752–756

Fukui Y, Hata M, Takahashi S, Matsubara K (1980) A new method for detecting diatoms in human organs. Forensic Sci Int 16:67–74

Ginellivá A, Farkaš D, Iannaccone SF, Vyhnálková V (2016) Unexpected fatal outcome of laparoscopic inguinal hernia repair. Forensic Sci Med Pathol 12:178–180

Goffin Y, Heyndrickx G (1974) Traumatic rupture of the right coronary artery with nine hours survival. Forensic Sci 4:135–144

Goldbach HJ, Hinüber H (1956) Lassen sich aus dem Zustand der elastischen Fasern der menschlichen Fußsohlenhaut Rückschlüsse auf eine eventuelle Liegezeit im Wasser ziehen? Zbl Path 95:105

Green ED, Simson LR, Kellerman HH, Horowitz RN, Sturner WQ (1980) Cardiac concussion following softball blow to the chest. Ann Emerg Med 9:155–157

Greene JF, Fitzwater JE, Burgess J (1974) Arterial lesions associated with neurofibromatosis. Am J Clin Pathol 62:481–487

Grellner W, Madea B (1996) Immunohistochemical characterization of alveolar macrophages and pulmonary giant cells in fatal asphyxia. Forensic Sci Int 79:205–213

Guan DA, Ohshima T, Jia JT, Kondo T, Li DX (1999) Morphological findings of “cardiac concussion” due to experimental blunt impact to the precordial region. Forensic Sci Int 100:211–220

Guan DW, Zhang XG, Zhao R, Lu B, Han Y, Hou ZH, Jia JT (2007) Diverse morphological lesions and serious arrhythmias with hemodynamic insults occur in the early myocardial contusion due to blunt impact in dogs. Forensic Sci Int 166:49–57

Hadley JA, Fowler DR (2003) Organ weight effects of drowning and asphyxiation on the lungs, liver, brain, heart, kidneys, and spleen. Forensic Sci Int 133:190–196

Haffner HAT, Graw M, Erdelkamp J (1994) Spleen findings in drowning. Forensic Sci Int 66:95–104

Harruff RC (1993) Subendocardial hemorrhages in forensic pathology autopsies. Am J Forensic Med Pathol 14:284–288

Hayashi T, Ishida Y, Mizunuma S, Kimura A, Kondo T (2009) Differential diagnosis between freshwater drowning and saltwater drowning based on intrapulmonary aquaporin-5 expression. Int J Legal Med 123:7–13

Hayashi T, AGo K, Ago M, Yamanouchi H, Bunai Y, Ogata M (2010) The infiltration of ‘primed’ neutrophils into multiple organs due to physical abuse to the elderly: an immunohistochemically study. Forensic Sci Int 202:17–25

Heath D, Edwards C, Harris P (1970) Post-mortem size and structure of the human carotid body. Thorax 25:129–140

Heinen M, Dotzauer G (1973) Problemfall: “Ertrinkungslunge”. Beitr Gerichtl Med 30:133

Heintz R (1961) Das Crushsyndrom. Arztl Fortbild 11:544–547

Hendey NI (1973) The diagnostic value of diatoms in cases of drowning. Med Sci Law 13:23–34

Henssge C, Wang H, Hoppe B (2002) Light microscopical investigations on structural changes of skeletal muscle as artifacts after post-mortem stimulation. Forensic Sci Int 125:163–171

Hewitt PL, Coren S, Steel GD (2001) Death from anorexia nervosa: age span and sex differences. Aging Ment Health 5:41–46

Hines GL, Lefkowitz L, Mothashemi M (2002) Infrarenal aortic rupture secondary to neurofibromatosis. Ann Vasc Surg 16:784–786

Holden HS, Crosfill JWL (1955) The significance of foreign bodies in the alveoli of apparently drowned. J Forensic Med 2:141–150

Hosemann W (1983) Die Exulceratio simplex Dieulafoy. Pathologe 4:41–43

Hughes DTD, Empey DW, Cameron JM, Sims BG, Taylor TH (1972) Immediate postoperative death associated with severe laryngeal obstruction. Med Sci Law 12:139–141

Hurlimann J, Feer P, Elber F, Niederberger K, Dirnhofer R, Wyler D (2000) Diatom detection in the diagnosis of death by drowning. Int J Legal Med 114:6–14

Ishikawa T, Zhu BL, Li DR, Zhao D, Michiue T, Maeda H (2007) Immunohistochemical investigation of ubiquitin and myoglobin in the kidney in medicolegal autopsy cases. Forensic Sci Int 171:136–141
Ito Y, Kimura H (1990) Histological examination of the temporal bone in medicolegal cases of asphyxia. Forensic Sci Int 44:135–142
Janssen W (1963) Riesenzellenbildung bei Erstickung. Dtsch Z Gerichtl Med 54:200–210
Janssen W (1977) Forensische Histologie. Schmidt-Römhild, Lübeck
Janssen W, Bärtschi G (1964) Vitale und supravitale Reaktionen der Alveolarzellen nach protrahiertem Sauerstoffmangel. Dtsch Z Gerichtl Med 55:47–60
Kakizaki E, Yukawa N (2015) Simple protocol for extracting diatoms from lung tissues of suspected drowning cases within 3 h: first practical application. Forensic Sci Int 251:179–185
Kampmann H, Bode G (1982) Traumatic infarction following stab wound of the heart. Z Rechtsmed 88:159–164
Kaplan JA, Karofsky PS, Volturo GA (1993) Commotio cordis in two amateur ice hockey players despite the use of commercial chest protectors: case reports. J Trauma 34:151–153
Karch SB, Billingham ME (1984) Morphologic effects of defibrillation: a preliminary report. Crit Care Med 12:920–921
Karkola K, Neittaanmaki H (1981) Diagnosis of drowning by investigations of left heart blood. Forensic Sci Int 18:149–153
Karofsky PS (1990) Death of a high school hockey player. Phys Sportsmed 18:99–103
Katragkou A, Dotis J, Kotsiou M, Tamiolaki M, Roilides E (2007) Scedosporium apiospermum infection after near drowning. Mycoses 50:412–421
Keil W, Berzlanovich A (2010) Suffocation with soft covers. Rechtsmedizin 20:519–528
Keil W, Rothämel T, Tröger HD (1991) Subendokardiale Hämorrhagien aus forensisch-medizinischer Sicht. Beitr Gerichtl Med 49:45–53
Kettner M, Schmidt P, Padosch SA (2007) Vascular rupture—a rare lethal complication of neurofibromatosis v Recklinghausen. Forensic Sci Med Pathol 3:206–209
Kohlhase C, Maxeiner H (2003) Morphometric investigation of emphysema aquosum in the elderly. Forensic Sci Int 134:93–98
Kouno A, Inoue H, Bajanowski T, Maseno Y, Iwasa M, Nakayama M, Nishi K, Brinkmann B, Matova R (2000) Development of haemoglobin subtypes and extramedullary haematopoiesis in young rats. Effects of hypercapnic and hypoxic environment. Int J Legal Med 114:66–70
Krous HE (1995) The international standardized autopsy protocol for sudden unexpected infant death. In: Rognum TO (ed) Sudden infant death syndrome. New trend in the nineties. Scand University Press, Oslo, pp 81–95
Kubo S, Ogata M, Kitamura O, Tsuda R, Orihara Y, Hirose W, Matsumoto H, Nakasono I (1994) Immunohistopathological investigations of autopsied carotid bodies and their application to diagnosing strangulation. Int J Legal Med 106:281–284
Kunz J (1960) Über die Verwertbarkeit des Zustandes der Lungenelastica zur Bestimmung der Liegezeit von Wasserleichen. Dtsch Z Gerichtl Med 50:559
Ladham S, Koehler SA, Woods P, Huston R, Dominick J, Fochtman FW, Wecht CH (2005) A case of a death by explosives: the keys to a proper investigation. J Clin Forensic Med 12:85–92
Laposata EA (1985) Collection of trace evidence from bombing victims at autopsy. J Forensic Sci 30:789–797
Lasczkowski G, Risse M, Gamerdinger U, Weiler G (2005) Pathogenesis of conjunctival petechiae. Forensic Sci Int 147:25–29
Liang Y, Tong F, Zhang L, Li W, Zhou Y (2016) Sudden death duo to rupture of the right internal carotid artery in neurofibromatosis type 1: case report. Legal Med 21:33–37
Lorente JA, Hernandez-Cueto C, Villanueva E, Luna JD (1990) The usefulness of lung surfactant phospholipids (LSP's) in the diagnosis of drowning. J Forensic Sci 35:1367–1372
Lunetta P, Modell JH (2005) Macroscopical, microscopical, and laboratory findings in drowning victims. In: Tsokos M (ed) Forensic pathology reviews, vol 3. Humana Press, Totowa, pp 3–77
Lunetta P, Penttilä A, Hällfors G (1998) Scanning and transmission electron microscopical evidence of the capacity of diatoms to penetrate the alveolo-capillary barrier in drowning. Int J Legal Med 111:229–237
Lunetta P, Modell JH, Sajantila A (2004) What is the incidence and significance of 'dry lungs' in bodies found in water? Am J Forensic Med Pathol 25:291–301
Malandrini A, Villanova M, Salvadori C, Gambelli S, Berti G, Di Paolo M (2001) Neuropathological findings associated with retained lead shot pellets in a man surviving two months after a suicide attempt. J Forensic Sci 46:717–721
Maron BJ, Poliac LC, Kapalan JA, Frederick OM (1995) Blunt impact to the chest leading to sudden death from cardiac arrest during sports activities. N Engl J Med 333:337–342
Maron BJ, Strasburger JF, Kugler JD, Bell BM, Brodkey FD, Poliac LC (1997) Survival following blunt chest impact-induced cardiac arrest during sports activities in young athletes. Am J Cardiol 79:840–841
Matsuda H, Seo Y, Takahama K (1997) A medico-legal approach to the myocardial changes caused by transthoracic direct current countershock. Nippon Hoigaku Zasshi 51:11–17
Maxeiner H (1983) Zum Beweiswert von Kehlkopfverletzungen. Arch Kriminol 171:33–44
Maxeiner H (1985) Weichteilblutungen im Kehlkopfinneren nach Strangulation. Z Rechtsmed 94:127–135
Maxeiner H (1987a) Posticusblutungen beim akuten Koronartod. Pathologe 8:221–226
Maxeiner H (1987b) Zur lokalen Vitalreaktion nach Angriff gegen den Hals. Z Rechtsmed 99:35–54

Maxeiner H (1996) The microscopical findings (early vital reactions) in bleedings of the laryngeal muscles after laryngeal injuries. In: Oehmichen M, Kirchner H (eds) The wound healing process—forensic pathological aspects, Research in legal medicine, vol 13. Schmidt-Römhild, Lübeck, pp 309–324

Mazzon D, Zanatta P, Curtolo S, Bernhardi V, Bosco E (1998) Upper airway obstruction by retropharyngeal hematoma after cervical spine trauma: report of a case treated with percutaneous dilational tracheostomy. J Neurosurg Anesthesiol 10:237–240

Mukaida M, Kimura H, Takada Y (1998) Detection of bathsalts in the lungs of a baby drowned in a bathtub: a case report. Forensic Sci Int 93:5–11

Neri M, Turillazzi E, Riezo I, Fineschi V (2007) The determination of firing distance applying a microscope quantitative method and confocal laser scanning microscopy for detection of gunshot residue particles. Int J Legal Med 121:287–292

Nishio H, Matusi K, Tsuji H, Tamura A, Suzuki K (2000) Immunohistochemical study of tyrosine phosphorylation signaling in the involuted thymus. Forensic Sci Int 110:189–198

Nogami M, Takatsu A, Endo N, Ishiyama I (2000) Immunohistochemical localization of P-selectin in the glomeruli from forensic autopsies. Legal Med 2:21–25

O'Donnell JJ, Birkinshaw R, Harte B (1997) Mechanical airway obstruction secondary to retropharyngeal haematoma. Eur J Emerg Med 4:166–168

Oehmichen M, Gerling I, Meißner C (2000) Petechiae of the baby's skin as differentiation symptom of infanticide versus SIDS. J Forensic Sci 45:602–607

Oehmichen M, Karren-Balting U, Saternus KS (1986) Reaktive Veränderungen bei Weichteilblutungen im Kehlkopfinneren. Beitr Gerichtl Med XLV:73–78

Ojala K, Lempinen M (1968) Die Initialphase der Muskelnekrose nach Schnittverletzung und ihr Identifizieren als vital im quergestreiften menschlichen Muskel. Dtsch Zschr Gerichtl Med 64:102–109

Ökrös S (1938) Annähernde Bestimmung der Todeszeit aus dem Hautzustand. Dtsch Z Ges Gerichtl Med 29:497

Ortmann C, Pfeiffer H, Brinkmann B (2001) Immunohistochemical alterations after intravital and post-mortem traumatic myocardial damage. Int J Legal Med 115:23–28

Ortmann C, Wüllenweber J, Brinkmann B, Fracasso T (2010) Fatal mycotic aneurysm caused by *Pseudallescheria boydii* after near drowning. Int J Legal Med 124:243–247

Otto H (1961) Über den Nachweis von Diatomeen in menschlichen Lungenstauben. Frankfurter Zschr Pathol 71:176–181

Paparo GP, Siegel H (1976) On the significance of posterior cricoarytenoid muscle hemorrhage. Forensic Sci 7:61–65

Parmley LF, Manion WC, Mattingly TW (1958) Nonpenetrating traumatic injury of the heart. Circulation 18:371–396

Peabody AJ (1980) Diatoms and drowning. A review. Med Sci Law 20:254–261

Pedal I, König HG (1983) Histologische Lungenbefunde nach Überfahrung mit unterschiedlicher Überlebenszeit. Beitr Gerichtl Med 41:271–277

Peter J, Kirchner A, Kuhlisch E, Menschikowski M, Neef B, Dreßler J (2006) The relevance of the detection of troponins to the forensic diagnosis of cardiac contusion. Forensic Sci Int 160:127–133

Piercecchi-Marti MD, Louis-Borrione CL, Bartoli C, Sanvoisin A, Panuel M, Pelissier-Alicot AL, Leonetti G (2006) Malnutrition, a rare form of child abuse: diagnostic criteria. J Forensic Sci 51:670–673

Piette MHA, de Letter EA (2006) Drowning: still a difficult autopsy diagnosis. Forensic Sci Int 163:1–9

Pinholster G (1994) SIDS paper triggers a murder charge. Science 264:197–198

Pollanen MS (1998) Diatoms and homicide. Forensic Sci Int 91:29–34

Pollanen MS (2016) Fatal rhabdomyolysis after torture by reverse hanging. Forensic Sci Med Pathol 12:170–173

Püschel K, Fechner G, Brinkmann B (1983) Zur Ultrastrukturpathologie der Ertrinkungslunge beim Menschen. Beitr Gerichtl Med 41:309–314

Püschel K, Lieske K, Schoof C (1987) Kindesvernachlässigungen mit Todesfolge. Pädiat Prax 35:17–27

Püschel K, Schulz F, Darrmann I, Tsokos M (1999) Macromorphology and histology of muscular hemorrhages in cases of drowning. Int. J Legal Med 112:101–106

Rajs J (1977) Left ventricular subendocardial haemorrhages. A study of their morphology, pathogenesis and prognosis. Forensic Sci Int 10:80–103

Rajs J, Thiblin I (2000) Histologic appearance of fractured thyroid cartilage and surrounding tissues. Forensic Sci Int 114:155–166

Reh H (1970) Diagnostik des Ertrinkungstodes und Bestimmung der Wasserzeit. Michael Triltsch Verlag, Düsseldorf

Reiter C (1984) Proof of death by drowning by smoker cells washed into the left heart blood. Z Rechtsmed 93:79–88

Riezzo I, Di Battista B, de Salvia A, Cantatore S, Neri M, Pomara C, Turillazzi E, Fineschi V (2014) Delayed splenic rupture: dating the sub-capsular hemorrhage as a useful task to evaluate causal relationships with trauma. Forensic Sci Int 234:64–71

Riße M, Rummel J, Tsokos M, Dettmeyer R, Büttner A, Lehmann H, Püschel K (2010) Verhungern und Verdursten. Rechtsmedizin 20:211–218

Ritter CH, Weiler G, Adebahr G (1985) Histomorphological lungs results in cases of long-term artificial respiration with special consideration of use of pure oxygen. Z Rechtsmed 94:41–49

Robbins RD, Sekhar HK, Siverls V (1988) Temporal bone histopathologic findings in drowning victims. Arch Otolaryngol Head Neck Surg 114:1020–1023

Rothschild MA, Maxeiner H (2000) Death caused by a letter bomb. Int J Legal Med 114:103–106

Rüchel R, Wilichowski E (1995) Cerebral *Pseudallescheria mycosis* after near-drowning. Mycoses 38:473–475
Sandooram D, Chandramohan AR, Radcliffe G (2000) Retropharyngeal haematoma causing airway obstruction: a multidisciplinary challenge. J Laryngol Otol 114:706–708
Saternus KS (1987) Traumatische Komplikationen bei der Reanimation. Der Notarzt 3:7–11
Scheers NJ, Dayton CM, Kemp JS (1998) Sudden infant death with external airways covered. Arch Pediatr Adolesc Med 152:540–547
Schleyer F (1951) Zur Histologie der Waschhaut. Dtsch Z Ges Gerichtl Med 40:680
Schmeling A, Fracasso T, Pragst F, Tsokos M, Wirth I (2009) Unassisted smothering in a pillow. Int J Legal Med 123:517–519
Schneider V (1972) Rasterelektronenoptische Untersuchungen zur Ertrinkungslunge. Beitr Gerichtl Med 29:26–274
Schollmeyer W (1961) Führt eine Blutung im Paraganglion caroticum den Tod herbei? Dtsch Z Ges Gerichtl Med 51:190–193
Schulz E (1968) Gefäßleukozytose bei gewaltsamen Tod. Blut 17:336–339
Schwaiblmair B, Höfling B (1997) Koronargefäßwandschädigung bei Thoraxtraumen. Dtsch Med Wschr 122:1043–1046
Seidl S (2005) Subendocardial hemorrhages. In: Tsokos M (ed) Forensic pathology reviews, vol 2. Humana Press, Totowa, pp 293–306
Sevitt S (1973) Coronary thrombosis following injury and burns. Med Sci Law 13:185–191
Sheehan HL (1940) Subendocardial hemorrhages in shock. Lancet 1:831–832
Shields L, Hunsaker DM, Hunsaker JC, Humbert KA (2003) Nonterrorist suicidal deaths involving explosives. Am J Forensic Med Pathol 24:107–113
Sidari L, DiNunno N, Costantinides F, Melato M (1999) Diatom test with Soluene-350 to diagnose drowning in sea water. Forensic Sci Int 103:61–65
Sigrist T (1986) Untersuchungen zur vitalen Reaktion der Skelettmuskulatur. Habilitationsschrift, St. Gallen
Sigrist T (1987) Untersuchungen zur vitalen Reaktion der Skelettmuskulatur. Beitr Gerichtl Med 45:87–101
Sigrist T, Germann U (1989) Homicide by asphyxia—yes or no? On the use of muscle histology. Z Rechtsmed 102:549–557
Sigrist T, Meier K, Zollinger U (1989) Traumatic carotid sinus reflex death. Beitr Gerichtl Med 47:257–266
Sivridis E, Pavlidis P, Fiska A, Pitsiava D, Giatromanolaki A (2011) Myocardial hypertrophy induces carotid body hyperplasia. J Forensic Sci 56(Suppl 1):S90–S94. https://doi.org/10.1111/j.1556-4029.2010.01582.x
Smith RP (1954) Subendocardial haemorrhages associated with intracranial lesions. J Pathol Bacteriol 68:327–334
Smith P, Jago R, Heath D (1982) Anatomical variation and quantitative histology of the normal and enlarged carotid body. J Pathol 137:287–304
Somers GR, Chiasson DA, Taylor GP (2008) Presence of periorbital and conjunctival petechial hemorrhages in accidental pediatric drowning. Forensic Sci Int 175:198–201
Spitz WU, Schneider V (1964) The significance of diatoms in the diagnosis of death by drowning. J Forensic Sci 9:11–18
Staak M (1968) Eine atypische posttraumatische Herzmuskelnekrose bei einem vierjährigen Knaben. Dtsch Zschr Gerichtl Med 62:14–19
Stiel M, Dettmeyer R, Madea B (2006) Explosiver "römischer" Fund. Arch Kriminol 217:36–44
Strunk T, Hamacher D, Schulz R, Brinkmann B (2010) Reaction patterns of pulmonary macrophages in protracted asphyxiation. Int J Legal Med 124:559–568
Tabata N (1998) Morphological changes in traumatized skeletal muscle: the appearance of 'opaque fibers'of cervical muscles as evidence of compression to the neck. Forensic Sci Int 96:197–214
Takeichi T, Kitamura O (2009) Detection of diatom in formalin-fixed tissue by proteinase K digestion. Forensic Sci Int 190:19–23
Tanegashima A, Yamamoto H, Yada I, Fukunga T (1999) Estimation of stress in child neglect from thymic involution. Forensic Sci Int 102:173–180
Tenzer ML (1985) The spectrum of myocardial contusion: a review. J Trauma 25:620–627
Thomas F, van Hecke W, Timpermann J (1961) The detection of diatoms in the bone marrow as evidence of death by drowning. J Forensic Med 8:142
Toklu AS, Alkan N, Gürel A, Cimsit M, Haktanir D, Körpinar S, Purisa S (2006) Comparison of pulmonary autopsy findings of the rats drowned at surface and 50 ft depth. Forensic Sci Int 164:122–125
Torre C, Varetto L (1985) Scanning electron microscope study of the lung in drowning. J Forensic Sci 30:456–461
Torre C, Varetto L, Tappi E (1983) Scanning electron microscopic ultrastructural alterations of the pulmonary alveolus in experimental drowning. J Forensic Sci 28:1008–1012
Tsai KJ, Huang YC (1999) Traumatic retropharyngeal hematoma: case report. J Trauma 46:715–716
Tsokos M, Paulsen F, Petri S, Madea B, Püschel K, Turk EE (2003) Histologic, immunohistochemical, and ultrastructural findings in human blast injury. Am J Respir Crit Care Med 168:549–555
Turillazzi E, Monaci F, Neri M, Pomara C, Riezzo I, Baroni D, Fineschi V (2010) Collection of trace evidence of explosive residues from the skin in a death due to a disguised letter bomb. The synergy between confocal laser scanning microscope and inductively coupled plasma atomic emission spectrometer analyses. Forensic Sci Int 197:e7–e12
Udermann H, Schuhmann G (1975) Eine verbesserte Methode zum Diatomeen-Nachweis. Z Rechtsmedizin 76:119–122
Uitdehaag S, Dragutinovic A, Kuiper I (2010) Extraction of diatoms from (cotton) clothing for forensic comparison. Forensic Sci Int 200:112–116

Valdes-Dapena M (1982) The pathologist and the sudden infant death syndrome. Am J Pathol 106:118–131

Varga M, Csabai G (1992) A suicidal death by explosives. Int J Legal Med 105:35–37

Vermeij E, Duvalois W, Webb R, Koeberg M (2009) Morphology and composition of pyrotechnic residues formed at different levels of confinement. Forensic Sci Int 186:68–74

Viano DC, Andrzejak DV, King AI (1992) Fatal chest injury by baseball impact in children. Clin J Sport Med 2:161–165

Wachholz (1907) Die Diagnose des Ertrinkungstodes. Vjschr Gerichtl Med 33:25

Wang Q, Ishikawa T, Michiue T, Zhu BL, Guan DW, Maeda H (2012) Intrapulmonary aquaporin-5 expression as a possible biomarker for discriminating smothering and choking from sudden cardiac death: a pilot study. Forensic Sci Int 220:154–157

Weiler G, Risse M (1988) Zum forensischen Beweiswert der nicht-traumatischen Posticusblutung. Beitr Gerichtl Med 46:237–240

Weinig E, Pfanz H (1951) Diagnosis of death by drowning through demonstration of diatoms in optically negative tissue sections. Dtsch Z Ges Gerichtl Med 40:664–668

Weinke H, Lang M, Lignitz E (2000) Über subendokardiale Blutungen. In: 9th spring meeting of the German Society of Forensic Medicine, Leipzig, 4–5 May 2000

Wilichowski E, Christen HJ, Schiffmann H, Schulz-Schaeffer W, Behrens-Baumann W (1996) Fatal *Pseudallescheria boydii* panencephalitis in a child after near drowning. Pediatr Infect Dis J 15:365–370

Zhu BL, Fujita MQ, Quan L, Ishida K, Oritani S, Fukita K, Kamikodai Y, Maeda H (1999) A sudden death due to cardiac conduction system injury from a blunt chest impact. Legal Med 1:26–29

Zhu BL, Ishida K, Fujita MQ, Maeda H (2000a) Immunohistochemical investigation of a pulmonary surfactant in fatal mechanical asphyxia. Int J Legal Med 113:268–271

Zhu BL, Ishida K, Quan L, Fujita MQ, Maeda H (2000b) Immunohistochemistry of pulmonary surfactant apoprotein A in forensic autopsy: reassessment in relation to the causes of death. Forensic Sci Int 113:193–197

Zhu BL, Ishida K, Quan L, Fujita MQ, Maeda H (2001) Immunohistochemistry of pulmonary surfactant-associated protein A in acute respiratory distress syndrome. Legal Med 3:134–140

Zhu BL, Ishida K, Quan L et al (2002) Pulmonary immunohistochemistry and serum levels of a surfactant-associated protein A in fatal drowning. Legal Med 4:1–6

Zhu BL, Quan L, Li DR et al (2003) Postmortem lung weight in drownings: a comparison with acute asphyxiation and cardiac death. Legal Med 5:20–26

4 Histopathology and Drug Abuse

Both acute and chronic drug consumption induce thousands of deaths, producing a variety of autopsy findings depending primarily on the duration of intravenous drug consumption (Gomez et al. 1989; Karch 2002; Schmidt et al. 2004). In addition to the consequences of the drug consumption itself, drug-associated diseases are often found, such as hepatitis and HIV, as well as other related infections (syringe abscesses, infected inguinal fistulas, thrombophlebitis, etc.). There are often drug-associated histopathological findings which, however, are not necessarily caused by the actual active ingredients in drugs. When immune status is impaired, immunological processes may also lead to histopathological findings in connection with other diseases (e.g., hepatitis, HIV, multiple syringe abscesses, injection of accompanying substances, etc.), all of which can also be observed independently of intravenous drug consumption. For this reason, this chapter is confined to clear and/or frequent drug-associated histopathological findings.

In the case of drug-induced lethal intoxication, massive pulmonary edema frequently weighing >1000 g per lung can be seen macroscopically (Levine and Grimes 1973). In cases of chronic and in particular intravenous drug consumption, histopathological findings are described, among others, in lung tissue, the heart, and the liver, as well as heroin-associated nephropathies (HAN). Substance-related histopathological findings are generally the result of chronic cocaine consumption with so-called cocaine cardiomyopathy and cocaine-induced organic infarction, as well as other complications. The fresh injection sites frequently found in drug-related deaths can be investigated immunohistochemically for the detection of morphine as well as for differentiation from insulin injection (Wehner et al. 1998, 2002). Injected substances are transported lymphogenically (Fig. 4.1) and hematogenically.

Histomorphological findings in the central nervous system (CNS) generally call for immunohistochemical techniques since drug-related CNS findings are often not visible with conventional staining. Excluding injection sites and syringe abscesses, drug-associated histopathological findings of the skin are comparatively rare. Findings in the gastrointestinal tract also occur only occasionally in the form of intestinal infarctions following cocaine consumption, while mucosal necrosis is possible during the transportation of incorporated drug containers ("body packing") when toxic drugs are excreted, particularly in the case of cocaine. Although histological investigations of the thyroid show slightly different functional conditions with evidence of intracolloidal resorption vacuoles and occasional signs of unspecific thyroiditis, postmortem investigations of endocrine organs in drug-related deaths show no obvious drug-associated histopathological lesions.

R. B. Dettmeyer, *Forensic Histopathology*, https://doi.org/10.1007/978-3-319-77997-3_4

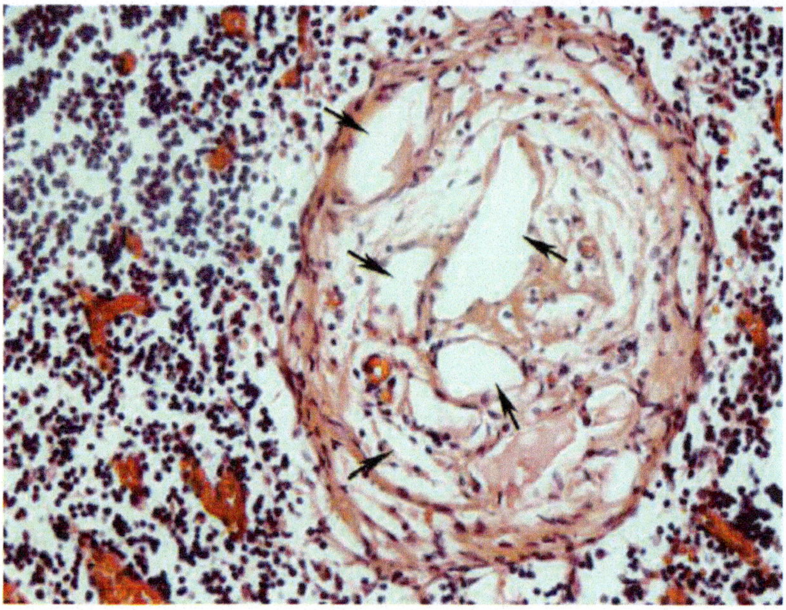

Fig. 4.1 Axillary lymph node with focal post-inflammatory fibrosis in the drainage area of multiple intravenous drug injections and embedded lymphatic ducts (*arrows*) (H&E ×200)

4.1 Pulmonary Histopathological Findings

Histopathological investigations of lung tissue in drug-related deaths can reveal a large number of findings which are primarily considered the result of drug-induced apnea or hypoxia (Gillet and Fort 1978). Initially, autopsy frequently reveals massive, relatively protein-rich pulmonary edema; microscopically, attention should be paid to microhemorrhages as well as pulmonary granulomatosis in the context of so-called junkie pneumopathy. In the case of protracted drug-induced pre-death morbidity, purulent bronchopneumonia may develop from a preexisting purulent bronchitis. Also, following many years of intravenous drug consumption, deposits of immunoglobulin and complement can be detected in the pulmonary interstitium (Smith et al. 1978), as well as in the glomeruli in the case of heroin-associated nephropathy (Dettmeyer et al. 2001, 2005).

4.1.1 Pulmonary Edema

The so-called toxic pulmonary edema associated with drug-related deaths is distinguished from others, in particular cardiac pulmonary edema (Carlson et al. 1979), and is discussed as a cause of sudden death, although its pathogenesis is not entirely understood (Addington et al. 1972; Dettmeyer et al. 2000). It involves edema with a histologically light eosin-red fluid in the alveolar spaces, partially penetrated with erythrocytes, thus a hemorrhagic pulmonary edema (Fig. 4.2). In the case of drug-related death, this pulmonary edema is particularly rich in proteins and can induce an excretion of foaming liquids from the respiratory orifices – the mouth and nose. The histopathological picture of pulmonary edema including extent and type has been used to estimate survival time after onset of intoxication: a short survival time of <1 h indicates a relatively slight edema, distinctive hemorrhages, as well as acute pulmonary emphysema; a survival time of 1–24 h indicates massive pulmonary edema with few hemorrhages and slight edema (Grellner et al. 1996). However, it is always essential to check whether the tissue samples are sufficiently representative in relation to the size of the lungs. Even when this is the case, estimating survival time according to histopathological findings alone appears to be unreliable in some cases. If purulent pneumonia developed shortly after intoxication, then a survival time of many hours, possibly more than 24 h, can be assumed.

Earlier investigations were able to show a considerable increase in pulmonary alveolocapillary

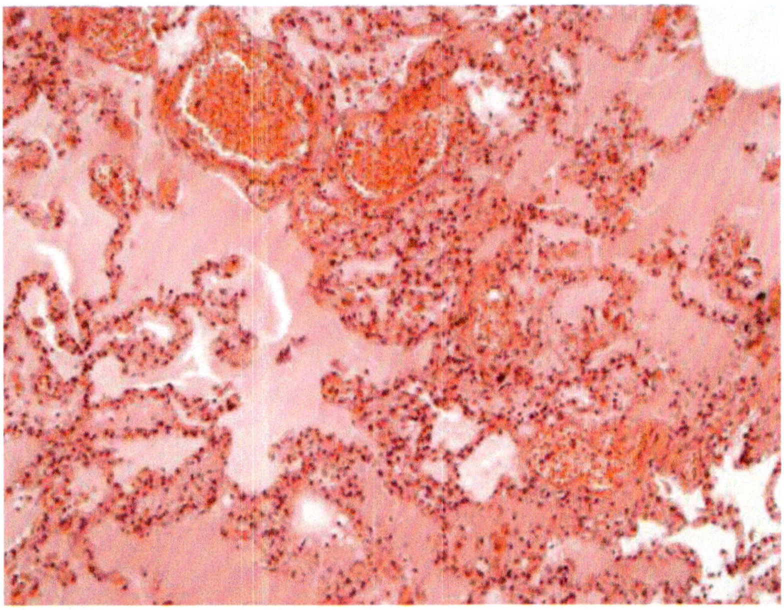

Fig. 4.2 Distinctive partially hemorrhagic and relatively protein-rich "toxic" pulmonary edema with eosin fluid in the pulmonary alveoli of a 32-year-old male drug-related death (H&E ×100)

permeability under the influence of heroin, together with a loss of albumins in the edema fluid (Katz et al. 1972). In such cases, primary toxic damage to the alveolocapillary basal membrane is considered. In the walls of the alveoli lie small alveolar cells (type I) extended in a membrane-like manner next to the upper alveolar cells (type II pneumocytes), which produce a fine phospholipid film ("surfactant"). These cells rest on an intact basal membrane. Elastic fibers, collagen fibers, and capillary networks run along the partitions between the alveoli. The capillary endothelia are nonporous, closed, and also rest on a basal membrane, which regularly merge with the basal lamina of the alveolar epithelial. The alveolar wall, as a wall between two alveoli, has alveolar pores measuring 10–20 µm. The alveolar septa with their fibrocytes form partitions in which immunocompetent cells are found (macrophages, lymphocytes, plasma cells).

In order to display the basal membranes, collagen IV (Fig. 4.3) and laminin (Fig. 4.4) have been represented immunohistochemically in the lung tissue of drug death victims. Collagen IV is a major constituent of the basal membrane. During this process, numerous ruptures of the alveolocapillary basal membranes were detected in the case of drug-induced pulmonary edema (Dettmeyer et al. 2000).

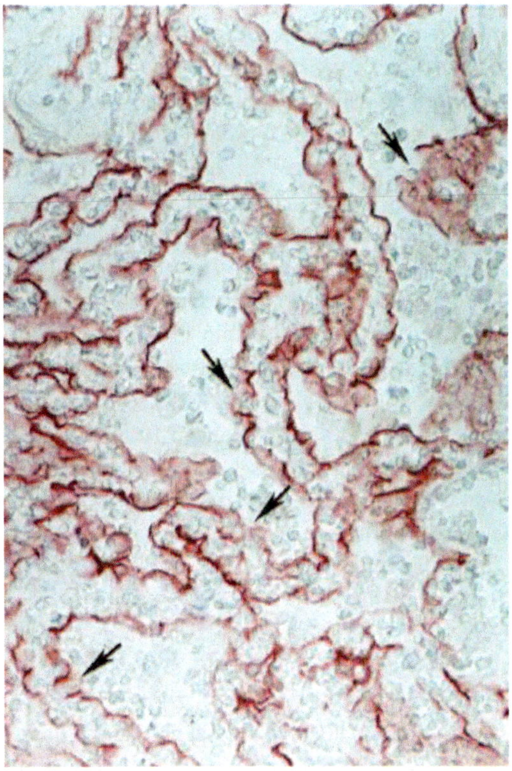

Fig. 4.3 A 28-year-old man who died of drug abuse: immunohistochemical representation of collagen IV in the alveolocapillary basal membrane with rupture sites (*arrows*) and excretion of erythrocytes into the alveolar space, as well as formation of a hemorrhagic pulmonary edema; lung weight 1080 g (×400)

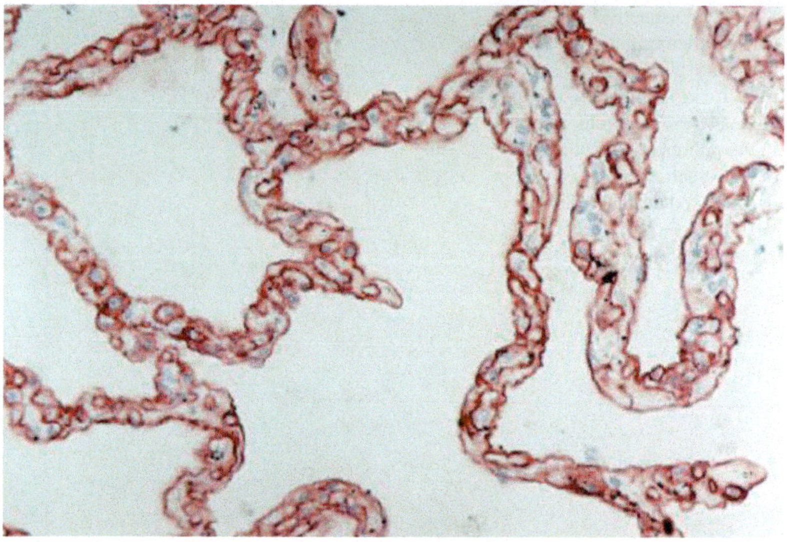

Fig. 4.4 Presentation of laminin in intact alveolocapillary basal membrane in a 27-year-old male traffic accident victim without pulmonary edema (×200)

The excretion of erythrocytes into the alveolar space is also displayed here and leads to a hemorrhagic pulmonary edema as observed in drug death victims. However, there are different explanations for this histopathological picture: apart from toxic damage, which cannot be proven microscopically, acute vascular congestion alone may lead to ruptures of the basal membrane mechanically since identical ruptures have also been observed in a control group with cardiac pulmonary edema (Dettmeyer et al. 2000). These findings are confirmed by the immunohistochemical demonstration of laminin in the basal membrane. Taken together, however, numerous ruptures of the basal membrane lead to considerable alveolocapillary damage (Matsubara et al. 1995). Similar damage has been observed in patients undergoing gold therapy for rheumatic disease and bronchiolo-alveolitis (Pääkkö et al. 1988). In the case of an allergic genesis of bronchiolo-alveolitis, antigens can sometimes be detected in lung tissue (Reijula and Sutinen 1985).

Microfocal accumulations of macrophages loaded with hemosiderin pigment are frequently found in the pulmonary interstitium of drug-related death victims (Fig. 4.5) (Lockemann and Pueschel 1993). These findings arouse the suspicion that transient microhemorrhages and hemorrhagic pulmonary edema must have occurred (and been survived) in the past. After resorption of the microhemorrhages, the siderophages remain, as shown in the Prussian blue reaction. In the differential diagnosis, distinction from a siderosis of the lung due to iron overload can be clearly made since the hemosiderin deposits in drug death victims without chronic vascular congestion are almost never in the alveolar macrophages but rather in a widened and fibrosed pulmonary interstitium.

In the case of allergic or anaphylactic reactions, an increased number of mastocytes in lung tissue is an indication of such reactions; however, it must be borne in mind that microscopic evaluation is more difficult with massive congestive hyperemia and pulmonary edema. Therefore, immunohistochemical identification of mastocytes and IgE-positive cells (Fig. 4.6) in the pulmonary interstitium is helpful (Fineschi et al. 2001b). In such cases, an anaphylactic reaction as the actual cause of death would be possible in spite of proven intoxication with relevant drugs (Berger et al. 1998; Edston and van Hage-Hamsten 1997). In individual cases, there are increased IgE-positive cells in the walls of peripheral branches of the bronchial tree (see Chap. 11).

In addition to focal deposits of hemosiderin-pigment-loaded macrophages, substances injected with the drug and carried embolically via the venous vascular system can be found. These can be a variety of substances which are used to dilute the drugs. If these substances get

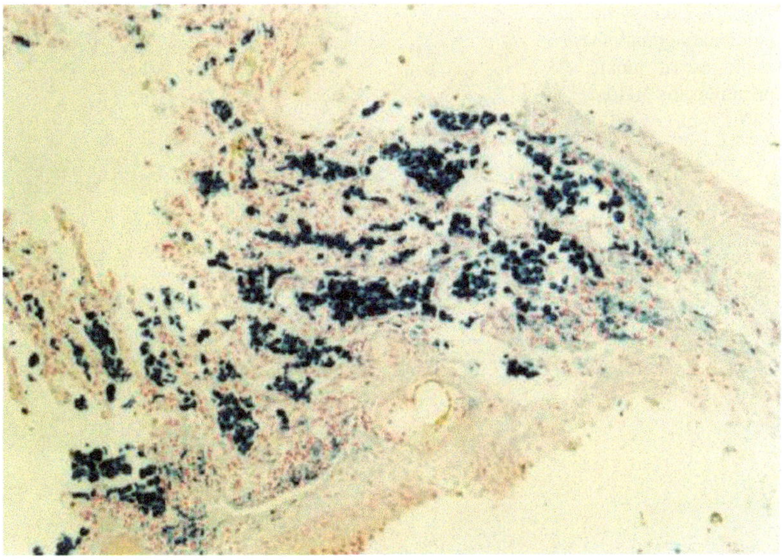

Fig. 4.5 Focal, fibrously widened pulmonary interstitium with an accumulation of siderophages as an indication of previous microhemorrhages in a 34-year-old man who died of drug abuse (Prussian blue ×200)

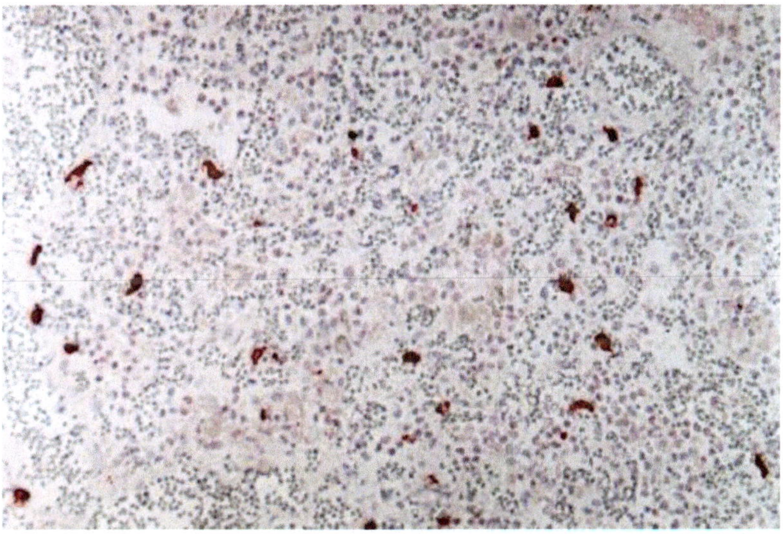

Fig. 4.6 Diffuse, loosely spread immunohistochemical IgE-positive mastocytes in the lung tissue of a 25-year-old man who died of drug abuse with acute congestive hyperemia and partially hemorrhagic pulmonary edema (×125)

caught in the capillary network of the pulmonary alveoli, a so-called junkie pneumopathy of varying severity may develop depending on the duration of intravenous drug consumption.

4.1.2 Pulmonary Granulomatosis (So-Called Junkie Pneumopathy)

"Junkie pneumopathy" describes full-blown pulmonary granulomatosis after many years of intravenous drug injection (Karch 2009; Müller 2004). These are accumulations of birefringent foreign material which entered the lung via the veins by means of embolism (Fig. 4.7). This foreign material is surrounded by perivascularly localized granulomas (Fig. 4.8) (Dettmeyer et al. 2009a; Püschel 1986; Püschel and Schoof 1987; Zeltner et al. 1982). In principal, spread into other organs via vascular anastomoses is also possible (Kringsholm and Christoffersen 1987a, b). The granulomas contain collagen fibers, a primarily lymphomonocytic inflammatory infiltrate and polynuclear foreign-body giant cells (Fig. 4.9). Depending on the genesis of the "junkie

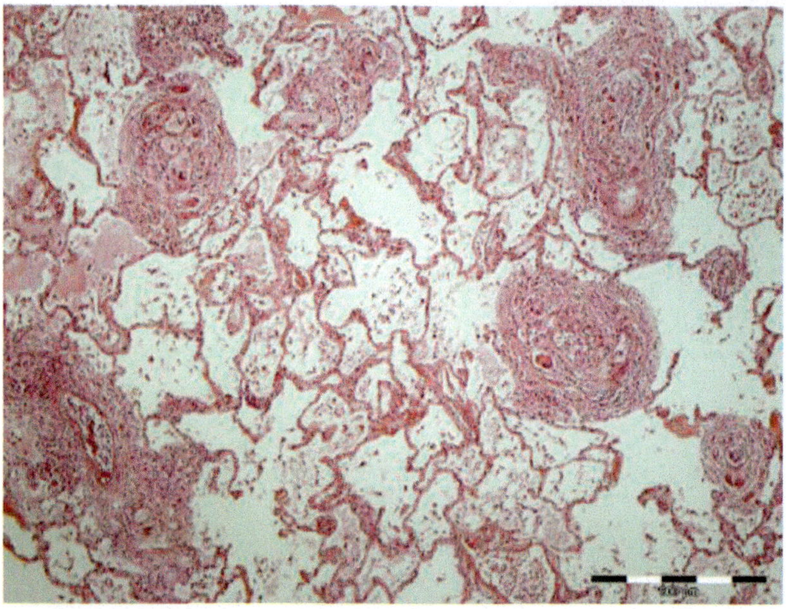

Fig. 4.7 Loosely spread pulmonary granulomas in the case of "junkie pneumopathy" (H&E ×40)

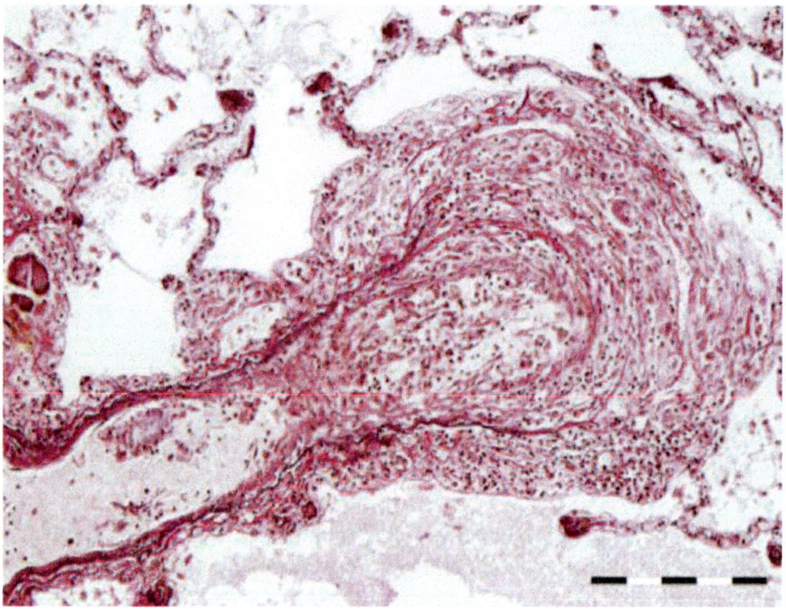

Fig. 4.8 Perivasal pulmonary granuloma with inflammation of the vascular wall; singular polynuclear foreign-body giant cell (*arrow*) (H&E ×200)

pneumopathy," granulomas can be found primarily perivascularly; birefringent foreign material can be visualized using polarization optics (Fig. 4.10) (Thomashefski and Hirsch 1980).

In extreme cases, junkie pneumopathy or pulmonary granulomatosis can include perivascular granulomas with subsequent and considerable right heart overload, resulting in right ventricular hypertrophy of the myocardium. In the literature, the term foreign-body angiitis is also used (Brinkmann et al. 1991), and the risk of microthrombosis formation is discussed (Hopkins 1972). It is always a condition that occurs after many years of intravenous drug consumption (Pare et al. 1984; Raijs et al. 1984). Very rarely, needle embolism is observed (Angelos et al. 1986; Lewis and Henry 1985; Thorne and Collins 1998). Talc components are more frequently seen (Crouch and Churg 1983; Gross 1973; Groth et al. 1972; Zientara and Moore 1970), as well as

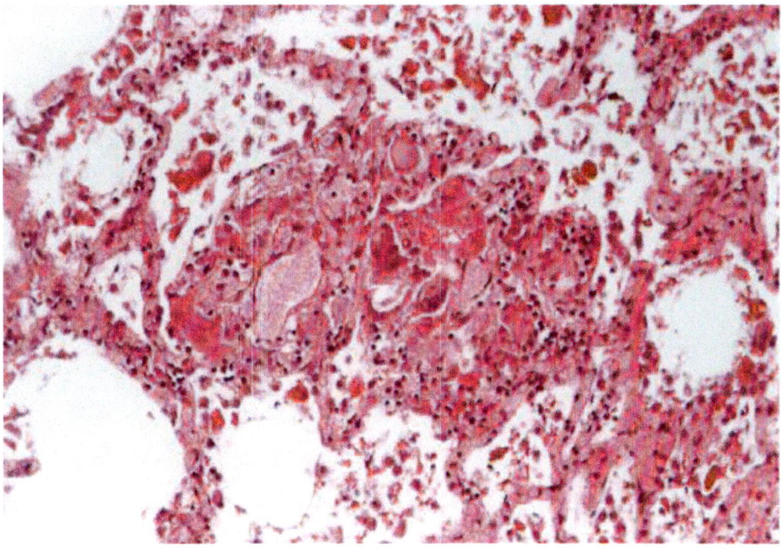

Fig. 4.9 Pulmonary granuloma with a polynuclear giant cell in a 36-year-old man with "junkie pneumopathy" (H&E ×400)

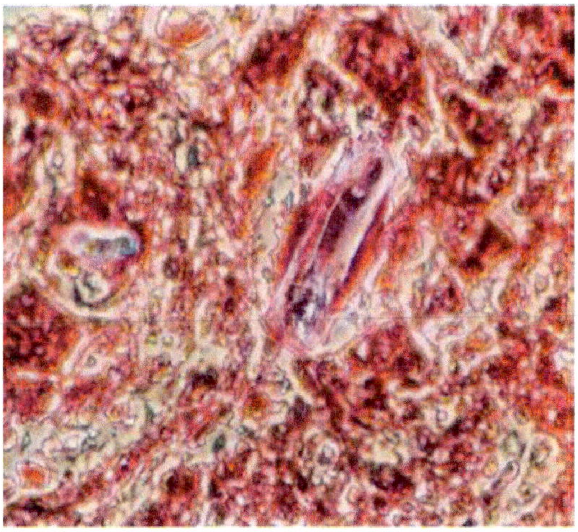

Fig. 4.10 Birefringent foreign material visualized using polarized light in a pulmonary granuloma of a 36-year-old man with "junkie pneumopathy" (H&E ×400)

other components which can partly be identified using electron microscopy (Dettmeyer et al. 2009b), even after the injection of a tablet suspension (Püschel 1988).

4.1.3 Pneumonia

The microscopic investigation of lung tissue in drug-related deaths frequently shows a more or less pronounced, partly acute, partly chronic tracheobronchitis, occasionally also a clear purulent bronchitis and pneumonia, sometimes due to aspiration of chyme (Fig. 4.11). Clearly, after a period agony, a purulent bronchopneumonia can develop relatively quickly following intravenous injection. The bronchopneumonia regularly shows fresh granulocytic infiltrates in the pulmonary alveoli and no advanced tissue repair processes. It is not unusual, however, for agonal aspiration of chyme to occur. Especially in the case of aspirated gastric acid with a low pH value, aspiration pneumonia may develop in some cases. If the lung tissue is additionally damaged by gastric acid, an inflammatory reaction can sometimes be detected, so-called gastromalacia acida (Karch 2009).

Occasionally, fungal infections, which may lead to fungal pneumonia even without accompanying HIV infection, develop following intravenous drug abuse, possibly promoted by impure street heroin. The following fungi come into consideration: *Aspergillus*, *Saccharopolyspora rectivirgula*, and *Thermoactinomyces vulgaris*, as well as *Candida albicans* (Collignon and Sorrell 1983; Karch 2009). The detection of fungal spores and fungal hyphae is carried out with Grocott staining, whereby fungal components are stained black-brown. In Central Europe, tuberculous pneumonia or miliary tuberculosis can only seldom be demonstrated in drug-related deaths. Acute eosinophilic pneumonia can occur following heroin inhalation (Brander and Tukiainen

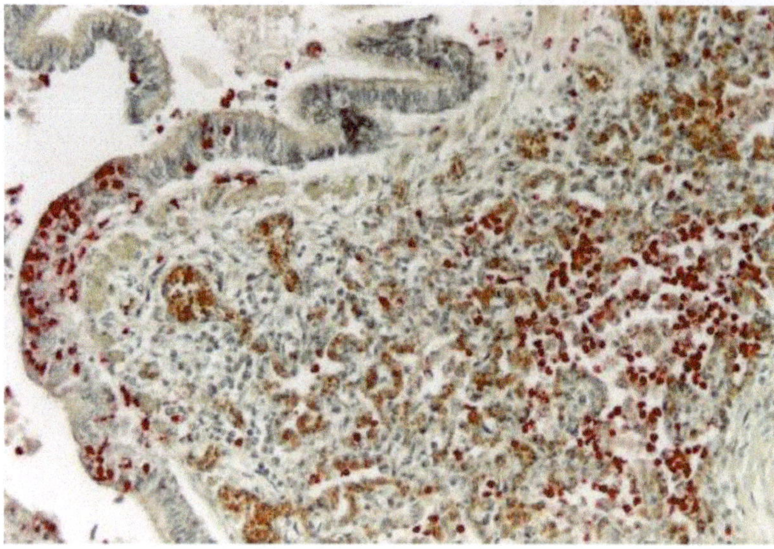

Fig. 4.11 Acute bronchitis (*left*) and pneumonia (*right*) due to aspiration of chyme in a 28-year-old male drug death victim after a period of agony of likely several hours according to patient history (ASD ×200)

1983). Microscopic criteria for scoring of chronic pulmonary alterations in intravenous drug addicts were suggested (Raijs et al. 1984).

4.2 Cardiac Histopathological Findings in Intravenous Drug Abuse

After many years of intravenous drug abuse, inflammatory as well as a toxic involvement of the myocardium must be considered. Animal experiments are helpful here, enabling us to differentiate the toxic effects of a substance from other influencing factors (Cerretani et al. 2008). This also applies to the independent toxic effect of any accompanying substances injected (Toth and Varga 2009). Inflammatory processes are significant due to the permanently activated immune status and the frequently preexisting viremia with hepatitis viruses B and C. Toxic processes are significant since injected drugs and toxins can lead to allergic eosinophilic myocarditis or to drug-induced cardiomyopathy, such as so-called cocaine cardiomyopathy. In addition, varying degrees of myofibrillar degeneration have been described; moreover, activation or degranulation of myocardial mastocytes and increased expression of TNF-alpha have also been cited (Perskvist et al. 2007). Bacterial and similar endocarditis is relatively seldom, at least in Central Europe, in spite of regular intravenous injections, but it is observed occasionally. Cardiopathologic findings have been described after long-term methamphetamine consumption (Islam et al. 2009).

4.2.1 Myocarditis

Investigations of the myocardium in drug-related deaths have shown that in cases where a chronically activated immune status is compared to a control group, more inflammatory cells can be detected in the myocardial interstitium (leukocytes, T-lymphocytes, macrophages), but it is not possible to diagnose myocarditis according to the Dallas criteria (Aretz 1987; Dettmeyer et al. 2009a). Likewise, an immunohistochemical qualification and quantification of interstitial leukocytes reveals higher cell counts only in individual cases, which may lead to the suspected diagnosis of myocarditis. Proinflammatory molecules may be increasingly expressed in the myocardium in drug-related deaths, for example, the MHC class II molecules (Fig. 4.12).

In cases where fresh interstitial lymphomonocytic infiltrates can be detected in the myocardium, this is an indication of viral myocarditis, and the most likely agents in drug-related deaths would be hepatitis viruses. However, in this context, no systematic investigations exist with an immunohistochemical diagnosis of myocarditis in combination

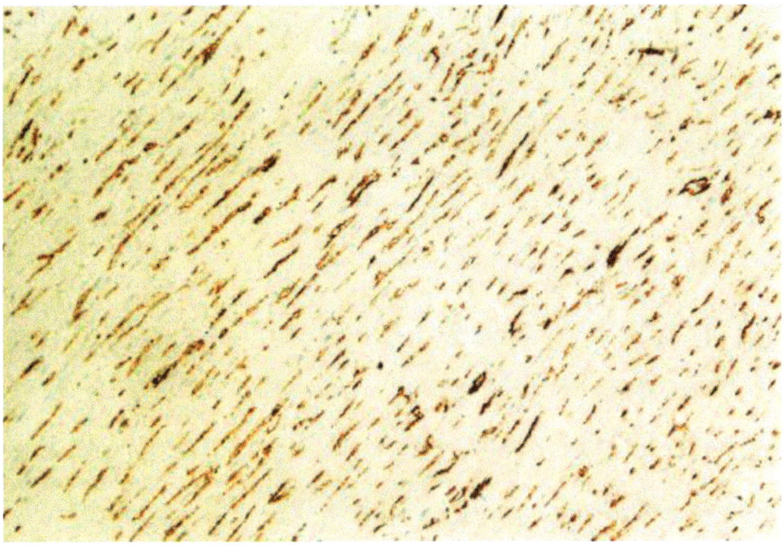

Fig. 4.12 Clear expression of proinflammatory MHC class II molecules in the myocardium after many years of intravenous drug abuse: A 36-year-old male drug death (×100)

with molecular genetic evidence of a viral genome from different viruses. Preexisting inflammatory involvement of the heart muscle in combination with further drug- and toxin-induced damage to the myocardium may explain why drug addicts in a state of intense excitement or with a so-called positional asphyxia seem to have an especially high risk for acute asystolia.

Eosinophilic myocarditis in the context of hypersensitivity myocarditis (Ferries and Rice 1979) can be reliably distinguished from toxic cardiomyopathies in that eosinophilic myocarditis:

- Occurs independently of dose
- Shows histopathological findings of the same age in all sections affected
- Rarely shows intramyocardial hemorrhage
- Generally does not induce myocardial necrosis

Many different drugs and medications can induce a more or less pronounced eosinophilic myocarditis (Fig. 4.13). The question frequently arises as to whether these findings are regarded as a disease. Ultimately, more pronounced eosinophilic inflammatory infiltrates in the myocardial interstitium cannot be excluded as an independent cause of death or at least as having contributed to death even with only small doses of the injected drugs.

The myocardium in drug-related deaths also frequently shows interstitial edema, interstitial and perivascular fibrosis, changes in caliber of cardiomyocytes, and differences in core size as well as myocardial single cell necrosis. Smaller areas of interstitial fibrosis, endocardial fibrosis, and occasionally fresh interstitial hemorrhage also occur. Major changes can be seen in so-called cocaine cardiomyopathy.

Increased expression of tumor necrosis factor (TNF-alpha) in the myocardium of acute drug-related fatalities is reported (Perskvist et al. 2007) and can be confirmed (Fig. 4.14). TNF-alpha is a cytokine involved in systemic inflammation and is a member of a group of cytokines stimulating acute phase reaction. TNF-alpha is able to induce apoptotic cell death and inflammation.

4.2.2 Cocaine-Induced Findings

There are a great number of reports on the effects of cocaine on the heart, although other drugs, such as amphetamines, can lead to toxic reactions and histopathological changes in the heart. The spectrum of cocaine-induced histopathological findings includes, among others:

- Cocaine cardiomyopathy
- Pulmonary anthracosis in "crack" smokers or "crack lung" (Forrester et al. 1989)

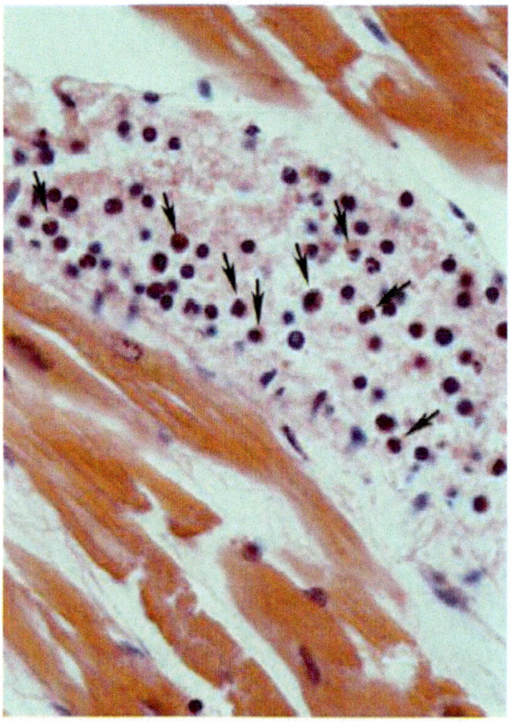

Fig. 4.13 Interstitial inflammatory infiltrates with eosinophilic granulocytes (*arrows*) in the myocardium of a 24-year-old man who died after simultaneous consumption of more than one drug (H&E ×400)

- Cocaine-associated dissecting aneurysms
- Changes in the pulmonary arteries and arterioles, particularly in association with cocaine-induced hypertrophy of the smooth muscle cells in the vascular walls and resulting hypertension
- An increased risk of micro- and macro-infarction of internal organs (Edgecombe and Milroy 2012)
- Cocaine-induced kidney disease (Gitmann and Singhal 2004)
- Effects of cocaine on the placenta (Cejtin et al. 1999)
- Occasionally, cerebral vasculitides occur after cocaine consumption

However, care must be taken when dealing with rare findings since cocaine users frequently consume additional substances and can have weakened immune status, while concomitant diseases can also cause or promote the occurrence of rare findings. Therefore, not all histopathological findings in cocaine users are the direct result of the effects of cocaine or its decomposition products (benzoylecgonine,

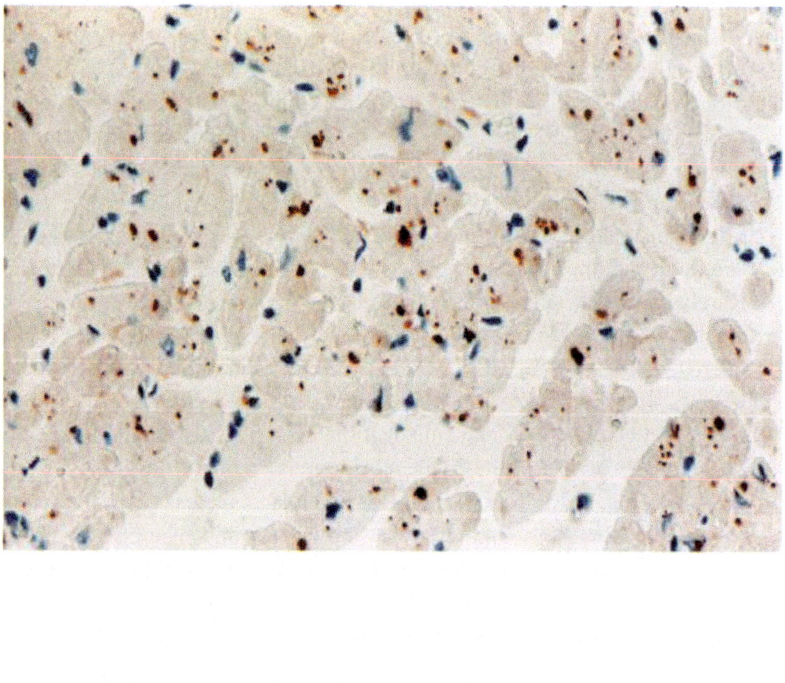

Fig. 4.14 Increased expression of TNF-alpha in the myocardium in a case of acute drug-related fatality (×200)

methylecgonine). It can be assumed, however, that there is a risk of developing cocaine cardiomyopathy (Karch 2005; Rajs and Falconer 1979; Tazelaar et al. 1987) or recurrent necroses in the myocardium (Fineschi et al. 1997). A number of reports have been published since 2010 on levamisole-related or levamisole-induced disease due to the addition of levamisole to cocaine. Levamisole-induced vasculitis, panniculitis, and immune complex glomerulonephritis have been reported (Karch et al. 2016; Lazareth et al. 2012). Vasculitis may be isolated to one organ, e.g., in the form of pulmonary vasculitis with intimal thickening and circular lymphatic infiltration, which can extend to perivascular areas and involve B-($CD20^+$) and T-($CD3^+$) lymphocytes (Karch et al. 2016). Separately to this, one may see other histological findings resulting from the parallel use of cocaine (e.g., hypercontraction of the cardiomyocytes with thickened Z-lines and short sarcomeres, myocardial necrosis). Acute coronary syndrome can be considered if toxicology tests detect levamisole and its metabolite aminorex (Michaud et al. 2014).

Cocaine Cardiomyopathy In cases of chronic cocaine consumption, a mainly left ventricular, yet overall concentric, myocardial hypertrophy can develop (Henning and Cuevas 2006; Karch et al. 1995); this is partly in the form of compensatory hypertrophy in the neighboring tissues of cocaine-induced myocardial necroses which are substituted for collagen scar tissue. In contrast to a larger myocardial infarction (>1 cm in diameter), small scars coalesced in a netlike manner are found with cocaine cardiomyopathy (Fig. 4.15). Preserved interstitial myocardial fibers show significant changes in dimension and enlarged hyperchromatic nuclei (Fineschi et al. 1997; Morris 1991). Knowledge on the effects of cocaine and cocaine-induced histopathological findings is partly based on animal experiments (Fineschi et al. 2001a; Tella et al. 1992).

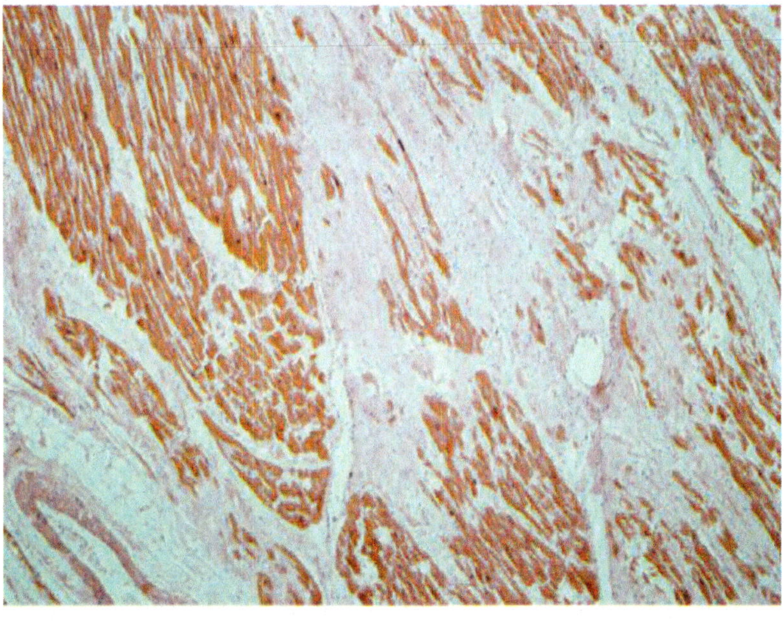

Fig. 4.15 Netlike myocardial fibrosis and compensatory interstitial hypertrophic cardiomyocytes with enlarged hyperchromatic nuclei in a 30-year-old man who died of cocaine cardiomyopathy (H&E ×40)

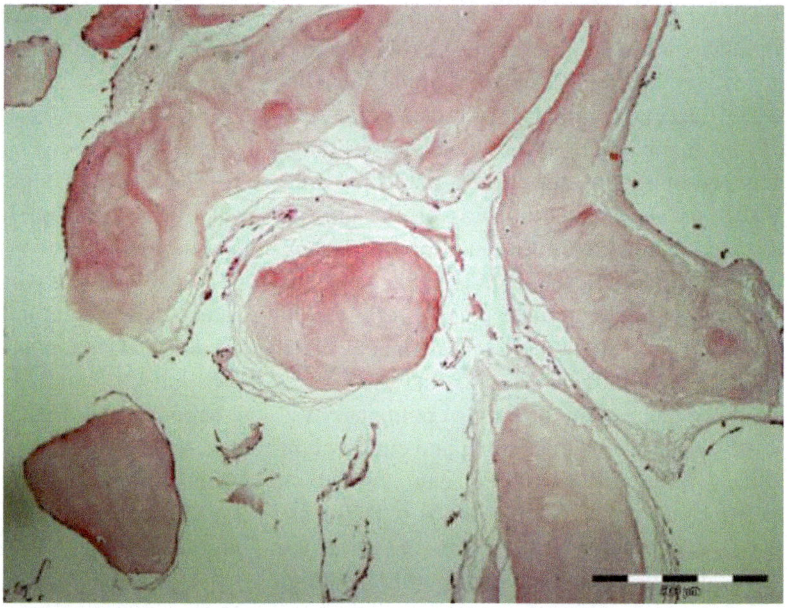

Fig. 4.16 Nonbacterial polypoid fibrous tricuspid valve endocarditis in a drug-related death (H&E ×200)

Based on the hypothesis that cocaine may lead to coronary spasms, it was postulated that myocardial infarction following exposure to cocaine can also be found in freely permeable and only slightly changed arteriosclerotic coronary arteries (Cregler and Mark 1985). Cocaine-induced myocardial damage leads to enhanced expression of myocardial infarction markers (Hollander et al. 1998). Parallel to this, there are isolated reports of methamphetamine-induced cardiomyopathy (Karch 2011). High case numbers have not been published to date, and individual studies tend to suggest a more rapid progression of coronary arteriosclerosis as a result of amphetamine or methamphetamine use (Karch 2009).

4.2.3 Endocarditis

Acute bacterial and nonbacterial endocarditis has become less frequent in intravenous drug-related deaths, one reason certainly being the increased purity of street heroin; however, they do still occur (Conway 1969; Dressler and Roberts 1989; Passarino et al. 2005; Hejna et al. 2014; Lapkus and Prahlow 2015). While in general the left ventricular heart valves, mitral valve, and aortic valve are most frequently affected, endocarditis in intravenous drug addicts occurs most frequently in the tricuspid valve (Fig. 4.16). The agents are for the most part *Streptococci* and *Staphylococcus aureus*, but in individual cases, a large number of agents are found (Mah and Shafran 1990). The probable supporting factor for endocarditis is drug-induced, discrete, and possibly temporary damage to the valve tissue (Karch 2009). In the acute phase, growths may be seen on the heart valve with thrombocytes toward the surface and more fibrin in the deep layers, while near the surface embedded accumulations of basophilic cocci in the form of bacterial colonies can be seen. The valve tissue is consistently edematous, while at the level of the growth, the endothelium has possibly undergone ulcerous destruction. Toward the base, subacute forms already show signs of cellular organization with sprouting, endothelially coated capillary blood vessels in the valve stroma, which is not usually vascularized.

Therefore, in the absence of an acute process, the detection of capillaries in the valve stroma is a clear indication of previous endocarditis. Post-inflammatory fibrous and hyalinized areas may calcify in the course of time (basophilic calcium salt deposits). The infection can heal with valve disorders, while the bacterial colonies can disappear after antibiotic treatment and may also calcify fibrously. Endocarditis can be the origin of lethal arterial and possibly infected embolisms; the heart, brain, kidneys, and spleen are frequently affected. In the case of infected microemboli, septicopyemic (micro-) abscesses can be detected and clinical sepsis exists. In individual cases, a Schönlein–Henoch purpura is described following staphylococci-induced endocarditis (Montoliu et al. 1987). If no infection of the damaged valve stroma occurs, nonbacterial polypoid endocarditis may result.

4.3 Drug-Associated Nephropathies

Regular intravenous consumption of drugs may lead to a wide range of histopathological findings in the kidneys (Eknoyan et al. 1973; Friedman et al. 1974; Kiloyne et al. 1972; Perazella 2005), including reversible drug-induced uremia (Friedman and Rao 1995; McGinn et al. 1970). The term used in the literature for such kidney disease is "heroin-associated nephropathy" (HAN), although it is generally other drugs and accompanying substances rather than the heroin itself which may lead to the damage of kidney tissue (Cunningham et al. 1980, 1983). However, intravenous drug consumption is an important factor in kidney failure (end-stage renal disease, ESRD) with subsequent dialysis treatment (Louria et al. 1967). Investigations of renal biopsies showed that histopathological findings can also be established in the case of asymptomatic drug consumers (Arruda et al. 1975; McGinn et al. 1974; Sameiro Faria et al. 2003; Zielezny et al. 1980). The spectrum of heroin-associated kidney diseases includes primarily acute kidney failure, glomerulopathies, such as focal segmental glomerulosclerosis (FSGS), and membranoproliferative glomerulonephritis (MPGN), frequently associated with chronic hepatitis B and C and less often with immune complex glomerulonephritis as a result of bacterial endocarditis or sepsis (Hill 1986). In addition, interstitial nephritis can be seen in various forms, while cases with renal amyloidosis in connection with "skin popping" are less frequently reported, and heroin-associated granulomatous nephritis is very rarely reported. At the same time, kidney lesions can occur in HIV-positive drug addicts; hence, their classification is HIV-associated nephropathies (HIVAN). Rarely and mainly in the case of cocaine consumption, renal infarctions can occur.

In the case of intravenous drug addicts, clinical symptoms vary from minimal abnormalities in the urine sediment with normal renal function to nephrotic syndrome with acute kidney failure, which can develop rapidly in some cases. Although the underlying morphological lesions are inconsistent, the following should be considered:

- Renal amyloidosis (Meador et al. 1979; Menchel et al. 1983; Neugarten et al. 1986; Scholer et al. 1979)
- Acute kidney failure in the case of drug-induced rhabdomyolysis (Blanco Garcia et al. 1999; Deighan et al. 2000; Welte et al. 2004)
- Granulomatous interstitial nephritis (rare; (McAllister et al. 1979)) or granulomatous glomerulonephritis following, for example, oxycodone (rare; Segal et al. 1998)
- Various glomerulopathies (Bakir et al. 1989; Grishman et al. 1976; Llach et al. 1979; Matalon et al. 1974; May et al. 1986; Salomon et al. 1972)

Various glomerular diseases have been described in relation to intravenous drug consumption, which can lead to chronic kidney failure within a few years following diagnosis. This is explained by the direct toxic effect of the injected drugs and/or accompanying substances (adulterants) (Cunningham et al. 1984; Hamilton et al. 2000). In addition, immunological processes play an important role in infections, particularly hepatitis forms B and C, as well as HIV infections (Freeman et al. 1974; Montoliu et al. 1987; Neugarten and Baldwin 1984; Shah et al. 1977). The infections mentioned above, however, can also lead to glomerulopathies unconnected to chronic intravenous drug consumption, as many studies have shown (Carbone et al. 1989;

Genderini et al. 1990; Johnson and Couser 1990; Johnson et al. 1993; Rollina et al. 1991; Romas et al. 1994; Rostoker et al. 1996; Soni et al. 1989; Sreepada Rao 1993; Sreepada Rao et al. 1984; Sreepada Rao and Friedman 1989; Stone and Appel 1994). In this context, immunological processes lead to glomerulopathies, the origin of which has still not been explained diagnostically (Brown et al. 1974); antigen–antibody reactions to bacteria, viruses, drugs, and/or accompanying substances are discussed.

4.3.1 Glomerulonephritis and Glomerulosclerosis

Proteinuric and nephrotic syndromes in intravenous heroin consumers were first described in the early 1970s. Minimal glomerular findings could be detected, in particular focal membranoproliferative glomerulonephritis (MPGN) accompanied by PAS-positive deposits in the glomerular loops and focal spreading of the glomerular basal membranes (Eknoyan et al. 1973; Erbersdobler et al. 1995; McGinn et al. 1970). Later studies using immunohistochemical techniques were able to detect increased levels of leukocytes and immunoglobulin (IgM) deposits in some deceased intravenous drug addicts, as well as complement factors in the glomeruli (Dettmeyer et al. 1998). There is no correlation between inflammatory activity and glomerular IgM deposits (Dettmeyer et al. 2001). This is in line with the observation that higher IgM concentrations in the serum of intravenous drug addicts decrease in the case of oral substitution with methadone. Normal IgM levels could be found in drug users inhaling heroin and cocaine (Bakir and Dunea 1996).

Focal Segmental Glomerulosclerosis (FSGS) Reports from the USA mention focal segmental glomerulosclerosis (FSGS) in African-American drug consumers with nephrotic syndrome who, to a large extent, were not intravenous consumers (Bakir and Dunea 1996; Friedman and Sreepada Rao 1983; May et al. 1986). FSGS showed deposits of IgM and complement C3 in the mesangium, damage to the epithelial podocytes, renal tubular atrophy, and interstitial fibrosis (Bakir et al. 1989; Sreepada Rao et al. 1974). African-American drug consumers with nephrotic syndrome showed more pronounced proteinuria, glomerulosclerosis (Fig. 4.17), and interstitial fibrosis compared to those drug addicts who consumed intravenously (Bakir et al. 1989). Thus, a genetic disposition is assumed here, as

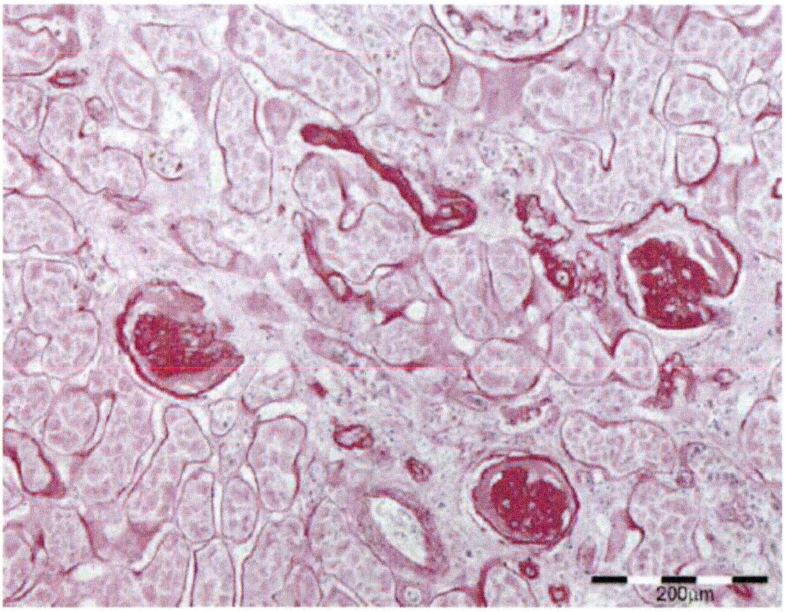

Fig. 4.17 Focal segmental glomerulosclerosis (FSGS) in a 28-year-old man who died after many years of intravenous drug abuse (PAS ×200)

has been shown in investigations into HLA association in heroin-associated nephropathy (Haskell et al. 1988).

Investigations by Singhal et al. (1992) indicate that the mesangial cells in the glomeruli are not able to metabolize heroin into morphine; morphine, however, can cause a widening of the mesangial matrix. A stimulation of mesangial cell proliferation due to morphine, an intensification of collagen synthesis, proline, and laminin, as well as an increase in immune complex deposits in the mesangium are suspected (Kapasi et al. 2000; Pan and Singhal 1994; Patel et al. 2003; Sagar et al. 1994; Singhal et al. 1992, 1997, 1998). Parallel damage to not only the mesangial but also the glomerular cells is assumed (Singhal et al. 1992).

Membranoproliferative Glomerulonephritis (MPGN) Type I In Europe, lymphomonocytic membranoproliferative glomerulonephritis (MPGN) type I is predominant in connection with heroin-associated nephropathy (HAN) (Erbersdobler et al. 1995). This MPGN can exist over a long period of time with no functional deficits. The quantification of immunohistochemically displayed leukocytes in the glomeruli can also show mild forms without being clinically regarded as a disease (Fig. 4.18). Empirical research indicates that more than three leukocytes per glomerulus as an average of 20 glomeruli counted can already mean increased cellular infiltration (Dettmeyer et al. 1998). Even without FSGS, deposits of PAS-positive immune complexes can be detected immunohistochemically (Fig. 4.19): IgM, IgG, C1q, and C4 complements could be found as deposits in the mesangium and in glomerular capillary walls (Fig. 4.20) (Dettmeyer et al. 2001). It is not clear, however, whether the detected immune complexes should be regarded as a reaction to the intravenous consumption of drugs and accompanying substances or whether they represent an immune reaction to hepatitis infection (Dettmeyer et al. 2001; Gonzalo et al. 1993; Horikoshi et al. 1993; Johnson et al. 1993; Kopfler and Paronetto 1965; Romas et al. 1994).

Renal Amyloidosis in Intravenous Drug Abuse Renal amyloidosis is rarely detected in long-term intravenous drug addicts. Using conventional histology, congo-red-positive amyloid deposits in the glomeruli, renal tubular atrophy, and amyloid deposits in renal tubular basal membranes can be seen. Peripheral arterial branches are frequently affected, while the renal interstitium can show focal fibrosis as well as focally inflammatory infiltrates. The amyloid deposits degrade only very slowly, if at all (Hill

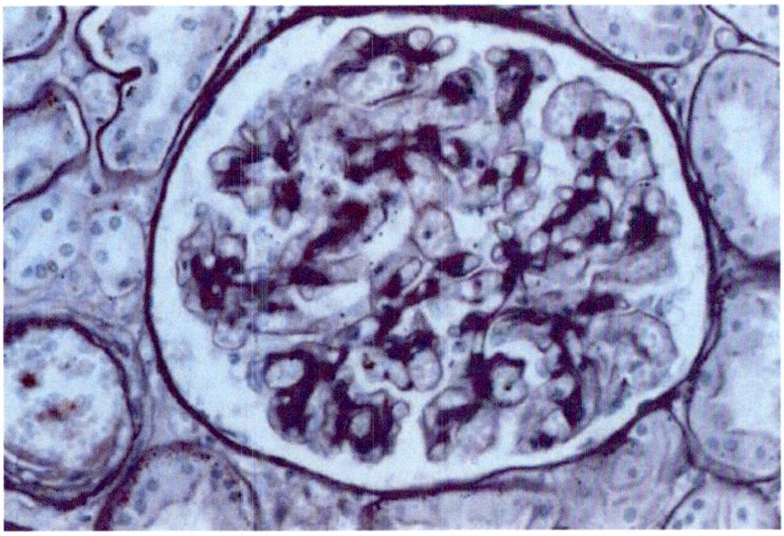

Fig. 4.18 Widespread PAS-positive deposits in the glomerular loops in heroin-associated nephropathy (PAS ×400)

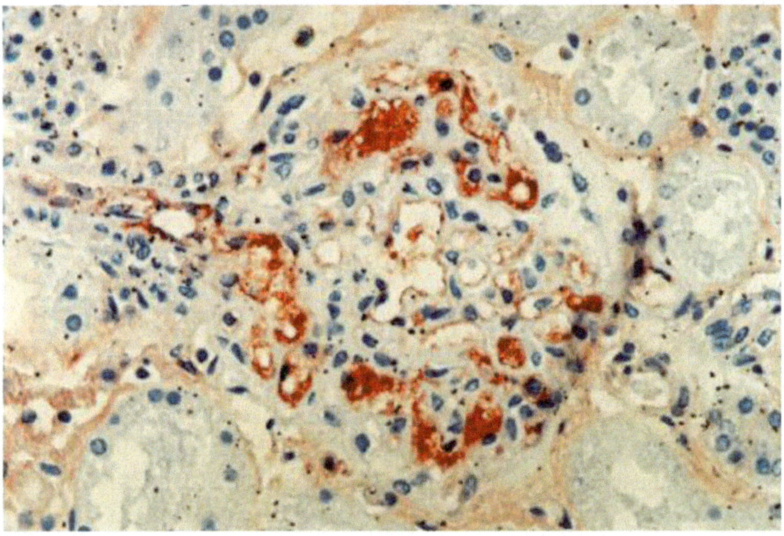

Fig. 4.19 Immunohistochemical IgM deposits in the glomeruli in heroin-associated nephropathy (×400)

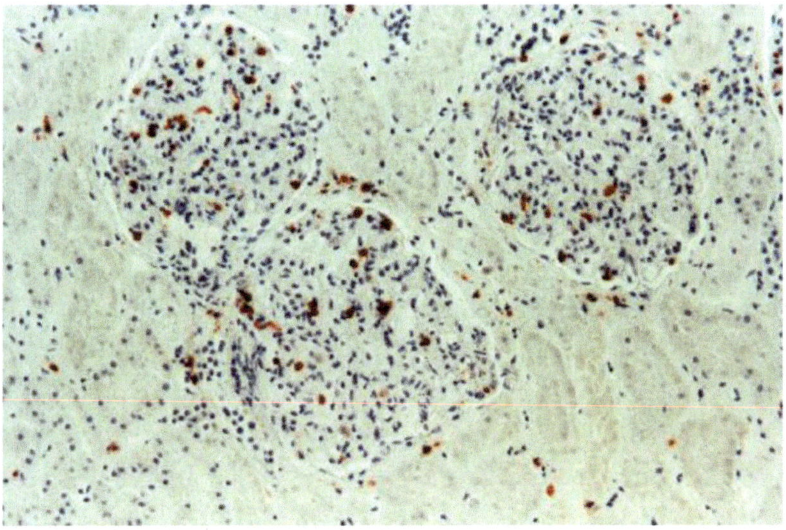

Fig. 4.20 Increased cellular infiltration of the glomeruli in heroin-associated nephropathy and MPGN; immunohistochemical representation of the leukocytes with leukocyte common antigen (LCA ×125)

1986). Chronic stimulation of the immune system due to regular drug injection is assumed to be the cause, possibly in conjunction with concomitant infection. Drug addicts with renal amyloidosis are, as a rule, relatively old, with a history of long-term drug abuse and cutaneous lesions, e.g., so-called syringe abscesses in the case of subcutaneous heroin injections ("skin popping") (Hill 1986). Amyloid deposits can almost always be found also in other organs, although in various forms.

Rhabdomyolysis Acute myoglobinuria was described for the first time in 1971 in a drug addict (Richter et al. 1971). It is meanwhile well-known that rhabdomyolysis not only occurs after heroin consumption but also promptly on absorption of other drugs, such as amphetamine (Kubat 2013; Ishigami et al. 2003; Scandting and Spital 1988), and in association with a compartment syndrome or muscle necrosis after drug abuse (Blanco Garcia et al. 1999; Deighan et al. 2000; Oehler et al. 2002). The prevalence of rhabdomyolysis in

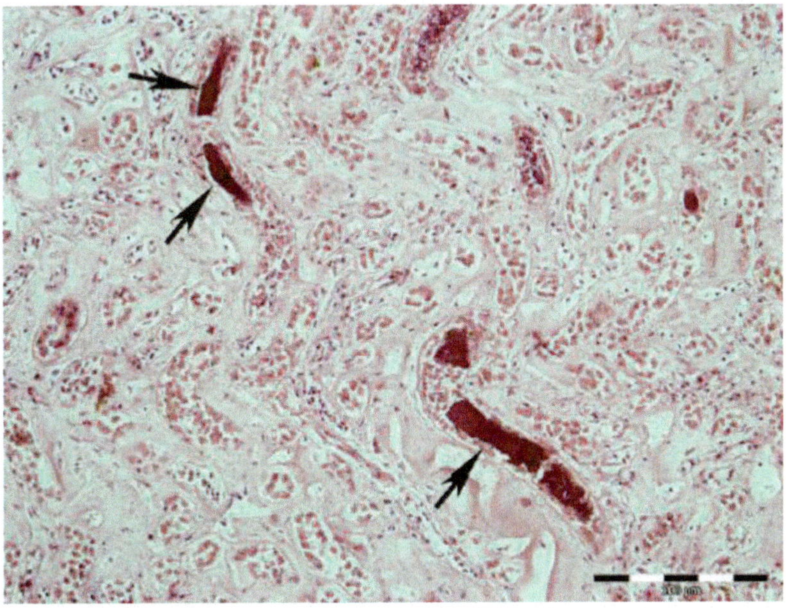

Fig. 4.21 Protein cylinders in the renal tubules after intravenous drug consumption and in the presence of clinically diagnosed rhabdomyolysis (H&E ×200)

drug-related deaths has been investigated (Kock and Simonsen 1994). In an immunohistochemical investigation, Welte et al. (2004) could show myoglobin deposits in renal tubules in comparison with a control group. A heroin overdose may result in myoglobin kidney failure (Rice et al. 2000). Even in H&E staining, protein cylinders can be proven in the renal tubules (Fig. 4.21), the character of which can be classified by means of immunohistochemical staining for myoglobin (Welte et al. 2004).

HAN and Hepatitis B and C Drug addicts often have hepatitis B or C (Blanck et al. 1979; Cunningham et al. 1980, 1983; Doutrelepont et al. 1993; Dubrow et al. 1985; Friedman et al. 1974; Gonzalo et al. 1993). However, viral hepatitis can also lead to morphological and functional damage to the kidneys, independent of drug consumption, in the case of both acute and chronic hepatitis with acute interstitial nephritis (Eknoyan et al. 1972; Ramirez et al. 1983). Both types of hepatitis infection can likewise be accompanied by focal widening of the glomerular basal membranes; an association with membranous glomerulonephritis is also described. Meanwhile, HBs, HBe, and HBc antigens have been observed in subepithelial deposits of the mesangium, while IgM sediments associated with hepatitis B or hepatitis C have also been found. The earliest report on an association between hepatitis C infection and membranous proliferative glomerulonephritis dates back to 1993 (Johnson et al. 1993); cryoglobulinemic MPGN and chronic infection with hepatitis C were described later (Rostoker et al. 1996).

HIV-Associated Nephropathy (HIVAN) Since the early 1990s, there have been few reports on heroin-associated nephropathy possibly because the quality or purity of street heroin has improved. Since that time, there have been studies on HIV-associated nephropathy (HIVAN); one reason undoubtedly being that the number of HIV-related deaths among drug addicts has increased intermittently (Busch et al. 1994; Casanova et al. 1995; Friedman and Rao 1995; Sreepada Rao et al. 1987). In the case of HIVAN, focal and segmental glomeruloscleroses, tubular necroses, even microcystic, tubulogenetic renal cortex cysts, inflammatory processes, and interstitial edema can be observed. These findings could not only be seen in HIV-positive drug addicts but also in HIV-positive homosexual men who did not take drugs (Cohen and Nast 1988). The glomerular findings of HIVAN,

Table 4.1 Drug additives used in intravenous drug injection, some of which cause embolic spread to the lungs (according to Lapachinske et al. (2015), Pawlik et al. (2015), Karch (2009), Dettmeyer et al. (2005), Pernegger et al. (2001), Hamilton et al. (2000), Cunningham et al. (1984))

Substance	Substance	Substance
Quinine	Mannitol	Lactose
Procaine	Caffeine	Inositol
Lidocaine	Starches	Methapyrilene
Sucrose	Acetyl procaine	Dextrose
Scopolamine	Sucrose	Tetracaine
Ephedrine	Phenylpropanolamine	Phentermine
Acetaminophen	Aminopyrine	Ascorbic acid
Aspirin	Boric acid	Diphenhydramine
Fentanyl	Niacinamide	Levamisole

however, should partly be differentiated from HAN (Chander et al. 1987; D'Agati et al. 1989). In the case of HIVAN in particular, immune complex glomerulonephritis has been described with a membranous proliferative and diffuse endocapillary component, as well as immunohistochemical evidence of IgA deposits (Sreepada Rao et al. 1987).

Designer Drugs and Drug Additives Both designer drugs and additives to intravenous injections are said to increase the risk of kidney failure (Cunningham et al. 1984; Pernegger et al. 2001). Up to 97% of an injection is said to consist of various additives including, among others, mannitol, lactose, dextrose, and scopolamine (Hamilton et al. 2000) (Table 4.1). The relevance of these additives for kidney failures has apparently decreased due to the increasing level of street heroin (Friedman and Rao 1995). Although renal histopathological findings in drug addicts can be described and classified, their exact genesis remains unclear.

4.4 Hepatic Histopathological Findings

With the exception of rare foreign-body-reactive granulomas in the liver, which may be suspicious for intravenous drug abuse, hepatitis B or C in particular are seen in drug-related deaths; after many years of drug abuse peliosis hepatis may also be seen. Macrophages with brown-pigmented, Fe-negative cytoplasm visualized in the hepatic portal fields can also be interpreted as a sign of long-term intravenous drug use (Fig. 4.22).

4.4.1 Hepatitis

In the liver, few findings taken in isolation indicate intravenous drug consumption, such as foreign-body granuloma, comparable with granulomas seen in the case of "junkie pneumopathy" or an increased number of macrophages with granular cytoplasm. However, previously serologically diagnosed hepatitis of varying intensities is frequently seen with: low activity and only light to moderate lymphomonocytic infiltration of the portal fields, dense inflammatory infiltration of the portal fields, and single hepatocellular necroses in the immediately adjacent liver tissue (Fig. 4.23). Isolated necrosis can be displayed well cytochemically using the orcein staining method (Bartok et al. 1976). In order to evaluate the inflammatory intensity of hepatitis C, a histological "liver cell damage index" has been proposed (Servais and Schiwy-Bochat 1998); Table 4.2): lymphoid infiltrates with florid germinal centers in the portal fields, which should be detectable in 50–84% of all hepatitis C cases, are not taken into consideration. Instead, attempts are made to record the damage of the liver parenchyma using histomorphological criteria, the characteristics of which are graduated and the diagnostic significance of which is evaluated: fatty liver, focal degeneration of the cytoplasm, single and zonal necroses, moth-eaten necrosis, and bridge necrosis. Another histological activity index also includes

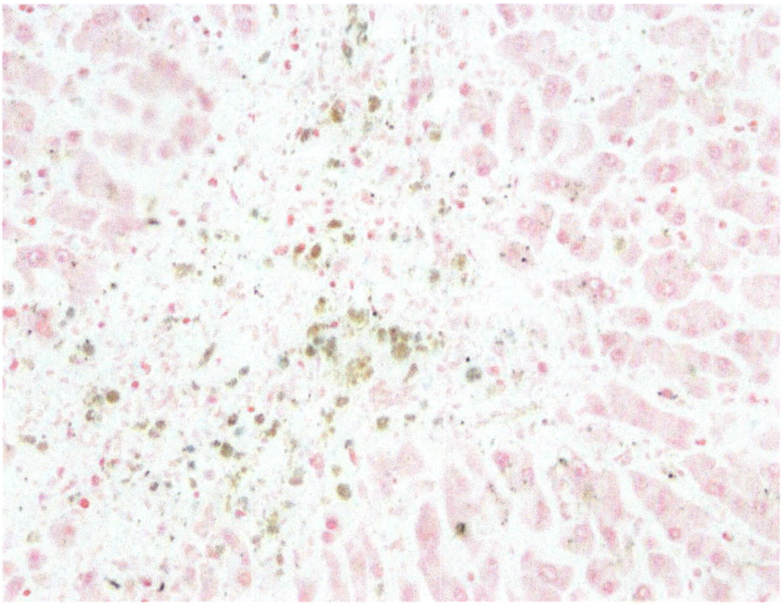

Fig. 4.22 Abundant pigmented, Fe-negative macrophages in the hepatic portal fields following long-term intravenous drug use (Prussian blue ×200)

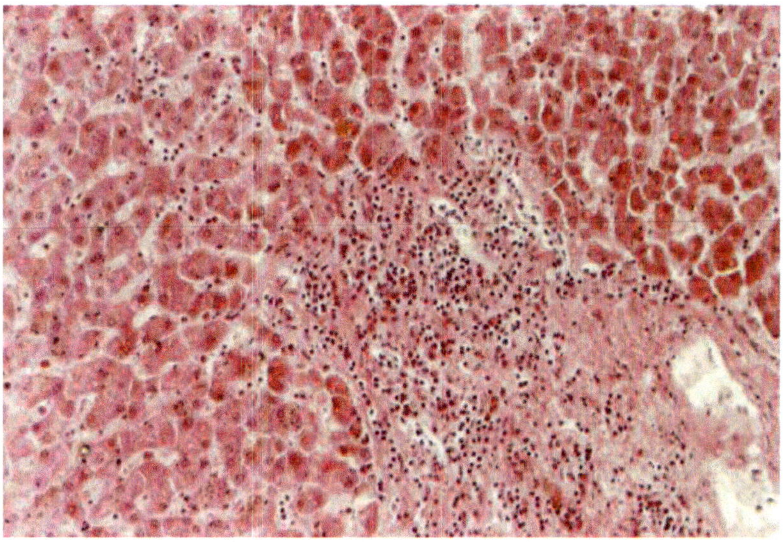

Fig. 4.23 Chronic hepatitis with spread of portal inflammatory cells to adjacent hepatocytes (H&E ×100)

Table 4.2 Index to classify the extent of current liver cell damage in the case of chronic hepatitis C (Servais and Schiwy-Bochat 1998)

Liver cell damage	Extent	Significance
Reversible damage		
Fatty liver	0–3	x 1
Focal degeneration of the cytoplasm	0–3	x 1
Irreversible damage		
Single necrosis	0–3	x 2
Zonal necrosis	0–3	x 2
Moth-eaten necrosis	0–3	x 2
Bridge necrosis	0–3	x 3
Total = index		

the irreversible long-term damage of chronic hepatitis C (fibrosis and cirrhosis) but, for this reason, classifies acute inflammatory activity less precisely (Dries et al. 2001; Knodell et al. 1981).

In some cases, it is possible to detect progressive and active hepatitis B with hepatitis B antigen, which can be identified immunohistochemically in numerous hepatocytes (Fig. 4.24). Otherwise, different conventional stains can be helpful including orcein staining (Bogomeletz 1976; Borchard and Gussmann 1979).

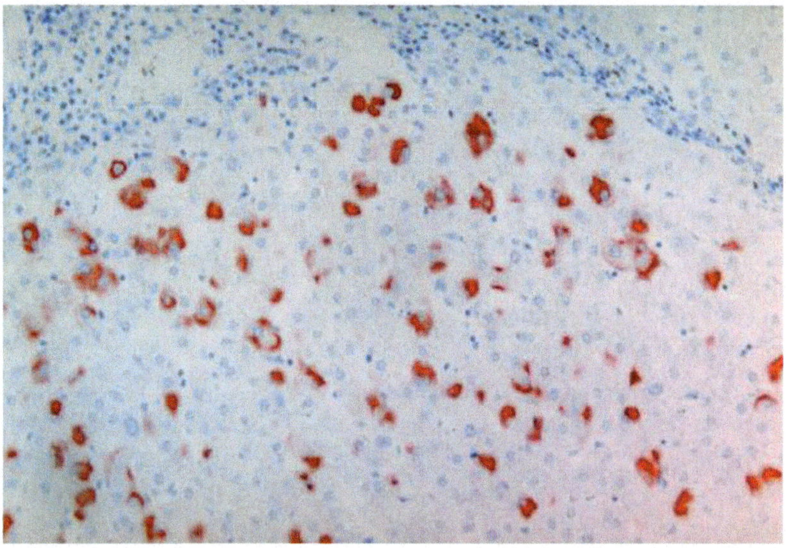

Fig. 4.24 Immunohistochemical identification of HBs antigen in numerous hepatocytes in the case of acute hepatitis B in a 30-year-old man who died of drug abuse (×200)

In the case of chronic hepatitis B, one can see only individual immunohistochemical hepatitis B-positive cells in the portal fields. An immunohistochemically negative result with markers against hepatitis B antigen is, in the case of hepatitis diagnosed using conventional histology in a drug-related death, an indication of hepatitis C; this is also easily verified serologically postmortem. Immunohistochemically, mainly CD45R0-positive T-lymphocytes infiltrate the portal fields of the liver in the case of a chronic hepatitis (Fig. 4.25).

While, in general, patients suffering from hepatitis seldom have an accompanying fatty liver, this is, based on personal experience, not unusual in the case of intravenous drug consumption due to a frequently occurring polytoxicomania and additional alcohol consumption.

4.4.2 Peliosis Hepatis

The literature indicates that peliosis hepatis, i.e., lake-like dilation of liver sinusoids with flattened hepatocyte trabeculae (Fig. 4.26), can also occur after many years of drug consumption (Tsokos and Erbersdobler 2005). Corresponding lesions in the liver may develop more often than assumed since attention is rarely focused on peliosis hepatis during drug death autopsies.

4.4.3 Amphetamine-Induced Liver Cell Necroses

In rare cases, the ingestion of amphetamines can have a hepatotoxic effect. Nonreactive hepatocellular single-cell necrosis, which is not accompanied by an inflammatory reaction at least in the acute phase, is particularly evident (Fig. 4.27). There appears to be a growing number of reports on the increased use of methamphetamine and the associated rise in the number of fatalities due to this drug (Trauer et al. 2015).

4.4.4 Ecstasy (MDMA)-Induced Malignant Hyperthermia and Rhabdomyolysis

Cardiac fatalities following 3,4-methylenedioxy methamphetamine (MDMA, ecstasy) use have been described, typically depending on the measured MDMA level at the time of death (Cerretani

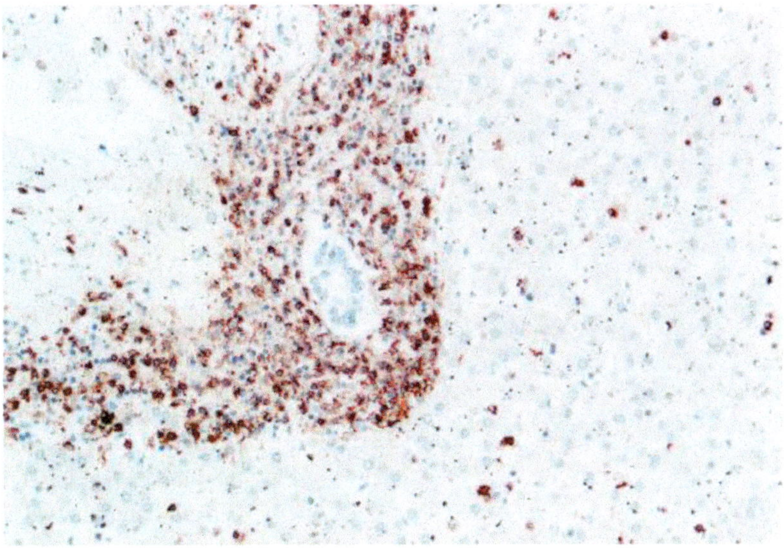

Fig. 4.25 Dense infiltration with CD45R0-positive T-lymphocytes in the portal fields of the liver in the case of chronic hepatitis B in a drug-related death (×200)

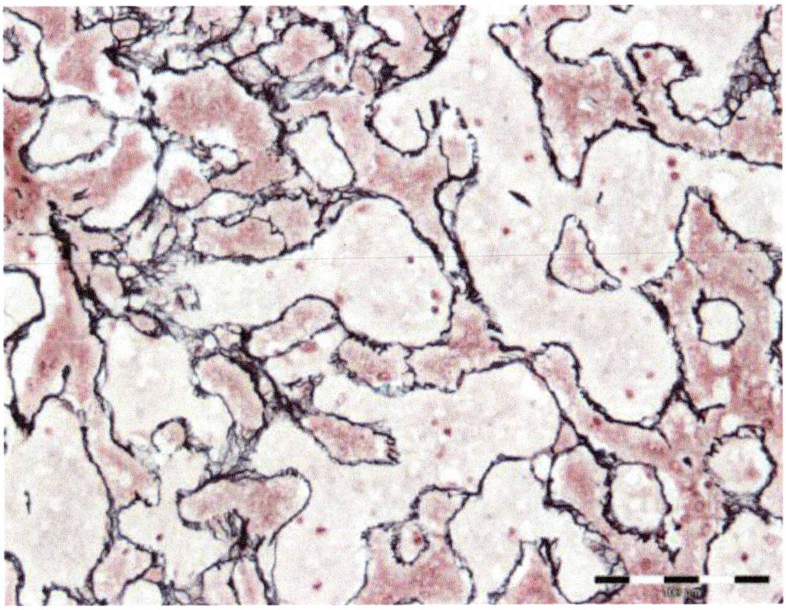

Fig. 4.26 Peliosis hepatis with small hepatocyte trabeculae after many years of drug abuse (Gomori ×400)

et al. 2008; Fineschi et al. 1999). In addition, MDMA use by genetically predisposed individuals can result in malignant hyperthermia accompanied by, e.g., rhabdomyolysis, liver cell necrosis, possible concomitant myocardial damage, and histological signs of increased functional thyroid activity (Lang et al. 2016; Gill et al. 2002; Screaton et al. 1992; Henry et al. 1992;). The literature describes amphetamine- and methamphetamine-related autopsy findings which, in the case of prolonged use, point to a cardiotoxic effect and an increased risk for coronary sclerosis (Karch 2009) or an increased risk for a toxic leukoencephalopathy (Mu et al. 2017). In the case of rhabdomyolysis, ubiquitous fresh necrotic foci in the smooth muscle skeletal muscles may be detected histologically, alongside marked eosinophilia, loss of cross-striation, and granular disintegration of muscle fibers (Fig. 4.28). Structural proteins of the muscular cytoskeleton (e.g., myo-

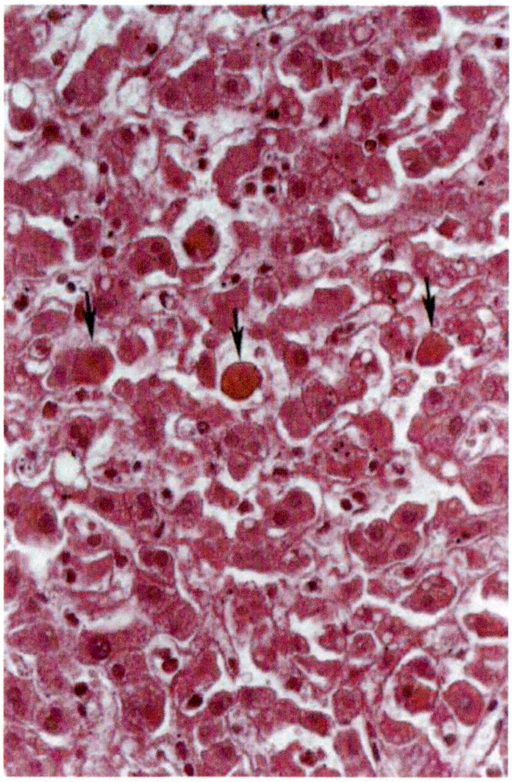

Fig. 4.27 Amphetamine-induced hepatocellular single-cell necrosis (*arrows*) without inflammatory reaction in the acute phase (H&E ×200)

globin, desmin) are expressed and flushed out. Depending on survival time, myoglobinuric kidney failure may develop, with immunohistochemically detected myoglobin in the renal tubules and a correspondingly visualizable loss of, e.g., myoglobin and desmin in the skeletal muscle fiber cytoplasm (Fig. 4.29a, b). Parallel to this, individual and group hepatocytic necrosis is seen in liver tissue, accompanied by loss of stainability of nuclei (Fig. 4.30). Depending on survival time, myocardial damage can exhibit less equivocal findings, e.g., isolated empty sarcolemma tubes (Fig. 4.31). At the same time, clinical laboratory tests reveal extremely elevated liver enzymes in the blood, particularly transaminases. Fulminant hepatic failure may develop in the further course, which can only be treated by liver transplant (Garbino et al. 2001). According to witness accounts, ecstasy-induced malignant hyperthermia is associated with uncontrollable muscle contractions, convulsions, confusion, and a sensation of heat. In some cases, behavior resembles that of drug-induced psychosis, and convulsion- and fall-related hematomas are seen in the setting of an apparent concomitant decrease in blood coagulability. Simultaneously, there is evidence of

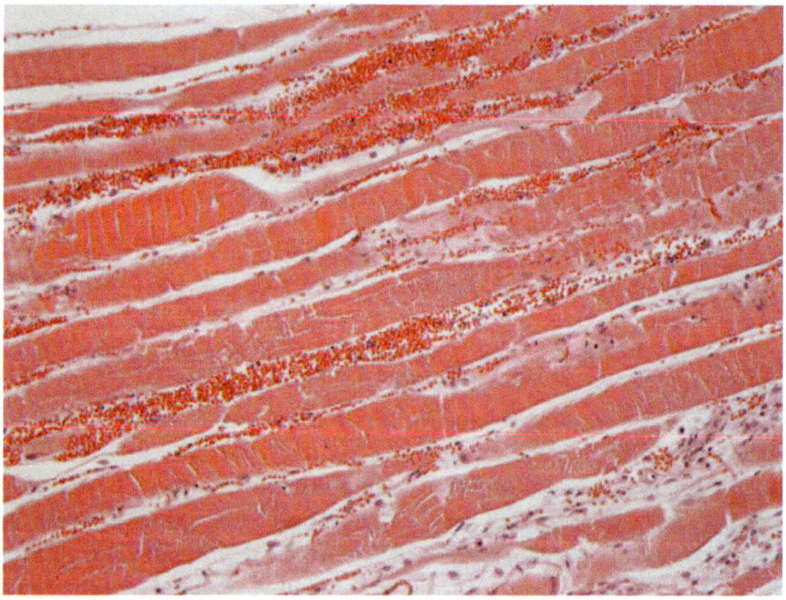

Fig. 4.28 MDMA (ecstasy)-induced rhabdomyolysis with ubiquitous breakdown of smooth muscle skeletal muscle fiber and accompanying hemorrhage (H&E ×100)

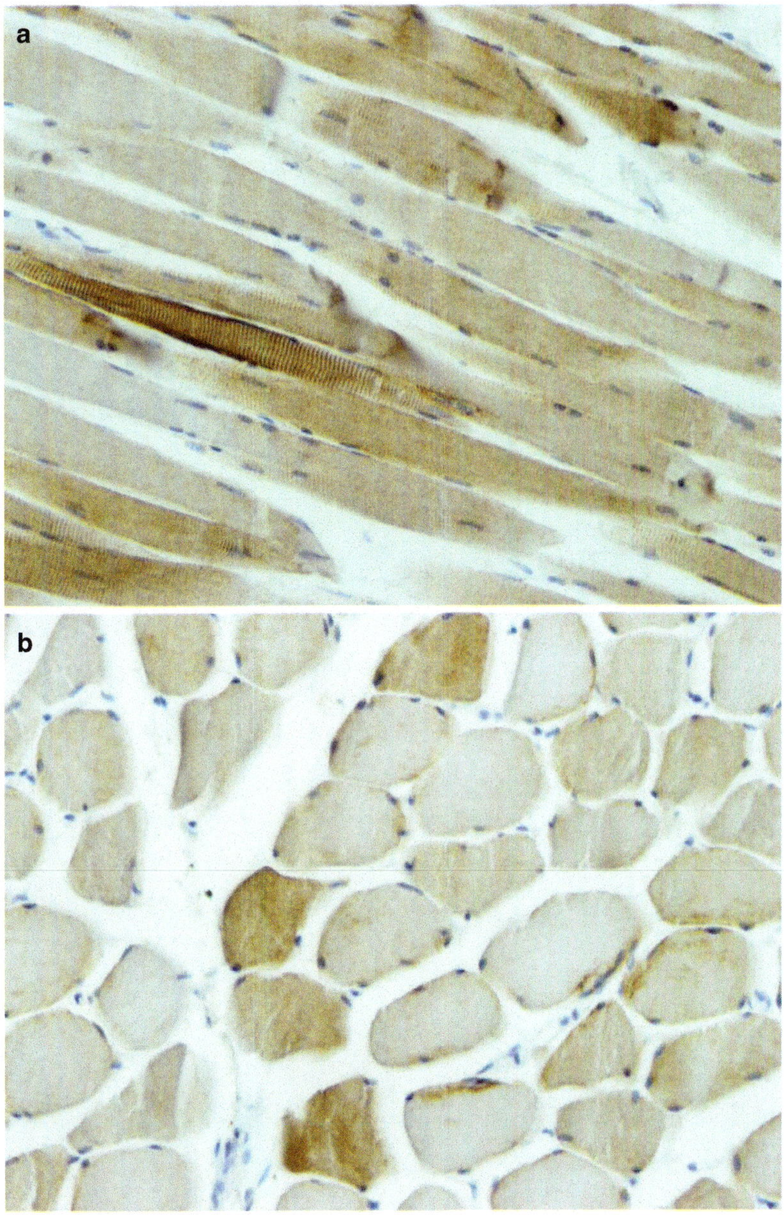

Fig. 4.29 (**a, b**) Immunohistochemically pronounced diffuse loss of desmin in skeletal muscle fibers in MDMA (ecstasy)-induced rhabdomyolysis (longitudinal view ×100; cross-sectional view ×200)

increased blood–brain barrier permeability in methamphetamine intoxication (Wang et al. 2014).

According to current knowledge, a genetic modification in the ryanodine receptor is believed to cause a predisposition to malignant hyperthermia (Li et al. 2017; Phillips et al. 1994). Besides MDMA, a number of volatile substances used in anesthesia, as well as muscle relaxants, come into question (Ellis et al. 1990). Therefore, malignant hyperthermia is a feared complication in anesthesia. The treatment of choice consists of administering Dantrolen®, a muscle relaxant, combined with steps to lower body temperature (which can rise to >43 °C): external cooling, administration of cold saline solution, and gastric

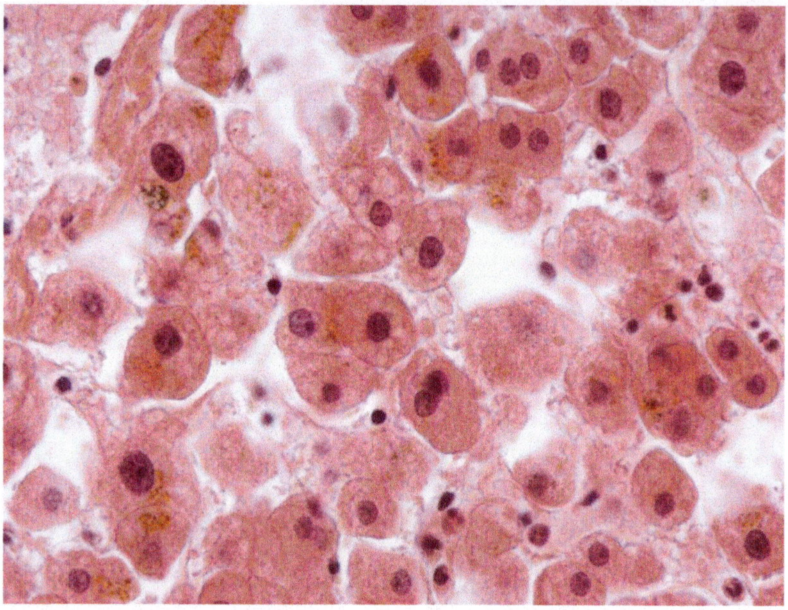

Fig. 4.30 Extensive MDMA (ecstasy)-induced liver cell necrosis with dissolution of cell nuclei and loss of stainability (H&E ×400)

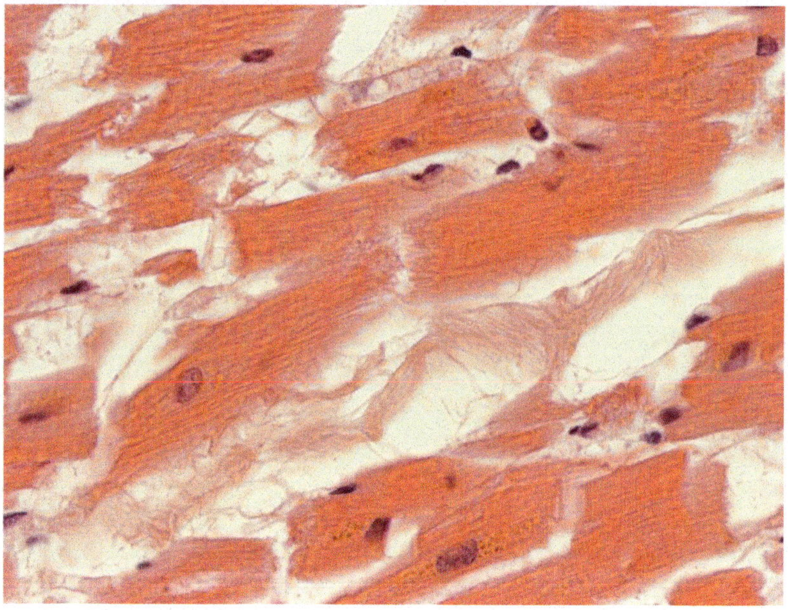

Fig. 4.31 The myocardium in malignant hyperthermia and rhabdomyolysis with isolated empty sarcolemma tubes (H&E ×400)

lavage with cold fluids (Dar and McBrien 1996; Tehan 1993; Larner 1993; Campkin and Davies 1993). Even in the case of optimal treatment, the mortality rate currently remains at around 5%. Hair analytical evidence of regular MDMA use in the case of malignant hyperthermia only after using high concentrations of MDMA indicates that there is clearly an MDMA threshold in individual cases that needs to be exceeded in order for malignant hyperthermia to develop (Lang et al. 2016).

4.4.5 Heroin-Related Rhabdomyolysis

Acute localized rhabdomyolysis is one of the rarer and lesser known complications of heroin intoxication (Oehler et al. 2002). Lower limb muscles, for example, can be – and apparently are more frequently – affected uni- or bilaterally (Rabl and Markwalder 1996). Extensive muscle necrosis may be clinically striking in the form of compartment syndrome and results in myoglobinuric kidney failure (Kathrein et al. 1983). However, the cause of muscle necrosis in heroin users – in contrast to MDMA use – is not necessarily considered to be a systemic effect of the heroin but rather local compression of, e.g., the supplying blood vessels and/or muscles, for instance, during a prolonged comatose state. Having said that, there is debate as to whether opioids have a direct toxic effect in the pathogenesis of rhabdomyolysis (Prendergast and George 1993; de Delcker et al. 1992; de Gans et al. 1985). Abundant protein conglomerates found in the renal tubules are considered a morphological equivalent of myoglobulinuric kidney and are already visible on conventional hemalaun-eosin staining (Fig. 4.32; see also Fig. 4.21). Immunohistochemically, this is myoglobulin (Fig. 4.33), which is found more frequently in the renal tubules in methamphetamine abusers (Ishigami et al. 2003). In the case of longer survival times, significantly more advanced rhabdomyolysis is seen histologically,

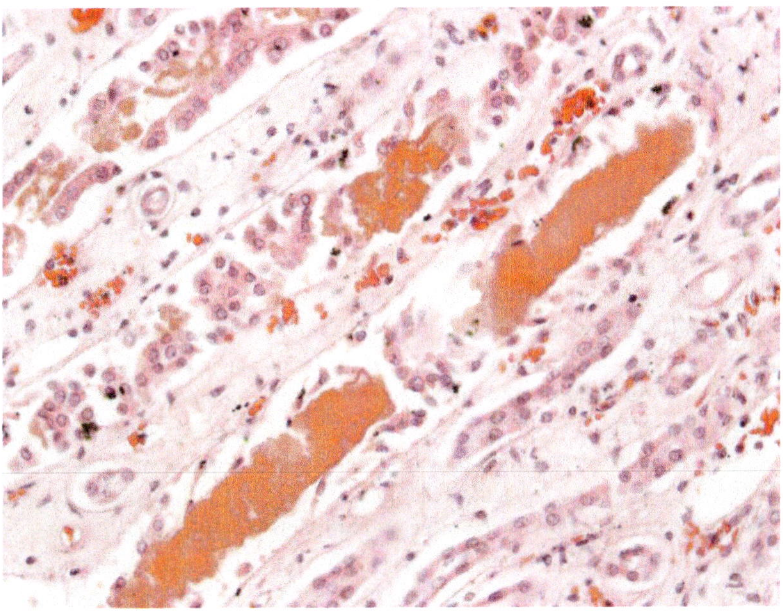

Fig. 4.32 Compact-appearing protein cylinders in the renal tubules in a case of myoglobinuric kidney failure in a heroin user (H&E ×200)

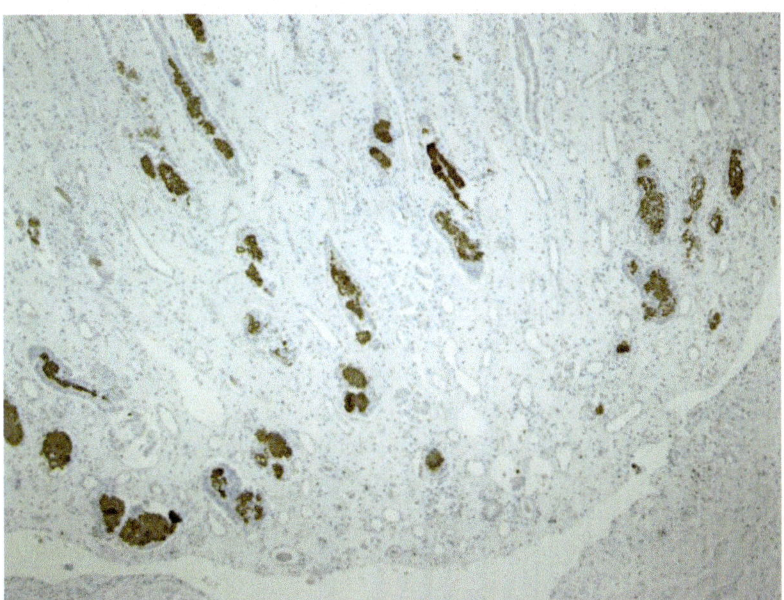

Fig. 4.33 Heroin-related rhabdomyolysis and myoglobinuric kidney failure: abundant myoglobin cylinders in the renal tubule lumina seen immunohistochemically (anti-myoglobin ×100)

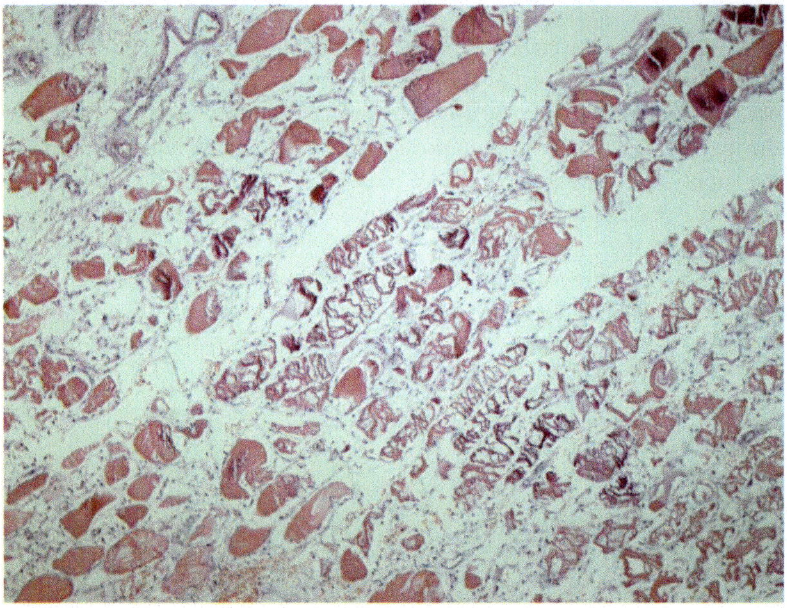

Fig. 4.34 Advanced rhabdomyolysis with empty skeletal muscle fibers and only coarsely preserved muscle cell remnants (H&E ×40)

with granular disintegration of the muscle fibers (Fig. 4.34). Myoglobinuric kidney failure develops parallel to this. Also in the case of a long-term comatose state due to drug abuse, fresh suppurative bronchopneumonia manifests after only a few hours.

The literature also reports on rhabdomyolysis following significant physical exertion and exsiccosis (in some cases under the effects of amphetamines or ecstasy), intensive sport activities (body building), or the administration of medication, e.g., isotretinoin, or due to torture by reverse hanging (Pollanen 2016; Cordner 2016).

4.4.6 Intravenous Injection of Methadone

The treatment of heroin addicts by means of a methadone substitution program is regulated strictly by law. Methadone has to be distributed in a prescription not suitable for parenteral application. Nevertheless, there are reports on intravenous usage of the oral preparation among drug addicts. In order to avoid this, additives are used, often a soluble colorant with yellow quinoline. In cases of intravenous application of this methadone, yellow pigments can be found in the liver (Fig. 4.35).

4.4.7 Rachacha Consumption

"Rachacha" is a homemade black paste produced using a decoction of poppy heads (*Papaver somniferum*). The paste, which contains various opium alkaloids (morphine, codeine, thebaine, papaverine, noscapine), is not considered particularly hazardous. There are only isolated reports of fatalities due to rachacha consumption in combination with alcohol use (Monteil-Ganiere et al. 2014). In addition to oral ingestion, the substance can also be added to cigarettes and consumed via inhalation. No specific histological findings have been reported; one sees the characteristic autopsy findings related to drug abuse (in particular, acute blood congestion, as well as brain and lung edema).

4.5 Neuropathological Findings

The effects of intravenous drug consumption on the central nervous system are described. Conventional histological findings are generally nonspecific. According to immunohistochemistry, axonal damage occurs (Büttner et al. 2006), in addition to hypoxic or hypoxemic pallidum lesions (Norheim Andersen and Skullerud 1999; Riße and Weiler 1984), as well as neurovascular complications after cocaine consumption (Daras et al. 1994). In cases of methamphetamine abuse, ubiquitin-positive

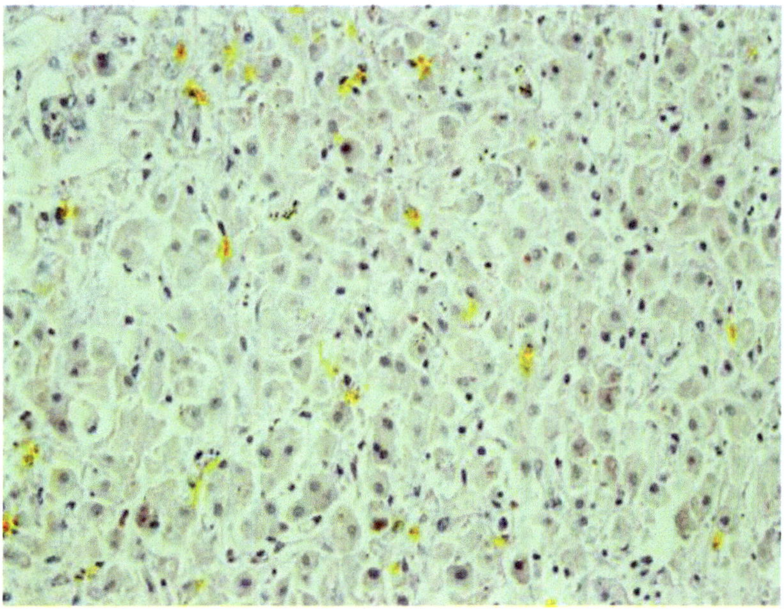

Fig. 4.35 Yellow pigment in the sinuses of the liver following intravenous injection of methadone containing a yellow colorant (H&E ×200)

structures can be found in the midbrain (Quan et al. 2005). When undergoing substitution therapy with methadone, this substance can be displayed immunohistochemically in the brain tissue (Wehner et al. 2000). Neurons of the central nervous system can express different kinds of opioid receptors, which, in the case of chronic opiate exposure, react adaptively with altered receptor density. Opioid receptors can be displayed immunohistochemically and by means of in situ hybridization. By this means, both "downregulation" and "upregulation" of receptor density have been observed (Schmidt et al. 1994, 1996).

Investigations of the hypophysis after drug abuse have shown an increase in the number but not in the size of follicles in the hypophyses in drug users which contain clusterin, an apolipoprotein which is well demonstrated using PAS staining (Ishikawa et al. 2007). This is presumed to be an expression of neurodegenerative processes, in particular in amphetamine users.

4.6 Organ Infarction After Drug Consumption

Infarctions of the internal organs, including renal infarctions, are described primarily in connection with the consumption of cocaine, although they represent relatively rare complications (Kramer and Turner 1993; Saleem et al. 2001). Cocaine consumption can lead to myoglobin-induced acute renal failure (Nzerue et al. 2000; Pogue and Nurse 1989) with immunohistochemically displayed myoglobin in the renal tubules. Ischemia of the intestines with ischemic colitis is also described (Brown et al. 1994; Gourgoutis and Das 1994; Nalbandian et al. 1985), as well as splenic infarctions (Novielli and Chambers 1991; Vaghjimal 1996), in individual cases with secondary infection and lethal sepsis (Dettmeyer et al. 2004). Cocaine-induced aortic dissections occur (Palmiere et al. 2004). Microinfarctions may be associated with cocaine-induced thrombotic processes (Heng and Haberfeld 1987) and may also affect the skin (Zamora-Quizada et al. 1988). Individual reports indicate an increased risk of spontaneous abortion following cocaine consumption in connection with nicotine abuse (Ness et al. 1999).

4.7 Injection-Related Tissue and Vascular Wall Damage

In the case of intravenous drug abuse, subcutaneous syringe abscesses (Fig. 4.36) can reoccur, sometimes on multiple occasions, with corresponding scarring after healing. Microscopically local purulent inflammation with abscesses in the

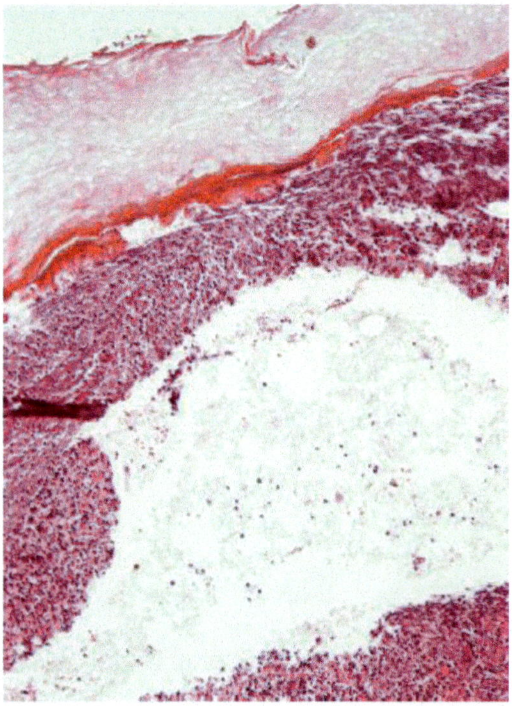

Fig. 4.36 Purulent subepidermal inflammation with abscess following intravenous drug injection, a so-called syringe abscess (H&E ×100)

subcutaneous soft tissue can be seen; rarely, phlegmonous purulent processes develop at the various injection sites (hands, forearms, neck, legs, back of penis, inguinal region, etc.). After many injections in the same location, the affected veins show vascular walls with thick scars and small residual lumen. Rarely, pyomyositis as an acute bacterial infection manifesting as pyemic abscess formation in the skeletal muscle can be observed in cases of intravenous drug abuse (Schalinski and Tsokos 2008).

Scar zones develop at the sites of multiple injections along the injection channels with deposits of hemosiderin-containing macrophages (siderophages); foreign-substance components may stay in the injection channel, and polynuclear foreign-body giant cells develop. According to own experience, this happens regularly in the case of multiple inguinal drug injections with the development of a fistula retracted in a funnel-like manner on the surface.

The macroscopic and microscopic findings in the case of inguinal fistulas (Fig. 4.37) following multiple injections are mentioned in Table 4.3.

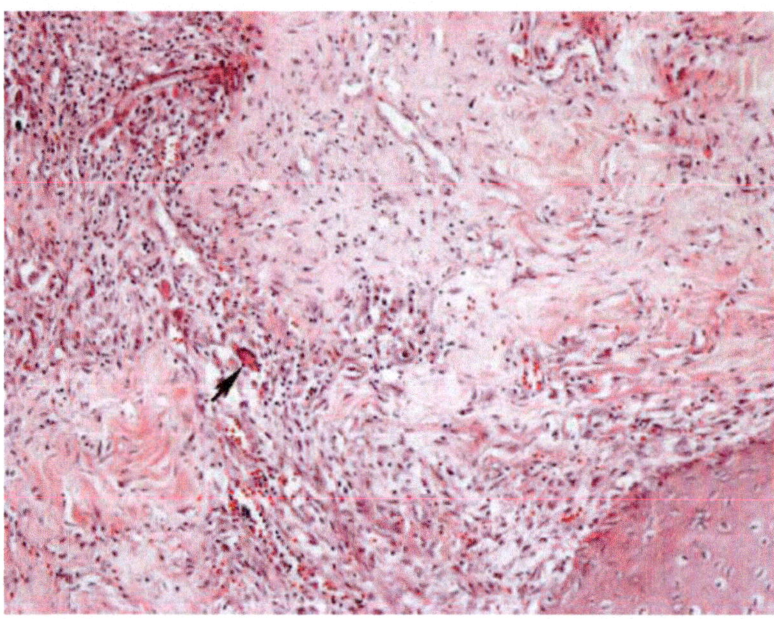

Fig. 4.37 Scarred inguinal fistulous tract after multiple drug injections with chronic fibrous inflammation, polynuclear foreign-body giant cells (*arrow*), and deposits of foreign substances in subepidermal areas (H&E ×100)

Table 4.3 Pathological findings in the case of inguinal fistulas following multiple drug injections

Macroscopical	Microscopical
A funnel-like depression at the surface	Central fistulous tract with circularly surrounding coarse fibrous wall
A coarse strand of connective tissue with embedded fistula up to the inguinal blood vessels	Embedded siderophages in the fistula wall as well as foreign substances and polynuclear foreign-body giant cells
Larger demarcated abscesses are macroscopically detectable	Microscopically small abscesses
Softened edematous tissue next to the fistula channel in the case of a soft tissue phlegmon	Phlegmonous purulent inflammation in the surrounding soft tissue
Fibrous peritonitis if inflammation has spread to the abdominal cavity	Fibrous peritonitis, various phases of the repair process depending on the duration of the inflammatory process
Extensive fresh hemorrhage in the inguinal soft tissue, possibly lethal bleeding into the abdominal cavity	In the case of targeted dissection: inflammatory arrosion of the vascular wall followed by bleeding; mechanical injury to the vascular wall during injection

In the case of abscesses and phlegmonous purulent processes (Fig. 4.38), arrosion of the arterial vascular wall can lead to lethal hemorrhage into the abdominal cavity or to lethal fibrous purulent peritonitis. In the case of phlegmonous purulent spread, scrotal soft tissue can also be affected with pronounced edematous swelling of the scrotum.

4.8 Necrotizing Myositis and Panniculitis Following Intravenous Drug Injection

If drugs are injected, the use of unsterile syringes and/or contaminated drugs may cause fatal infection in some cases (Dancer et al. 2002; Brayn 2000; Holmass et al. 1998; Passaro et al. 1998). Isolated cases of anthrax among drug abusers have been reported, e.g., by the National Anthrax Outbreak Control Team in Scotland. Cases of necrotizing myositis due to *Clostridium perfringens* are also seen following apparent intramuscular or subcutaneous drug injection. A finding of

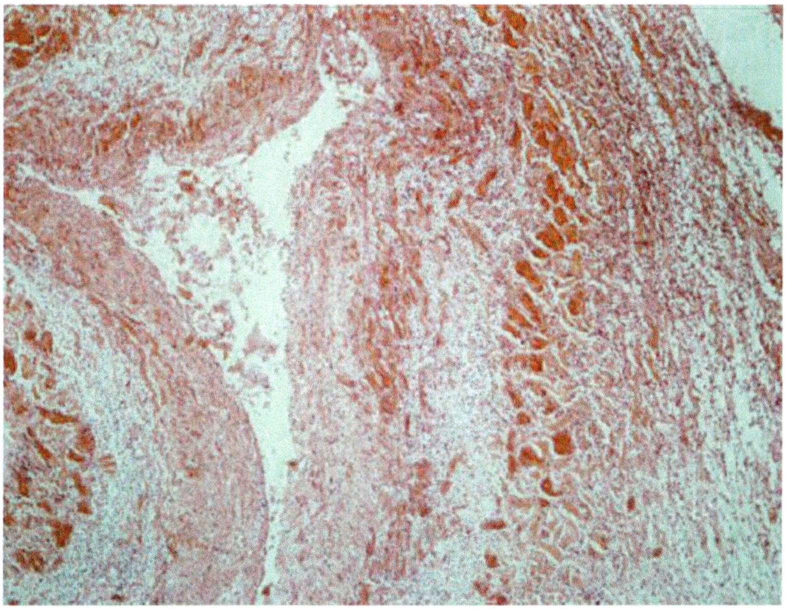

Fig. 4.38 Purulent infection of an inguinal fistula with purulent softening of the arterial wall. A 31-year-old man who died of drug abuse with acute arterial bleeding into the inguinal soft tissue and abdominal cavity (H&E ×40)

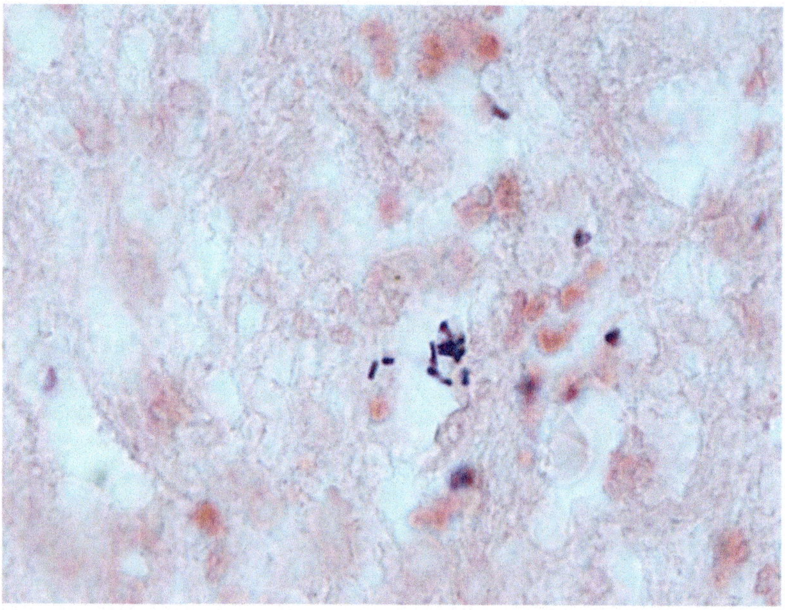

Fig. 4.39 Necrotizing panniculitis following the injection of drugs contaminated with gram-positive anthrax pathogens/*Bacillus anthracis* (×1000)

crepitus caused by gas is made in the necrotic zone of the affected skeletal muscle, while more or less abundant gram-positive rod-shaped bacteria are observed histologically (Mahfoud et al. 2002).

Contaminated heroin can also cause anthrax infection with *Bacillus anthracis* in heroin users, referred to as "injection anthrax" (Grunow et al. 2012; National Anthrax Outbreak Control Team 2011). The gram-positive, spore-forming, and encapsulated bacterium *Bacillus anthracis* is the pathogen that causes anthrax. Infection among humans occurs via the skin in 95% of cases. Pronounced redness and swelling develop at and around the injection site. *Bacillus anthracis* toxins trigger immunomodulatory and cytolytic processes in the cell, among other effects. The mortality rate for injection anthrax is put at around 30%, at around 50% for pulmonary anthrax and intestinal anthrax, and at around 5% for cutaneous anthrax (Grunow et al. 2012). Priority is given to detecting *Bacillus anthracis* by means of blood culture or by using serological or molecular genetic techniques. Like other bacteria, *Bacillus anthracis* can also be isolated directly from the heroin (Grass et al. 2016).

Both clinically and at autopsy, the affected body region may show a macroscopic picture of subcutaneous phlegmonous/purulent infection following injection of contaminated heroin. From a histological perspective, several specimens from the affected soft tissue region should be analyzed. The suspicion of *Bacillus anthracis* infection is supported if gram-positive rods are detected microscopically (Fig. 4.39). As a matter of principle, anthrax pathogens can also be inhaled via the respiratory tract and cause pulmonary anthrax. This potential resulted in the classification of *Bacillus anthracis* as a biological weapon (Inglesby et al. 2002; Schorle 2002).

References

Addington WW, Cugell DW, Bazley ES, Westerhoff TR, Shapiro B, Smith RT (1972) The pulmonary edema of heroin toxicity – an example of the stiff lung syndrome. Chest 62:199–205

Angelos MG, Sheets CA, Zych PR (1986) Needle emboli to lung following intravenous drug abuse. J Emerg Med 4:391–396

Aretz TH (1987) Myocarditis – the Dallas criteria. Hum Pathol 18:619–624

Arruda JAL, Kurtzman NA, Pillay VKG (1975) Prevalence of renal disease in asymptomatic heroin addicts. Arch Intern Med 135:535–537

Bakir A, Dunea G (1996) Drugs of abuse and renal disease. Curr Opin Nephrol Hypertens 5:122–126

Bakir AA, Bazilinski NG, Rhee LH, Ainis H, Dunes G (1989) Focal segmental glomerulosclerosis. A common entity in nephrotic black adults. Arch Intern Med 149:1802–1804

Bartok I, Remenar E, Toth J (1976) Demonstration of hepatitis B surface antigen by orcein staining in paraffin sections of cirrhotic liver. Virchows Arch A Pathol Anat Histol 369:239–248

Berger P, Walls AF, Marthan R, Tunon-de-Lara JM (1998) Immunoglobulin E-induced passive sensibilization of human airways. Am J Respir Crit Care Med 157:610–616

Blanck RR, Ream N, Conrad M (1979) Hepatitis B antigen and antibody in heroin users. Am J Gastroenterol 71:164–167

Blanco Garcia S, Martinez Ubieto J, Sanchez Tirado JA, Laglera Trebol S, Gomez Munoz C, Garcia Laborda C, Urieta Solanas A (1999) Rhabdomyolysis and compartment syndrome associated with drug abuse. Rev Esp Anestesiol Reanim 46:46–47

Bogomeletz WV (1976) Orcein staining of hepatitis B antigen in conventional paraffin sections of liver biopsies. Acta Hepatogastroenterol 23:412–414

Borchard F, Gussmann V (1979) Detection of HBsAg containing cells in liver biopsies by different stains and classification of positively reacting ground-glass hepatocytes. Virchows Arch A Pathol Anat Histol 384:245–261

Brander PE, Tukiainen P (1983) Acute eosinophilic pneumonia in a heroin smoker. Eur Respir J 6:750–752

Brayn C (2000) Gangrene bug killed 35 heroin users. Br Med J 320:1690

Brinkmann B, Kollmeier J, Müller KM (1991) Fremdkörper-Endangiitis bei Fixerpneumopathie. Atemwegs Lungenkr 17:282–283

Brown SM, Stimmel B, Taub RN, Kochwa S, Rosenfeld RE (1974) Immunologic dysfunction in heroin addicts. Arch Intern Med 134:1001–1006

Brown DN, Rosenholtz MJ, Marshall JB (1994) Ischemic colitis related to cocaine abuse. Am J Gastroenterol 89:1558–1561

Busch HW, Riechman S, HEyen P, Heidenreich S, Kaufman CC, Rahn KH, Zidek W (1994) Albuminuria in HIV-infected patients. AIDS Res Hum Retroviruses 10:717–719

Büttner A, Rohrmoser K, Mall G, Penning R, Weis S (2006) Widespread axonal damage in the brain of drug abusers as evidenced by accumulation of beta-amyloid precursor protein (beta-APP): an immunohistochemical investigation. Addiction 101:1339–1346

Campkin NJ, Davies UM (1993) Treatment of "ecstasy" overdose with dantrolene. Anaesthesia 48:82–83

Carbone L, D'Agati V, Cheng JT, Appel GB (1989) Course and prognosis of human immunodeficiency virus-associated nephropathy. Am J Med 67:389–395

Carlson RW, Schaeffer RC, Michaels SG, Weil MH (1979) Pulmonary edema fluid. Spectrum of features in 37 patients. Circulation 60:1161–1169

Casanova S, Mazzucco G, Barbiano del Belgiojoso G, Motta M, Boldorini R, Genderini A, Monga G (1995) Pattern of glomerular involvement in human immunodeficiency virus-infected patients: an Italian study. Am J Kidney Dis 26:446–453

Cejtin HE, Young SA, Ungaretti J, Anciaux D, Imam S, Teopengco E, Sander CM (1999) Effects of cocaine on the placenta. Pediatr Dev Pathol 2:143–147

Cerretani D, Riezzo I, Fiaschi AI, Centini F, Giorgi G, D'Errico S, Fiore C, Karch SB, Neri M, Pomara C, Turillazzi E, Fineschi V (2008) Cardiac oxidative stress determination and myocardial morphology after a single ecstasy (MDMA) administration in a rat model. Int J Legal Med 122:461–469

Chander P, Soni A, Suri A, Bhagwat T, Yoo J, Treser G (1987) Renal ultrastructural markers in AIDS-associated nephropathy. Am J Pathol 126:513–526

Cohen AH, Nast CC (1988) HIV-associated nephropathy – a unique combined glomerular, tubular, and interstitial lesion. Mod Pathol 1:87–97

Collignon PJ, Sorrell TC (1983) Disseminated candidiasis: evidence of a distinctive syndrome in heroin abusers. Br Med J 287:861–862

Conway N (1969) Endocarditis in heroin addicts. Br Heart J 31:543–545

Cordner S (2016) A rare report of fatal torture. Forensic Sci Med Pathol 12:204–205

Cregler LL, Mark H (1985) Relation of acute myocardial infarction to cocaine abuse. Am J Cardiol 56:794

Crouch E, Churg A (1983) Progressive massive fibrosis of the lung secondary to intravenous injection of talc. A pathologic and mineralogic analysis. Am J Clin Pathol 80:520–526

Cunningham EE, Brentjens JR, Zielezny MA, Andres GA, Venuto RC (1980) Heroin nephropathy – a clinicopathologic and epidemiologic study. Am J Med 68:47–53

Cunningham EE, Zielezny MA, Venuto RC (1983) Heroin-associated nephropathy – a nationwide problem. JAMA 250:2935–2936

Cunningham EE, Venuto RC, Zielezny MA (1984) Adulterants in heroin/cocaine: implications concerning heroin-associated nephropathy. Drug Alcohol Depend 14:19–22

D'Agati V, Suh J, Carbone L, Cheng JT, Appel G (1989) Pathology of HIV-associated nephropathy: a detailed morphologic and comparative study. Kidney Int 35:1358–1370

Dancer SJ, McNair D, Finn P, Kolsto AB (2002) Bacillus cereus cellulitis from contaminated heroin. J Med Microbiol 51:278–281

Dar KJ, McBrien ME (1996) MDMA induced hyperthermia: report of a fatality and review of current therapy. Intensive Care Med 22:995–996

Daras M, Tuchman AJ, Koppel BS, Samkoff LM, Weitzner I, Marc J (1994) Neurovascular complications of cocaine. Acta Neurol Scand 90:124–129

de Gans J, Stam J, van Wijngaarden GK (1985) Rhabdomyolysis and concomitant neurological lesions after intravenous heroin abuse. J Neurol Neurosurg Psychiatry 48:1057–1059

Deighan CJ, Wong KM, McLaughlin KJ, Harden P (2000) Rhabdomyolysis and acute renal failure resulting from alcohol and drug abuse. J Med 93:29–33
Delcker A, Dux R, Diener HC (1992) Acute plexus lesions in heroin dependence. Nervenarzt 63:240–243
Dettmeyer R, Wessling B, Madea B (1998) Heroin-associated nephropathy – a post mortem study. Forensic Sci Int 95:109–116
Dettmeyer R, Schmidt P, Musshoff F, Dreisvogt C, Madea B (2000) Pulmonary edema in fatal heroin overdose: immunohistological investigations with IgE, collagen IV and laminin – no increase of defects of alveolar-capillary membranes. Forensic Sci Int 110:87–96
Dettmeyer R, Stojanovski G, Madea B (2001) Pathogenesis of heroin-associated glomerulonephritis. Correlation between the inflammatory activity and renal deposits of immunoglobulin and complement? Forensic Sci Int 113:227–231
Dettmeyer RM, Schlamann MB, Madea B (2004) Cocaine-associated abscesses with lethal sepsis after splenic infarction in a 17-year-old woman. Forensic Sci Int 140:21–23
Dettmeyer R, Preuß J, Wollersen H, Madea B (2005) Heroin-associated nephropathy. Expert Opin Drug Saf 4:19–28
Dettmeyer R, Friedrich K, Schmidt P, Madea B (2009a) Heroin-associated myocardial damages – conventional and immunohistochemical investigations. Forensic Sci Int 187:42–46
Dettmeyer R, Verhoff MA, Brückel B, Walter D (2009b) Widespread pulmonary granulomatosis following long time intravenous drug abuse – a case report. Forensic Sci Int 197:e27–e30
Doutrelepont JM, Adler M, Willems M, Durez P, Yap SH (1993) Hepatitis C infection and membranoproliferative glomerulonephritis. Lancet 341:317
Dressler FA, Roberts WC (1989) Infective endocarditis in opiate addicts: analysis of 80 cases studied at necropsy. Am J Cardiol 63:1240–1257
Dries V, Odenthal M, Schirmacher P, Dienes HP (2001) Liver biopsy in chronic hepatitis C. Histopathology, molecular diagnostic analysis, and implications for therapeutic management. Pathologe 22:362–368
Dubrow A, Mittman N, Ghali V, Flamenbaum W (1985) The changing spectrum of heroin-associated nephropathy. Am J Kidney Dis 5:36–41
Edgecombe A, Milroy C (2012) Sudden death from superior mesenteric artery thrombosis in a cocaine user. Forensic Sci Med Pathol 8:48–51
Edston E, van Hage-Hamsten M (1997) Anaphylactoid shock – a common cause of death in heroin addicts. Allergy 52:950–954
Eknoyan G, Györkey F, Dichoso C, Martinez-Maldonado M, Suki WN, Györkey P (1972) Renal morphological and immunological changes associated with acute viral hepatitis. Kidney Int 1:413–419
Eknoyan G, Györkey F, Dichoso C, Hyde SE, Györkey P, Suki WN, Martinez-Maldonada M (1973) Renal involvement in drug abuse. Arch Intern Med 132:801–806
Ellis FR, Halsall PJ, Christian AS (1990) Clinical presentation of suspected malignant hyperthermia during anaesthesia in 402 probands. Anaesthesia 45:838–841
Erbersdobler A, Wullbrand A, Kneissler U, Helmchen U (1995) Heroin-assoziierte membranoproliferative Glomerulonephritis Typ I: Eine neue Entität? Verh Dtsch Ges Pathol 79:459
Ferries JAJ, Rice J (1979) Drug-induced myocarditis: a report of two cases. Forensic Sci Int 13:261–265
Fineschi V, Wetli CV, Di Paolo M, Baroldi G (1997) Myocardial necrosis and cocaine – a quantitative morphologic study in 26 cocaine-associated deaths. Int J Legal Med 110:193–198
Fineschi V, Centini F, Mazzeo E, Turillazzi E (1999) Adam (MDMA) and Eve (MDEA) misuse: an immunohistochemical study on three fatal cases. Forensic Sci Int 104:65–74
Fineschi V, Baroldi G, Centini F, Cerretani D, Fiaschi AI, Micheli L, Parolini M, Turillazi E, Giorgi G (2001a) Markers of cardiac oxidative stress and altered morphology after intraperitoneal cocaine injection in a rat model. Int J Legal Med 114:323–330
Fineschi V, Cecchi R, Centini F, Paglicci Reattelli L, Turillazzi E (2001b) Immunohistochemical quantification of pulmonary mast-cells and post-mortem blood dosages of tryptase and eosinophil cationic protein in 48 heroin-related deaths. Forensic Sci Int 120:189–194
Forrester JM, Steele AW, Waldron JA, Parsons PE (1989) Crack lung: an acute pulmonary syndrome with a spectrum of clinical and histopathologic findings. Am Rev Respir Dis 142:462–467
Freeman BC, Kreps EM, Ronsheim NJ, Lejano RF, Sommers SC (1974) Poststaphylococcal glomerulonephritis in heroin addicts. N Y State J Med 74(12):2241–2243
Friedman EA, Rao TKS (1995) Disappearance of uremia due to heroin-associated nephropathy. Am J Kidney Dis 25:689–693
Friedman EA, Sreepada Rao TK (1983) Why does uremia in heroin abusers occur predominantly among blacks? JAMA 250:2965–2966
Friedman EA, Rao TKS, Nicastri AD (1974) Heroin-associated nephropathy. Nephron 13:421–426
Garbino J, Henry JA, Mentha G, Romand JA (2001) Ecstasy ingestion and fulminant hepatic failure: liver transplantation to be considered as a last therapeutic option. Vet Hum Toxicol 43:99–102
Genderini A, Bertani T, Bertoli S, Scorza D, Barbiano di Belgiojoso G (1990) HIV-associated nephropathy: a new entity. A study of 12 cases. Nephrol Dial Transplant 1:84–87
Gill JR, Hayes JA, De Souza IS, Marker E, Stajic M (2002) Ecstasy (MDMA) deaths in New York City: a case series and review of the literature. J Forensic Sci 47:121–126
Gillet DG, Fort GT (1978) Drug-induced lung disease. In: Thurlbeck WM, Abell MR (eds) The lung: structure, function and disease. Williams and Wilkins, Baltimore, pp 21–42

Gitmann MD, Singhal PC (2004) Cocaine-induced renal disease. Expert Opin Drug Saf 3:441–448

Gomez A, Stockert JC, Mosquera RM, del Castillo P, Tena G, Sancho M (1989) Chronic intoxication by heroin: histopathological effects on seminiferous tubules. Forensic Sci Int 43:97–101

Gonzalo A, Barcena R, Mampaso F, Zea A, Ortuno J (1993) Membranoproliferative glomerulonephritis and hepatitis C virus infection. Nephron 63:475–476

Gourgoutis G, Das G (1994) Gastrointestinal manifestations of cocaine addiction. Int J Clin Pharmacol Ther 32:136–141

Grass G, Ahrens B, Schleenbecker U, Dobrzykowski L, Wagner M, Krüger C, Wölfel R (2016) Technical note: simple, scalable, and sensitive protocol for retrieving Bacillus anthracis (and other live bacteria) from heroin. Forensic Sci Int 259:32–35

Grellner W, Madea B, Sticht G (1996) Pulmonary histopathology and survival period in morphine-involved deaths. J Forensic Sci 41:433–437

Grishman E, Churg J, Porush JG (1976) Glomerular morphology in nephrotic heroin addicts. Lab Investig 35:415–424

Gross EM (1973) Talc embolism: sudden death following intravenous injection of phenyltoloxamine. Forensic Sci Int 2:475–480

Groth HD, McKay R, Crable JV, Cochran TH (1972) Intravenous injection of talc in a narcotic addict. Arch Pathol 94:171–178

Grunow R, Verbeek L, Jacob D, Holzmann T, Birkenfeld G, Wiens D, von Eichel-Streiber L, Grass G, Reischl U (2012) Injection anthrax – a new outbreak in heroin users. Dtsch Ärztebl Int 109:843–848

Hamilton RJ, Perrone J, Hoffman R et al (2000) A descriptive study of an epidemic of poisoning caused by heroin adulterated with scopolamine. J Toxicol Clin Toxicol 38:597–608

Haskell LP, Glicklich D, Senitzer D (1988) HLA associations in heroin-associated nephropathy. Am J Kidney Dis 12:45–50

Hejna P, Janík M, Dobiáš M (2014) Tricuspid valve endocarditis complicated by septic pulmonary embolism in an intravenous drug user. Forensic Sci Med Pathol 10:126–129

Heng MC, Haberfeld G (1987) Thrombotic phenomenon associated with intravenous cocaine. J Am Acad Dermatol 16:462–468

Henning RJ, Cuevas J (2006) Cocaine activates calcium/calmodulin kinase II and causes cardiomyocyte hypertrophy. J Cardiovasc Pharmacol 48:802–813

Henry JA, Jeffreys KJ, Dawling S (1992) Toxicity and deaths from 3,4-methylenedioxymeth-amphetamine ("ecstasy"). Lancet 340:384–387

Hill GS (1986) Drug-associated glomerulopathies. Toxicol Pathol 14:37–44

Hollander LMA, Young GP, Briglia E, Wetle CV, Gawad Y (1998) Effect of recent cocaine use on the specificity of cardiac markers for diagnosis of acute myocardial infarction. Am Heart J 135:245–252

Holmass G, Gilhus NE, Gjerde IO, Lund-Tonnessen S, Langorgen J (1998) Wound botulism in heroin addiction. Tiddsskr Nor Laegeforen 118:4357–4359

Hopkins GB (1972) Pulmonary angiothrombotic granulomas in drug offenders. JAMA 221:909–911

Horikoshi S, Okada T, Shirato I, Inokuchi S, Ohmuro H, Tomino Y, Koide H (1993) Diffuse proliferative glomerulonephritis with hepatitis C Virus-like particles in paramesangial dense deposits in a patient with chronic hepatitis C Virus hepatitis. Nephron 64:462–464

Inglesby TV, O'Toole T, Henderson DA et al (2002) Anthrax as a biological weapon. Updated recommendations for management. JAMA 287:2236–2252

Ishigami A, Tokunaga I, Gotohda T, Kubo S (2003) Immunohistochemical study of myoglobin and oxidative injury-related markers in the kidney of methamphetamine abusers. Legal Med 5:42–48

Ishikawa T, Zhu BL, Miyaishi S, Ishizu H, Maeda H (2007) Increase in clusterin-containing follicles in the adenohypophysis of drug abusers. Int J Legal Med 121:395–402

Islam MN, Jesmine K, Molh AKS, Hasnan J (2009) Histopathological studies of cardiac lesions after long term administration of methamphetamine in high dosage – part II. Legal Med 11:S147–S150

Johnson RJ, Couser WG (1990) Hepatitis B infection and renal disease: clinical, immunopathogenic and therapeutic considerations. Editorial review. Kidney Int 37:663–676

Johnson RJ, Gretch DR, Yamabe H, Hart J, Bacchi CE, Hartwell P, Couser WG, Corey L, Wener MH, Alpers CE, Willson R (1993) Membranoproliferative glomerulonephritis associated with hepatitis C virus infection. N Engl J Med 328:465–470

Kapasi AA, Gibbons N, Mattana J, Singhal PC (2000) Morphine stimulates mesangial cell TNF-alpha and nitrite production. Inflammation 24:463–476

Karch SB (2002) Pathology of drug abuse, 3rd edn. CRC Press, Boca Raton, pp 91–106

Karch SB (2005) Cocaine cardiovascular toxicity. South Med J 98:794–799

Karch SB (2009) Karch's pathology of drug abuse, 4th edn. CRC Press, Boca Raton, pp 523–533

Karch SB (2011) The unique histology of methamphetamine cardiomyopathy: a case report. Forensic Sci Int 212:e1–e4

Karch SB, Green GS et al (1995) Myocardial hypertrophy and coronary artery disease in male cocaine users. J Forensic Sci 40:591–595

Karch SB, Busardó FP, Vaiano F, Portelli F, Zaami S, Bertol E (2016) Levamisole adulterated cocaine and pulmonary vasculitis: presentation of two lethal cases and brief literature review. Forensic Sci Int 265:96–102

Kathrein H, Kirchmair W, Konig P, von Dittrich P (1983) Rhabdomyolysis with acute kidney failure after heroin poisoning. Dtsch Med Wochenschr 108:464–467

Katz S, Aberman A et al (1972) Heroin pulmonary edema. Evidence for increased pulmonary capillary permeability. Am Rev Respir Dis 106:472–474

Kiloyne MM, Gocke DJ, Meltzer JI, Daly JJ, Thomson GE, Hsu KC (1972) Nephrotic syndrome in heroin addicts. Lancet 1:17–20

Knodell RG, Ishak KG, Black WC, Chen TS, Craig R, Kaplowitz N, Kiernan TW, Wollman J (1981) Formulation and application of numerical scoring system for assessing histological activity in asymptomatic chronic active hepatitis. Hepatology 1:431–435

Kock KF, Simonsen KW (1994) Renal myoglobin in drug addicts: occurrence and significance in a postmortem study. Forensic Sci Int 65:113–119

Kopfler D, Paronetto F (1965) Immunofluorescent localization of immunoglobulins, complement and fibrinogen in human diseases. II. Acute, subacute and chronic glomerulonephritis. J Clin Invest 44:1665–1671

Kramer RK, Turner RC (1993) Renal infarction associated with cocaine use and latent protein C deficiency. South Med J 86:1436–1438

Kringsholm B, Christoffersen P (1987a) Lung and heart pathology in fatal drug addiction. A consecutive autopsy study. Forensic Sci Int 34:39–51

Kringsholm B, Christoffersen P (1987b) The nature and the occurrence of birefringent material in different organs in fatal drug addiction. Forensic Sci Int 34:53–62

Kubat B (2013) Drugs, muscle pallor, and pyositis. Forensic Sci Med Pathol 9:564–567

Lang J, Dettmeyer R, Henn V, Birngruber CG, Veit F (2016) Fatal ecstasy-induced malignant hyperthermia with rhabdomyolysis. A case report. Rom J Legal Med 24:212–215

Lapachinske SF, Okai GC, dos Santos A, Valle de Bairros A, Yonamine M (2015) Analysis of cocaine and its adulterants in drugs for international trafficking seized by the Brazilian Federal Police. Forensic Sci Int 247:48–53

Lapkus M, Prahlow JA (2015) Infective endocarditis in an intravenous drug abuser. Forensic Sci Med Pathol 11:609–613

Larner AJ (1993) Dantrolene and "ecstasy" overdose. Anaesthesia 48:179–180

Lazareth H, Peytavin G, Poliovka L, Dupin N (2012) The hairy-print for levamisole-induced vasculitis. Br Med J Case Rep. https://doi.org/10.1136/bcr-2012-006602

Levine SB, Grimes ET (1973) Pulmonary edema and heroin overdose in Vietnam. Arch Pathol 95:330–332

Lewis TD, Henry DA (1985) Needle embolus: a unique complication of intravenous drug abuse. Ann Emerg Med 14:906–908

Li W, Zhang L, Liang Y, Tong F, Zhou Y (2017) Sudden death due to malignant hyperthermia with a mutation of RYR1: autopsy, morphology and genetic analysis. Forensic Sci Med Pathol 13:444–449

Llach F, Descoeudres C, Massry SG (1979) Heroin-associated nephropathy: clinical and histological studies in 19 patients. Clin Nephrol 11:7–12

Lockemann U, Pueschel K (1993) Siderophages in the lung of drug addicts. Forensic Sci Int 59:169–175

Louria DB, Henslet T, Rose J (1967) The major medical complications of heroin addiction. Ann Intern Med 67:1–22

Mah MW, Shafran SD (1990) Polymicrobial endocarditis with eight pathogens in an intravenous drug abuser. Scand J Infect Dis 22:735–737

Mahfoud B, Heinemann A, Gehl A, Püschel K (2002) Nekrotisierende Myositis durch Clostridium perfringens nach intravenöser Heroinapplikation. Rechtsmedizin 12:109–111

Matalon R, Katz L, Gallo G, Waldo E, Cabaluna C, Eisinger RP (1974) Glomerular sclerosis in adults with nephrotic syndrome. Ann Intern Med 80:488–495

Matsubara O, Tamura A, Ohdama S, Mark EJ (1995) Alveolar basement membrane breaks down in diffuse alveolar damage: an immunohistochemical study. Pathol Int 45:473–482

May D, Helderman H, Eigenbrodt EH, Silva FG (1986) Chronic sclerosing glomerulopathy (heroin-associated nephropathy) in intravenous T's and blues abusers. Am J Kidney Dis 8:404–409

McAllister CJ, Horn R, Havron S, Abramson JH (1979) Granulomatous interstitial nephritis: a complication of heroin abuse. South Med J 72:162–165

McGinn JT, McGinn TG, Hoffman RS (1970) Nephrotic syndrome in heroin (HER) and cocaine (COC) addicts. Clin Res 18:699

McGinn JT, McGinn TG, Cherubin CE, Hoffman RS (1974) Nephrotic syndrome in drug addicts. N Y State J Med 74(1):92–95

Meador KH, Sharon Z, Lewis EJ (1979) Renal amyloidosis and subcutaneous drug abuse. Ann Intern Med 91:565–567

Menchel S, Cohen D, Gross E, Frangione B, Gallo G (1983) AA protein-related renal amyloidosis in drug addicts. Am J Pathol 112:195–199

Michaud K, Grabherr S, Shiferaw K, Doenz F, Augsburger M, Mangin P (2014) Acute coronary syndrome after levamisole-adulterated cocaine abuse. J Forensic Legal Med 21:48–52

Monteil-Ganiere C, Gaulier JM, Chopineaux D, Barrios L, Pineau A, Dailly E, Clément R (2014) Fatal anoxia due to rachacha consumption: two cases reported. Forensic Sci Int 245:e1–e5

Montoliu J, Miró JM, Campistol JM, Trilla A, Mensa J, Torras A, Revert L (1987) Henoch-Schönlein purpura complicating staphylococcal endocarditis in a heroin addict. Am J Nephrol 7:137–139

Morris DC (1991) Cocaine heart disease. Hosp Pract 26:81–90

Mu J, Li M, Guo Y, Lv B, Qiu M, Dong H (2017) Methamphetamine-induced toxic leukoencephalopathy: clinical, radiological and autopsy findings. Forensic Sci Med Pathol 13:362–366. https://doi.org/10.1007/s12024-017-9893-2

Müller KM (2004) Fixerpneumopathie. Pneumologie 58:552

Nalbandian H, Sheth N, Dietrich R et al (1985) Intestinal ischemia caused by cocaine ingestion: report of two cases. Surgery 97:374–376

National Anthrax Outbreak Control Team (2011) An outbreak of anthrax among drug users in Scotland,

December 2009 to December 2010. Health Protection Scotland, Glasgow, pp 1–117

Ness RB, Grisso JA, Hirschinger N, Markovic N, Shaw LM, Day NL, Kline J (1999) Cocaine and tobacco use and the risk of spontaneous abortion. N Engl J Med 340:333–339

Neugarten J, Baldwin DS (1984) Glomerulonephritis in bacterial endocarditis. Am J Med 77:297–304

Neugarten J, Gallo G, Buxbaum J, Katz LA, Rubinstein J, Baldwin DS (1986) Amyloidosis in subcutaneous heroin abusers ("skin poppers' amyloidosis"). Am J Med 81:635–640

Norheim Andersen S, Skullerud K (1999) Hypoxic/ischaemic brain damage, especially pallidal lesions, in heroin addicts. Forensic Sci Int 102:51–59

Novielli KD, Chambers CV (1991) Splenic infarction after cocaine use. Ann Intern Med 114:251–252

Nzerue CM, Hewan-Lowe K, Riley LJ (2000) Cocaine and the kidney: a synthesis of pathophysiologic and clinical prospectives. Am J Kidney Dis 35:783–795

Oehler U, Sinicina I, Helpap B (2002) Ausgedehnte bilaterale Unterschenkelmuskelnekrosen nach nasaler Heroinapplikation. Pathologe 23:318–320

Pääkkö P, Sutinen S, Anttila S, Autio-Harmainen H, Sormunen R (1988) Bronchiolo-alveolitis with pulmonary basal lamina injury in a rheumatoid patient during gold treatment. Pathol Res Pract 183:46–53

Palmiere C, Burkhardt S, Staub C, Hallenbarter M, Pizzolato G, Dettmeyer R, La Harpe R (2004) Thoracic aortic dissection associated with cocaine abuse. Forensic Sci Int 141:137–142

Pan CO, Singhal PC (1994) Coordinate and independent effects of cocaine, alcohol, and morphine on accumulation of IgG aggregates in the rat glomeruli. Proc Soc Exp Biol Med 205:29–34

Pare JP, Cote G, Fraser RS (1984) Long-term follow-up of drug abusers with intravenous talcosis. Am Rev Respir Dis 139:233–241

Passarino G, Ciccone G et al (2005) Histopathological findings in 851 autopsies of drug addicts, with toxicologic and virologic correlations. Am J Forensic Med Pathol 26:106–116

Passaro DJ, Werner SB, McGee J, McKenzie WR, Vugia DJ (1998) Wound botulism associated with black tar heroin among injecting drug users. JAMA 279:859–863

Patel J, Manjappan N, Bhat R, Mehrotra P, Bhaskaran M, Singhal PC (2003) Role of oxidative stress and heme oxygenase activity in morphine-induced glomerular epithelial cell growth. Am J Physiol Renal Physiol 285:F861–F869

Pawlik E, Mahler H, Hartung B, Plässer G, Daldrup T (2015) Drug-related death: adulterants from cocaine preparations in lung tissue and blood. Forensic Sci Int 249:294–303

Perazella MA (2005) Drug-induced nephropathy: an update. Expert Opin Drug Saf 4:689–706

Pernegger TV, Klag MJ, Whelton PK (2001) Recreational drug use: a neglected risk factor for end-stage renal disease. Am J Kidney Dis 38:49–56

Perskvist N, Söderberg C, van Hage M, Edston E (2007) Pathogenetic role of cardiac mast cell activation/degranulation, TNF-alpha, and cell death in acute drug related fatalities. Vasc Health Risk Manag 3:1053–1062

Phillips MS, Khanna VK, De Leon S, Frodis W, Britt BA, MacLennan DH (1994) The substitution of Arg for Gly2433 in the human skeletal muscle ryanodine receptor is associated with malignant hyperthermia. Hum Mol Genet 3:2181–2186

Pogue VA, Nurse HM (1989) Cocaine-associated acute myoglobinuric renal failure. Am J Med 86:183–186

Pollanen MS (2016) Fatal rhabdomyolysis after torture by reverse hanging. Forensic Sci Med Pathol 12:170–173

Prendergast BD, George CF (1993) Drug-induced rhabdomyolysis-mechanisms and management. Postgrad Med J 69:333–336

Püschel K (1986) Fremdkörpergranulome nach i.v. Drogenapplikation. Beitr Path 102:400–401

Püschel K (1988) Pulmonales Mikroemboliesyndrom durch Injektion einer Tablettensuspension. In: Bauer G (ed) Gerichtsmedizin. Festschrift für Wilhelm Holczabek. Franz Deuticke, Wien, pp 163–166

Püschel K, Schoof W (1987) Zur Morphogenese hämatogen entstandener Fremdkörpergranulome im Lungenparenchym. Beitr Gerichtl Med 45:121–128

Quan L, Ishikawa T, Michiue T, Li DR, Zhao D, Oritani S, Zhu BL, Maeda H (2005) Ubiquitin-immunoreactive structures in the midbrain of methamphetamine abusers. Legal Med 7:144–150

Rabl W, Markwalder C (1996) Fatal posture- and heroin-related intestinal infarction and leg muscle necrosis after snorting heroin. A case report. Am J Forensic Med Pathol 17:163–166

Raijs J, Harm T, Ormstad K (1984) Postmortem findings of pulmonary lesions of older datum in intravenous drug addicts. A forensic-pathologic study. Virchows Arch A Pathol Anat Histopathol 402:405–414

Rajs J, Falconer B (1979) Cardiac lesions in intravenous drug addicts. Forensic Sci Int 13:193–209

Ramirez G, Stinson JB, Zawada ET, Moatamed F (1983) Acute interstitial nephritis associated with chronic active hepatitis. South Med J 76:391–394

Reijula K, Sutinen S (1985) Detection of antigens in lung biopsies by immunoperoxidase staining in extrinsic allergic bronchiolo-alveolitis (EABA). Acta Histochem 76:121–125

Rice EK, Isbel NM, Becker GJ, Atkins RC, McMahon LP (2000) Heroin overdose and myoglobinuric acute renal failure. Clin Nephrol 54:449–454

Richter RW, Challenor YB, Pearson J, Kagen L, Hamilton LL, Ramsey W (1971) Acute myoglobinuria associated with heroin addiction. JAMA 216:1172–1176

Riße M, Weiler G (1984) Heroinsucht als seltene Ursache einer symmetrischen Pallidumnekrose. Z Rechtsmed 93:227–235

Rollina C, Roccatello D, Giachino O, Basolo B, Piccoli G (1991) Hepatitis C virus infection and membranous glomerulonephritis. Nephron 59:319–320

Romas E, Power DA, Machet D, Powell H, D'Apice AJF (1994) Membranous glomerulonephritis associated with hepatitis C virus infection in an adolescent. Pathology 26:399–402

Rostoker G, Pawlotsky A, Bastie A, Weil B, Dhumeaux D (1996) Type I membranoproliferative glomerulonephritis and HCV infection. Nephrol Dial Transplant 11:22–24

Sagar S, Sorbi D, Arbeit LD, Singhal PC (1994) Morphine modulates 72-kDa matrix metalloproteinase. Am J Phys 267:F654–F659

Saleem TM, Singh M, Murtaza M, Singh A, Kasubhai M, Gnanasekaran I, Freudenberger RS, Cappell MS, Hutt DA (2001) Renal infarction: a rare complication of cocaine abuse. Am J Emerg Med 19:528–529

Salomon MI, Poon TP, Goldblatt M, Tchertkoff V (1972) Renal lesions in heroin addicts. A study based on kidney biopsies. Nephron 9:356–363

Sameiro Faria M, Sampaio S, Faria V, Carvalho E (2003) Nephropathy associated with heroin abuse in Caucasian patients. Nephrol Dial Transplant 18:2308–2313

Scandting J, Spital A (1988) Amphetamine-associated myoglobinuric renal failure. South Med J 75:237–240

Schalinski S, Tsokos M (2008) Fatal pyomyositis: a report of 8 autopsy cases. Am J Forensic Med Pathol 29:131–135

Schmidt P, Schröder H, Maderspach K et al (1994) Immunohistochemical localization of kappa opioid receptors in the human frontal cortex. Brain Res 654:223–233

Schmidt P, Wevers A, Maderspach K et al (1996) Cerebrocortical delta-opioid receptor mRNA expression in morphine addicts. Soc Neurosci Abstr 22:823

Schmidt P, Padosch SA, Dettmeyer R, Madea B (2004) Rechtsmedizinische Aspekte des Drogentodes. Med Welt 55:199–205

Scholer J, Derosena R, Appel GB, Jao W, Boyd MT, Pirani CL (1979) Amyloidosis in chronic heroin addicts with the nephrotic syndrome. Ann Intern Med 91:26–29

Schorle H (2002) Anthrax. Die keimende Gefahr. Pathologe 23:167–169

Screaton GR, Singer M, Cairns HS, Thrasher A, Sarner M, Cohen SL (1992) Hyperpyrexia and rhabdomyolysis after MDMA ("ecstasy") abuse. Lancet 339:677–678

Segal A, Dowling JP, Ireton HJ, Rhodes H, Thomas GW, Kerr PG, Spagnolo DV (1998) Granulomatous glomerulonephritis in intravenous drug users: a report of three cases in oxycodone addict. Hum Pathol 29:1246–1249

Servais D, Schiwy-Bochat KH (1998) Beurteilung der Entzündungs-Intensität einer Hepatitis C-Virus Infektion mit Hilfe eines histologischen "Leberzellschaden-Index". Rechtsmedizin 8:229–231

Shah SV, Madhavan T, Saeed S, Levin NW, Quinn EL (1977) Focal glomerulonephritis and interstitial nephritis in methicillin-treated, heroin-related infective endocarditis. South Med J 70:1132–1134

Singhal PC, Gibbons N, Abramovici M (1992) Long term effects of morphine on mesangial cell proliferation and matrix synthesis. Kidney Int 41:1560–1570

Singhal PC, Sharma P, Gibbons N, Franki N, Kapasi A, Wagner JD (1997) Effect of morphine on renomedullary interstitial cell proliferation and matrix accumulation. Nephron 77:225–234

Singhal PC, Sharma P, Sanwal V, Prasad A, Kapasi A, Ranjan R, Franki N, Reddy K, Gibbons N (1998) Morphine modulates proliferation of kidney fibroblasts. Kidney Int 53:350–357

Smith WR, Glauser FL, Dearden LC, Wells ID, Novey HS, McRae DM, Reid JS, Sand BA, Newcomb KA (1978) Deposits of immunoglobulin and complement in the pulmonary tissue of patients with "Heroin Lung". Chest 73:471–475

Soni A, Agarval A, Chander P, Yoo J, Singhal D, Salomon N, Robinson B, Treser G (1989) Evidence for an HIV-related nephropathy: a clinico-pathological study. Clin Nephrol 31:12–17

Sreepada Rao TK (1993) A decade of human immunodeficiency virus-associated nephropathy (HIVAN). Transplant Proc 25:2439–2440

Sreepada Rao TK, Friedman EA (1989) AIDS (HIV)-associated nephropathy. Does it exist? Am J Nephrol 9:441–453

Sreepada Rao TK, Nicastri AD, Friedman EA (1974) Natural history of heroin-associated nephropathy. N Engl J Med 290:19–23

Sreepada Rao TK, Filippone EJ, Nicastri AD, Landesman SH, Frank E, Chen CK, Friedman EA (1984) Associated focal and segmental glomerulosclerosis in the acquired immunodeficiency syndrome. N Engl J Med 310:669–673

Sreepada Rao TK, Friedman EA, Nicastri AD (1987) The types of renal disease in the acquired immunodeficiency syndrome. N Engl J Med 316:1062–1068

Stone DS, Appel RG (1994) Human immunodeficiency virus-associated nephropathy: current concepts. Am J Med Sci 307:212–217

Tazelaar HD, Karch SB, Stevens BG, Billingham ME (1987) Cocaine and the heart. Hum Pathol 18:195–199

Tehan B (1993) Ecstasy and dantrolene. Br Med J 306:146

Tella SR, Schindler CW, Goldberg SR (1992) Cardiovascular effects of cocaine in conscious rats: relative significance of central sympathetic stimulation and peripheral neuronal monoamine uptake and release mechanism. J Pharmacol Exp Ther 262:602–610

Thomashefski JF Jr, Hirsch CS (1980) The pulmonary vascular lesions of intravenous drug abuse. Hum Pathol 11:133–145

Thorne LB, Collins KA (1998) Speedballing with needle embolization: case study and review of the literature. J Forensic Sci 43:1074–1076

Toth AR, Varga T (2009) Myocardium and striated muscle damage caused by licit or illicit drugs. Legal Med 11:S484–S487

Trauer H, Günzel A, Dreßler J (2015) Methamphatin-assoziierte Todesfälle bei gerichtlichen Sektionen im Bereich Leipzig/Chemnitz. Rechtsmedizin 25:350–351

Tsokos M, Erbersdobler A (2005) Pathology of peliosis. Forensic Sci Int 149:25–33
Vaghjimal A (1996) Splenic infarction related to cocaine use. Postgrad Med J 72:768
Wang Q, Ishikawa T, Michiue T, Zhu BL, Guan DW, Maeda H (2014) Molecular pathology of brain matrix metalloproteases, claudin5, and aquaporins in forensic autopsy cases with special regard to methamphetamine intoxication. Int J Legal Med 128:469–474
Wehner F, Mittmeyer HJ, Wehner HD, Schieffer MC (1998) Insulin – or morphine-injection? Immunohistochemical contribution to the elucidation of a case. Forensic Sci Int 95:241–246
Wehner F, Wehner HD, Schieffer MC, Subke J (2000) Immunohistochemical detection of methadone in the human brain. Forensic Sci Int 112:11–16
Wehner F, Mittmeyer HJ, Wehner HD (2002) Immunhistochemischer Morphinnachweis an der subkutanen Injektionsstelle. Rechtsmedizin 1:10–12
Welte TB, Bohnert M, Pollak S (2004) Prevalence of rhabdomyolysis in drug deaths. Forensic Sci Int 139:21–25
Zamora-Quizada JC, Dinerman H, Stadecker MJ et al (1988) Skin infarction after free-basing cocaine (crack). Ann Intern Med 108:564–566
Zeltner TB, Nussbaumer U, Rudin O, Zimmermann A (1982) Unusual pulmonary vascular lesions after intravenous injections of microcrystalline cellulose. Virchows Arch Pathol Anat 395:207–216
Zielezny MA, Cunningham EE, Veuto RC (1980) The impact of heroin abuse on a regional end-stage renal disease program. Am J Public Health 70:829–831
Zientara M, Moore S (1970) Fatal talc embolism in a drug addict. Hum Pathol 1:324–327

5 Toxin- and Drug-Induced Pathologies

There is a long history of histopathological findings induced by toxins and medication. A comprehensive list of iatrogenic histopathological findings is reported in the literature, e.g., incidents involving radiopaque substances and findings following radiation (e.g., Vock 1984; Lau 2005). Some iatrogenic histopathological findings, e.g., thorotrastosis, are rare today, while side effects of new medications have become more relevant. The literature on treating iatrogenic or drug-induced (medicamentous) injuries has become almost overwhelming, and the forensic literature also contains numerous case histories.

In forensic medical practice, toxin- and drug-induced histopathological findings are primarily used to determine cause of death, but occasionally a plausible explanation of clinical symptoms can only be provided after a forensic chemical toxicological analysis. Often, forensic autopsy yields nonspecific signs of intoxication, e.g., high-grade swelling of the brain and acute blood congestion of the viscera. Toxin-induced but in themselves nonspecific histopathological findings resulting from a reaction to legal or illegal substances are not uncommon, e.g., in the myocardium or in the striated skeletal musculature (Tóth and Varga 2009). Although numerous other substances can be readily determined in toxicological analysis, it is often the case that possible correlating histopathological findings cannot be causally and conclusively attributed to the ingested substances. Only in the case of sometimes patent overdoses is it possible to identify morphological findings in individual organs and attribute these to an active substance. For example, acetaminophen, an analgesic and antipyretic, can have hepatotoxic effects (Kubic et al. 2009). Moreover, one must bear in mind that histopathologically detectable findings are not necessarily the result of the use of a single substance, but rather that only the combined use of two or more substances can cause pathological changes, e.g., if a relevant but (as yet) unknown genetic disposition is present. It is by no means the case that only ever synthetic substances are involved—naturally occurring substances can of course also have a toxic effect depending on the dosage of herbs or other plant constituents (Gilbert et al. 2014; Byard and Musgrave 2010). A number of medications can cause (albeit it rarely or extremely rarely) severe toxic reactions involving the development of toxic agranulocytosis (e.g., carbimazole, a drug used for hyperthyroidism; Lynch and Woodford 2008).

Uncharacteristic histopathological findings have been described in inhaled or aspirated ingestion of acidic, alkaline, and volatile substances, such as necrosis, hemorrhage, and inflammatory reactions, sometimes in the form of chemical burns to the surfaces of the respiratory system and mostly the upper gastrointestinal tract (Amadasi et al. 2015; Advenier et al. 2014), similar to detergents (Kawamoto et al. 2013). Anticoagulant drugs are known to trigger internal bleeding, in particular phenprocoumon, which can also have a hepatotoxic effect (see Fig. 5.7), as well as

R. B. Dettmeyer, *Forensic Histopathology*, https://doi.org/10.1007/978-3-319-77997-3_5

various heparins (Ventura et al. 2014). Antibiotics and other drugs are believed to account for possible incidental findings of microscopic focal lymphocytic infiltrates and eosinophilic infiltrates in the myocardium (Zhang et al. 2013). Administering a substance in an unauthorized mode can also cause toxic reactions: for instance, the injection (combined with inhalation) of chloroform resulted in a systemic inflammatory reaction consistent with systemic inflammatory response syndrome (SIRS) (Dettling et al. 2016).

In addition to identifying clinical, symptomatic, acute, and long-term effects of medication and other pollutants (excluding illicit drugs in the narrower sense; see Chap. 4), e.g., heavy metals, microscopic examinations may be suitable to:

- Strengthen the chemical toxicological evidence of substances
- Provide grounds to conduct targeted toxicological analyses
- Lead to a diagnosis or explanation of findings which have been hitherto unclear
- Aid in determining cause of death
- Identify unknown bodies or body parts
- Prove iatrogenic injury
- Provide evidence of medication particles (Hecht and Lamprecht 2010)
- Establish relevance to insurance law in connection with chronic medication abuse (Markwalder 1983)

With the exception of allergic anaphylactic reactions, histomorphological findings are less expected in acute types of intoxication that cause death rapidly and are associated with lethal intoxication after a latent period of several hours, days, or even months.

In cases of intoxication caused by heavy metals, blood count changes have been characterized, e.g., toxic granulation of granulocytes or basophilic dotting of erythrocytes in lead and thallium poisoning. Acidophile intranuclear embedding in epithelia of the renal tubules may indicate survived lead intoxication. Intoxication caused by phosphoric acid ester and thiophosphoric acid ester can be shown by blocking the histochemically demonstrable acetylcholinesterase, together with the effects of blocking on unspecified esterases in blood monocytes (Oehmichen and Besserer 1982). However, these detection methods currently play a minor role in forensic practice in relation to intoxication caused by heavy metals.

In other cases, histomorphological findings are present but alone not specific to a defined intoxication. At the same time, intoxication may mimic natural disease patterns. The effect of toxins can also differ significantly: direct cytotoxic injury, secondary toxic-acting cell decomposition products, disruption of the cardiac circulatory system, decreased blood clotting, permeability injuries, imbalance of electrolytes, etc.

There is a wide spectrum of possible effects and side effects of drugs and medication. For this reason, it is necessary to restrict detection methods to essential, forensically relevant, and relatively frequent histopathological findings. Numerous iatrogenically caused findings can be macroscopically and histomorphologically demonstrated; however, they are rarely acutely relevant to cause of death, e.g.:

- Tissue calcification in the case of vitamin D therapy overdose (von Kossa staining)
- Silicon-induced splenomegaly
- Postoperative foreign-body-reactive granuloma (e.g., talcum powder granuloma)
- Tissue damage following radiation
- Dialysis-dependent analgesic nephropathy, e.g., phenacetin abuse (Markwalder 1983; Mihatsch et al. 1978, 1979)

In both general and specialized pathology, the topic of toxin- or medication-induced findings draws little attention. Depending on substance and genetic disposition, toxins may cause histomorphological changes in different organs (organotrophy) and cause undesired side effects (Table 5.1). Microscopic findings are often nonspecific but can, in part, demonstrate a toxic effect; sometimes, these findings alone, or in combination with toxicological analyses, enable an interpretation of results. Many substances cause microscopically demonstrable changes only after prolonged use, while some cause pathological findings with only one exposure.

Table 5.1 Forensically relevant histopathological drug-induced findings (selection)

Substance	Possible organotrophy and relatively common histopathological findings (list incomplete)
Accidental intrathecal injection of vincristine	Extensive necrosis of all spinal cord cells (see Chap. 1)
Allopurinol	Toxic epidermal necrolysis (Lyell's syndrome; Figs. 5.44 and 5.45); also described in connection with acetylsalicylic acid, phenacetin, barbiturate acid derivative, other analgesics, and antibiotics – Penicillin; Stevens–Johnson syndrome
Amiodarone	Lipofuscin deposits in the cornea
Anthraquinone-containing laxatives	Pseudomelanosis coli et recti (Fig. 5.2)
Antibiotics	Pseudomembranous colitis (Figs. 5.42 and 5.43)
Anticonvulsives	Epithelioid-cell granuloma in the liver parenchyma (Fig. 5.9)
Chloroform injection	Systemic inflammatory response syndrome (SIRS)
Contraceptives and anabolic steroids	Hepatic peliosis, focal nodular hyperplasia (FNH; Figs. 5.10, 5.11, and 5.12)
Cytostatics	Pulmonary hyaline membranes
Digoxin	Central pontine myelinolysis
Halothane	Liver necrosis
Herbicides, insecticides, solvents, aflatoxins, acetylsalicylic acid (ASS), valproinate	Fatty degeneration of internal organs, encephalopathy (Reye's syndrome)
Nonsteroidal antirheumatics (NSAR), e.g., diclofenac	Erosions and ulcers of the stomach mucosa
Olanzapine, carbimazole	Toxic agranulocytosis
Phenacetin	Suspicion of necrosis of the papilla tip of the kidneys with capillary sclerosis, so-called phenacetin kidney
Phenacetin, aminophenazone, or chlorpromazine abuse	Hepatocellular lipofuscin, pronounced at the center of the lobule, lipofuscin of Kupffer stellate cells following necrosis of lipofuscin-containing hepatocytes
Propoxur (2-isopropoxyphenyl-N-methylcarbamate), an insecticide	Intraalveolar, partially hemorrhagic pulmonary edema; varying degrees of hepatic steatosis; polymorphic cell nuclei in the hepatocytes with nuclear vacuoles; small, diffusely distributed glycogen droplets in the hepatocytes; necrosis of the renal tubular epithelial cells with predilection for the straight nephron segments; cloudy swelling and nuclear pyknosis of the renal tubular epithelial cells with marginal nucleoli; single and group hepatocyte necrosis depending on survival time (Pfordt et al. 1987)
Thorotrast	Polarization optical, birefringent deposits of thorium dioxide in the hypophysis, pulmonary interstitium, Kupffer stellate cells of the liver, spleen, lymph nodes, and renal pelvis
Thallium	Kidneys: swelling, vacuolization, coagulative necrosis, and autolysis in proximal convoluted tubules (Li et al. 2015)
Various medications, e.g., clozapine, diclofenac, penicillin, carbamazepine, ranitidine, etc.	Drug-induced myocarditis, often with eosinophilic granulocytes (Figs. 5.14, 5.15, 5.16, 5.17, 5.18, 5.19, 5.20, 5.21, 5.22, 5.23, 5.24, and 5.25)
Yellow phosphorus (ingestion of firecrackers)	Liver: massive necrosis around the portal region, acute inflammatory cells, macrophage, and bile duct proliferation with pseudoglandular formation, depending on survival time (Yilmaz et al. 2015)

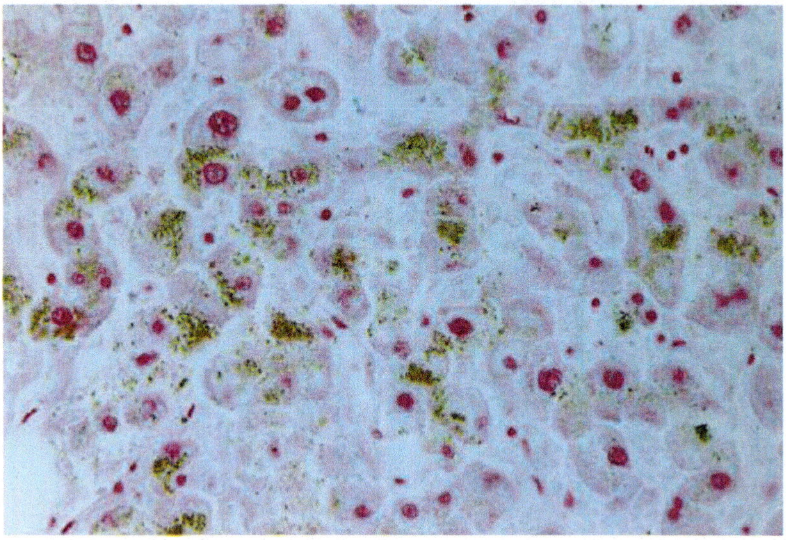

Fig. 5.1 Marked drug-induced hepatocellular lipofuscin in a 28-year-old female patient (Prussian blue ×100)

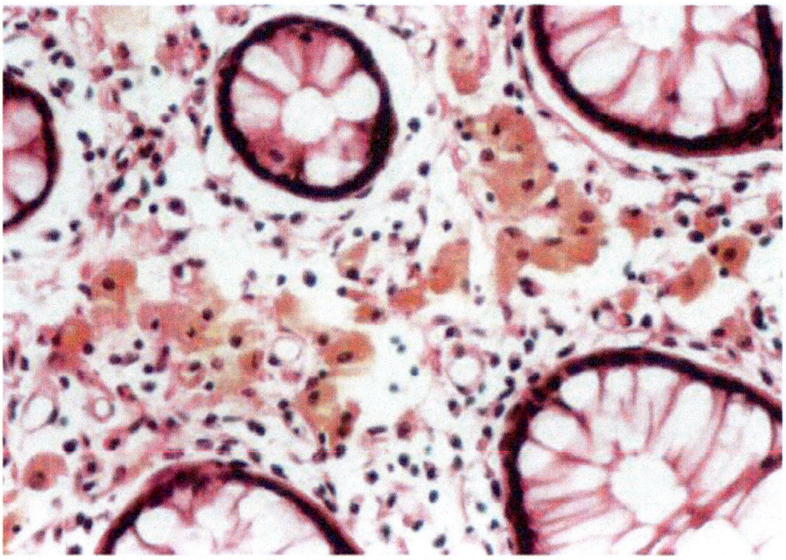

Fig. 5.2 Numerous macrophages in the mucosa of the large intestine with blackish-brownish pigments following anthraquinone-containing laxative abuse of many years' standing (H&E ×400)

For example, one result of long-term use of medication is a symptomless development of lipofuscinosis of the liver (Fig. 5.1), or pseudomelanosis coli et recti following long-term intake of anthraquinone-containing laxatives (Fig. 5.2), choleretics, or weight loss aids. One of the mild, nonspecific toxin- or medication-induced reactions is (often discrete) drug-induced hepatitis with intrahepatic cholestasis (Fig. 5.3). Finally, there are isolated reports of histopathological findings such as central pontine myelinolysis following digoxin use in severe vomiting (Unuma et al. 2010). In the case of drugs used on a large scale, there needs to be more than merely one case study on histopathologically detectable findings before a causal link between drug administration and the described findings can be assumed.

Some findings, although not discussed in detail here, should nevertheless be mentioned: phenacetin kidney (Gloor 1982); olanzapine-induced, toxic bone marrow depression (Dettling et al. 1999; Meissner et al. 1999; Naumann et al. 1999; Steinwachs et al. 1999); lethal liver necrosis following halothane narcosis (Wilbert and Creutzfeld 1967); and Lyell's syndrome and

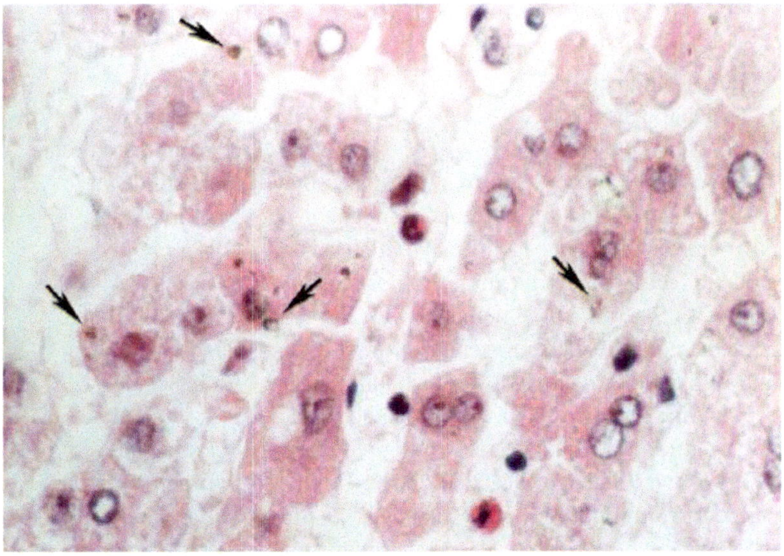

Fig. 5.3 Mild drug-induced hepatitis with discrete cholestasis (*arrows*) and without iron deposits (Prussian blue ×400)

Stevens–Johnson syndrome following allopurinol, as well as numerous other substances (Halevy et al. 2008). There are also rare cases of drug-induced necrotizing granulomatous arteritis (Symmers 1962), as well as random cases of pulmonary hyaline membranes following cytostatic therapy (Ulrich et al. 1982).

From the large spectrum of toxic and iatrogenic drug-induced histopathological findings, those most often described in the literature of forensic medicine should be mentioned, both in relation to individual organs and to the systemic effects or special type of application. The liver and kidneys are most commonly affected (see, e.g., Zimmerman and Ishak 2002; Shaohua et al. 2010; Gloor 1978).

5.1 Hepatotoxic Histopathological Findings

The liver belongs to the group of organs which most frequently show histopathological findings following ingestion of medications, drugs, and various toxins (Safrai 2007; Kasper et al. 2006; Zimmerman and Ishak 2002; Teschke 2001; Weber 1985; Machnik 1985; Rubin 1980; Zimmerman 1978). Mention should be made here of substances that necessarily cause generally dose-dependent liver damage (e.g., carbon tetrachloride), while others are harmful to the liver only in isolated cases in an unpredictable manner (e.g., hepatitis following halothane anesthetic, hepatocellular single-cell necrosis following oxyphenisatin and α-methyldopa use, cholestasis following chlorpromazine administration). Various histological findings may be seen depending on the type of toxin: hepatic steatosis, hepatocyte necrosis, cholestasis, bile duct lesions, fibrosis, and hepatic vein occlusions. Other findings include intralobular or portal infiltrations with lymphocytes, monocytes, and eosinophilic or neutrophilic granulocytes, as well as proliferation and/or hypertrophy of sinus endothelial cells, accompanied by prominent Kupffer cells. Eosinophilic leukocytes in particular are often found in patients with generalized hypersensitivity but also in the context of viral hepatitis or mechanical obstructive jaundice. Drug-induced liver damage may be caused by overdose, toxic metabolic processes, as well as allergic and immunological reactions. Risk factors, which can only be described in relation to the use of individual medications, include:

- Age
- Gender
- Genetic disposition (pharmacogenetic disposition)
- Body weight

- Fasting
- Ingestion of alcohol, drugs, etc.
- Renal dysfunction
- Metabolic disorder

Repeated exposure to a toxic substance may result in a new and severe reaction; alcohol or other enzyme-inducing agents may initiate a hepatotoxic reaction to medication. In most cases, a toxic reaction was not anticipated with the first administration, except in connection with a known overdose. An overdose of isoniazid, mercaptopurine (Thierauf et al. 2009), methotrexate, tetracyclines, and paracetamol will predictably result in liver damage (Teschke 2001). In most cases of drug-induced liver damage, a life-threatening progression is not anticipated. However, a selection of medicines is mentioned in the literature that may lead to granulomatous hepatitis, toxic liver cell necrosis, and lethal hepatic coma (according to Teschke 2001):

Allopurinol
Amiodarone
Amoxicillin plus clavulanic acid
Amphotericin B
Aurothiopropanol/-malate
Benoxaprofen
Carbromal
Carbimazole
Chlorpromazine
Clozapine
Cyproterone
Dacarbazine
Dactinomycin
Dantrolene
Desipramine
Dihydralazine
Disulfiram
Enflurane
Erythromycin
Flutamide
Halothane
Imipramine
Iproclozide
Indomethacin
Iproniazid
Isocarboxazid
Isoniazid
Mercaptopurine
α-Methyldopa
Minocycline
Natrium perchlorate
Nimesulide
Nortriptyline
Ofloxacin
Paracetamol
Phenylbutazone
Phenytoin
Probenecid
Propylthiouracil
Pyrazinamide
Pyrimethamine
Sulfasalazine
Tetracycline
Tiabendazole
Tolbutamide
Troglitazone
Valproic acid

Guidelines for the histological evaluation of drug-induced liver damage were published as early as 1975 (Bianchi et al. 1975). The main features of possible drug-induced findings in the liver can be found in Table 5.2.

5.1.1 Nonspecific Drug-Induced Hepatitis

Drug-induced liver damage includes a series of morphological findings. In the case of drug-induced or otherwise toxic hepatitis, the following are present:

- Hepatocellular single and/or group necrosis
- Granulomatosis of the liver
- Partially portal, partially lobular inflammatory reactions
- Often prominent Kupffer stellate cells and accompanying cholestasis of varying intensity
- Toxin-induced hepatic steatosis
- Accompanying eosinophilia
- Hepatocellular lipofuscin (Abrahams et al. 1964)

Table 5.2 Possible toxin- and drug-induced histological findings in the liver following ingestion of selected substances

Substance or medication	Histological findings	Staining method
Allopurinol	Nonspecific hepatitis, epithelioid-cell granuloma (Fig. 5.9)	H&E
Amphetamines (see Chap. 4)	Ubiquitous hepatocellular, areactive single-cell necrosis	H&E
Contraceptives, anabolic steroids (Thaler 1987; Baumgarten et al. 1981; Bagheri and Boyer 1974)	Hepatic peliosis, FNH	H&E, Gomori
Cortisone, cortisone derivate, tetracycline in therapeutic doses, tuberculostatics, phenylbutazone, ethanol (Thaler 1987; Altmann and Klinge 1972; Dölle and Martini 1962)	Intracytoplasmic, diffuse hepatic steatosis with fine and coarse nodules	Hematoxylin and eosin (H&E), fat staining, e.g., Sudan III
Phenacetin, aminophenazone, or chlorpromazine abuse (Thaler 1987; Altmann and Klinge 1972; Berneis and Studer 1967; Abrahams et al. 1964)	Hepatocellular lipofuscin: granular lipofuscin deposits in the cytoplasm of hepatocytes, more marked at lobule center, possibly lipofuscin of Kupffer stellate cells	H&E, Prussian blue to eliminate siderosis
Plasticizers in, e.g., silicone hoses and dialyzers (in hemodialysis patients) (Bommer et al. 1981, 1983)	Multiple granular foreign-body giant cells in the portal fields with embedded foreign material	H&E, polarization optical, birefringence
Prolonged glucocorticoid therapy (Itoh et al. 1977)	Vacuolar degeneration of the hepatocytes, hepatic steatosis, alcoholic hyaline, hepatic peliosis, FNH	H&E, Mallory staining, fat staining (e.g., Sudan III)
Prolonged ingestion of anticonvulsive agents (Hübner 1976)	Epithelioid-cell granulomatosis of the liver parenchyma	H&E
Transfusion siderosis (Oliver 1959; Morningstar 1955; Muirhead et al. 1949)	Iron pigment deposits in Kupffer stellate cells, possibly in hepatocytes (DD: hemochromatosis)	Prussian blue
Valproic acid (anticonvulsive agent)	Diffuse hepatic steatosis, possibly with necrosis to hepatic coma (in children: Reye's syndrome)	H&E, fat staining (e.g., Sudan III)

While cholestasis is strongly induced by canalicular bile thrombi, it is difficult to demonstrate both discrete intracellular deposits of bile pigments in the hepatocytes and Kupffer stellate cells using H&E staining. However, this dual staining can be performed using Prussian blue with a light counterstaining. In addition, it is possible to differentiate from iron pigment deposits (Bianchi et al. 1975). Cholestasis by itself is not an evidence of a toxic reaction to medication. The toxic reaction is apparent in inflammatory reactive hepatitis intralobularly and also with varying degrees of infiltration of the portal fields via lymphocytes, histiocytes, eosinophilic or neutrophilic granulocytes, and prominent sinus endothelial cells. The bile duct epithelium can be completely free of inflammation, but bile duct lesions are also possible. There are severe forms of necrosis (Fig. 5.4), cell decomposition, Councilman bodies, as well as diffuse vacuolization and hydropic swelling as an expression of degenerative changes of hepatocytes. In addition, Kupffer stellate cells are activated. On the one hand, there is no reliable differentiation of microscopic findings in cases of progressed autolysis and early decomposition, while on the other, there are intense inflammatory processes with the result that acute viral hepatitis must be considered in the differential diagnosis, e.g., if marked infiltration of T-lymphocytes can be determined (Fig. 5.5). Concomitant hepatic steatosis counterindicates viral hepatitis (exception: drug addicts). In addition, Kupffer stellate cells are typically activated, which can be clearly shown at the margin of liver sinusoids (Fig. 5.6). The degree of expression of drug-induced hepatitis may vary drastically and may be significant in individual cases (Fig. 5.7). Diagnostic reliability

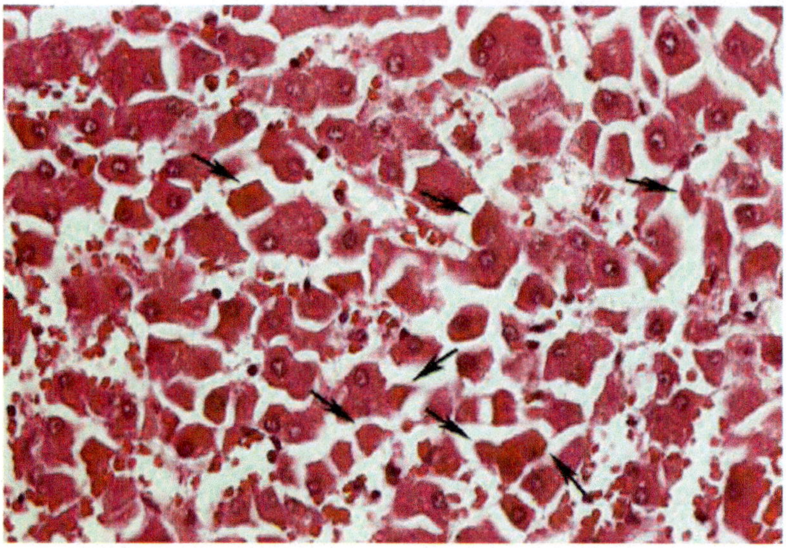

Fig. 5.4 Evenly pronounced metamizole-related, drug-induced hepatitis with hepatocellular single-cell necrosis (*arrows*) showing a homogenous, eosinophilic cytoplasm – clinically known as metamizole intolerance (H&E ×400)

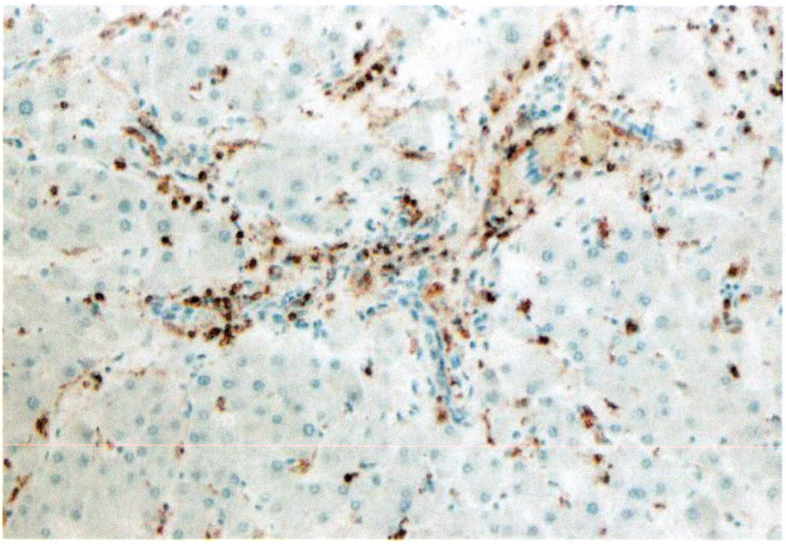

Fig. 5.5 Immuno histochemically CD45-positive T-lymphocytic inflammatory infiltrates in the liver with nonspecific drug-induced hepatitis; in the differential diagnosis, consideration should be given to viral hepatitis, which was eliminated here with the help of serological examinations (×200)

for the purpose of differentiating from postmortem autolytic changes gradually increases with the number of microscopically examined samples.

Hepatic steatosis may occur as a reaction to medication, including toxic fatty liver, for example, when caused by medications which adversely impact mitochondrial β-oxidation, such as valproic acid, aspirin, or tetracycline (Krähenbühl and Kaplowitz 1996). One reason for the variation in findings is seen in the differing pharmacogenetic conditions, although certain empirical data exist. It is known, for example, that chlorpromazine causes cholestasis with a relatively mild portal or lobular inflammatory reaction, whereas other medications cause hepatic changes (Bianchi et al. 1975). Halothane anesthesia may lead to precisely demarcated necrotic zones in the liver, whereas numerous other medications can show the clinical picture of granulomatous hepatitis. The histological diagnosis of drug-induced cholestasis is, ultimately, a diagnosis of exclusion. The commonly used Marcumar, for example, can cause nonspecific drug-induced hepatitis, as does

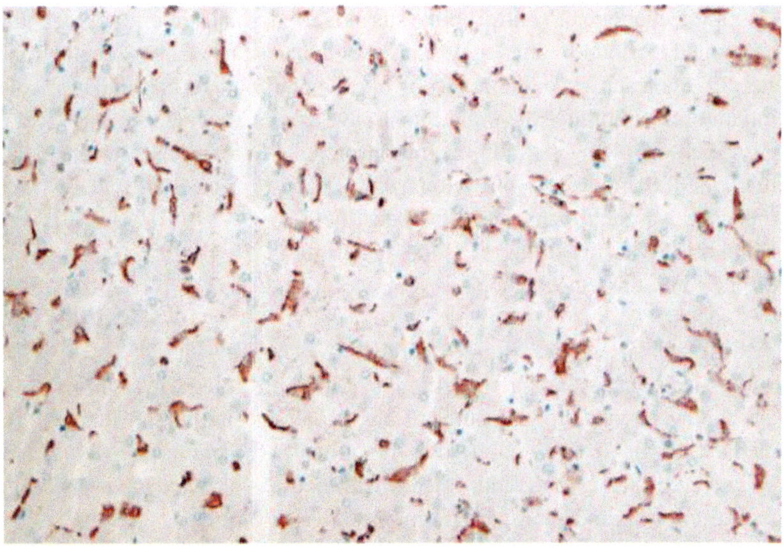

Fig. 5.6 Immuno histochemically marked detection of Kupffer stellate cells in the liver with the macrophage marker CD68 – clinically known as metamizole intolerance (×200)

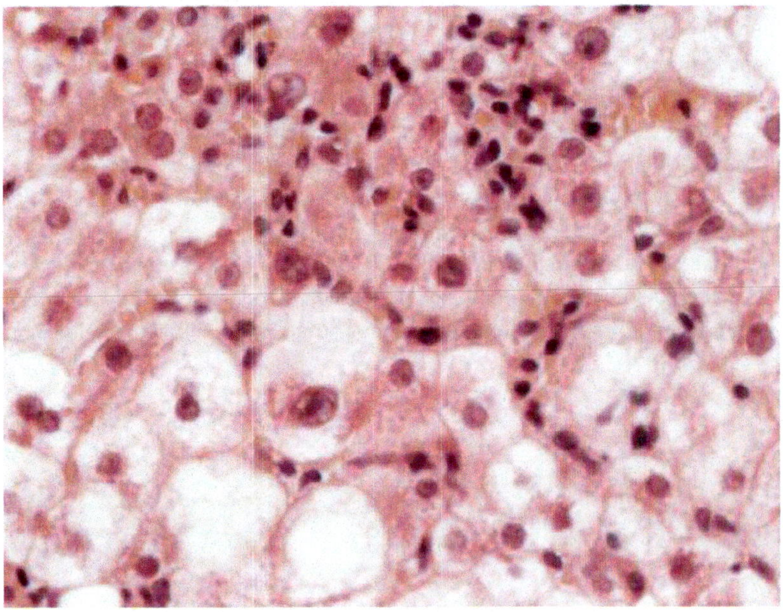

Fig. 5.7 Drug-induced hepatitis following phenprocoumon (Marcumar®) ingestion (H&E ×400)

metamizole. In certain cases, nonalcoholic hepatic steatosis may be caused by medication therapy, e.g., long-term glucocorticoid therapy (Itoh et al. 1977).

Liver damage caused by medication can occur within several days (e.g., unwanted repeated exposure, tetracycline, halothane), over several weeks (e.g., chlorpromazine, C-17 alkyl steroids), or months (e.g., α-methyldopa). Drug-induced liver damage is also possible several weeks after the medication has been ceased. Combinations of medicines can also have a hepatotoxic effect, e.g., when simultaneously ingested with herbal preparations. Some Chinese herbal mixtures are said to contain potentially hepatotoxic medicines. Substances which cause cytochrome P450 2E1 induction may promote liver damage (particularly alcohol); St. John's wort may induce cytochromes P450 3A4 and 1A2 (active component: hypericin).

Taking anabolic or contraceptive steroids for a prolonged period of time may cause so-called steroid cholestasis, possibly with intralobular inflammation. Intrahepatic granulomas have been described following the administration of halothane, sulfonamides, or phenylbutazone. Drug-induced vascular changes include hepatic peliosis, as well as forms of Budd–Chiari syndrome (e.g., thrombosis, hepatic vein occlusion, or stenosis).

Case reports on lethal intoxication cover a wide spectrum, including in particular children and the deceased following suicidal ingestion of medication or toxins. Numerous functionally effective medicines may cause death with acute ingestion of toxic dosing without morphological changes, especially antiarrhythmics, such as pilsicainide and atenolol (Hikiji et al. 2008). This may also be valid for β-blockers, even though an unspecific fine-vacuolar transformation in the cytoplasm of hepatocytes was observed with regular overdosing and finally lethal β-blocker intoxication (own findings as yet unpublished; Fig. 5.8). It would appear, however, that strychnine intoxication does not necessarily produce histopathological changes (Prat et al. 2015).

Epithelioid-cell granulomas and epithelioid-cell granulomatous hepatitis are rarely demonstrated and described, e.g., after ingestion of anticonvulsive agents or allopurinol (Fig. 5.9).

In particular, steroids may lead to changes in the liver, such as focal nodular hyperplasia (FNH) and peliosis hepatis (PH), after long-term ingestion.

5.1.2 Hepatic Peliosis and Focal Nodular Hyperplasia

A great number of medications, substances (including illicit drugs), and diseases may cause hepatic peliosis, as well as focal nodular hyperplasia. However, in general, these findings are rare.

Hepatic Peliosis This is a rare entity, histologically characterized by the presence of scattered, small, blood-filled cystic spaces throughout the liver parenchyma (Figs. 5.10 and 5.11). Over the years, reports have been published linking hepatic peliosis to many underlying pathological conditions.

The primary triggers of hepatic peliosis include anabolic or ovulation-inhibiting steroids – excluding, however, hormone-producing granular cell

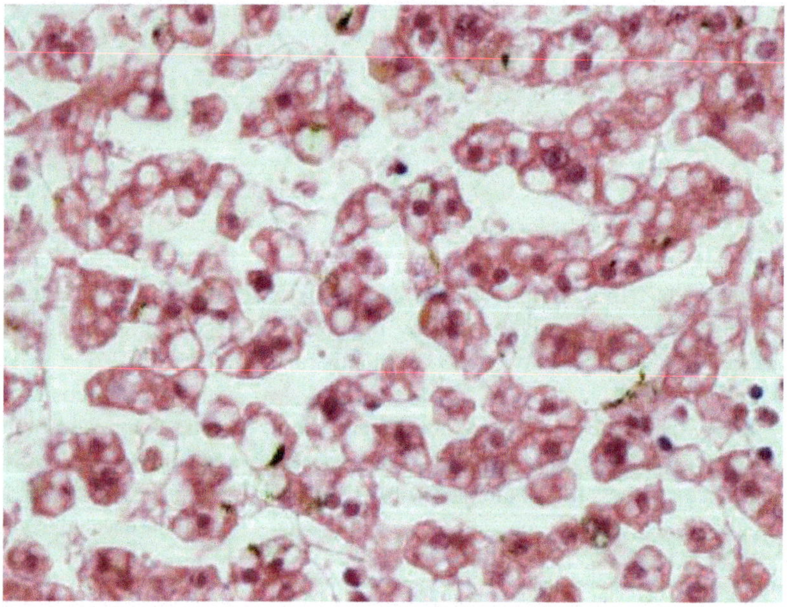

Fig. 5.8 Intra cytoplasmic, unspecified microvacuolar transformation of hepatocytes in chronic β-blocker intoxication proven using hair analysis in a female with no cardiac disease and no medical indication for β-blocker administration. No lipid-containing vacuoles in Sudan III staining (H&E ×200)

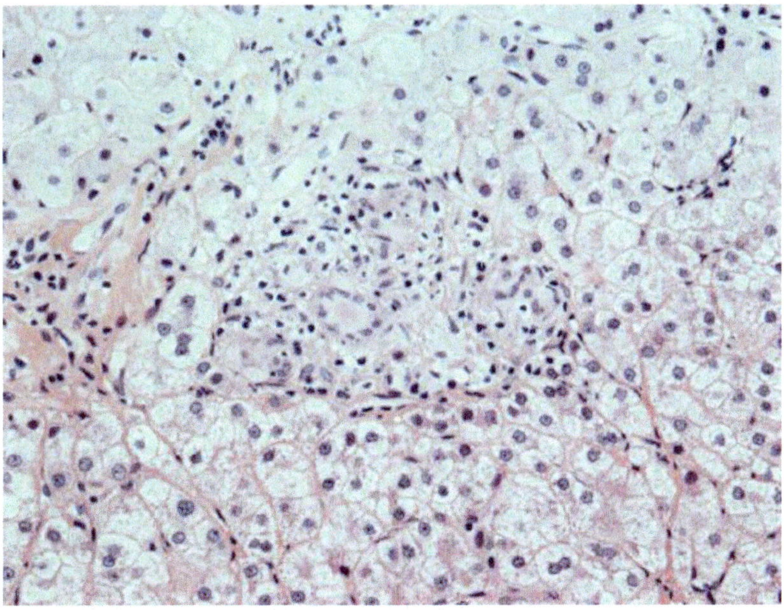

Fig. 5.9 Epithelioid-cell granulomatosis of the liver after ingestion of allopurinol (H&E ×400)

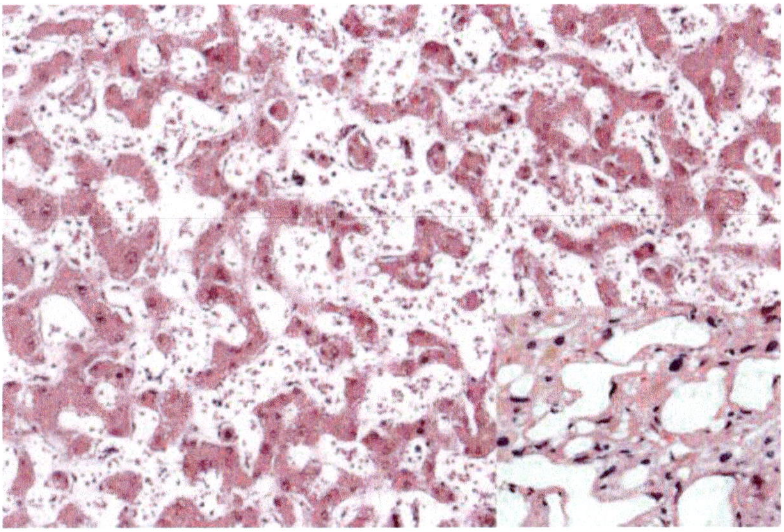

Fig. 5.10 Hepatic peliosis with enlarged liver sinusoids and rarefied liver cell trabeculae (H&E ×200; H&E ×400)

tumors (Tzirogiannis et al. 2006; Tsokos and Erbersdobler 2005; Knudsen 2002; Nuzzo et al. 1985; Schonberg 1982; Asano et al. 1982; Kalra et al. 1976; Bagheri and Boyer 1974; Burger and Marcuse 1952). In some cases, generalized hepatic peliosis may appear (van Erpecum et al. 1988). Hepatic peliosis has also been mentioned in connection with tuberculosis (Zak 1959), as well as with long-term intravenous drug use.

The enlarged liver sinusoids are linked via central veins or sublobular veins (Thaler 1987; Valla and Benhamou 1988). The developing stagnant blood or cavities have a diameter ranging from several millimeters up to 5 cm. The rupture of subcapsular peliosis centers may cause acute lethal hemoperitoneum; however, children are rarely affected (Karger et al. 2005). Although the pathogenesis of hepatic peliosis remains unclear, local destruction of the perisinusoidal mesh fiber network, which is better demonstrated using Gomori's staining, has been suggested.

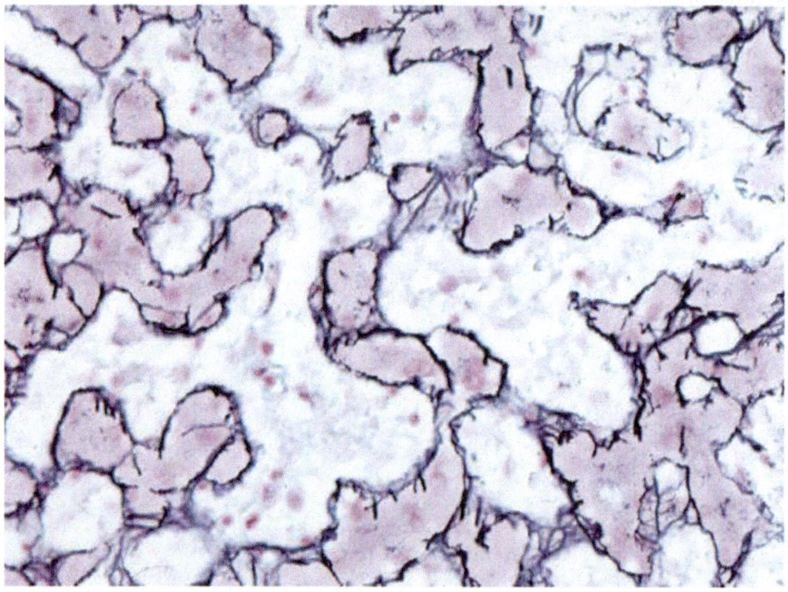

Fig. 5.11 Hepatic peliosis (same case as in Fig. 5.10) in Gomori's stain (×400)

Hepatic peliosis can be detected in focal nodular hyperplasia (FNH), a centralized change to liver tissue which may also appear following ingestion of oral contraceptives, anabolic steroids, and/or glucocorticoids (Wittstock 1983). Isolated peliosis of the spleen, characterized by the gross appearance of multiple cyst-like, blood-filled cavities on the cut surface of the organ, is a very rare pathological entity (Tsokos and Püschel 2004).

Focal Nodular Hyperplasia (FNH) This knot-shaped hyperplasia of up to 5 cm in size is not encapsulated but can be macroscopically detected due to its brown-red or yellow-red color with a sharp border to neighboring liver tissue. The hyperplastic parenchyma of FNH has nodular subsections connected with larger areas and often contains elevated glycogen or fat; cholestatic changes may also occur. The septa leading to the knotty subsection often show inflammatory infiltration, significant capillarization, and may contain bile duct proliferates (Thaler 1987) (Fig. 5.12). Oral contraceptives may cause FNH, in addition to hepatic vein thrombosis (Asbeck et al. 1972).

5.1.3 Hepatic Lipofuscin

As in other organs, lipofuscin deposits can be found in hepatocytes with increasing age, albeit with great variability (so-called brown atrophy of the liver). An unusually pronounced deposit of lipofuscin pigment in the cytoplasm of hepatocytes in relation to age may occur in the setting of side effects caused by medication (Abrahams et al. 1964). Medicines mentioned in this context include phenacetin, aminophenazone, and chlorpromazine. Rather coarse granular deposits of lipofuscin are involved, and the lobular center is typically more affected than the lobular periphery. If hepatocytes are destroyed, lipofuscin in Kupffer stellate cells can also be observed (Fig. 5.1).

5.1.4 Transfusion Siderosis of the Liver

Iron overload may occur, in particular, when numerous blood transfusions are administered, yielding the microscopic diagnosis of transfusion siderosis (Oliver 1959; Morningstar 1955;

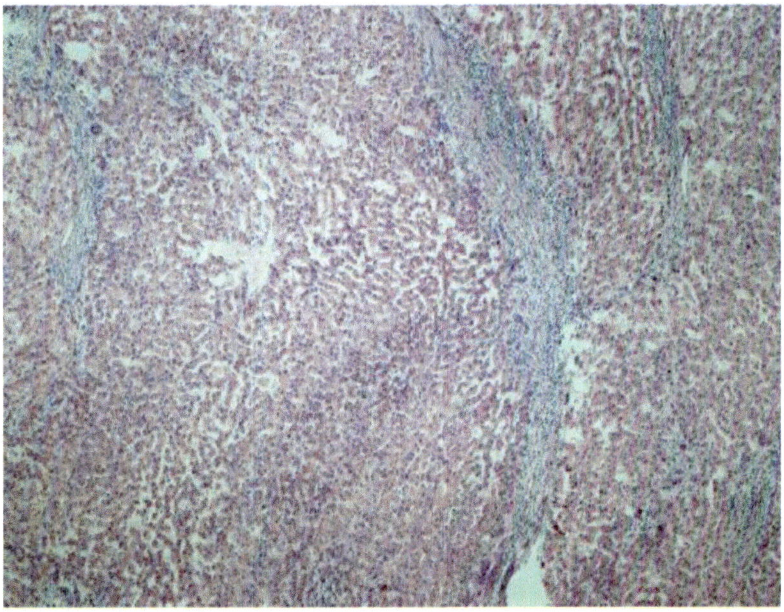

Fig. 5.12 Microscopic focal nodular hyperplasia in liver tissue after long-term contraceptive use (H&E ×200)

Muirhead et al. 1949): using Prussian blue staining, strong stellate cell siderosis with less-intense accompanying hemosiderin deposits in the cytoplasm of the hepatocytes can be observed in the liver in cases of mild to moderate expression (Fig. 5.13a). If iron overload continues, hepatocytes will eventually be entirely filled with hemosiderin. In such cases, differential diagnostic consideration should be given to hereditary hemochromatosis (Fig. 5.13b). Siderosis of the myocardium rarely occurs following administration of multiple transfusions (Thurner 1970).

Failed transfusions or the use of incompatible blood types may lead to phagocytosis of foreign erythrocytes (erythrophagia).

In forensic practice, both long-term side effects of medications or toxins and acute intoxication caused by substances ingested unknowingly, knowingly, or with suicidal intent (e.g., quinine, colchicine, fungal poison, heavy metal intoxication, arsenobenzene intoxication, among others) or administered (potentially with intent to harm) should be evaluated when establishing the cause of death. Accidental poisoning can occur in connection with fungal poison, e.g., *Amanita* and the leaves and flowers of other plants found in nature, such as meadow saffron, laburnum, or red foxglove.

5.2 Histopathology of the Cardiotoxic Effects of Selected Medications: Drug-Induced Myocarditis

Cardiotoxic medications may cause acute death even in the absence of abnormalities in the patient history (Lewis and Silver 2001). Histological examinations may result in clarification when the cause of death cannot be macroscopically explained. Drug-induced myocarditis is shown by eosinophilic leukocytes (Fig. 5.14), not seldom accompanied by a lymphomonocytic inflammatory infiltrate, myocardial single-cell necrosis, and cardiomyocytes which in some cases reveal a homogeneous, eosinophilic cytoplasm.

The histological picture does not allow a conclusion in regard to the triggering medication, but it may provide a rationale to conduct toxicologic examinations, e.g., hair analysis to check for long-term ingestion of foreign substances. In regard to

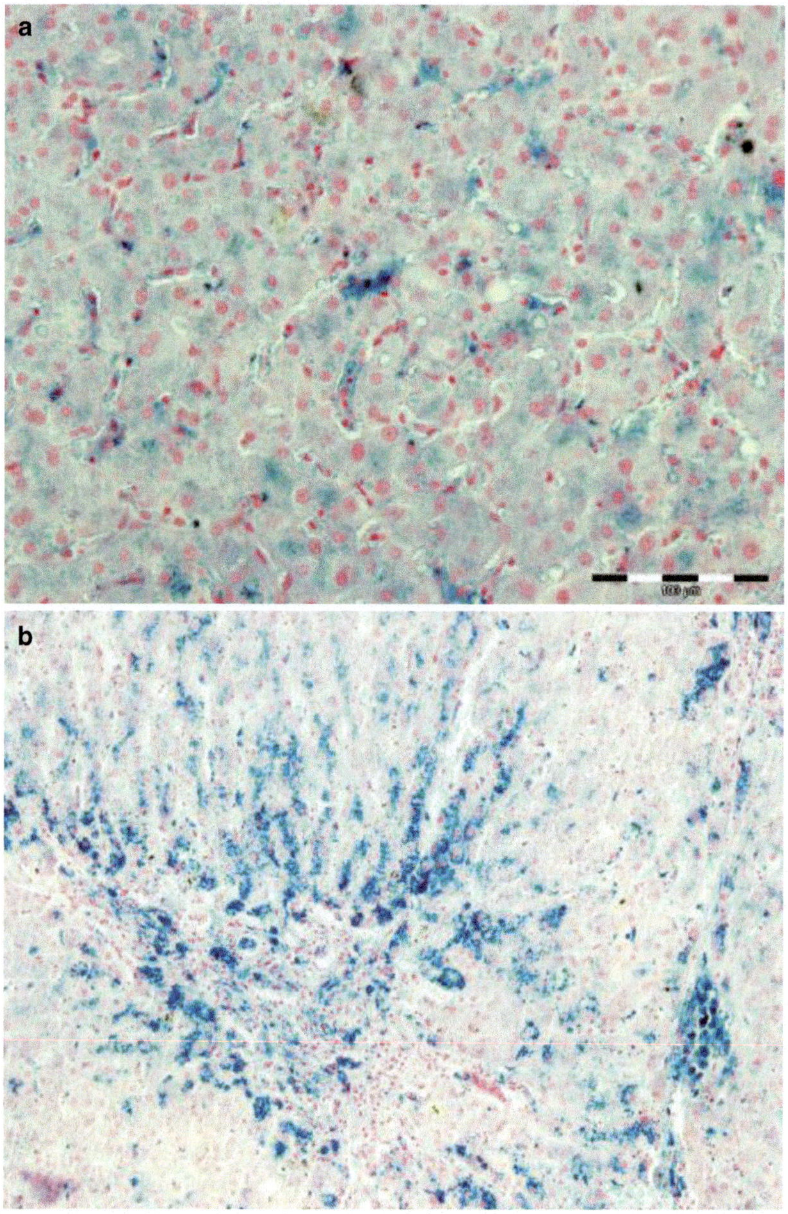

Fig. 5.13 Transfusion siderosis of the liver with overload of hepatocytes and Kupffer stellate cells (**a**) and a case of hereditary hemochromatosis (**b**) (Prussian blue ×200)

sudden unexpected death of psychiatric patients ingesting atypical neuroleptics, drug-induced myocarditis must also be considered; however, there may also be other causes (Gradinger et al. 2008). Although often the case, eosinophilic leukocytes are not always predominant. Rarer substances, e.g., paraphenylenediamine (PPD), an aromatic derivative of aniline frequently used as an ingredient in cosmetics, can also trigger toxic myocarditis in some cases (Jedidi et al. 2016). There are also individual reports of acute lymphocytic myocarditis following monoclonal antibody treatment (adalimumab) and development of biventricular cardiac decompensation (Arzneimittelkommission der Deutschen Ärzteschaft 2016). Drugs such as carbamazepine and ranitidine can also cause toxic myocarditis in extremely rare cases (Arsenovic et al. 2010).

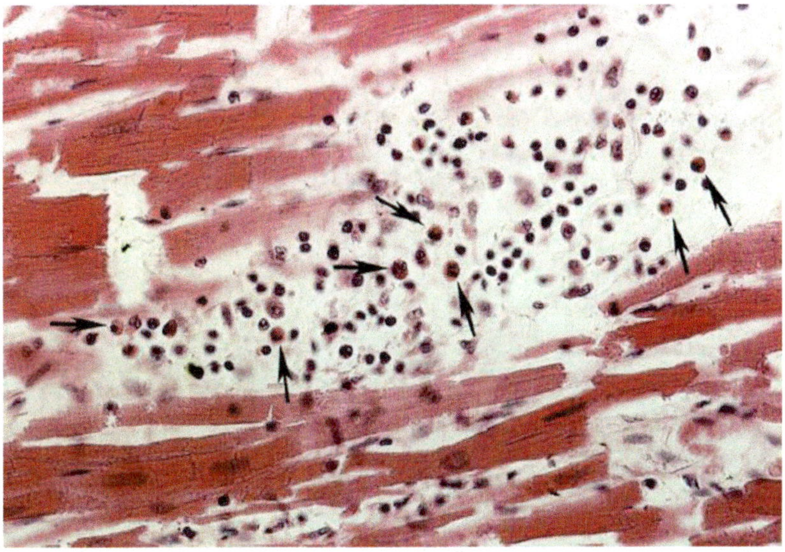

Fig. 5.14 Suspected drug-induced myocarditis with eosinophilic leukocytes (*arrows*) and accompanying lymphocytes and macrophages (H&E ×400)

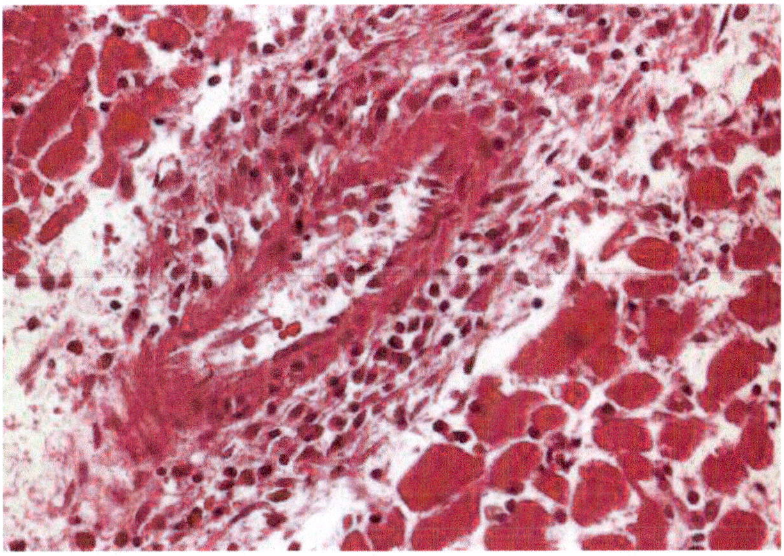

Fig. 5.15 Marked intramyocardial inflammatory infiltrate in the perivascular area in a case of clozapine-induced myocarditis (H&E ×400)

Clozapine Myocarditis Clozapine is a valuable drug for patients with treatment-resistant schizophrenia. Myocarditis is the most publicized cardiac complication of clozapine treatment, but cardiomyopathy and pericarditis have also been reported (Layland et al. 2009). Drug-induced myocarditis has been described particularly in cases of clozapine (an atypical neuroleptic) administration (Kakar et al. 2006; Razminia et al. 2006; Merrill et al. 2005, 2006; Fitzsimons et al. 2005; Pieroni et al. 2004; Wehmeier et al. 2005; Kilian et al. 1999).

In cases of clozapine-induced myocarditis, a lymphomonocytic inflammatory infiltrate may be present, particularly in the perivascular region (Fig. 5.15), and there may even be septum-like extension to the myocardium (Fig. 5.16). The endothelium of peripheral arterioles shows expression of the proinflammatory marker E-selectin (Fig. 5.17), as well as the MHC class II molecules (Fig. 5.18). T-lymphocytes (Fig. 5.19) and macrophages (Fig. 5.20) can, in part, be detected in large quantities, and myocardial

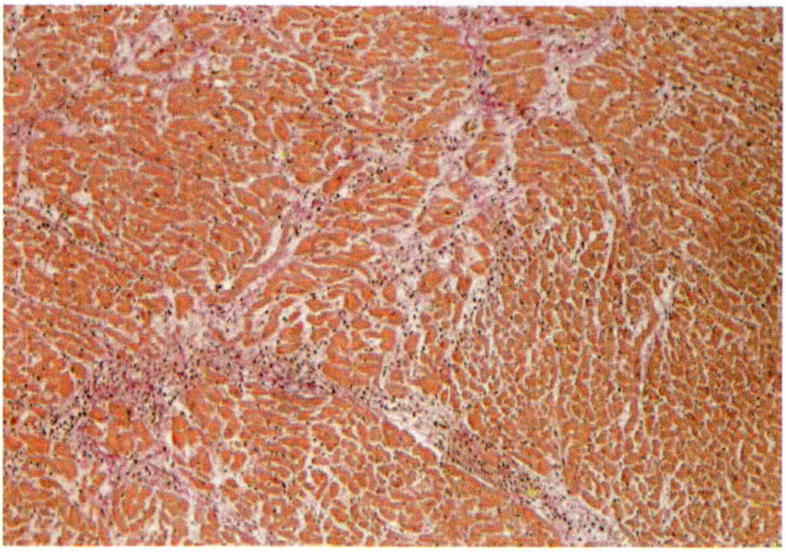

Fig. 5.16 Septum-like extension of the inflammatory infiltrate to the myocardium in clozapine myocarditis (EvG ×100)

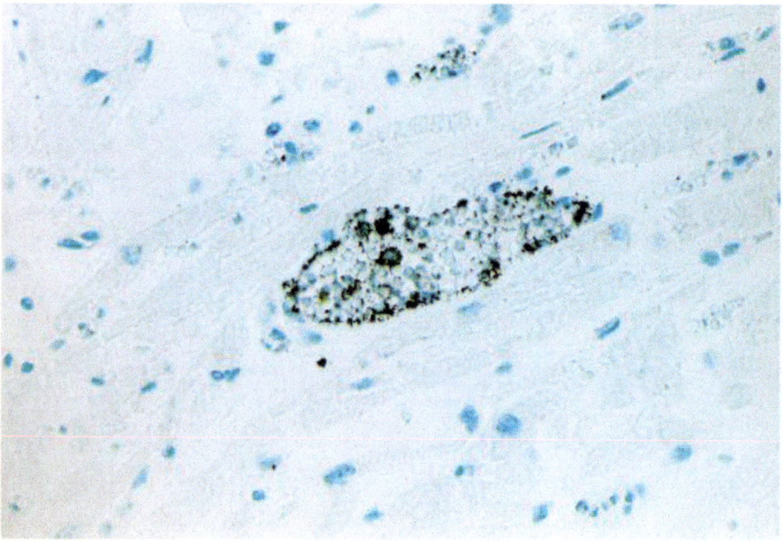

Fig. 5.17 Expression of proinflammatory E-selectin in the endothelium of intramyocardial arterioles and capillaries in clozapine myocarditis detected postmortem (×400)

necrosis, also as single-cell necrosis, can be detected with the necrosis marker C5b-$9_{(m)}$ (Fig. 5.21). As little as one-off use of clozapine can cause death, albeit extremely rarely (Stanworth et al. 2012).

The morphological picture of drug-induced myocarditis may in fact vary. While clozapine-induced myocarditis shows perivascular septal enlargement, myocarditis may show a different histological picture due to the analgesic diclofenac, a nonsteroidal antirheumatic agent (NSAR).

Diclofenac Myocarditis In the case of the rarely occurring diclofenac-induced myocarditis, localized inflammatory infiltrates can be found with myocardial necrosis and focal, relatively well-demarcated inflammatory necrosis advancing toward the myocardium. Neighboring cardiomyocytes are destroyed or show homogeneous eosinophilia. Between inflammatory cells and neighboring areas, e.g., in the subepicardial fatty tissue, loosely distributed eosinophilic leukocytes can be observed (Figs. 5.22, 5.23, 5.24, and 5.25).

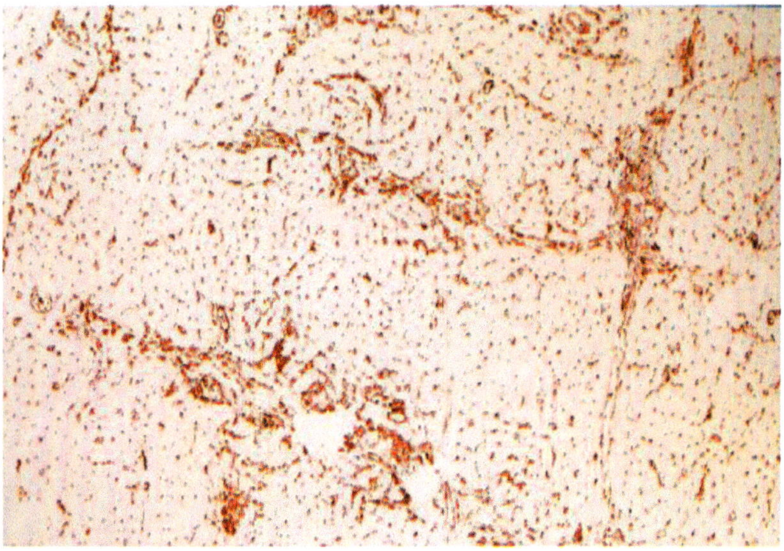

Fig. 5.18 Marked expression of MHC class II molecules in clozapine myocarditis (×100)

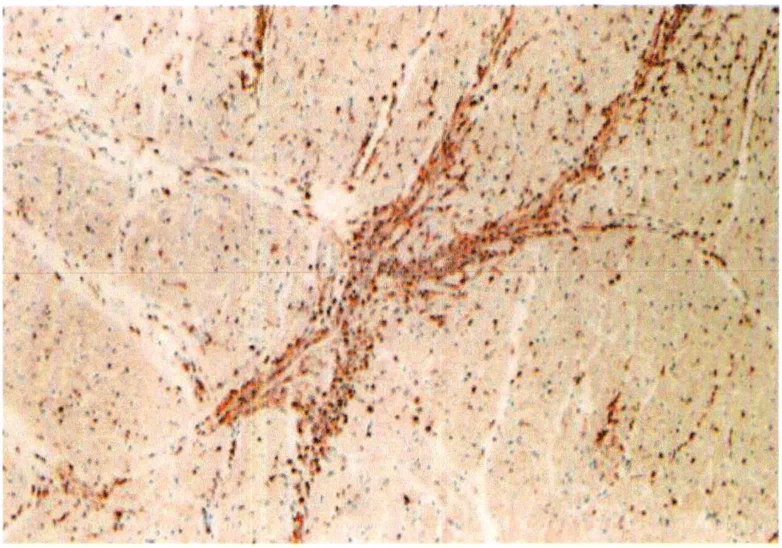

Fig. 5.19 Inflammatory infiltrate with involvement of abundant CD45R0-positive T-lymphocytes in clozapine myocarditis (×100)

Ultimately, histological findings may vary in cases of drug-induced myocarditis and show diverse pictures depending on stage, with flowing transitions between varying forms. Findings shown with the help of optical microscopy include eosinophilic, homogeneous degeneration, as well as atrophy and hypertrophy of cardiomyocytes. In addition to varying cell and nucleus sizes, myocardial necrosis, fibrosis, and vacuolar transformation of the cytoplasm of cardiomyocytes are described; an uneven arrangement of heart muscle fibers and accompanying edema, as well as the appearance of resorptive processes with granulation tissue containing branched capillary blood vessels, has also been described.

The suspicion of drug-induced, lethal myocarditis may be raised solely on the basis of microscopic findings. However, if possible, toxicological evidence of a triggering agent is required, as well as the exclusion of a competing cause of death and, most crucially, a corresponding patient

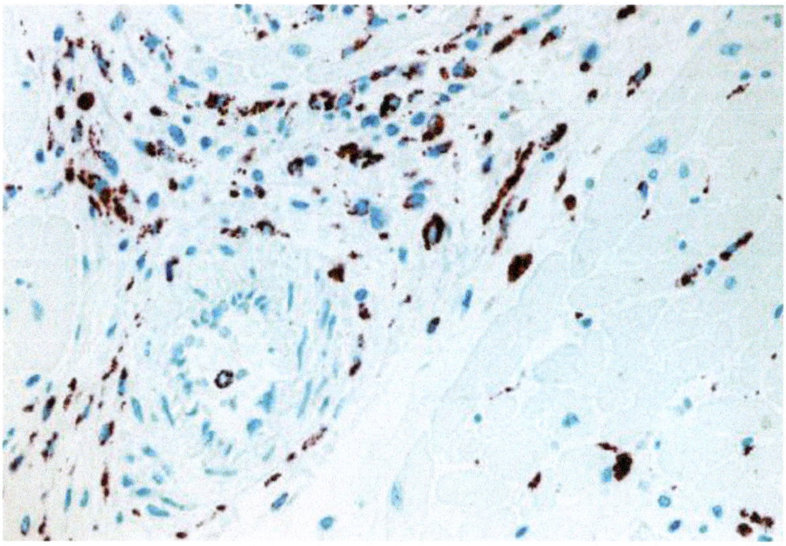

Fig. 5.20 Clozapine myocarditis with abundant perivascular macrophages (CD68 ×400)

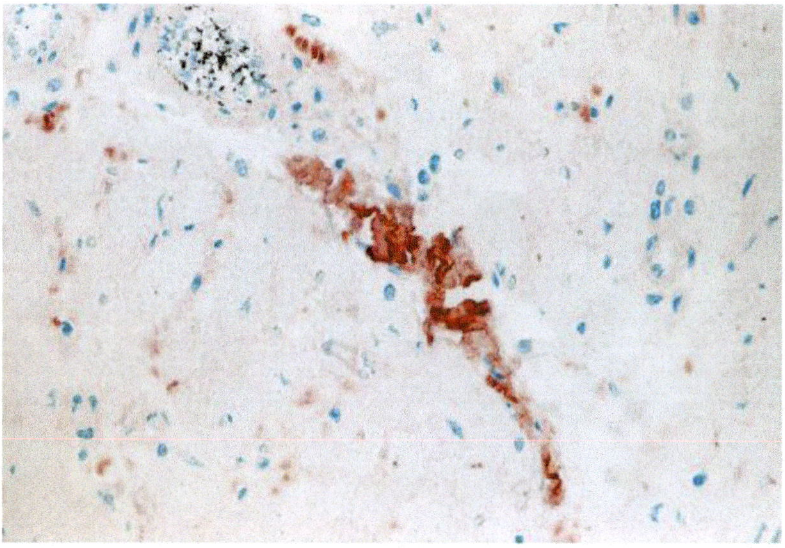

Fig. 5.21 Isolated myocardial necrosis demonstrated with the necrosis marker C5b-$9_{(m)}$ (×400)

history demonstrating relatively recent ingestion of the medication.

Naturally, numerous other drugs can cause rare, isolated cases of often eosinophilic hypersensitivity myocarditis; this has been described for, e.g., carbamazepine (Arsenovic et al. 2010), paraphenylenediamine (Brahmi et al. 2006), and ranitidine (Kendell et al. 1995).

In addition to rare fatal side effects, such as drug-induced myocarditis, toxic reactions to drugs are also seen primarily in the liver and kidneys. The literature refers in particular to psychotropic drugs. For example, evidence of serotonin toxicity or neuroleptic malignant syndrome (NMS) following intoxication with fluvoxamine and lithium has been seen, involving the development of a hyperthermic state, apparently mild rhabdomyolysis, and myoglobin proteins in the kidneys (Mannou et al. 2014).

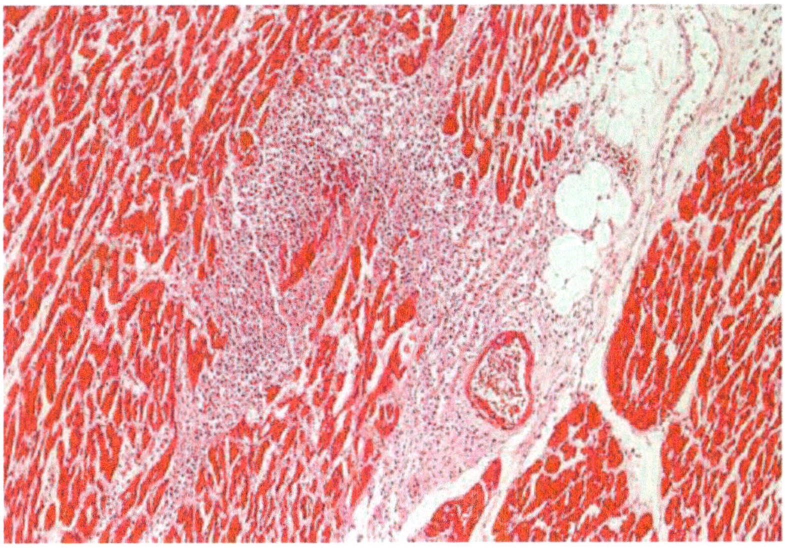

Fig. 5.22 Prompt onset of myocarditis after first ingestion of diclofenac, as proven by toxicological examinations, with focal lymphomonocytic infiltration and necrosis (H&E ×100)

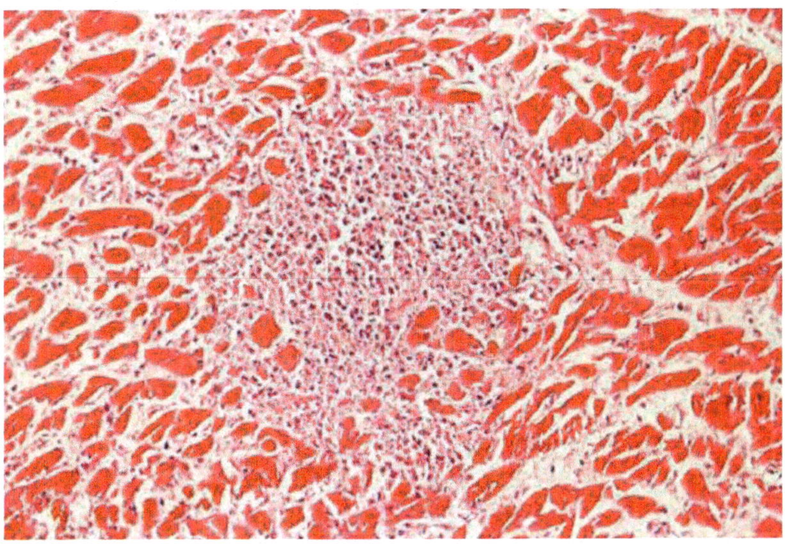

Fig. 5.23 Focal, relatively well-demarcated inflammatory necrosis advancing toward the myocardium in a case of diclofenac-induced myocarditis (H&E ×200)

5.3 Histopathology of Other Special Intoxications

Many microscopic findings may point to intoxication but do not allow for additional precise statements concerning the cause of findings. Alternately, intoxications may lead to histopathological findings which diagnostically point to particular substances or prove the ingestion of a specific substance. A number of reports point to histopathological findings detected following oral use of toxic substances depending on survival time. These can be synthetic or plant toxins. Findings such as necrosis, inflammation, and resorption responses in the mucosa of the mouth, esophagus, and gastrointestinal tract have been described especially in children following (accidental) ingestion of solvents or disinfection agents, e.g., 35% hydrogen peroxide or acids (Indurato et al. 2014; Advenier et al. 2014; Aquila et al. 2014; Meatherall and Oleschuk 2015).

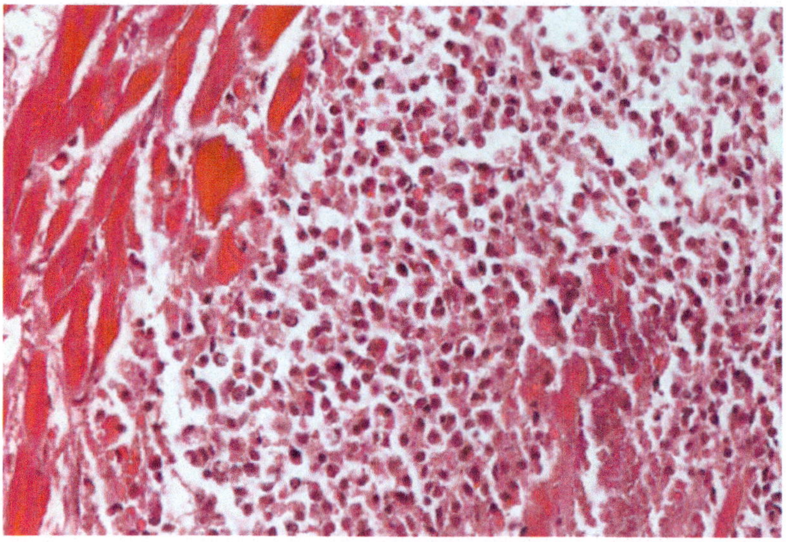

Fig. 5.24 Localized inflammatory destruction of the cardiomyocytes with necrosis and partially homogenous eosinophilia of the cytoplasm – diclofenac myocarditis (H&E ×400)

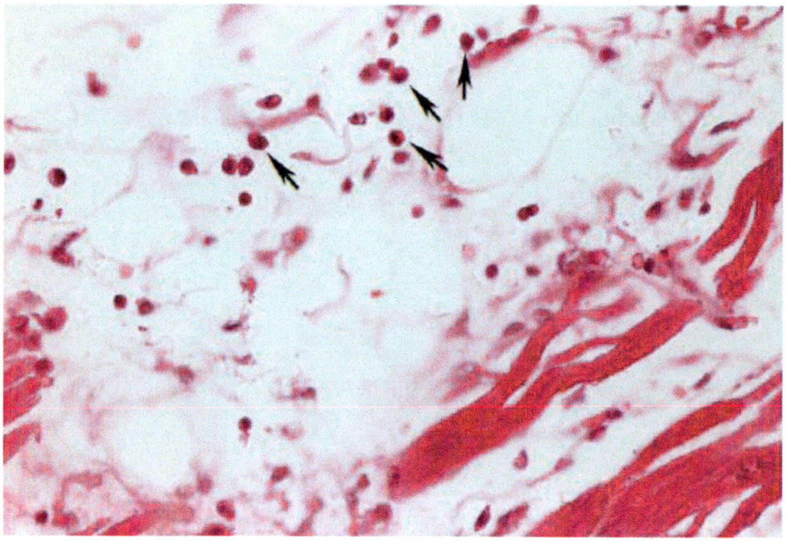

Fig. 5.25 Loosely distributed eosinophilic granulocytes (*arrows*) in the subepicardial fatty tissue in a case of diclofenac myocarditis (H&E ×400)

5.3.1 Special Histopathology in the Case of Colchicine Intoxication

Lethal intoxication with colchicine, e.g., following accidental ingestion of tea made with bear's garlic leaves (Wollersen et al. 2009a) (Fig. 5.26), shows a comparable histopathological picture to other intoxications with fine-vacuolar transformation of hepatocyte cytoplasm and sometimes nuclear vacuoles. This histopathological finding in the liver is similar to that previously described for other substances, e.g., following pesticide intoxications (Saleki et al. 2007). According to personal experience, it is found relatively often in connection with various toxins (e.g., also in chronic intoxication with β-blockers).

Colchicine is a liposoluble alkaloid of meadow saffron (*Colchicum autumnale*) but is also found in bear's garlic (*Allium ursinum*). The similarity

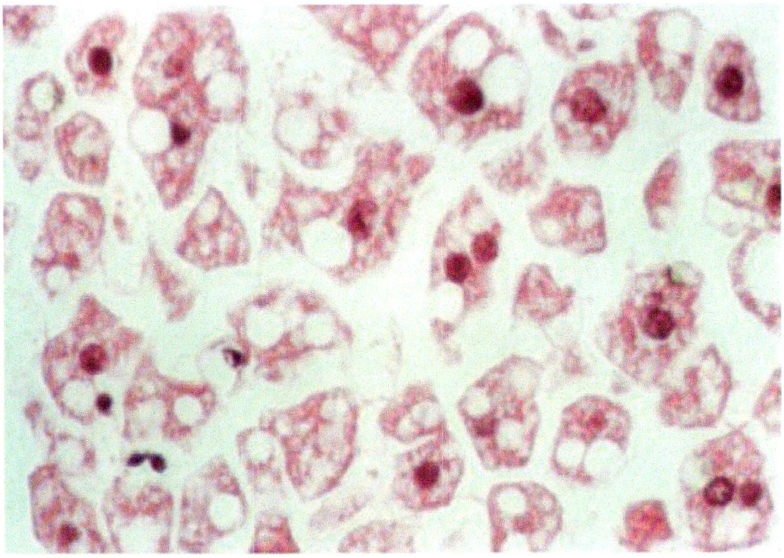

Fig. 5.26 Fine-vacuolar intracytoplasmic transformation of the hepatocytes in lethal colchicine intoxication – colchicine concentration of 65 ng/mL in femoral vein blood (H&E ×200)

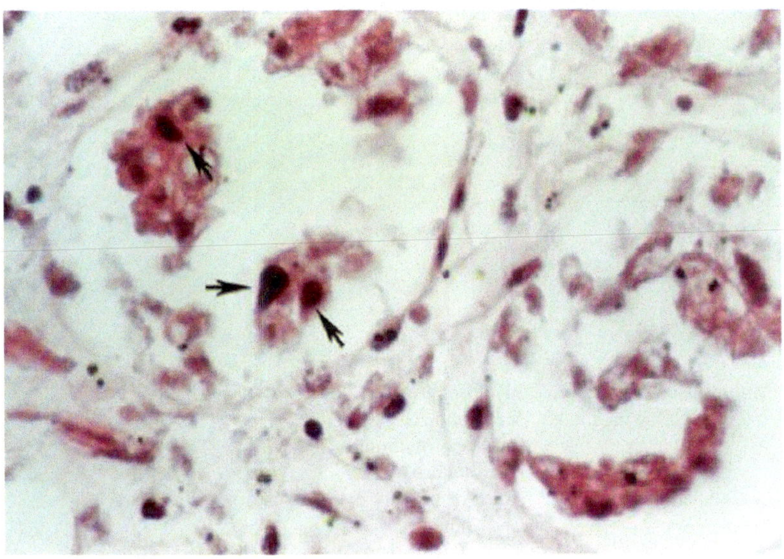

Fig. 5.27 Despite advanced autolysis, clear evidence of unevenly enlarged and hyperchromatic cell nuclei (*arrows*) in the epithelium of the intestinal mucosa in cases of colchicine intoxication (H&E ×400)

between the two plants may lead to misidentification (Wollersen et al. 2009a). Colchicine has an antimitotic effect and causes an increased number of reactive mitoses on intoxication. These reactive mitoses can be proven at autopsy in non-keratinizing squamous epithelium of the esophagus and in gland epithelium of the gastrointestinal tract, depending on autolysis or decomposition (Sannohe et al. 2002; Gilbert and Byard 2002; Iacobuzio-Donahue et al. 2001; Stemmermann and Hayashi 1971; Roll and Klintschar 1999; Klintschar et al. 1999; Yamada et al. 1998; McIntyre et al. 1994; Clevenger et al. 1991; Allender 1982).

In addition, it is possible to show unevenly enlarged, hyperchromatic cell nuclei in the surface epithelium, particularly of the gastrointestinal tract (Fig. 5.27). Clinical symptoms and histological findings are listed in Table 5.3. Differential diagnostic consideration should be given to intoxication with aconitine (Pullela et al. 2008).

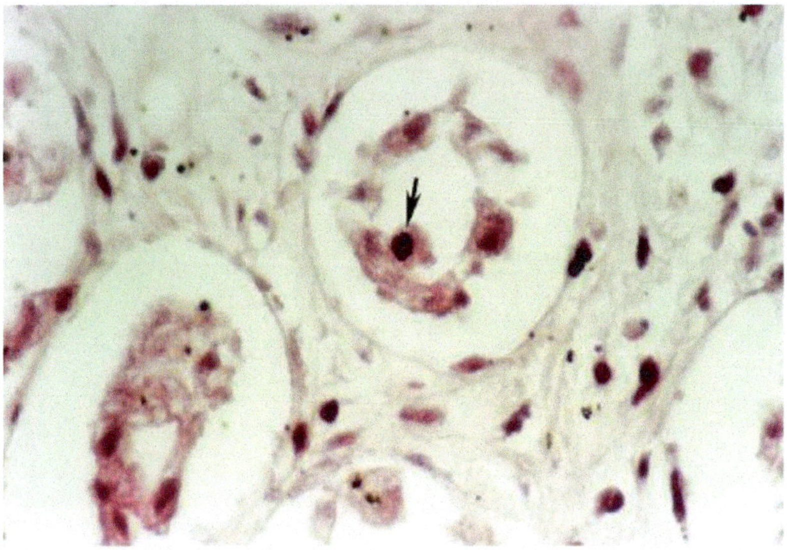

Fig. 5.28 Single mitoses (*arrow*) in the intestinal epithelium can be seen with marked autolysis in cases of colchicine intoxication (H&E ×400)

Table 5.3 Clinical symptoms and histopathological findings in colchicine intoxication with a phase-like course

Phase	Clinical symptoms	Histopathological findings
Gastrointestinal phase: 0–24 h following intake	Nausea, vomiting, abdominal pain, bloody diarrhea, electrolyte imbalances, hypovolemia, tachypnea, leukocytosis, salivation	• Herbal components in stomach contents • Focal hepatocellular necrosis • Increased number of mitoses in: • Basal cell layers of non-keratinizing squamous epithelium of the esophagus • Mitosis in the respiratory epithelium of the bronchi • Mitosis in the gland epithelium of the gastrointestinal tract (Fig. 5.28) • Fine-vacuolar transformation in hepatocyte cytoplasm
Multiorgan dysfunction: 1–7 days following intake	Myelosuppression Metabolic acidosis Cardiac arrhythmia Heart failure Acute respiratory distress syndrome Liver failure Kidney failure Impaired coagulation Secondary sepsis Impaired consciousness Neurological symptoms, including cramps and paralysis	

Cases of iatrogenic overdose are seen. For example, colchicine is used in the treatment of gout, as well as familial Mediterranean fever and Behçhet disease. Since colchicine has a narrow therapeutic index, fatalities following its medical prescription have been described (Mullins et al. 2011; Finkelstein et al. 2010; Yamazaki et al. 2013).

5.3.2 Special Histopathology in Cases of Ethylene Glycol Intoxication

Ethylene glycol is sweet and odorless; ingestion may be accidental, as a substitute for ethanol, or with suicidal intent (Takahashi et al. 2008; Lovrić et al. 2007; Leth and Gregersen 2005; Hantson et al. 2002; Cavender and Sowinski 2001), but seldom in connection with cases of intentional homicide (Armstrong et al. 2006). The abusive consumption of ethylene glycol may cause severe or lethal intoxication depending on the quantity consumed (Leth and Gregersen 2005; Hantson et al. 2002; Ammar and Heckerling 1996; Aderjan and Joachim 1988). Symptoms of intoxication are uncharacteristic: vomiting, dizziness, cramps, mild hypotonia, tachycardia, and light fever. Also described are nystagmus, ophthalmoplegia, and papilla edema, followed by atrophy of the optical nerve, weakening reflexes, generalized or focal cramp attacks, and tetanic contractions. Initially, moderate leukocytosis with an increased number of polymorphonuclear cells, proteinuria, and microhematuria are seen. Calcium oxalate crystals can be found relatively early in urine (Jacobsen et al. 1982). Severe intoxication with ethylene glycol will lead to death within 24–48 h in most cases. Reports of longer survival times are seldom (Takahashi et al. 2008). Characteristic histopathological findings following ethylene glycol intoxication are found particularly in the kidneys and brain (Parry and Wallach 1974) in the form of crystalline deposits of oxalates (oxalosis) (Frohberg et al. 2006). There are extremely rare reports of oxalate crystal deposits in cardiomyocytes, accompanied by fibrosing myocarditis (Pikula et al. 1973). Additional histopathological findings are described in Table 5.4.

In cases of ethylene glycol intoxication, the characteristic deposits of calcium oxalate crystals may undergo postmortem decomposition via autolytic decomposition processes, whereupon depending on the level of severity, it may no longer be possible to prove their presence.

Even without special staining, crystalline deposits are detectable with H&E staining (Fig. 5.29) and can substantiate the suspicion of ethylene glycol intoxication (Wollersen et al. 2009b). Calcium oxalate crystals are visible using the von Kossa staining as black-brown deposits, also without polarimetric diagnosis (Figs. 5.30 and 5.31).

Following initial survival of ethylene glycol intoxication, the calcium oxalate crystals may persist, particularly in the brain (Fig. 5.32) and in renal tissue (chronic oxalosis; Fig. 5.33), leading to protracted kidney failure (Desilva and Mueller 2009). In such cases, massive birefringent crystalline deposits can be seen (Nizze et al. 1997), particularly in the proximal renal tubules (Hovda et al. 2010; McMartin 2009). There are reports of single cases of intracerebral, bipallidal hemorrhage (Caparros-Lefebvre et al. 2005), while laser scanning microscopy investigations were conducted by Pomara et al. (2008). In rare cases, histopathological findings such as those found following ethylene glycol intoxication can be induced by consuming xylitol (Pfeiffer et al. 2004; Heye et al. 1991; Ludwig et al. 1984; Evans et al. 1973; Thomas et al. 1972).

Table 5.4 Histopathological findings in cases of ethylene glycol intoxication

Sample	Findings
Blood	Increased number of polymorphonuclear cells
Urine	Calcium oxalate crystals
Heart	Petechial hemorrhage, subepicardial, subendocardial, and intramyocardial; rarely, oxalate crystals in cardiomyocytes and fibrosing myocarditis
Lung	Pulmonary edema, subpleural and intrapulmonary hemorrhages, bronchopneumonia
Kidney	Dilated proximal renal tubules, intratubular calcium oxalate crystals, intracellular crystals, especially in the proximal renal tubules, no definite glomerular damages
	With longer periods of survival: progressive interstitial fibrosis, tubular atrophies, deposit of polarization optical, birefringent crystals
Brain	Edema, acute congestion hyperemia, petechial hemorrhage, calcium oxalate crystals in the vessel walls of intracerebral and meningeal vessels, also perivascular and rarely bilateral hemorrhage in the pallid globe (Caparros-Lefebvre et al. 2005)
Other	Vessel walls of other internal organs may also show crystalline calcium oxalate deposits

5.3.3 Lethal Death Cap Intoxication

Death caps (*Amanita phalloides*) are highly poisonous mushrooms, leading to the rapid destruction of liver tissue (toxic hepatosis), the development of blood clotting disorders (general hemorrhagic diathesis), and sudden death with development of toxic brain edema, similar to that

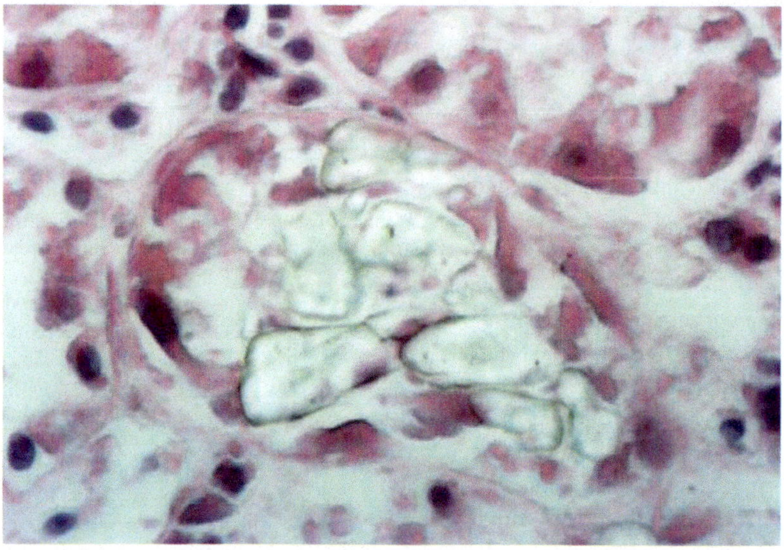

Fig. 5.29 Crystalline deposits visible intratubular in H&E stained kidney section following ethylene glycol intoxication (H&E ×400)

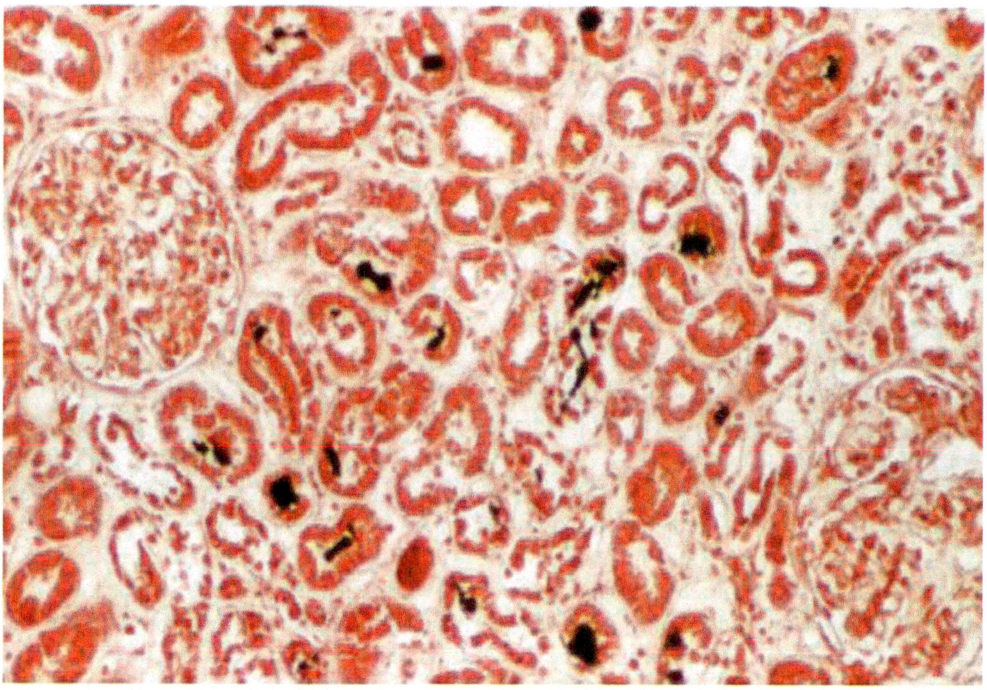

Fig. 5.30 Calcium oxalate crystals inside the lumina of the renal tubules (von Kossa ×100)

seen in connection with other poisonous mushrooms (Magdalan et al. 2009; Barthel and Gerber 1962; Wölkart et al. 1954). With the white and green death cap, liver tissue undergoes significant destruction between the third and fifth day following fungal toxin ingestion.

In some cases, histological examinations of the contents of the stomach and intestines may show plant-based components of the mushroom, as well as fungal conidia on the gastric or intestinal mucosa (Figs. 5.34 and 5.35). The epithelial cells of the gastric and intestinal mucosa may

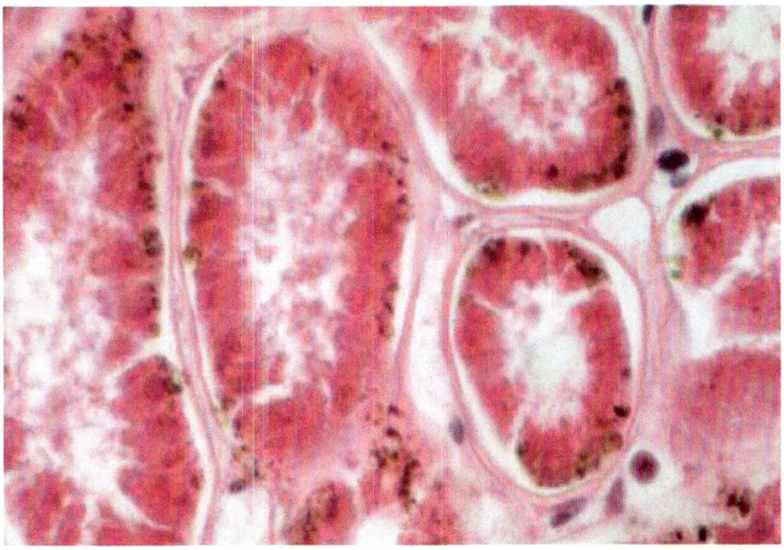

Fig. 5.31 Calcium oxalate crystals in basal parts of the renal tubular epithelium (von Kossa ×400)

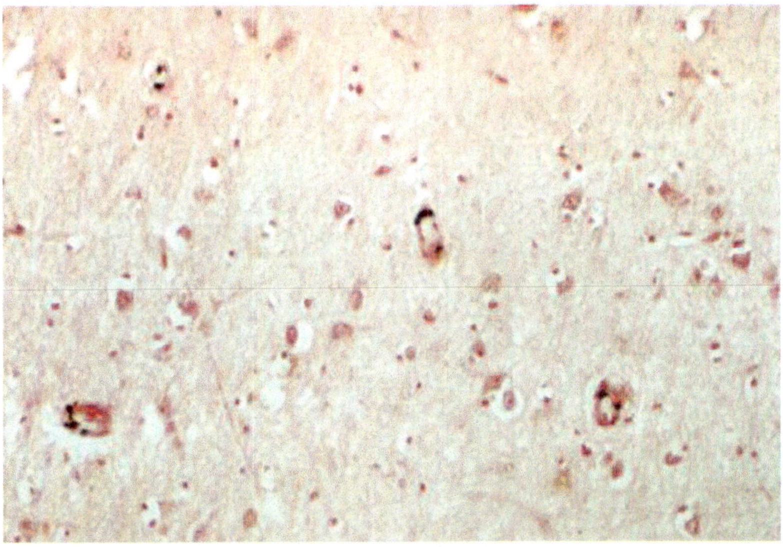

Fig. 5.32 Calcium oxalate crystals in the walls of intracerebral vessels (von Kossa ×100)

show significant cell and nucleus polymorphy (Fig. 5.36). As a consequence of the failing blood clotting system, laminar hemorrhage can be seen both at autopsy and histologically, e.g., in the gastric mucosa (Fig. 5.37). It is possible that at the time of death, fungal conidia are found in the interstitium of the lamina mucosae. At the time of death, the liver tissue has been largely destroyed and is necrotic with hemorrhage. The functional structure of the liver tissue is dissolved; in addition to intracytoplasmic vacuolization, there are deformed hepatocytes with pyknotic, hyperchromatic nucleoli. There may also be single and group hepatocyte necrosis, Kupffer stellate cell necrosis, and diffuse coarse nodular hepatic steatosis (Figs. 5.38 and 5.39). Similar histological findings in the liver may be found with phosphorus and tetrachloride carbon intoxication: the histological findings are not specific to lethal death cap intoxication. In cases of tetrachloride carbon intoxication, there may be additional fat embolism (Lahl 1973).

The ingestion of plant-based foodstuff components as such can be microscopically demonstrated

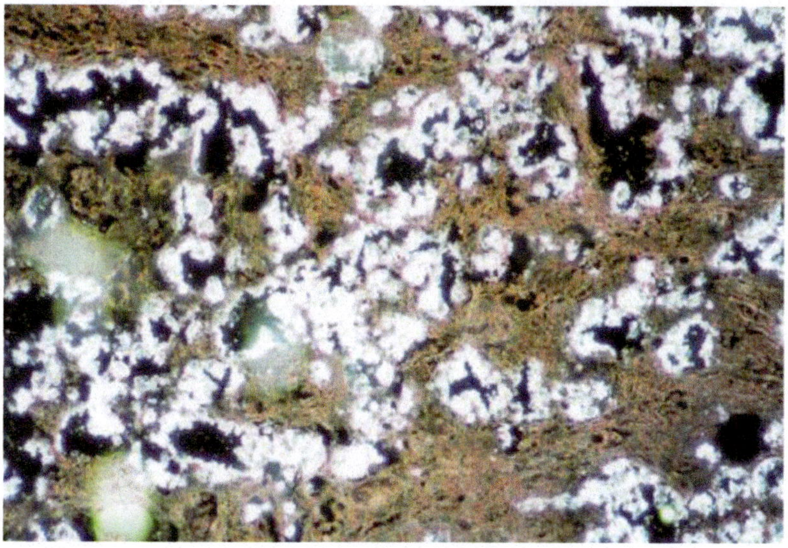

Fig. 5.33 Multiple polarization optical, birefringent oxalate crystals in chronic oxalosis (×200)

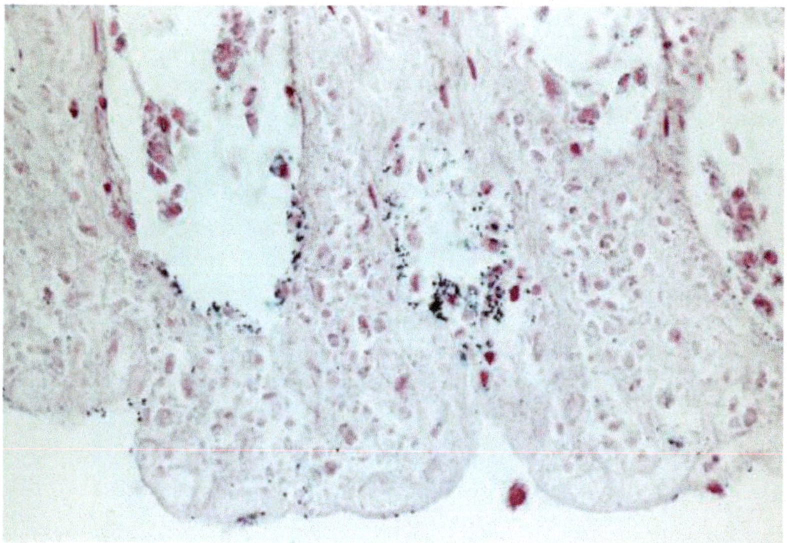

Fig. 5.34 Autolytic stomach mucosa with deposited fungal components (fungal conidia) following accidental ingestion of death cap in food (Grocott ×400)

in cases where death occurs promptly and where corresponding findings can be seen in the esophagus, stomach, or small intestine (Fig. 5.40).

Histologically identified plant components only seldom enable a conclusion on toxicity or even on the type of plant consumed. This may be possible only in individual cases when very characteristic plant components can be found to support the suspicion of a particular form of intoxication, e.g., the detection of yew needles in stomach contents. The use of herbal polypharmacy, even in the context of traditional herbal medicine, can cause acute liver necrosis in isolated cases, at least as described in a case of preexisting chronic hepatitis B (Gilbert et al. 2014).

5.3.4 Histopathological Findings in Anabolic Abuse

After prolonged use of oral anabolic steroids, severe cardiovascular side effects may develop, including myocardial infarction, stroke, enlargement of

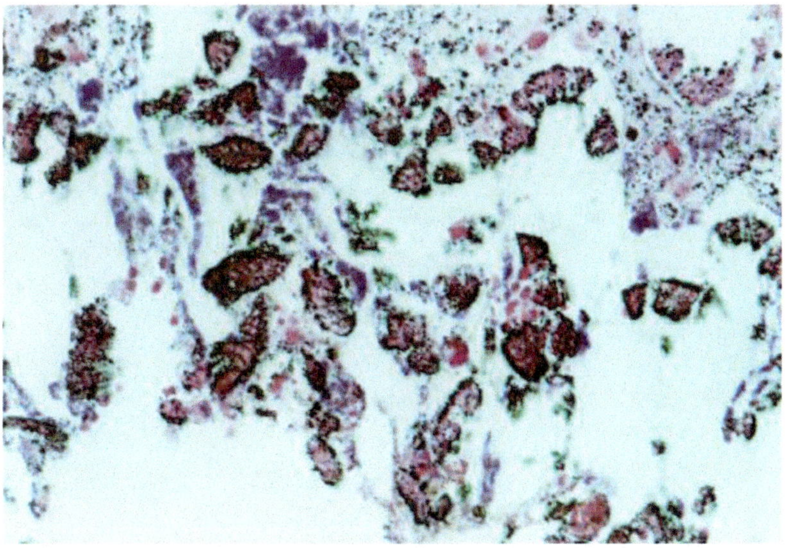

Fig. 5.35 Intestine mucosa with retained fungal components in death cap poisoning (Grocott ×400)

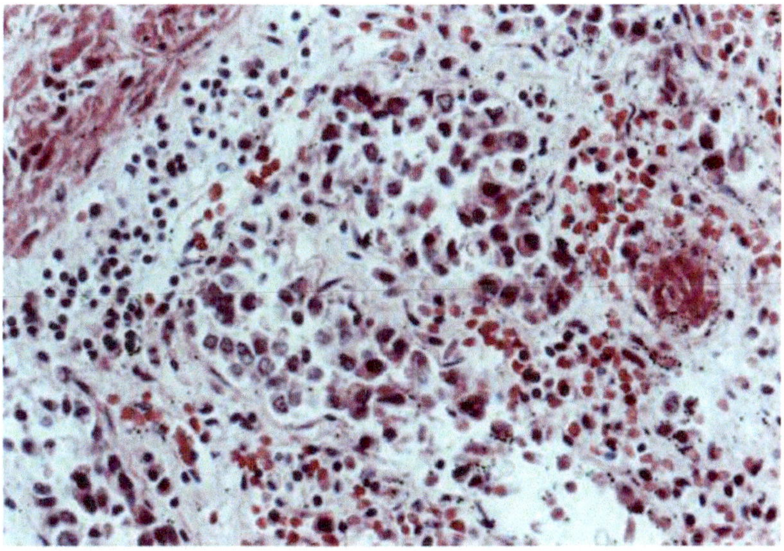

Fig. 5.36 Significant cell and nucleus polymorphy of gastric mucosa epithelial cells following death cap intoxication (H&E ×400)

internal organs, and severe atherosclerosis (Table 5.5) (Darke et al. 2014; Welder and Melchert 1993; Bowman et al. 1989; Hallagan et al. 1989; McKillop et al. 1986; Behrend 1977). There are many descriptions of sudden death with macroscopic and histopathological findings, typically following a long period of anabolic abuse (Fineschi et al. 2007; Hausmann 2004; Westaby et al. 1977). Most deaths are related to cardiac causes, including myocardial infarction (Lüderwald et al. 2008; Tischer et al. 2003; Thiblin et al. 2000; La Rosée et al. 1997; Kennedy 1993; Kennedy and Lawrence 1993; Ferenchick and Adelman 1992; Lynberg 1991; Luke et al. 1990; Bowman 1989; McNutt et al. 1988), in particular when the critical weight of the heart, 500 g, is exceeded (Montisci et al. 2012; Maron et al. 1996; McKillop et al. 1986) (Fig. 5.41). Anabolic androgenic steroids increase the risk of liver cell adenomas and liver cell carcinomas (Socas et al. 2005; Creagh et al. 1988; Overly et al. 1984), including FNH, as described in relation to oral contraceptive use (Omer et al. 1978). In addition, there is an increased risk for coronary ectasias and coronary thrombosis (Tischer et al. 2003). In cases of

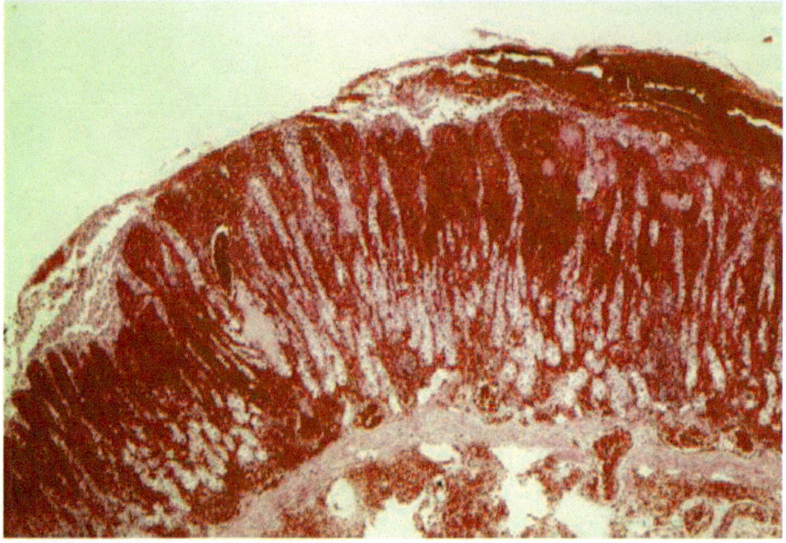

Fig. 5.37 Extensive fresh hemorrhage in the gastric mucosa following death cap intoxication (H&E ×200)

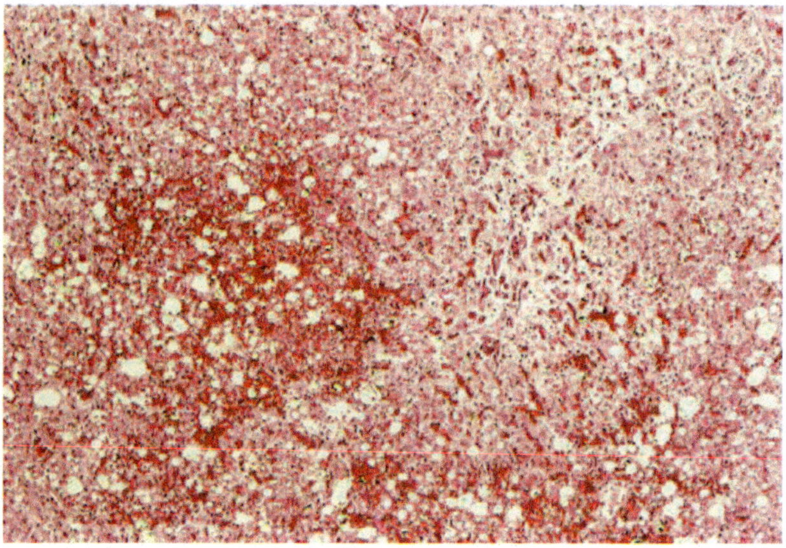

Fig. 5.38 Extensive destruction and hemorrhage in hepatic tissue in acute death cap intoxication (H&E ×100)

anabolic abuse, fine nodular hepatic steatosis of varying severity has been described (Lüderwald et al. 2008), as well as nuclear vacuoles in hepatocyte nuclei. There are also reports of peliosis hepatis following anabolic abuse, and a rare case of pulmonary peliosis has been reported (Vougiouklakis et al. 2009). The risk of cerebral infarction is also increased (Frankle et al. 1988; Mochizuki and Richter 1988), while steroid acne has also been reported (Plewig and Jansen 1998). Adrenal cortex hypotrophy following abuse of a combination of anabolic steroids and ephedrine has been reported (Thiblin et al. 2009).

5.3.5 Reye's Syndrome

In 1963, Reye et al. described a clinical picture in children: acute encephalopathy and fatty degeneration of the internal organs (Reye et al. 1963). In Anglo-Saxon countries, Reye's syndrome was said to be one of the most

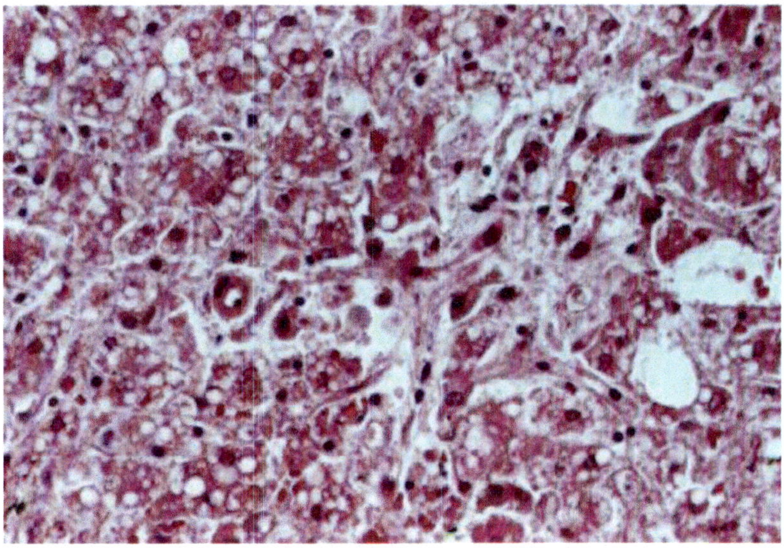

Fig. 5.39 Necrotic liver tissue with vacuolated cytoplasm, partly pyknotic, partly hyperchromatic hepatocyte nucleoli in death cap intoxication (H&E ×400)

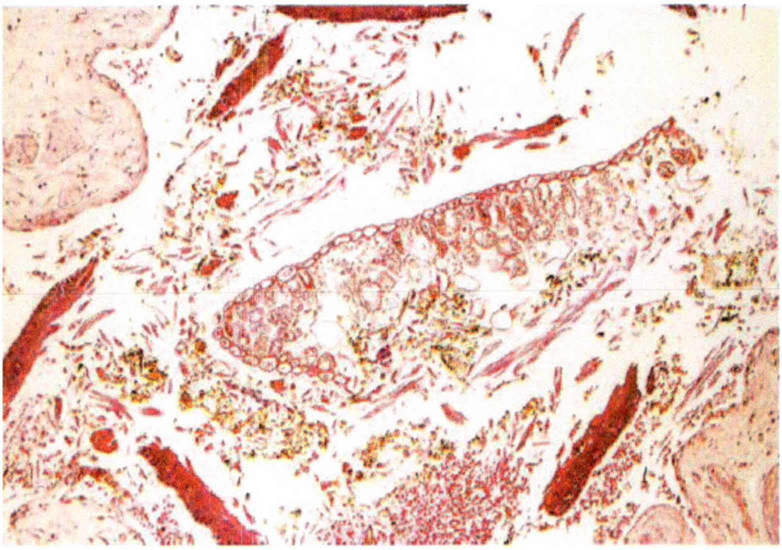

Fig. 5.40 Plant-based foodstuff components next to squamous non-keratinizing epithelium of the esophageal mucosa (H&E ×100)

frequent causes of liver failure in childhood (Wagner-Thiessen 1985). Children between the ages of 5 months and 16 years are typically affected, while adults are rarely affected (Movat 1983).

Viral infections are thought to be the main cause but also toxins such as herbicides, insecticides, solvents, and aflatoxin. An association with the medication acetylsalicylic acid (ASS) is also suspected, as with the anticonvulsive agent valproate (Zimmerman and Ishak 1982). The following histopathological findings are mentioned:

- Pleomorphic mitochondria seen on electron microscopy
- Hepatocytes with a partially oncocytic appearance
- Plurivacuolar hepatic steatosis
- Hypertrophy of the flat endoplasmic reticulum seen on electron microscopy
- Depletion of glycogen
- Fatty degeneration of epithelial cells with fine nodules in the renal tubules, cardiomyocytes, and cross-striated skeletal muscles
- Massive hepatocellular necrosis, mostly in the lobules (rare)

Table 5.5 Histopathological findings after long-term anabolic steroid abuse

Organ	Findings
Heart	Ventricular myocardial hypertrophy: caliber fluctuations in cardiomyocytes, variations in nucleus size, interstitial fibrosis, dehiscence of intercalated disks, myocardial necrosis, and signs of coronary insufficiency following recurrent myocardial ischemia, myocardial infarctions
Coronary arteries	Coronary sclerosis, coronary thrombosis (prothrombotic effect of anabolic steroids)
Liver	Hepatomegaly, hepatic steatosis (triglyceride), but also fat-free nuclear vacuoles, intrahepatic and mainly centrilobular cholestasis, hepatic peliosis, periportal fibrosis, increased hepatocellular adenomas, and carcinomas
Lungs	Capillary hyperemia, platelet aggregations in pulmonary arteries, possibly so-called heart failure cells
Kidney	Possibly increased risk of kidney tumors, fibrin plugs in renal blood vessels (fibrin staining according to Weigert!)
Brain	Increased risk of stroke (rare)
Mammary gland tissue	Gynecomastia
Testes	Testicular atrophy
Adrenal glands	Adrenal cortex hypotrophy
Skin	Steroid-induced acne (so-called steroid acne); virilization in women; possible injection site abscess in the case of i.v. administration
Muscular system	Muscle hypertrophy, rarely muscle and tendon ruptures

- Possible increase in peripheral proliferation of small bile ducts
- Pancreatitis (rare)

Reye's syndrome is assigned to the group of mitochondrial diseases, even though an infectious or toxic substance is regarded as the trigger. Histopathologically, Reye's syndrome is similar to hepatic steatosis in pregnancy and tetracycline-induced hepatic steatosis, both clinical pictures also showing encephalopathy with fatty degeneration of internal organs.

5.3.6 Antibiotic-Induced Pseudomembranous Colitis

Pseudomembranous colitis is a life-threatening complication of broad-spectrum antibiotic therapy caused by *Clostridium difficile*. Untreated, the disease can lead to severe and, in many cases, fatal complications such as peritonitis due to colonic wall perforation, shock as a consequence of volume depletion, toxic megacolon, or massive lower gastrointestinal hemorrhage.

Pseudomembranous enterocolitis was first described by Billroth in 1867. Since the 1950s, there have been reports of diarrhea and colitides after administration of a broad-spectrum antibiotic (Hoberman et al. 1976; Munk et al. 1976). In addition to antibiotics, other medications have also been linked to colitis, including chloramphenicol, aminoglycoside (e.g., gentamicin), metronidazole, and cefotaxime. The clinical course may lead to toxic colon dilation (toxic megacolon). Anticholinergics, narcotics, and barium enemas have also been linked to toxic megacolon (Norland and Kirsner 1969). In the case of pseudomembranous antibiotic-induced colitis, erosions on the surface of the large intestine mucosa with a coating of fibrin, mucus, and granulocytes, creating an overlying pseudomembrane, are histologically observed (Figs. 5.42 and 5.43). Enlarged crypts and fragmented muscularis mucosa in the case of edematous submucosa may appear deep within the mucosa. An inflamed infiltrate consisting of granulocytes, lymphocytes, and plasma cells of varying composition is primarily found in the mucosa (Medline et al. 1976; Summer and Tedesco 1975). Lethal processes may also occur in relatively young patients, but fatal complications mostly occur in elderly people with a high degree of comorbidity (Türk et al. 2002).

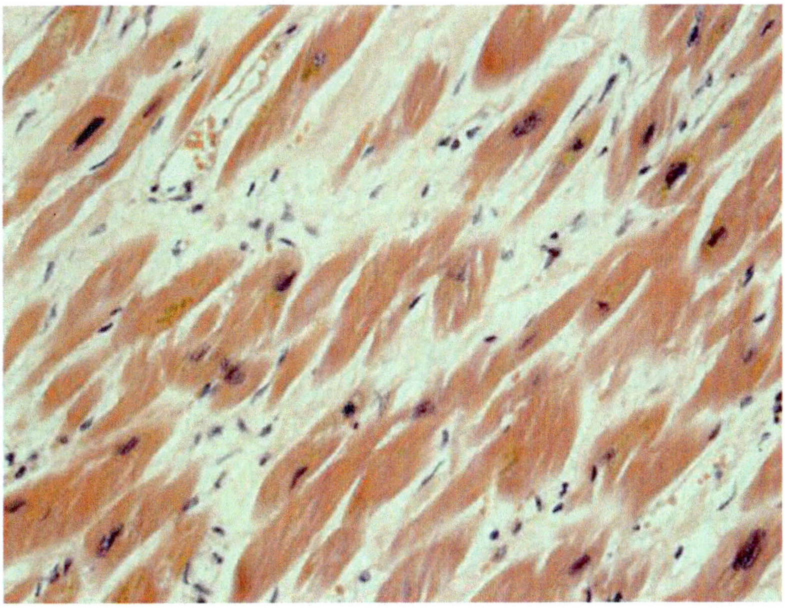

Fig. 5.41 Diffuse interstitial fibrosis in the myocardium with hypertrophy of the cardiomyocytes, enlarged cell nuclei, and interstitial fibrosis after long-term anabolic steroid abuse with a heart weight of 580 g (H&E ×100)

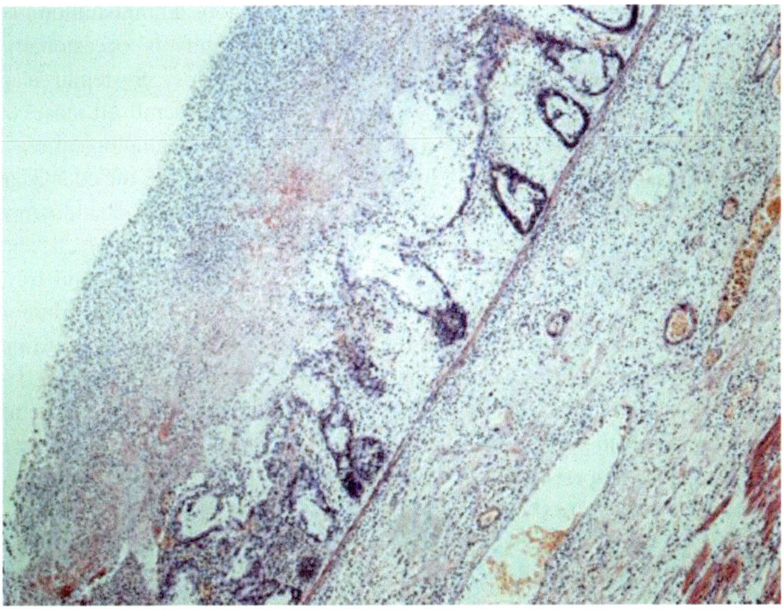

Fig. 5.42 Striated fibrin threads interspersed with granulocytes on mucosa of the colon in antibiotic-induced pseudomembranous colitis (H&E ×100)

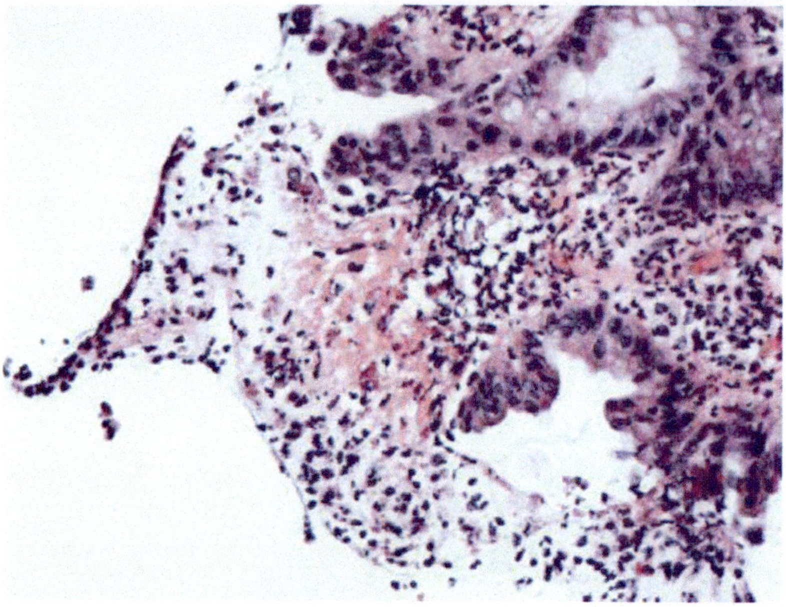

Fig. 5.43 Antibiotic-induced pseudomembranous colitis with erosion of the mucosa crest and overlying fibrin eschar (H&E ×400)

5.3.7 Acute Drug-Induced Anaphylaxis (Anaphylactic Shock)

As a cause of death, acute drug-induced reactions are macroscopically more visible with epidermal necrolysis (toxic epidermal necrolysis or Lyell's syndrome), also referred to as burned skin syndrome (Dämmrich and Ormanns 1982; Metter and Schulz 1978). Here, one may observe hemorrhagic cleft formation with blistery detachment of the epidermis, running through the subepidermal corium in a striated manner (Fig. 5.44). The hemorrhage reaches the partially destroyed epidermal basal membrane. Particularly in the basal layers of the epidermis, flat epithelial cells show polymorphic, hyperchromatic cell nuclei and sporadically vacuolized cytoplasm (Fig. 5.45).

In other cases, clinical examinations prior to death indicated toxic processes caused by medication, such as excessive increase in liver values. With drug-induced death, one may observe partially increased numbers of pulmonary mast cells as an expression of an assumed anaphylactic reaction (Fineschi et al. 2001).

In the context of adverse medical events, including negligence, acute death during intravenous administration of therapeutic and diagnostic agents is occasionally encountered in forensic autopsy. Systemic anaphylaxis occurs as a result of generalized mast cell degranulation caused by an immunological reaction. At autopsy, laryngeal and epiglottic edema can be found, as well as common acute death symptoms, but no specific findings of anaphylactic shock (Pumphrey and Roberts 2000; Delage and Irey 1972). Elevated levels of histamine and immunoglobulin E (IgE) are classic indicators for confirming an anaphylactic reaction (Yunginger et al. 1991; Shepherd 2003).

Using fluorescein angiography, Fineschi et al. (1999) observed mast cell levels fivefold greater than normal in the lungs of an anaphylaxis victim. Various physical conditions of nonallergic reactions can affect tryptase values, e.g., amniotic fluid embolism (Nishio et al. 2002), myocardial infarction (Edston and van Hage-Hamsten 1995), and hyperthermia (Nishio and Suzuki 2005).

Thus, also in medication-induced anaphylactic reactions, there is a classic IgE-mediated hyper-

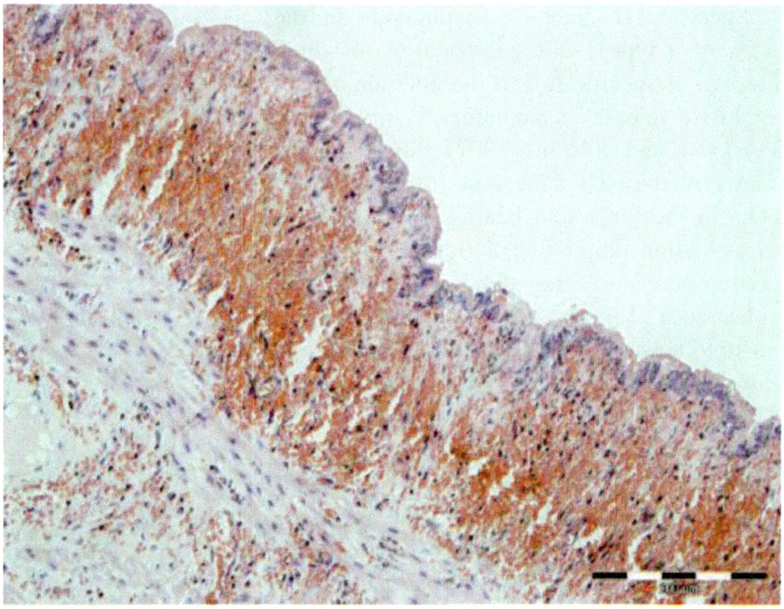

Fig. 5.44 Acute drug-induced dermatitis with subepidermal hemorrhage in the superficial corium and blistery detachment of the epidermis (H&E ×100)

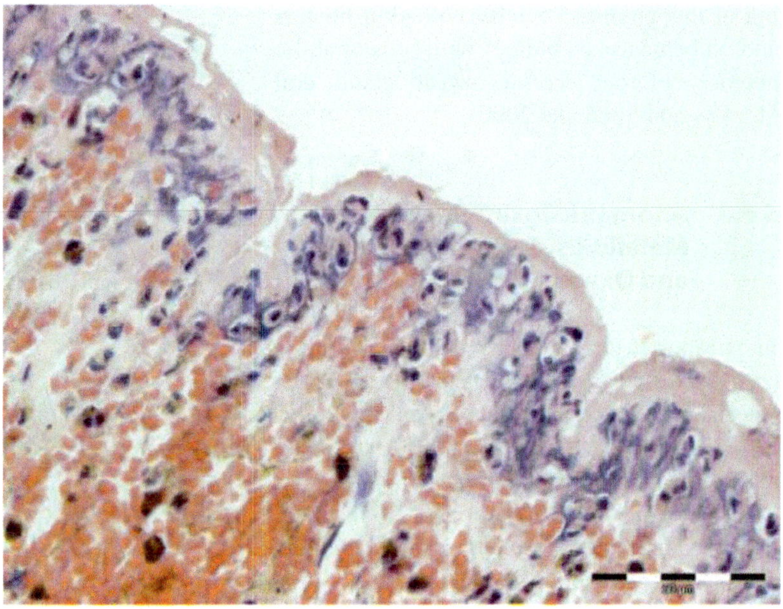

Fig. 5.45 Acute drug-induced dermatitis with partially hemorrhagic destruction of the epidermal basal membrane, as well as significant cell and nuclear polymorphism and sporadic cytoplasmic vacuolization of the mainly flat basal epithelial cells (H&E ×400)

sensibility with tryptase as an indicator (Osawa et al. 2008; Schwartz et al. 1987). An immediate hypersensitivity is involved. This may result in a systemic degranulation of activated mast cells (Trani et al. 2008). Tryptase and chymase are regarded as postmortem-stable compared to histamine and are thus used for the serological diagnosis of anaphylactic shock (Trani et al. 2008; Edston and Hage-Hamsten 1998; Schwartz et al. 1987).

Specific IgE induces anaphylaxis in the form of a type 1 allergic reaction in which binding of specific IgE to the allergen causes explosive release of mediators by mast cells. Perskvist and Edston (2007) noted significantly increased numbers of infiltrated mast cells in the lungs and heart. In an extensive investigation employing a double immunostaining procedure, they demonstrated that the appearance of tryptase-negative and chymase-positive mast cells was specific to those sections associated with fatal anaphylaxis. Therefore, clinical laboratory indicators and immunohistochemical results are possible markers of postmortem diagnosis of anaphylaxis (Osawa et al. 2008; Fineschi et al. 2001). Additionally, in cases of fatal anaphylaxis, diffuse perifollicular and endosinusoidal eosinophilia was found in the spleen (Trani et al. 2008). Rare cases concern fatal poisoning of theophylline toxicity with skin blisters and subepidermal bullae with eosinophilic necrosis of the eccrine sweat gland coil (Tsokos and Sperhake 2002).

5.3.8 Anorganic Toxins, Metals, Metalloids, Carbon Monoxide, and Oxygen

Intoxication with anorganic substances shows partially acute symptoms and histologically detectable changes, including chronic intoxications with varying clinical symptoms and gradually appearing histomorphological findings. Detectable histological findings will be mentioned with keywords, while toxins are alphabetically listed in Table 5.6. Additional information can be found in the relevant literature.

Without a verified patient history, the histological findings alone are in general nonspecific – they can be observed in other forms of intoxication and in a number of various illnesses.

Following beryllium, magma, and silver nitrate intoxication, only nonspecific histological findings are made. In addition, acute and chronic arsenic intoxications show no specific microscopic findings.

Table 5.6 Histological findings in intoxication with selected anorganic substances

Substance	Histological finding
Hydrogen cyanide	Rapidly lethal enzyme poison with no histological findings. Nonspecified, microscopic abnormality seen only in peracute course, possible brain and hepatocyte necrosis, similar to that seen in hypoxic damage of other causes; myocarditis (Janssen and Burger 1968), as well as myocardial infarction (Salomone and Scorsone 1961)
Lead	*Chronic intoxication*
	Kidneys: proximal epithelial (principal) cells of the kidney: round, intense eosinophilic inclusions in the cell nuclei (Lesch 1968; Zollinger 1953), tubular degeneration, focal and diffuse interstitial fibrosis, partially inflamed infiltrate (Galle and Morel-Maroger 1965; Morgan et al. 1966). Cell nucleus inclusions may remain for up to 10 years after lead exposure has ended (Janssen 1977; Totović 1964)
	Possible multiple renal adenoma – “lead tumors” (Franke and Kyrieleis 1976)
	Liver: Homogeneous eosinophilic nuclear inclusions in hepatocytes (Lesch 1968)
	Bone marrow: Initial reactive hyperplasia followed by osteomyelofibrosis to sclerosis
	Electron microscopic: Eosinophilic nuclear inclusions equate to typical corpuscular elements with fine granular, as well as mycel-like, filamentous components (Totović 1964)
Boric acid	Intracytoplasmic inclusions in the epithelial cells of the exocrine pancreas, diameter 2–10 μm, marginal in the acinus cells (Janssen 1977)
Cadmium	*Acute intoxication* (Chang et al. 2012; Peter 1955)
	Gastroenteritis, necrotic tracheobronchitis, hemorrhagic infarcts of the lung, possibly myocarditis
	Liver: Centrilobular necrosis
	Chronic intoxication
	Kidney: Chalk nephrosis, desquamation of the proximal tubular epithelial cells, vacuolization, granulation, nuclear decomposition (Axelsson and Piscator 1966)
	Lungs: “Cadmium fume pneumopathy” with expanded mesenchymal cell reaction in the interalveolar septa, closure of the alveoli, loss of normal lung structure (Fruscella 1963)
	Myocardium: Cloudy swelling of cardiomyocytes, partial vacuolization of cells of the cardiac conduction system, in addition to ECG changes (Janssen 1977)

Table 5.6 (continued)

Substance	Histological finding
Fluorine-containing compounds	*Acute intoxication*
	Corrosion with oral and inhaled ingestion, hemorrhagic gastritis, lung edema (Greendyke and Hodge 1964), development of fat-free vacuoles, and mixed nodular hepatocyte steatosis
	Heart: Pancarditis (Calderon and Cualla 1964), necrosis of the heart muscle fibers, and interstitial edema (Pribilla 1966)
Carbon monoxide (CO)	*Acute intoxication*: No specific histologically demonstrable findings
	(Initially) survived intoxication
	Histological findings only for longer periods of survival as an indirect result of CO intoxication, perhaps as a consequence of hypoxia
	Heart: Necrobiosis and necrosis of cardiomyocytes (Klavis and Schulz 1966; Frommhold 1964), hemorrhage, necrosis, and fatty degeneration of the myocardium (Korb and David 1962), extremely rare myocardial infarction
	Brain: Pallidum necrosis, mostly bilateral (Bianco and Floris 1996; Ali-Cherif et al. 1984; Janssen 1977; Krug 1965)
	Liver: Fat-free vacuolization, marked periportal degeneration of hepatocytes (Meier 1962)
	Case histories: Chronic myositis with atrophy and degeneration of the skeletal muscles, kidney findings same as in crush syndrome, acute kidney insufficiency (Burck and Potwich 1964), changes in the hematopoietic system (Janssen 1977, with additional evidence), intrauterine death (Müller and Graham 1955)
Phosphorus	*Liver*: Initial swelling and diffuse microvacuolar hepatocyte steatosis, hyperemia of the liver sinus, followed by centrilobular steatosis with increasingly fine nodules and average to large nodules in the intermediary zone, necrosis, early regeneration starting in portal fields with bile duct proliferation, inflammatory cell infiltration mainly with lymphocytes and plasma cells; later, either postnecrotic liver cirrhosis or progression to almost complete destruction of the liver tissue
	Kidneys: Fine nodular fatty degeneration in renal tubule epithelium
	Heart: Fine nodular fatty degeneration in cardiomyocytes (Janssen 1977, with additional evidence; Hallermann and Pribilla 1959)
Mercury	*Kidneys*: Light-microscopic changes after approximately 24 h; proximal renal tubules show nuclear pyknosis, vacuolization, cell necrosis, and, later, extensive dystrophic calcification, including microcalcification in the interstitium of the medullary cone (so-called sublimate kidney). Acute sublimate intoxication leads to argyrophilic by-products in the kidney. Timm's sulfide silver method is recommended for detection (Timm 1958, 1961, 1962), but the histological finding is also characteristic in H&E staining
Oxygen	Particularly in cases of hyperbaric oxygen therapy in the form of iatrogenic injury with changes in the lungs (so-called artificial respirator lung; Ritter et al. 1985)
	Lungs: Bronchopulmonary dysplasia in newborns, especially in preterm infants, hypertrophy of wall muscles in peripheral branches of the bronchial tree, narrow glands of the bronchial mucosa, dedifferentiated respiratory epithelium, partial necrosis and desquamation of alveolar epithelial cells, enlarged alveolar septa, increase in collagenous fibers in the interstitium, swelling and necrosis of endothelial cells in septal capillaries, development of so-called hyaline membranes, lung edema (Giusti and Gentile 1974; Molz 1971)
	Brain: Necrotic zones
	Myocard: Enlarged interstitium, focal inflammatory reactions
Thallium	*Liver*: Fatty degeneration of hepatocytes
	Central nervous system: Polyneuritis with destruction of the myelin sheaths up to myelin sheath failure, endothelial swelling, edema of the vascular media, adventitial cell proliferation, glial cell proliferation in the spinal ganglia, atrophy and pyknosis of Nissl substance
	Skeletal muscles: Muscle fiber necrosis, increase in muscle cell nuclei, perivascular inflammatory infiltrate
	Hair: Stratified inclusions in hair are possible but may be absent
	Thallium can be detected histochemically using Timm's (1958) sulfide silver method

5.3.9 Intoxication by Medication (Sleep Medications, Analgesics, Anesthetics, Etc.), Organic Poisons, Solvents, Pesticides (Herbicides, Fungicides, Etc.), and Other Selected Poisons

Intoxication caused by organic solvents or poisons occurs occasionally, e.g., tetrachloride carbon (CCl_4) (Lahl 1973), ethylene trichloride, benzene, and alcohols. In a case of tetrachloroethylene intoxication, intratubular and periglomerular calcium salt deposits were described in the kidneys (alizarin red stain), as well as contraction band necrosis in the myocardium and leukostasis of polymorphonuclear leukocytes (Amadasi et al. 2015). Pesticides such as E 605 or the herbicide paraquat are primarily ingested with suicidal intent, while accidental nicotine poisoning can occur in young children. The types of intoxication mentioned are relatively rare, and histological findings are not always present; for this reason, only a selection of important types of intoxication is discussed here.

Some toxic substances or medications, e.g., barbiturates, may lead to cutaneous blister formation. Nevertheless, cutaneous blisters on a corpse are not only of forensic interest regarding their etiology and genesis but also in regard to the time of origin (there is potential for vital, agonal, supravital, or postmortem occurrence of cutaneous blisters) (Riße et al. 1998).

E 605 Unusually marked hyperemia of the internal organs is described in cases of intoxication caused by E 605 (Adebahr 1963, 1976). In Pickworth's benzidine staining, the kidneys in particular show enlarged blood vessels in the arterial, capillary, and venous vessels. In addition, there are bulging, blood-filled capillary loops in the glomeruli. After a survival time of only 15 min, there is intense granulation of the cytoplasm, hyperchromatosis of the walls of the cell nucleus, clumping and reduction of chromatin, as well as marginal nucleoli. The epithelial cells of the renal tubules show increased pyknotic cell nuclei after a survival time of approximately 30 min (Adebahr 1960) (Fig. 5.46).

In other internal organs, additional cell nuclear polymorphisms are described in conventional stainings; however, this does not include necrosis in the case of generally short survival times (<1 h).

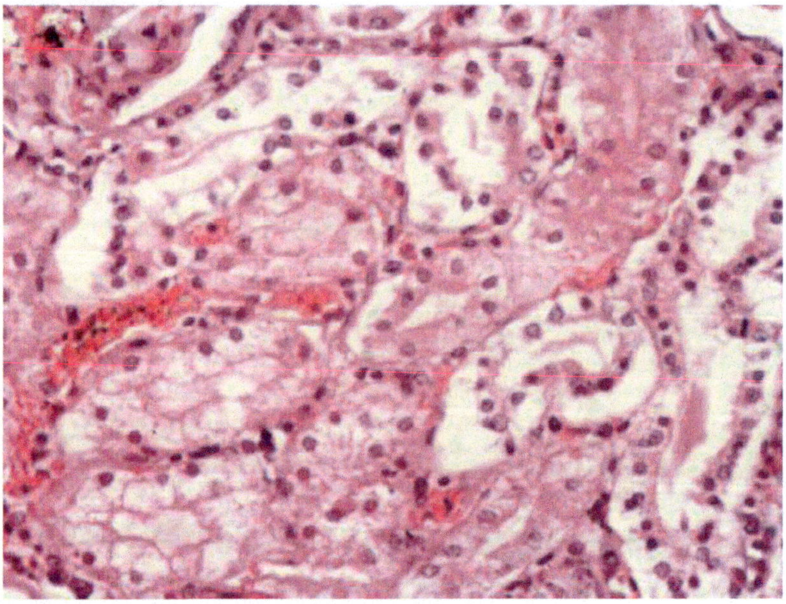

Fig. 5.46 Tubular necroses in the kidney after short survival of E 605 intoxication with suicidal intent: some cases show destruction of the cell nuclei, detachment of the tubular epithelium, as well as pyknotic and destroyed cell nuclei (H&E ×250)

Pyramidon Histological findings have been described in the small number of cases of pyramidon intoxication:

- Detachment of vascular endothelial cells
- Blackish granules in endothelial cells, leukocytes, and vascular walls
- Decomposition of leukocytes
- Increased eosinophilic leukocytes
- Occurrence of hepatocytes in liver veins (liver cell mobilization)
- Enlarged cell nuclei and mitoses, chromatin-rich hepatocytes, as well as epithelial cells of the seminiferous tubules in the kidneys (Fazekas 1957).

In addition, there is a certain lipid discharge in the adrenal cortex. Clinical observations include neurological failure (Hallermann and Illichmann-Christ 1951). The described findings were interpreted as an expression of toxic shock syndrome in association with the release of histamine (Fazekas 1957).

Methyl Parathion In cases of intoxication caused by parathion, the histological findings depend on survival time. After a survival time of 2 h, marked brain and lung edema is seen, accompanied by hyperemia. After 20 h, pulmonary hemorrhage and degenerative changes occurred, including cellular fatty degeneration. After 20–24 h, fragmented heart muscle cells were observed, together with the destruction of liver cells. In addition, partial detachment of endothelial cells is seen (Fazekas 1971).

Paraquat Paraquat is the active agent in a widely used herbicide. After oral ingestion with suicidal intent (in most cases) and survival of several days, marked necrosis of the pulmonary alveoli may develop followed by connective tissue transformation in lung tissue (Teare 1976; Carson and Carson 1976). In this context, interstitial hemorrhage may occur, together with edema and eosinophilic hyaline membranes in the early phase of injury, particularly involving the basal membranes. Aneurysmal ectasias of the alveolar capillaries have also been mentioned (von der Hardt and Cardesa 1971). Toxic lung fibrosis also affects the lumina of the alveoli and bronchioles (Borchard et al. 1974; Eisenmenger et al. 1974); corresponding changes were observed in animal models (Ishida et al. 2006). Bronchopneumonic sources are possible, including proliferation of the epithelia of the terminal bronchioles (Herczeg and Reif 1968). Reports include necrosis of the skeletal muscles following paraquat ingestion (Kibler 1973). The accompanying fibrinous exudate in the lung contains numerous lymphocytes and plasma cells and relatively few granulocytes. Following initial survival following oral ingestion, ulcerations in the throat and mouth region may occur, together with ulcerous glossitis, laryngitis, and esophagitis (Fischer and Kahler 1979). In animal experiments the immunohistochemical administration of paraquat especially in the stomach and the esophagus was possible (Nagao et al. 1993).

Nicotine There are no characteristic histomorphological findings using conventional staining in nicotine poisoning. Swelling of vascular walls has been described, with tearing of the internal elastic membrane, which has a strongly wavy appearance in median to small arteries. The endothelial cell nuclei are also said to show marked palisade formation. The remaining histological findings for internal organs are nonspecific for poisoning by nicotine (Adebahr and Voigt 1963; Adebahr 1960, 1963).

Aconitine A diterpenoid alkaloid, aconitine is found in the monkshood plant. It is known as one of the most potent phytotoxins and causes bradyarrhythmia. Lethal intoxication may cause massive pulmonary hemorrhage and pulmonary edema (Pullela et al. 2008).

Lidocaine Lidocaine is an antiarrhythmic, and at toxic levels, serious symptoms associated with the central nervous system and cardiac system are noted (Amitai et al. 1986; Kalin and Brissie 2002). In rare cases of oral ingestion of lidocaine, histological examination reveals generalized stasis. In the myocardium, segmentation of the myocardial cells and/or widening of intercalated disks and associated group of hypercontracted myocardial cells with "square" nuclei in line with hyperdistended ones can be found. Non-eosinophilic bands of hypercontracted sarcomeres alternating with stretched, often apparently separated sarcomeres are described, as well as small foci of paradiscal contraction band necrosis and perivascular fibrosis (Centini et al. 2007).

Taxus Poisoning Case reports of suicides have presented fatal poisoning with *Taxus baccata*, an evergreen shrub, the toxicity of which has long been known. The postmortem evaluation of acute *Taxus* poisoning is usually unremarkable. Visible abnormalities are often absent, and microscopic lesions are rarely observed. Nevertheless, *Taxus* leaves can be identified in the stomach or duodenum content (Pietsch et al. 2007; Sinn and Porterfield 1991; van Ingen et al. 1992) (Fig. 5.47). The toxicity of *Taxus baccata*, which varies according to season, is based primarily on a mixture of different alkaloids. There are reports not only of fatal courses but also of survived intoxications (Grobosch et al. 2013).

Phosphine Poisoning Phosphides of aluminum and zinc are two pesticides commonly used in agriculture. In cases of fatal phosphine poisoning, major histopathological findings involve the liver with mild to severe sinusoidal congestion. Central vein congestion and centrilobular necrosis are possible, as well as nuclear fragmentation in the hepatocytes. Fine isomorphic cytoplasmic lobules were observed, mainly distributed uniformly in all hepatic zones; no remarkable portal inflammation was observed (Cochran and Watson 1969; Saleki et al. 2007).

Petrol Exposure Dermal lesions following postmortem petrol exposure have been described with the earliest onset of skin changes within 2 h of exposure. Swelling and wrinkling with detachment of the upper layers of skin were observed (positive Nikolsky's sign). The lesions appeared as non-vital acantholyses, located in the prickle cell layer with formation of intraepidermal bullae (Bux et al. 2006). Other histopathological findings are described following death caused by arsenobenzene (Fazekas and Dósa 1953, 1954).

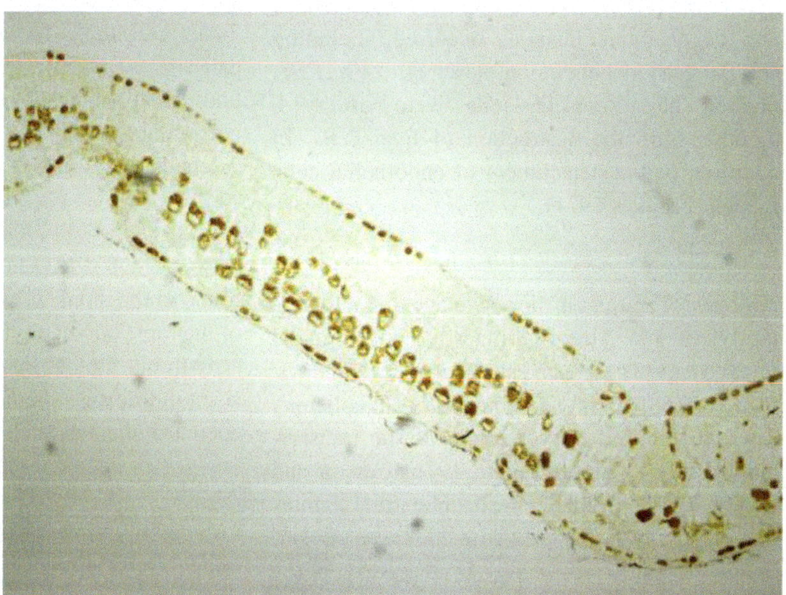

Fig. 5.47 A conifer fragment from English yew (*Taxus baccata*) found in the duodenal lumen and cleaned at autopsy in a case of fatal *Taxus* poisoning (H&E ×40)

There are reports of additional, mainly nonspecific histopathological findings involving acute as well as chronic intoxication with various substances, e.g., benzol, arsenic, bromcarbamide, hydrogen phosphide, inhalation of quicksilver steam, petroleum injection, inhalation of polytetrafluoroethylene, cyanides, ozone, halothane, chloroform, crotarbital, barium polysulfide, fluoride, and strychnine. However, in specific cases, some of the indicated substances may cause severe histomorphological injury.

5.3.10 Further Fatal Adverse Drug Reactions and Medical Errors

Iatrogenic deaths associated with the administration of medications involve:

- Drug-induced anaphylactic reactions (e.g., penicillin allergies), medication-induced myocarditis (see above), as well as Stevens–Johnson syndrome/toxic epidermal necrolysis from, e.g., penicillin, sulphonamides, barbiturates, salicylates, or antimalarials
- Drug-induced malignant syndromes, including malignant hyperthermia
- Toxic reactions to medications with or without overdose: necrosis of the liver with intrahepatic cholestasis, toxic cardiomyopathies, tubulointerstitial nephritides, etc. (Lau 1995a, b).

Lethal reaction may be an unavoidable side effect of medication or the result of an error by the physician, whereby the number of possible medications causing lethal reaction is almost overwhelming (Gelven et al. 1996; Lau 1995a, b; Adebahr 1976).

The erroneous administration of a medicine, such as excessively rapid intravenous injection or incorrect dilution of medication, may cause death. Mix-up of medicines may also occur. The spectrum of possible errors is enormous, and specific histopathological findings are rare. Mostly nonspecific findings are involved, which may be interpreted as a medication error (in detail: Lau 2005).

In addition, there are relatively rare and often undiagnosable intoxications and side effects caused by medication, particularly barbiturates, corticoids, cytostatic agents, antibiotics (e.g., antibiotic-associated pseudomembranous colitis; see above), and pain medication [e.g., those belonging to the phenacetin group (phenacetin kidney), pyrazole, salicylic acid derivatives, strychnine, paracetamol, and others] (Figs. 5.48, 5.49, and 5.50). Severe side effects are known for nonsteroidal anti-inflammatory (NSAI) agents, especially in the gastrointestinal tract, including

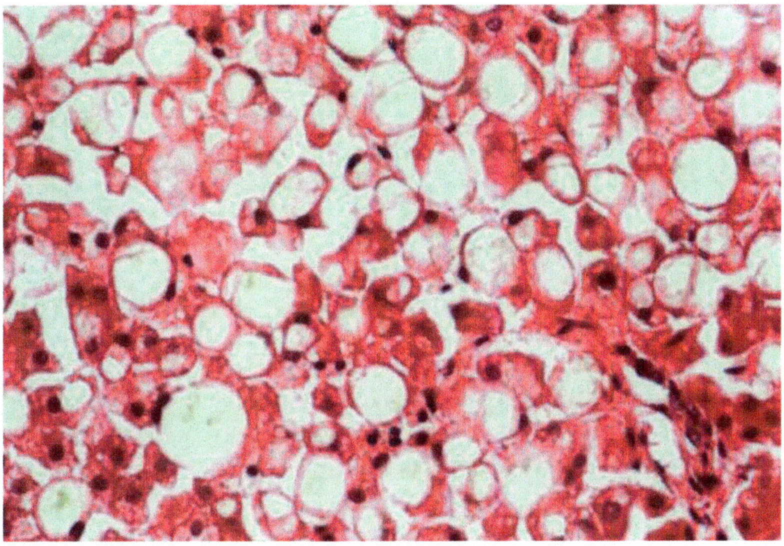

Fig. 5.48 Microvacuolar transformation of hepatocytes in a case of strychnine intoxication, similar findings as in cases of colchicine intoxication (see Fig. 5.26) (H&E ×400)

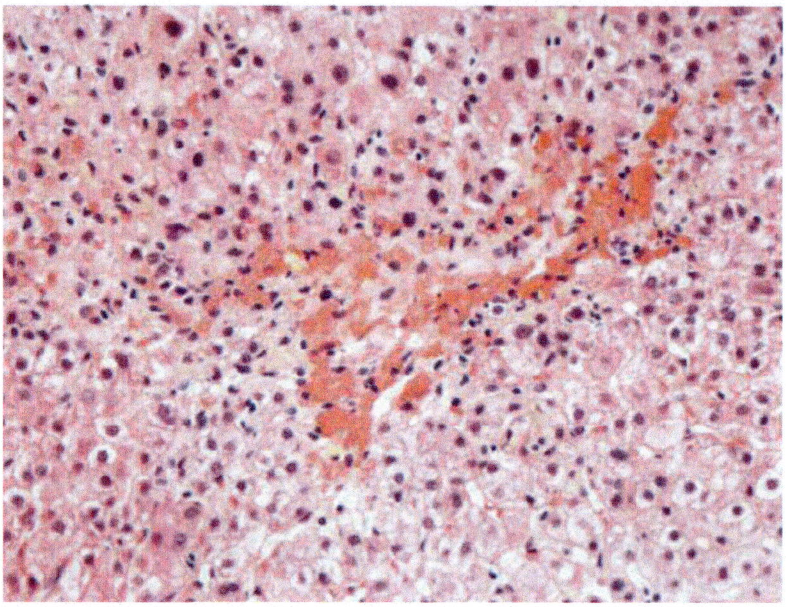

Fig. 5.49 Liver cell necrosis due to paracetamol (H&E ×100)

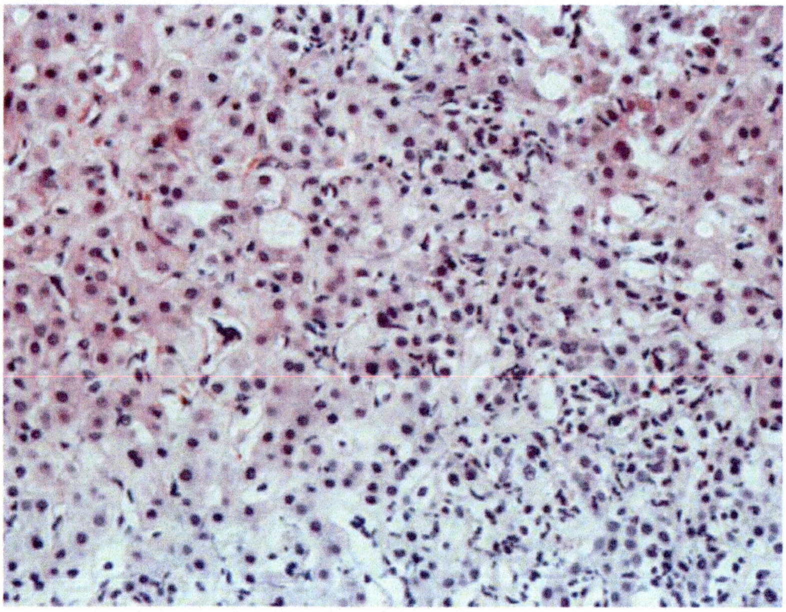

Fig. 5.50 Liver cell necrosis and inflammatory reaction in the liver due to cytostatica (H&E ×100)

the development of ulcers. This may cause lethal hemorrhage in certain cases.

There often are only case histories for individual substances. For necrosis in various organs, histological findings can also describe uncharacteristic changes, such as vacuole-like transformation in the hepatocyte cytoplasm, changes to epithelial cells in the renal tubules, as well as changes in the ventricular walls. In terms of injury pattern, some substances show a certain organotrophy. The relevant literature may serve as a source of reference.

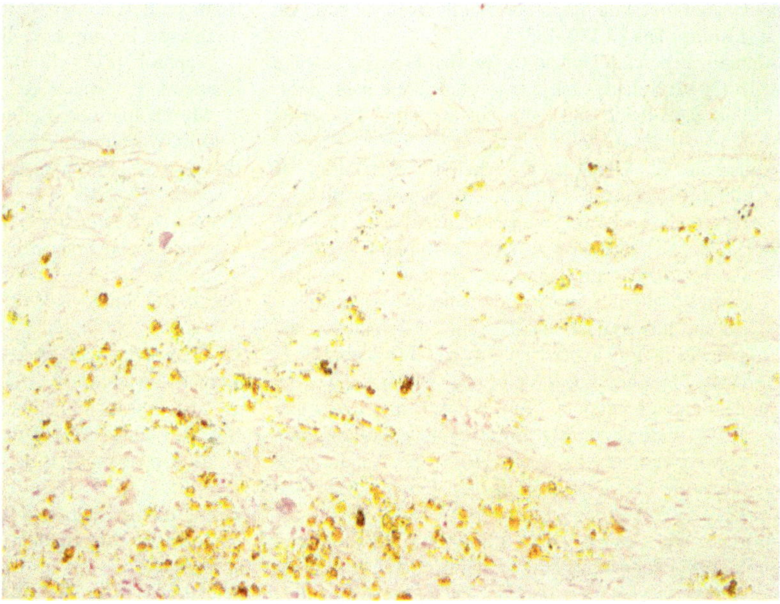

Fig. 5.51 Ocher-yellowish pigment deposits in the skin, predominantly in the upper layers and between the keratin lamellae following long-term nicotine use (H&E ×100)

5.3.11 Toxin-Induced Histopathological Findings of the Skin

Not all histopathological skin findings are necessarily the result of intoxication due to the intake of substances via the gastrointestinal tract or respiratory system. Moreover, there are findings that can be caused both ante- and postmortem. For example, washing the skin with bleach causes erosive detachment of the epidermis, and hair shafts may detach from the hair follicles, which give the striking optical impression of being empty (Adair et al. 2007). In the case of long-term nicotine use, ocher-yellowish deposits may be macroscopically visible on the skin of the finger used to hold a cigarette. Discoloration of this kind can also be seen using microscopy (Fig. 5.51).

References

Abrahams C, Wheatley A, Rubenstein AH, Stables D (1964) Hepatocellular lipofuscin after excessive ingestion of analgesics. Lancet 2:621–622

Adair TW, Dobersen MJ, Lear-Kaul K (2007) Appearance of chemical burns resulting from the washing of a deceased body with bleach. J Forensic Sci 52:709–711

Adebahr G (1960) Nierenveränderungen bei der E 605-Vergiftung des Menschen. Arch Toxikol 18:107

Adebahr G (1963) Leberveränderungen bei der E 605-Vergiftung des Menschen. Beitr Gerichtl Med 22:1

Adebahr G (1976) Zur Pathologie der Organschäden nach diagnostischen und therapeutischen Eingriffen. Z Rechtsmed 78:173

Adebahr G, Voigt GE (1963) Morphologische Veränderungen bei der akuten tödlichen Nicotinvergiftung. Dtsch Z f gerichtl Med 54:304

Aderjan R, Joachim H (1988) Ethylene glycol intoxication with fatal outcome. Z Rechtsmed 100:199–206

Advenier AS, Dorandeu A, Charlier P, Lorin de la Grandmaison G (2014) Microscopic acute lesions after caustic exposure. Forensic Sci Int 234:57–63

Ali-Cherif A, Royere ML, Gosset A, Poncet M, Salomon G, Khalil R (1984) Behavior and mental activity disorders after carbon monoxide poisoning. Bilateral pallidal lesions. Rev Neurol 140:401–405

Allender WJ (1982) Colchicine poisoning as a mode of suicide. J Forensic Sci 27:944–947

Altmann HW, Klinge O (1972) Morphologische Reaktionen menschlichen Lebergewebes auf Pharmaka. Verh Dtsch Ges Pathol 56:194–214

Amadasi A, Mastrolucca L, Marasciuolo L, Caligara M, Sironi L, Gentile G, Zoja R (2015) Death due to acute tetrachloroethylene intoxication in a chronic abuser. Int J Legal Med 129:487–493

Amitai Y, Withesell L, Lovejoy FH (1986) Death following accidental overdose in a child. N Engl J Med 314:182–183

Ammar KA, Heckerling PS (1996) Ethylene glycol poisoning with a normal anion gap caused by concurrent

ethanol ingestion: importance of the osmolal gap. Am J Kidney Dis 27:130–133
Aquila I, Pepe F, di Nunzio C, Ausania F, Serra A, Ricci P (2014) Suicide case due to phosphoric acid ingestion: case report and review of literature. J Forensic Sci 59:1665–1667
Armstrong EJ, Engelhart DA, Jenkins AJ, Balraj EK (2006) Homicidal ethylene glycol intoxication: a report of a case. Am J Forensic Med Pathol 27:151–155
Arsenovic N, Sheehan L, Clark D, Moreira R (2010) Fatal carbamazepine induced fulminant eosinophilic (hypersensitivity) myocarditis: emphasis on anatomical and histological characteristics, mechanisms and genetics of drug hypersensitivity and differential diagnosis. J Forensic Legal Med 17:57–61
Arzneimittelkommission der Deutschen Ärzteschaft (2016) Fulminante Myokarditis mit akuter kardialer Dekompensation nach Erstgabe von Adalimumab (Humira®) bei Colitis ulcerosa. Deutsches Ärzteblatt 113:B579–B580
Asano S, Wakasaka H, Kaise S, Nishimaki T, Kasukawa R (1982) Peliosis hepatis. Report of two autopsy cases with a review of literature. Acta Pathol Jpn 32:861–877
Asbeck F, Joist H, Löhrs U (1972) Lebervenenthrombose und Ovulationshemmer. Ein weiterer Fall von Budd-Chiari-Syndrom nach Einnahme eines oralen Kontrazeptivums. Med Klin 67:82
Axelsson B, Piscator M (1966) Nierenschädigung nach längerer Cadmiumexposition. Experimentelle Untersuchungen. Arch Environ Health 12:360
Bagheri SA, Boyer JL (1974) Peliosis hepatis associated with androgenic-anabolic steroid therapy. Ann Intern Med 81:610–680
Barthel J, Gerber HU (1962) Ein Beitrag zur Vergiftung mit Wasserschierling (Cicuta virosa L.) bei Kindern. Kinderärztl Prax Sonderdruck 12:543–547
Baumgarten R, Fengler JD, Bartke D, Roschlau G, May D (1981) Peliosis hepatis – eine seltene Form der arzneimittelinduzierten Leberschädigung. Dtsch Gesundh Wes 23:629–631
Behrend H (1977) Myocardial cell lesions caused by an anabolic hormone. Cell Tissue Res 181:423–426
Berneis K, Studer A (1967) Vermehrung von Lipofuscin in der Leber als Folge von Phenacetinabusus. Zentrifugation von menschlicher und tierischer Leber im Dichtegradienten. Virchows Arch Pathol Anat 343:75–80
Bianchi L, De Groote J, Desmet V, Gedigk P, Korb G, Popper H, Poulsen H, Scheuer PJ, Schmid M, Thaler H, Wepler W (1975) Richtlinien für die histologische Beurteilung arzneimittelbedingter (medikamentöser) Leberschäden. Dtsch Med Wochenschr 100:1746–1750
Bianco F, Floris R (1996) MRI appearance consistent with haemorrhagic infarction as an early manifestation of carbon monoxide poisoning. Neuroradiology 38(suppl 1):S70
Bommer J, Waldherr R, Gastner M, Lemmes R, Ritz E (1981) Iatrogenic multiorgan silicone inclusions in dialysis patients. Klin Wochenschr 59:1149–1157
Bommer J, Waldherr R, Ritz E (1983) Silicone storage disease in long-term hemodialysis patients. Contrib Nephrol 36:115–126
Borchard F, Grabensee B, Jax W, Huth F (1974) Morphologische Befunde bei Paraquatvergiftungen. Klin Wochenschr 52:657
Bowman SJ (1989) Anabolic steroids and infarction. Br Med J 299:632
Brahmi N, Kouraichi N, Blei Y et al (2006) Acute myocarditis and myocardial infarction induced by paraphenylenediamine poisoning. Int J Cardiol 113:93–95
Burck HC, Potwich F (1964) Akute Niereninsuffizienz nach schwerer Kohlenmonoxyd-Intoxikation. Frankfurt Z Path 73:520
Burger R, Marcuse P (1952) Peliosis hepatis: report of a case. Am J Clin Pathol 2:569–573
Bux R, Stengel PD, Schnabel A (2006) Dermal lesions after post mortem petrol-exposure. Forensic Sci Int 163:115–118
Byard RW, Musgrave I (2010) Herbal medicines and forensic investigations. Forensic Sci Med Pathol 6:81–82
Calderon JJ, Cualla U (1964) Ein interessanter Fall von Fluorvergiftung. Rev Med Legae Colomb 17(89):145
Caparros-Lefebvre D, Policard J, Sengler C, Benabdallah E, Colombani S, Rigal M (2005) Bipallidal haemorrhage after ethylene glycol intoxication. Neuroradiology 47:105–107
Carson DJ, Carson ED (1976) The increasing use of paraquat as a suicidal agent. Forensic Sci 7:151–160
Cavender FL, Sowinski EJ (2001) Glycols. In: Bingham E, Cohrssen B, Powell CH (eds) Pattys toxicology, 5th edn. Wiley, New York, pp 1–71
Centini F, Fiore C, Riezzo I, Rossi G, Fineschi V (2007) Suicide due to oral ingestion of lidocaine: a case report and review of the literature. Forensic Sci Int 171:57–62
Chang Y, Wen J, Cai J, Xiao-ying W, Yang L, Guo Y (2012) An investigation and pathological analysis of two fatal cases of cadmium. Forensic Sci Int 220:e5–e8
Clevenger CV, August TF, Shaw LM (1991) Colchicine poisoning: report of a fatal case with body fluid analysis by GC/MS and histopathologic examination of post-mortem tissues. J Anal Toxicol 15:151–154
Cochran AJ, Watson AA (1969) Leberveränderungen bei einem Patienten nach Behandlung mit Cytostatica, ähnlich denjenigen bei akuter Phosphorvergiftung. Med Sci Law 9:202
Creagh TM, Rubin A, Evans DJ (1988) Hepatic tumors induced by anabolic steroids in an athlete. J Clin Pathol 41:441–443
Dämmrich J, Ormanns W (1982) Lyell-Syndrom und nekrotisierende granulomatöse Arteriitis als gleichzeitige, arzneimittelbedingte Reaktionen. Pathologe 3:352–358
Darke S, Torok M, Duflou J (2014) Sudden or unnatural deaths involving anabolic-androgenic steroids. J Forensic Sci 59:1025–1028
Delage C, Irey NS (1972) Anaphylactic deaths: a clinicopathologic study of 43 cases. J Forensic Sci 17:525–540

Desilva MB, Mueller PS (2009) Renal consequences of long-term, low-dose intentional ingestion of ethylene glycol. Ren Fail 31:586–588

Dettling A, Stadler K, Eisenbach C, Skopp G, Haffner HT (2016) Systemic inflammatory response due to chloroform intoxication – an uncommon complication. Int J Legal Med 130:401–404

Dettling M, Cascorbi I, Hellweg R, Deicke U, Weise L, Müller-Oerlinghausen B (1999) Genetic determinants of drug-induced agranulocytosis: potential risk of olanzapine? Pharmacopsychiatry 32:110–112

Dölle W, Martini GA (1962) Zusammenstellung von Arzneimitteln, die Leberschädigung mit und ohne Gelbsucht verursachen können. Acta Hepatol Splen 9:74–85

Edston E, van Hage-Hamsten M (1995) Immunoglobulin E, mast cell-specific tryptase and the complement system in sudden death from coronary artery thrombosis. Int J Cardiol 52:77–81

Edston E, van Hage-Hamsten M (1998) Beta-Tryptase measurements post-mortem in anaphylactic deaths and in controls. Forensic Sci Int 93:135–142

Eisenmenger W, Henn R, Beckmann G (1974) Klinische und pathologisch-anatomische Befunde der Paraquat-Vergiftung. Beitr Ger Med 32:262–266

Evans GW, Philipps G, Mukherjee TM, Snow MR, Lwarence JR, Thomas DW (1973) Identification of crystal deposits in brain and kidney after xylitol administration by biochemical, histochemical, and electron diffraction methods. J Clin Pathol 26:32–36

Fazekas IG (1957) Tödliche Pyramidonvergiftung bei einem Säugling mit besonderer Berücksichtigung der histologischen Veränderungen. Dtsch Z f gerichtl Med 47:374

Fazekas IG (1971) Über die makroskopischen und mikroskopischen Veränderungen bei der Wofatox-Vergiftung (Methyl-Parathion). Z Rechtsmed 68:189–194

Fazekas IG, Dósa A (1953) Sektionserfahrungen bei Arsenobenzoltodesfällen. Arch f Dermatol Syph 196:288–304

Fazekas IG, Dósa A (1954) Histologische Veränderungen bei Arsenobenzoltodesfällen und ihre Bewertung. Arch f Dermatol Syph 197:436–448

Ferenchick GS, Adelman S (1992) Myocardial infarction associated with anabolic steroids use in a previously healthy 37-year-old weight lifter. Am Heart J 124:507–508

Fineschi V, Monasterolo G, Rosi R, Turillazzi E (1999) Fatal anaphylactic shock during a fluorescein angiography. Forensic Sci Int 100:137–142

Fineschi V, Cecchi R, Centini F, Reattelli LP, Turillazzi E (2001) Immunohistochemical quantification of pulmonary mast-cells and post-mortem blood dosages of tryptase and eosinophil cationic protein in 48 heroin-related deaths. Forensic Sci Int 120:189–194

Fineschi V, Riezzo I, Centini F, Silingardi E, Licata M, Beduschi G, Karch SB (2007) Sudden cardiac death during anabolic steroid abuse: morphologic and toxicologic findings in two fatal cases of bodybuilders. Int J Legal Med 121:48–53

Finkelstein Y, Aks SE, Hutson JR et al (2010) Colchicine poisoning; the dark side of an ancient drug. Clin Toxicol (Phila) 48:407–414

Fischer H, Kahler J (1979) Zur tödlichen Paraquatvergiftung. Z Rechtsmed 84:61–67

Fitzsimons J, Berk M, Lambert T, Bourin M, Dodd S (2005) A review of clozapine safety. Expert Opin Drug Saf 4:731–744

Franke W, Kyrieleis C (1976) Gewerbliche Bleivergiftung als Todesursache. Med Welt 27:233

Frankle MA, Eichberg R, Zachariah SB (1988) Anabolic androgenic steroids and a stroke in an athlete: case report. Arch Phys Med Rehabil 69:632–633

Frohberg K, Dorion RP, McMartin KE (2006) The role of calcium oxalate crystals deposition in cerebral vessels during ethylene glycol poisoning. Clin Toxicol 44:315–318

Frommhold H (1964) Licht- und fluoreszenzmikroskopische Untersuchungen am Herzmuskel nach akut-tödlicher Kohlenoxydvergiftung. Med Diss. zitiert nach: Janssen 1977, Hamburg

Fruscella FDER (1963) Experimentelle Cadmiumpneumopathie: ein histologischer Beitrag. Rass Med Industr 32:537. (zitiert nach: Janssen 1977)

Galle P, Morel-Maroger (1965) Nierenveränderungen bei klinischer und experimenteller Bleivergiftung. Nephron 2:273

Gelven PL, Cina SJ, Lee JD, Nichols CA (1996) Massive hepatic necrosis and death following repeated isoflurane exposure. Case report and review of the literature. Am J Forensic Med Pathol 17:61–64

Gilbert JD, Byard RW (2002) Epithelia cell mitotic arrest – a useful post-mortem histologic marker in cases of possible colchicine toxicity. Forensic Sci Int 126:150–152

Gilbert JD, Musgrave IF, Hoban C, Byard RW (2014) Lethal hepatocellular necrosis associated with herbal polypharmacy in a patient with chronic hepatitis B infection. Forensic Sci Int 241:138–140

Giusti GV, Gentile V (1974) Hyaline membrane disease in adults after artificial ventilation: a histopathologic study. Forensic Sci 4:207

Gloor F (1978) Changing concepts in pathogenesis and morphology of analgesic nephropathy as seen in Europe. Kidney Int 13:27–33

Gloor F (1982) Die Kapillarosklerose in den ableitenden Harnwegen bei Schmerzmittel-(Phenazetin)-Mißbrauch. Pathologe 3:132–136

Gradinger R, Jung C, Reinhardt D, Mall G, Figulla HR (2008) Toxic myocarditis due to oral ingestion of hydrofluoric acid. Heart Lung Circ 17:248–250

Greendyke RM, Hodge HC (1964) Unfallbedingte Todesfälle durch Fluorwasserstoff. J Forensic Sci 9:383

Grobosch T, Schwarze B, Felgenhauer N, Riesselmann B, Roscher S, Binscheck T (2013) Eight cases of fatal and non-fatal poisoning with *Taxus baccata*. Forensic Sci Int 227:118–126

Halevy S, Ghislain PD, Mockenhaupt M et al (2008) Allopurinol is the most common cause of Stevens-

Johnson syndrome and toxic epidermal necrolysis in Europe and Israel. J Am Acad Dermatol 58:25–32
Hallagan JB, Hallagan LF, Snyder MB (1989) Anabolic-androgenic steroid use by athletes. N Engl J Med 321:1042–1045
Hallermann W, Illichmann-Christ A (1951) Die Pathologie der akuten tödlichen Ditonalvergiftung beim Kinde. Zugleich ein Beitrag zur Frage der akuten Pyramidonvergiftung und zur Entstehung kreislaufbedingter Schäden am Gehirn. Dtsch Z gerichtl Med 40:511–552
Hallermann W, Pribilla O (1959) Tödliche Vergiftungen mit Phosphorwasserstoff. Arch Toxikol 17:219
Hantson P, Vanbinst R, Mahieu P (2002) Determination of ethylene glycol tissue content after fatal oral poisoning and pathologic findings. Am J Forensic Med Pathol 23:159–161
Hausmann R (2004) Long-term effects of anabolic-androgenic-steroid abuse. Morphological findings associated with fatal outcome. In: Tsokos M (ed) Forensic pathology reviews, vol 2. Humana, Totowa, pp 273–289
Hecht L, Lamprecht A (2010) Intramuskuläre Applikation von Depotmedikamenten. Rechtsmedizin 20:510–514
Herczeg E, Reif A (1968) Lungenveränderungen bei tödlich verlaufender Paraquatvergiftung. Zentralbl All Pathol 111:325–328
Heye N, Zimmer C, Terstegge K, Sirtl C, Cervos-Navarro J (1991) Oxalate-induced encephalitis after infusions of sugar surrogates. Intensive Care Med 17:432–434
Hikiji W, Kudo K, Nishida N, Ishida T, Usumoto Y, Tsuji A, Ikeda N (2008) Acute fatal poisoning with pilsicainide and atenolol. Int J Legal Med 122:503–506
Hoberman LJ, Eigenbrodt EH, Kilman WJ, Hughes LR, Norgaard RP, Fordtran JS (1976) Colitis associated with oral clindamycin therapy. Dig Dis Sci 21:1–17
Hovda KE, Guo C, Austin R, McMartin KE (2010) Renal toxicity of ethylene glycol results from internalization of calcium oxalate crystals by proximal tubule cells. Toxicol Lett 192:365–372
Hübner K (1976) Morphologie der Arzneimittelschäden der Leber. Therapiewoche 26:590–604
Iacobuzio-Donahue CA, Lee EL, Abraham SC, Yardley JH, Wu TT (2001) Colchicine toxicity: distinct morphologic findings in gastrointestinal biopsies. Am J Surg Pathol 25:1067–1073
Indurato F, Raffino C, Tropea FM, Barbera N, Grieco A, Bartolini G (2014) Fatal accidental ingestion of 35% hydrogen peroxide by a 2-year-old female: a case report and literature review. Forensic Sci Med Pathol 10:443–447
Ishida Y, Takayasu T, Kimura A, Hayashi T, Kakimoto N, Miyashita T, Kondo T (2006) Gene expression of cytokines and growth factors in the lungs after paraquat administration in mice. Legal Med 8:102–109
Itoh S, Igarashi M, Tsukada Y, Ichinoe A (1977) Nonalcoholic fatty liver with alcoholic hyaline after long-term glucocorticoid therapy. Acta Hepatogastroenterol Stuttg 24:415–418
Jacobsen D, Akesson J, Shefter E (1982) Urinary calcium oxalate monohydrate crystals in ethylene glycol poisoning. Scand J Clin Lab Invest 146:121–234
Janssen W (1977) Forensische histologie. Schmidt-Römhild, Lübeck
Janssen W, Burger E (1968) Ungewöhnliche Art einer tödlichen Vergiftung durch Kaliumzyanid mit außergewöhnlichem Organbefund. Arch Kriminol 141:99
Jedidi M, Bel Hadj M, Masmoudi T, Abdelkarim SB, Mlayeh S, Dhiab MB, Souguir MK (2016) Fatal toxic myocarditis induced by paraphenylene diamine. A case report. Rom J Leg Med 24:17–20
Kakar P, Millar-Craig M, Kamaruddin H, Burn S, Loganathan S (2006) Clozapine induced myocarditis: a rare but fatal complication. Int J Cardiol 112:e5–e6
Kalin JR, Brissie RM (2002) A case of homicide by lethal injection with lidocaine. J Forensic Sci 47:1135–1138
Kalra TM, Mangla JC, DePapp EW (1976) Benign hepatic tumors and oral contraceptive pills. Am J Med 61:871–877
Karger B, Varchmin-Schultheiß K, Fechner G (2005) Fatal hepatic haemorrhage in a child-peliosis hepatis versus maltreatment. Int J Legal Med 119:44–46
Kasper MR, Drebber U, Hirsch I, Dienes H (2006) Morphologische Veränderungen der medikamenten-induzierten Leberschädigung. Pathologe 27:175–181
Kawamoto O, Ishikawa T, Oritani S, Kuramoto Y, Michiue T, Maeda H (2013) Death following the ingestion of detergent: an autopsy case with special regard to the histochemical findings. Forensic Sci Med Pathol 9:208–213
Kendell KR, Day JD, Hruban RH et al (1995) Intimate association of eosinophils to collagen bundles in eosinophilic myocarditis and ranitidine-induced hypersensitivity myocarditis. Arch Pathol Lab Med 119:1154–1160
Kennedy MC (1993) Myocardial infarction in association with misuse of anabolic steroids. Ulster Med J 62:172–174
Kennedy MC, Lawrence C (1993) Anabolic steroid abuse and cardiac death. Med J Aust 158:346–348
Kibler WB (1973) Skeletal muscle necrosis secondary to parathion. Toxicol Appl Pharmacol 25:117
Kilian JG, Kerr K, Lawrence C, Celermajer DS (1999) Myocarditis and cardiomyopathy associated with clozapine. Lancet 354:1841–1845
Klavis G, Schulz L (1966) Herzschäden bei der akuten Kohlenmonoxyd-Vergiftung. Arch Toxikol 21:250
Klintschar M, Beham-Schmidt C, Radner H, Henning G, Roll P (1999) Colchicine poisoning by accidental ingestion of meadow saffron (Colchicum autumnale): pathological and medicolegal aspects. Forensic Sci Int 106:191–200
Knudsen AH (2002) Peliosis hepatis as the cause of liver affection in a patient treated with immunosuppressive agents. Ugeskr Laeger 164:3215–3216
Korb G, David H (1962) Fluoreszenzmikroskopische und elektronenoptische Untersuchungen am Herzmuskel

der Ratte nach Leuchtgasvergiftungen. Dtsch Zschr f gerichtl Med 52:549
Krähenbühl S, Kaplowitz N (1996) Drug-induced hepatotoxicity: clinical presentation, pathogenesis, risk factors, diagnosis and treatment. In: Schmidt R, Bianchi L, Blum HE, Gerok W, Maier KP, Stalder GA (eds) Acute and chronic liver diseases. Molecular biology and clinics. Kluwer, Dordrecht, pp 147–158
Krug H (1965) Die Hirnkonsistenz bei tödlicher Kohlenmonoxydvergiftung. Dtsch Z ges gerichtl Med 56:74
Kubic A, Burda AM, Bockewitz E, Wahl M (2009) Hepatotoxicity in an infant following supratherapeutic dosing of acetaminophen for twenty-four hours. In: Santa Cruz DJ, Leikin JB, (eds) Seminars in diagnostic pathology. Toxicologic/Environmental Pathology. vol 26:pp 7–9
La Rosée K, Schulz A, Böhm M, Erdmann E (1997) Kardiale Dekompensation eines bodybuilders. Dtsch Med Wochenschr 122:1586–1590
Lahl R (1973) Fettembolien nach experimenteller Tetrachlorkohlenstoffintoxikation. Z Ges Inn Med 28:367
Lau G (1995a) A fatal case of drug-induced multi-organ damage in a patient with Hansen's disease: dapsone syndrome or rifampicin toxicity? Forensic Sci Int 73:109–115
Lau G (1995b) Iatrogenic-related, fatal hemorrhage occurring in end-stage renal failure: a series of three cases. Forensic Sci Int 73:117–124
Lau G (2005) Iatrogenic injury. A forensic perspective. In: Tsokos M (ed) Forensic pathology reviews, vol 3. Humana Press, Totowa, pp 351–439
Layland JJ, Liew D, Prior DL (2009) Clozapine-induced cardiotoxicity: a clinical update. Med J Aust 190:192
Lesch R (1968) Histologische und histoautoradiographische Befunde bei der experimentellen chronischen Bleivergiftung. Verh Dtsch Ges Path, p 542
Leth PM, Gregersen M (2005) Ethylene glycol poisoning. Forensic Sci Int 155:179–184
Lewis W, Silver MD (2001) Effects of drugs on the cardiovascular system. In: Silver MD, Gotlieb AI, Schoen FJ (eds) Cardiovascular pathology, 3rd edn. Churchill Livingstone, New York, pp 541–561
Li S, Huang W, Duan Y, Xing J, Zhou Y (2015) Human fatality due to thallium poisoning: autopsy, microscopy, and mass spectrometry assays. J Forensic Sci 60:247–251
Lovrić M, Granić P, Čubrilo-Turek M, Lalić Z, Sertić J (2007) Ethylene glycol poisoning. Forensic Sci Int 170:213–215
Lüderwald S, Zinka B, Thieme D, Eisenmenger W (2008) Missbrauch von anabolen androgenen Steroiden. Rechtsmedizin 18:183–188
Ludwig B, Schindler E, Bohl J, Pfeiffer J, Kremer G (1984) Reno-cerebral oxalosis induced by xylitol. Neuroradiology 26:517–521
Luke JL, Farb A, Virmani R, Sample RH (1990) Sudden cardiac death during exercise in a weight lifter using anabolic androgenic steroids: pathological and toxicological findings. J Forensic Sci 35:1441–1447
Lynberg K (1991) Myocardial infarction and death of a body builder after using anabolic steroids. Ugeskr Laeger 153:587–588
Lynch ML, Woodford NWF (2008) Fatality complicating agranulocytosis in the setting of carbamazole therapy. Forensic Sci Med Pathol 4:246–249
Machnik G (1985) Morphological reaction patterns of the liver induced by drugs. Zentralbl Allg Pathol 130:491–507
Magdalan J, Ostrowska A, Podhorska-Okolow M, Piotrowska A, Izykowska I, Nowak M, Dolinska-Krajewska B, Zabel M, Szelag A, Dziegiel P (2009) Early morphological and functional alterations in canine hepatocytes due to a-amanitin, a major toxin of amanita phalloides. Arch Toxicol 83:55–60
Mannou H, Ikemura M, Nakagawa Y, Nata M, Inoue H (2014) An autopsy case of serotonin toxicity resulting from suicidal administrations of fluvoxamine and lithium. Rom J Leg Med 22:59–62
Markwalder C (1983) Zum morphologischen Nachweis des Mißbrauchs phenacetin-haltiger Analgetica. Beitr Gerichtl Med 41:63–66
Maron BJ, Shirani J, Poliac LC, Mathenge R, Roberts WC, Müller FO (1996) Sudden death in young competitive athletes. JAMA 276:199–204
McIntyre IM, Ruszkiewicz AR, Crump K, Drummer OH (1994) Death following poisoning. J Forensic Sci 39:280–286
McKillop G, Todd IC, Ballantyne D (1986) Increased left ventricular mass in a body builder using anabolic steroids. Br J Sports Med 20:151–152
McMartin K (2009) Are calcium oxalate crystals involved in the mechanism of acute renal failure in ethylene glycol poisoning? Clin Toxicol 47:859–869
McNutt RA, Ferenchick GS, Kirhn PC, Hamlin NJ (1988) Acute myocardial infarction in a 22-year-old worldclass weight lifter using anabolic steroids. Am J Cardiol 62:164
Meatherall R, Oleschuk C (2015) Suicidal fatality from azide ingestion. J Forensic Sci 60:1666–1667
Medline A, Shin DH, Medline NM (1976) Pseudomembranous colitis associated with antibiotics. Hum Pathol 7:693–703
Meier W (1962) Experimentelle Untersuchungen zur Bedeutung der vacuoligen Umwandlung der Leber für die Diagnostik der Kohlenmonoxydvergiftung. Dtsch Z ges gerichtl Med 52:258
Meissner W, Schmidt T, Kupsch A, Trottenberg T, Lempert T (1999) Reversible leucopenia related to olanzapine. Mov Disord 14:872–873
Merrill DB, Dec GW, Goff DC (2005) Adverse cardiac effects associated with clozapine. J Clin Psychopharmacol 25:32–41
Merrill DB, Ahmari SE, Bradford JM, Lieberman JA (2006) Myocarditis during clozapine treatment. Am J Psychiatry 163:204–208
Metter D, Schulz E (1978) Tödliche Verbrühung oder Lyell-Syndrom? Z Rechtsmed 81:329–334

Mihatsch MJ, Torhorst J, Amsler B, Zollinger HU (1978) Capillarosclerosis of the lower urinary tract in analgesic (phenacetin) abuse. Virchows Arch Pathol Anat 381:41–47

Mihatsch MJ, Torhorst J, Steinmann E, Hofer H, Stickelberger M, Bianchi L, Berneis K, Zollinger HU (1979) The morphologic diagnosis of analgesic (phenacetin) abuse. Pathol Res Pract 164:68–79

Mochizuki RM, Richter KJ (1988) Cardiomyopathy and cerebrovascular accident associated with anabolic-androgenic steroid use. Phys Sportsmed 16:108–114

Molz G (1971) Pneumopathien bei Neugeborenen nach langfristiger intratrachealer Druckbeatmung mit hochgespanntem Sauerstoff. Beitr Gerichtl Med 28:66

Montisci M, El Mazloum R, Cecchetto G, Terranova C, Ferrara SD, Thiene G, Basso C (2012) Anabolic androgenic steroids abuse and cardiac death in athletes: morphological and toxicological findings in four fatal cases. Forensic Sci Int 217:e13–e18

Morgan JM, Hartley MW, Miller RE (1966) Nephropathie bei chronischer Bleivergiftung. Arch Intern Med 118:17

Morningstar WA (1955) Exogenous hemochromatosis. Arch Pathol 59:355–358

Movat AP (1983) Reye's syndrome: 20 years on. Br Med J 286:1999–2000

Muirhead EE, Crass G, Jones F, Hill JM (1949) Iron overload (Hemosiderosis) aggravated by blood transfusions. Arch Intern Med 83:477–501

Müller GL, Graham S (1955) Intrauteriner Fruchttod durch Kohlenmonoxydvergiftung. N Engl J Med 252:1075

Mullins M, Cannarozzi AA, Bailey TC, Ranganathan P (2011) Unrecognized fatalities related to colchicine in hospitalized patients. Clin Toxicol (Phila) 49:648–652

Munk JF, Collopy BT, Connell JL, McTeigue JJ, Hughes JF, Hood RN, Breen KJ (1976) Lincomycin-clindamycin-associated pseudomembranous colitis. Med J Aust 2:95–97

Nagao M, Zhang W, Itakura Y, Kobayashi M, Yamada Y, Yagi K, Oono T, Takatori T (1993) Immunohistochemical localization and dynamics of paraquat in the stomach and esophagus of rats. Int J Legal Med 106:142–144

Naumann R, Felber W, Heilemann H, Reuster T (1999) Olanzapine-induced agranulocytosis. Lancet 354:566–567

Nishio H, Suzuki K (2005) Three cases of suspected hyperthermia with remarkable elevation of serum mast cell tryptase. Forensic Sci Int 149:51–55

Nishio H, Matsui K, Miyazaki T, Tamura A, Iwata M, Suzuki K (2002) A fatal case of amniotic fluid embolism with elevation of serum mast cell tryptase. Forensic Sci Int 126:53–56

Nizze H, Schwabbauer P, Brachwitz C, Lange H (1997) Fatal chronic oxalosis after sublethal ethylene glycol poisoning. Pathologe 18:328–334

Norland CC, Kirsner JB (1969) Toxic dilatation of colon (toxic megacolon): etiology, treatment and prognosis in 42 patients. Medicine 48:229–250

Nuzzo JL, Manz HJ, Maxted WC (1985) Peliosis hepatis after long-term androgen therapy. Urology 25:518–519

Oehmichen M, Besserer K (1982) Forensic significance of acetylcholinesterase histochemistry in organophosphate intoxication. Original investigations and review of the literature. Z Rechtsmed 89:149–165

Oliver RAM (1959) Siderosis following transfusions of blood. J Pathol Bacteriol 77:171–194

Omer FB, Iozzo RV, Casetti P, Dellarole AC (1978) Focal nodular hyperplasia of the liver and contraceptive steroids. Acta Hepatogastroenterol 25:319–321

Osawa M, Satoh F, Horiuchi H, Tian W, Kugota N, Hasegawa I (2008) Postmortem diagnosis of fatal anaphylaxis during intravenous administration of therapeutic and diagnostic agents: evaluation of clinical laboratory parameters and immunohistochemistry in three cases. Legal Med 10:143–147

Overly WL, Dankhoff JA, Wank BK, Singh VD (1984) Androgens and hepatocellular carcinoma in an athlete. Ann Intern Med 100:158–159

Parry MF, Wallach R (1974) Ethylene glycol poisoning. Am J Med 57:143–150

Perskvist N, Edston E (2007) Differential accumulation of pulmonary and cardiac mast cell-subsets and eosinophils between fatal anaphylaxis and asthma death: a post-mortem comparative study. Forensic Sci Int 169:43–49

Peter H (1955) Organbefunde nach akuter Cadmiumvergiftung. Verh Dtsch Ges Path, p 225

Pfeiffer H, Weiss FU, Karger B, Aghdassi A, Lerch MM, Brinkmann B (2004) Fatal cerebro-renal oxalosis after appendectomy. Int J Legal Med 118:98–100

Pfordt J, Magerl H, Vock R (1987) Fatal intoxications with propoxur. Z Rechtsmed 98:43–48

Pieroni M, Cavallaro R, Chimenti C, Smeraldi E, Frustaci A (2004) Clozapine-induced hypersensitivity myocarditis. Chest 126:1703–1705

Pietsch J, Schulz K, Schmidt U, Andresen H, Schwarze B, Dreßler J (2007) A comparative study of five fatal cases of Taxus poisoning. Int J Legal Med 121:417–422

Pikula B, Plamenac P, Ćurčić B, Nikulin A (1973) Myocarditis caused by primary oxalosis in a 4-year-old child. Virch Arch A Path Anat 358:99–103

Plewig G, Jansen T (1998) Acneiform dermatoses. Dermatology 196:102–107

Pomara C, Fiore C, D'Errico S, Riezzo I, Fineschi V (2008) Calcium oxalate crystals in acute ethylene glycol poisoning: a confocal laser scanning microscope study in a fatal case. Clin Toxicol 46:322–324

Prat S, Hoizey G, Lefrancq T, Saint-Martin P (2015) An unusual case of strychnine poisoning. J Forensic Sci 60:816817

Pribilla O (1966) Tödliche Vergiftungen mit Salzen der Kieselfluorwasserstoffsäure. In: Gerchow J (ed) An den Grenzen von Medizin und Recht. Enke, Stuttgart

Pullela R, Young L, Gallagher B, Avis S, Randell EW (2008) A case of fatal aconitine poisoning by monkshood ingestion. J Forensic Sci 53:491–494

Pumphrey RS, Roberts IS (2000) Postmortem findings after fatal anaphylactic reactions. J Clin Pathol 53:273–276

Razminia M, Salem Y, Sivasubramaniam D, Shah N, Khosla S (2006) Clozapine induced myocarditis. Early recognition improves clinical outcome. Am J Ther 13:274–276

Reye RDK, Morgan G, Baral J (1963) Encephalopathy and fatty degeneration of the viscera. A disease entity in childhood. Lancet 2:749–752

Riße M, Türker T, Weiler G (1998) Postmortale Differentialdiagnose und forensische Relevanz kutaner Blasenbildungen. Rechtsmedizin 8:141–146

Ritter C, Weiler G, Adebahr G (1985) Histomorphological lung results in cases of long-term artificial respiration with special consideration of use of pure oxygen. Z Rechtsmed 94:41–49

Roll P, Klintschar M (1999) Two cases of poisoning resulting from accidental ingestion of Meadow Saffron (Colchicum autumnale). Proceedings of the international association of forensic sciences 15th triennial meeting, The International Association of Forensic Sciences, Los Angeles, 22–28 Aug 1999

Rubin E (1980) Iatrogenic hepatic injury. Hum Pathol 11:312–331

Safrai A (2007) Morphological changes in toxic hepatitis. Forensic Sci Int/Abstracts 169S:2

Saleki S, Ardalan FA, Javidan-Nejad A (2007) Liver histopathology of fatal phosphine poisoning. Forensic Sci Int 16:190–193

Salomone L, Scorsone A (1961) Myocardinfarkt als Folge einer Blausäurevergiftung. Folia Med Napoli 44:609. (zitiert nach: Janssen 1977)

Sannohe S, Makino Y, Kita T, Kuroda N, Shinozuka T (2002) Colchicine poisoning resulting from accidental ingestion of meadow saffron (Colchicum autumnale). J Forensic Sci 47:1391–1396

Schonberg LA (1982) Peliosis hepatis and oral contraceptives. A case report. J Reprod Med 27:753–756

Schwartz LB, Metcalfe DD, Miller JS, Earl H, Sullivan T (1987) Tryptase levels as an indicator of mast-cell activation in systemic anaphylaxis and mastocytosis. N Engl J Med 316:1622–1626

Shaohua Z, Ananda S, Ruxia Y, Liang R, Xiaorui C, Liang L (2010) Fatal renal failure due to Chinese herb "GuanMu Tong" (Aristolochia manshuriensis): autopsy findings and review of the literature. Forensic Sci Int 1999:e5–e7

Shepherd GM (2003) Hypersensitivity reactions to drugs: evaluation and management. Mt Sinai J Med 70:113–125

Sinn LE, Porterfield JF (1991) Fatal taxine poisoning from yew leaf ingestion. J Forensic Sci 36:599–601

Socas L, Zumbado M, Perez-Luzardo O et al (2005) Hepatocellular adenomas associated with anabolic androgenic steroid abuse in bodybuilders: a report of two cases and review of the literature. Br J Sports Med 39:27–31

Stanworth D, Hunt NCA, Flanagan RJ (2012) Clozapine – a dangerous drug in a clozapine-naïve subject. Forensic Sci Int 214:e23–e25

Steinwachs A, Grohmann R, Pedrosa F, Rüther E, Schwerdtner I (1999) Two cases of olanzapine-induced reversible neutropenia. Pharmacopsychiatry 32:154–156

Stemmermann GN, Hayashi T (1971) Colchicine intoxication: a reappraisal of its pathology based on a study of three fatal cases. Hum Pathol 2:321–332

Summer HW, Tedesco FJ (1975) Rectal biopsy in clindamycin-associated colitis. Arch Pathol 99:237–241

Symmers WSC (1962) The occurrence of angiitis and other generalized diseases of connective tissues as a consequence of the administration of drugs. Proc R Soc Med 55:20–28

Takahashi S, Kanetake J, Kanawaku Y, Funayama M (2008) Brain death with calcium oxalate deposition in the kidney: clue to diagnosis of ethylene glycol poisoning. Legal Med 10:43–45

Teare RD (1976) Poisoning by paraquat. Med Sci Law 16:9–12

Teschke R (2001) Toxische Leberschäden durch Arzneimittel. Dtsch Ärztebl 40:B-2220–B-2225

Thaler H (1987) Leberkrankheiten, 2nd edn. Springer, Heidelberg, New York, Tokio

Thiblin I, Lindquist O, Rajs J (2000) Cause and manner of death among users of anabolic androgenic steroids. J Forensic Sci 45:16–23

Thiblin I, Mobini-Far H, Frisk M (2009) Sudden unexpected death in a female athlete, with a possible connection to the use of anabolic androgenic steroids (AAS) and ephedrine. Forensic Sci Int 184:e7–e11

Thierauf A, Gnann H, Bohnert M, Vennemann B, Auwärter V, Weinmann W (2009) Suicidal poisoning with mercaptodimethur – morphological findings and toxicological analysis. Int J Legal Med 123:327–331

Thomas DW, Edwards JB, Gilligan JE, Lawrence JR, Edwards RG (1972) Complications following intravenous administration of solutions containing xylitol. Med J Aust 1:1238–1246

Thurner J (1970) Iatrogene pathologie. Urban & Schwarzenberg, München

Timm F (1958) Zur Histochemie der Schwermetalle. Das Sulfidsilberverfahren. Dtsch Z ges gerichtl Med 46:706

Timm F (1961) Der histochemische Nachweis der Sublimatvergiftung. Beitr Gerichtl Med 21:195

Timm F (1962) Zur Histochemie der chronischen Quecksilbervergiftung. Beitr Gerichtl Med 22:321

Tischer KH, Heyny von Haussen R, Mall G, Doenecke P (2003) Koronarthrombosen und –ektasien nach langjähriger Einnahme von anabolen Steroiden. Z Kardiol 92:326–331

Tóth AR, Varga T (2009) Myocardium and striated muscle damage caused by licit and illicit drugs. Legal Med 11:S484–S487

Totović V (1964) Elektronenmikroskopische Befunde in der Niere bei chronischer Bleivergiftung der Ratte. Verh Dtsch Ges Path 339:193

Trani N, Bonetti LR, Gualandri G, Barbolini G (2008) Immediate anaphylactic death following antibiotics injection: splenic eosinophilia easily revealed by pagoda red stain. Forensic Sci Int 181:21–25

Tsokos M, Erbersdobler A (2005) Pathology of peliosis. Forensic Sci Int 149:25–33
Tsokos M, Püschel K (2004) Isolated peliosis of the spleen: report of 2 autopsy cases. Am J Forensic Med Pathol 25:251–254
Tsokos M, Sperhake J (2002) Coma blisters in a case of fatal theophylline intoxication. Am J Forensic Med Pathol 23:292–294
Türk EE, Sperhake JP, Tsokos M (2002) Pseudomembranous colitis with fatal outcome in a 43-year-old man. Legal Med 4:246–250
Tzirogiannis KN, Papadimas GK, Kondyli VG, Kourentzi KT, Demonakou MD, Kyriakou LG, Mykoniatis MG, Hereti RI, Panoutsopoulos GI (2006) Peliosis hepatis: microscopic and macroscopic type, time pattern, and correlation with liver cell apoptosis in a model of toxic liver injury. Dig Dis Sci 51:1998–2006
Ulrich W, Schwarz HP, Aiginger P, Grabner G, Kumpan W, Seidl G (1982) Pulmonale hyaline Membranen nach Zytostatikatherapie. For Pathol 3:195–197
Unuma K, Harada K, Nakajima M, Eguchi H, Tsushima K, Ito T, Shintani-Ishida K, Kojima H, Yoshida K (2010) Forensic Sci Int 194:e5–e8
Valla D, Benhamou JP (1988) Drug-induced vascular and sinusoidal lesions of the liver. Baillières Clin Gastroenterol 2:481–500
Van Erpecum KJ, Janssens AR, Kreuning J, Ruiter DJ, Kroon HM, Grond AJ (1988) Generalized peliosis hepatis and cirrhosis after long-term use of oral contraceptives. Am J Gastroenterol 83:572–575
van Ingen G, Visser R, Peltenburg H, van der Ark AM, Voortman M (1992) Sudden unexpected death due to Taxus poisoning. A report of five cases with review of the literature. Forensic Sci Int 56:81–87
Ventura F, Bonsignore A, de Stefano F, Pizzorno E, Palmiere C (2014) Fatal intrahepatic hemorrhage after nadroparin use for total hip arthroplasty. Forensic Sci Med Pathol 10:619–622
Vock R (1984) Iatrogene histopathologische Befunde – eine systematische Zusammenstellung. Z Rechtsmed 92:1–25
von der Hardt H, Cardesa A (1971) Die histopathologischen Frühveränderungen nach Paraquat-Intoxikation. Klin Wochenschr 49:544–550
Vougiouklakis T, Mitselou A, Batistatou A, Boumba V, Charalabopoulos K (2009) First case of fatal pulmonary peliosis without any other organ involvement in a young testosterone abusing male. Forensic Sci Int 186:e13–e16
Wagner-Thiessen E (1985) Das Reye-syndrom. Pathologe 6:220–223
Weber W (1985) Genesis of atraumatic liver hemorrhages. Z Rechtsmed 95:145–152
Wehmeier PM, Heiser P, Remschmidt H (2005) Myocarditis, pericarditis and cardiomyopathy in patients treated with clozapine. J Clin Pharm Ther 30:91–96
Welder AA, Melchert RB (1993) Cardiotoxic effects of cocaine and anabolic-androgenic steroids in the athletes. J Pharmacol Toxicol Methods 29:61–68
Westaby D, Ogle SJ, Paradinas FJ, Randell JB, Murray-Lyon IM (1977) Liver damage from long-term methyltestosterone. Lancet 2:262–263
Wilbert L, Creutzfeld W (1967) Wiederholter Ikterus mit tödlicher Lebernekrose nach zweimaliger Halothan-Narkose. Dtsch Med Wochenschr 13:597–600
Wittstock G (1983) Focal nodular hyperplasia of the liver. Zbl Allg Pathol 127:135–143
Wölkart N, Soos E, Rankl W (1954) Zur Klinik und Pathologie der Knollenblätterpilzvergiftung. Wien klinische Wochenschr Sonderabdruck 16:273–276
Wollersen H, Erdmann F, Risse M, Dettmeyer R (2009a) Accidental fatal ingestion of colchicine-containing leaves – toxicological and histological findings. Legal Med 11:S498–S499
Wollersen H, Erdmann F, Risse M, Dettmeyer R (2009b) Oxalate-crystals in different tissues following intoxication with ethylene glycol: three case reports. Legal Med 11:S488–S490
Yamada M, Nakagawa M, Haritani M, Kobayashi M, Furuoka H, Matsui T (1998) Histopathological study of experimental acute poisoning of cattle by autumn crocus (Colchicum autumnale L.) J Vet Med Sci 60:949–952
Yamazaki A, Iranami H, Nishikawa K (2013) Severe colchicine intoxication after self-administration of colchicine concomitantly with loxoprofen. J Anesth 27:483–484
Yilmaz R, Yilmaz E, Ozdemir V, Can M, Pakis I, Piskin IE, Dokgoz H, Ozer E, Numanoglu KV (2015) An evaluation of childhood deaths in Turkey due to yellow phosphorus in firecrackers. J Forensic Sci 60: 648–652
Yunginger JW, Nelson DR, Squillace DL, Jones RT, Holley KE, Hyma BA et al (1991) Laboratory investigations of deaths due to anaphylaxis. J Forensic Sci 36:857–865
Zak F (1959) Peliosis hepatis. Am J Pathol 26:1–15
Zhang M, Tavora F, Zhang Y, Ripple M, Fowler D, Zhao Z, Burke A (2013) The role of focal myocardial inflammation in sudden unexpected cardiac and non-cardiac deaths – a clinicopathological study. Int J Legal Med 127:131–138
Zimmerman HJ (1978) Drug-induced liver disease. Drugs 16:25–45
Zimmerman HJ, Ishak KG (1982) Valproate induced hepatic injury. Analysis of 23 fatal cases. Hepatology 2:591–597
Zimmerman HJ, Ishak KG (2002) Hepatic injury due to drugs and toxins. In: MacSween RNM, Burt AD, Portmann BC, Ishak KG, Scheuer PJ, Anthony PP (eds) Pathology of the liver, 4th edn. Churchill Livingstone, London, pp 621–709
Zollinger HU (1953) Durch chronische Bleivergiftung erzeugte Nierenadenome und –carcinome bei Ratten und ihre Beziehungen zu den entsprechenden Neubildungen des Menschen. Virchows Arch Path Anat 323:694

6 Alcohol-Related Histopathology

Chronic alcohol consumption leads to a multitude of histopathological findings, particularly in the advanced stages of alcoholism. The liver is by no means the only organ affected by alcohol consumption. Pathological changes are routinely observed where collagen connective tissue is replaced by toxic, damaged liver tissue; this process begins with truncation and fibrosis of the portal fields, leading to liver fibrosis and the development of pseudolobules demarcated by connective tissue in the case of fine- to medium-coarse nodular portal liver cirrhosis. In addition, alcohol-induced pathological changes of the pancreas can occur. When portal congestion is present, splenomegaly will also develop, and varices of the esophagus may be seen. Alcoholic cardiomyopathy should be mentioned separately; with regard to differential diagnoses, inflammatory cardiomyopathy must be considered in connection with dilative cardiomyopathy (see Chap. 13). The intracerebral reduction in Purkinje cells, which may be detected morphometrically, leads to the diagnosis of chronic alcohol abuse (Schuck 1983). In cases of death with a relatively low blood alcohol concentration, cardiomyocytic microvesicular steatosis and lipid droplet discharge in the adrenal cortex at the time of death have been reported surprisingly often (Bschor and Keilbach 1968). Fracasso et al. (2008) reported clotted blood as a sign of alcohol intoxication. Poisoning with alcohols or chemically related substances besides ethyl alcohol (ethanol), e.g., methanol, propanol, or ethyl glycol (see Chap. 5), is occasionally reported. In addition to histopathological findings in brain tissue, methanol can also cause extensive necrosis of the esophageal and gastric mucosa (Cascalla et al. 2012).

6.1 Alcoholic Liver Pathology

Changes to the liver tissue due to chronic alcohol consumption detectable using conventional histology enable classification of the degree of severity of findings. In the early stage, the dominant finding is steatosis with accompanying portal fibrosis (Fig. 6.1), but alcoholic and nonalcoholic steatohepatitis show an almost identical morphology: a combination of steatosis, hepatocellular injury (ballooning degeneration, apoptosis, necrosis), perivenular and pericellular fibrosis, and inflammation (Denk et al. 2001; Dancygier 1997; Diehl et al. 1988). Nonalcoholic steatohepatitis is mainly associated with adipositas, diabetes type II, hyperlipidemia, and complete parenteral nutrition or rarely drug associated (e.g., amiodarone, perhexiline maleate, chloroquine, glucocorticoids). A proposal for grading and staging of histological lesions in cases of nonalcoholic steatohepatitis was made (Brunt et al. 1999).

With additional alcohol use, the degree of fibrosis may increase, and the liver may already show fatty liver macroscopically (Fig. 6.2) if >50% of the hepatocytes are fatty. This is usually

R. B. Dettmeyer, *Forensic Histopathology*, https://doi.org/10.1007/978-3-319-77997-3_6

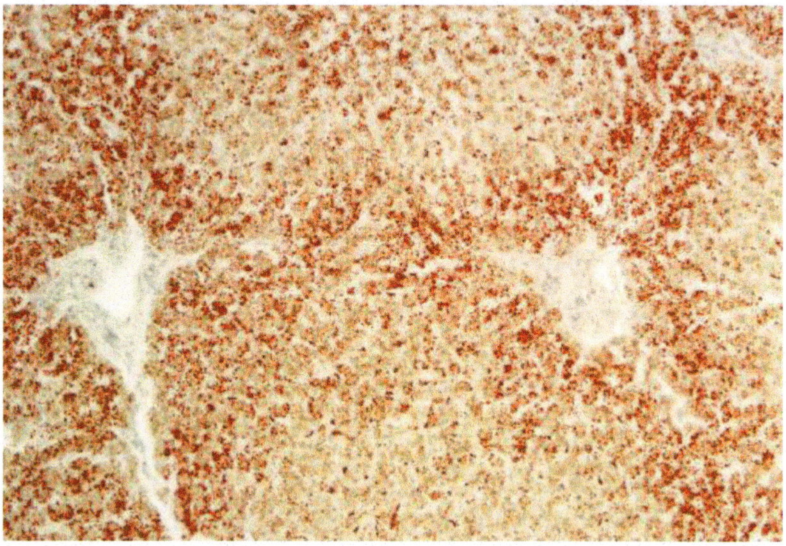

Fig. 6.1 Distinct alcoholic and nutrition-/toxin-related steatosis around the portal fields. Stage 3 hepatic steatosis (Sudan III ×100)

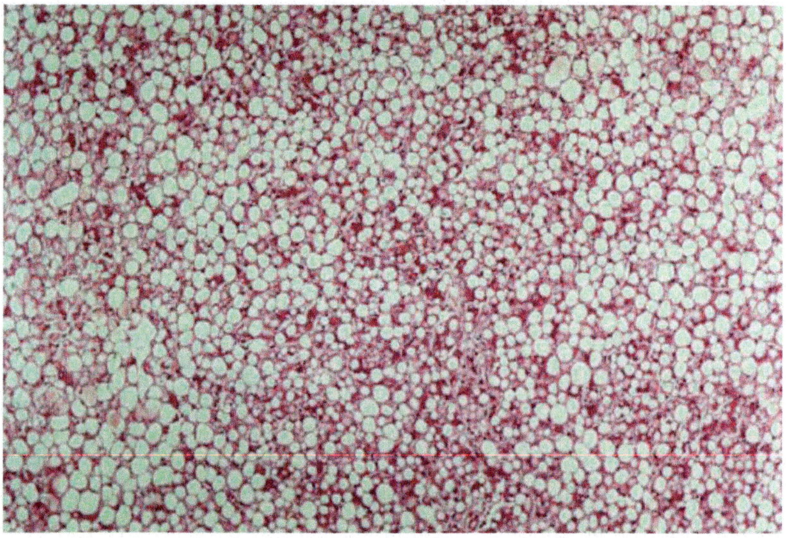

Fig. 6.2 Alcoholic hepatic steatosis with no inflammatory activity and no fibrosis in a 58-year-old alcoholic, found dead in the kitchen (H&E ×100)

microvesicular adiposis of hepatocytes, which may be of varying etiology. Due to steatosis, the liver can weigh up to 4000 g compared to its normal weight of approximately 1500 g. Unlike fibrosis and cirrhosis, steatosis is always reversible and may quickly regress within 3 or 4 weeks once the person stops alcohol consumption. In advanced stages, portal liver cirrhosis with pseudolobules occurs, often showing adipose hepatocytes (Fig. 6.3). Notable bile duct proliferation can be observed in areas of cirrhotic transformation (Fig. 6.4), and the risk of hepatocellular and/or cholangiocellular liver carcinoma is increased (see Table 6.1). Activated stellate cells play a significant role in the genesis of liver fibrosis and cirrhosis, although there is not always a clear correlation between histologically detectable fibrosis and stellate cell activation. Kupffer cells secrete cytokines (TNF-alpha, IL-6, TGF-ß 1), thereby stimulating collagen synthesis (Denk et al. 2001; McClain et al. 1999; Tsukamoto et al. 1990). At the same time, hepatic cell destruction via apoptosis is believed to play a role in alcohol-related damage to liver tissue. Thus, the number of apoptotic cells in alcoholic hepatic steatosis should be as elevated as in animal models using

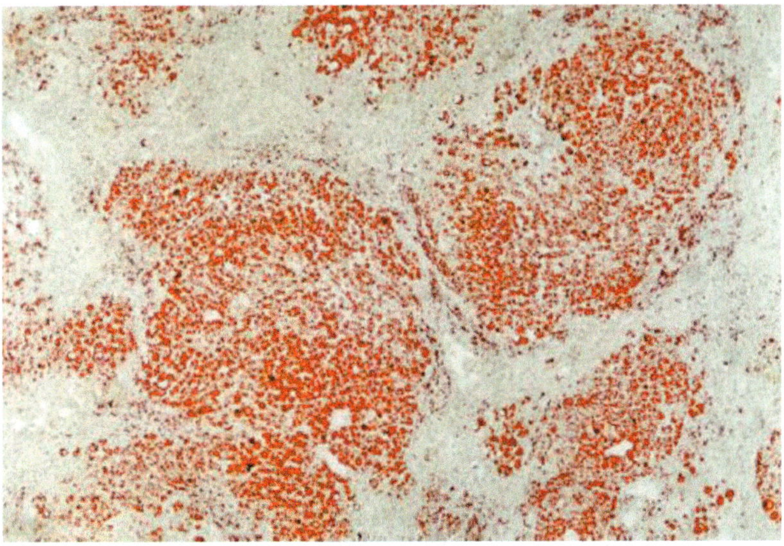

Fig. 6.3 Established alcoholic liver cirrhosis with diffuse fine- to medium-coarse nodules with hepatic steatosis (Sudan III ×100)

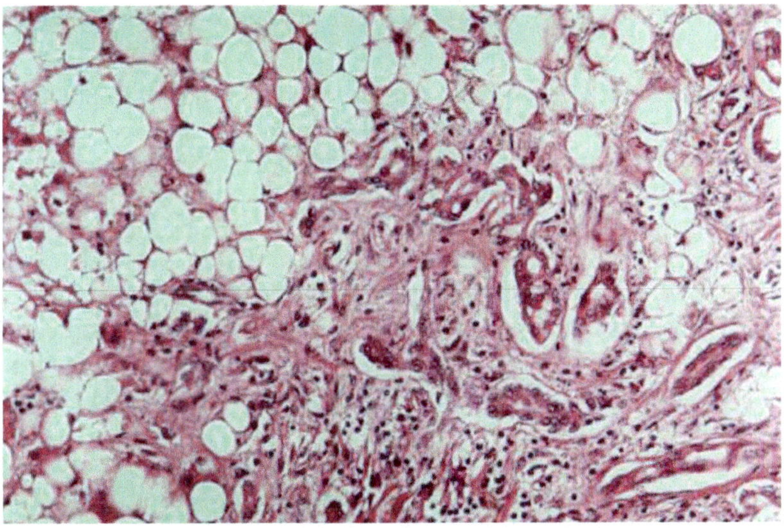

Fig. 6.4 Alcoholic liver cirrhosis with abundant bile duct proliferation, stage 4 hepatic steatosis, and low inflammatory activity (H&E ×200)

rats, in which chronic alcohol administration was intended to increase apoptotic hepatic cells (Day 2001; Natori et al. 2001; Nanji 1998).

Steatosis may be accompanied by an inflammatory response, which has led to the term "acute alcoholic hepatitis." Here, chronically or acutely inflamed, infiltrated portal fields may be observed, consisting mainly of lymphocytes and histiocytes. In the case of fatty liver hepatitis, the bile ducts are not affected. There is occasionally a suspicion of viral hepatitis in response to the histologic picture with moderate or severe inflammatory infiltrates (grade 2 or 3), associated with an absence of increased collagen fibers and no significant fatty transformation. In such cases, Councilman bodies may be present, and serologic investigations are helpful to clarify the cause of inflammatory infiltrates, which can also be an indication of chronic alcohol addiction.

Councilman Bodies Councilman, an American pathologist, discovered eosinophilic bodies, now termed Councilman bodies. Also known as Councilman hyaline bodies or eosinophilic globules, Councilman bodies are indicative of an hepatocyte undergoing apoptosis. Councilman

Table 6.1 Classification of alcoholic histopathological findings in liver tissue (According to Ferries and Thompson 1981)

Degree	Fibrosis/cirrhosis	Degree of steatosis (%)	Inflammatory activity
0	No pathological finding	0–5	No increase in infiltrates
1	Mild fibrosis of the portal fields; from the differential diagnostic perspective, a condition following hepatitis or ascending cholangitis should be considered	5–25	Mild increase in lymphocytes and monocytes at portal field margins
2	Portal field fibrosis with connective tissue-like branching into the hepatic sinus; however, no communication between branches (pre-cirrhotic restructuring of liver parenchyma)	25–50	Lymphocytic and monocytic infiltrates in the portal fields and around neighboring liver parenchyma
3	Thin fibrotic strands, which arise from the portal fields and continue along the hepatic lobules, coalesce while developing pseudolobules which surround intact liver tissue	50–75	Dense infiltrates with lymphocytes and monocytes in the portal fields and in the liver parenchyma
4	Wide fibrotic strands surround small pseudolobules with sparsely remaining intact hepatocytes, intense bile duct proliferation, inflammatory infiltrates with hepatocellular necrosis	75–100	"Fatty liver hepatitis" with hepatocellular necrosis and hyaline (Mallory bodies)

Steatosis = % of hepatocytes with intracytoplasmic fatty vacuoles with fine and coarse droplets

bodies are small, hyaline, round, or oval eosinophilic inclusions in the cytoplasm of hepatic cells; in yellow fever, they are believed to represent necrosis around viral particles. Councilman bodies may also be seen in other forms of toxic or viral hepatitis and more rarely in bacterial or parasitic infections. Both Councilman bodies and Mallory bodies can be accompanied by ballooned hepatocytes.

Mallory–Denk Bodies Mallory, also an American pathologist, first described ballooned hepatocytes, which contain a large lipid vacuole and a blue, amorphous body in the cytoplasm (Mallory 1911) (Fig. 6.5). The bodies are also termed both Mallory bodies and Mallory–Denk bodies, since Denk, a pathologist from Austria, described further findings on these bodies (Zatloukal et al. 2007; Denk et al. 2000). Immunohistochemically, Mallory–Denk bodies (alcoholic hyaline) can present with increased expression of cytokeratins (Strnad et al. 2008) and are primarily seen in cases of alcoholic steatohepatitis. Hepatocytes also present with larger mitochondria in the ballooned cells.

However, alcoholic hyaline (Mallory–Denk bodies) is rarely seen, and its appearance is not evidence of alcohol consumption. It appears as cloudy, acidophilic deposits with a round, elongated shape and poorly demarcated margins around the nucleus. Balloon cells often (but not always) contain Mallory–Denk bodies, which are irregular cytoplasmic inclusions consisting of keratins and nonkeratin components, including ubiquitin and chaperones (heat shock protein, HSP), particularly HSP 70 and HSP 25. Under electron microscopy, Mallory–Denk bodies comprise irregularly arranged, unbranched tubular elements with an irregular surface measuring approximately 10 nm in diameter (Denk et al. 2001). Therefore, antibodies against ubiquitin can be used to detect Mallory–Denk bodies by immunohistochemistry (Fig. 6.6).

Alcoholic hyaline does not only occur in alcohol-damaged hepatocytes; nonalcoholic fatty liver with alcoholic hyaline has also been described after long-term glucocorticoid therapy (Itoh et al. 1977). This toxic response of the liver tissue is potentially genetically determined. For example, no alcoholic hyaline could be found in Japanese alcoholics (Ichida 1970; Kagawa 1970). The detection of Mallory–Denk bodies, combined with a corresponding alcohol anamnesis, is an indication that the liver is currently being affected by alcohol. Steatosis and acute alcoholic

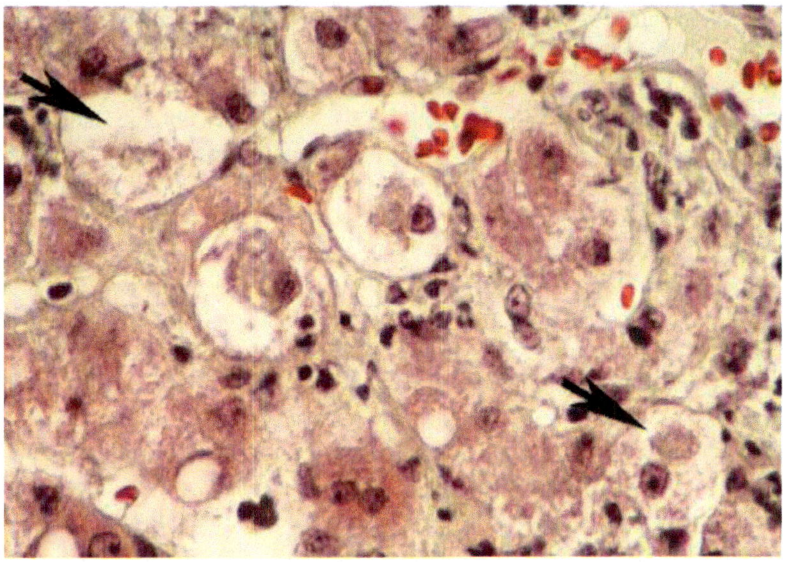

Fig. 6.5 Liver tissue with alcoholic hyaline, Mallory–Denk bodies (*arrows*) (orcein ×500)

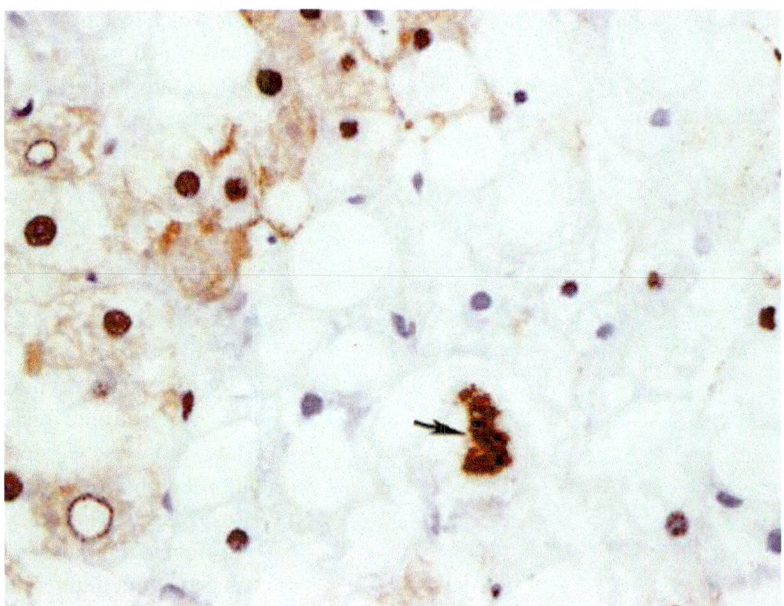

Fig. 6.6 Mallory–Denk body detected immunohistochemically using an antibody against ubiquitin (*arrow*) (×400)

hepatitis are reversible if alcohol consumption is stopped. If not, there will be an increase in reticulin and collagen fibers which surround single hepatocytes or groups of hepatocytes like a mesh, termed wire mesh fibrosis. Wire mesh fibrosis is also a characteristic of alcoholic liver damage; however, differential diagnostic consideration should be given to Morbus Wilson disease, primary and biliary liver cirrhosis, as well as phosphorus intoxication (Janssen 1977).

The assumption that hepatitis must be present when the portal fields do not contain alcoholic inflammatory infiltrates and in the absence of adiposis of the liver does not fully apply. Particularly with regard to polytoxic drug addicts, there may be significant adiposis of the liver as a result of concurrent alcohol consumption despite florid hepatitis. Otherwise, inflamed cells can be found in the vicinity of hepatocellular necrobioses.

As a result of alcohol consumption, enlarged and multiplied Kupffer stellate cells may also appear, often containing iron pigments and termed "alcoholic's iron."

In the advanced stage of liver cirrhosis with signs of decompensation, intrahepatic cholestasis is seen along with bile pigment deposits in the cytoplasm of remaining hepatocytes as well as retained bile thrombi in smaller bile ducts in some cases. As a rule, autopsy reveals icterus of the skin, eyelid connective tissue, mucous membranes, and vessel intima in all body regions. Epithelial cells of the renal tubules may reabsorb bile pigment, leading to the histopathological picture of the so-called cholemic nephrosis (Fig. 6.7).

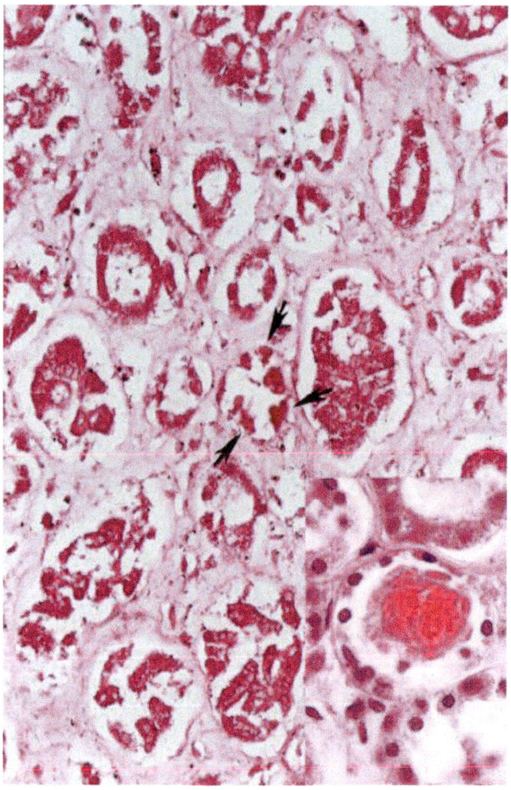

Fig. 6.7 Microphotographs from two cases of death in hepatic coma with cholemic nephrosis due to chronic alcohol abuse: autolytic epithelium of the renal tubules with reabsorbed bile pigment (*arrows*) (H&E ×200); high magnification (H&E ×500)

6.2 The Pancreas

Alcohol-related damage to pancreas tissue is usually chronic damage (Böcker and Seifert 1972). Fibrosis and lipomatosis of the pancreas with perilobular and intralobular fibrosis may develop, along with atrophy of the parenchyma and moderate inflammatory infiltration. Advanced stages show thickened, fibrous walls of the gland excretory ducts with flattened epithelial cells and an often loose lymphocytic inflammatory infiltrate in the context of unspecific chronic fibrous pancreatitis (Fig. 6.8). In addition, duct ectasia is present in which retained secretion may accumulate, as well as microscopically small concrements. In the case of severe damage, there may be predigestion of the surrounding tissue. In this case, one may observe tryptic fatty tissue necrosis which resembles candle grease spots (Fig. 6.9) and which may calcify in the future (Fig. 6.10). There are isolated reports of (tryptic) fat tissue necrosis in acute pancreatitis beyond the immediately adjacent peripancreatic region. For example, steatonecrosis was observed in the subepicardial fat tissue adjacent to the myocardium in a case of exacerbation of chronic pancreatitis (Roncati et al. 2012).

The morphological changes may manifest via steatorrhea and glucose intolerance; maldigestion and malabsorption syndrome may also occur. In optoelectronic–microscopic studies of pancreatic biopsies in alcoholics, findings included fibrotic changes, accumulation of fatty droplets (triglyceride) in the cytoplasm, shrinkage of the zymogen granules, and enlargement of the endoplasmic reticulum with myelin-like figures in the vesicles (Noronha et al. 1982).

6.3 Alcoholic Cardiomyopathy

Toxic myocardial damage caused by prolonged alcohol abuse yielding electron microscopic findings (Alexander 1967) results in alcoholic cardiomyopathy falling into the category of secondary cardiomyopathies. Histologically, cardiomyocytes

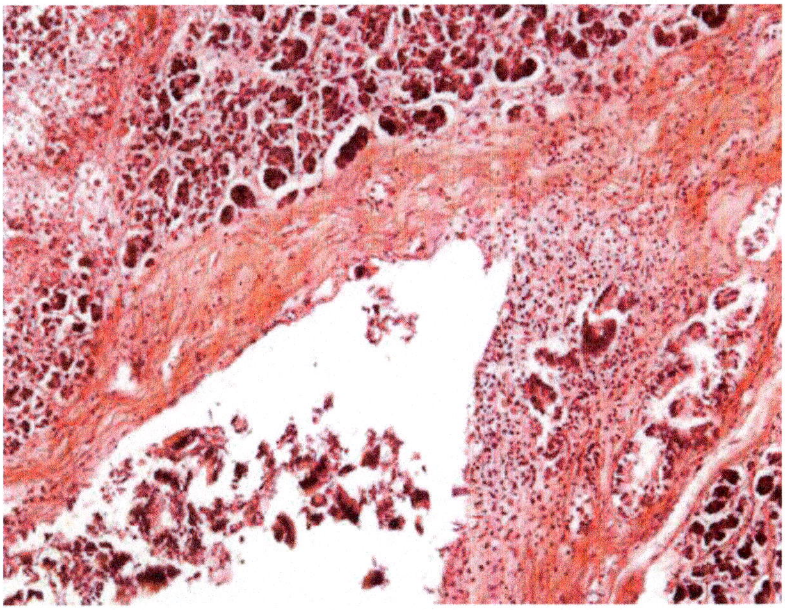

Fig. 6.8 Nonspecific chronic fibrous pancreatitis in the case of chronic alcohol abuse: fibrosis of the pancreas, duct ectasia, and lymphocytic infiltrate in the wall of the excretory duct of the gland (H&E ×100)

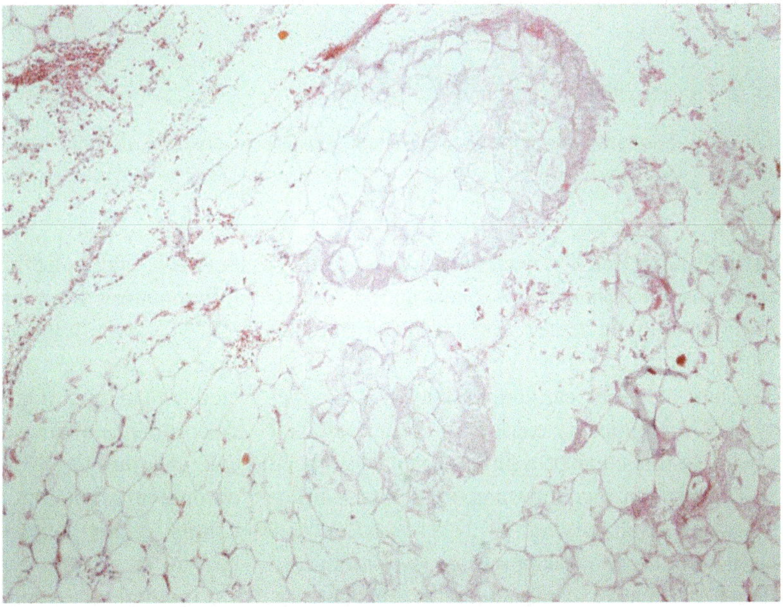

Fig. 6.9 Tryptic fat tissue necrosis in peripancreatic fat tissue in chronic alcohol abuse (H&E ×40)

are partially hypertrophic, partially degenerated. Interstitial fibrosis zones may appear, along with patchy endocardial fibrosis. The clinical and morphological presentation corresponds to dilative cardiomyopathy, which may lead to sudden death in the case of chronic alcohol abuse (Clark 1998; Copeland 1985; Riesner and Janssen 1978). However, in the case of sudden death of an alcoholic, other causes should also be discussed, e.g., alcoholic ketoacidosis (Kadis et al. 1999). Alcohol-related effects on skeletal muscle have also been examined in regard to an association with alcoholic cardiomyopathy (Rubin 1979).

There are often other histological findings which correspond to alcohol consumption, particularly in the liver (Frenzel et al. 1988; Ferries and Thompson 1981). Excessive alcohol consumption can apparently lead to impairment of

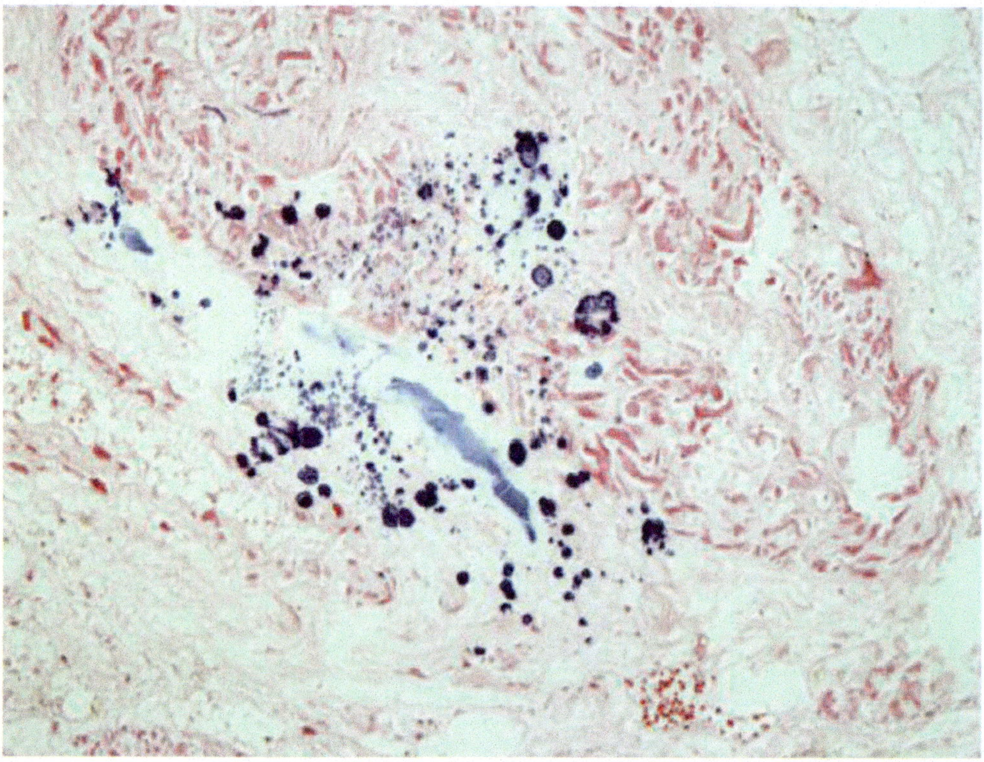

Fig. 6.10 Basophilic concrements in chronic fibrous pancreatitis after alcohol abuse of many years' standing (H&E ×100)

cardiac pump function even in people who otherwise abstain from alcohol consumption, potentially resulting in acute lethal cardiac arrhythmia (Spodick et al. 1979; Ettinger et al. 1978).

Thus, alcoholic cardiomyopathy is a dilative-type cardiomyopathy caused by chronic alcohol abuse. In this context, a differentiation has been made between alcoholic and idiopathic cardiomyopathy (Bulloch et al. 1972). The toxic effects of alcohol are first taken into consideration as a cause of dilative cardiomyopathy (Richardson et al. 1986; Regan et al. 1969), but the volume effects linked to beer consumption on the cardiovascular system have also been discussed as a cause (Morin and Daniel 1967).

In addition to alcohol-related etiology, there is controversy as to whether, in some cases, a primarily nonalcohol-related, dilative cardiomyopathy in the form of an inflammatory cardiomyopathy or chronic myocarditis may be present. Here, the question is whether it is even possible to differentiate solely morphologically between alcoholic cardiomyopathy and the inflammatory form of dilative cardiomyopathy (DCMi), even with descriptions of histological findings that were interpreted as being associated with alcohol (Ogbuihi 1989) (see Chap. 13). According to own investigations, both histological and immunohistochemical criteria of a chronic inflammatory process indicate that associating dilative cardiomyopathy directly with alcohol as a cause is not always valid. Rather, chronic immune suppression caused by alcohol consumption may lead to the development of chronic myocarditis (Dettmeyer et al. 2002).

Increased numbers of cells of LCA-positive leukocytes, T-lymphocytes, and macrophages point to a chronic progressive process, without excluding the chronic toxic effects of alcohol as a single or additional cause. Single-cell myocardial necrosis may lead to an immunohistochemically detectable histiocytic reaction with CD68-positive macrophages (Fig. 6.11). At present, this problem cannot be definitively evaluated. The immunohis-

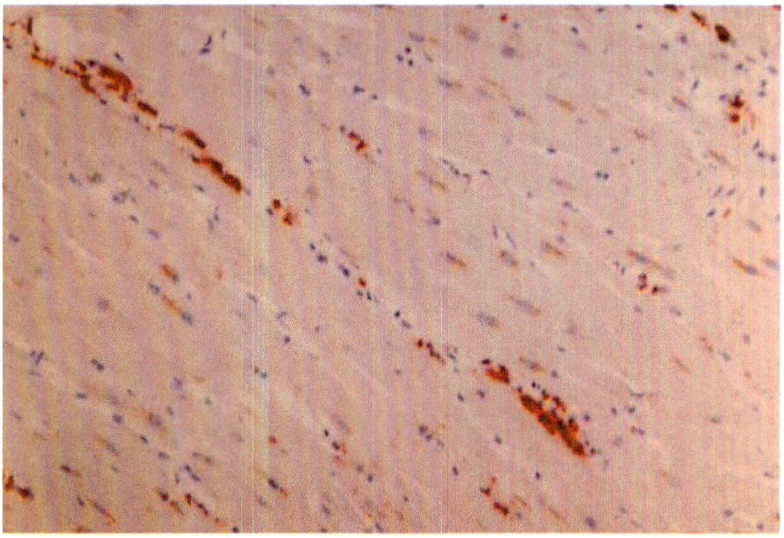

Fig. 6.11 Striated arrangement of CD68-positive macrophages along myocardial necrosis (×200). Note: endothelial tenascin expression may serve as an internal control for the detection of immunohistochemical tenascin (Fig. 6.12)

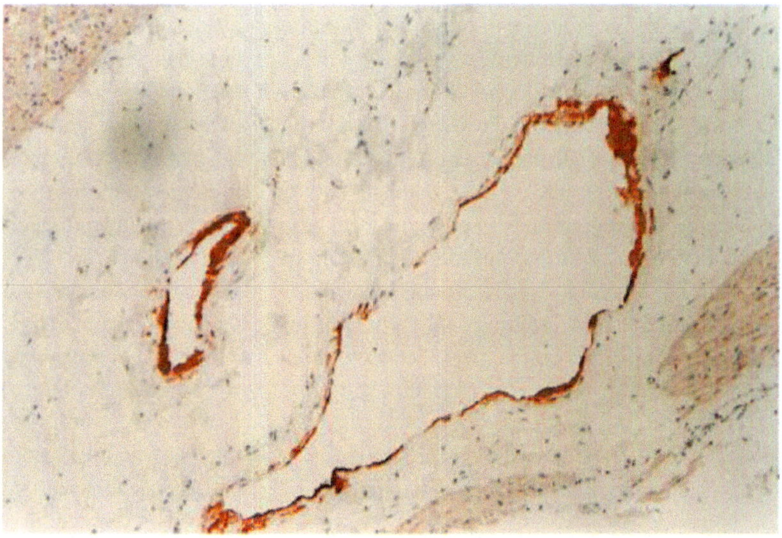

Fig. 6.12 Physiological endothelial expression of tenascin in a case of suspected alcoholic cardiomyopathy (×100)

tochemical expression of tenascin may be considered a sign of progressive myocardial fibrosis.

There is increased tenascin expression at the margin of interstitial fibrosis in the myocardium, as described in patients with dilative cardiomyopathy (Tamura et al. 1996) and shown in cases of alcoholics with dilative cardiomyopathy (Dettmeyer et al. 2002) (Fig. 6.13).

More specifically, alcoholic cardiomyopathy is a toxic cardiomyopathy, whereby ethanol and other forms of alcohol function as the toxic substances triggering cardiomyopathy. However, macroscopic findings in the heart alone do not substantiate the diagnosis "alcoholic cardiomyopathy"; alcohol anamnesis of the deceased and – if present – other alcohol-related pathological findings, in particular in the liver and pancreas, must also be considered.

Conventional histological examinations do not permit a reliable differential diagnosis, since ventricular dilatation of the myocardial fibers, partially interstitial and partially perivascular fibrosis of varying degrees, as well as varying sizes of myocardial cell nuclei can regularly be seen. Fiber breakage and empty sarcolemma tubes may also occur. Due to a histiocytic reaction, myocardial single-cell necrosis may be filled with macrophages in the context of a

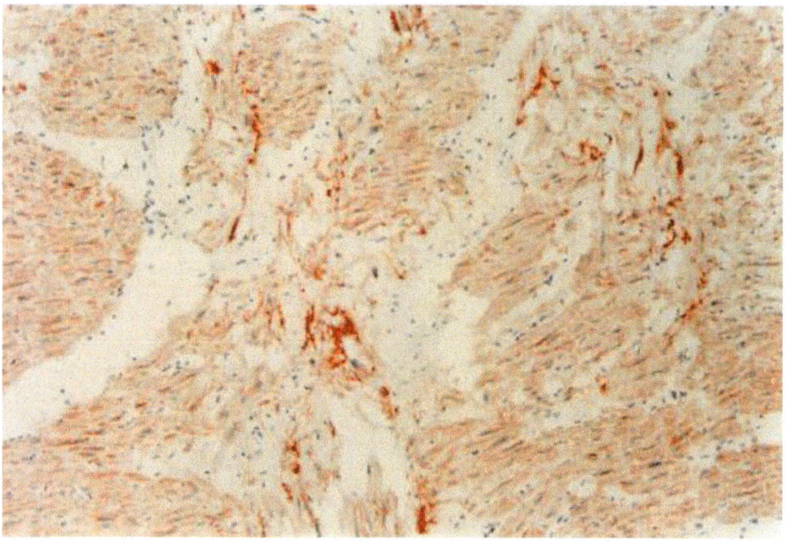

Fig. 6.13 Diffuse interstitial myocardial fibrosis with marked expression of tenascin at the margins of cardiomyocytes in a case of alcoholic cardiomyopathy (×100)

removal reaction, which can be shown immunohistochemically (see above).

In cases of lethal alcohol intoxications, the expression of fibronectin and C5b-$9_{(m)}$ was compared to groups of different causes of death. It was shown that fresh cardiac damage can be detected at both ventricles in cases of fatal ethanol intoxication with an antibody against fibronectin. The damages were found prevalently localized in the myocardium of the right ventricle (Fracasso et al. 2011).

6.4 Other Alcohol-Associated Histopathological Findings

Nervous System Although alcohol-related damage to the central nervous system shows no specific histomorphological findings, it produces (occasionally severe) deviations from the norm compared with control brains (Schuck 1983). Notable among these is Wernicke encephalopathy, which is clinically associated with Korsakov's psychosis, eye muscle palsy, and ataxia. There are morphological changes within the margins of the third and fourth ventricle and the aqueduct involving glial cell proliferation, accompanied by branched capillary blood vessels presenting with thickened vascular walls (Janssen 1977). The clinical picture resembles inflammation but affects less than 1% of all alcoholics (Torvik et al. 1982). Red wine consumption is more likely to result in central pontine myelinolysis (Marchiafava syndrome). With the consumption of fusel alcohol, particularly methanol, neurological symptoms may appear, including cerebral hemorrhage and necrosis (Fontenot and Pelak 2002; Glazer and Dross 1993). Other histomorphological changes are described in the neuropathology literature (Oehmichen et al. 2006).

Kidneys A handful of publications describe subnuclear vacuolization of renal tubular epithelial cells consistent with Armanni–Ebstein cells. This picture is known in diabetic ketoacidosis (see Fig. 6.3). In diabetes, the vacuoles also contain at least glycogen – in alcoholic ketoacidosis, however, they contain fats without concomitant hyperglycemia. Elevated acetone levels were measured parallel to this. Similarly, Armanni–Ebstein cells were found in a case of poisoning with isopropanol, which converts to acetone (Parai et al. 2012). Therefore, the detection of Armanni–Ebstein cells is not specific for diabetic ketoacidosis. Detecting these changes in the cytoplasm of renal tubular epithelial cells supports the diagnosis of alcoholic ketoacidosis (possibly as a cause of death) in nondiabetics with a history of alcohol abuse (Brinkmann et al. 1998; Thomsen et al. 1995).

However, other causes of death, e.g., hypothermia (Zhou and Byard 2011), can also result in the Armanni–Ebstein lesion.

Bone Marrow With chronic alcohol abuse, alcohol-induced impairment of hemopoietic bone marrow is seen in the form of vacuolized bone marrow cells at an early stage of erythropoiesis and leukopoiesis (Pribilla et al. 1966). However, the entire hemopoietic system may be affected, also as a result of lack of folic acid and vitamin B12. The result is megaloblastic anemia, genetically determined to sideroblastic anemia. Macrocytosis may disclose concealed alcohol abuse.

Oral Cavity, Esophagus, and Gastrointestinal Tract With chronic alcohol consumption, mucous membrane inflammation of the oral cavity often appears, including caries, parodontosis, and also carcinoma of the tongue, hypopharynx, and larynx. Chronic esophagitis leads to an increased incidence of esophageal cancer. Gastritis of varying degrees of severity is also found more frequently with chronic alcohol consumption. Advanced liver cirrhosis causes hypertension in the portal circulation, and esophageal varices develop, causing the feared and often fatal complication of esophageal variceal bleeding. Histologically, these varices can in places be seen close beneath the non-keratinized squamous epithelium of the esophageal mucosa (Fig. 6.14).

Mallory–Weiss Syndrome With repeated vomiting, there may be longitudinal tears in the cardia region of the stomach with associated bleeding (Mallory–Weiss syndrome) (Türk et al. 2002). This syndrome is an upper gastrointestinal hemorrhage due to longitudinal mucosal lacerations in the esophagogastric junction (Fig. 6.15).

Boerhaave Syndrome Complete rupture of the esophageal wall may also be seen in (very rare) cases other than Mallory–Weiss syndrome. Boerhaave syndrome (spontaneous rupture of the esophagus) is similarly associated with excessive food and alcohol intake. Acute vomiting is frequently (>95%) the cause of spontaneous rupture of the esophageal wall; other causes, such as asthma, epilepsy, straining during defecation, and gastrointestinal gas, are also seen (<5%) (Hecser et al. 2011). The majority of esophageal wall tears run in a longitudinal direction, despite the fact that Boerhaave's original description was of a lesion running in a transverse direction. Wall tears measure between 0.5 and 20 cm in length and are predominantly localized in the left posterior to

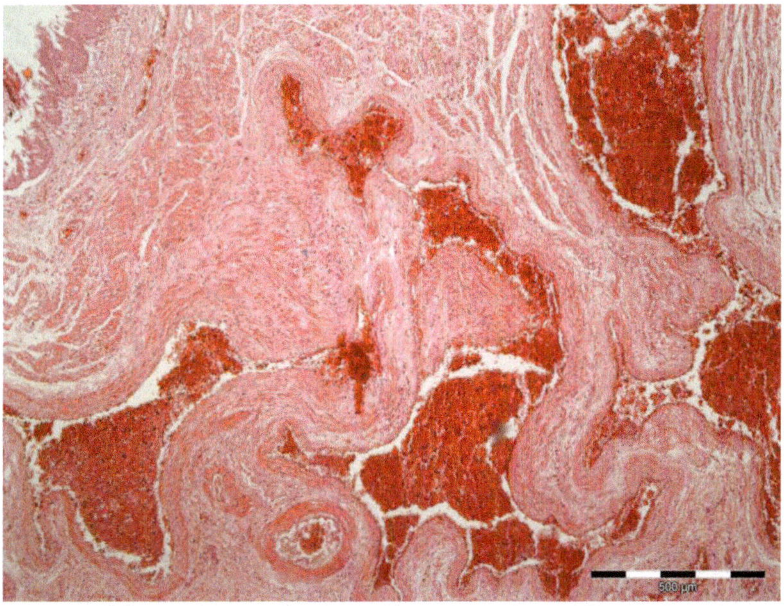

Fig. 6.14 Esophageal varices in alcoholic liver cirrhosis lying close beneath the non-keratinized squamous epithelium (*top left*) of the esophagus (H&E ×40)

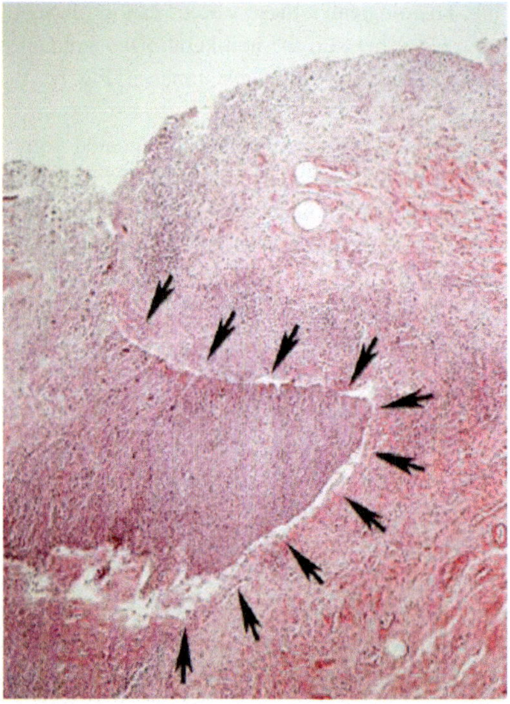

Fig. 6.15 Longitudinal tear (*arrows*) in the esophagogastric junction following repeated vomiting in a case of chronic alcoholism with fatal bleeding (Mallory–Weiss syndrome) (H&E ×200)

lateral esophageal wall, approximately 2–6 cm above the diaphragm (in 80% of cases) (Hecser et al. 2011; Johnson 2008; Griffin and Lamb 2008). Histologically, one sees hyperemia and inflammation in the area of the esophageal rupture; phlegmonous purulent mediastinitis and lethal sepsis develop in the further course.

Gastritis: Gastric Ulcer In the case of gastritis, hemorrhagic erosive inflammation is dominant, similar to that seen following acetylsalicylic acid consumption. It would appear that alcohol consumption tends to increase the risk for ventricular or duodenal ulcer.

Ethylene glycol intoxication leads to neurological deficits (Morgan et al. 2000; Maier 1983) and microscopically visible deposits of oxalate crystals (see Chap. 5).

Although alcohol undoubtedly leads to functional deficits, e.g., in the small intestine and other organs such as the kidney, there are, as a rule, no characteristic conventional histological findings. Severe alcohol-induced changes appear with heavy alcohol abuse that may lead to testicular atrophy. In forensic practice, the effects of alcohol on the liver, pancreas, and heart are highly significant in terms of determining cause of death.

Rhabdomyolysis Very few case studies report rhabdomyolysis and myoglobinuric kidney failure (following, e.g., heroin or ecstasy use; see Chap. 4) as a result of binge drinking in the setting of chronic alcohol abuse and lying unassisted in a vulnerable situation for a protracted period of time, culminating in delirium tremens. Pressure necrosis due to immobile positioning on a hard surface has been discussed as causal in localized rhabdomyolysis. Urine is described as abnormally red-brownish in color, while kidney failure is attributed to toxic damage to the renal tubules due to myoglobin cleaved in the acidic environment (Gerhard et al. 1989).

Black Esophagus The diagnosis of "black esophagus" requires the exclusion of other causes of sudden death and must be based on histological examination. Black esophagus is a rare pathological condition of unknown etiology. Macroscopically, a full length, circumferential black discoloration of the entire esophageal mucosa can be observed. Histologically, the esophageal mucosa is completely necrotic and demarcated by a leukocytic infiltrate in the upper mucosa (Fig. 6.16) (Brennan 1967; Goldenberg et al. 1990; Day and Sayegh 2010; Altenburger et al. 2011; Tsokos 2011; Tsokos and Herbst 2005). Individual reports suggest that this phenomenon is seen more frequently in alcohol abusers but possibly also in diabetics (Keresztesi et al. 2016; Unuma et al. 2011). Black esophagus can be deemed the cause of death in individual cases (Venara et al. 2013). The unusual appearance of black esophagus in a case of fatal hypothermia is mentioned in the literature (Živković and Nikolić 2013).

Table 6.2 lists diseases and histologically detectable findings that occur in conjunction with chronic alcohol abuse

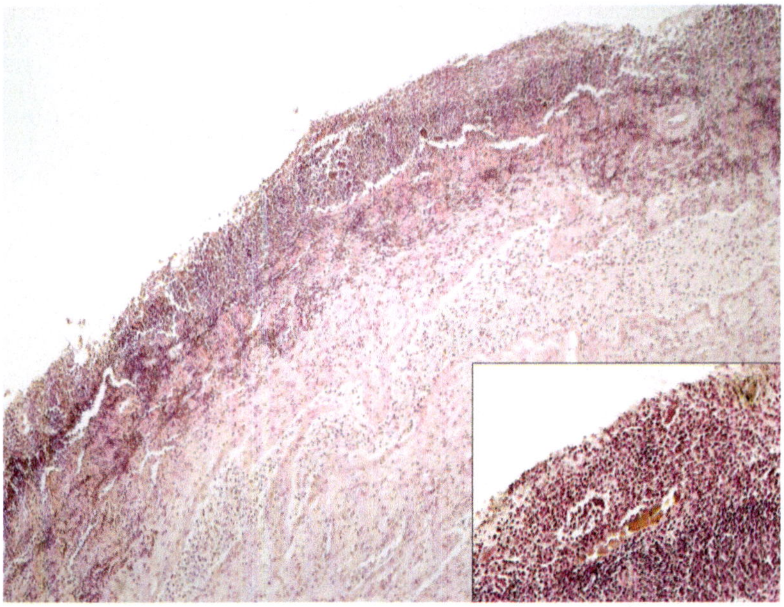

Fig. 6.16 The so-called black esophagus: the esophageal mucosa is completely necrotic and demarcated by a leukocytic infiltrate in the upper mucosa (H&E ×40; H&E ×200)

Table 6.2 The main histopathological findings following chronic alcohol abuse (excluding congener alcohols)

Organ	Histopathological finding
Esophagus	Submucosal esophageal varices; Mallory–Weiss syndrome; Boerhaave syndrome; possibly a higher risk of circular mucosal necrosis ("black esophagus")
Stomach	Erosive and/or atrophic gastritis; high risk of gastric ulcer
Duodenum	High risk of duodenal ulcer
Liver	Grade I–IV nutritional toxic hepatic steatosis
	Portal fibrosis, precirrhosis, and cirrhosis of the liver with cholestasis, bile duct proliferation, concomitant inflammation, and increased risk of hepato- or cholangiocellular cancer Mallory–Denk bodies (so-called alcoholic hyaline)
Pancreas	Acute necrotizing pancreatitis Chronic fibrosing pancreatitis (more common) with fibrosis, chylous disorder, duct ectasia, and peripancreatic tryptic fat tissue necrosis
Spleen	Portal congested spleen in advanced liver cirrhosis
Heart	Alcoholic cardiomyopathy (most important differential diagnosis: inflammatory dilated cardiomyopathy; DCMi)
Skeletal musculature	Muscle atrophy (in advanced-stage alcohol addiction, then extremely rarely evident position-related rhabdomyolysis)
Central nervous system	Wernicke encephalopathy (in advanced-stage alcohol addiction; Olds et al. 2014)

References

Alexander CS (1967) Electron microscopic observations in alcoholic heart disease. Br Heart J 29:200–206

Altenburger DL, Wagner AS, Caravaglia J (2011) A case of black esophagus with histopathologic description and characterization. Arch Pathol Lab Med 135:797–798

Böcker W, Seifert G (1972) Zur Pathologie der Alkohol-Pankreatitis. Dtsch Med Wochenschr 97:803

Brennan JL (1967) Case of extensive necrosis of the oesophageal mucosa following hypothermia. J Clin Pathol 20:581–584

Brinkmann B, Fechner G, Karger B, DuChesne A (1998) Ketoacidosis and lactic acidosis – frequent causes of death in chronic alcoholics? Int J Legal Med 111:115–119

Brunt EM, Janney CG, Di Bisceglie AM, Neuschwander-Tetri BA, Bacon BR (1999) Nonalcoholic steatohepatitis: a proposal for grading and staging the histological lesions. Am J Gastroenterol 94:2467–2474

Bschor F, Keilbach H (1968) Die Bedeutung chronischer Organschäden für die tödliche Alkoholvergiftung. Dtsch Z Gesamte Gerichtl Med 62:183
Bulloch RT, Pearce MB, Murphy ML, Jenkins BJ, Davis JL (1972) Myocardial lesions in idiopathic and alcoholic cardiomyopathy. Study by ventricular septal biopsy. Am J Cardiol 29:15
Cascalla JL, Gordo V, Montes R (2012) Severe necrosis of oesophageal and gastric mucosa in fatal methanol poisoning. Forensic Sci Int 220:e9–e12
Clark JC (1998) Sudden death in the chronic alcoholic. Forensic Sci Int 36:105–111
Copeland AR (1985) Sudden death in the alcoholic. Forensic Sci Int 29:159–169
Dancygier H (1997) "Alkoholische" Leberschäden bei Nichtalkoholikern. Dtsch Med Wochenschr 122:1183–1188
Day CP (2001) Apoptosis in alcoholic hepatitis: a novel therapeutic agent? J Hepatol 34:330–333
Day A, Sayegh M (2010) Acute oesophageal necrosis: a case report and review of the literature. Int J Surg 8:6–14
Denk H, Stumptner C, Zatloukal K (2000) Mallory bodies revisited. J Hepatol 32:689–702
Denk H, Stumptner C, Fuchsbichler A, Zatloukal K (2001) Alcoholic and nonalcoholic steatohepatitis. Histopathologic and pathogenetic considerations. Pathologe 22:388–398
Dettmeyer R, Reith K, Madea B (2002) Alcoholic cardiomyopathy versus chronic myocarditis – immunohistological investigations with LCA, CD3, CD68 and tenascin. Forensic Sci Int 126:57–62
Diehl AM, Goodman Z, Ishak KG (1988) Alcohol-like liver disease in nonalcoholics. A clinical and histologic comparison with alcohol-induced liver injury. Gastroenterology 95:1056–1062
Ettinger PO, Wu CF, de la Cruz C, Weisse AB, Ahmed SS, Regan TJ (1978) Arrhythmias and the 'holiday heart'. Alcohol-associated cardiac rhythm disorders. Am Heart J 95:555
Ferries JAJ, Thompson PJ (1981) A histological assessment of the incidence of alcoholic cardiomyopathy in subjects with alcohol associated liver disease. Can Soc Forensic Sci J 14:113–133
Fontenot AP, Pelak VS (2002) Development of neurologic symptoms in a 26-year-old woman following recovery from methanol intoxication. Chest 122:1436–1439
Fracasso T, Brinkmann B, Breike J, Pfeiffer H (2008) Clotted blood as a sign of alcohol intoxication: a retrospective study. Int J Legal Med 122:157–161
Fracasso T, Pfeiffer H, Köhler H, Wieseler S, Hansen SD, Jentgens L, Sauerland C, Schmeling A (2011) Immunohistochemical expression of fibronectin and C5b-9 in the myocardium in cases of fatal ethanol intoxication. Int J Legal Med 125:537–542
Frenzel H, Roth H, Schwartzkopff B (1988) Alkohol und Herz-Kreislaufsystem. Z Gastroenterol 26(suppl 3):84–96
Gerhard H, Graben N, Risse M, Scharafinski HW (1989) Rhabdomyolyse und akutes myoglobinurisches Nierenversagen nach Alkohol-Intoxikation und Delirium Tremens. Akt Neurol 16:XXVII
Glazer M, Dross P (1993) Necrosis of the putamen caused by methanol intoxication: MR findings. Am J Roentgenol 160:1105–1106
Goldenberg SP, Wain SL, Marignani P (1990) Acute necrotizing esophagitis. Gastroenterology 98:493–496
Griffin SM, Lamb PJ (2008) Spontaneous rupture of the esophagus. Br J Surg 95:1115–1120
Hecser L, Siklodi KP, Csiki G, Lungu MF, Jung H, Buda O (2011) Boerhaave syndrome. A case report. Rom J Leg Med 19:281–286
Ichida F (1970) Morphologische Befunde bei chronischer Alkoholintoxikation in Japan. Therapiewoche 20:2351
Itoh S, Igarashi M, Tsukada Y, Ichinoe A (1977) Nonalcoholic fatty liver with alcoholic hyaline after long-term glucocorticoid therapy. Acta Hepatogastroenterol (Stuttg) 24:415–418
Janssen W (1977) Forensische Histologie. Schmidt-Römhild, Lübeck
Johnson SB (2008) Esophageal trauma. Semin Thorac Cardiovasc Surg 20:46–51
Kadis P, Balazic J, Ferlan-Marolt V (1999) Alcoholic ketoacidosis: a cause of sudden death of chronic alcoholics. Forensic Sci Int 103:53–59
Kagawa M (1970) Histopathologische Leberuntersuchungen an unausgewählten Sektionsfällen. Überprüfung des Vorkommens von "Mallory-Körpern", Fett-Cirrhosen und "acidophilen Einschlüssen". Jap J Leg Med 24:427
Keresztesi AA, Asofie G, Chinezu L, Jung H (2016) Acute esophageal necrosis ("black esophagus"): case series in forensic autopsies casuistry. Rom J Leg Med 24:87–91
Maier W (1983) Cerebral computed tomography of ethylene glycol intoxication. Neuroradiology 24:175–177
Mallory FB (1911) Cirrhosis of the liver. Five different types of lesions from which it may arise. Bull Johns Hopkins Hosp 22:69–75
McClain CJ, Barve S, Deaciuc I, Kugelmans M, Hill D (1999) Cytokines in alcoholic liver diseases. Semin Liver Dis 19:205–219
Morgan BW, Ford MD, Follmer R (2000) Ethylene glycol ingestion resulting in brainstem and midbrain dysfunction. J Toxicol Clin Toxicol 38:445–451
Morin Y, Daniel P (1967) Quebec beer-drinkers cardiomyopathy etiological considerations. Can Med Ass J 97:926–928
Nanji AA (1998) Apoptosis and alcoholic liver disease. Semin Liver Dis 18:187–190
Natori S, Rust C, Stadheim LM, Srinivan A, Burgart LJ, Gores GJ (2001) Hepatocyte apoptosis is a pathologic feature of human alcoholic hepatitis. J Hepatol 34:248–253
Noronha M, Salgadinho A, Ferreira de Almeida MJ (1982) Alcohol and pancreas: clinical associations and histopathology of minimal pancreatic inflammation. Am J Gastroent 77:827–832

Oehmichen M, Auer RN, König HG (2006) Forensic neuropathology and associated neuropathology. Springer, Berlin Heidelberg/New York/Tokio

Ogbuihi S (1989) Zur Pathomorphologie chronischer alkohol-assoziierter Myokardveränderungen. Z Rechtsmed 102:231–239

Olds K, Langlois NEI, Blumbergs P, Byard RW (2014) The pathological features of Wernicke encephalopathy. Forensic Sci Med Pathol 10:466–468

Parai JL, Kodikara S, Milroy CM, Pollanen MS (2012) Alcoholism and the Armanni-Ebstein lesion. Forensic Sci Med Pathol 8:19–22

Pribilla W, Härtel G, Albrecht M (1966) Veränderungen des Knochenmarks bei chronischem Alkoholismus. Med Klin 61:1031

Regan TJ, Levinson GE, Oldewurtel HA, Frank MJ, Weisse AB, Moschos CB (1969) Ventricular function in non-cardiacs with alcohol fatty liver. Role of ethanol in production of cardiomyopathy. J Clin Invest 48:397–407

Richardson PJ, Wodak AD, Atkinson L, Saunders JB, Jewitt DE (1986) Relation between alcohol intake, myocardial enzyme activity and myocardial function in dilated cardiomyopathy. Evidence for the concept of alcohol induced heart-muscle disease. Br Heart J 56:165–170

Riesner K, Janssen W (1978) Alkoholbedingte Kardiomyopathie und plötzlicher Herztod. Beitr Gerichtl Med 36:352–358

Roncati L, Gualandri G, Fortuni G, Barbolini G (2012) Sudden death and lipomatous infiltration of the heart involved by fat necrosis resulting from acute pancreatitis. Forensic Sci Int 217:e19–e22

Rubin E (1979) Alcoholic cardiomyopathy in heart and skeletal muscle. N Engl J Med 301:28

Schuck M (1983) Vergleichende, quantitative, makroskopische und mikroskopische Untersuchungen an Alkoholiker- und Kontrollgehirnen. Habil Schrift München

Spodick DH, Pigott VM, Chirife R (1979) Preclinical cardiac malfunction in chronic alcoholism. N Engl J Med 287:677–680

Strnad P et al (2008) Mallory-Denk bodies: lessons from keratin-containing hepatic inclusion bodies. Biochim Biophys Acta 1782:764–774

Tamura A, Kusachi S, Nogami K, Yamanishi A, Kajikawa Y, Hirohata S, Tsuji T (1996) Tenascin expression in endomyocardial biopsy specimens in patients with dilated cardiomyopathy: distribution along margin of fibrotic lesions. Heart 75:291–294

Thomsen JL, Felby S, Theilde P, Nielsen E (1995) Alcoholic ketoacidosis as a cause of death in forensic cases. Forensic Sci Int 75:163–171

Torvik A, Lindboe CF, Rodge S (1982) Brain lesions in alcoholics. A neuropathological study with clinical correlation. J Neurol Sci 56:233–248

Tsokos M (2011) Black esophagus. Forensic Sci Med Pathol 7:374–376

Tsokos M, Herbst H (2005) Black oesophagus: a rare disorder with potentially fatal outcome. A forensic pathological approach based on five autopsy cases. Int J Legal Med 119:146–152

Tsukamoto H, Gaal K, French SW (1990) Insights into the pathogenesis of alcoholic liver necrosis and fibrosis: status report. Hepatology 12:599–608

Türk EE, Anders S, Tsokos M (2002) Mallory-Weiss syndrome as the cause of sudden, unexpected death. Arch Kriminol 209:36–44

Unuma K, Harada K, Funakoshi T, Uemura K (2011) Sudden death of an alcoholic elderly man with acute esophageal necrosis (black esophagus). Forensic Sci Int 212:e15–e17

Venara A, Pavageau AH, Maillart CR, Jousset N (2013) Sudden death due to black esophagus: a case report. Am J Forensic Med Pathol 34:16–17

Zatloukal K et al (2007) From Mallory to Mallory-Denk bodies: what, how and why? Exp Cell Res 313:2033–2049

Zhou C, Byard RW (2011) Armanni-Ebstein phenomenon and hypothermia. Forensic Sci Int 206:e82–e84

Živković V, Nikolić S (2013) The unusual appearance of black esophagus in a case of fatal hypothermia: a possible underlying mechanism. Forensic Sci Med Pathol 9:613–614

7 Heat, Fire, Electricity, Lightning, Radiation, and Gases

The effects of heat, electricity, radiation, and burn injuries from open fire, inhalation of hot air or gases, as well as whole-body hyperthermia can have a lethal course and partly be detected microscopically (Fineschi et al. 2005; Bohnert 2004; Karger and Teige 2002; Myers et al. 1999; Pioch 1966a, b). Thus, pulmonary changes following heat or fire have long been the subject of histological investigations (Zinck 1940; Foerster 1934, 1932; Olbrycht 1927). Electricity can leave current marks on the skin and can even directly damage the myocardium. Initially, the impact of heat leads to injury of the locally affected tissue. In the case of higher-degree burns, the entire body is affected (burn disease). Special forms, such as heat inhalation trauma, may lead to specific injury to the respiratory tract. In the case of lightning, injuries include striated skin and organ damage between the site of entry and the site of exit of the lightning; thus, organ damage can be detected histologically and immunohistochemically. From a macroscopic perspective, one should be particularly alert to Lichtenberg dust figures, as well as to skin burns, scorched hair, and thermal damage to metal parts on clothing (Zack et al. 2013).

7.1 Heat and Fire

The effect of heat and open fire on the organism can lead to injuries of varying severity to death. Heat effects occur in particular as a result of scalding, burns from open flames, and contact with hot (e.g., metallic) objects. The skin is particularly exposed. In animal studies, varying degrees of damage could be differentiated, e.g., after postmortem exposure to kerosene in rats (Hieda et al. 2004).

7.1.1 The Effects of Heat on the Skin

Heat damage to the skin is graduated depending on the depth of injury and can be investigated histologically. Not all histological or cytological findings need to be present. In the case of death due to scalding, all degrees and forms of thermal epidermis damage can be found:

- Peeling of the epidermis (Fig. 7.1).
- Intra- and subepidermal gap formation.
- Partially palisade position of basal epithelial cells.
- Thermal coagulative necrosis of the corium to the subcutaneous fatty tissue and the musculature (Fig. 7.2).
- Connective tissue fibers may be homogenized and broadened, partly with destruction of the nuclear chromatin.
- Fat lying in extracellular spaces can build up in the subcutis.
- Pseudo cyst-like spaces may occur in the epidermis and corium.
- Intravascular proteins also show heat-related denaturation, and cellular debris, lumps, homogenization, and microthrombi may occur (Brinkmann et al. 1979).

R. B. Dettmeyer, *Forensic Histopathology*, https://doi.org/10.1007/978-3-319-77997-3_7

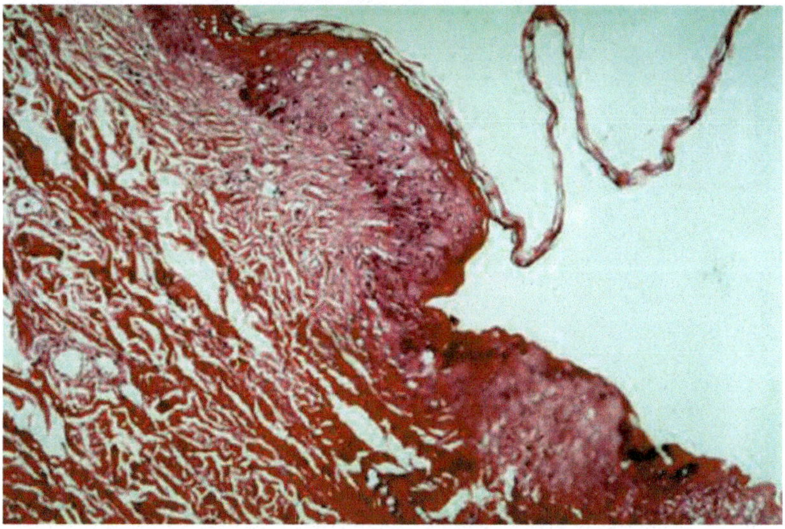

Fig. 7.1 Burn blister with parchment-like thin flaking of keratin lamellae and upper layer of the epidermis, as well as heat injury to adjacent squamous epithelial cells (H&E ×40)

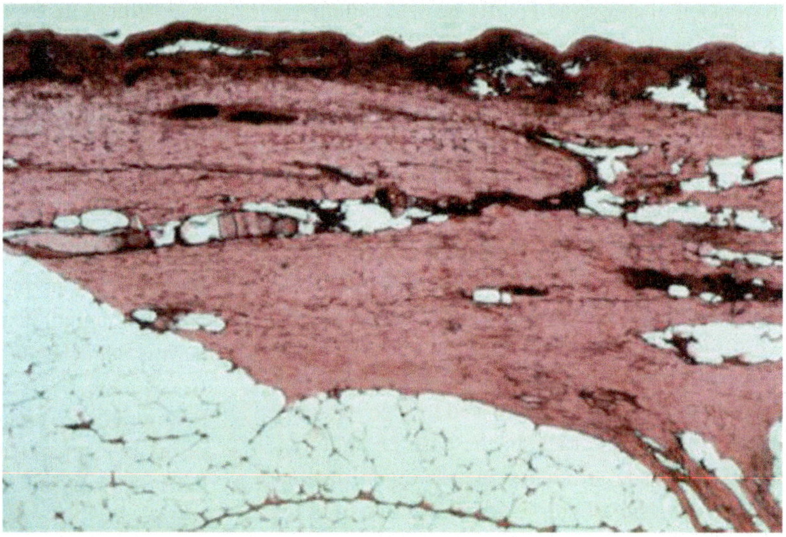

Fig. 7.2 Heat injury with epidermal coagulation and homogenization of fibrous structures in the corium (H&E ×40)

Related to the question of detection and classification of heat injury is the problem of vitality, i.e., whether heat injury developed while the patient was still alive (Bohnert et al. 2003). A massive intravascular concentration of Sudan III-positive fats can be regarded as a vital sign in the case of heat injury. Investigations including the detection of small fat concentrations after experimental postmortem application of heat (Schollmeyer 1962) do not oppose this.

Histological findings in the case of thermal damage to the skin and soft tissue according to the degree of damage are shown in Table 7.1.

Please note: the presence of fibrin and leukocytes in the blister content is considered evidence of a vital reaction to heat. In the case of prolonged exposure to slowly heated water, there have been reports on two- to three-degree burns to the skin and the formation of small skin blisters, the content of which has a jellylike consistency. Histologically, one sees subepidermal blisters with a partially fluid and partially firm content (Pircher et al. 2016). Immunohistochemical investigations showed increased expression of heat shock proteins (HSP) not only in heat-damaged skin (Kowall-Vern et al. 2000), but also in the

Table 7.1 Histological findings according to the degree of heat damage to the skin and subcutaneous soft tissue (Modified according to Janssen (1977))

Extent	Heat-damaged structures
1. Erythema	Erythema and swelling with reactive ectasia lasting only a few days and hyperemia of capillary blood vessels in the papillary stratum of the cutis in particular, accompanied by edema
2. Blistering	*Serous blister*. Mostly serous blister with one chamber (with few lymphocytes, polymorphonuclear, seldom eosinophilic, neutrophilic granulocytes, monocytes). In the case of serous blister content, the floor of the blister passes the basal stratum of the epidermis, which forms the floor of the blister, occasionally with overlying fibrin strings. An inflammatory reaction in the papillary stratum and superficial corium is possible; reactive hyperemia and edema are, however, more likely. Epithelial cells along the edge can show faded cell nuclei, as well as single necrosis. The adjacent segments of the epidermis show a basilar elongation of the cell nuclei
	Hemorrhagic blister. If the entire epidermis, including the germinative stratum, is affected, the floor of the blister consists of partially damaged papillary stratum. The capillary blood vessels contained therein are initially contracted; later they are dilated and hyperemic with agglutinated, fragmented erythrocytes in the vascular opening. Beneath the blister, the collagen fibers show pronounced basophiles
	Differential diagnoses:
	Blister following barbiturate intoxication or other foreign substances (Riße et al. 1998): a predominant lack of basophils in collagen fibers, agglutination of erythrocytes, and nuclear elongation of the basal epidermis cells at the edge (Schollmeyer 1961)
	Blister due to putrefaction: peeling of the entire epidermis, no hyperemia, no inflammation, cell-free blister content
3. Necrosis	Heat-related necrosis of the skin and subcutaneous tissue: coagulative necrosis with destroyed epidermis and a peripheral comb-like pattern, followed by lengthwise protrusions of cells and cell nuclei (palisade position). In addition, swelling of the cells and cell nuclei, intracytoplasmic vacuole formation including basophils, pyknosis of cell nuclei, loss of granulation in the cytoplasm, and karyorrhexis (=early necrobiosis) are also described. There is also deferred loss of nuclear dyeability in the skin appendages (after approximately 12–24 h). Collagen and elastic fibers can remain visible for several days. Particularly with deep heat injuries, there is a delayed appearance of inflammatory cells (after 6–24 h) in the form of densely populated leukocytes
4. Deep burn injuries + charring	Necrosis and charring to the bones (primarily due to direct impact of fire); charring due to scalding alone is not possible

According to current knowledge, immunohistochemical findings in skin samples after heat injury are helpful as vitality markers but alone cannot assess the degree of damage or age of heat impact

respiratory tract and lung tissue in the context of heat inhalation trauma (Marschall et al. 2006).

Burnt Bones Microradiographic investigations were able to reveal changes to bone structure due to the effects of heat (Imaizumi et al. 2014).

7.1.2 Heat Inhalation Trauma

The inhalation of hot gases or air (heat inhalation trauma) leads to extensive damage to the respiratory tract epithelium (Brinkmann and Püschel 1978; Foerster 1933) up to the second- and third-order bronchi, as well as injury to lung tissue. This leads to partial flaking of the respiratory epithelium and vacuolar transformation of epithelium cells (Fig. 7.3); a fine layer of soot dust is often seen microscopically on the vocal cords (Fig. 7.4).

While the interpretation of individual findings should be done cautiously, the overall picture of heat injury to the respiratory tract can be treated as a vital sign, demonstrating that the patient was alive at the time of fire outbreak. If the patient initially survives heat inhalation trauma, effects (Table 7.2) develop with increasing survival time (Sochor and Mallory 1963). Respiratory tract mucous membrane with heat-related necrosis is a breeding ground for secondary bacterial infections, and simultaneously, mucinous mucus is

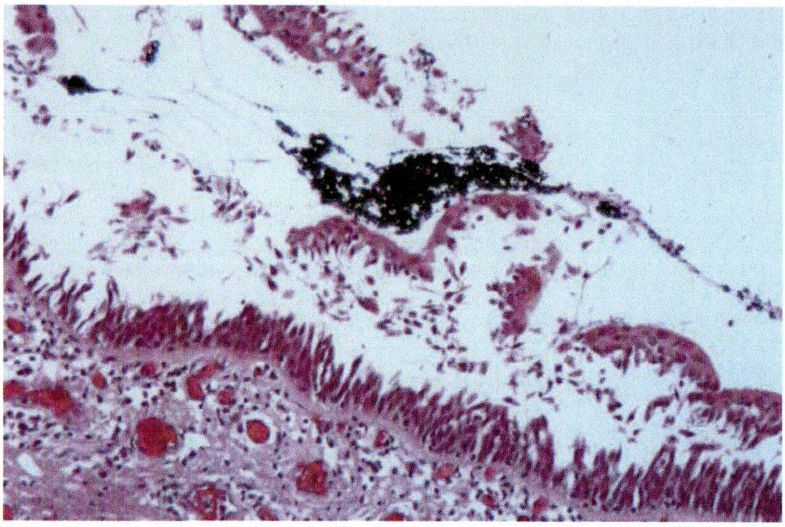

Fig. 7.3 Heat injury to the respiratory epithelium with elongated cylinder epithelia, elongated cell nuclei, reactive hyperemia in the subepithelial tissue, and peripheral soot particles following heat inhalation trauma (H&E ×100)

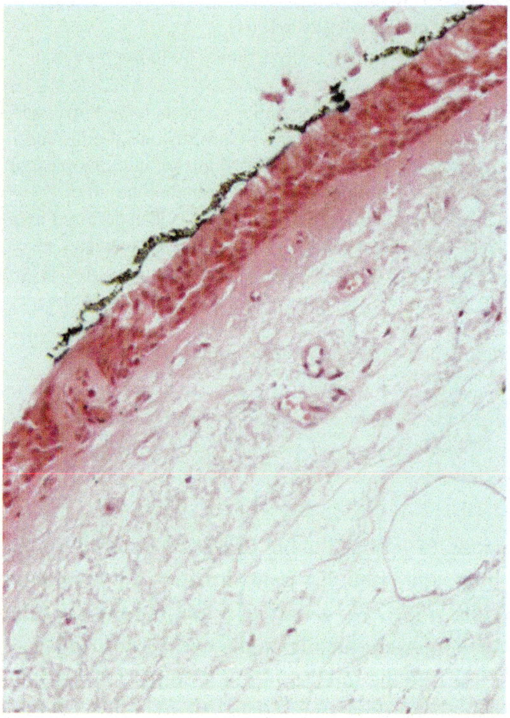

Fig. 7.4 A fine layer of soot dust on the non-keratinized squamous epithelium of the vocal cords (H&E ×20)

Table 7.2 Histologically detectable early and late sequelae of heat inhalation trauma

Early findings	Late findings
• Loss of the ciliated border	• Pseudomembranous tracheobronchitis
• Basal vacuolization of the respiratory epithelium	• Purulent bronchitis and bronchiolitis
• Elongated cell nuclei in palisade position	• Interstitial and alveolar hemorrhage
• Swelling and coagulative necrosis of the cylinder epithelium	• Fibrin thrombi in peripheral arteries and arterioles of the lung tissue
• Reactive hyperemia in subepithelial tissue	• Pulmonary atelectases of varying degrees
• Protrusions of superficial mucous glands (glandulae mucosae)	• Areas of acute focal emphysema
• Peripheral soot dust particles, partly embedded in mucus	• Purulent bronchopneumonia
• Edema of the submucosa	• Decay products in cells lead to protein cylinders in the renal tubules
	• Stress ulcers, particularly in the gastric mucosa (shock equivalent)

produced, which cannot effectively be coughed up. There are case reports showing desquamative loss of respiratory epithelium up to the middle bronchi, while the bronchial lumen was filled with clumps of mucopurulent secretions mixed with necrotic epithelial cells; the cause of death was delayed asphyxia due to an inhalation/aspiration injury (Fracasso and Schmeling 2011; Cox et al. 2008).

Parts of the body directly exposed to fire may char. With protrusion of the tongue, which frequently occurs in fire victims, "heat blisters" can be seen histologically, sometimes with incorporated soot particles (Fig. 7.5). Deeply aspirated fine soot particles can be detected microscopically in lung tissue; however, this is not always the case due to particle size (Fig. 7.6).

In addition, there are further findings in burn disease that can be presented histologically, including almost all internal organs in the case of burn shock. Burn shock findings correspond in part with findings in a shock event in general (see Chap. 15). In the case of intravital heat impact to the lungs, damage is said to be evenly distributed in the lung tissue; in the case of postmortem heat injury, damage is found macroscopically only in peripheral parts of the lung (Foerster 1933).

Long-term survival after carbon monoxide intoxication has been accepted for a long time as pathognomonic for elective cerebral tissue damage, especially in cases of isolated symmetrical necrosis of the globus pallidus. Meanwhile, different causes of symmetrical necrosis of the globus pallidus are identified (Riße and Weiler 1984).

Immunohistochemical investigations of lung tissue in fire victims could provide evidence of injury by detecting the expression of fibronectin and heat shock protein 70 (hsp 70) (Bohnert et al. 2010; Marschall et al. 2006); other investigations included the expression of ubiquitin (Shoji 1997). Such investigations help to answer

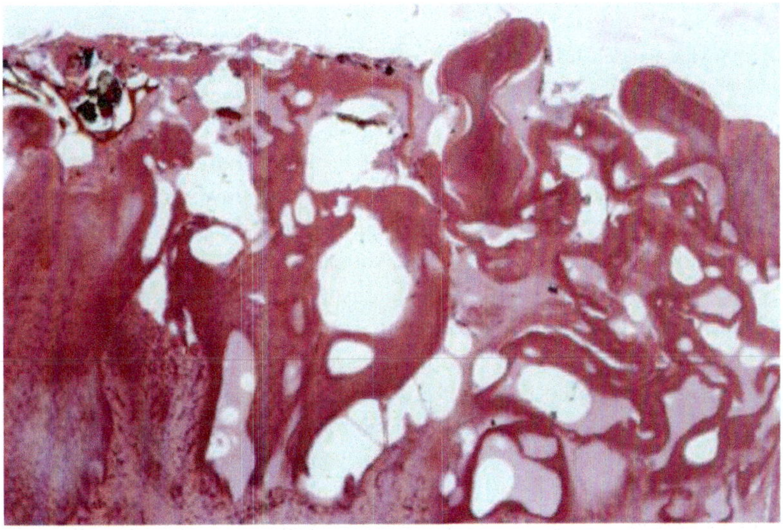

Fig. 7.5 Fire victim with comb-like heat damage to the tongue (heat blisters) and incorporated soot particles – these findings alone do not prove that the deceased was alive at the time of the outbreak of fire (H&E ×125)

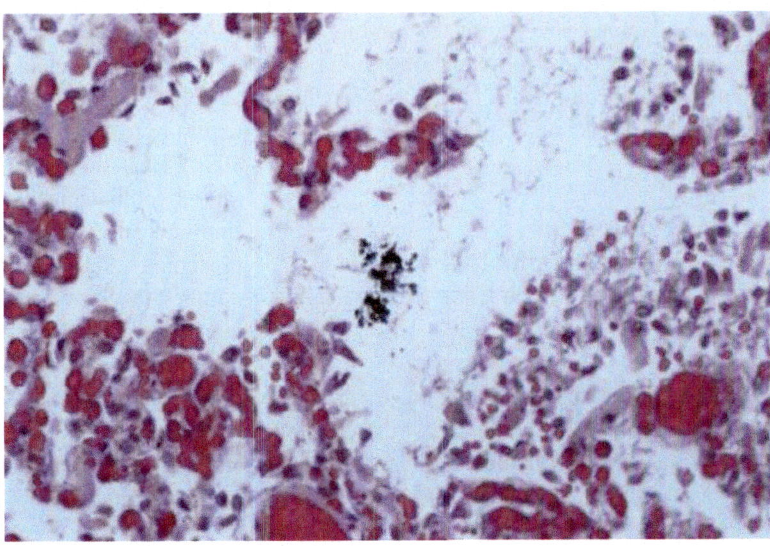

Fig. 7.6 Histologically detectable soot particles following deep soot aspiration in the lung tissue (H&E ×400)

Table 7.3 Vital signs in the case of heat impact

Vital signs	Histological findings
Serous blister	Detection of fibrin and leukocytes in the blister content
Heat inhalation trauma	Detection of early heat injury (see above) to the respiratory epithelium in the absence of direct heat- or fire-related opening of and damage to the respiratory tracts
Pulmonary fat embolism	Intravascular branched and wormlike Sudan III-positive neutral fats
Soot dust in the respiratory tract	Histological detection of soot dust particles in deeper layers of the respiratory tracts which did not open due to fire embedded in mucus
Soot particles in the pulmonary alveoli	Depending on particle size, very fine soot dust can get into the peripheral branches of the bronchial tree (bronchioles) and into the pulmonary alveoli

Even if vital signs are histologically clear, one should not dispense with a determination of the carbon monoxide concentration in the blood

the well-known question of whether there are vital reactions in the lung following the inhalation of hot air (Goldbach 1956). Heat shock proteins protect the human epithelium against nitric oxide-mediated cytotoxicity (Wong et al. 1997). To clarify the question of whether the patient was alive at the time of the fire outbreak, all findings mentioned in Table 7.3 should be scrutinized.

A note on taking samples: tissue samples from all levels of the tracheobronchial tree and from all pulmonary lobes, both central and peripheral, are necessary. Among the protracted findings are long-term damage due to inhalation trauma and findings in connection with burn shock, such as stress ulcers (Drüner and Grözinger 1972).

7.1.3 Histological and Immunohistochemical Findings in the Case of Burn Shock

Depending on the survival time of the victim, conventional histological findings show the reaction of the organism to heat inhalation trauma and heat- or fire-related tissue necrosis. For example, histology can show reactive hyperemia in submucosal capillaries of the respiratory tract, a cellular histiocytic reaction along the margin of necrotic areas, microthrombi, purulent tracheobronchitis, and organization of tissue damage in internal organs, in particular, in lung tissue (Janssen 1977; Reh 1960). Depending on survival time, other internal organs also respond to extended heat injury, in particular, the kidneys, liver, adrenals, brain, and pancreas (Table 7.4). A massive attack of cells and cellular decay products may lead to acute kidney failure with histological detection of protein cylinders in the renal tubules.

Immunohistochemical investigations of lung tissue in fire victims were performed to stain adhesion molecules. In 73% of fire fatalities, the endothelium of the peribronchial vessels could be stained with antibodies to von Willebrand factor, 66% with anti-CD62P (P-selectin), and CD31 (PECAM-1) showed a differential distribution pattern (Weis and Bohnert 2008). These investigators found statistically significant differences between the study group with cases of burn shock and the control group with hemorrhagic shock with strong staining for P-selectin, particularly in the lumina of the blood vessels, and von Willebrand factor in the specimens of burn shock victims. Otherwise, expression of PECAM-1 was lower in lungs from burn shock than in those from hemorrhagic shock fatalities.

Heatstroke Heatstroke is defined as a core body temperature that rises above 40.6 °C and is accompanied by mental status abnormalities such as delirium, convulsions, or coma resulting from exposure to environmental heat (Ng'walali et al. 1998). Heatstroke induces c-fos expression in the rat hypothalamus (Tsay et al. 1999). Immunohistochemistry of the brain showed that preceding ethanol administration increased the number of c-fos-immunoreactive neurons, as a marker of neuronal activation, in the central amygdaloid nucleus, which is involved in thermoregulation (Kibayashi et al. 2009).

Knowledge about hyperthermia-specific changes in internal organs is partly based on animal experiments, whereby relevant findings

Table 7.4 Significant histological findings in internal organs in the case of burn shock

Organ	Findings and their severity depending on survival time
Lungs	Diffuse interstitial edema, focal intra-alveolar edema relatively rich in proteins, focal hemorrhage, microthrombi containing fibrin in peripheral arteries and arterioles, focal atelectases, focal bronchopneumonia, areas of emphysema, necrotizing bronchiolitis (agents: in particular staphylococci, streptococci, or gram-negative rods). Later development of so-called shock lung or ventilation lung
Heart	Interstitial edema, focal pallors, homogeneous cytoplasm of cardiomyocytes [more pronounced in the right ventricle than in the left; Janssen (1977)]; later disseminated perivascular myocardial necrosis with cellular histiocytic reaction, fat, or Sudan III-negative vacuolization in the cytoplasm of cardiomyocytes, extremely elastic venules, swelling of endothelial cells
Brain	Pronounced edema, swelling, and homogenization of ganglion cells, vacuolar degeneration, loss of cellular processes; dentate nucleus, olive cells, Purkinje cells, pons, and cerebral cortex are particularly affected (Zinck 1940)
Pancreas	Concomitant reaction in the context of burn shock, with necrosis of single parenchymal cells, group necrosis, and thrombi containing fibrin in the capillaries and arterioles (Janssen 1977)
Gastrointestinal tract	Concomitant reaction in the case of burn shock with erosions and "stress ulcers"
	Cave: bleeding to death due to a preexisting ventricular ulcer or duodenal ulcer; for this reason histological determination of ulcer age to differentiate from a preexisting chronic ulcer. This shows a clear wall of connective tissue (van Gieson stain) at the margin and a partly fibrous ulcer base
	Histological differentiation from a fresh medication-induced ulcer (e.g., cortisone ulcer, ulcer after the administration of nonsteroidal antirheumatics—NSAID ulcer) is rarely possible
Kidneys	Necrotic cells or decay products in cells (rhabdomyolysis) may lead to protein cylinders and hemoglobin cylinders in the renal tubules and to acute dialysis-dependent renal failure; hyaline-drop degeneration of the distal tubular cells, apparently cell-rich glomeruli, possible necrotizing nephrosis, hyperemia of the renal medullary zone, cloudy swelling of proximal tubular epithelia
Adrenals	After several hours, hyperplasia of the external layer of the adrenal cortex may develop, which may later also reach the internal layer of the adrenal cortex with decreased lipid content (lipid storage in the adrenal cortex). After 2–4 days, dystrophic changes (Janssen 1977), hemorrhage, and necrosis of the adrenal cortex also occur (Olbrycht and Ramult 1924)
Liver	Pronounced hydropic vacuolization of hepatocytes, leukocytosis in the hepatic sinus, phagocytosis in cells of the reticulohistiocytic system, acute vascular congestion, intravascular spread of hepatocytes, coagulation products, and cell detritus in the hepatic sinus as PTAH-positive particles (Brinkmann et al. 1979)

The histology of burn shock can partly mimic the histomorphology of shock with varying causes

could not as yet been extrapolated to the forensic practice of investigating human tissue and organ samples (Kibayashi et al. 2009). Ethanol intake is a well-known predisposing factor in heatstroke. Immunohistochemical investigations found that hyperthermia combined with ethanol administration induces c-fos expression in the central amygdaloid nucleus of the mouse brain (Kibayashi et al. 2009).

Heat shock protein (hsp) response in the central nervous system following hyperthermia is also well known (Westman and Sharma 1998), and hsp70 leads to the activation of natural killer cells (Multhoff 2002). Immunohistochemical staining of ubiquitin (an hsp) in the midbrain in fire fatalities revealed increased intranuclear ubiquitin reactivity in the pigmented neurons of the substantia nigra (Quan et al. 2001). Other studies found a heat-induced immunoreactivity of tau protein in neocortical neurons in fire fatalities (Kibayashi and Shojo 2003).

In lung tissue in cases of fire death, immunohistochemical investigations also revealed a significantly higher expression of surfactant protein A along the alveolar interior surface and on the interface of the intra-alveolar effusion in comparison with controls including CO intoxication due to non-fire-related causes. Also, aggregated granular deposits were found in the intra-alveolar spaces, usually observed in the atelectatic areas. It has also been suggested that pulmonary surfactant protein A may be increased due to various fatal stresses and may indicate an advanced pulmonary alveolar injury (Zhu et al. 2001a; 1997).

Further investigations of the respiratory tract and lungs of fire victims revealed a statistically significant enhanced expression of hsp70 in the epiglottis, trachea, and both the main and peripheral bronchi compared to a control group (Marschall et al. 2006). The authors concluded that their results suggest a vital or supravital reaction due to the inhalation of hot fire fumes.

Depending on the extent of heat-related necrosis, cellular decay products can be found in the bloodstream; in some cases, rhabdomyolyses are possible, and acute kidney failure may develop (McCaninch et al. 1964; Pinchuk et al. 1964). Histopathologically, pronounced general hyperemia is apparent as well as cloudy swelling and hyaline-drop degeneration of the distal tubular cells. Protein or hemoglobin cylinders and a broadened Bowman's capsule can be found. The distal tubular cells may be separated from the basal membrane. In addition to regressive changes in the distal tubular cells, extensive necrotizing nephrosis may develop. The glomeruli are relatively cell-rich; they can degenerate, and in some cases even granulocytic infiltrates may accrue (in the case of sepsis) (Janssen 1977; Reh 1960). More extensive necrosis can be seen in patients with fixed hypertension and existing nephrosclerosis in the case of relatively low-grade burns (Pinchuk 1964).

7.2 Electricity and Lightning Stroke

Accidental death by electricity occurs in the home and at work, occasionally also as suicide. In rare cases, electricity is used to kill a human being, for example, a hairdryer in a water-filled bathtub (Stolt 2005). In this case, attention should be paid to a possible linear mark of the skin caused by the electricity at the point where air and water meet (Weiler and Riße 1985).

There may be a significant difference in damage patterns involving accidents with electricity depending on the intensity of the power source (low-voltage power, high-voltage power, etc.) and the type of surface that makes contact with the victim's body (Zhang and Cai 1995; Fish 1993a, b). When the surface of the power source is large, for example, a power line in the water, skin must not show morphological findings. In the case of a lightning strike, however, large burns will be recognizable on the skin, as well as injury to internal organs. In addition to heat-induced areactive necrosis in cases of acute death, histological findings will vary depending on survival time following electric shock or lightning strike.

7.2.1 Electrocution

Histological findings of current marks were the subject of several investigations in both animal and human studies (Üzün et al. 2008; Takamiya et al. 2001; Danielsen et al. 1978; Pioch 1968, 1967, 1966c).

The histomorphological representation of (usually small) current marks consists of a central depression and marginally preserved epidermis (keratinizing squamous epithelium); the basal cell layers are accentuated, and the epidermis shows elongated cell formations with elongated cell nuclei (Fig. 7.7). The nuclei-containing keratin

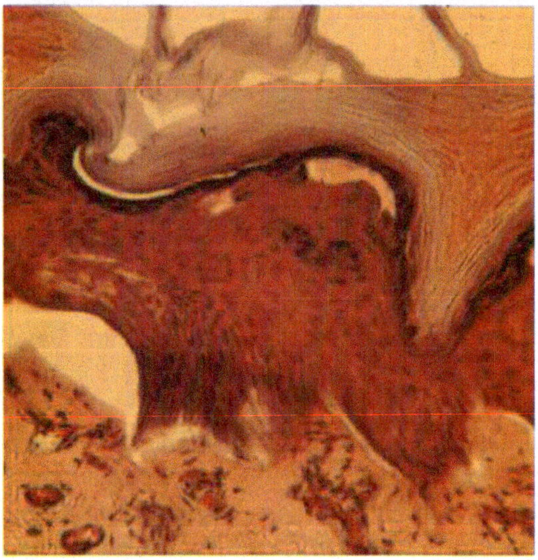

Fig. 7.7 Current marks with elongated epidermis cells and elongated cell nuclei emphasized at the base (H&E ×200)

lamellae (keratinocytes) are also partly elongated. Epidermal nuclear elongation is one of the most important signs for the diagnosis of electrical injury. In the case of a body under the influence of low-voltage current for 7 days, hypercontraction bands of the intercostal muscles and coagulative changes of the perineurium of peripheral nerves have been found (Anders et al. 2001).

Separations may form in the epidermis at the edge of the current mark – intraepidermal separation in electrocution (Saukko and Knight 2004). Cells of the skin appendages in the superficial corium may show similar damage. Formation of subepidermal separations is rarer (Üzün et al. 2008). In addition, epidermal coagulation necrosis and eosinophilic condensed tissue may occur (Üzün et al. 2008; Wankhede and Sariya 2006). Examinations based on animal models support the assumption that electricity, as well as heat, causes the skin to expand and that this mechanical effect of expansion is the cause of histologically visible cell and nucleus elongation (Bellini et al. 2016; Üzün et al. 2008; Takamiya et al. 2001). This thesis is supported by investigations involving mechanical damage to cadaver skin where cell and nucleus elongation was produced, as well as cluster-type arrangements or compressions of the subepidermal connective tissue. In this way, histological findings involving current exposure or current marks can be simulated (Schwerd and Höchel 1966).

A note on taking samples: when removing damaged skin samples for suspected current marks, the surrounding region of skin and the subepidermal soft tissue, including the muscle tissue below, should be included (Janssen 1984). This trend is valid when results involving animal models are considered: intraepidermal separation is most frequent in electrical lesions, and subepidermal separation is the most frequent finding in naked flame burns; a combination of both is most likely to be caused by electricity (Üzün et al. 2008).

When the skin is exposed to electricity for an extended period of time, e.g., when someone commits suicide using electricity, coagulation necrosis of the subepidermal soft tissue occurs, which appears edematous and swollen. When the corium is small, hypodermic fatty tissue may appear to be cooked and display a homogenous, golden color, while the cells of the top layers of the epidermis may show a current mark (Fig. 7.8).

Likewise, with prolonged exposure of the skin to electricity, a metallic conductor may cause blackish carbonization of the epidermis and the subepidermal soft tissue (Jacobsen 1997). Embedded in the blackish carbonized area, one may find microscopically small, blackish particles, termed "electrical metallization" (Böhm 1967b, 1968a, b) (Fig. 7.9). "Thermal metallization" can be differentiated from "electrical metallization": in the case of "electrical metallization," blackish particles are often found at the margin of the injury, while in "thermal metallization," they are also found in all areas at the center of the injury (Böhm 1967a).

Death by electric shock is caused by acute cardiac arrest when the conduction system of the

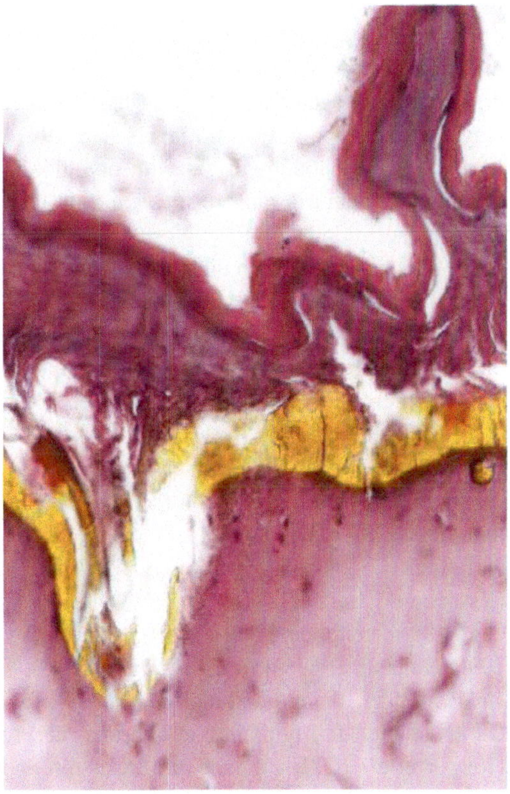

Fig. 7.8 Effects on skin exposed to electricity for an extended period of time with edematous coagulation necrosis of soft tissue found deep inside, cooked subepidermal tissue with golden yellow color, and damage to epidermal cells caused by electricity (H&E ×40)

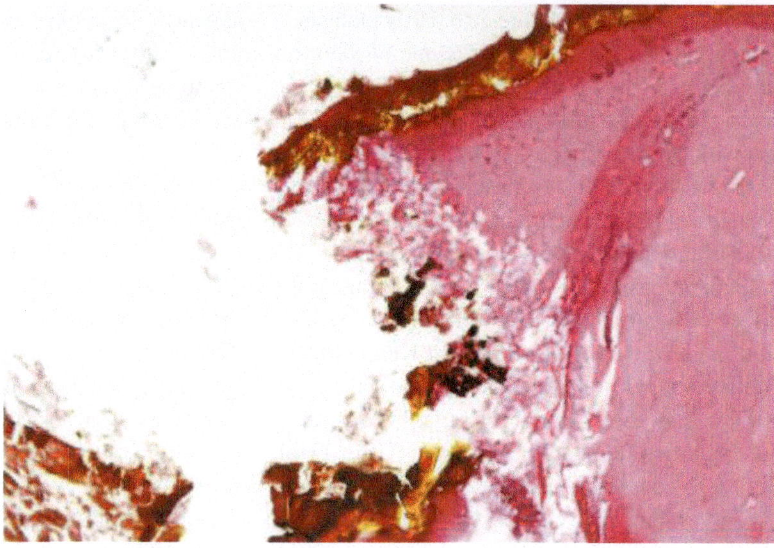

Fig. 7.9 *Blackish* particles of a metallic conductor—"electrical metallization"—at the level of the current mark (H&E ×100)

heart is interrupted during a vulnerable phase. Evidence of a histomorphological correlate is not needed. With higher voltages, findings in the myocardium are described that lead to myocardial infarction; accidents involving high voltage may cause rhabdomyolysis (Franzius et al. 1997). In addition to rhabdomyolysis with myoglobinuria, hemoglobinuria may result as a long-term consequence (Cooper 1980; Yost and Holmes 1974; Zhu et al. 2001b); in this case, there may be protein or rather myoglobin cylinders, and hemoglobin cylinders may be found in the tubules. The effect of electricity on the myoglobin content in skeletal muscle has also been examined (Keil et al. 1984).

There are various hypotheses (Table 7.5) on the thermal–electrical effect on the myocardium that can be based in part on clinical processes and partly on histopathological findings (Vianello 1997; Zack et al. 1997; Lichtenberg et al. 1993; Xenopoulos et al. 1991; James et al. 1990; Ku et al. 1989; Wright and Davis 1980). A small number of publications mention "electrical petechiae" and tympanic membrane rupture (Karger et al. 2002; Cooper 1980; Castren and Kytila 1963). Case reports on pregnant women who suffered electric shock exist (Chan and Sivasamboo 1972; Rees 1965). Bundles of hypercontracted myocytes and bundles of hyperdistended myocardial cells, as well as separation of sarcomeres in myofibers connected to contracted ones, were detected before death (Fineschi et al. 2006; Baroldi et al. 2005). Following exposure to electricity, the skeletal musculature can also show hemorrhage with hypercontraction bands, pathological longitudi-

Table 7.5 Hypotheses on the causes of myocardial damage in electrical or high-voltage accidents

Hypothesis	Histopathological finding
Electrical damage	Electrical damage or interruption of the cardiac conduction system function with lethal cardiac arrhythmia with no opportunity to identify specific structural findings histopathologically
Direct thermal–electrical damage	Diffusely distributed myocardial necrosis and hemorrhage with cellular reaction and signs of organization depending on survival time
Vascular causes	Localized distribution pattern of myocardial damage due to thermal–electrical damage to the vascular wall myocytes with local microthrombi, vascular wall ruptures, and focal hemorrhage
Vasospasm	Thermally/electrically induced vasospasms of the coronary arteries—with and without structural changes to the vascular walls—will result in localized disturbances in myocardial perfusion (myocardial infarct)

Cardiopulmonary resuscitation with frequent defibrillation should be taken into consideration as a cause for histological or immunohistochemical findings

nal striation, and segmental as well as discoid degeneration of muscle fibers; PTAH staining is recommended (Anders et al. 2000).

In addition to the proposed direct electrical injury to the myocardium in high-voltage accidents, it is assumed that electrically induced vasospasm of the coronary arteries occurs, leading to myocardial infarction (Franzius et al. 1997). Reliable histomorphological correlates following application of electric shock devices (Tasers) have not yet been described (Banaschak et al. 2001).

7.2.2 Lightning

Although humans may survive direct lightning strikes, neurological injuries often remain (Stütz et al. 2006; Koeppen 1965; Krauland 1951). The tissue damaged by lightning shows severe burns and necrosis, which may also involve internal organs depending on the direction of the lightning strike (Zack et al. 2013, Dettmeyer et al. 2007, Fineschi et al. 2006, Lederer et al. 2002, Zack et al. 1997, Lichtenberg et al. 1993). In cases of prolonged survival, areas of skin necrosis including the epidermis are infiltrated by inflammation with participation of granulocytes (Fig. 7.10).

Varying levels of necrosis may be detectable in internal organs. Depending on survival time, inflammatory reactions and elimination reactions of varying intensity may occur (Fig. 7.11). In this case, the border between lightning strike-induced necrosis and damage-free tissue may be easily visible (Fig. 7.12). Focal damage to the central nervous system can often be seen, and with early autopsy following the lightning strike, hemorrhage is at least detectable (Fig. 7.13).

7.3 Malignant Hyperthermia

Malignant hyperthermia is a rare pharmacogenetic disorder first described in 1960 (Denborough and Lovell 1960). The disorder is triggered by volatile anesthetic agents and depolarizing muscle relaxants in the context of a heterogenous genetic disposition (Allen and Brubaker 1998; Gronert 1980; Britt et al. 1974). Histological examination demonstrates fragmentation of the muscle fibers of the heart and focal necrosis in acute up to mixed resorptive stages in the skeletal muscles: sarcolysis with lumpy breakdown, phagocytosis of myoglobin, fatty infiltration of the muscle, sarcolysis with hole-like defects, and longitudinal striation from clumped myofibrils (Karger and Teige 2002). In addition, alveolar lung edema, small alveolar macrophages, and abundant clots containing myoglobin in small lung vessels and in dilated distal renal tubules are

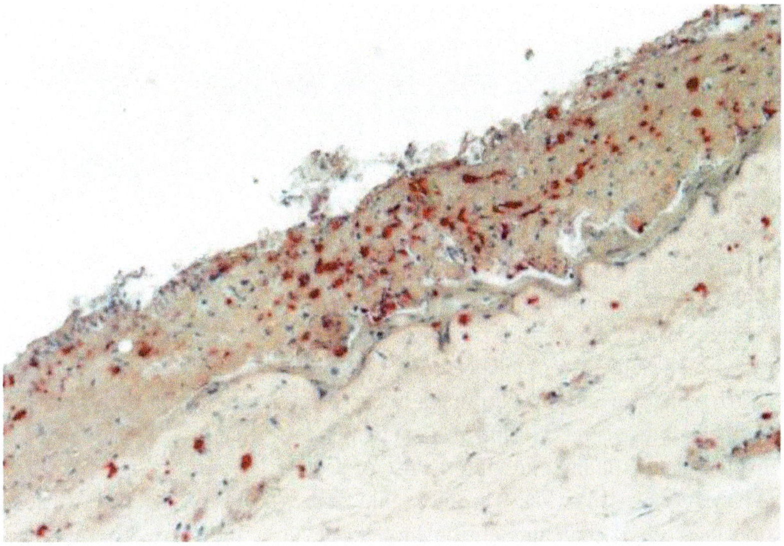

Fig. 7.10 A 35-year-old man died 4 days after surviving a lightning strike and reanimation; laminar skin necrosis and early dense infiltration of the residual epidermis damaged by granulocytes (ASD ×200)

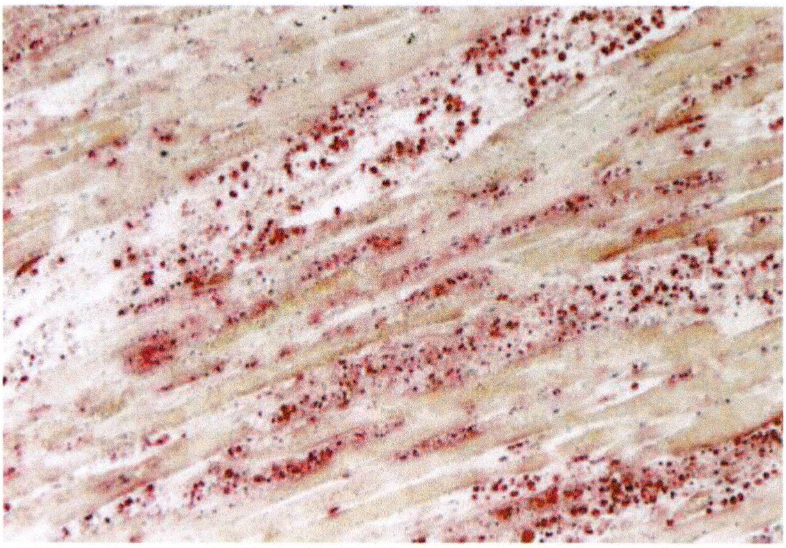

Fig. 7.11 Intensive, ASD-positive, granulocytic infiltration of the myocardium after initial survival of a lightning strike (ASD ×200)

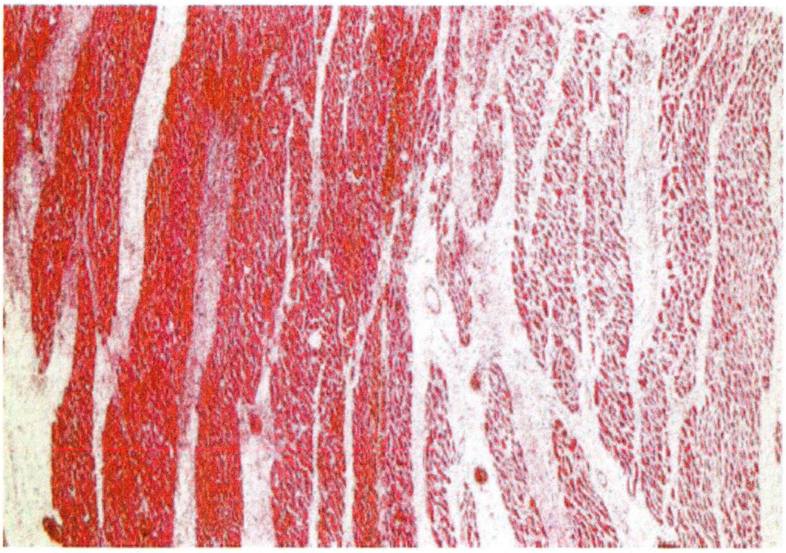

Fig. 7.12 Well-demarcated damage to the myocardium caused by a lightning strike (*left*), as distinct from damage-free myocardial tissue (*right*) (H&E ×40)

described (Karger and Teige 2002; Abe et al. 2001). In cases of malignant hyperthermia, the forensic diagnosis has to rely on microscopic examinations with regard to the clinical history (Püschel and Brinkmann 1978; Brinkmann and Püschel 1977; Maresch 1973). Postmortem urinary myoglobin levels can be found (Zhu et al. 2001b). In rare cases, malignant hyperthermia and rhabdomyolysis develop in genetically predisposed individuals following the use of ecstasy (MDMA) (see Chap. 4). Chromogranin expression in the hypothalamus and adenohypophysis as a stress marker has been reported in the context of hyperthermia (as well as hypothermia) (Yoshida et al. 2011).

Hyperthermia and Sudden Infant Death Syndrome The role of hyperthermia in sudden infant death has long been discussed. Many authors have called attention to the preterminal sweating of infants during sleep (Wilske 1984), and in 1983 Beal reported preterminal nocturnal sweating in 38% of sudden infant death cases (Beal 1983). Profuse sweating during sleep may therefore be regarded as an indication of an increased risk of sudden infant death (Kahn et al.

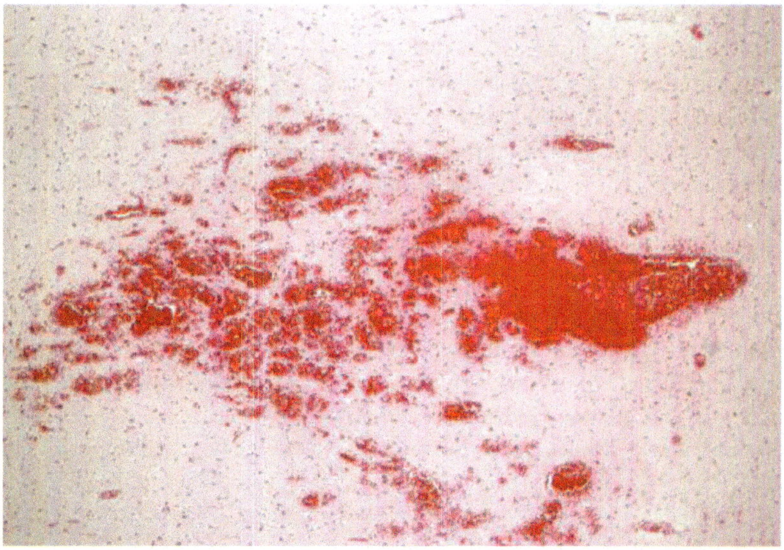

Fig. 7.13 Focal fresh hemorrhage within the cerebral cortex following a lightning strike (H&E ×40)

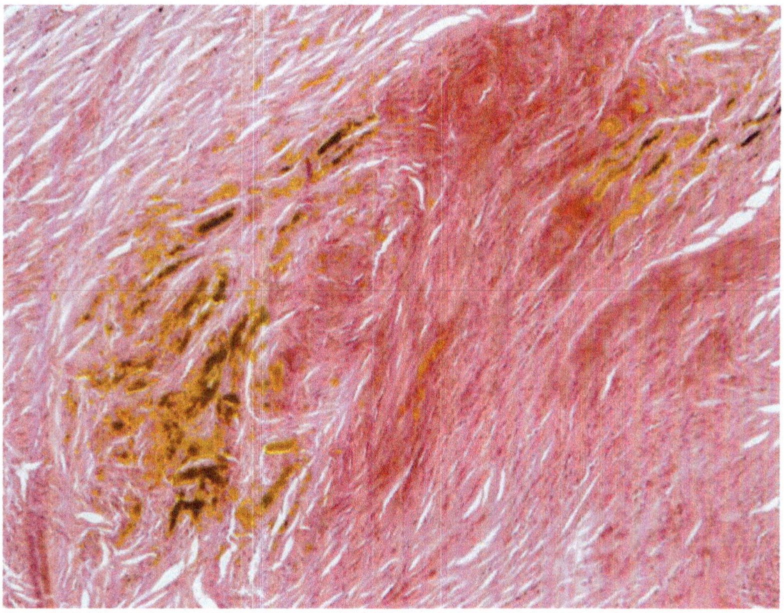

Fig. 7.14 Thermally coagulated tissue following the use of thermal cautery (H&E ×100)

1990; Wilske 1984). Nevertheless, there are no histological and immunohistochemical findings indicating hyperthermia in cases of suspected sudden infant death syndrome, since there are no specific microscopic lesions typical for hyperthermia. From an immunohistochemical perspective, the question arises as to whether heat shock protein is expressed in SIDS victims compared with controls. Heat shock proteins are primarily shock proteins whose increased expression in response to a significant rise in temperature is assumed to enable survival for a certain period of time even at increased temperatures. Tests conducted at moderate heat stress in gene expression studies suggest differences between SIDS cases and controls (Rohde et al. 2013).

Iatrogenic Heat Damage The use of electrothermal tissue coagulation in the tissue concerned can produce characteristic histological findings. Rarely, one finds "thermogranulomas," which have a granuloma-like, round/oval structure. Tissue may also have undergone necrotic fibrosis and show yellowish-beige necrosis (Fig. 7.14).

7.4 Radiation

Damage caused by radiation is very rare in forensic medicine. It may involve, for example, allegations of medical malpractice on the basis of erroneously indicated radiation therapy which led to the injury. Histological investigation may reveal ulceration of the skin surface or thin atrophic epidermis. The corium shows a poor cell count in parts with areas of fibrosis, as well as few accompanying fibrocytes and fibroblasts with potentially swollen cell nuclei and minimal chromatin. The subepidermal small vessels show fibrosis and hyalinosis of the intima with narrowing of the vascular spaces. In addition, there may be ectatic vessels. A lymphocytic inflammatory infiltrate of varying density may also appear; this is minimal at an advanced stage such that the overall picture points to radiodermatitis (Fig. 7.15).

As a rule, one should always anticipate cell and tissue damage following exposure to ionizing radiation (Oehlert 1970). In the early phase, the cell reacts by a lifting of the outer lamella of the nuclear membrane, which can only be proven electron-microscopically and with vacuole expansion of the intramembranous space. The results are loss of chromatin, swelling of

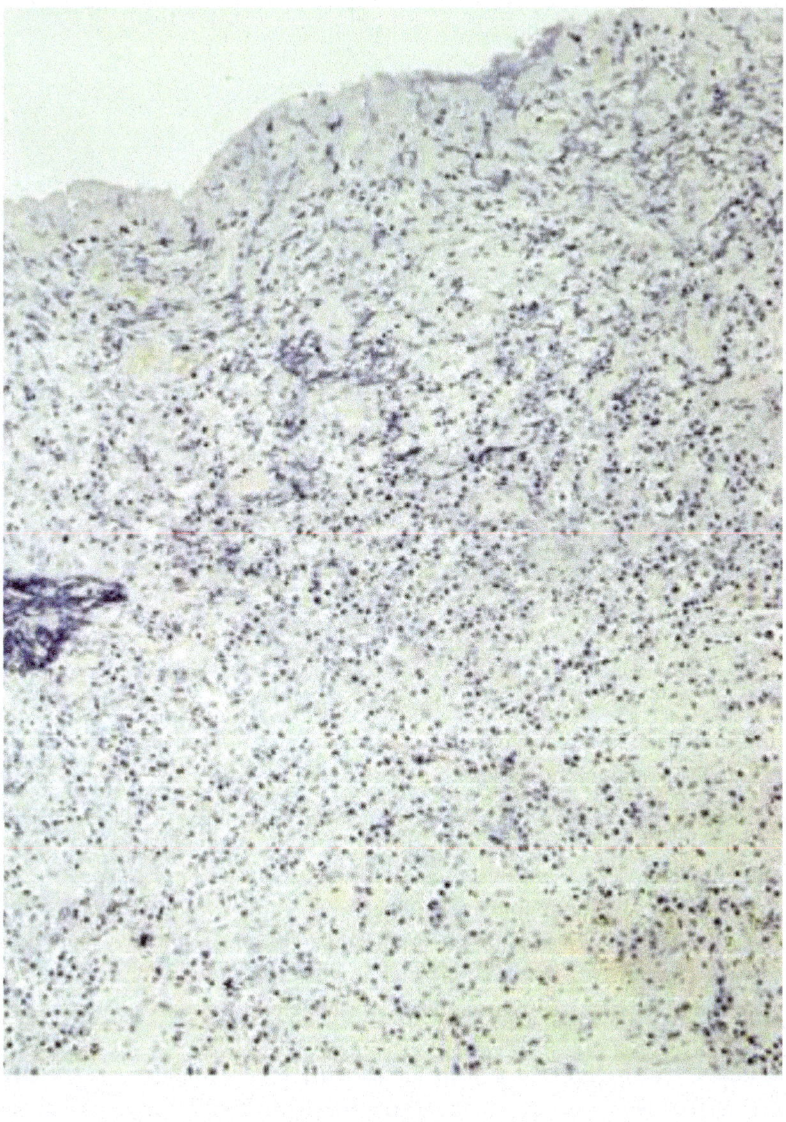

Fig. 7.15 Skin damage caused by radiation, i.e., radiodermatitis (Giemsa ×40)

cell nuclei, plication of the nuclear membrane, and formation of giant cells, followed by nuclear pyknosis, karyolysis, and karyorrhexis (Bergeder 1963).

The first morphologically detectable reaction in radiation-exposed tissue is a reactive expansion of capillaries; hours later, swelling develops in the nuclei and cytoplasm of endothelial cells. Perinuclear vacuoles then develop with depression of the nuclei and detachment of entire endothelial sections. It is possible that endothelial proliferates may develop with bizarre, pyknotic cell nuclei. Inside larger blood vessels, fibrinoid coagulation and macrophages with vacuolized cytoplasm may be found (Zollinger 1960).

In addition to radiodermatitis of the skin, the skeleton may also be damaged (osteoradionecroses), as well as the bone marrow and the musculature of the heart and skeleton (actinic myocardiopathy) with cloudy swelling of cardial myocytes (Thurner 1970; Werthemann 1930). There are other descriptions of histomorphological findings following radiation to joints, the central nervous system (radiation necrosis of the brain), and peripheral nerves (radiogenic peripheral neuropathy). Damage to the liver (Reed and Cox 1966), kidneys, and lungs has also been demonstrated (Villiers and Gross 1967). Radiation embryopathy and thorotrast damage are special cases (Steiner and Brinkmann 1974; Gehrmann et al. 1963) with histologically detectable radioactive thorium dioxide.

7.5 Selective Internal Radiotherapy (SIRT)

In rare cases, patients undergo autopsy following selective internal radiotherapy (SIRT), in particular for liver tumors and liver metastases. SIRT involves injecting minute radioactive beads (microspheres, SIRT particles) measuring approximately 40 μm in diameter (around a third of the size of a human hair) into the vessels supplying the tumor through a catheter via the femoral artery. Radioactive yttrium-90 has a half-life of approximately 64 h. The procedure uses beta radiation with a maximum range of 1 cm and an extremely high local effect. Therefore, in the case of autopsy shortly after the administration of yttrium-90, those performing the autopsy are at risk of possible radiation exposure when dissecting the liver. If carefully sought, the yttrium-90 beads can be visualized microscopically (Fig. 7.16).

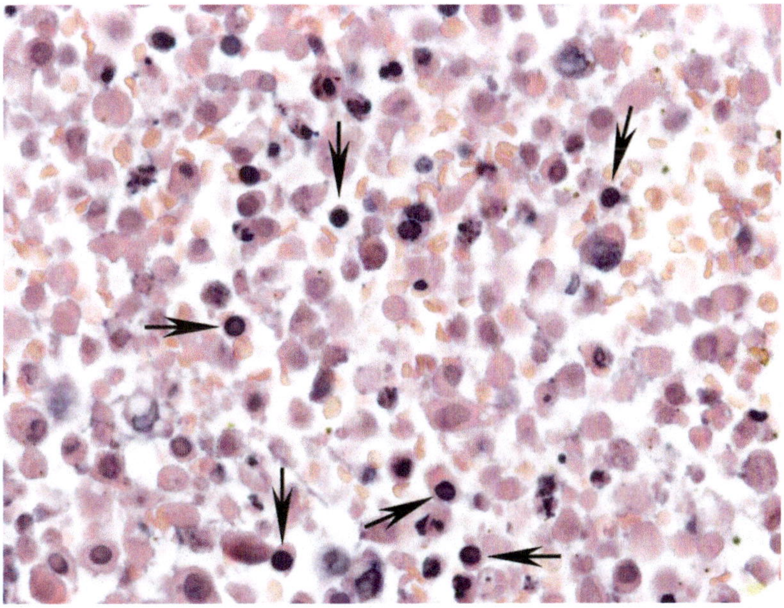

Fig. 7.16 Yttrium-90 beads (*arrow*) and surrounding necrotic tissue following SIRT: patient with metastasized adenocarcinoma (H&E ×400)

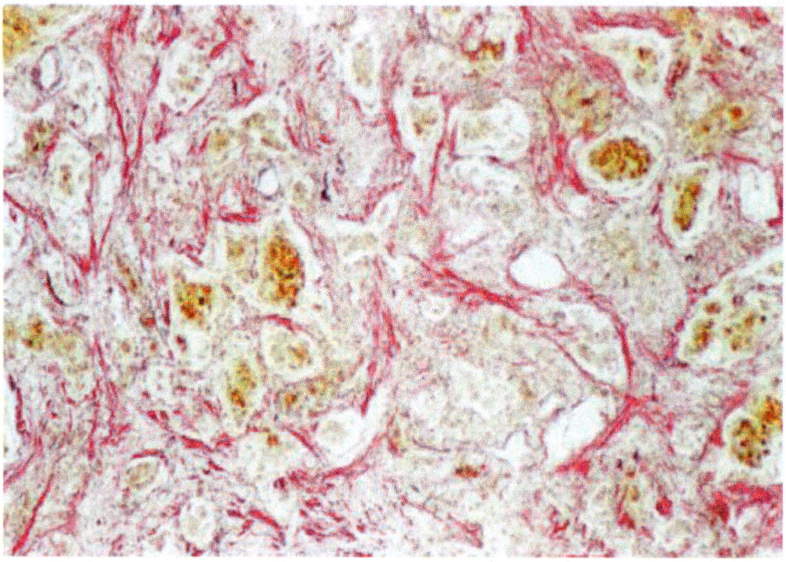

Fig. 7.17 At 13 days after survival of an accident involving chlorine gas with toxic damage to the pulmonary tissue and posttraumatic pulmonary fibrosis (H&E ×100)

7.6 Gases

Burns, the inhalation of carbon monoxide (CO) and/or other toxic gases, and a lack of atmospheric oxygen are accepted to be the major lethal factors in fires (Zhu et al. 2001b; Gormsen et al. 1984). Gases often lead to rapid death, e.g., carbon monoxide and decomposition gases in decomposition towers. In relation to rapid death, reports include acute pulmonary emphysema, sometimes accompanied by massive pulmonary edema (Oesterhelweg et al. 2006).

Inhalation of gases may lead to severe injury to the respiratory system and lungs (see Chap. 11). In most cases, accidents (e.g., industrial accidents) are involved. In the case of initial accident survival, resulting damage to the lungs may manifest, ultimately leading to death. In the case of accidents involving chlorine gas, severe pulmonary injuries are described with multiple hemorrhages and posttraumatic fibrosis, which partially resembles carnified pneumonia (Fig. 7.17). Siderin deposits are found in the Prussian blue compound as residuals of intrapulmonary hemorrhages. Carbon monoxide poisoning with a fatal outcome can evidently cause brain injury, including apoptotic responses and brain tissue necrosis, prior to death. Laminar necrosis, edema, cell pyknosis, eosinophilic degeneration, accentuated perineural spaces, spongiosis, and congestion have been reported (Uemura et al. 2001). At the same time, there is evidence that fibronectin is expressed in the myocardium, as is the necrosis marker C5b-9 (Fracasso et al. 2011).

Combined inhalation of carbon monoxide and formic acid resulted in loss of respiratory epithelium of the trachea, subepithelial lymphoplasmacellular infiltration, reactive hyperemia, and alveolar pulmonary edema. Erythrocyte extravasation and microthrombi in small vessels have also been described. Hepatic microsteatosis has been reported in the liver, while the liver sinus was filled with bloated erythrocytes (Bakovic et al. 2016).

References

Abe M, Saitoh H, Sato Y, Hamaguchi K, Kiuchi M (2001) Immunohistochemical study of the kidneys after severe muscular injury. Int J Legal Med 114:232–236

Allen GC, Brubaker CL (1998) Human malignant hyperthermia associated with desflurane anaesthesia. Anaesth Analg 86:1328–1331

Anders S, Schulz F, Tsokos M (2000) Intramuskuläre Hämorrhagien bei letaler suizidaler Strombeibringung. In: 9th spring meeting of the German society of forensic medicine – northern region, Leipzig, Germany, 4–5 May 2000

Anders S, Matschke J, Tsokos M (2001) Internal current mark in a case of suicide by electrocution. Am J Forensic Med Pathol 22:370–373

Bakovic M, Nestic M, Mayer D (2016) Suicidal chemistry: combined intoxication with carbon monoxide and formic acid. Int J Legal Med 130:723–729
Banaschak S, Milbradt H, Humpert M, Roll P, Madea B (2001) Zum Nachweis der Anwendung von Elektroschockgeräten. Arch Kriminol 208:149–158
Baroldi G, Silver MD, Parolini M, Pomara C, Turillazzi E, Fineschi V (2005) Myofiber break-up: a marker of ventricular fibrillation in sudden cardiac death. Int J Cardiol 100:435–441
Beal SM (1983) Some epidemiological factors about sudden infant death syndrome (SIDS) in South Australia. In: Tildon JT, Roeder LM, Steinschneider A (eds) Sudden infant death syndrome. Academic, New York, pp 15–28
Bellini E, Gambassi G, Nucci G, Benvenuti M, Landi G, Gabbrielli M, Vanezis P (2016) Death by electrocution: histological technique for copper detection on the electric mark. Forensic Sci Int 264:24–27
Bergeder HD (1963) Grundlagen der biologischen Strahlenwirkung und Strahlenschäden. Ergebn Allgem Path 42:1
Böhm E (1967a) Differentialdiagnostisch bedeutsame Unterschiede zwischen Strom- und Wärmemarken. Dtsch Z Gesamte Gerichtl Med 61:128–136
Böhm E (1967b) Untersuchungen über die Gestalt oberflächlicher Metallisationen der Haut. Dtsch Z Gesamte Gerichtl Med 59:26–34
Böhm E (1968a) Die Versilberungsmethode nach Timm als Nachweisreaktion für elektrische Metallisation. Dtsch Z Gesamte Gerichtl Med 62:26–31
Böhm E (1968b) Zur Frage der Differentialdiagnose zwischen thermischen und elektrischen Verbrennungen. Dtsch Z Gesamte Gerichtl Med 63:149–153
Bohnert M (2004) Morphological findings in burned bodies. In: Tsokos M (ed) Forensic pathology reviews, vol I. Humana, Totowa, pp 3–27
Bohnert M, Werner CR, Pollak S (2003) Problems associated with the diagnosis of vitality in burned bodies. Forensic Sci Int 135:197–205
Bohnert M, Anderson J, Rothschild MA, Böhm J (2010) Immunohistochemical expression of fibronection in the lungs of fire victims proves intravital reaction in fatal burns. Int J Legal Med 124:583–588
Brinkmann B, Püschel K (1977) Zur Histomorpologie der Herz- und Skelettmuskulatur bei maligner Hyperthermie. Z Rechtsmed 80:117–133
Brinkmann B, Püschel K (1978) Heat injuries to the respiratory system. Virchows Arch A Pathol Anat Histol 379:299–311
Brinkmann B, Kleiber M, Koops E, Püschel K (1979) Vitale Reaktionen bei akutem Verbrühungstod. Z Rechtsmed 83:1–16
Britt BA, Web GE, LeDuc C (1974) Malignant hyperthermia induced by curare. Can Anaesth Soc J 21:371–375
Castren JA, Kytila J (1963) Eye symptoms caused by lightning stroke. Acta Ophthalmol 41:139–143
Chan YF, Sivasamboo R (1972) Lightning accidents in pregnancy. J Obstet Gynaecol Br Commonw 79:761–762
Cooper MA (1980) Lightning injuries: prognostic signs for death. Ann Emerg Med 9:134–138
Cox RA, Mlcak RP, Chinkes DL, Jacob S, Enkhbaatar P, Jaso J, Parish LP, Traber DL, Jeschke ML, Herndon DN, Hawkins HK (2008) Upper airway mucus deposition in lung tissue of burn trauma victims. Shock 29:356–361
Danielsen L, Thomsen HK, Nielsen O, Aalund O, Nielsen KG, Karlsmark T, Genefke IK (1978) Electrical and thermal injuries in pig skin-evaluated and compared by light microscopy. Forensic Sci Int 12:211–225
Denborough MA, Lovell RRH (1960) Anaesthetic deaths in a family. Lancet 2:45
Dettmeyer R, Preuß J, Madea B (2007) 4 Tage überlebter Blitzschlag nach erfolgreicher Renanimation. 15th spring meeting of the German society of forensic medicine, Hamburg, Germany
Drüner HE, Grözinger KH (1972) Streß-Ulzera nach Verbrennungen. Med Welt 23:707
Fineschi V, D'Errico S, Neri M, Panarese F, Ricci P, Turillazzi E (2005) Heat stroke in an incubator: an immunohistochemical study in a fatal case. Int J Legal Med 119:94–97
Fineschi V, Karch SB, D'Errico S, Pomara C, Riezzo I, Turillazzi E (2006) Cardiac pathology in death from electrocution. Int J Legal Med 120:79–82
Fish R (1993a) Electric shock. Part I: nature and mechanisms of injury. J Emerg Med 11:309–312
Fish R (1993b) Electric shock. Part II: nature and mechanisms of injury. J Emerg Med 11:457–462
Foerster A (1932) Über Veränderungen der Luftröhrenschleimhaut bei Verbrannten. Dtsch Z Gesamte Gerichtl Med 19:293–301
Foerster A (1933) Experimentelle Untersuchungen über Veränderungen an den Atmungsorganen bei plötzlicher Einwirkung hoher Temperaturen. Dtsch Z Gesamte Gerichtl Med 20:445–461
Foerster A (1934) Mikroskopische Untersuchungen über das Verhalten der Alveolen bei Verbrannten. Dtsch Z Gesamte Gerichtl Med 23:281–288
Fracasso T, Schmeling A (2011) Delayed asphyxia due to inhalation injury. Int J Legal Med 125(2):289–292
Fracasso T, Pfeiffer H, Michaud K, Köhler H, Sauerland C, Schmeling A (2011) Immunohistochemical expression of fibronection and C5b-9 in the myocardium in cases of monoxide poisoning. Int J Legal Med 125:377–384
Franzius C, Meyer-Hofmann H, Lison AE (1997) Myokardinfarkt und Rhabdomyolyse nach einem Hochspannungsunfall mit erfolgreicher Reanimation. Dtsch Med Wochenschr 122:400–406
Gehrmann G, Schäfer EL, Wunder M (1963) Klinische und radiologische Befunde bei Thorotrastschädigungen. Dtsch Med Wochenschr 88:2050
Goldbach HJ (1956) Gibt es vitale Reaktionen der Lunge nach Heißlufteinatmung? Dtsch Z Gesamte Gerichtl Med 45:394
Gormsen H, Jeppesen N, Lund A (1984) The causes of death in fire victims. Forensic Sci Int 24:107–111

Gronert GA (1980) Malignant hyperthermia. Anesthesiology 53:395–423

Hieda Y, Tsujino Y, Xue Y, Takayama K, Fujihara J, Kimura K, Dekio S (2004) Skin analysis following dermal exposure to kerosene in rats: the effects of post-mortem exposure and fire. Int J Legal Med 118:41–46

Imaizumi K, Taniguchi K, Ogawa Y (2014) DNA survival and physical and histological properties of heat-induced alterations in burnt bones. Int J Legal Med 128:439–446

Jacobsen H (1997) Electrically induced deposition of metal on the human skin. Forensic Sci Int 90:85–92

James TN, Riddick L, Embry JH (1990) Cardiac abnormalities demonstrated post-mortem in four cases of accidental electrocution and their potential significance relative to nonfatal electrical injuries of the heart. Am Heart J 120:143–157

Janssen W (1977) Forensische Histologie. Schmidt-Römhild, Lübeck

Janssen W (1984) Injuries caused by heat and cold. In: Janssen W (ed) Forensic histopathology. Springer, New York, pp 234–260

Kahn A, Wacholder A, Winkler M, Rebuffat E (1990) Prospective study on the prevalence of sudden infant death and possible risk factors in Brussels: preliminary results (1987–1988). Eur J Pediatr 149:284–286

Karger B, Teige K (2002) Fatal malignant hyperthermia – delayed onset and atypical course. Forensic Sci Int 129:187–190

Karger B, Suggeler O, Brinkmann B (2002) Electrocution – autopsy study with emphasis on "electrical petechiae". Forensic Sci Int 126:210–213

Keil W, Yoshida H, Ishiyama I (1984) Untersuchungen zur Wirkung von Elektrizität auf den Myoglobingehalt humaner Herz- und Skelettmuskulatur. Z Rechtsmed 91:185–193

Kibayashi K, Shojo H (2003) Heat-induced immunoreactivity of tau protein in neocortical neurons of fire fatalities. Int J Legal Med 117:282–286

Kibayashi K, Nakao K, Shojo H (2009) Hyperthermia combined with ethanol administration induces c-fos expression in the central amygdaloid nucleus of the mouse brain. A possible mechanism of heatstroke under the influence of ethanol intake. Int J Legal Med 123:371–379

Koeppen S (1965) Personenschäden durch Blitzeinwirkung. Med Klin 60(35):1390–1394

Kowall-Vern A, Goral J, Gamelli RL, McGill V, Clancy J (2000) Hsp 70, Hsp 32, and Grp 78 are increased in thermally injured skin with and without antithrombin (human) concentrate infusion. J Burn Care Rehabil 21:213–219

Krauland W (1951) Schäden und Todesfälle durch Blitzschlag. Dtsch Z Gesamte Gerichtl Med 40:298–312

Ku CS, Lin SL, Hsu TL, Wang SP, Chang MS (1989) Myocardial damage associated with electrical injury. Am Heart J 118:621–624

Lederer W, Wiedermann FJ, Baubin MA, Kroesen G (2002) Blitzschlagverletzung und kardiopulmonale Reanimation. Notfall & Rettungsmedizin 5:474–479

Lichtenberg R, Dries D, Ward K, Marshall W, Scanlon P (1993) Cardiovascular effects of lightning strikes. J Am Coll Cardiol 21:531–536

Maresch W (1973) Maligne hyperthermie. Beitr Gerichtl Med 30:289–296

Marschall S, Rothschild MA, Bohnert M (2006) Expression of heat-shock protein 70 (HSP 70) in the respiratory tract and lungs of fire victims. Int J Legal Med 120:355–359

McCaninch J, Matter P, Lynch JB, Lewis SR, Blocker TG (1964) Renal pathophysiology in severe burns: five year review of kidney pathology in fatal burns. Tex Rep Biol Med 22:348

Multhoff G (2002) Activation of natural killer cells by heat shock protein 70. Int J Hyperth 18:576–585

Myers SL, Williams JM, Hodges JS (1999) Effects of extreme heat on teeth with implications for histologic processing. J Forensic Sci 44:805–809

Ng'walali PM, Kibayashi K, Yonemitsu K, Ohtsu Y, Tsunenari S (1998) Death as a result of heat stroke in a vehicle: an adult case in winter confirmed with reconstruction and animal experiments. J Clin Forensic Med 5:183–186

Oehlert W (1970) Pathologische Veränderungen in Organen und Geweben nach Applikation von Radioisotopen und Kontrastmitteln. Langenbecks Arch Chir 327:229

Oesterhelweg L, Kaufmann R, Hornborstel G, Bostelmann J, Schulz F, Püschel K (2006) Todesfälle im Zusammenhang mit Biogas. Kriminalistik 10:594–598

Olbrycht J (1927) Mikroskopische Untersuchungen von Lungen verbrannter Neugeborener zum Nachweis ihres Gelebthabens, nebst Bemerkungen über die forensische Bedeutung der histologischen Lungenprobe. Dtsch Z Gesamte Gerichtl Med 9:529

Olbrycht J, Ramult M (1924) Der Einfluß der Verbrühung, des anaphylaktischen Schocks und der parenteralen Zufuhr verschiedener Eiweißstoffe auf das histologische Bild der Nebennieren. Dtsch Z Gesamte Gerichtl Med 3:401

Pinchuk VM (1964) Morphological changes of the kidneys during the first period of burn. Arch Path (Mosk) 26(6):40

Pioch W (1966a) Die histochemische Untersuchung thermischer Hautschäden und ihre Bedeutung für die forensische Praxis. Schmidt-Römhild, Lübeck

Pioch W (1966b) L'image histologique des lèsions vitales et post-mortem causèes par brûlures. Extrait des Acta Medicinæ Legalis et Socialis XIX:327–333

Pioch W (1966c) Histologisch-histochemische Untersuchungen zur Identifizierung von Strommarken. Dtsch Z Gesamte Gerichtl Med 57:165–169

Pioch W (1967) Zur Diagnostik polytypischer Strommarken. Vorträge im Landeskriminalpolizeiamt Niedersachsen (Sonderdruck) Naturwissenschaftliche Kriminalistik, p 39–48

Pioch W (1968) Zur gerichtsmedizinischen Untersuchung von Tötungsdelikten durch elektrischen Strom. Arch Kriminol 142:143–152

Pircher R, Pollak S, Vogt S, Epting T, Kramer L, Geisenberger D (2016) A special type of scald caused by prolonged exposure to slowly heated water. Forensic Sci Int 263:158–163

Püschel K, Brinkmann B (1978) Tod durch maligne Hyperthermie. Ätiologie, Pathophysiologie, Epidemiologie und Pathomorphologie. Med Welt 29:522–531

Quan L, Zhu BL, Oritani S, Ishida K, Fujita MQ, Maeda H (2001) Intranuclear ubiquitin immunoreactivity in the pigmented neurons of the substantia nigra in fire fatalities. Int J Legal Med 114:310–315

Reed GB, Cox AJ (1966) The human liver after radiation injury. A form of veno-occlusive disease. Am J Path 48:597

Rees WD (1965) Pregnant woman struck by lightning. Br Med J 1:103–104

Reh H (1960) Spättod nach Einwirkung von Kontaktwärme (55-60°C) auf die Haut in einem Heißluftbad, zugleich ein Beitrag zur pathologischen Anatomie der Verbrennungskrankheit. Dtsch Z Gesamte Gerichtl Med 49:703

Riße M, Weiler G (1984) Heroin addiction as a rare cause of symmetrical necrosis of the globus pallidus. Z Rechtsmed 93:227–235

Riße M, Türker T, Weiler G (1998) Postmortale Differentialdiagnose und forensische Relevanz kutaner Blasenbildungen. Rechtsmedizin 8: 141–146

Rohde MC, Corydon TJ, Hansen J, Pedersen CB, Schmidt SP, Gregersen N, Banner J (2013) Heat stress and sudden infant death syndrome – stress gene expression after exposure to moderate heat stress. Forensic Sci Int 232:16–24

Saukko P, Knight B (2004) Knight's forensic pathology, 3rd edn. Edward Arnold, London, pp 319–331

Schollmeyer W (1961) Zur histologischen Differentialdiagnose der Hautblasen nach Hitzeeinwirkung und nach Barbituratvergiftung. Dtsch Z Gesamte Gerichtl Med 51:180

Schollmeyer W (1962) Zur Frage der Fettembolie des Lungengewebes bei postmortal Verbrannten. Acta Med Leg Soc 15:77

Schwerd W, Höchel K (1966) Vortäuschung von Strommarken. Arch Kriminol 138:1–7

Shoji T (1997) Demonstration of heat shock protein, ubiquitin, in fire death autopsy cases by immunohistochemical study (in Japanese). Nippon Hoigaku Zasshi 51:70–76

Sochor FM, Mallory KG (1963) Lung lesions in patients dying of burns. Arch Pathol 75:303

Steiner D, Brinkmann B (1974) Mitursächlichkeit eines Thorotrastschadens bei Tod durch stumpfe Gewalt. Z Rechtsmed 75:213

Stolt FD (2005) Stromtodesfälle. Kriminalistik 5:297–299

Stütz N, Weiss D, Reichert B (2006) Verletzungen durch Blitzschlag. Unfallchirurg 109:495–498

Takamiya M, Saigusa K, Nakayashiki N, Aoki Y (2001) A histological study on the mechanism of epidermal nuclear elongation in electrical and burn injuries. Int J Legal Med 115:152–157

Thurner J (1970) Iatrogene Pathologie. Urban & Schwarzenberg, München Berlin Wien

Tsay HJ, Li HY, Lin CH, Yang YL, Yeh JY, Lin MT (1999) Heatstroke induces c-fos expression in the rat hypothalamus. Neurosci Lett 262:41–44

Uemura K, Harada K, Sadamitsu D, Tsuruta R, Takahashi M, Aki T, Yasuhara M, Maekawa T, Yoshida K (2001) Apoptotic and necrotic brain lesions in a fatal case of carbon monoxide poisoning. Forensic Sci Int 116:213–219

Üzün I, Akyildiz E, Akif Inanici M (2008) Histopathological differentiation of skin lesions caused by electrocution, flame burns and abrasion. Forensic Sci Int 178:157–161

Vianello F (1997) A man in the thunderstorm: coronary injuries and electric shock. Cardiology 8:486

Villiers AJ, Gross P (1967) Radiation pneumonitis X-ray induced lesions in hamsters and rats. Arch Environ Health 15:650

Wankhede GA, Sariya DR (2006) An electrocution by metal kite line. Forensic Sci Int 163:141–143

Weiler G, Riße M (1985) Tötung durch elektrischen Strom in der Badewanne. Beweisführung durch eine geformte lokale sowie eine lineare Strommarke. Arch Kriminol 176:82–88

Weis A, Bohnert M (2008) Expression patterns of adhesion molecules P-selectin, von Willebrand factor and PECAM-1 in lungs. A comparative study in cases of burn shock and hemorrhagic shock. Forensic Sci Int 175:102–106

Werthemann A (1930) Experimentelle Röntgenschädigung des Herzmuskels. Strahlentherapie 38:702

Westman J, Sharma HS (1998) Heat shock protein response in the central nervous system following hyperthermia. Prog Brain Res 115:207–239

Wilske J (1984) Der plötzliche Säuglingstod (SIDS). Springer, Berlin

Wong HR, Ryan M, Mendez IY, Denenberg A, Wispe JR (1997) Heat shock protein induction protects human respiratory epithelium against nitric-oxide-mediated cytotoxicity. Shock 8:213–218

Wright RK, Davis JH (1980) The investigation of electrical deaths: a report of 20 fatalities. J Forensic Sci 25:514–521

Xenopoulos N, Movahed A, Hudson P, Reeves WC (1991) Myocardial injury in electrocution. Am Heart J 122:1481–1484

Yoshida C, Ishikawa T, Michiue T, Quan L, Maeda H (2011) Postmortem biochemistry and immunohistochemistry of chromogranin a as a stress marker with special regard to fatal hypothermia and hyperthermia. Int J Legal Med 125:11–20

Yost JW, Holmes FF (1974) Myoglobinuria following lightning stroke. JAMA 228:1147–1148

Zack F, Hammer U, Klett I, Wegener R (1997) Myocardial injury due to lightning. Int J Legal Med 110:326–328

Zack F, Raphael T, Kupfer J, Jokuszies A, Vogt PM, Büttner A, Püschel K, Schalke B, Todt M, Dettmeyer R (2013) Four fatalities due to lightning on a golf course. Rechtsmedizin 23:114–118

Zhang P, Cai S (1995) Study on electrocution death by low voltage. Forensic Sci Int 76:115–119

Zhu BL, Oritami S, Nagai K, Imura M, Fukita K, Maeda H (1997) Immunohistochemical investigation of pulmonary surfactant in fatalities due to fire. Legal Med 1997:405–407

Zhu BL, Ishida K, Oritani S, Quan L, Taniguchi M, Li DR, Fujita MO, Maeda H (2001a) Immunohistochemical investigation of pulmonary surfactant-associated protein a in fire victims. Legal Med 3:23–28

Zhu BL, Ishida K, Quan L, Taniguchi M, Oritani Y, Kamikodai Y, Fujita MQ, Maeda H (2001b) Postmortem urinary myoglobin levels with reference to the causes of death. Forensic Sci Int 115:183–188

Zinck KH (1940) Pathologische Anatomie der Verbrennung. Veröffentlichungen aus der Konstitutions- und Wehrpathologie. Fischer, Jena, zit nach: Janssen 1977

Zollinger HU (1960) Radio-histologie und radio-histopathologie. In: Handb d Allgem Path 10, Teil 1:127. Springer, Berlin

Hypothermia

8

Pathophysiological investigations of hypothermia-induced changes in the human body were first described toward the end of the nineteenth century, initially with Wischnewski spots in the gastric mucosa (Ehrlich 2004; Wischnewski 1895). Later findings described changes in the gastrointestinal tract (Tidow 1943; Büchner 1943). In the 1940s, hypothermia-induced changes were investigated in tumor patients (Sano and Smith 1940), and atrocious medical experiments relating to hypothermia were carried out on concentration camp inmates (Eckart and Vondra 2004; Berger 1990). Observational studies based on accidental hypothermia have been published over the course of several decades (Pavlic et al. 2004; Oehmichen 2004; Danzl and Pozos 1994; Bourne et al. 1986; Coe 1984; Coniam 1979; Mant and Path 1969, Mant 1967, 1964; Brendel et al. 1968; Read et al. 1961; Duguid et al. 1961; Emslie-Smith 1958; Müller et al. 1943), some following experimental hypothermia (Fisher et al. 1957).

The macroscopic morphological findings in the case of local frostbite and general hypothermia ("systemic hypothermia"—cooling of the human body below 35 °C or 95 °F) are known as local blistering and widespread necrosis, while generalized hypothermia leads to cold erythema (Fig. 8.1) (perniones) in the form of acute congestive hyperemia in the subcutaneous soft tissue and to characteristic erosions of the gastric mucosa with Wischnewski spots (Wischnewski 1895). These spots may also occur in the ectopic gastric mucosa (Preuß et al. 2007a). Although the diagnostic relevance of Wischnewski spots as evidence of death due to hypothermia was confirmed in later studies, it has nevertheless been the subject of some critical discussion (Bright et al. 2013; Türk et al. 2005; Sperhake et al. 2004; Mizukami et al. 1999; Wolf et al. 1999; Takada et al. 1991; Birchmeyer and Mitchell 1989; Hirvonen 1976, 1977; Hirvonen and Elfving 1974; Cali et al. 1965). Histopathological findings in the event of death due to hypothermia correspond with macroscopically visible damage, such as cold erythema and Wischnewski spots. Microscopically, cold erythemas show pronounced vascular hyperemia in subepidermal soft tissue. Probably, cooling of the body in the setting of cold ambient temperatures leads to circumscribed hemorrhages of the gastric glands in the agonal period. Subsequently, due to autolysis, erythrocytes are destroyed, and hemoglobin is released. Following exposure to gastric acid, hemoglobin is hematinized, leading to the typical blackish–brownish appearance of Wischnewski spots seen at gross examination (Tsokos et al. 2006).

Wischnewski spots (Fig. 8.2), blackish erosions of the gastric mucosa, can be clearly recognized histologically due to their characteristic coloring; immunohistochemically, a high incidence of hemoglobin can be detected at these sites, likewise in cold erythemas (Türk et al. 2006).

The cause of further findings in hypothermic death can be found in microcirculation disorders,

R. B. Dettmeyer, *Forensic Histopathology*, https://doi.org/10.1007/978-3-319-77997-3_8

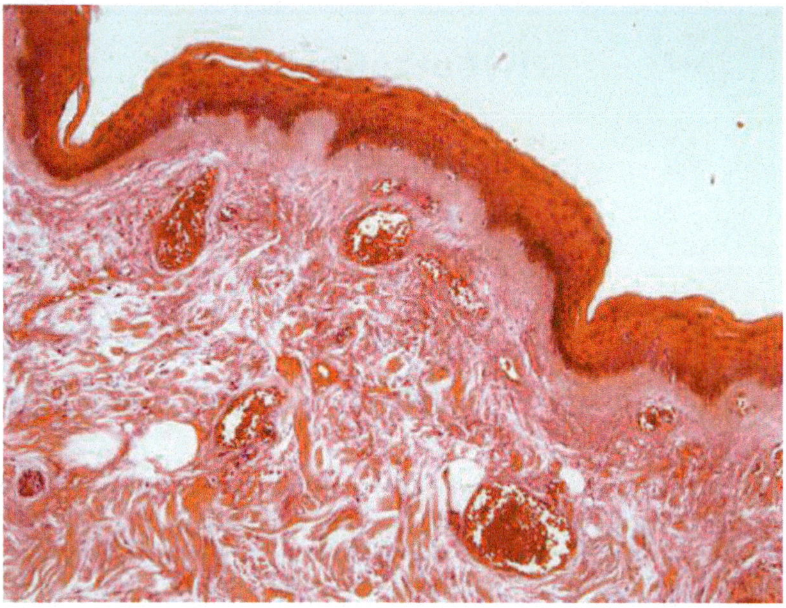

Fig. 8.1 Cold erythema with pronounced vascular hyperemia in subepidermal soft tissue (H&E ×200)

partly at the base of hypothermia-related (micro-) thrombi (Fig. 8.3).

Intestinal segment infarctions caused by microthrombi were found to be the result of circulation disorders (Stoddard 1962), as well as thrombosis of the portal vein in the case of hypothermia (Wolf et al. 1999). In addition, there are reports that fatty degeneration of the renal tubular epithelial cells (Fig. 8.4) occurs more often in hypothermic deaths (Preuß et al. 2004; Thrun 1992).

Simultaneous alcohol consumption significantly promotes fatty degeneration of the renal tubules (Bockholdt et al. 2004). In addition to renal tubular epithelial cells, hypothermia can also result in varying degrees of fatty degeneration of the cardiomyocyte cytoplasm (Fig. 8.5). Intracytoplasmic lipid vacuoles, which can be detected using lipid staining, must be differentiated histologically from lipofuscin deposits, which are primarily found near both nuclear poles of cardiomyocyte nuclei (Preuß et al. 2006).

There are also indications of cell vacuolization in the anterior pituitary gland due to hypothermia (Yoshida et al. 2011; Ishikawa et al. 2008, 2004), as well as damage to the pancreas (Preuß et al. 2007b; Hirvonen 1977).

Immunohistochemical investigations may reveal pronounced HSP70 expression in kidneys in hypothermic death (Preuß et al. 2008); others report expression of ubiquitin (Shimizu et al. 1997). Few immunohistochemical studies of hypothermic deaths have addressed the detection of adrenocorticotropic hormone, while other studies investigated the hippocampus in the central nervous system (Kitamura et al. 2005). Further immunohistochemical investigations on the expression of, e.g., MMP-2, MMP-9, ICAM-1, Claudin-5, AQP-1, and AQP-5 reveal trends in the diagnostic context (Wang et al. 2013). Additionally, decrease in body temperature activates the function of most of the endocrine glands which histologically may present intracytoplasmic vacuoles, e.g., in the pancreas, and signs of an increased activation of the glandula thyroidea.

Pancreas Pancreatic changes in hypothermia are described (Preuß et al. 2007b). Sano and Smith (1940) described focal or diffuse pancreatitis in the case of therapeutic hypothermia; microhemorrhage (Fig. 8.6) and fatty tissue necrosis may also occur (Hirvonen 1976; Mant and Path 1969; Duguid et al. 1961). Occasionally, fine vacuolization is apparent intracytoplasmically (Fig. 8.7); however, its differentiation from

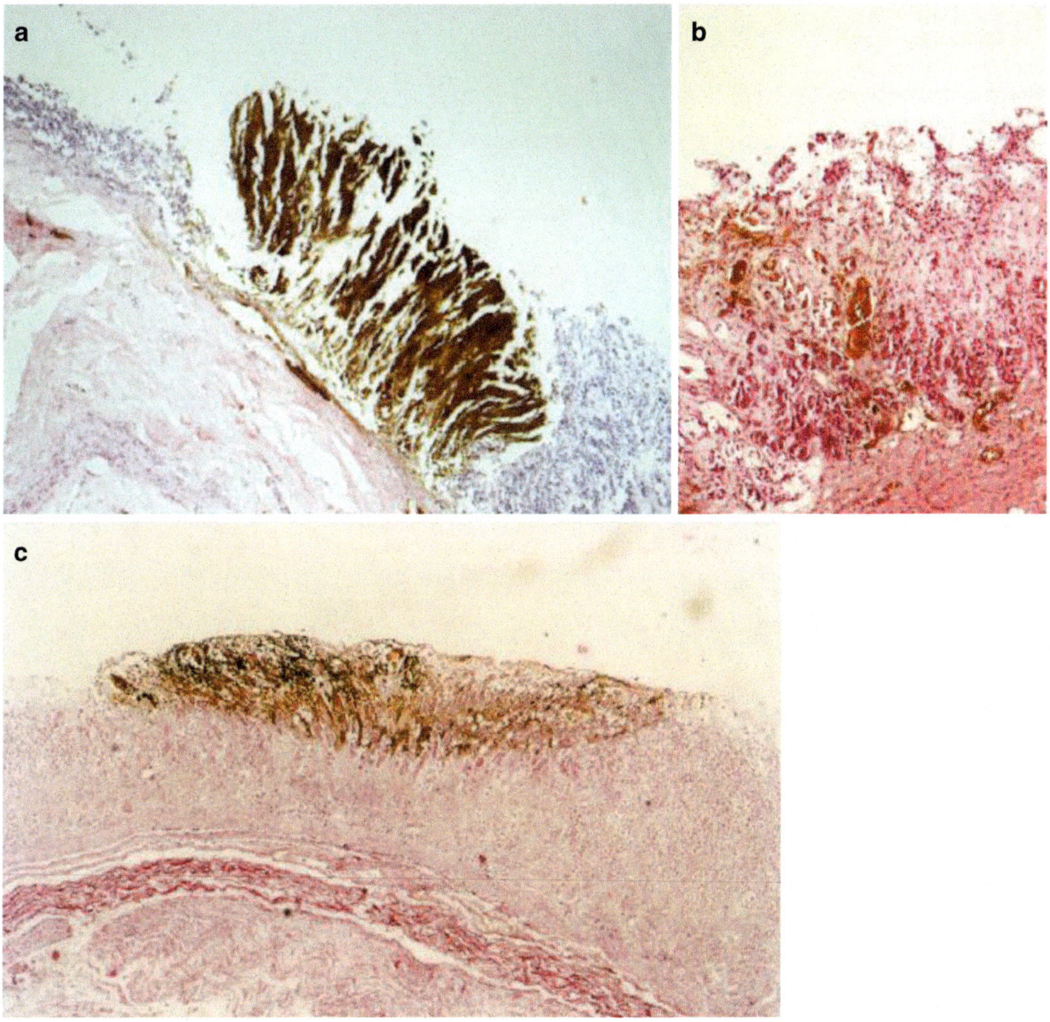

Fig. 8.2 Different forms of Wischnewski spots: (**a**) almost v-shaped Wischnewski spot with characteristic coloring of the erosion in the gastric mucosa (×40) (**b**) incomplete Wischnewski spot (×100) (**c**) superficial Wischnewski spot (×100)

changes due to alcohol is the subject of discussion (Preuß et al. 2007b).

Kidneys The phenomenon seen in diabetic ketoacidosis of subnuclear, vacuolar deposit of glycogen and lipids in the clinical picture of Armanni–Ebstein cells (see Chap. 16) evidently also occurs in hypothermia (Zhou and Byard 2011). Best's carmine or PAS stain should be performed to make a differential diagnostic distinction from glycogen-containing vacuoles. As a basic principle, one should consider the possibility of decompensated diabetes as the possible cause of both ketoacidosis and hypothermia. Complementary biochemical tests may be helpful in the postmortem diagnosis of hypothermia (Bańka et al. 2014; Palmiere et al. 2013; Bańka et al. 2013). Of course, one also frequently sees intoxications that are able to explain an individual's hypothermic state (Armbrust et al. 2010). Other causes of ketoacidosis may also be associated with the Armanni–Ebstein lesion, e.g., alcoholic ketoacidosis (Parai et al. 2012; see Chap. 6). The phenomenon referred to as "black

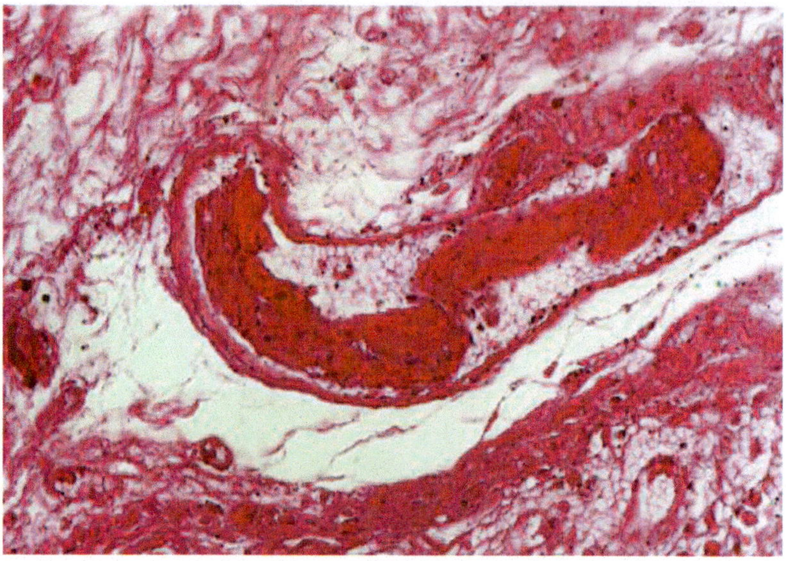

Fig. 8.3 Peripheral vascular branches can be partially or completely closed by developed microthrombi with infarction in the downstream supply area; microthrombi in mesenteric blood vessels are shown here (H&E ×200)

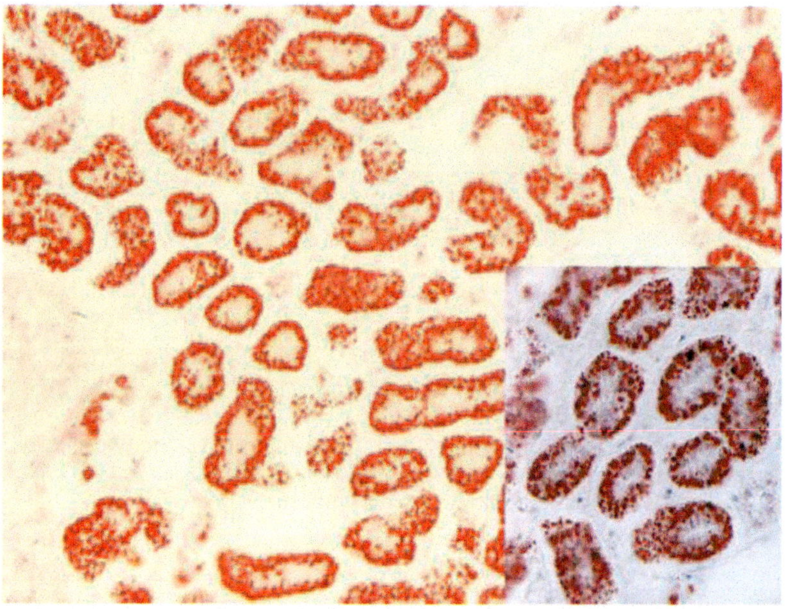

Fig. 8.4 Marked fatty degeneration of the renal tubular epithelial cell cytoplasm in hypothermic death (Sudan III ×100; ×200)

esophagus" is also described in both chronic alcohol abuse and lethal hypothermia (Živković and Nikolić 2013).

Thyroid Marked colloid depletion in the follicular lumen of the thyroid gland has been observed histologically in isolated cases; systematic studies with large numbers of cases are not available as yet (Fig. 8.8).

Individual studies using animal models (adult rats) describe histopathological findings in the myocardium, brain tissue, adrenal glands, as well as in the anterior pituitary following induced fatal hyperthermia. The findings are dominated by structural loss in the preexisting organoid tissue, vacuolation, and hemorrhage (Elshama et al. 2016).

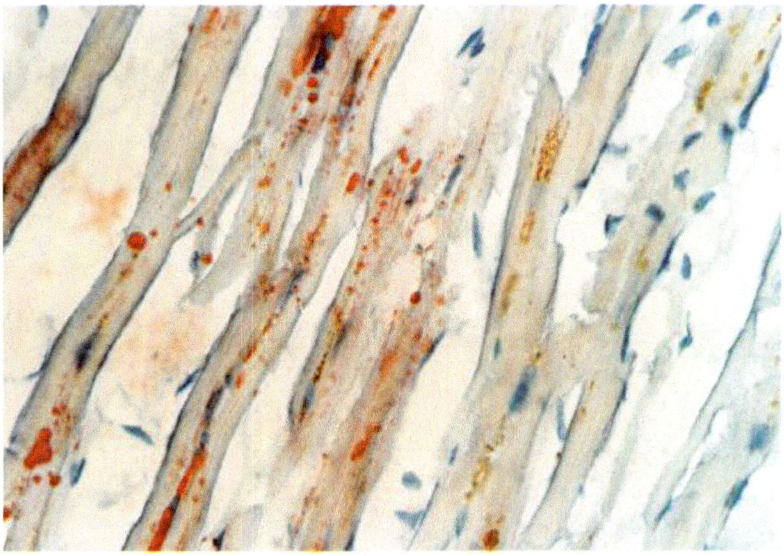

Fig. 8.5 Microvacuolar intracytoplasmic fatty degeneration in cardiomyocytes in hypothermic death (Sudan III ×200)

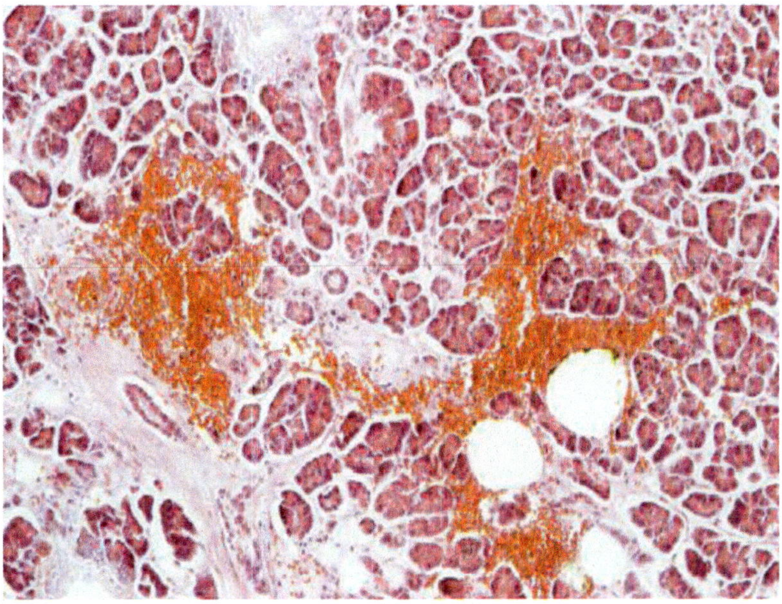

Fig. 8.6 Microhemorrhages in the pancreatic tissue (H&E ×100)

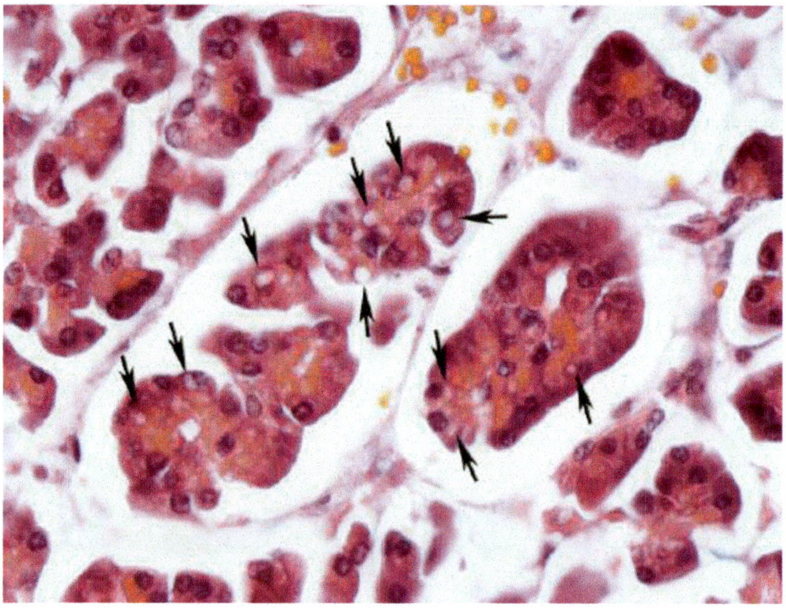

Fig. 8.7 Death due to hypothermia with optically empty vacuoles adjacent to the cell core (*arrows*) in adenoid cells of the pancreas (H&E ×400)

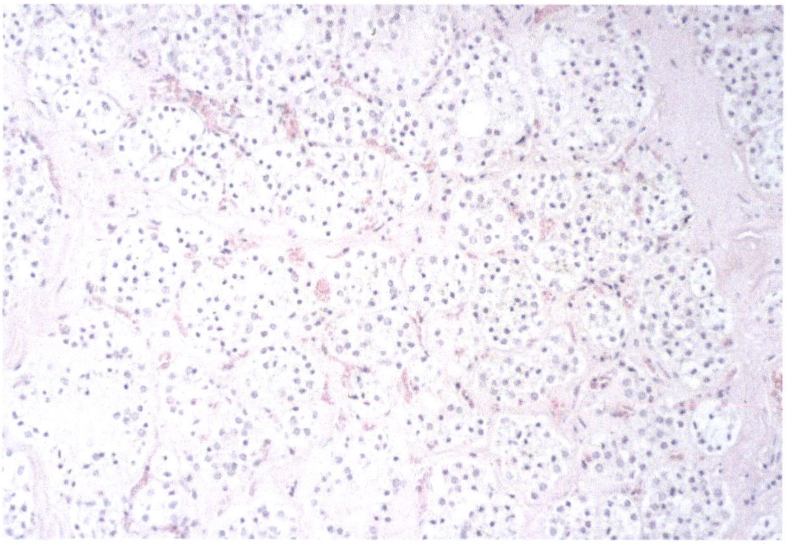

Fig. 8.8 Colloid-depleted thyroid follicle in death due to hypothermia (H&E ×100)

References

Armbrust S, Nikischin W, Rochholz G, Franzelius C, Bielstein A, Kramer HH (2010) Hypothermia in a combined intoxication with doxepin and moclobemide in an adolescent. Forensic Sci Int 195:e1–e3

Bańka K, Teresiński G, Buszewicz G (2014) Free fatty acids as markers of death from hypothermia. Forensic Sci Int 234:79–85

Bańka K, Teresiński G, Buszewicz G, Mądro R (2013) Glucocorticosteroids as markers of death from hypothermia. Forensic Sci Int 229:60–65

Berger RL (1990) Nazi science – the Dachau hypothermia experiments. N Engl J Med 322:1435–1440

Birchmeyer MS, Mitchell EK (1989) Wischnewski revisited: the diagnostic value of gastric mucosa ulcers in hypothermic deaths. Am J Forensic Med Pathol 10:28–30

Bockholdt B, Maxeiner H, Müllter S (2004) Death due to hypothermia in the city of berlin: circumstances, post mortem findings, specific features. In: Oehmichen M (ed) Hypothermia. Clinical, pathomorphological and forensic features. Research in legal medicine, vol 31. Schmidt-Römhild, Lübeck, pp 85–103

Bourne MH, Piepkorn MW, Clayton F, Leonard LG (1986) Analysis of microvascular changes in frostbite injury. J Surg Res 40:26–35

Brendel W, Müller C, Messmer K, Reulen HJ (1968) Der klinische Tod in Hypothermie. Z Gesamte Exp Med 146:189–205

Bright F, Winskog C, Byard RW (2013) Wischnewski spots and hypothermia: sensitive, specific, or serendipitous? Forensic Sci Med Pathol 9:88–90

Büchner F (1943) Die Pathologie der Unterkühlung. Klin Wochenschr 22:89–92

Cali JR, Glaubitz JP, Crampton RS (1965) Gastric necrosis due to prolonged local gastric hypothermia. JAMA 191:154–155

Coe JL (1984) Hypothermia: autopsy findings and vitreous glucose. J Forensic Sci 29:289–395

Coniam WS (1979) Accidental hypothermia. Anaesthesia 34:250–256

Danzl DF, Pozos RS (1994) Accidental hypothermia. N Engl J Med 331:1756–1760

Duguid H, Simpson G, Stowers J (1961) Accidental hypothermia. Lancet 2:1213–1219

Eckart WU, Vondra H (2004) Disregard for human life: hypothermia experiments in the Dachau concentration camp. In: Oehmichen M (ed) Hypothermia. Clinical, pathomorphological and forensic features. Research in legal medicine, vol 31. Schmidt-Römhild, Lübeck, pp 19–31

Ehrlich E (2004) Wischnewski's spots. A new sign of death from hypothermia. The translated text of the original Russian article from 1885. In: Oehmichen M (ed) Hypothermia. Clinical, pathomorphological and forensic features, research in legal medicine, vol 31. Schmidt-Römhild, Lübeck, pp 205–210

Elshama SS, Osman HEH, El-Kenawy AEM (2016) Postmortem diagnosis of induced fatal hypothermia in adult albino rats. Rom J Leg Med 24:106–114

Emslie-Smith D (1958) Accidental hypothermia. Lancet 2:492–495

Fisher ER, Fedor EJ, Fisher B (1957) Pathologic and histochemical observations in experimental hypothermia. AMA Arch Surg 75:817–827

Hirvonen J (1976) Necropsy findings in fatal hypothermia cases. Forensic Sci 8:155–164

Hirvonen J (1977) Systemic and local effects of hypothermia. In: Tedeschi CG, Eckert WG, Tedeschi LG (eds) Forensic medicine, vol 1. Saunders Company, Philadelphia, pp 758–774

Hirvonen J, Elfving R (1974) Histamine and serotonin in the gastric erosions of rats dead from exposure to cold: a histochemical and quantitative study. Z Rechtsmed 74:273–281

Ishikawa T, Miyaishi S, Tachibana T, Ishizu H, Zhu BL, Maeda H (2004) Fatal hypothermia related vacuolation of hormone-producing cells in the anterior pituitary. Legal Med 6:157–163

Ishikawa T, Quan L, Li DR, Zhao D, Michiue T, Hamel M, Maeda H (2008) Postmortem biochemistry and immunohistochemistry of adrenocorticotropic hormone with special regard to fatal hypothermia. Forensic Sci Int 179:147–151

Kitamura O, Gotohda T, Ishigami A, Tokunaga I, Kubo S, Nakasono I (2005) Effect of hypothermia on postmortem alterations in MAP 2 immunostaining in the human hippocampus. Legal Med 7:24–30

Mant AK (1964) Some post-mortem observations in accidental hypothermia. Med Sci Law 4(1):44–46

Mant AK (1967) The pathology of hypothermia. In: Simpson K (ed) Modern trends in forensic medicine, vol 2. Butterworths, London, pp 224–232

Mant AK, Path FC (1969) Autopsy diagnosis of accidental hypothermia. J Forensic Med 16:126–129

Mizukami H, Shimizu K, Shiono H, Uezono T, Sasaki M (1999) Forensic diagnosis of death from cold. Legal Med 1:204–209

Müller E, Rotter W, Carow G, Kloos KF (1943) Über Untersuchungsergebnisse bei Todesfällen nach allgemeiner Unterkühlung des Menschen in Seenot. Beitr Pathol Anat 108:552–589

Oehmichen M (2004) Hypothermia. Clinical, pathomorphological and forensic features. Research in legal medicine, vol 31. Schmidt-Römhild, Lübeck

Palmiere C, Bardy D, Letovanec I, Mangin P, Augsburger M, Ventura F, Iglesias K, Werner D (2013) Biochemical markers of fatal hypothermia. Forensic Sci Int 226:54–61

Parai JL, Kodikara S, Milroy C, Pollanen MS (2012) Alcoholism and the Armanni-Ebstein lesion. Forensic Sci Med Pathol 8:19–22

Pavlic M, Grubwieser P, Rabl W (2004) Death in snow avalanches: hypoxia – blunt trauma – hypothermia. In: Oehmichen M (ed) Hypothermia. Clinical, pathomorphological and forensic features. Research in legal medicine, vol 31. Schmidt-Römhild, Lübeck, pp 141–152

Preuß J, Dettmeyer R, Lignitz E, Madea B (2004) Fatty degeneration in renal tubule epithelium in accidental hypothermia victims. Forensic Sci Int 141:131–135

Preuß J, Dettmeyer R, Lignitz E, Madea B (2006) Fatty degeneration of myocardial cells as a sign of death due to hypothermia versus degenerative deposition of lipofuscin. Forensic Sci Int 159:1–5

Preuß J, Thierauf A, Dettmeyer R, Madea B (2007a) Wischnewski's spot in an ectopic stomach. Forensic Sci Int 169:220–222

Preuß J, Lignitz E, Dettmeyer R, Madea B (2007b) Pancreatic changes in cases of death due to hypothermia. Forensic Sci Int 166:194–198

Preuß J, Dettmeyer R, Poster S, Lignitz E, Madea B (2008) The expression of heat shock protein 70 in kidneys in cases of death due to hypothermia. Forensic Sci Int 176:248–252

Read AE, Emslie-Smith D, Gough KR, Holmes R (1961) Pancreatitis and accidental hypothermia. Lancet 2:1219–1221

Sano ME, Smith CW (1940) Fifty post-mortem patients with cancer subjected to local or generalized refrigeration. J Lab Clin Med 26:443

Shimizu K, Ohtani S, Shiono H, Fukusima T, Sasaki M (1997) Expression of ubiquitin protein in each organ at death from hypothermia. Forensic Sci Int 86:61–68
Sperhake JP, Rothschild MA, Riße M, Tsokos M (2004) Histomorphology of Wischnewski's spots: a contribution to the forensic histopathology of fatal hypothermia. In: Oehmichen M (ed) Hypothermia. Clinical, pathomorphological and forensic features. Research in legal medicine, vol 31. Schmidt-Römhild, Lübeck, pp 211–220
Stoddard JC (1962) Mesenteric infarction during hypothermia. Br J Anaesth 34:825–830
Takada M, Kusano I, Yamamoto H, Shiraishi T, Yatani R, Haba K (1991) Wischnewski's gastric lesions in accidental hypothermia. Am J Forensic Med Pathol 12:300–305
Thrun C (1992) Verfettung der Tubulusepithelien der Niere – ein Hinweis für Hypothermie? Rechtsmedizin 2:55–58
Tidow R (1943) Kälteschäden des Magendarmkanals unter besonderer Berücksichtigung der Abkühlung. Münch Med Wochenschr 90:597–600
Tsokos M, Rothschild MA, Madea B, Rie M, Sperhake JP (2006) Histological and immunohistochemical study of Wischnewski spots in fatal hypothermia. Am J Forensic Med Pathol 27:70–74
Türk EE, Sperhake JP, Pueschel K, Tsokos M (2005) An approach to the evaluation of fatal hypothermia. Forensic Sci Med Pathol 1:31–35
Türk EE, Sperhake JP, Madea B, Preuß J, Tsokos M (2006) Immunohistochemical detection of hemoglobin in frost erythema. Forensic Sci Int 158:131–134
Wischnewski SM (1895) Neues Merkmal des Todes bei Unterkühlung. Informationsblatt der Hygiene, gerichtliche und praktische Medizin 3:11–20
Wang Q, Ishikawa T, Michiue T, Zhu BL, Guan DW, Maeda H (2013) Molecular pathology of pulmonary edema in forensic autopsy cases with special regard to fatal hyperthermia and hypothermia. Forensic Sci Int 228:137–141
Wolf DA, Aronson JF, Rajaraman S, Veasey SP (1999) Wischnewski ulcers and acute pancreatitis in two hospitalized patients with cirrhosis, portal vein thrombosis, and hypothermia. J Forensic Sci 44:1082–1085
Yoshida C, Ishikawa T, Michiue T, Quan L, Madea H (2011) Postmortem biochemistry and immunohistochemistry of chromogranin a as a stress marker with special regard to fatal hypothermia and hyperthermia. Int J Legal Med 125:11–20
Zhou C, Byard RW (2011) Armanni-Ebstein phenomenon and hypothermia. Forensic Sci Int 206:e82–e84
Živković V, Nikolić S (2013) The unusual appearance of black esophagus in a case of fatal hypothermia: a possible underlying mechanism. Forensic Sci Med Pathol 9:613–514

9 Thrombosis and Embolism

Thrombosis and embolism are frequent autopsy findings in forensic practice (Kaufmann and Keresztes 1967; Knight 1966), often as a post-traumatic diagnosis (Foedisch and Kloos 1966; Greendyke 1964). Fatal pulmonary embolism is extremely rare in infants and children (de la Grandmaison and Durigon 2002). Evidence of an embolism is considered a sign of life, i.e., an event which occurs while the subject is still alive, since continuous blood circulation is the prerequisite for embolism. Exceptions include embolic processes under reanimation conditions, which need to be taken into consideration during the interpretation of findings (Schneider and Klug 1971). In the case of thromboembolism, the original cause requires clarification; in individual cases, the age of a thromboembolism may be of interest. Various iatrogenic embolisms may occur (Sowell et al. 2007; Röding and Röse 1967). Fatal pulmonary embolism leads to an intolerable increase in pressure in the lesser circulation and consequently to acute right heart failure. Even in cases of non-fatal pulmonary embolism, signs of ischemic injury are detectable in the right and left ventricular myocardium. Fatal venous thrombosis without embolism may be seen in the form of coronary thrombosis, as well as thrombosis of large mesenteric veins, e.g., the superior mesenteric vein accompanied by hemorrhagic infarction of the associated intestinal segment and gastrointestinal bleeding (Watanabe et al. 2016). Air embolism due to severe electrical injury is unusual (Kitulwatte and Pollanen 2009).

9.1 Thrombosis

The causes of thrombosis (thrombogenesis) are described using Virchow's triad:

- Alterations in the vascular wall
- Reduction in bloodstream velocity
- Increased likelihood of blood coagulation

For this reason, in the case of thromboembolism of the lung artery detected at autopsy, it is important to investigate whether previous—caused by a third party and/or legally relevant—trauma may have led to damage of the vascular wall at the level of the detected thrombosis, whether immobility caused by previous trauma or an accident has helped increase the likelihood of thrombosis, and whether a preexisting disorder of the coagulation physiology is present or rather can be excluded. For example, it has long been known that the use of oral contraceptives increases the risk of thrombosis (Reutter et al. 1965).

Thromboses should be completely stabilized and repaired together with the affected vascular segment (Orth's solution facilitates the separation of blood components). Including the vascular wall in histological investigations, with adventitia and surrounding soft tissue, may clarify the question of whether primary, genuine vascular wall damage is present (phlebitis, arteritis), or whether trauma has caused the vascular wall damage, and thus also the thrombosis. Among

R. B. Dettmeyer, *Forensic Histopathology*, https://doi.org/10.1007/978-3-319-77997-3_9

other things, attention should be paid to iron deposits—macrophages loaded with hemosiderin pigment—and multinucleated foreign-body giant cells.

A differentiation is made between red thrombi and white thrombi; however, white or mixed thrombi occur more often.

Red thrombi (homogeneous dark red) are created by hypercoagulability or simply by a decrease in bloodstream velocity. They may expand relatively quickly within a larger vein system. In the early stage, they do not present with wall-adhering elements. Histologically, a relatively homogeneous distribution of erythrocytes is noticeable, while layering within the thrombus is not detectable (Fig. 9.1).

In the case of a fresh red thrombus, local trauma causing vascular wall damage is generally absent, while a forensically relevant trauma-based, general immobility may exist. Red thrombi, for example, develop in the intracranial dural venous sinuses when significant hypoxic brain injury is present and may be found there during autopsy, e.g., following determination of brain death, often together with marked autolysis of brain tissue and clear signs of pressure to the brain. For differential diagnostic purposes, histological examination of a wall-adherent portion of the thrombus is of particular significance for the differentiation from a white thrombus.

White thrombi ("white" or "gray" color of the thrombi) are histologically distinctive due to their alternating layers consisting of fibrin and corpuscular blood elements (mainly leukocytes). The fibrin-rich areas appear more homogeneous and result in a slightly undulated surface due to their alternation with denser corpuscular areas (Fig. 9.2).

The white thrombus has a wall-adherent or fixed tail, and in particular here it displays the microscopically detectable layering described above, while the so-called tail end of the thrombus may resemble a red thrombus both macroscopically and microscopically. When thrombus specimens from this area are examined under microscope, a differential diagnosis between red and white thrombus may be impossible.

Thrombi may increase gradually as well as expand retrogradely. The literature occasionally differentiates between different types of growth (Janssen 1977):

- Isolated growth of thrombus: the section between two vein branches is not exceeded.
- Intermittent thrombus growth: various vein segments are involved.
- So-called continuous growth thrombus: multicentric thrombus expansion.

In practice, mainly "mixed" thrombi are present, which are those with a "white-gray" wall-

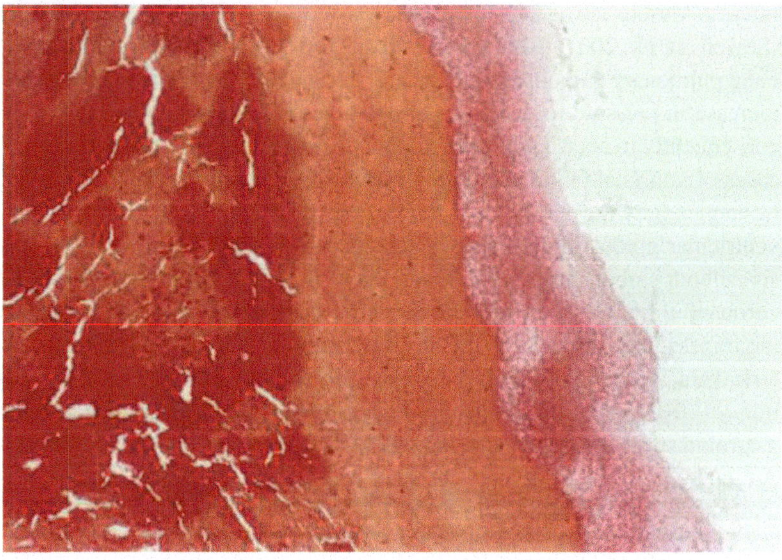

Fig. 9.1 Fresh red thrombosis with homogeneous distribution of erythrocytes and without detectable layering (H&E ×100)

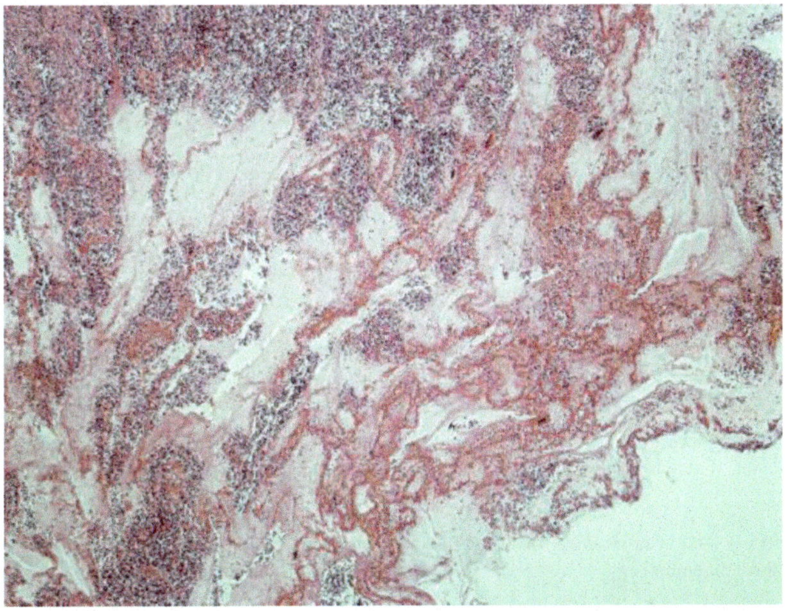

Fig. 9.2 White thrombus with alternating layers consisting of fibrin threads and embedded leukocytes (H&E ×200)

adherent and "red" tail. Histologically, sections of onion peel-like and garland-shaped structures also occur. The portion of the thrombus located against the bloodstream has the appearance of a mixed thrombus, while the portion of the thrombus freely floating in the bloodstream—the tail—has the appearance of a red coagulation thrombus.

The most frequently found at autopsy are deep vein and pelvic vein thromboses. Differentially diagnosing a thrombus and a postmortem blood clot (cruor) at autopsy is sometimes challenging (Table 9.1). Although the macroscopic examination is the determining factor, histological and immunohistochemical examination may be helpful in specific cases (Uekita et al. 2008).

Deep vein and pelvic vein thrombosis have particular practical and forensic relevance, as well as thrombosis of the coronary artery, brain stem arteries, carotid arteries, traumatic aneurysm, and rarely the portal vein. Arterial thrombosis regularly develops over preexisting arteriosclerosis. Only microscopically detectable thrombi (microthrombi) are found in the case of shock of varying causes but also in the case of, e.g., death by hypothermia (see Chap. 8). Therefore, in the case of shock (or in the case of Sanarelli–Shwartzman syndrome, e.g.), hyaline thrombi can be differentiated from macroscopically visible thrombosis or thromboembolism. Consumptive coagulopathy, which results from a dysfunction in coagulation physiology occurring during shock, leads to the development of homogeneous thrombi in the capillary flow bed.

The term "parietal thrombosis" is used in different ways: on the one hand, in a broader sense for all wall-adherent thromboses while on the other only for parietal, layered thrombosis in trauma- or nontrauma-based aneurysms.

Thrombosis populated by bacteria is also known as infected thrombosis, which may result in infected (septic) embolism.

The literature provides details on the organism's reaction to thrombosis or thromboembolism. In this context, the chronology of a thrombus' organization and decomposition is examined, enabling an approximate estimation of age (Table 9.2) (Maffeis et al. 2017; Nosaka et al. 2011, 2012, 2013, 2015, 2017; Fineschi et al. 2009a, b, 2012; Ro et al. 2008; Steiner 2007; Leu and Leu 1989). The organization of a thrombus first occurs at the vascular wall with the dissolution of the basal membrane from the vascular intima and migration of fibroblasts and macrophages, among others (Fig. 9.3). Subsequently, branched-off capillary blood ves-

Table 9.1 Differential diagnosis between thrombus and cruor (postmortem blood clot)

	Thrombus	Cruor/"buffy coat"
Macroscopic	"Red" thrombus: dry-damp, smooth surface, somewhat elastic, wall-adherent, and livid in its progression	Fluid-rich, also somewhat elastic, smooth and more reflective surface, never wall-adherent, partially livid, partially gray to gray-yellowish (leukocytes deposited at stasis)
	"White" thrombus: dry, partially brittle, finely striated surface, partially wall-adherent, partially gray-white, partially gray-red portions with a border unrelated to the position of the body	If the body has not been moved, a clear, often horizontal border is present between the red and gray portions
Microscopic	Somewhat organized with more compact, layered thrombocyte aggregates, partially garland-shaped arrangement, fibrin threads and embedded erythrocytes—partially reticulated, wall adherence is a sign of (early) organization	Rather loose fibrin fiber meshwork, leukocytes, depending on the direction of the incision, leukocytes positioned unidirectionally according to the force of gravity, occasional thrombocytes, no signs of organization

In cases where predominantly erythrocytes are found, with few fibrin fibers, few thrombocytes, and no deposited leukocytes, it may be impossible to make a differential diagnosis between thrombus and cruor

Table 9.2 Chronology of the histologically microscopically detectable organization of a thrombus or thromboembolism

Phase	Histological diagnosis
I. Day 2 (days 1–3)	No reaction between vascular endothelium and thrombus. Continuity of basal membrane and endothelium is present. In the center of the thrombus, there are embedded, more densely layered erythrocytes, with somewhat looser erythrocytes peripherally. There are also leukocytes and fibrin threads (partially meshwork-like) and thrombocytes
II. Day 5 (days 3–8)	Endothelium branches originating at the vascular endothelium, early "endothelialization" of the thrombus surface, centrally originating "hyalinization" of the thrombotic material. Incorporated leukocytes become pyknotic, and monocytes appear enlarged and lighter in color. Cracks caused by atrophy begin to appear within the periphery
III. Day 10 (days 4–20)	Inside the thrombus, originating in the macroscopic wall-adherent portion, migrated fibroblasts, fibrocytes, mesenchymal cells, and hemosiderin pigment-laden macrophages (Prussian blue reaction) are found, as well as branched endothelium-wrapped capillaries. Marked swelling of monocytes, occasional leukocyte-type core debris
IV. Week 3–4 (8 days–2 months)	Pronounced capillarization, collagen, and argyrophile fibers (fibroplasia). Also, shadowlike, leukocytic core debris within hyalinized areas, after 8–17 days no more monocytic swelling
V. Month 6 (months 2–8)	Only a few cellular elements, single capillaries, denser argyrophilic, collagen, and also single elastic fibers. In hyalinized areas, unusual acicular cholesterin crystals (in the area of the incision, there are visibly empty, spindle-shaped caverns). In specific cases, capillary blood vessels beginning at the adventitia may be detected. Perfused, sinusoidal cavities (early rechanneled residual thrombus) may appear in the center
VI. Older than 6–12 months	Completed recanalization, elements of an original residual thrombus are no longer detectable, collagenized connective tissue with low cell numbers, residual iron deposits, partially as macrophages, e.g., inside "rope ladderlike" tissue clamps of the pulmonary artery intima

Modified according to Irninger (1963)

sels and increasing deposits of hemosiderin pigment-laden macrophages can be seen (Fig. 9.4), followed by changes to the connective tissue of the thrombus with appearance of neovessels and myofibroblasts (Nosaka et al. 2010b) (Fig. 9.5).

Determining the age of thrombosis or thromboembolism histologically is challenging; specimens from multiple sections must be regularly examined microscopically (recommendation, six specimens, longitudinal incision, and lateral incision; dye, H&E, Elastica van Gieson, and Prussian blue reaction). Even then, the determination of only an approximate age is possible. This uncertainty is increased when the possible minimum and maximum age of the thrombus is to be determined. In this case, and in a departure from Table 9.3, a narrowing down to three stages is more appropriate: 1st to 7th day, 5th day to 8th week, and older than 8 weeks (see also Fineschi et al. 2009b).

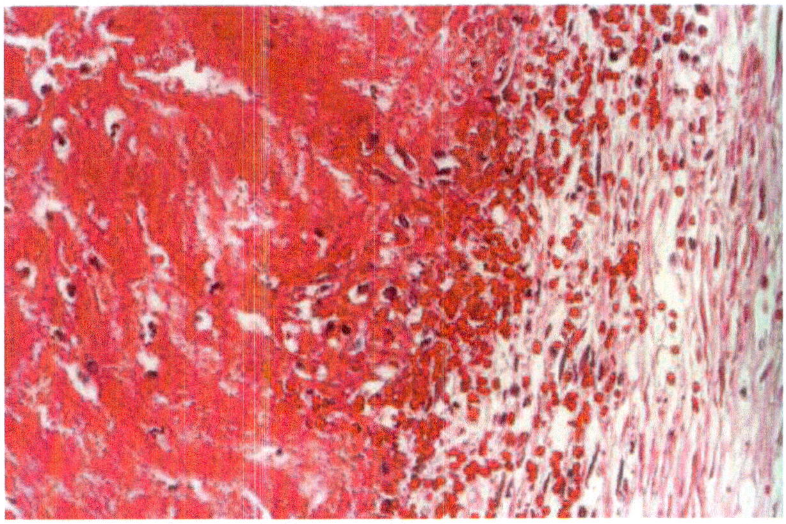

Fig. 9.3 Early thrombus organization with dissolution of the basal membrane of the vascular intima and migrating fibroblasts, as well as macrophages (H&E ×400)

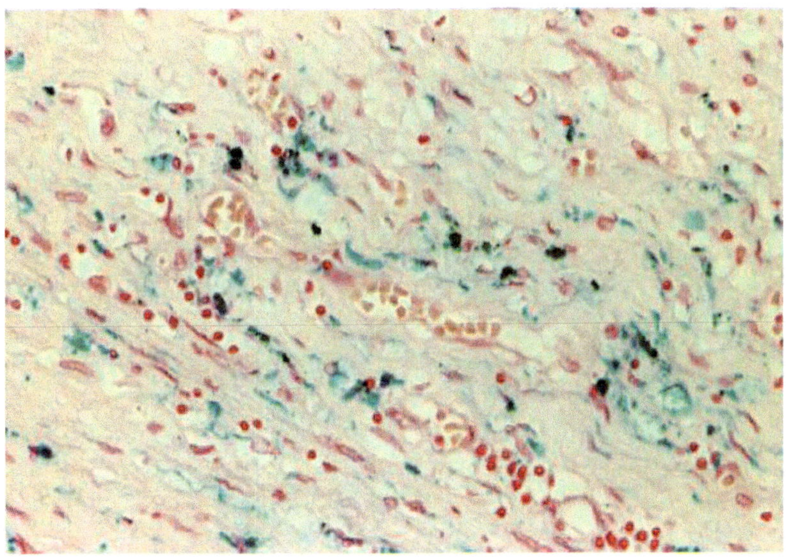

Fig. 9.4 Advanced thrombus organization with branched capillary blood vessels and hemosiderin pigment-laden macrophages (Prussian blue ×400)

Attempts at more precise thrombus age determination are correlated to the intrathrombotic ratio of neutrophilic leukocytes to macrophages; for approximately the first 7 days after thrombus development, a mouse model showed a continual decrease in neutrophilic leukocytes, while macrophages increased in parallel (Nosaka et al. 2009). The mouse model also showed immunohistochemically, and with the help of semiquantitative analyzes, a continuous intrathrombotic increase in the expression of metalloproteinases MMP-2 and MMP-9 until approximately day 14 after thrombosis development (Nosaka et al. 2010a).

It is possible to survive local thrombosis with total or local occlusion of the vessel lumen. Once thrombus organization is complete, the histological picture of an old, organized, and partially recanalized thrombosis may persist (Fig. 9.6). In the case of coronary thrombosis, an old myocardial infarction scar is often found in the downstream supply area in the cardiac muscle.

If the patient history indicates sepsis, or in the case of thrombosing, mostly polypoid endocarditis with secondary bacterial infection, embolic displacement of an infected thrombus is possible. In this case, histology may detect bacterial colonies within the thrombotic material, mostly a col-

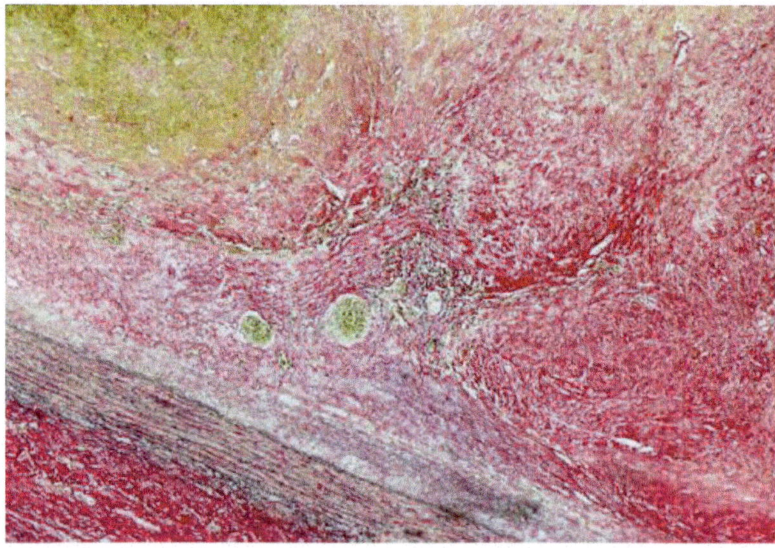

Fig. 9.5 Connective tissue-like organization of a thrombus (H&E ×40)

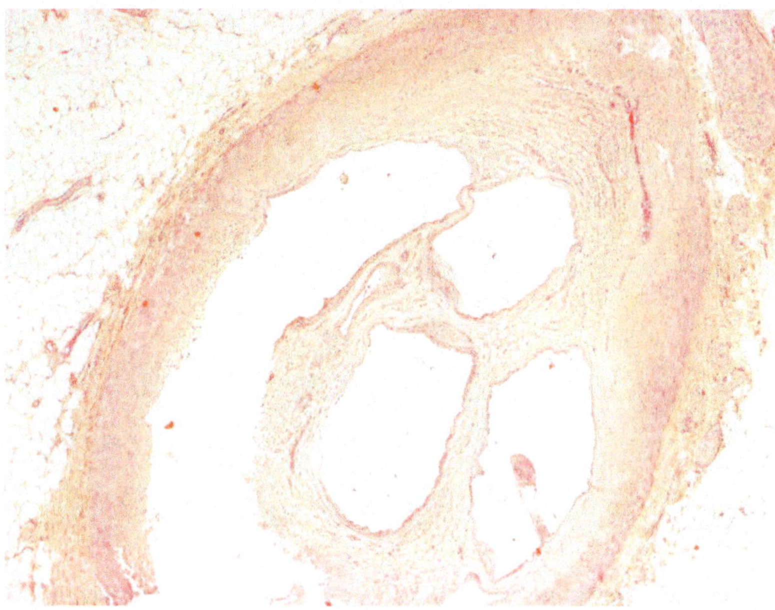

Fig. 9.6 Old, organized, and partially recanalized coronary thrombosis (H&E ×200)

lection of basophilic cocci but possibly also rod-shaped bacteria.

9.2 Embolism

Embolism, i.e., the partial, subtotal, or total blockage of a vessel (obturation) due to an embolus or embolically spread material, is frequent depending on the type. On the one hand, there are preexisting, macroscopically diagnosable embolisms, like most thromboembolisms (see above), while on the other hand, there are embolisms, which in the context of an autopsy and given the patient history and circumstances of death, need to be included in the overall expert opinion (Türk and Tsokos 2003). The spectrum of (forensically relevant) embolisms is given in Table 9.3. Thromboembolism resulting from natural causes, posttraumatic embolism (fat and

Table 9.3 Forensically relevant embolisms

Type of embolism	Possible causes or relevance to an expert opinion (examples)
Acute or recurrent pulmonary arterial thromboembolism	For example, patients confined to bed following trauma (recent or older traffic accident?) Spontaneous thrombosis and thromboembolism? Proper anticoagulation? Infected thrombus?
Fat embolism (in lung arterioles and septal capillaries, in renal glomeruli, intracerebral)	Posttraumatic (Décollement)? Death due to hypothermia? Status post liposuction? Preexisting disease, such as fatty liver?
Amniotic fluid embolism	Death during pregnancy? During birth?
Megakaryocyte embolism	Shock—final shock situation due to various causes
Foreign-body embolism following intravenous drug abuse	"Junkie pneumopathy" (see Chap. 4)
Gas embolism: air embolism, nitrogen embolism	Particularly following cut throat injuries with opening of larger veins, suicidal venous injection of air, nitrogen embolism in the case of caisson disease (decompression sickness)
Bone marrow embolism	Posttraumatic in the case of fractures of large long bones (e.g., traffic accidents), shock, intraoperative, above all in the case of implantation of a femoral head endoprosthesis
Tissue embolism	Embolic spread of specific organic tissue (parenchyma embolism)
Arterial embolism	Normally thromboembolism, originating from (occasionally infected) parietal thrombi in the left heart (atrium thrombus) of the heart valves, the endocardium, or after traumatic damage to the vascular intima (Atrial fibrillation? Endocarditis? Thrombosed myocardial aneurysm?)
Cholesterol crystal embolism	Rare, arterial-embolic spread of cholesterol crystals from atherosclerotic plaques (Donohue et al. 2003; Wongprasartsuk et al. 2001)
Parasitic embolism	Rare, embolic spread of parasites or parasite components
Bacterial embolism	Bacterial spread in the presence of sepsis, such as focal nephritis in the case of bacterial endocarditis lenta, septic or infected (thrombo-) embolus
Tumor embolism	Rare, embolic spread of tumor cells (Janík and Hejna 2015)
Other foreign-body emboli	For example, embolically spread projectile after a gunshot wound
Traumatic embolism	Embolism caused directly by trauma, e.g., cerebral embolism following trauma to the carotid artery, dissection, and thrombosis of the carotid or vertebral artery following chiropractic therapy
Lime cement embolism	In the case of, e.g., total endoprosthesis (Palacos® embolism)
Silicone embolism syndrome	Rare: in cosmetic surgery, following silicone implant placement, or sub- and intracutaneous injection of liquid silicone
Metallic/mercury embolism	Extremely rare: postmortem computer tomography may be helpful; 1 to 2 mm particles surrounded by fibrosis in the case of long survival times have been described (Makino et al. 2015)
Embolism of cyanoacrylate	Extremely rare: fatal pulmonary embolism of cyanoacrylate glue following endoscopic gastric variceal injection (Burke et al. 2017)
Other iatrogenic embolisms	For example, TUR syndrome with intraoperative embolic spread of rinsing fluid via the open veins of the prostatic venous plexus (see Chap. 1); embolism following puncture; thromboembolism due to venous or arterial vascular catheters; air embolism upon removal of a central venous catheter (Wild et al. 2013); during transbronchial biopsy (Strange et al. 1987); and during coronary angiography (Türk et al. 2007).

Paradox embolism = Place of origin of the embolus in a vein of the systemic circulation, spread by means of foramen ovale or arteriovenous anastomosis into the arterial circulation (Holczabek 1968; Huber 1965; Young et al. 1948)

bone marrow embolism; Büchner 1964) and shock-induced megakaryocyte embolism are predominant in the field of forensic autopsy. Less common are air embolism (Bowen and Sycamore 1976), amniotic fluid embolism (Kössling 1963; Duda and Papilian 1962; Haynes 1956; Obersteg 1949), tumor, and other tissue embolism (Gilbert and Borchard 1980;

Stoltenburg-Didinger and Vogel 1980; Wilhelmi and Hildebrand 1972; Bschor 1963), such as liver tissue embolism (Schulz et al. 1992), as well as foreign-body embolism (Brettel and Lutz 1973; Althoff 1967; Konwaler 1950), such as a projectile (Sivanesan 1976). More pronounced embolism leads to hemodynamically relevant right heart strain, which in turn leads to an increase in intramyocardial CD68-positive macrophages in the right ventricular myocardium (Iwadate et al. 2003). The rise in pressure in the lesser circulation may lead to right heart failure in the case of both thromboembolism and fat embolism with myocardial single and group necroses in the right ventricular myocardium. Immunohistochemically, this myocardial necrosis can be detected using antibodies against fibronectin, an early necrosis marker, and $C5b\text{-}9_{(m)}$, a necrosis marker which responds slightly later, whereby detection is more pronounced in the right ventricle than in the left (Fracasso and Varchmin-Schultheiß 2009; Fracasso et al. 2010, 2011, 2015). Iatrogenic fat embolism is rare but does occur (Watanabe et al. 2007; Pragst et al. 2007), e.g., following liposuction (Senen et al. 2009; Costa et al. 2008; Shairkh et al. 2008).

Histological investigations can help clarify numerous questions, such as:

- Localization of the origin of a thrombosis or thromboembolism
- Classification of intensity of a pulmonary fat embolism
- Attributing megakaryocyte and bone marrow embolism to trauma, surgical intervention, or shock event
- Determining survival time after a preceding embolism, as well as age of thrombus and thromboembolism
- Determining the age of other embolisms
- Detection of residuals following a preceding embolism
- Clarification of the traumatic cause of an embolism

Iatrogenic embolisms are not uncommon, e.g., in the form of bone marrow embolism during or shortly after the implantation of a femoral head endoprosthesis or transurethral resection (TUR) syndrome in the setting of prostate surgery (Dettmeyer et al. 1999).

9.2.1 Thromboembolism

Histologically, thromboembolism (most frequently due to deep vein and pelvic vein thrombosis) shows a layered structure with a partially central erythrocyte column surrounded by an alternating dense fibrin fiber net in which red erythrocytes are also embedded. The organization of a thrombosis located close to a vascular wall begins at the endothelium with a histologically documentable chronology (see above). Macroscopically, residuals of a pulmonary thromboembolism appear with delicate, liftable, partially rope ladderlike flaps in the vascular intima of the pulmonary branch arteries. Histologically, these tissue flaps contain deposits of iron pigment detectable in Prussian blue preparation (Fig. 9.7).

Hereditary thrombophilia increases the risk of thrombosis and thromboembolism (Ely and Gill 2005).

9.2.2 Fat and Bone Marrow Embolism

Alongside thromboembolism, fat embolisms are the most frequently observed (Wehner 1968), in particular following trauma, such as traffic accidents (Emson 1958; Säker 1955). In very rare cases, child abuse has resulted in nonfracture-associated fatal fat embolism (Nichols et al. 1990). Fat, bone marrow, and megakaryocyte embolisms (Figs. 9.8, 9.9, and 9.10), as well as other embolisms, are considered to be a vital reaction. Possible causes could include polytrauma; preexisting internal diseases, such as fatty liver (Schulz and Tsokos 2004); and shock of various origins, thus traumatic and nontraumatic causes (Wirth and Staak 1972). Fat embolism was observed in fire-related deaths (Schollmeyer 1965) and in cases of frostbite (Hardmeier 1963). Pulmonary fat embolism can

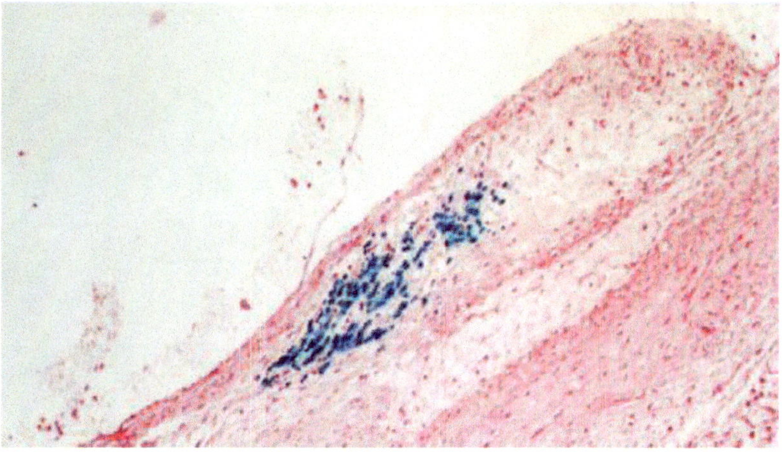

Fig. 9.7 Old organized and resorbed thromboembolism with residual iron deposits (Prussian blue ×40)

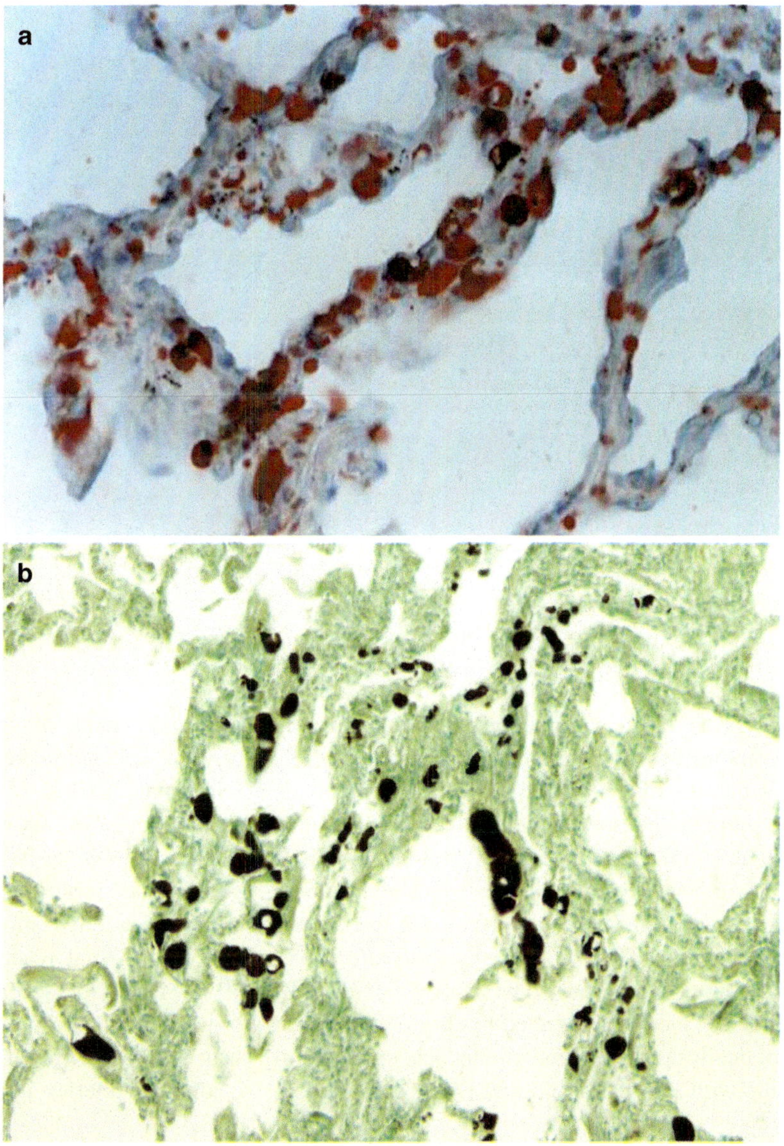

Fig. 9.8 Pulmonary fat embolism with fat droplets in the capillaries of the alveolar septa—a polytrauma patient after a traffic accident with a survival time of approximately 9 h (**a**) Sudan III ×400 and (**b**) Osmium ×200)

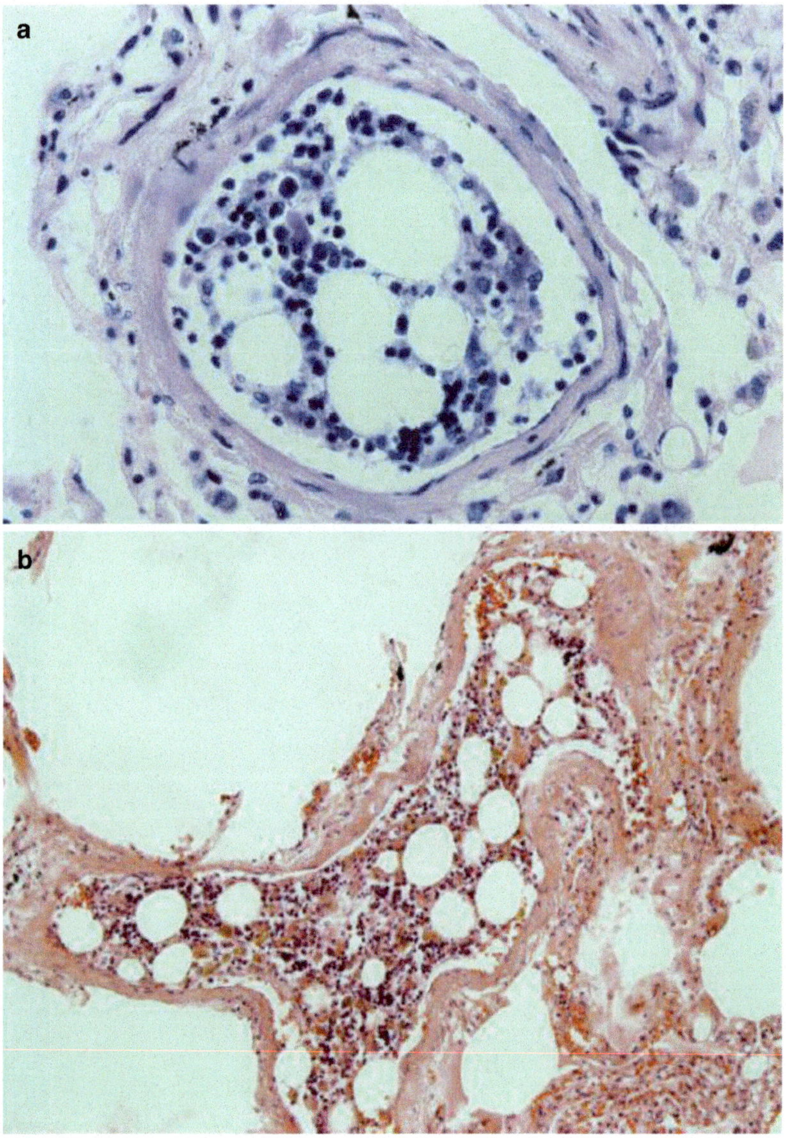

Fig. 9.9 Pulmonary bone marrow embolism—death on the operating table during implantation of a femoral head endoprosthesis following femoral neck fracture (**a**) (H&E ×200) and (**b**) H&E ×100)

be observed in polytrauma patients, frequently combined with cerebral fat embolism (Fig. 9.11). In the case of nonlethal pulmonary fat embolism, the lipids are resorbed into the lung tissue (Gigon et al. 1966). In the case of cerebral fat embolism, lipids, which can be identified using staining, were detected in the capillaries but also in the epithelium of the choroid plexus (Sperr 1968). The lipids can be viewed well using the Sudan III staining method. Extracted lipids are represented optically as voids; immunohistochemical staining with anti-CD61 and anti-fibrinogen antibodies should enable diagnosis of a fat embolism in cerebral and pulmonary arteries and capillaries (Neri et al. 2010).

In cases where an embolism is considered to be caused by intensive reanimation measures, in particular with rib fractures and fat or soft tissue compression, such embolisms are not reliable evidence of a vital reaction (Schneider and Klug 1971). Primarily ischemic and secondarily hemorrhagic pulmonary infarctions due to fat embolism can occur when fat emboli get past the contractile arteries in the lung, which is more

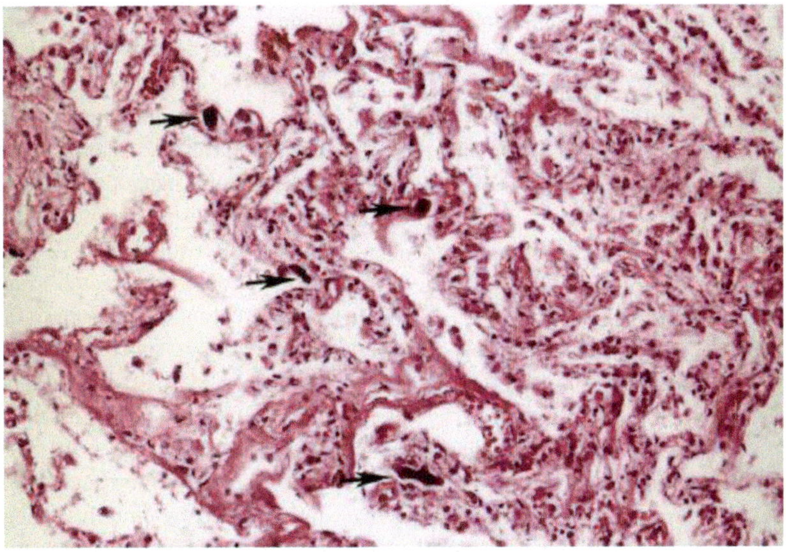

Fig. 9.10 Pulmonary megakaryocyte embolism (*arrows*) due to septic shock (H&E ×100)

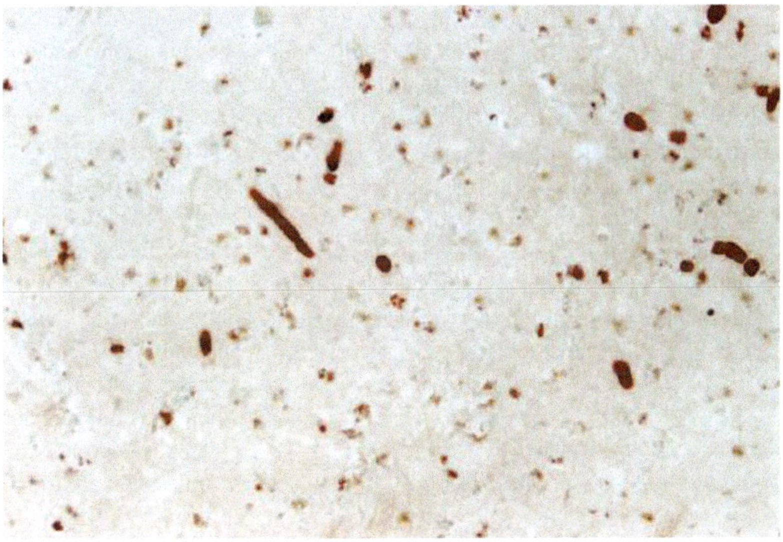

Fig. 9.11 Cerebral fat embolism in a polytrauma patient with a survival time of approximately 9 h (Sudan III ×400)

likely to happen under high pressure (Adebahr 1979). The pulmonary artery and vein, which belong to the functional circulation of the lung, are a terminal artery and vein, respectively; they have no precapillary anastomoses. The bronchial artery and vein, on the other hand, show arterioarterial and venovenous anastomoses. Branches of the pulmonary artery anastomose with branches of the bronchial artery; between lie very strong contractile arteries. It has occasionally been suggested that the gas pressure in decomposing bodies may cause the liquefied fat to be pressed into the pulmonary vessels. As a rule, an intravital fat embolism can be reliably identified and—depending on storage conditions of the corpse—can still be detected months later (Schollmeyer 1965; Henn and Spann 1965). Macroscopically, fat embolisms cannot be reliably diagnosed. Fat and bone marrow embolisms are forensically relevant in the following instances:

- Serious traffic accidents, in particular those involving extensive detachment injury (Saternus 1975)

- Occupational accidents involving polytrauma
- Occasionally in the case of liposuction
- Fat embolism in fire-related deaths
- Fat embolism in cases of hypothermia
- In the case of death on the operating table associated with the surgical treatment of fractures
- In cases of intraoperative and postoperative death of a patient following insertion of a femoral head endoprosthesis (TEP-OP); here it is important to pay attention to the temporal relation to the so-called Palacos phase

Not all embolisms or fat embolisms have such hemodynamic relevance, whereby acute right heart failure due to a sudden pressure rise can be easily explained. In order to evaluate the extent of a fat embolism, Falzi et al. (1964) proposed a classification (Table 9.4). Fat embolism diagnostics are based on the selection of a sufficient number of specimens from different pulmonary lobes and various parts of the lungs (central, medial, peripheral). Based on personal experience, taking two samples from each pulmonary lobe, central and peripheral, is advisable.

In the case of pulmonary fat embolism, saturated triglycerides from the trauma site generally predominate (in addition to cholesterol, fatty acids, and cholesterol esters). In cases of pronounced fatty tissue compression or contusion due to detachment caused by a traffic accident, the extent of fat embolism correlates, according to the literature, with survival time following serious accidents, acute deaths ($n = 300$) showed pulmonary fat embolism in approximately 20% of cases, in 96% with a survival time of 6 h, and after more than 12 h, a pulmonary fat embolism could be detected in all cases (100%). Thus, the extent of pulmonary fat embolism increased parallel to survival time.

Table 9.4 Classification of pulmonary fat embolism, evaluation at 100× magnification

Extent of fat embolism	Form of fat embolism	Localization of fat embolism
I = mild fat embolism	Teardrop-like	Scattered but at 25-fold magnification in every field of vision
II = distinct fat embolism	Lake- or sausage-shaped	Multiple fat emboli, disseminated in every field of vision
III = massive fat embolism	Fat emboli with antler-like configuration	Visible in huge numbers in all regions, no field of vision without fat emboli
0 = no fat embolism	Punctiform where relevant	Possibly visible in isolation, never in all fields of vision

According to Falzi et al. (1964), modified from Janssen (1977)

Microscopic evidence of pulmonary fat embolism should be assessed critically and in consideration of all findings: accompanying microhemorrhages, microthrombi, shock (bone marrow embolus? megakaryocytes?), damage to the capillary wall, perivascular edema, fat embolism in other organs (kidney? brain?), condition following trauma including fractures and soft tissue contusions, and condition following intensive cardiopulmonary reanimation.

Pulmonary fat embolism is sometimes also referred to as primary fat embolism, while further embolic spread of lipids into other organs is referred to as secondary fat embolism. The latter affects the heart muscle, brain, and kidneys in particular. Differences between neutral fats and fatty acids could be seen on Sudan III staining in an animal model (Takada et al. 2015). Isolated cases of systemic fat embolism have been seen when oil is injected during cosmetic surgery, e.g., gluteal injections of vitamin E (Mendoza-Morales et al. 2016).

Renal Fat Embolism Given that the kidneys absorb a considerable amount of blood volume, it is understandable that fat emboli in the systemic circulation likely enter glomerular capillaries (Fig. 9.12). In severe cases, a large number of glomeruli can be affected by fat embolism, unless renal blood supply is reduced as part of a peripheral shutdown. Fat emboli in the interlobar arteries as well as the afferent and efferent arterioles can rarely be detected. Fat emboli are also seldom between the capillary loops of the glomeruli and the Bowman's capsule, as well as in the renal tubules. These fat emboli are said to show cloudy swelling; fat vacuoles are only visible in the

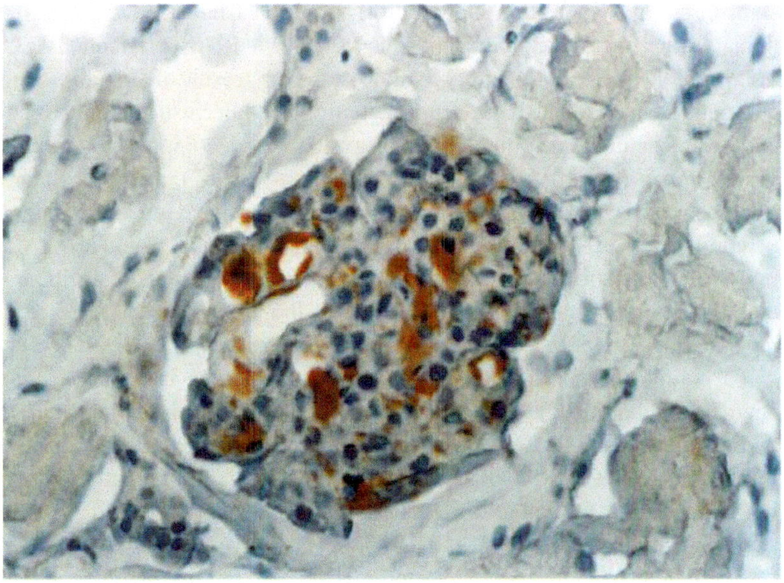

Fig. 9.12 Renal glomerular fat embolism in a polytrauma patient—a traffic accident victim with a survival time of approximately 9 h (Sudan III ×400)

ascending branches of Henle's loop. Fat emboli in the glomerular capillaries are accompanied by fibrin deposits.

Cerebral Fat Embolism Fat embolism with brain involvement develops after negotiating or avoiding the pulmonary capillary bed on the one hand, or via arteriovenous anastomoses (Holczabek 1968), and an open foramen ovale (paradox embolism) on the other. According to investigations by Henn and Spann (1965), it is most likely that cerebral fat embolism develops considerably later than pulmonary fat embolism (exception: anatomically open foramen ovale). Firstly, fat carried through from the pulmonary capillaries is absorbed, and secondly, posttraumatic circulation reactions through to shock reactions reduce embolic spread to the brain. In the case of higher trauma-related pressure, earlier cerebral fat embolism may be possible.

Cerebral fat emboli can be found in the cerebral cortex in particular; here, ring or ball hemorrhage—as in the case of cerebral air embolism—can be seen; a peripheral vessel branch (arterioles, capillaries) lies in the center and can be surrounded in a ring shape by hemorrhage into the brain tissue. With increasing survival time, microscopic necrosis develops (elective parenchymal necrosis) with a lipophage removal reaction. Fresh cerebral fat embolism does not necessarily have to show ring hemorrhage and cellular reactions.

In cases of cerebral fat embolism, fat embolic petechiae of the lid conjunctiva are also described, in particular of the lower eyelids (Wehner 1968). These embolically spread fats can produce pronounced and extensive petechiae as seen in neck compression due to violence. In this context, fresh fat emboli can also cause petechiae of the ocular fundus. Massive fat embolism in the systemic circulation can lead to extensive petechial skin hemorrhage. Fat embolism in other internal organs is possible, such as the spleen, liver, and kidneys.

When looking at the relevance of fat embolism as a cause of death, other organ diseases need to be considered, in particular organic heart disease. According to Falzi et al. (1964), fat embolism of the third degree can usually be accepted as a direct cause of death; however, it must form part of a causal chain, which can vary depending on the individual case. Less pronounced fat and pulmonary artery thromboembolism can lead to acute right heart failure when preexisting cardiac damage has been defined morphologically. The following should be included in the overall picture of findings: signs of preexisting right heart strain, hypertrophy and dilatation of the right atrium and right ventricle, signs of chronic congestion (nutmeg liver?), pulmonary artery ectasia, lipoidosis of the vascular intima of the pulmonary artery branches, right ventricular endocardial fibrosis and flattening of cardiac trabeculae, size of the pulmonary and tricuspid valve, extent of coronary artery atherosclerosis, diseases of the myocardium in the form of coronary insufficiency or myocardial infarction scars, interstitial and perivascular myocardial fibrosis, and inflammatory reactions in the myocardium.

Fat embolism can lead to single-cell and group necrosis in other internal organs, in particular the myocardium. It is often not possible to attribute this necrosis to fat embolism, since other competing causes can come into consideration, such as stenosing coronary sclerosis. If fat and bone marrow embolism can already be detected in a small number of tissue sections in the lung, the detection of further embolism in other organs depends on the extent of specimens taken and the number of tissue sections. In addition to fat embolism, detection of bone marrow embolism in the myocardium can also be possible in the form of a paradox embolism or via vascular anastomoses in polytrauma patients and/or during hip endoprosthesis implantation (see Chap. 1). Fat embolism following intoxication is rare but was detected following experimental carbon tetrachloride intoxication (Lahl 1973).

9.2.3 Air Embolism

Although venous and arterial air embolisms both occur, venous air embolism occurs much more often in forensic practice, where it is important to take the macroscopic evidence of an air embolism into account (Keil and Berzlanovich 2007; Bajanowski et al. 1998; Schneider et al. 1983; Patzelt et al. 1978; Brinkmann et al. 1976; Schubert 1952a, b, 1954; Loeschke 1950; Rössle 1944), e.g., after a stab wound to the neck with opening of large veins. Air embolisms have also been detected, however, after stab wounds to the lungs (Henßge and Madea 1991) or in the form of iatrogenic air embolism (Cheng et al. 2010; Cha et al. 2010; Mennim et al. 1992; Weiler 1976; Westcott 1973; Christmann 1969), as a result of sexual practices involving transvaginal air insufflation (Hendry 1964), in the case of decompression sickness (Seemann and Wandel 1967), and after illegal abortion (Wojahn 1970). Surviving an air embolism can mean that neurological damage of varying degrees of severity may remain. In the case of severe neurological deficit, a histological correlate can be expected during autopsy: cerebral cortex atrophy, perivascular borders of lipophages, and hemosiderin pigment-laden macrophages (Wojahn 1970; Janssen 1967). In cases of arterial air embolism in animal experiments, spaces in the form of air bubbles could be detected in the arteries and veins of the ocular fundus after a few minutes (Krause and Klein 1969).

Venous Air Embolism Venous air embolism, particularly when relevant to the cause of death and hemodynamically, is primarily a macroscopic diagnosis. Histological findings in the blood following air embolism are critically discussed (Adebahr et al. 1984; Adebahr and Kupffer 1967; Adebahr 1952, 1953, 1954, 1960). In addition, apparently empty spaces in the blood of the right heart, partly in the blood of the large veins, in the coronary veins, and in the blood of the pulmonary artery, can be detected. These “embolized air bubbles” are surrounded by leukocytes and thrombocyte aggregates with few fibrin strings. However, these histological findings could not be verified (Janssen 1977).

Arterial Air Embolism Following arterial air embolism, vesicular spaces in the erythrocyte columns close to the endothelium (with a sharp border and otherwise clear acute congestive hyperemia) may be detected primarily in the capillaries and arterioles of brain tissue (Fig. 9.13; Janssen 1977; Greiner 1954), but also in the myocardium (Hung et al. 2002; Harter 1947; Hausbrandt 1938). However, investigations of the myocardium are not suitable for microscopic identification of air embolism. Perivascularly, apparently empty areas, unevenly distended in a

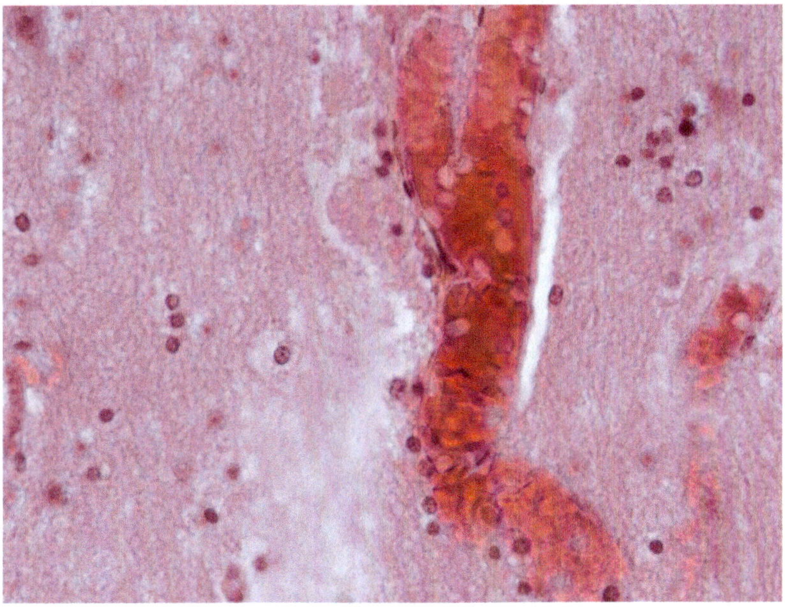

Fig. 9.13 Microscopically small, air bubble-like spaces in the peripheral vascular branches of brain tissue in macroscopically proven air embolism (H&E ×400)

bubble-like manner, are observed. A differentiation from artifacts depending on other factors (postmortem interval, etc.), however, prompts a recommendation to evaluate these histological findings very cautiously; they cannot be considered as sufficiently specific. Animal experiments with arterial air embolism (and fat embolism) showed evidence of lipid deposits and necrosis in the heart muscle and liver, partially within minutes or hours, accompanied by eosinophilic leukocytes (Schoenmackers 1950).

Macroscopically, cerebral purpura is marked in cases of cerebral air embolism; ring and ball hemorrhage can be seen microscopically already after a survival time of 30 min (Fig. 9.14) (Janssen 1967, 1977; Köhn 1952, 1953). Viewed in cross section, they show a centrally located blood vessel with a smaller surrounding area of presumably necrotic brain cells and adjacent circular brain hemorrhage.

Leukocytic reactions are rarely reported. In this process, vascular wall necrosis may be observed, along with intravascular microthrombi. In cases of longer survival time, more extensive necrosis, in particular of the cerebral cortex, is described with a histologically detectable histiocytic reaction.

In practice, however, it can be assumed that histological findings of an air embolism after a certain survival time lead, at best, to sufficiently characteristic changes in the brain. The absence of appropriate findings does not exclude an air embolism.

9.2.4 Amniotic Fluid Embolism

In the case of amniotic fluid embolism, the amniotic fluid itself and corpuscular components contained therein breach the venous spaces of the uterus, for example, as a result of a pregnancy termination procedure, medical malpractice, or injury following a traffic accident (Rainio and Penttilä 2003). It is rarely also fatal (Jecmenica et al. 2011; Nadjem et al. 2001). The risk of amniotic fluid embolism is higher in cases of multiparity, early placental abruption, protracted birth, and hypertonic uterine contractions intrapartum (Lau and Chui 1994; Nadesam and Jayalakshimi 1997). A precondition for amniotic fluid embolism is a defect in the chorion, in particular in connection with placental detachment. Epithelial cells of the epidermis, mucus, lanugo hair, meconium (Kearney 1999), components of

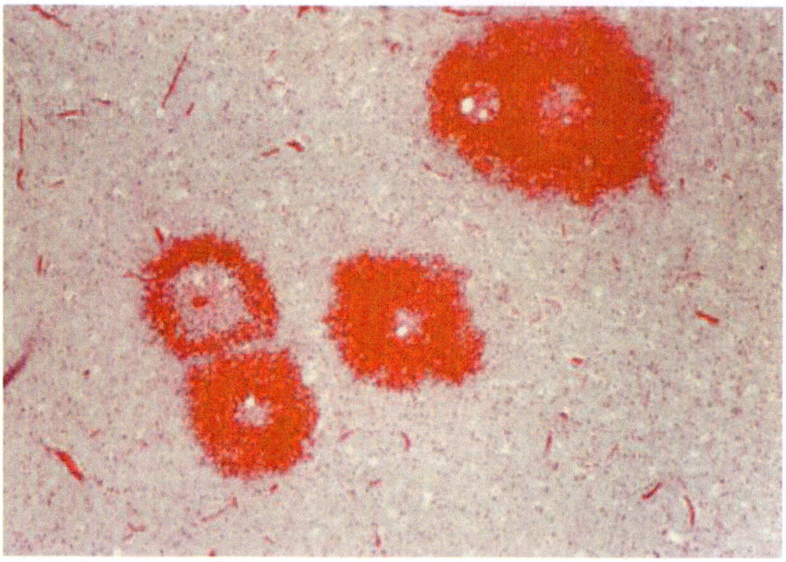

Fig. 9.14 Ring bleeding in the case of cerebral air embolism (H&E ×40)

the decidua, or even of the chorion swim in the amniotic fluid. Postmortem evidence for amniotic fluid embolism is based on the identification of amniotic fluid components, mainly in the capillaries of the pulmonary circulation, but also in other organs (Balažic et al. 2003), including resultant retinal ischemia (Fischbein 1969). Histologically, the peripheral pulmonary artery branches are filled with leukocytes and cell detritus with homogeneous parts, which can be seen in conventional histology using the mucicarmine staining method, the PAS reaction, and fibrin staining according to Weigert (Lau 2005; Rämsch 1960).

In cases where the pulmonary circulation is breached—or in the case of an open foramen ovale (paradox embolism)—amniotic fluid embolism may also develop in the arterial circulation. In the differential diagnosis, the histological findings on giant cells in particular must take shock-induced megakaryocyte embolism into account, in which case trophoblast giant cells are absent (Lunetta and Penttilä 1996). According to immunohistochemistry, embolically spread epidermal cells and other amniotic fluid components can be detected in the pulmonary capillaries—as in the case of amniotic fluid aspiration in newborns (see Chap. 11)—by means of the cytokeratin staining method (Fig. 9.15; Marcus et al. 2005; Garland and Thompson 1983).

In addition, immunohistochemical evidence of glycoproteins in amniotic fluid is described (Kobayashi et al. 1997; Ohi et al. 1993), as well as quantification of pulmonary mast cell tryptase in the case of amniotic fluid embolism (Turillazzi et al. 1998). Investigations to detect pulmonary amniotic fluid embolism depending on survival interval showed that amniotic fluid embolism can be detected microscopically for at least 36 h (Sinicina et al. 2010). If histologically marked tissue repair processes in the form of fibroblasts and newly built capillary blood vessels are casuistically described (Yamamoto et al. 1989), then a much longer detectability of amniotic fluid embolism can be assumed. Thus, amniotic fluid embolism could be identified in one case even after 36 days (Attwood and Delprado 1988). The spectrum of changes that can be identified immunohistochemically is the subject of scientific studies, including degranulation of activated mast cells with increased serum tryptase concentrations (Fineschi et al. 2009a; Nishio et al. 2002), in line with anaphylactic reactions in the case of amniotic fluid embolism (Aguilera et al. 2002). In addition, disseminated intravascular coagulation (DIC) may develop, which can be attributed to the activating effect of mucins (Cyr et al. 1998; Lau 1994). For example, it is not unusual to detect microthrombi in the capillary blood vessels in fatal amniotic fluid embolism (Fig. 9.16).

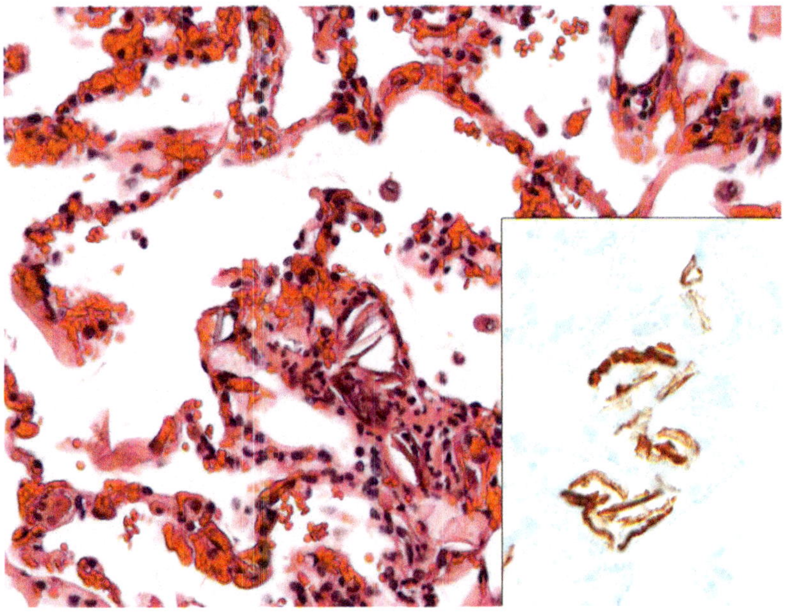

Fig. 9.15 Pulmonary septal capillaries with nonnucleated keratin lamellae in the vascular lumina in fatal amniotic fluid embolism (H&E ×200; anti-cytokeratin ×400; images kindly provided by Dr. K. Varchmin-Schultheiß, Münster, Germany)

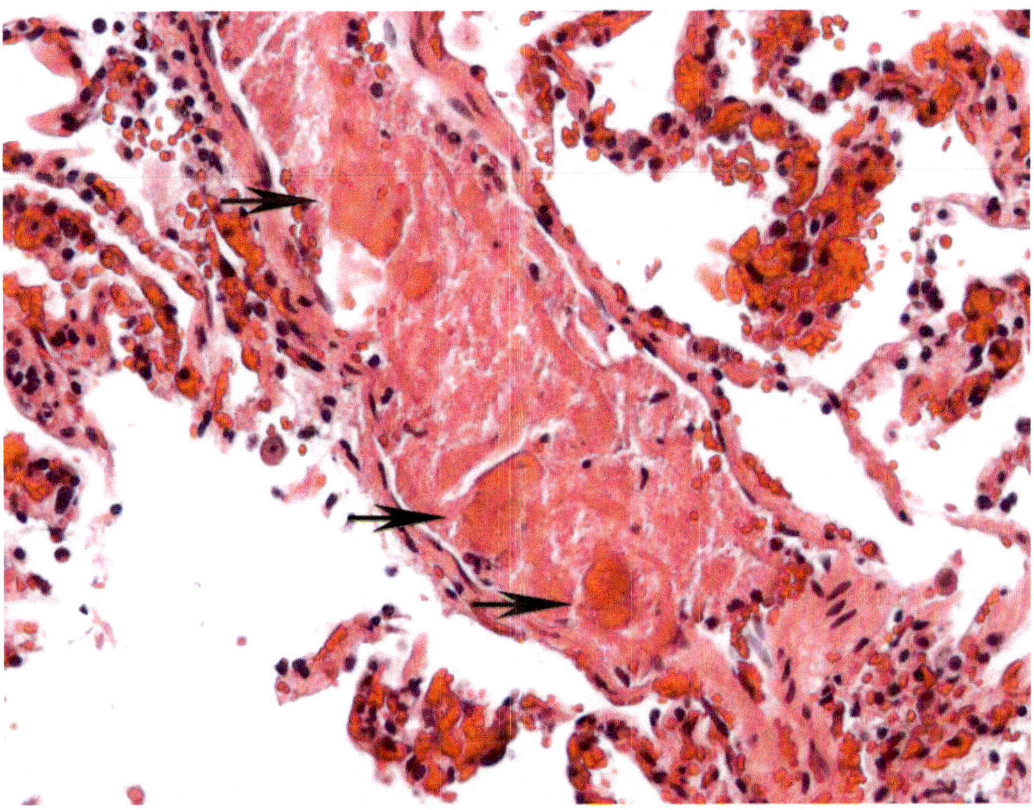

Fig. 9.16 Amniotic fluid embolism with microthrombi in pulmonary vascular branches (H&E ×200; image kindly provided by Dr. K. Varchmin-Schultheiß, Münster, Germany)

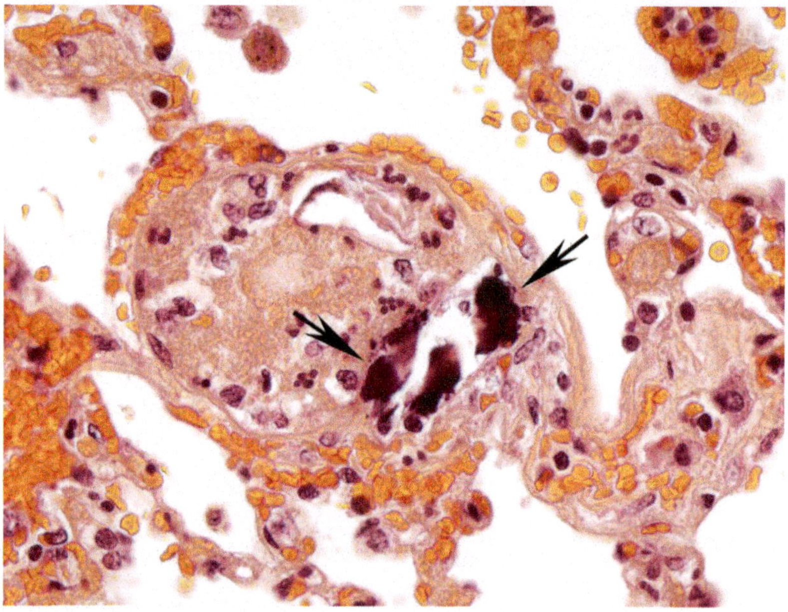

Fig. 9.17 Pulmonary amniotic fluid embolism with meconium particles in the vascular lumina (H&E ×400; image kindly provided by Dr. K. Varchmin-Schultheiß, Münster, Germany)

Occasionally, the spread of microscopically small particles of meconium is seen if amniotic fluid contains meconium in the setting of amniotic fluid embolism (Fig. 9.17). Embolisms with amniotic fluid particles may also be detected within the wall of the uterus. Zinc coproporphyrin-I (ZnCP-I) and sialyl-Tn (STN) are known components of meconium; both substances should be detectable by serological or histological analysis in amniotic fluid embolism (Hikiji et al. 2013). The immunohistochemical detection of meconium has also been described (Furuta et al. 2012). Differential diagnoses include Sanarelli–Shwartzman phenomenon and hemorrhagic hypovolemic shock, e.g., in the case of late diagnosis of atonic secondary postpartum hemorrhage in the uterine cavity.

9.2.5 Iatrogenic Embolism

In addition to the iatrogenic embolism mentioned earlier, microembolism following angiography and intravenous infusion has been described (Schubert et al. 1972). Dissection of the carotid, vertebral, and basilar arteries with thrombosis and cerebral embolism can also develop following chiropractic therapy (Smith et al. 2003; Rossetti et al. 2001; Lorenz and Vogelsang 1972). It is not uncommon to see—often non-fatal—Palacos® embolization, e.g., following prosthetic replacement of the femoral head or vertebroplasty. Silicone embolism syndrome in the context of cosmetic procedures, on the other hand, is far rarer.

Palacos® Embolism In general, embolic spread of low viscosity Palacos® (bone cement), which is injected at relatively high pressure into well vascularized areas and enters the blood circulation via venous vessels, can occur already during the surgical procedure (Amberg et al. 2015, Kunar et al. 2014, Monticelli et al. 2004). Only severe Palacos® embolism causes a hemodynamically relevant increase in pressure, particularly on the right heart, and may then be the triggering event that causes death. Pulmonary cement embolism is often asymptomatic (Apergis et al. 2011). Cement embolism can be seen in conventionally stained sections (Fig. 9.18), as well as using spectroscopy (Zheng et al. 2013).

Silicone Embolism Syndrome (SES) SES is the embolic spread of silicone, a highly stable liquid polymer. Silicone has been in use for decades, e.g., in the form of implants for cosmetic breast augmentation surgery or liquid silicone for sub-

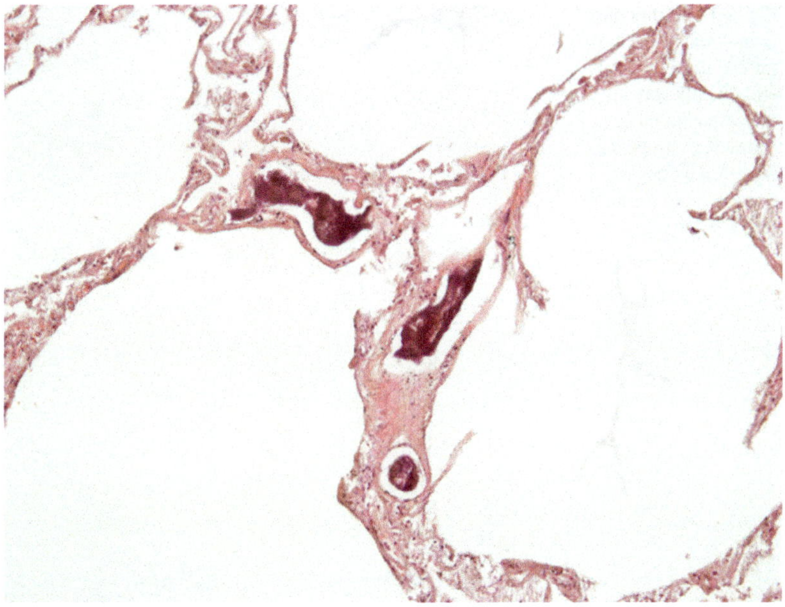

Fig. 9.18 Cement embolism with cement particles in the peripheral pulmonary branches (H&E ×100)

or intracutaneous injection (Kim et al. 2013; Schnabel et al. 1998; Rodriguez et al. 1989; Vilde et al. 1983; Preiß et al. 1977; Wilkie 1977). A small number of publications report silicone embolism following cosmetic surgery (Schmid et al. 2005), whereby pulmonary embolism is found to be predominant in this context. Since silicone does not react with the usual stains, it cannot be visualized using histological staining. Added to this is the fact that the embedding solutions used (e.g., xylene) dissolve both silicone and fats. There are isolated reports that Sudan staining of frozen sections under phase contrast shows silicone anti-foaming agent embolisms (Frick 1974). Silicone embolism is also reported to be visualizable as light pink mottling when using oil red O staining (Penry et al. 1960). Using microscopy, optically empty cavities have been described in the affected connective tissue, some of which are coalesced and exhibit a granulomatous inflammatory reaction at the margin involving foreign-body giant cells. Ectatic, optically empty areas have been reported in the pulmonary septal capillaries of the glomerular loops in the case of pulmonary and renal silicone embolism (Schnabel et al. 1998). A lipid stain (Sudan III staining of frozen sections) is required in order to differentiate a silicone embolism from a fat embolism (Frick 1974). However, histological findings alone are unlikely to be sufficiently characteristic—reliable diagnosis is only possible in combination with toxicological results.

9.2.6 Other Embolisms

A further embolism that should be taken into consideration is "junkie pneumopathy" with embolic spread of "cut" drug mixtures into the pulmonary circulation (Córdova and Alfageme 2014; see Chap. 4). Here, perivascular granulomas with birefringent foreign material and polynuclear foreign-body giant cells develop (Fig. 9.19). The granulomas are partially palpable in the lung tissue, while the foreign material (such as talc crystals) can be detected within the granulomas using polarization, with accompanying fibrosis and a loose lymphomonocytic inflammatory infiltrate.

Lethal tumor embolism is rare (Fracasso and Varchmin-Schultheiß 2009); similarly, there are few reports of embolic spread of projectiles (Sivanesan 1976; Hiebert and Gregory 1974). There is also only one reported case of pulmonary polyacrylamide hydrogel embolism as a fatal consequence of an illegal cosmetic vaginal tightening procedure (Duan et al. 2014). The inadvertent

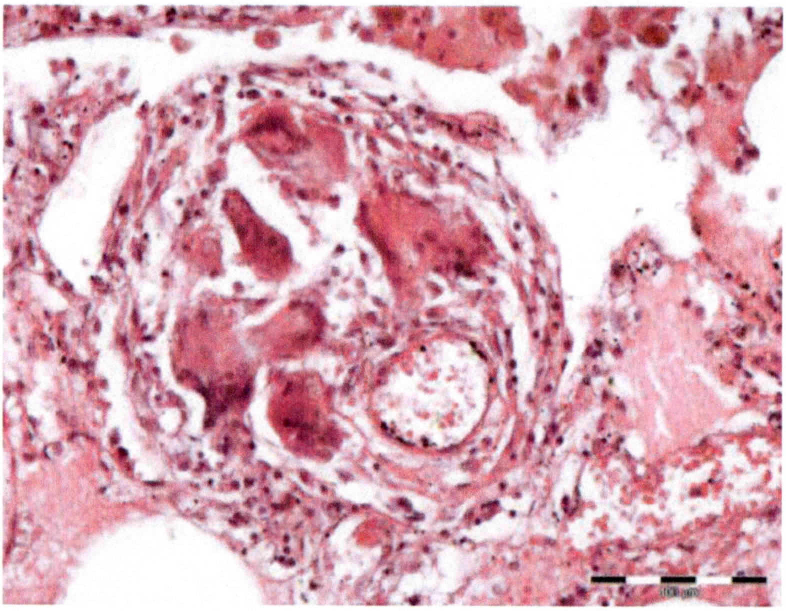

Fig. 9.19 Pulmonary granuloma in the case of junkie pneumopathy: embolically spread foreign material following intravenous injection with a foreign-body reaction (H&E ×400)

injection of liquid nutrition into a vascular catheter resulted in microscopically detectable particles (liquid nutrition emboli) in the lungs; embolic spread of liquid nutrition to the coronary artery branches and subsequent myocardial necrosis are also possible. A case of fatal foreign-body granulomatous pulmonary embolization due to microcrystalline cellulose in a patient receiving total parenteral nutrition is reported in the literature (Strickland et al. 2015).

Embolism Following Trauma Case studies show that embolic spread of vascular wall components may develop after trauma with injury to the vascular wall; cerebral embolisms may develop following carotid or vertebral artery trauma (Sigrist et al. 1997). The fat and bone marrow embolisms seen relatively frequently are also usually trauma-related (Bollinger et al. 2011). A case of fatal thromboembolism following physical restraint in a psychiatric patient has been reported (Cecchi et al. 2012).

References

Adebahr G (1952) Luftembolie im großen Kreislauf (Herz und Gehirn). (Sonderabdruck) Zbl Allg Path Anat 89: 216–222

Adebahr G (1953) Studien zum anatomischen Nachweis der Luftembolie unter besonderer Berücksichtigung der morphologischen Verhältnisse des Herzblutes. Virchows Arch 323:155–173

Adebahr G (1954) Beobachtungen und experimentelle Untersuchungen zum anatomischen Nachweis der Luftembolie. (Sonderabdruck) Zbl All Path Anat 92: 53–58

Adebahr G (1960) Anatomischer Nachweis der Luftembolie im Herzblut. Zbl Allg Path Anat 101: 347–352

Adebahr G (1979) Die Bedeutung von Sperrarterien für die Entstehung von Blutungen und kleinen hämorrhagischen Infarkten in der Lunge des Menschen bei Fettembolie. Z Rechtsmed 83:291–302

Adebahr G, Kupffer A (1967) Morphologischer Nachweis der Luftembolie im Herzblut. Abwandlung des Befundes in der Barbituratvergiftung beim Kaninchen. Dtsch Z gerichtl Med 61:1–12

Adebahr G, Weiler G, Risse M (1984) Die Bedeutung der mikroskopischen Untersuchung der mittleren und kleinen Äste der Arteria pulmonalis für die Diagnose der Luftembolie. Z Rechtsmed 92:127–135

Aguilera LG, Fernandez C, Plaza A, Gracia J, Gomar C (2002) Fatal amniotic fluid embolism diagnosed histologically. Acta Anaesthesiol Scand 46:334–337

Althoff H (1967) Fremdkörperembolie in das Gehirn nach Betriebsunfall. Monatsschr Unfallheilkde 70:124

Amberg R, Kernbach-Wighton G, Madea B (2015) Palacos® embolization following vertebroplasty. Rechtsmedizin 25:556–560

Attwood HD, Delprado WJ (1988) Amniotic fluid embolism: fatal case confirmed at autopsy five weeks after delivery. Pathology 20:381–382

Apergis G, Lagzdins M, Soueidan A (2011) Asymptomatic pulmonary cement emboli. Chest 140:8A

Bajanowski T, West A, Brinkmann B (1998) Proof of fatal air embolism. Int J Legal Med 111:208–211

Balažic J, Rott T, Jančigaj T, Popovič M (2003) Amniotic fluid embolism with involvement of the brain, lungs, adrenal glands, and heart. Int J Legal Med 117:165–169

Bollinger SA, Muehlematter K, Thali MJ, Ampanozi G (2011) Correlation of fat embolism severity and subcutaneous fatty tissue crushing and bone fractures. Int J Legal Med 125:453–458

Bowen DA, Sycamore E (1976) Traumatic air embolism. Med Sci Law 16:56–58

Brettel HF, Lutz FU (1973) Die Knorpelembolie als Sonderform vitaler Reaktionen. Z Rechtsmed 72:161

Brinkmann B, Borgner M, Bülow M (1976) Die Fettembolie der Lungen als Todesursache – Ätiologie, Pathogenese und Beweisführung. Z Rechtsmed 78:255

Bschor F (1963) Fettleber und Fettembolie. Dtsch Med Wschr 88:1112

Büchner C (1964) Traumatische Knochenmarksembolie der Lungen. Dtsch Med Wschr 89:1390–1394

Burke MP, O'Donnell C, Baber Y (2017) Death from pulmonary embolism of cyanoacrylate glue following gastric vein endocopic injection. Forensic Sci Med Pathol 13:82–85

Cecchi R, Lazzaro A, Catanese M, Mandarelli G, Ferracuti S (2012) Fatal thromboembolism following physical restraint in a patient with schizophrenia. Int J Legal Med 126:477–482

Cha S, Kwon CI, Seon HG, Ko KH, Hong SP, Hwang SG, Park PW, Rim KS (2010) Fatal biliary-systemic air embolism during endoscopic retrograde cholangiopancreatography: a case with multifocal liver abscesses and choledochoduodenostomy. Yonsei Med J 51:287–290

Cheng HM, Chiang KH, Chang PY, Chou YF, Huang HW, Chou AS, Yen PS (2010) Coronary artery air embolism: a potentially fatal complication of CT-guided percutaneous lung biopsy. Br J Radiol 83:e83–e85

Christmann W (1969) Nil nocere! Koronare Luftembolie bei internistischem Eingriff (Komplikationen beim Absaugen eines Pneumothorax). Münch Med Wschr 16:938–941

Córdova A, Alfageme I (2014) Foreign-body pulmonary embolism. Chest 145:508A

Costa AN, Mendes DM, Toufen C, Arrunategui G, Caruso P, de Carvalho CR (2008) Adult respiratory distress syndrome due to fat embolism in the postoperative period following liposuction and fat grafting. J Bras Pneumol 34:622–625

Cyr PV, Shuhaibar H, Kay JM (1998) Spontaneous duodenal-caval fistula with embolization of intestinal contents. Hum Pathol 29:1165–1166

de la Grandmaison G, Durigon M (2002) Pulmonary embolism. A rare cause of sudden infant death. Am J Forensic Med Pathol 23:257–259

Dettmeyer R, Schmidt P, Grellner W, Madea B (1999) "Einschwemmungs-Syndrom" (TUR-Syndrom) mit letalem Verlauf – morphologische und arztrechtliche Aspekte. Rechtsmedizin 10:39–42

Donohue KG, Saap L, Falanga V (2003) Cholesterol crystal embolization: an atherosclerotic disease with frequent and varied cutaneous manifestations. J Eur Acad Dermatol Venereol 17:504–511

Duan Y, Zhang L, Li S, Yang Y, Xing J, Li W, Wang X, Zhou Y (2014) Polyacrylamide hydrogel pulmonary embolism – a fatal consequence of an illegal cosmetic tightening procedure: a case report. Forensic Sci Int 238:e6–e10

Duda E, Papilian VV (1962) Exitus post partum durch Fruchtwasserembolie. Zbl Gynäk 84:690

Ely SF, Gill JR (2005) Fatal pulmonary thromboembolism and hereditary thrombophilias. J Forensic Sci 50:411–418

Emson HE (1958) Fat embolism studied in 100 patients dying after injury. J Clin Pathol 11:28–35

Falzi G, Henn R, Spann W (1964) Über pulmonale Fettembolien nach Traumen mit verschieden langer Überlebenszeit. Münch Med Wschr 106:978

Fineschi V, Riezzo I, Cantatore S, Pomara C, Turillazzi E, Neri M (2009a) Complement C3a expression and tryptase degranulation as promising histopathological tests for diagnosing fatal amniotic fluid embolism. Virchows Arch 454:283–290

Fineschi V, Turillazzi E, Neri M, Pomara C, Riezzo I (2009b) Histological age determination of venous thrombosis: a neglected forensic task in fatal pulmonary thrombo-embolism. Forensic Sci Int 186: 22–28

Fineschi V, Bafunno V, Bello S, de Stefano F, Margaglione M, Neri M, Riezzo I, Turillazzi E, Bonsignore A, Vecchione G, Ventura F, Grandone E (2012) Fatal pulmonary thromboembolism. A retrospective autopsy study: searching for genetic thrombophilias (Vactor V Leiden (G1691A) and FII (G20210A) gene variants) and dating the thrombus. Forensic Sci Int 214: 152–158

Fischbein F (1969) Ischemic retinopathy following amniotic fluid embolization. Am J Ophthalmol 67: 351–357

Foedisch HJ, Kloos K (1966) Thrombotische Verschlüsse im Stromgebiet der Arteria carotis nach stumpfen Schädelhalstraumen. Hefte Unfallheilkde 88:1

Fracasso T, Varchmin-Schultheiß K (2009) Sudden death due to pulmonary embolism from right atrial myxoma. Int J Legal Med 123:157–159

Fracasso T, Karger B, Pfeiffer H, Sauerland C, Schmeling A (2010) Immunohistochemical identification of prevalent right ventricular ischemia causing right heart failure in cases of pulmonary fat embolism. Int J Legal Med 124:537–542

Fracasso T, Pfeiffer H, Sauerland C, Schmeling A (2011) Morphological identification of right ventricular failure in cases of fatal pulmonary thromboembolism. Int J Legal Med 125:45–50

Fracasso T, Schrag B, Sabatasso S, Lobrinus JA, Schmeling A, Mangin P (2015) Different degrees of ischaemic injury in the right and left ventricle in cases of severe, nonfatal, pulmonary embolism. Int J Legal Med 129:525–529

Frick R (1974) Über die histologische Differenzierung von Fettembolie und Silikonembolie nach extrakorporalem Kreislauf mit dem Beuteloxygenator. Beitr Pathol 152:408–417
Furuta N, Yaguchi C, Itoh H, Morishima Y, Tamura N, Kato M, Uchida K, Suzuki K, Sugihara Y, Kawabata N, Suzuki T, Sasaki K, Horiuchi K, Kanayama N (2012) Immunohistochemical detection of meconium in the fetal membrane, placenta and umbilical cord. Placenta 33:24–30
Garland IW, Thompson WD (1983) Diagnosis of amniotic fluid embolism using an antiserum to human keratin. J Clin Pathol 36:625–627
Gigon JP, Enderlin F, Scheidegger S (1966) Über das Schicksal infundierter Fettemulsionen in der menschlichen Lunge. Schweiz Med Wschr 96:71–75
Gilbert P, Borchard F (1980) Hautembolie der Lunge. Pathologe 1:161–163
Greendyke RM (1964) Fat embolism in fatal automobile accidents. J Forensic Sci 9:201–208
Greiner H (1954) Histologische Befunde bei arterieller Luftembolie. Dtsch Z Gerichtl Med 43:415–523
Hardmeier T (1963) Schwere Fettembolie bei Erfrierungen an beiden unteren Extremitäten. Schweiz Med Wschr 93:465
Harter L (1947) Über Zirkulationsstörungen des Zentralnervensystems bei experimenteller Fett- und Luftembolie. Virchows Arch Path Anat 314:211
Hausbrandt F (1938) Beitrag zur Frage der kombinierten Luftembolie des kleinen und des großen Kreislaufs nach Abtreibungsversuchen. Dtsch Z Gerichtl Med 30:19
Haynes DM (1956) Cerebral hypoxia from air embolus following attempted abortion. Am J Obstet Gynecol 71:1111–1113
Hendry WT (1964) An unusual case of air embolism. Med Sci Law 4:179–181
Henn RHE, Spann W (1965) Untersuchungen über die Häufigkeit der cerebralen Fettembolie nach Trauma mit verschieden langer Überlebenszeit. Monatsschr Unfallheilkde 12:513–522
Henßge C, Madea B (1991) Luftembolie bei iatrogener Lungenstichverletzung. In: Schütz H, Kaatsch HJ, Thomsen H (eds) Medizinrecht – psychopathologie – rechtsmedizin. Springer, Heidelberg, pp 393–400
Hiebert CA, Gregory FJ (1974) Bullet embolism from the head to the heart. JAMA 299:442–443
Hikiji W, Tamura N, Shigeta A, Kanayama N, Fukunaga T (2013) Fatal amniotic fluid embolism with typical pathohistological, histochemical and clinical features. Forensic Sci Int 226:e16–e19
Holczabek W (1968) Das Verhalten der arterio-venösen Anastomosen bei der Lungenfettembolie. Dsch Z Gerichtl Med 62:170
Huber R (1965) Bedeutung der Lungenembolie für gekreuzte Embolien bei offenem Foramen ovale. Schweiz Med Wschr 95:963–969
Hung MJ, Kuo LT, Wang CH, Cherng WJ (2002) Irreversible myocardial damage after coronar air embolism. Angiology 53:213–216
Irninger W (1963) Histologische Altersbestimmung von Thrombosen und Embolien. Virch Arch Path Anat 336:220–237
Iwadate K, Doi M, Tanno K, Katsumura S, Ito H, Sato K, Yonemura I, Ito Y (2003) Right ventricular damage due to pulmonary embolism: examination of the number of infiltrating macrophages. Forensic Sci Int 134:147–153
Janík M, Hejna P (2015) Renal cell carcinoma pulmonary embolism: a rare cause of sudden death. Forensic Sci Med Pathol 11:468–471
Janssen W (1967) Zur Pathogenese und forensischen Bewertung von Hirnblutungen nach cerebraler Luftembolie. Dtsch Z Gesamte Gerichtl Med 61:62–80
Janssen W (1977) Forensische Histologie. Schmidt-Römhild Verlag, Lübeck, pp 111–150
Jecmenica D, Baralic I, Alempijevic D, Pavlekic S, Kiurski M, Terzic M (2011) Amniotic fluid embolism – apropos two consecutive cases. J Forensic Sci 56:S247–S251. https://doi.org/10.1111/j.1556-4029.2010.01588.x
Kaufmann F, Keresztes A (1967) Bericht über die fulminante, tödliche Lungenembolie des Obduktionsmaterials der Jahre 1952 bis 1965. Wiener Klin Wochenschr 79:155–161
Kearney MS (1999) Chronic intrauterine meconium aspiration causes fetal lung infarcts, lung rupture, and meconium embolism. Pediatr Dev Pathol 2:544–551
Keil W, Berzlanovich A (2007) Luftembolie. Rechtsmedizinische Aspekte. Rechtsmedizin 17:403–414
Kim HJ, Seides B, Mulaikal E, Mukherjee V, Eiss B, Patrawalla P (2013) Silicone embolism syndrome (SES): still out there. Chest 144:912A
Kitulwatte I, Pollanen MS (2009) Electrical injury of the neck and cardiac air embolism: a novel mechanism of death. Forensic Sci Med Pathol 5:32–35
Knight B (1966) Fatal pulmonary embolism: factors of forensic interest in 400 cases. Med Sci Law 6:150–154
Kobayashi H, Ooi H, Hayakawa H, Arai T, Matsuda Y, Gotoh K, Tarao T (1997) Histological diagnosis of amniotic fluid embolism by monoclonal antibody TKH-2 that recognizes NeuAc alpha 2-6GalNAc epitope. Hum Pathol 28:428–433
Köhn K (1952) Kritische Bemerkungen zur histologischen Diagnostik der arteriellen Luftembolie des Gehirns. Frankf Z Pathol 63:360–374
Köhn K (1953) Zum Nachweis der arteriellen Luftembolie des Gehirns. Dtsch Z Gerichtl Med 42:301–307
Konwaler BE (1950) Pulmonary emboli of cotton fibers. Am J Clin Pathol 20:385–389
Kössling FK (1963) Zur Pathologie der Fruchtwasserembolie. Geburtsh Frauenheilkde 8:707–720
Krause D, Klein S (1969) Tierexperimentelle Untersuchungen zur postmortalen ophthalmoskopischen Diagnostik der arteriellen Luftembolie. Dtsch Z Gesamte Gerichtl Med 65:22–27
Kunar N, Malviya M, De Meireles M (2014) It should not be here! A strange case of pulmonary cement embolism following balloon kyphoplasty. Chest 143: 559A

Lahl R (1973) Fettembolien nach experimenteller Tetrachlorkohlenstoffintoxikation. Z Gesamte Inn Med 28:367
Lau G (1994) Amniotic fluid embolism as a cause of sudden maternal death. Med Sci Law 34:213–220
Lau G (2005) Iatrogenic injury, a forensic perspective. In: Tsokos M (ed) Forensic pathology reviews, vol 3, pp 351–439
Lau G, Chui PP (1994) Amniotic fluid embolism: a review of 10 fatal cases. Singapore Med J 35:180–183
Leu AJ, Leu HJ (1989) Spezielle Probleme bei der histologischen Altersbestimmung von Thromben und Emboli. Pathologe 10:87–92
Loeschke H (1950) Über zerebrale Luftembolien und ihren Nachweis bei der Sektion. Z Gesamte Inn Med 5:631–633
Lorenz R, Vogelsang HG (1972) Thrombose der Arteria basilaris nach chiropraktischen Maßnahmen an der Halswirbelsäule. Dtsch Med Wschr 123:1389–1399
Lunetta P, Penttilä A (1996) Immunohistochemical identification of syncytiotrophoblastic cells and megakaryocytes in pulmonary vessels in a fatal case of amniotic fluid embolism. Int J Legal Med 108:210–214
Maffeis V, Nicolè L, Rago C, Fassina A (2017) Histological criteria for age determination of fatal venous thromboembolism. Int J Leg Med, https://doi.org/10.1007/s00414-017-1705-4
Makino Y, Abe H, Yokoyama M, Torimitsu S, Chiba F, Yokota H, Oka T, Iwase H (2015) Mercury embolism of the lung and right ventricle revealed by postmortem computed tomography and X-ray analytic microscopy. Forensic Sci Med Pathol 11:464–467
Marcus BJ, Collins KA, Harley RA (2005) Ancillary studies in amniotic fluid embolism: a case report and review of the literature. Am J Forensic Med Pathol 26:92–95
Mendoza-Morales RC, Camberos-Nava EV, Luna-Rosas A, Garcés-Ramírez L, de la Cruz F, García-Dolores F (2016) A fatal case of systemic fat embolism resulting from gluteal injections of vitamin E for cosmetic enhancement. Forensic Sci Int 259:e1–e4
Mennim P, Coyle CF, Taylor JD (1992) Venous air embolism associated with removal of central venous catheter. Br Med J 305:171–172
Monticelli F, Meyer HJ, Tutsch-Bauer E (2004) Fatal pulmonary cement embolism following percutaneous vertebroplasty (PVP). Forensic Sci Int 149:35–38
Nadesam K, Jayalakshimi P (1997) Sudden maternal deaths from amniotic fluid embolism. Ceylon Med J 42:185–189
Nadjem H, Bohnert M, Pollak S (2001) A case of fatal amniotic fluid embolism. Arch Kriminol 207:89–96
Neri M, Riezzo I, Dambrosio M, Poimara C, Turillazzi E, Fineschi V (2010) CD61 and fibrinogen immunohistochemical study to improve the post-mortem diagnosis in a fat embolism syndrome clinically demonstrated by transesophageal echocardiography. Forensic Sci Int 202:e13–e17
Nichols GR II, Corey TS, Davis GJ (1990) Nonfracture-associated fatal fat embolism in a case of a child abuse. J Forensic Sci 35:493–499
Nishio H, Matsui K, Miyazaki T, Tamura A, Iwata M, Suzuki K (2002) A fatal case of amniotic fluid embolism with elevation of serum mast cell tryptase. Forensic Sci Int 126:53–56
Nosaka M, Ishida Y, Kimura A, Kondo T (2009) Time-dependent appearance of intrathrombus neutrophils and macrophages in a stasis-induced deep vein thrombosis model and its application to thrombus age determination. Int J Legal Med 123:235–240
Nosaka M, Ishida Y, Kimura A, Kondo T (2010a) Immunohistochemical detection of MMP-2 and MMP-9 in a stasis-induced deep vein thrombosis model and its application to thrombosis age estimation. Int J Legal Med 124:439–444
Nosaka M, Ishida Y, Kimura A, Kondo T (2010b) Time-dependent organic changes of intravenous thrombi in stasis-induced deep vein thrombosis model and its application to thrombus age determination. Forensic Sci Int 195:143–147
Nosaka M, Ishida Y, Kimura A, Kuninaka Y, Inui M, Mukaida N, Kondo T (2011) Absence of IFN-γ accelerates thrombus resolution through enhanced MMP-9 and VEGF expression in mice. J Clin Invest 121:2911–2920
Nosaka M, Ishida Y, Kimura A, Kondo T (2012) Immunohistochemical detection of uPA, tPA, and PAI-1 in a stasis-induced deep vein thrombosis model and its application to thrombus age estimation. Int J Legal Med 126:421–425
Nosaka M, Ishida Y, Kimura A, Kondo T (2013) Immunohistochemical detection of intrathrombotic macrophage-derived cytokines and its application to thrombus age estimation in murine deep vein thrombosis model. Int J Legal Med 127:937–942
Nosaka M, Ishida Y, Kimura A, Hama M, Kawaguchi T, Yamamoto H, Kuminaka Y, Shimada E, Kondo T (2015) Immunohistochemical detection of intrathrombotic IL-6 and its application to thrombus age estimation. Int J Legal Med 129:1021–1025
Nosaka M, Ishida Y, Kimura A et al (2017) Immunohistochemical detection of intrathrombotic fibrocytes and its application to thrombus age estimation in murine deep vein thrombosis model. Int J Legal Med 131:179–183
Obersteg J (1949) Die Luftembolie bei kriminellem Abort. Dtsch Z Gerichtl Med 39:646–687
Ohi H, Kobayashi H, Terao T (1993) A new histologic diagnosis for amniotic fluid embolism by means of monoclonal antibody TKH-2 that recognizes mucin-type glycoprotein, a component in meconium. Nippon Sanka Fujinka Gakkai Zasshi 44:813–819
Patzelt D, Lignitz E, Keil W, Takatsu A (1978) Zur Problematik der Diagnose Luftembolie an der Leiche. Beitr Ger Med XXXVII:401–405

Penry JK, Cordell AR, Johnston FR, Netsky MG (1960) Cerebral embolism by antifoam A in a bubble oxygenator system. Surgery 47:784–794

Pragst F, Correns A, Priem F, Herre S, Martin H (2007) A sudden death with lung embolism after inadvertent infusion of zinc oxide shake lotion. Forensic Sci Int 170:207–212

Preiß G, Brunner P, Tulusan AH (1977) Die pulmonale Silikonembolie. Virchows Arch A Pathol Anat Histopathol 373:55–65

Rainio J, Penttilä A (2003) Amniotic fluid embolism as cause of death in a car accident – a case report. Forensic Sci Int 137:231–234

Rämsch R (1960) Tödliche Fruchtwasserembolie. Zbl Allg Path 101:470–474

Reutter F, Siebenmann R, Wegmann T (1965) Tödliche Lungenembolie bei Verabreichung eines oralen Ovulationshemmers. Schweiz Med Wschr 95:303–305

Ro A, Kageyama N, Tanifuji T, Fukunaga T (2008) Pulmonary thromboembolism: overview and update from medicolegal aspects. Legal Med 10:57–71

Röding H, Röse W (1967) Iatrogene Embolien. Dtsch Gesundheitsw 34:1585–1591

Rodriguez MA, Martinez MC, Lopez-Artiquez M, Soria ML, Bernier F, Repetto M (1989) Lung embolism with liquid silicon. J Forensic Sci 34:504–510

Rossetti AO, Combrement PC, Bogousslavsky J (2001) Dissections artérielles lors de manipulations cervicales: attention, danger! Schweiz Ärztezeitung 82: 495–497

Rössle R (1944) Über die Luftembolie der Capillaren des großen und kleinen Kreislaufes. Virchows Arch 313:1–27

Saternus KS (1975) Plötzlicher Tod am Unfallort bei Fußgängern. Kriminalistik 11:498–501

Säker G (1955) Fettembolie bei Verkehrsunfällen. Münch Med Wschr 97:625–628

Schmid A, Tzur A, Leshko L, Krieger BP (2005) Silicone embolism syndrome: a case report, review of the literature, and comparison with fat embolism syndrome. Chest 127:2276–2281

Schnabel A, Röhrich J, Schmidt K, Kavert G, Bratzke H (1998) Zur forensischen Beweisführung bei einer Silikonembolie durch Kombination histologischer und toxikologischer Untersuchungsmethoden. Rechtsmedizin 8:147–152

Schneider V, Klug E (1971) Fettembolie der Lungen nach äußerer Herzmassge. Beitr Ger Med 28:76

Schneider V, Klug E, Phillip W (1983) Die Luftembolie im kleinen Kreislauf – ihr Nachweis an der Leiche. Pathologe 4:97–102

Schoenmackers J (1950) Die markierte arterielle Luftembolie im Kaninchenversuch (Luft-Fettembolie). Virchows Arch 318:234–249

Schollmeyer W (1965) Über die Fettembolie des Lungengewebes nach Verbrennung. Forum der Kriminalistik 5:32–34

Schubert W (1952a) Über das Ergebnis einer Reihen- und Gruppenuntersuchung an 150 Leichen zur Prüfung auf arterielle Luftembolien im großen Kreislauf. Virchows Arch 322:472–487

Schubert W (1952b) Über einen makroskopischen Nachweis von Luftembolien im Organgewebe durch Fixierung im Unterdruckraum in Formalin im Anschluss an die Sektion. Virchows Arch 322:494–502

Schubert W (1954) Weitere Erfahrungen bei Druckstoß von Explosionen und Spontanluftembolien aus der Lunge. Virchows Arch 325:57–69

Schubert GE, Reifferscheid P, Flach A (1972) Mikroembolien von Fremdmaterial nach Angiographien und intravenösen Infusionen. Dtsch Med Wschr 97: 1745–1748

Schulz F, Hildebrand E, Graß H (1992) Ein ungewöhnlicher Fall von traumatischer Leberruptur mit Lebergewebsembolie der Lungen. Rechtsmedizin 2:152–155

Schulz F, Tsokos M (2004) Fettleber und Fettembolie. Rechtsmedizin 14:463–466

Seemann K, Wandel A (1967) Der Taucherunfall mit Überdehnung der Lunge und Luftembolie. Münch Med Wschr 42:2168–2175

Senen D, Atakul D, Erten G, Erdogan B, Lortlar N (2009) Evaluation of the risk of systemic fat mobilization and fat embolus following liposuction with dry and tumescent technique: an experimental study on rats. Aesthetic Plast Surg 33:730–737

Shairkh N, Hanssens Y, Kettern MA, Deleu D, Ruiz-Miyares F, Mesraoua B (2008) Cerebral fat embolism as a rare complication of liposuction with abdominoplasty. Rev Neurol 47:277–278

Sigrist T, Markwalder C, Gstrein G (1997) Seltene Form einer cerebralen Embolie nach Karotistrauma. Rechtsmedizin 7:90–94

Sinicina I, Pankratz H, Bise K, Matevossian E (2010) Forensic aspects of post-mortem histological detection of amniotic fluid embolism. Int J Legal Med 124:55–62

Sivanesan S (1976) Bullet embolism to the heart. Med Sci Law 16:59–61

Smith WS, Johnston SC, Skalabrin EJ et al (2003) Spinal manipulative therapy is an independent risk factor for vertebral artery dissection. Neurology 60: 1424–1428

Sowell MW, Lovelady CL, Brogdon BG, Wecht CH (2007) Infant death due to air embolism from peripheral venous infusion. J Forensic Sci 52:183–188

Sperr W (1968) Sudanophile Veränderungen am Plexus chorioideus. Dtsch Z Gesamte Gerichtl Med 62:20–25

Steiner I (2007) Pulmonary embolism-temporal changes. Cardiovasc Pathol 16:248–251

Stoltenburg-Didinger G, Vogel M (1980) Kleinhirngewebsembolie nach Beckenendlage bei einem Neugeborenen (Falldemonstration). Berliner Gesellsch für Pathologie (e.V.) 189. wissenschaftliche Sitzung – 11. 03.1980, Tagungsberichte, p 189

Strange C, Heffner JE, Collins BS, Brown FM, Sahn SA (1987) Pulmonary hemorrhage and air embolism complicating transbronchial biopsy in pulmonary amyloidosis. Chest 92:367–369

Strickland S, Pena E, Walker AE (2015) Fatal foreign-body granulomatous pulmonary embolism due to microcrystalline cellulose in a patient receiving total parenteral nutrition: all crystals are not what they seem. Forensic Sci Med Pathol 11:255–261

Takada M, Chiba S, Nagai T, Takeshita H, Kanno S, Ikawa T, Sakamoto K, Sagi M, Ichiba K, Mukai T (2015) Inflammatory responses to neutral fat and fatty acids in multiple organs in a rat model of fat embolism syndrome. Forensic Sci Int 254:126–132

Turillazzi E, Gambassi R, Gheradi M, Fineschi V (1998) The diagnosis of amniotic fluid embolism: an immunohistochemical study for the quantification of pulmonary mast cell tryptase. Int J Legal Med 111:238–243

Türk EE, Tsokos M (2003) Sudden infant death due to pulmonary embolism. Am J Forensic Med Pathol 24:106

Türk E, Schulz N, Püschel K (2007) Air embolism during coronary angiography. Rechtsmedizin 17:215–217

Uekita I, Ijiri I, Nagasaki Y, Haba R, Funamoto Y, Matsunaga T, Jamal M, Wang W, Kumihashi M, Ameno K (2008) Medicolegal investigation of chicken fat clot in forensic cases: immunohistochemical and retrospective studies. Legal Med 10:138–142

Vilde F, Arkwright S, Galliot M, Galle P, Labrousse J, Lissac J (1983) Fatal pneumopathy linked to subcutaneous injections of liquid silicone into soft tissue. Ann Pathol 3:307–325

Watanabe S, Terazawa K, Matoba K, Yamada N (2007) An autopsy case of intraoperative death due to pulmonary fat embolism-possibly caused by release of tourniquet after multiple muscle-release and tenotomy of the bilateral lower limbs. Forensic Sci Int 171:73–77

Watanabe M, Unuma K, Makino Y, Noritake K, Yamada A, Iwase H, Uemura K (2016) An autopsy case of acute massive hematochezia caused by superior mesenteric vein thrombosis: a first report in forensic medicine. J Forensic Sci 61:271–273

Wehner W (1968) Die Fettembolie. VEB Verlag Volk und Gesundheit, Berlin

Weiler G (1976) Zur venösen Gasembolie bei diagnostischen und therapeutischen Eingriffen unter besonderer Berücksichtigung des Pneumoperitoneums. Beitr Gerichtl Med 34:9–14

Westcott J (1973) Air embolism complicating percutaneous needle biopsy of the lung. Chest 63:108–110

Wild U, Defosse JM, Wappler F, Sakka SG (2013) Luftembolie nach ZVK-Entfernung. Anästhesiol Intensivmed Notfallmed Schmerzther 48:28–31

Wilhelmi F, Hildebrand E (1972) Tödliche Lungenembolie nach Aortenaneurysma-Ruptur in die Vena cava caudalis. Z Rechtsmed 71:246

Wilkie TF (1977) Late development of granuloma after liquid silicone injections. Plast Reconstr Surg 60: 179–188

Wirth E, Staak M (1972) Untersuchungen zur Frage des Auftretens der Fettembolie bei Todesfällen aus traumatischer und nichttraumatischer Ursache. Beitr Ger Med XXIX:98–103

Wojahn H (1970) Klärung einer Abtreibung mit zentraler Luftembolie nach 4 Jahren. Beitr Ger Med XXVII:97–100

Wongprasartsuk S, Finlay M, Perry GJ (2001) Cholesterol emboli to the kidney: an immunoperoxidase study. Pathology 33:157–162

Yamamoto K, Yamamoto Y, Watanabe H, Fujimiya T, Okae M, Ukita K (1989) A case of sudden death by decidual cell embolism. Z Rechtsmed 102:415–416

Young RL, Derbyshire RC, Cramer OS (1948) Paradoxic embolism. Arch Pathol 46:3–48

Zheng N, Liang M, Zhang HD, Zhu SH, Yang TT, Zhuo L, Wang GF, Liu HX, Liu L (2013) Fatal extensive bone cement embolism: histological findings confirmed by Fourier transform infrared spectroscopy. Forensic Sci Int 229:e23–e25

10 Vitality, Injury Age, Determination of Skin Wound Age, and Fracture Age

The determination of vitality, i.e., whether an injury was incurred during life, and age of an internal injury or skin wound is a fundamental issue in forensic medicine (Fronczek et al. 2015a, b; Cecchi 2010; Kondo and Ishida 2010; Grellner et al. 1997, 2000, 2005; Dreßler et al. 1997a, b, 1999a, 2001; Wyler 1996; Lorente 1996; Kondo and Ohshima 1996b; Betz 1995a, b, Betz et al. 1992a, c, 1993e, 1995; Fechner et al. 1991; Oehmichen et al. 1989; Raekallio 1965a, 1970, 1980a, b; Lindner 1962, 1967, 1980; (Berg and Bonte 1971; Lindner and Huber 1973). This examination includes the comparison of injuries incurred while alive with postmortem injuries (Vieira 1996; Oehmichen and Kirchner 1996; Oehmichen 1990a; Oehmichen and Cröpelin 1995; Oehmichen et al. 1988a, b; Naeve and Bause 1974), while epidermal esterase activity following blunt force trauma has been previously investigated (Pioch 1969).

In this context, internal injuries and skin wounds are of interest, as well as bony or skeletal injuries, particularly in terms of determining vitality (Nakajima et al. 2006; Fechner et al. 1991). Investigations of subcutaneous hematomas (Tutsch-Bauer et al. 1981), including intravascular aggregation of thrombocytes and formation of microthrombi at the wound margin (Thomsen 1996), have been performed in order to determine injury age. In some cases, the age of a wound or hemorrhage may be of interest in the context of an intracranial injury, particularly the age of epi- and subdural hematomas or of brain contusions (see Chap. 20).

Keeping an overview of today's literature on age determination of injuries or wounds is challenging, since there are also many articles from other specialties (see, e.g., Oehmichen and Kirchner 1996). Investigations on age determination of skin wounds and brain tissue injuries predominate, while investigations of other injuries or biological responses to inflammatory processes with respect to age determination are relatively rare but include burns (Castagnoli et al. 1994; Mulligan et al. 1994), injection via cannulas (Püschel et al. 1996; Schaeffer-Schulz et al. 1996; Friebel and Woohsmann 1968), or age determination in cases of peritonitis, pleurisy, or pericarditis. A smaller number of investigations deal with histological findings in scar tissue, such as in connection with melanocyte migration (Dreßler et al. 2001). Investigating the appearance of the injury may already enable a general conclusion on the age of injury due to:

- Hemorrhagic wound margins
- Edema and swelling in the injured region
- Coagulated blood in or on the wound
- Signs of wound healing, such as hyperemia of the wound margins and a fibrin scab that covers the wound
- Clearly pronounced granulation tissue
- Scar tissue

R. B. Dettmeyer, *Forensic Histopathology*, https://doi.org/10.1007/978-3-319-77997-3_10

The color of a hematoma and its demarcation from the vicinity are relatively uncertain criteria but may enable a statement on whether an injury is "fresh" or "not fresh." The rough macroscopic evaluation of injury age can be improved by means of conventional histological and immunohistochemical investigations.

Conventional histology shows cellular reactions with routine staining methods (e.g., H&E, PAS, Prussian blue, EvG, trichrome). These findings can only be seen, however, after a survival time or wound age of approximately 30 min. Only neutrophil infiltration can start earlier; the detection of new collagen fibers and the formation of granulation tissue occur later. In spite of numerous studies on wound age determination, conventional histological wound age determination remains the basis of all wound age diagnostics.

Enzyme histochemical methods established in the 1960s and 1970s are based on the detection of increased activity in cells or of different enzymes in the wound area, in particular fibroblasts (Betz 1994; Raekallio 1960, 1964, 1965b, 1972, 1973; Raekallio and Mäkinen 1967). Enzyme histochemical reactions can be detected earlier than cellular wound reactions (with the exception of the invasion of neutrophil granulocytes, which can be detected relatively early). Hence, a wound age of only a few hours can be seen more precisely with these methods (Table 10.1).

Since the late 1980s, attempts have been made to narrow the age range of injuries or wounds by detecting specific cellular and extracellular antigens by means of immunohistochemical investigations. The focus lies here on the determination of cell adhesion molecules or cytokines at the injury margin (Ninggou et al. 2006; Dreßler et al. 1997a, b; Flad 1996; Betz et al. 1993a, g, 1995; Mauch et al. 1994; Fries et al. 1993; Dachum and Jiazhen 1992; McKay and Leigh 1991; Blitstein-Willinger 1991; Mackie et al. 1988).

Numerous experimental investigations have been based on animal models and therefore cannot necessarily be extrapolated to human wounds. This also applies to the validity of tissue samples taken during autopsy. Even during autopsy of a body cold-stored shortly after death, age-related effects on injuries are already present, such as drying out of wound margins. For this reason, histological and immunohistochemical investigations on wound age must always consider postmortem reliability of findings with increasing postmortem intervals. Statements on the vitality of an injury need to be differentiated from statements on injury age.

When evaluating injury or wound age, a number of influencing factors must be considered, including, for example, temperature and medication consumption (Bode et al. 1979, 1980). There are a number of publications on the influence of endogenous and exogenous factors with respect to wound healing, including:

- Age of decedent (Nerlich and Bosch 1988; Berg 1975; Raekallio and Mäkinen 1974).
- Medication, e.g., barbiturates (Bode et al. 1979), or other medications (Mann and Bednar 1977).
- Chronic and acute effects of alcohol (MacGregor et al. 1988; Berg and Elbel 1969; Schollmeyer 1965).

Table 10.1 Occurrence of enzyme histochemical reactions

Vital wound age	ATPase	Esterase	Aminopeptidase	Acid phosphatase	Alkaline phosphatase	Many polymorphonuclear cells	Many mononuclear cells
>16 h	+	+	+	+	+	+	+
>8 h	+	+	+	+	+	+	
>4 h	+	+	+	+			
>2 h	+	+	+				
>1 h	+	+					

Raekallio (1960, 1964, 1965a, b, 1970, 1972, 1973), according to Dürwald (1987)

- Temperature (Maxeiner 1994; Bode et al. 1980).
- Localization and type of injury (Oehmichen 1990b; Nerlich and Bosch 1988).
- It is unclear to what extent genetic disposition affects the speed of wound healing.

A summary of factors influencing age determination of internal injuries and skin wounds can be seen in Table 10.2.

Due to the strict standards applied in criminal law, the age determination of injuries and wounds

Table 10.2 Factors influencing age determination of internal injuries and skin wounds

Influencing factor	Significance
Postmortem period	During the postmortem period, autolytic processes occur, as well as hypostasis phenomena and potential wound colonization with maggots; drafts or ambient temperature may cause the wound to dry out. Therefore, postmortem stability in a wound region, as well as for all immunohistochemical markers, must be scrutinized
Draft, ambient temperature, submersion in water, etc.	Environmental conditions to which the body has been exposed can influence wound age diagnosis
Circumstances of death	If, depending on the circumstances of death and autopsy results, a longer agonal period can be assumed, impaired responsiveness of the body to a peripheral wound must be considered, e.g., shock-related circulatory centralization
Preexisting disease	In individual cases, it is possible that preexisting diseases [e.g., leukemia, agranulocytosis, thrombocytopenia, disseminated intravascular coagulation (DIC), sepsis, diabetes mellitus, uremia, malignant tumors, liver cirrhosis] may affect wound healing and thus also the determination of wound age
Previous medication	The influence of medication must be considered in specific cases, such as drugs that impair blood coagulation and/or immunosuppressive drugs, as well as sleeping pills, cytostatic drugs, etc.
Previous alcohol and drug consumption	The influence of chronic alcohol and drug consumption on the wound healing process is difficult to assess
Localization of tissue samples taken at autopsy	Since wound healing reactions of the body—thrombocyte aggregates, cellular infiltration, etc.—do not start in the hemorrhagic center or center of tissue necrosis, tissue samples from peripheral regions of an injury are more meaningful
Number of tissue samples examined per injury	The assumption that the infliction of an injury would trigger the same reaction at the same time in all peripheral regions of the body has not yet been conclusively proven by systematic investigations. In the case of smaller peripheral skin wounds with identical perfusion distribution in all peripheral wound regions, a certain homogeneity in the wound reaction can be assumed
Selection of conventional histological staining methods	The staining methods selected must allow for an evaluation of all relevant parameters necessary for the age determination of wounds. The following are routinely required: H&E, EvG, and Prussian blue staining, each of which gives the experienced examiner valid insights. Less experienced examiners are recommended to also use ASD staining as the specific enzyme histochemical staining for granulocytes
Evaluating tissue sections	When evaluating tissue sections, technical errors and artifacts must be excluded or at least identified
Selection of immunohistochemical markers (in particular adhesion molecules)	Insofar as specific immunohistochemical markers have been shown by previous investigations to be technically reproducible and helpful in determining minimum wound age, these markers should be selected. In the case of immunohistochemical staining methods, technical errors and artifacts must also be considered
Evaluation	Vitality: easy to affirm if a conventional histological wound reaction is obvious or if immunohistochemical markers accepted among experts are absent
	Minimum wound age: if a certain time must have passed until evidence of some findings is reliable, a minimum wound age may be stated (with an associated degree of probability)
	Maximum wound age: if, depending on the circumstances and other findings, certain histological or immunohistochemical findings are expected but cannot be detected, this may at least provide evidence that a wound must be younger or older than the detection interval for the microscopic criterion chosen

In specific cases, a combination of immunohistochemical markers that are accepted among experts should be chosen for wound age diagnostics. If the findings can be interpreted, they must be seen within the context of all findings before making statements on the probable skin wound age

is still not of particular use in court because of the large number of influencing factors and the unproven transferability of results gained in animal experiments to humans. However, histological, enzyme histochemical, and immunohistochemical findings may be indicative of and support a certain wound age, negate it, or, in some cases, exclude it completely. Scientific studies on immunohistochemical age determination of wounds previously focused on skin wounds and brain tissue injuries and not on other injuries to internal organs (Beneke 1972).

10.1 Vitality of an Injury or Skin Wound

In forensic medicine, histomorphological findings which prove that an injury has been inflicted during life are of interest. This implies that certain changes cannot be inflicted postmortem. In this context, the following have been investigated (according to Betz 1996a):

- The excretion of fibrin, which begins almost immediately following injury but which can also be observed postmortem.
- Thrombocyte aggregates, which are difficult to recognize and can also occur in the early postmortem phase.
- A massive mast cell discharge can be observed after approximately 2–4 h, while single-cell discharge can be observed earlier; however, this phenomenon is difficult to detect microscopically (Amon et al. 1996).
- Metachromasy in toluidine blue was shown to be an artifact, and extracellular PAS-positive mucopolysaccharide release sediments are of little significance, since an enrichment of proteoglycans is also possible postmortem.
- Other methods relate to longer periods of time after wound incurrence (signs of active responses of the body, such as inflammation, resorption, and wound repair processes).

Currently, conventional histology remains the basis for approximate wound age determination. Here, the focus lies on cellular reactions: the occurrence of neutrophil granulocytes, lymphocytes, macrophages, and collagen fiber tissue (fibroblasts, fibrocytes). Phagocytic reactions lead to the formation of lipophages, siderophages, and erythrophages.

Traumatic internal injury to tissue must be differentiated from injury to organs as well as from skin wounds. In cases where internal injuries are associated with hemorrhage and tissue necrosis, the severity of the body's reaction can be used to determine the approximate injury age, similar to the determination of heart attack age. In the case of medical malpractice allegations where fibrinous and purulent peritonitises have been overlooked in a postoperative setting or diagnosed too late, the age of peritonitis is of interest.

The same approach applies to skin wounds, but the degree of re-epidermalization of the skin surface, the formation of an intact basal membrane, and the reaction of skin appendages may provide further insights (Pierce et al. 1994; Ortonne et al. 1981).

Since the 1960s, enzyme histochemical investigations into the role of different enzymes in determining wound age have been conducted (Raekallio 1976), followed by the biochemical determination of serotonin and histamine in wound margins (Berg and Bonte 1971; Berg et al. 1968). Immunohistochemical diagnostics opened up new opportunities in determining wound age by identifying growth factors and cytokines, as well as cellular and extracellular proteins such as various forms of extracellular collagen (Betz et al. 1992a, b, c, d, 1993a, b; ten Dijke and Iwata 1989; Eisenmenger et al. 1988).

Forensic cytological diagnosis may be helpful in determining the posttraumatic survival time. Here, the quantity and quality of cellular reactions to an injury or wound are taken into consideration, e.g., the mast cell reactivity at the margin of human skin wounds as early cell marker of wound survival (Oehmichen et al. 2009). However, cellular reactions of blood cells do not occur simultaneously. Erythrophagia preceded by hemorrhage and siderin formation both occur in the brain after approximately 70 h (Oehmichen and Raff 1980); erythrophagia was observed in the lungs after 30 min, and siderin was detected after 17 h (Oehmichen 1984). A clear cellular reaction was seen after survival times of approximately 1 h following compression trauma to the neck (Maxeiner 1987) (see Chap. 3).

Due to the large number of influencing factors, specifying wound age on the basis of conventional histological investigations alone should be treated with reserve. In some cases, it is possible to narrow down wound age further by means of conventional staining. Initially, however, indications relating to wound age should be restricted to the periods of time mentioned in Table 10.3.

In individual cases, it is possible to further narrow down wound age, sometimes by making use of enzyme histochemical and immunohistochemical investigations. With representative samples that have been appropriately obtained but show no wound healing reaction, reliable statements on vitality or wound age are not possible.

10.2 Wound Age in the Case of Tissue Injuries

Chronological histopathological alterations characterize the different phases of wound healing and can be applied to wound age determination; however, the cellular repair reaction is particularly dependent on the extent of the injury. Neutrophils are initially recruited at the injury site, followed by macrophages, according to the post-infliction interval. In general, many biological reactions are of importance in the wound healing process:

- Degenerative changes to injured cells (e.g., muscle cells)
- Local reaction of the blood circulation
- Reactions of noninjured parenchyma
- Presence of necrosis or fatty degeneration of damaged cells
- Appearance of polymorphic nucleated leukocytes
- Appearance of iron pigment
- Changes in the size of nuclei
- Mitoses in parenchymatous and connective tissue cells in proximity to the injury, indicating proliferation
- Appearance of newly formed mucopolysaccharides, collagen, and elastic fibers

It is impossible to use only one of these histological criteria. As many criteria as possible

Table 10.3 Possible terminological statements on vitality and indicative time specifications on the approximate wound age based on conventional histological staining of appropriately obtained tissue samples

Statement	Histological findings
Wound incurred shortly before or after death	Wound without indication of an active immune reaction or active wound healing: no conclusion as to vitality or wound age possible
Vital wound, i.e., inflicted during lifetime	Signs of an active immune reaction, in particular invasion of neutrophil granulocytes (so-called capturing, first contact between the endothelium and neutrophil granulocytes, induced by selectins, integrins; Zarbock and Ley 2008), invading macrophages, and fibroblasts
	Hemorrhage, fibrin deposition, and thrombocyte aggregates alone are not sufficient to assume a vital injury; this also applies to detectable peripheral hyperemia (supposedly reactive) at the wound margin
Fresh vital injury (hours to a few days)	Clear signs of a body reaction with invasion of neutrophil granulocytes and signs of an early wound repair process: macrophages, fibroblasts, branched capillary blood vessels, siderin deposits, and polynuclear foreign-body giant cells. Fibrin deposition and thrombocyte aggregates alone do not permit a reliable statement on wound age
Vital wound, no longer fresh (few days to weeks, in the single-digit range)	Signs of resorption and wound repair spreading from the wound margin to the deep recesses of the wound, clear collagen fiber tissue (fibroblasts, fibrocytes), invading macrophages and lymphocytes, hemosiderin pigment-laden macrophages, polynuclear foreign-body giant cells, granulation tissue with endothelially coated capillary blood vessels, scarred areas with few cells
Vital injury, not very old (weeks to months)	Repaired wound with scar tissue, partly vascularized containing loosely spread lymphocytes and macrophages
Vital, old, healed injury (many months to years)	Dense collagen scar tissue without leukocytes, no or few embedded blood vessels, residual siderin pigment deposits; basophilic calcium salt deposits can occur in old and dense bradytrophic scar tissue

Considerable intra- and interindividual variations possible

must be compared and correlated with the conditions under which the injury was inflicted (Beneke 1972).

Contrary to previous expectations, the determination of enzyme histochemical reactions has met with only limited acceptance in forensic practice. Age determination of injuries is still primarily performed with conventional histological staining methods; this includes injuries to subcutaneous soft tissue as well as to deeper muscles. Injury to internal organs as well as skin wounds must be considered separately.

The chronology of the healing process of injuries has been described histopathologically by means of conventional histological staining methods as well as enzyme histochemical and immunohistochemical reactions. The results gained in this way enable an approximate classification of injuries in time. Information given in the literature on conventional age determination of injuries is listed in Table 10.4. In view of the abovementioned rationale, the specification of wound age should be treated with reserve, however, and should be limited to the periods of time mentioned in Table 10.3.

Many other investigations deal with age determination of injuries, and new insights are frequently gained from animal experiments (Yu et al. 2010). Otherwise, studies have shown that bruises in children were present for at least 30 h without a leucocyte infiltrate (Byard et al. 2008).

10.2.1 Invasion of Granulocytes

The fact that the invasion of granulocytes is the hallmark of an early cellular wound reaction is widely acknowledged. Although overall conditions must be considered, a very fresh injury can be assumed in the case of completely areactive

Table 10.4 Chronology of injury healing

Time following injury	Histological findings and enzyme histochemical reactions
<20 min–1 h	Hemorrhage with destroyed tissue and cells but with no cellular reaction, in particular no signs of granulocytic invasion
<1 h	Neutrophil granulocytes, partly marginalized at the inner vascular wall, partly amoeboid migration into the tissue
1 h	Fresh hemorrhage, tissue edema, local acidosis, single polymorphonuclear leukocytes, evidence of ATPase, unspecific esterase, aminopeptidase, increased histamine, serotonin, α-esterases
2 h	Degranulation of mast cells, infiltration of polymorphonuclear leukocytes, fiber necrosis, ground substance segregation, extracellular activation of fermentation—glucosidase, monoamine oxidase
2–4 h	Invasion of monocytic cells, phagocytic reactions
4–6 h	Peripherally increasing reactive hyperemia, fibrin deposition, peripheral formation of a leukocyte wall, also involving granulocytes
6–8 h	Necrobiosis of cells and tissue, pronounced inflammatory demarcation, increasing phagocytosis
8–12 h	Increase in and further activation of mononuclear cells and histiocytes, invasion of single macrophages, evidence of alkaline phosphatase, cytochrome oxidase, and phosphorylases
12–16 h	Gradually, mononuclear cells predominate, leukocyte decomposition
16–32 h	Mobilized histiocytic cell elements, formation of collagen fibers with fibroblasts and fibrocytes, angioneogenesis with first branched capillary blood vessels
32–72 h	Formation of granulation tissue with collagen fiber tissue and capillary blood vessels, embedded macrophages (siderophages, lipophages)
3–4 days	Ground substance formation, denser collagen fiber tissue, potential decrease in the number of macrophages, new formation of mast cells, possibly polynuclear foreign-body giant cells
4–10 days	Decrease of histochemical reactions in collagen fiber tissue, densification of scar tissue, decrease in the number of leukocytes and macrophages, possible persistence of siderophages
>10 days	Denser scar tissue with fewer cells, decreasing vascularization, potential persistence of siderin deposits; after a very long time, basophilic calcium salt deposits are also possible

Modified according to Janssen (1977)
Considerable variations or deviations are possible

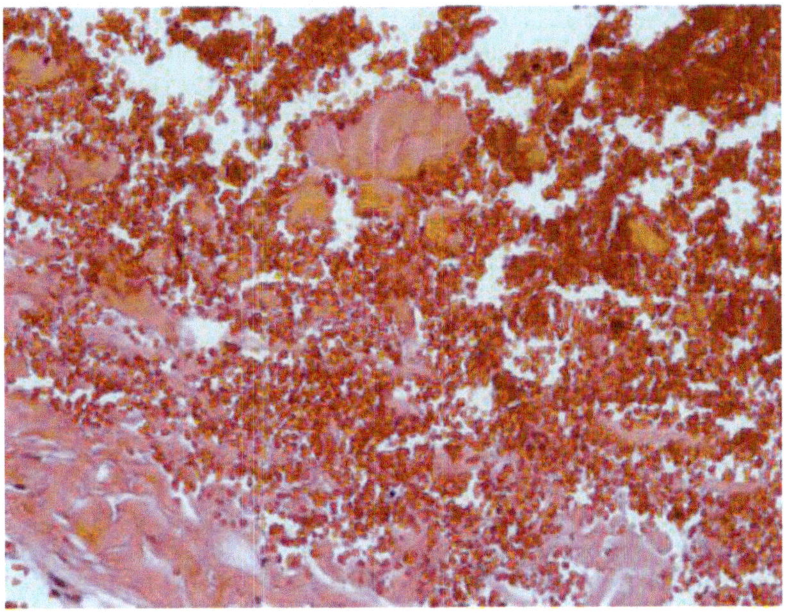

Fig. 10.1 Fresh areactive hemorrhage in soft tissue without any sign of granulocyte invasion despite cell and tissue destruction after a survival time of approximately 10 min (H&E ×200)

hemorrhage in the tissue, in particular when signs of granulocyte invasion are absent despite histologically visible cell and tissue destruction (Fig. 10.1).

Granulocytes can be clearly seen in H&E staining; however, a more specific granulocyte stain may be useful. A marginalization of granulocytes on the endothelium of the inner vascular wall (Tannenberg margination) can be seen, as well as invading granulocytes in the wound margin. However, uninjured tissue can also show increased numbers of granulocytes at the wound margin, which invaded through endothelial gaps due to amoeboid migration (Fig. 10.2). This process is controlled by chemotactic stimuli in the wound region (denatured proteins, lymphokines, leukotrienes, thromboxanes, etc.) (Helpap 1987). A marginalization of granulocytes on the endothelium of the inner vascular wall has been described in the literature (Walcher 1936). Frequently, however, it is not possible to differentiate this marginalization from an artificial accumulation of cells or a hypostatic phenomenon. For this reason, these findings alone may not be useful (Betz 1996a; Berg 1972, 1975). It should be noted that statements in the literature on the time of the first occurrence of granulocytes vary

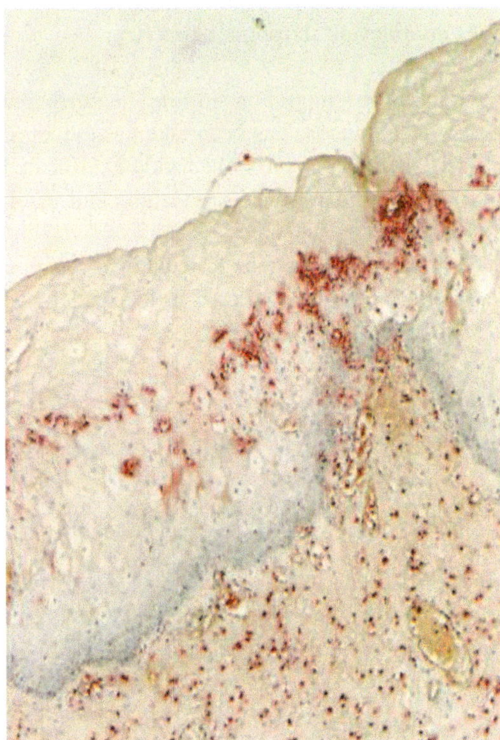

Fig. 10.2 Abundant intra- and extravascular neutrophil granulocytes in the nonkeratinizing squamous epithelium of the upper lip and subepithelial soft tissue following laceration from a blow; reported survival time, 4–6 h (ASD ×40)

considerably, from 10 min up to over 12 h (Betz 1996b). Interobserver variability undoubtedly plays a role here, but the varying results also show that interpretation of microscopic findings in regard to wound age must be treated with reserve. Evidence of an invasion of granulocytes is crucial, i.e., granulocytes should be proven outside the vascular lumen and distal from hemorrhage. The detection of at least three to four granulocytes is required (Janssen 1977); other authors assume extravascular granulocytes to be evidence of vitality and a reaction initiation (Oehmichen 1990a). In cases where numerous granulocytes occur in the tissue of the wound margin, it can be safely assumed that the injury was inflicted during life and that the person survived for only a short time (Fig. 10.3). Including the number of granulocytes to estimate the approximate wound age has to be treated with reserve but can be taken as an indication. The following indications are relevant in forensic practice:

- Granulocyte migration in the hemorrhagic laryngeal mucosa has been taken as evidence of vitality if a person choked and/or suffocated to death (Maxeiner 1987; Oehmichen et al. 1987).
- Following stab wounds, a leukocyte reaction has been described after 6 h due to delayed wound healing (Berg 1975).
- Thermal injuries may cause more delayed wound healing than mechanical injuries (Helpap and Cremer 1972).

As with conventional histological methods, immunohistochemical staining methods enable potential differentiation between acute and chronic inflammation (Abe et al. 1996).

10.2.2 Occurrence of Macrophages

Macrophages are transformed monocytes or histiocytes and have a partly peripheral round to oval cell nucleus and vacuolar cytoplasm. Microscopic evidence in H&E staining, however, requires experience with respect to cellular differentiation. During the initial wound repair process, macrophages appear later in the wound margin than neutrophil granulocytes and are considerably involved in cellular histiocytic reactions by means of phagocytosis of denatured proteins or necrotic tissue (Leibovich and Wiseman 1988). The transformed monocytes migrate—frequently together with lymphocytes—into the wound region and act as phagocytic macrophages. Since phagocytic substances are of different origin, the following types of phagocytes can be differentiated: lipophages, siderophages, and erythrophages. If polynuclear cells generate following phagocytosis of nonde-

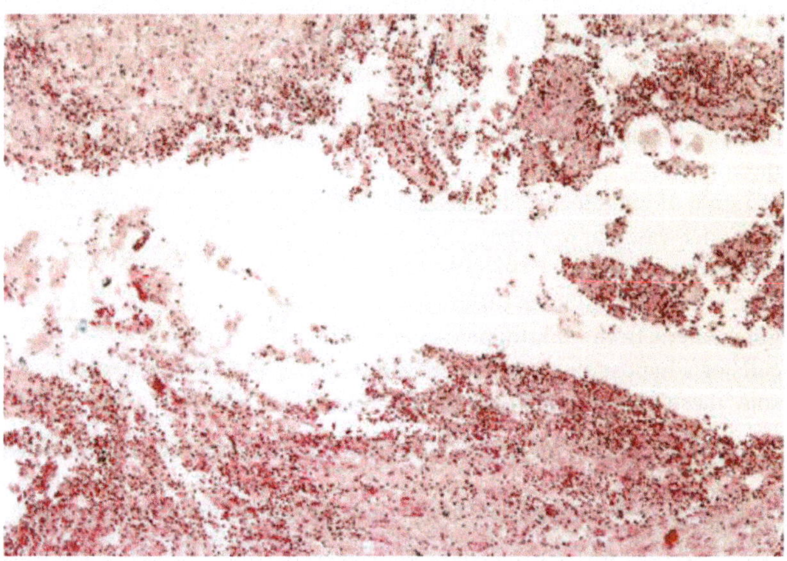

Fig. 10.3 Stab wound track with intense enzyme histochemical granulocytic infiltration along the stab wound wall as evidence of vitality and short-term survival of the stab wound (ASD ×100)

gradable foreign material, the occurrence of these polynuclear foreign-body giant cells must also be considered. In specific cases, birefringent foreign material with polarization effects may be detectable.

Reports on the first occurrence of macrophages vary between 2 and 7–9 h, while other reports give time periods of 12–16 or 16–24 h before enough cells are present for reliable evidence. In order to explain the different time periods, methodological aspects must be considered, as well as an increased interobserver variability in conventional staining.

10.2.3 Granulation Tissue Formation

Following macrophage invasion to the injured tissue, fibroblast migration can be observed (Radzun 1996; Betz et al. 1992c; Ross 1968), as well as migration of fibrocytes and angiocytes with formation of initially loose and later dense collagen fiber tissue (Willems et al. 1996; Müller and Brinckmann 1996). Capillary endothelial blood vessels are often embedded herein (Joseph-Silverstein and Rifkin 1990), which leads to the formation of granulation tissue. Frequently, lymphocytes, monocytes, and scant granulocytes with differential spreading can be seen, decreasing gradually in number with increasing scar formation. Capillarization of collagen fiber tissue also decreases until ultimately a dense scar tissue with few cells has been formed. Siderophages, however, can be found in scar tissue for a long time. Conventional histological staining methods (H&E, EvG, Prussian blue) help to further narrow down the age of granulation tissue to fresh or no longer fresh and older, almost scarred granulation tissue. The density of fiber tissue is important, as well as the number of branched capillaries and the intensity of cellular infiltration. As soon as the granulation tissue has been completely transformed into dystrophic scar tissue, hyalinized areas with few cells can be seen, which are sparsely vascularized and contain, at most, siderophages or siderin deposits. Over an extended period of time (years), dystrophic basophilic calcium salt deposits may occur in scar tissues.

10.2.4 Inflammation Age in the Case of Fibrinous and Purulent Peritonitis, Pleurisy, and Pericarditis

In the case of medical malpractice allegations with a fibrinous and purulent peritonitis diagnosed too late, the age of the peritonitis may be of interest. Usually, fibrinous and purulent peritonitises have a point of origination, and the inflammation gradually spreads into the abdomen until a so-called four-quadrant peritonitis occurs. As a result, areas with older peritonitis, adjacent to areas with fresher, predominantly fibrinous peritonitis, may also occur. The older areas are considered to be in the vicinity of the origination point of the inflammation, such as intestinal perforation. In specific cases, tissue samples from this location should be examined, as well as samples from the remaining sections of the peritoneum. To my knowledge, no systematic histological and immunohistochemical age determinations of peritonitis have been performed. Statements on the age of a fibrinous and purulent peritonitis would only be possible if the fibrin layers showed signs of wound repair on the peritoneum (missing mesothelial cell boundaries, fibroblast activation, granulation tissue, etc.). Even then, it may not be possible to exclude the microscopic detection of a local, postoperative "physiological" peritonitis caused by previous medical treatment. For this reason, reliable microscopic diagnostics for the age determination of fibrinous and purulent peritonitis are not yet possible. Thus, when statements on the age of peritonitis are made, they must be based on various criteria, in particular on clinical data. This also applies to the age determination of fibrinous pleurisy. In the case of fibrinous pericarditis, indicative statements on inflammation age are more likely to be made, since the fibrinous inflammation process spreads relatively quickly over an anatomically limited area. Thus, a similar reaction of the inflammation repair process is also expected at different localizations. Microscopic evaluation using conventional histological staining is restricted to the classifications "fresh," "not fresh," and "old." In the case of fresh fibrinous inflammation (hours to several days), villiform fibrin components can be seen on the surface, sometimes with still fresh signs of the repair process, as well as a leukocytic inflammatory infiltrate (Fig. 10.4a). Inflammatory processes that are no longer fresh show a smoother surface and signs of fibrous organization with migrated fibrocytes, fibroblasts, branched capillary blood vessels, and macrophages, potentially also siderophages. The inflammatory infiltrate is already loosened (Fig. 10.4b). Older epicarditis in the process of healing and lacking inflammation but with post-inflammatory collagen fiber tissue shows a completely smooth surface and capillary vascularization (Fig. 10.4c).

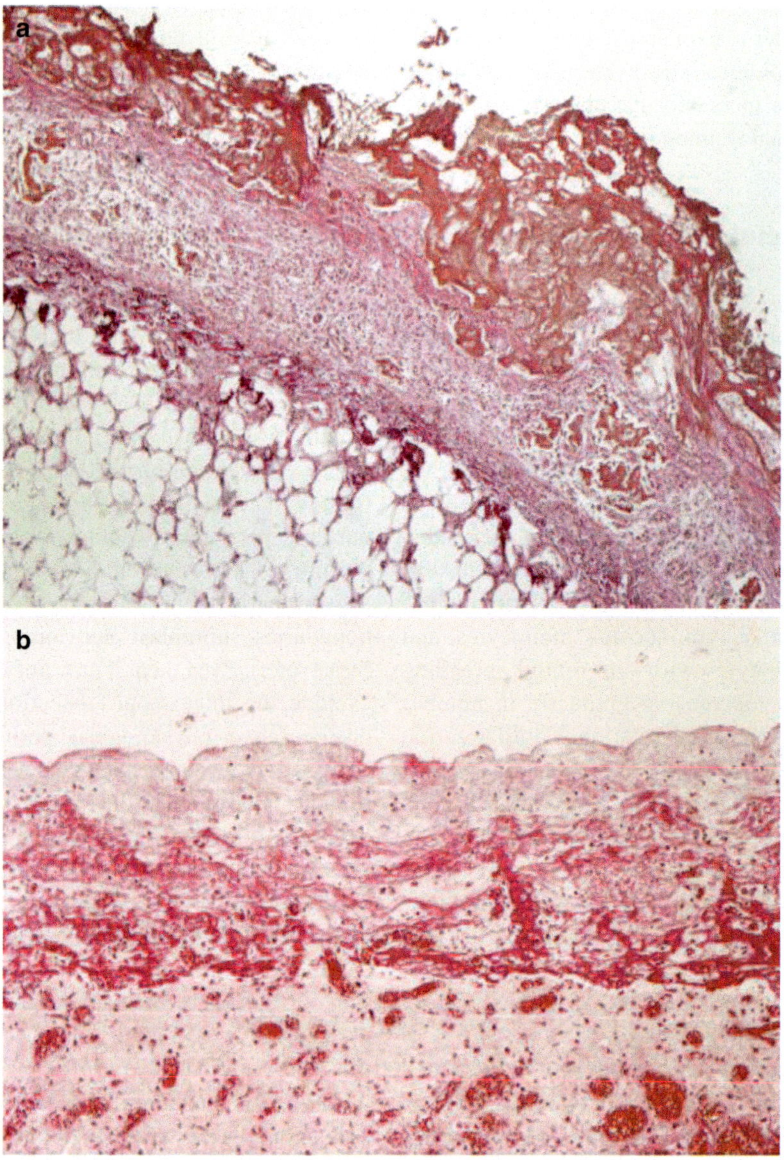

Fig. 10.4 (**a**) Fibrinous epicarditis and pericarditis (several days old) with villiform fibrin strings on the epicardium, few branched capillary blood vessels, signs of fibrous organization, and a relatively dense lymphomonocytic inflammatory infiltrate in the area between subepicardial fat tissue and fibrinous villi (Elastica van Gieson ×200). (**b**) Fibrinous pleurisy, no longer fresh, with an already smooth surface and remaining residuals of fibrin components in the repair process, as well as loosely spread lymphocytes and histiocytes (H&E ×200). (**c**) Older and largely organized and healed epicarditis (H&E ×40)

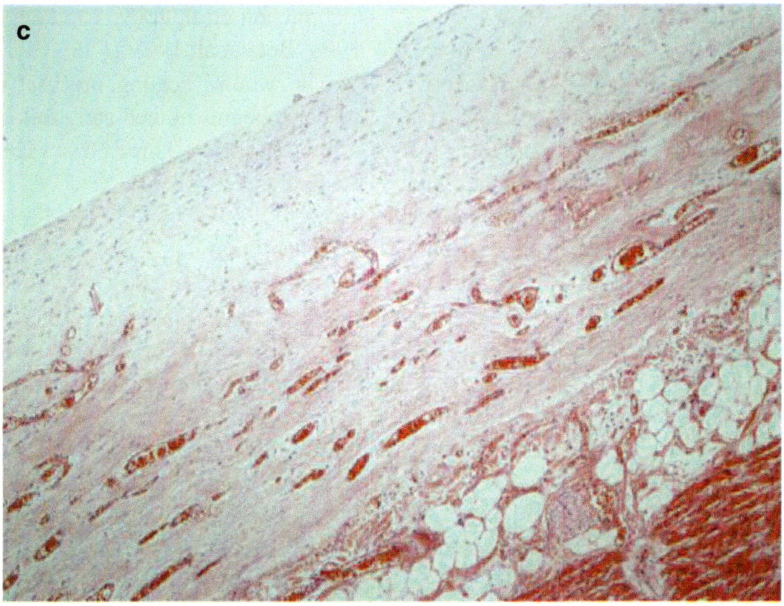

Fig. 10.4 (continued)

10.2.5 Injury Age of Muscle Trauma

Posttraumatic damage to the fiber texture of skeletal muscle fibers with long fibrillar structures can be detected posttraumatically after approximately 30 min at 1100× magnification. Shortly after trauma, findings such as changes in hypercontraction bands and rupture zones can be detected with electron microscopy (Fechner et al. 1990, 1991; Fechner 1995).

Following muscle trauma, an accumulation of muscle proteins (e.g., actin, myosin, desmin, myoglobin) and non-muscle proteins (e.g., fibrin, fibrinogen, fibronectin) occurs within the first hour. At 1 h posttrauma, necrosis factor C5b-9(m) can be determined (Fechner 1995). For further information on vitality determination of skeletal muscle trauma, see Chap. 3. An animal model showed that the expression of MyoD and Pax7 in injured skeletal muscle can be detected depending on the age of the wound (Tian et al. 2016); the expression of troponin I mRNA in contused skeletal muscle appears to be less helpful (Sun et al. 2010). However, when interpreting histological findings in skeletal muscles obtained using light microscopy, it is important to bear in mind that artifacts inflicted postmortem can be erroneously interpreted as vital injuries. Evidently, artifacts of this kind can be caused in particular during the supravital postmortem phase, e.g., by external blunt trauma to the muscles. In these cases, one sees findings such as muscle destruction, loss of muscle fiber integrity, invagination, and contraction bands (Henssge et al. 2002). Analysis of this kind reveals a fundamental weak point in investigations to date on the vitality and age of skin lesions or tissue injury. There are no comparative studies on impacts, skin lesions, and tissue damage not inflicted until the early postmortem interval in a targeted manner. Without this type of investigation, the question arises in some cases of whether a suspected vital, i.e., antemortem, injury could possibly be attributed to an early postmortem effect. For example, contusions to the subcutaneous upper arm muscles suspected of having occurred antemortem could also have been caused by vigorous gripping of the upper arms during transportation of the body.

10.3 Skin Wounds

There are numerous investigations on the chronology of the skin wound healing process. Many studies have been published in nonforensic journals. Particularly in the early posttraumatic interval, conventional histological age determination of skin wounds, including iatrogenic injections (Schollmeyer 1965), is not reliable. Immunohistochemical findings show overall tendencies, but there is a lack of certainty in regard to:

- The number of skin tissue samples that should be investigated.
- The selection of immunohistochemical markers to be investigated.
- The influence of individual or constitutional factors on the injured person.
- Evaluating the significance of other influencing factors, such as temperature, humidity, or postmortem changes (Maxeiner 1994).
- In connection with microscopic age determination of skin wounds for the detection of endogenous and exogenous influencing factors, it is sometimes forgotten that uninjured skin in the relevant body region must also be investigated, above all to exclude the effect of wound location as well as inter- and intraindividual differences.
- Autolytic or putrefactive changes to the skin can show—depending on the postmortem interval—different immunohistochemical findings (Betz et al. 1993e).

Although immunohistochemical wound age determination of skin wounds can provide reproducible results in clinical settings (animal experiments: Kondo and Ohshima 1996b; Murakami et al. 1989; Ordmann and Gillmann 1966), results are not transferable to human skin wounds or to the reliability requirements in criminal proceedings (Bai et al. 2008).

However, histological and immunohistochemical investigations of skin wounds can provide indicative results and can be helpful both in determining the vitality of an injury and in reconstructing the chronology in combination with other information (Fronczek et al. 2015a, b; Oehmichen et al. 2009; Ishida et al. 2009; Betz 1994; Betz et al. 1993f).

The wound healing process, including skin wounds, begins immediately following the infliction of an injury. Three phases can be differentiated here:

- Inflammation
- Proliferation
- Maturation

During the inflammatory phase, an aggregation of thrombocytes can be seen, followed by an infiltration of leukocytes with participation of neutrophil granulocytes, macrophages, and T-lymphocytes, originating from the wound margins or wound base. Next, re-epithelization or re-epidermization is initiated on the surface, and the wound will be closed by newly formed granulation tissue with fibroblasts, fibrocytes, and endothelially coated capillary blood vessels. Angiogenesis is indispensable for sustaining granulation tissue. Many cytokines, growth factors, proteases, etc. are closely involved in the wound healing process (Singer and Clark 1999; Martin 1997; Amberg 1996). As a rule, the first siderophages in the wound region cannot be expected before the 3rd day postinjury. However, single siderophages can be seen earlier (Betz and Eisenmenger 1996). In the case of intravital blunt injuries, an enzyme histochemical positive α-naphthyl-esterase reaction can be detected in human skin, even with very short survival times. An increasing interval of 15–30 min until death shows a stronger and more obvious reaction failure compared to more immediate fatal skin injuries (animal experiments and autopsy material; Pioch 1969). According to investigations by Oehmichen et al. (1989), in the case of intravital skin injuries, immunohistochemically detected proteinase inhibitors can show an enrichment in the corium parallel to the wound surface. Investigations into wound age of iatrogenic skin punctures due to syringe needles resulted in the chronology presented in Table 10.5.

It is important to note that in immunohistochemical diagnostics, positive and negative controls must be processed along with the section to

Table 10.5 Chronology of the skin wound healing process with conventional histological staining in the case of iatrogenic injection punctures

Time	Histological findings
<4 h	Gaping injection channel, surrounding hemorrhage, scant early cellular infiltration
6 h	Stronger leukocyte infiltration with leukocytes, lymphocytes, macrophages, fibroblasts; a clot closes the wound; degenerative changes in the epidermis next to the wound margins
8–16 h	Injection channel largely closed, a clot seals the injection channel on the outside
Circa 24 h	Stronger cellular infiltration; demarcation of the clot with inflammatory cells, producing a bowl-like appearance
Circa 36 h	The "bowl" is included in the clot, which now exceeds skin level; division of epidermis at the germinal layer
Circa 48 h	Formation of epithelial tissue beneath separated epidermis, termed definite epithelium; an upper and lower epidermis develops
Circa 72 h	Gradual degeneration of cellular infiltration in the injection channel
72–96 h	Early detachment of the clot with "bowl," including upper and lower epidermis
120–124 h	Clot rejection, sparse cellular infiltrates
>124 h	Earliest possibility of total recovery, epidermis at skin level

According to Schollmeyer (1965)

be investigated. The following include observations on some immunohistochemical markers:

Collagen Various subtypes of collagen replace necrotic tissue by forming a netlike structure with embedded fibroblasts. The formation of the collagen fiber net takes some time, i.e., collagen subtypes can be proven immunohistochemically after 2–4 days (Betz et al. 1993c, d). A quantification of collagen types I and II in histological paraffin sections has also been described (Ogbuihi et al. 1988).

Fibronectin Fibronectin, as a cell adhesion protein, is integrated in the wound healing process and involved in the adhesion of fibroblasts, keratinocytes, and endothelial cells. Only a few minutes after wound infliction, fibronectin can be detected immunohistochemically (Betz et al. 1992b). However, according to investigations in porcine skin, postmortem wound infliction can also lead to the detection of fibronectin (Grellner et al. 1998; Kondo and Ohshima 1996a). A wound age probability scoring system, based on the immunohistochemical expression levels of fibronectin, CD62p, and factor VIII in wound hemorrhage, was developed (van de Goot et al. 2014).

Adhesion Molecules The migration of leukocytes via an interaction with vascular endothelial cells is controlled via adhesion molecules, which include P-selectin, E-selectin, the intercellular adhesion molecule (ICAM)-1, and the vascular endothelial adhesion molecule (VCAM)-1. While P-selectin can appear already after only a few minutes, other adhesion molecules are not detectable immunohistochemically until after 1–3 h (Dreßler et al. 1997a, b, 1999a, b).

In terms of wound age determination, information gained not from only the earliest detection of all immunohistochemical markers is relevant, but also the duration of detection and the longest detection period are relevant, since some markers can disappear relatively quickly, some after only hours (Table 10.6).

Other authors, who investigated the time-dependent detection of transforming growth factors (TGF-α and TGF-β1), came to different conclusions (Kekow and Gross 1996; Grellner et al. 2005). Numerous other immunohistochemical markers have been used to determine wound age, including MRP8, MRP14, defensin, α1-chymotrypsin, α2-macroglobulin, and lysozyme (Fieguth et al. 1994, 2003), but also IL1β, IL-6, and TNF-α (Grellner 2002; Grellner et al. 2000), VEGF (Hayashi et al. 2004) as well as ubiquitin (Kondo et al. 2002) and apoptosis-related factors in cell signaling during incised skin wound healing in mice (Zhao et al. 2009).

Table 10.6 Immunohistochemical markers and earliest appearance

Marker	Earliest appearance after infliction	Reference
CD 14	1–5 days	Yagi et al. (2016)
Collagen I	4–6 days	Betz et al. (1993a, 1995) and Betz (1996b)
Collagen III	2–3 days	Betz et al. (1993b) and Betz (1996b)
Collagen IV	4 days	Betz et al. (1992a, d)
Collagen V	3 days	Betz et al. (1993b) and Betz (1996b)
Collagen VI	3 days	Betz et al. (1993a) and Betz (1996b)
Collagen VII	4 days	Betz et al. (1992a)
Endothelial progenitor cells (EPCs)	Average number >20 = 7–12 days Average number <15 = 14–21 days	Ishida et al. (2015a, b)
Laminin in myofibroblasts	1.5–4 days	Betz et al. (1992a)
HSPG in myofibroblasts	1.5–4 days	Betz et al. (1992a)
Fibronectin	10–20 min	Betz et al. (1992b) and Betz (1996b)
α-Actin in myofibroblasts	5 days	
Laminin—basement membrane components	4–8 days	Betz (1996b)
MMP-2$^+$ macrophages	Semiquantitative >20 = 7–12 days	Ishida et al. (2015a, b)
MMP-9$^+$ macrophages	Semiquantitative >30 = 3–14 days	Ishida et al. (2015a, b)
P-selectin	Several minutes–7 h	Dreßler et al. (1999a)
E-selectin	1 h–17 days	Dreßler et al. (1997a, b, 1999a, b)
ICAM-1	1.5 h–3 days	Dreßler et al. (1997a, b, 1999a, b)
VCAM-1	3 h–3.5 days	Dreßler et al. (1997a, b, 1999a, b)
TGF-α	Circa 10 min	Grellner et al. (2005)
TGF-β1	Several minutes	Grellner et al. (2005)
SMC-actin	5 days	Betz (1995a)
Keratin 5—complete staining of basal cell layer	13 days	Betz et al. (1993b) and Betz (1995b)

Modified and supplemented by Kondo (2007), selection; in detail: Cecchi (2010)
Collagen IV and VII, laminin, and heparin soleplate proteoglycan (HSPG) are basement membrane components

The occurrence of apoptotic keratinocytes in skin wounds from a wound age of around 120 min has also been described, whereas noninjured skin controls were negative for apoptosis (Suárez-Penarada et al. 2002). It was also possible to demonstrate in a murine model the benefit of immunohistochemical wound age determination for an interval of up to 24 h using numerous immunohistochemical markers [E-selectin, P-selectin, fibronectin, interleukin 1 alpha, transforming growth factor beta 1 (TGF-ß1), collagen I and II, vascular endothelial growth factor (VEGF)] (Kara et al. 2016). A number of studies report an increased number of immunohistochemically marked cells depending on wound age, meaning a minimum wound age can be inferred from a particular cell count, e.g., of matrix metalloproteinase-2 (MMP-2) and MMP-9 (see Table 10.6) (Ishida et al. 2015a, b). Although the first occurrence of a series of immunohistochemically detectable markers following an injury can be well determined, there is less (reliable) information on the last detectable point in time of wound healing. Some studies noted that, following increased expression of immunohistochemical markers over a certain time period, a decline was observed with increasing wound age, e.g., of endothelial progenitor cells (EPCs) in human skin injuries (Ishida et al. 2015a, b). Individual studies refer to the phenomenon of "autophagy" as a marker for a vital wound reaction (Kimura et al. 2015) or the use of fibronectin and P-selectin expression as a vitality marker (Capatina et al. 2013)—not, however, for wound age determination. Other murine models have been used to investigate wound healing and determine the time-dependent expression and distribution of monoacylglycerol lipase in skin wounds (Ma et al. 2011). Immunohistochemical investigation of aquaporin AQP1 and AQP3 was performed in human skin wounds obtained from forensic autopsy cases to support the accuracy of wound age determination (Ishida et al. 2017).

When interpreting immunohistochemical findings, the relationship between positive and negative reactions within the tissue sections can also be used to draw conclusions on wound age (Hausmann et al. 1998). Finally, the interpretation of immunohistochemical staining can also differentiate between injured and uninjured skin (Betz et al. 1992a, b, 1993d). Currently, immunohistochemical age diagnostics of skin wounds combined with the use of immunohistochemical markers only enables reliable conclusions in the case of wounds that are no longer fresh (older than 30 h)—with 95% probability. Reliable immunohistochemical wound age determination for the early posttraumatic interval has not been established as yet. This does not preclude, however, that immunohistochemical findings may have an important indicative significance for wound age determination in specific cases.

To date, the most useful methods for age determination of skin wounds with a survival time of a few days include the detection of hemosiderin and the immunohistochemical localization of different collagen subtypes (Betz et al. 1992d; Eisenmenger et al. 1988; Betz and Eisenmenger 1996). However, in all forensic medical cases, the use of histological techniques can be limited by autolytic decomposition of morphological structures. Immunohistochemistry, in particular, has been assumed to be relatively sensitive to tissue decay due to decomposition of the relevant antigens, whereas enzyme histochemistry of the skin is characterized by considerable resistance to putrefaction. In skin already showing microscopic alteration of the tissue structure, fibronectin and collagen type III could not be reliably localized. The distribution of laminin and cytokeratin 5, however, was well preserved (Betz et al. 1993e).

Differentiation of Vital Skin Wounds from Postmortem Injuries When evaluating the vitality of an injury, immunohistochemical diagnosis can provide reliable information, in particular by examining endothelial adhesion molecules. For further specific information, please refer to the relevant literature.

If, according to conventional histology, an evaluation of the vitality of skin wounds is not possible, or if the result requires confirmation by means of further investigations, immunohistochemical markers can be helpful. Clear endothelial expression of P- and E-selectin can be detected in vital skin wounds, while no or minimal expression of this marker can be seen in postmortem injuries (Dreßler et al. 1999a). An autolytic postmortem degradation of P- and E-selectin, as well as VCAM-1, is barely visible (Dreßler et al. 1999b; Grellner et al. 1997). However, the point in time of the latest possible antigen detection times must be taken into consideration. Further immunohistochemical markers for evaluating vitality, as mentioned in Table 10.6, can be used to determine whether an injury was inflicted during life or not. The same markers, also in combination, only allow for probability statements with respect to wound age determination.

A progressive increase in TNF-alpha-containing mast cell numbers was found 1 h after trauma in skin lesions, while samples from postmortem lesions had significantly fewer mast cells and fewer TNF-alpha-positive cells (Bacci et al. 2006).

10.4 Bone Fractures and Fracture Healing

A fracture is a complete or incomplete disruption of bone tissue continuity. In addition to primary fracture healing without callus formation, a fracture triggers a regular tissue reaction with the aim of restoring bone continuity (Klotzbach et al. 2003; Table 10.7). Although fracture healing depends on the age of the individual and their nutritional status, age does not play an important role once adulthood has been reached. Rib fractures may be associated with non-accidental injury (NAI) in infancy (Weber et al. 2009). The histological finding can demonstrate particular features in fractures following blast trauma such

Table 10.7 Stages of fracture healing

Time frame	Histological findings
1 day	Hematoma and traumatic inflammation: acute hemorrhage at the point of fracture secondary to vessel rupture, formation of a fusiform hematoma surrounding and joining the ends of the bone
1–2 days	Organization: fibrin is deposited in the hematoma, an inflammatory response with edema is seen, continuing fibrin deposition, accumulation of large numbers of polymorphonuclear cells
2–3 days	Appearance of fibroblasts, mesenchymal cells, gradual development of granulation tissue; necrosis of the bone adjacent to the fracture becomes evident; empty lacunar spaces due to death of osteocytes; clear line between dead bone (empty lacunae) and live bone
3–6 days	Provisional fibrous callus (Figs. 10.5 and 10.6), originating from Periosteum Endosteum Havers channels Blood vessels in the bone marrow space and musculature
	After approximately 3 days, the devitalized bone fragments begin to be reabsorbed
	The periosteum is composed of an outer fibrous layer and an inner osteogenic layer: marked proliferation of the cells in the deep layer of the periosteum and the cells of the endosteum
7–14 days	Provisional bony callus (Fig. 10.7): morphology of the connective tissue cells is undergoing modification. A homogeneous osteoid matrix is being deposited between the proliferating cells. Transformation of fibrous callus into provisional bony callus: connective tissue cells form ground substance and collagen fibers; fibroblasts transform into osteoblasts and produce osteoid, the organic matrix of the bone; chondroblasts are involved; islets of cartilage develop in the fibrous stroma; bone formation, remodeling into lamellar bone (this bone forms the final callus) by means of osteoclasts and osteoblasts
2–3 weeks	Callus reaches its maximum size
3–4 weeks	Hard bony callus, bone formed from periosteal and endochondral ossification
>4 weeks	Rearrangement of callus and bony union: remodeling of the new bone from a woven appearance to mature bone; histologically, ossification and new bone can be found (Fig. 10.8)

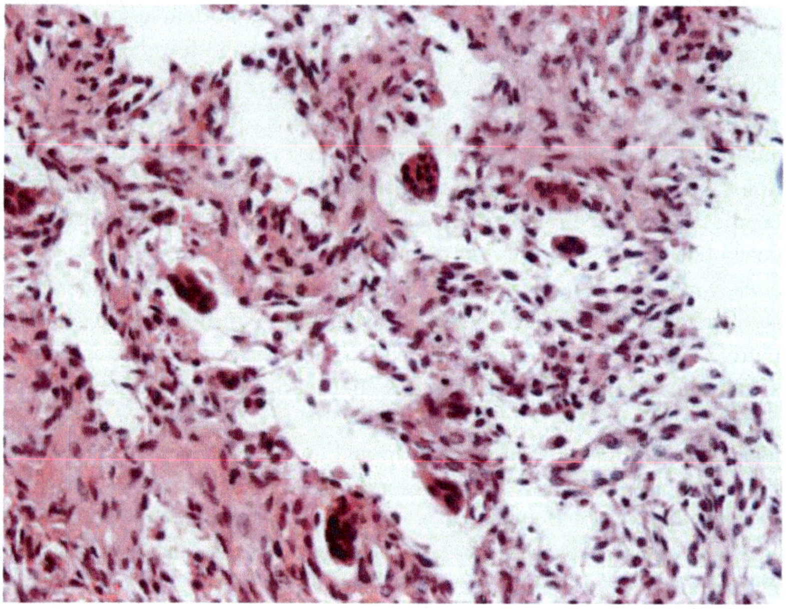

Fig. 10.5 Provisional fibrous callus with osteoblasts and fibroblasts (H&E ×200)

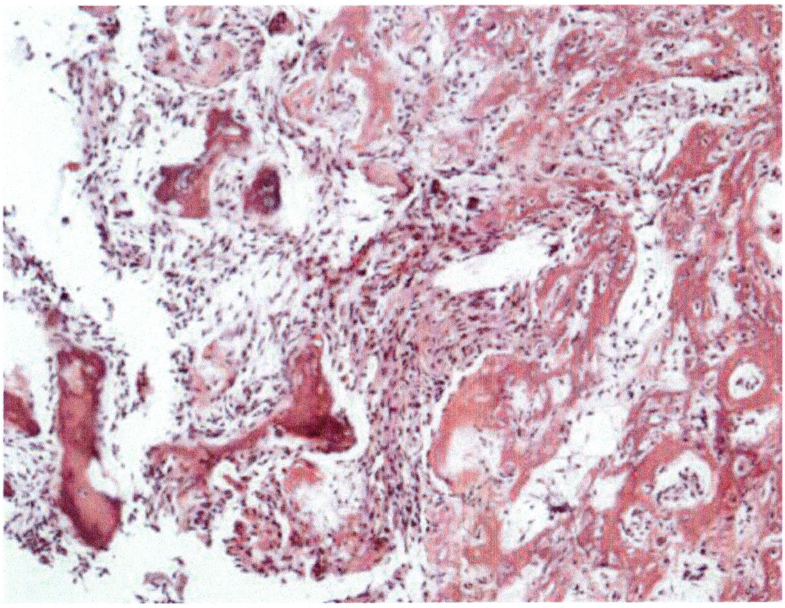

Fig. 10.6 Fracture zone with necrosis consisting of dead bone fragments (*left*) and fibrous callus with single osteoblasts (H&E ×100)

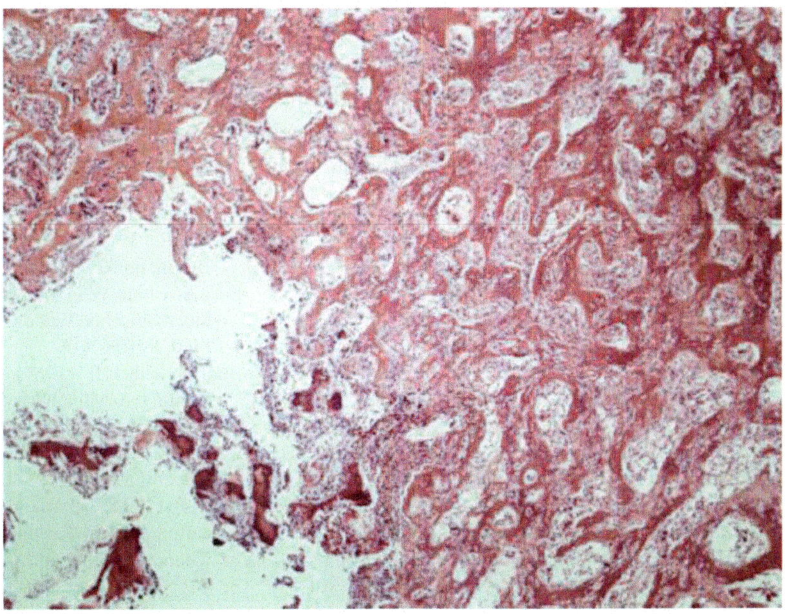

Fig. 10.7 Completed formation of a provisional bony callus with microscopic residual necrotic fragments (H&E ×40)

as fractures lines through the Haversian canal (Pechníková et al. 2015). The bone changes of vitamin D deficiency rickets have been invoked as an alternative explanation for child abuse-related fractures, but a histologic comparison shows the maturation disturbance in the growth plate that occurs in rickets is a distinctive entity that cannot be confused histologically with healing fractures, including the classical metaphyseal lesion (Kepron and Pollanen 2015; Pinsker et al. 2016; Rolvien et al. 2016).

During the stages of granulation tissue growth and early calcification of the callus, any twisting or shearing motion will lead to tissue injury. Persistence of such injury leads to the formation of large amounts of cartilage. If cartilaginous and bony calluses are replaced by more yielding fibrous tissue, once mature, it will not revert to

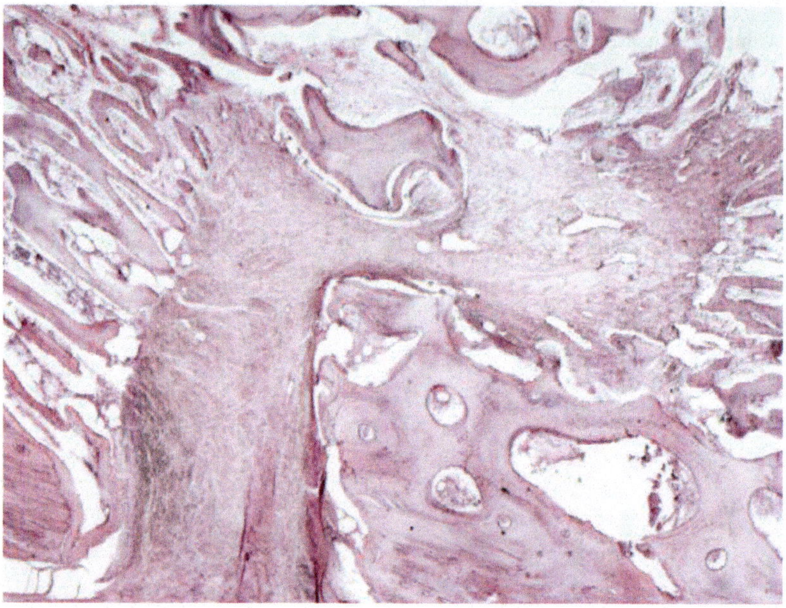

Fig. 10.8 Later in fracture healing with ossification into the fracture gap (H&E ×100)

bone. In such cases, fracture results in fibrous union, and no evidence of reparative changes remains. Occasionally, a pseudarthrosis results, and cartilage covers each fractured bone end, and an articular cavity lined by synovial membrane will be formed.

References

Abe Y, Sugisaki K, Dannenberg AM Jr (1996) Rabbit vascular endothelial adhesion molecules: ELAM 1 is most elevated in acute inflammation, whereas VCAM-1 and ICAM-1 predominate in chronic inflammation. J Leukoc Biol 60:692–703

Amberg R (1996) Time-dependent cytokine expression in cutaneous wound repair. In: Oehmichen M, Kirchner H (eds) The wound healing process – forensic pathological aspects, Research in legal medicine, vol 13. Schmidt-Römhild, Lübeck, pp 107–121

Amon U, Gibbs BF, Wolff HH (1996) Mast cells: mediators and aspects of wound healing. In: Oehmichen M, Kirchner H (eds) The wound healing process – forensic pathological aspects, Research in legal medicine, vol 13. Schmidt-Römhild, Lübeck, pp 173–202

Bacci S, Romagnoli P, Norelli GA, Forestieri AL, Bonelli A (2006) Early increase in TNF-alpha-containing mast cells in skin lesions. Int J Legal Med 120:138–142

Bai R, Wan L, Shi M (2008) The time-dependent expressions of IL-1β, COX-2, MCP-1 mRNA in skin wounds of rabbits. Forensic Sci Int 175:193–197

Beneke G (1972) Altersbestimmung von Verletzungen innerer Organe. Z Rechtsmed 71:1–16

Berg S (1972) The timing of skin wounds. Z Rechtsmed 70:121–135

Berg S (1975) Vitale Reaktionen und Zeitschätzungen. In: Mueller B (ed) Gerichtliche Medizin, vol 1. Springer, Berlin, pp 327–340

Berg S, Bonte W (1971) Praktische Erfahrungen mit der biochemischen Wundaltersbestimmung. Beitr Gerichtl Med 28:108–114

Berg S, Elbel R (1969) Altersbestimmung subcutaner Blutungen. Münch Med Wochen 111:1185–1190

Berg S, Ditt J, Friedrich D, Bonte W (1968) Möglichkeiten der biochemischen Wundaltersbestimmung. Dtsch Z Gerichtl Med 63:183–198

Betz P (1994) Histological and enzyme histochemical parameters for the age estimation of human skin wounds. Int J Legal Med 107:60–68

Betz P (1995a) Forensische Altersbestimmung menschlicher Hautwunden. In: Bratzke H, Schröter A (eds) Immunhistochemie in der Rechtsmedizin. Hänsel-Hohenhausen, Egelsbach, pp 37–100

Betz P (1995b) Immunohistochemical parameters for the age estimation of human skin wounds. Am J Forensic Med Pathol 16:203–209

Betz P (1996a) Collagen subtypes – markers for the healing of skin wounds. In: Oehmichen M, Kirchner H (eds) The wound healing process – forensic pathological aspects, Research in legal medicine, vol 13. Schmidt-Römhild, Lübeck, pp 247–256

Betz P (1996b) Neue Methoden zur histologischen Altersbestimmung menschlicher Hautwunden. Schmidt-Römhild, Lübeck

Betz P, Eisenmenger W (1996) Morphometrical analysis of hemosiderin deposits in relation to wound age. Int J Legal Med 108:262–264

Betz P, Nerlich A, Wilske J, Tubel J, Wiest I, Penning R et al (1992a) The time-dependent rearrangement of the epithelial basement membrane in human skin wounds – immunohistochemical localization of collagen IV and VII. Int J Legal Med 105:93–97

Betz P, Nerlich A, Wilske J, Tubel J, Wiest I, Penning R et al (1992b) Immunohistochemical localization of fibronectin as a tool for the age determination of human skin wounds. Int J Legal Med 195:21–26

Betz P, Nerlich A, Wilske J, Tübel J, Penning R, Eisenmenger W (1992c) Time-dependent appearance of myofibroblasts in granulation tissue of human skin wounds. Int J Legal Med 105:99–103

Betz P, Nerlich A, Wilske J, Tübel J, Wiest I, Penning R, Eisenmenger W (1992d) Time-dependent pericellular expression of collagen type IV, laminin, and heparin sulfate proteoglycan in myofibroblasts. Int J Legal Med 105:169–172

Betz P, Nerlich A, Tübel J, Penning R, Eisenmenger W (1993a) Localization of tenascin in human skin wounds – an immunohistochemical study. Int J Legal Med 105:325–328

Betz P, Nerlich A, Tübel J, Penning R, Eisenmenger W (1993b) The time-dependent expression of keratins 5 and 13 during the reepithelialization of human skin wounds. Int J Legal Med 105:229–232

Betz P, Nerlich A, Wilke J, Tubel J, Penning R, Eisenmenger W (1993c) Analysis of the immunohistochemical localization of collagen type III and V for the time-estimation of human skin wounds. Int J Legal Med 105:329–332

Betz P, Nerlich A, Wilske J, Tubel J, Penning R, Eisenmenger W (1993d) Immunohistochemical localization of collagen types I and VI in human skin wounds. Int J Legal Med 106:31–34

Betz P, Nerlich A, Wilske J, Tubel J, Penning R, Eisenmenger W (1993e) The immunohistochemical analysis of fibronectin, collagen type III, laminin, and cytokeratin 5 in putrified skin. Forensic Sci Int 61:35–42

Betz P, Nerlich A, Wilske J, Tübel J, Penning R, Eisenmenger W (1993f) The immunohistochemical localization of alpha1-antichymotrypsin and fibronectin and its meaning for the determination of the vitality of human skin wounds. Int J Legal Med 105:223–227

Betz P, Nerlich A, Wilske J, Tübel J, Penning R, Eisenmenger W (1993g) The time-dependent localization of Ki-67 antigen positive cells in human skin wounds. Int J Legal Med 106:35–40

Betz P, Tübel J, Eisenmenger W (1995) Immunohistochemical analysis of markers for different macrophage phenotypes and their use for a forensic wound age estimation. Int J Legal Med 107:197–200

Blitstein-Willinger E (1991) The role of growth factors in wound healing. Skin Pharmacol 4:175–182

Bode G, Garbe G, Stöckigt W, Förster B (1979) Der Einfluss von Schlafmitteln auf die Entwicklung der morphologischen und biochemischen Wundreaktion. Z Rechtsmed 82:337–347

Bode G, Garbe G, Ick D (1980) Der Einffluss von Kälte bzw. Tod durch Erfrieren auf die frühen Wundheilungsvorgänge an Hautschnitten. Beitr Gerichtl Med 38:119–124

Byard RW, Wick R, Gilbert JD, Donald T (2008) Histologic dating of bruises in moribund infants and young children. Forensic Sci Med Pathol 4: 187–192

Capatina CO, Ceaușu M, Hostiuc S (2013) Usefulness of fibronectin and P-selectin as markers for vital reaction in uncontrolled conditions. Rom J Leg Med 21:281–286

Castagnoli C, Stella M, Magliacani G, Ferrone S, Momigliano Richiardi P (1994) Similar ectopic expression of ICAM-1 and HLA-class II molecules in hypertrophic scars following thermal injury. Burns 20:430–433

Cecchi R (2010) Estimating wound age: looking into the future. Int J Legal Med 124:523–536

Dachum W, Jiazhen Z (1992) Localization and quantification of the non-specific esterase in injured skin for timing of wounds. Forensic Sci Int 53:203–213

Dreßler J, Bachmann L, Kasper M, Hauck JG, Müller E (1997a) Time dependence of the expression of ICAM-1 (CD 54) in human skin wounds. Int J Legal Med 110:299–304

Dreßler J, Bachmann L, Müller E (1997b) Enhanced expression of ICAM-1 (CD54) in human skin wounds: diagnostic value in legal medicine. Inflamm Res 46:434–435

Dreßler J, Bachmann L, Koch R, Müller E (1999a) Enhanced expression of selectins in human skin wounds. Int J Legal Med 112:39–44

Dreßler J, Bachmann L, Koch R, Müller E (1999b) Estimation of wound age and VCAM-1 in human skin. Int J Legal Med 112:159–162

Dreßler J, Busuttil A, Koch R, Harrison DJ (2001) Sequence of melanocyte migration into human scar tissue. Int J Legal Med 115:61–63

Dürwald W (1987) Gerichtliche Medizin, 3rd edn. J.A. Barth, Leipzig, p 87

Eisenmenger W, Nerlich A, Glück D (1988) Die Bedeutung des Kollagens bei der Wundaltersbestimmung. Z Rechtsmed 100:79–100

Fechner G (1995) Immunhistochemische Untersuchungen bei Muskeltraumen. In: Bratzke H, Schröter A (eds) Immunhistochemie in der Rechtsmedizin. Hänsel-Hohenhausen, Egelbach, pp 22–36

Fechner G, Petkovits T, Brinkmann B (1990) Zur Ultrastruktur-Pathologie mechanischer Skelettmuskelschädigungen. Z Rechtsmed 103:291–299

Fechner G, Hauser R, Sepulchre MA, Brinkmann B (1991) Immunohistochemical investigations to dem-

onstrate vital direct traumatic damage of skeletal muscle. Int J Legal Med 104:215–219
Fieguth A, Kleemann WJ, Tröger HD (1994) Immunohistochemical examination of skin wounds with antibodies against alpha-1 chymotrypsin, alpha-2-macroglobulin and lysozyme. Int J Legal Med 107:29–33
Fieguth A, Feldbrügge H, Gerich T, Kleemann WJ, Tröger HD (2003) The time-dependent expression of fibronectin, MRP8, MRP14 and defensin in surgically treated human skin wounds. Forensic Sci Int 131:156–161
Flad HD (1996) Chemokines and proinflammatory cytokines in wound healing. In: Oehmichen M, Kirchner H (eds) The wound healing process – forensic pathological aspects, Research in legal medicine, vol 13. Schmidt-Römhild, Lübeck, pp 49–57
Friebel L, Woohsmann H (1968) Die Altersbestimmung von Kanüleneinstichen mittels enzymhistochemischer Methoden. Dtsch Z Gerichtl Med 62:252–260
Fries JWU, Williams AJ, Atkins RC, Newman W, Lipscomb MF, Collins T (1993) Expression of VCAM-1 and E-selectin in an in vivo model of endothelial activation. Am J Pathol 143:725–737
Fronczek J, Lulf R, Korkmaz HI, Witte BI, de Goot a, Begieneman PV, Schalkwijk CG, Krijnen PAJ, Rozendaal L, Niessen HWM, Reijnders UJL (2015a) Analysis of inflammatory cells and mediators in skin wound age in living subjects in forensic medicine. Forensic Sci Int 247:7–13
Fronczek J, Lulf R, Korkmaz HI, Witte BI, van de Goot FRW, Begieneman PV, Krijnen PAJ, Rozendaal L, Niessen HWM, Reijnders UJL (2015b) Analysis of morphological characteristics and expression levels of extracellular matrix proteins in skin wounds to determine wound age in living subjects in forensic medicine. Forensic Sci Int 246:86–91
Grellner W (2002) Time-dependent immunohistochemical detection of proinflammatory cytokines (IL-1β, IL-6, TNF-α) in human skin wounds. Forensic Sci Int 130:90–96
Grellner W, Ester-Bode T, Köhler L, Staak M (1997) Zur Rolle von Adhäsionsmolekülen für die frühe Wundaltersschätzung. In: 6. Frühjahrstagung – Region Nord – der Deutschen Gesellschaft für Rechtsmedizin. Berlin, 23. und 24. Mai 1997
Grellner W, Dimmeler S, Madea B (1998) Immunohistochemical detection of fibronectin in postmortem incised wounds of porcine skin. Forensic Sci Int 97:109–116
Grellner W, Georg T, Wilske J (2000) Quantitative analysis of proinflammatory cytokines (IL-1β, Il.6, TNF-α) in human skin wounds. Forensic Sci Int 113:251–264
Grellner W, Vieler S, Madea B (2005) Transforming growth factors (TGF-α and TGF-β1) in the determination of vitality and wound age: immunohistochemical study on human skin wounds. Forensic Sci Int 153:174–180
Hausmann R, Nerlich A, Betz P (1998) The time-related expression of p53 protein in human skin wounds – a quantitative immunohistochemical analysis. Int J Legal Med 111:169–172
Hayashi T, Ishida Y, Kimura A, Takayasu T, Eisenmenger W, Kondo T (2004) Forensic application of VEGF expression to skin wound age determination. Int J Legal Med 118:320–325
Helpap B (1987) Leitfaden der allgemeinen Entzündungslehre. Springer, Berlin
Helpap B, Cremer H (1972) Zellkinetische Untersuchungen zur Wundheilung der Mäuseleber. Virchows Arch B Cell Pathol 10:134–144
Henssge C, Wang H, Hoppe B (2002) Light microscopical investigations on structural changes of skeletal muscle as artifacts after postmortem stimulation. Forensic Sci Int 125:163–171
Ishida Y, Kimura A, Takayasu T, Eisenmenger W, Kondo T (2009) Detection of fibrocytes in human skin wounds and its application for wound age determination. Int J Legal Med 123:299–304
Ishida Y, Kimura A, Nosaka M, Kuminaka Y, Shimada E, Yamamoto H, Nishiyama K, Inaka S, Takayasu T, Eisenmenger W, Kondo T (2015a) Detection of endothelial progenitor cells in human skin wounds and its application for wound age determination. Int J Legal Med 129:1049–1054
Ishida Y, Kuninaka Y, Nosaka M, Kimura A, Kawaguchi T, Hama M, Sakamoto S, Shinozaki K, Eisenmenger W, Kondo T (2015b) Immunohistochemical analysis on MMP-2 and MMP-9 for wound age determination. Int J Legal Med 129:1043–1048
Ishida Y, Kuminaka Y, Furukawa F, Kimura A, Nosaka M, Fukami M, Yamamoto H, Kato T, Shimada E, Hata S, Takayasu T, Eisenmenger W, Kondo T (2017) Immunohistochemical analysis on aquaporin-1 and aquaporin-3 in skin wounds from aspects of wound age determination. Int J Legal Med 132:237–242. published online 28 October 2017
Janssen W (1977) Forensische Histologie. Schmidt-Römhild, Lübeck
Joseph-Silverstein J, Rifkin DB (1990) Endothelial cell growth factors and the vessel wall. In: Oehmichen M (ed) Die Wundheilung. Springer, Berlin
Kara S, Akbaba M, Kul S, Bakir K (2016) Is it possible to make early wound age estimation by immunohistochemical methods? Rom J Leg Med 24:92–99
Kekow J, Gross WL (1996) Role of TGFβ in wound healing. In: Oehmichen M, Kirchner H (eds) The wound healing process – forensic pathological aspects, Research in legal medicine, vol 13. Schmidt-Römhild, Lübeck, pp 59–68
Kepron C, Pollanen MS (2015) Rickets or abuse? A histologic comparison of rickets and child abuse-related fractures. Forensic Sci Med Pathol 11:78–87
Kimura A, Ishida Y, Nosaka M, Shiraki M, Hama M, Kawaguchi T, Kuminaka Y, Shimada E, Yamamoto H, Takayasu T, Kondo T (2015) Autophagy in skin wounds: a novel marker for vital reactions. Int J Legal Med 129:537–541
Klotzbach H, Delling G, Richter E, Sperhake J, Püschel K (2003) Post-mortem diagnosis and age estimation of infant's fractures. Int J Legal Med 117:82–89

Kondo T (2007) Timing of skin wounds. Legal Med 9:109–114
Kondo T, Ishida Y (2010) Molecular pathology of wound healing. Forensic Sci Int 203:93–98
Kondo T, Ohshima T (1996a) Experimental study on the estimation of skin wound age after injury by immunostaining interleukin 1a, collagen type I and fibronectin. In: Oehmichen M, Kirchner H (eds) The wound healing process – forensic pathological aspects, Research in legal medicine, vol 13. Schmidt-Römhild, Lübeck, pp 123–132
Kondo T, Ohshima T (1996b) The dynamics of inflammatory cytokines in the healing process of mouse skin wound: a preliminary study for possible wound age determination. Int J Legal Med 108:231–236
Kondo T, Tanaka J, Ishida Y, Mori R, Tykayasu T, Ohshima T (2002) Ubiquitin expression in skin wounds and its application to forensic wound age determination. Int J Legal Med 116:267–272
Leibovich SJ, Wiseman DM (1988) Macrophages, wound repair and angiogenesis. In: Growth factors and other aspects of wound healing: biological and clinical implications. Alan R Liss, New York, pp 131–145
Lindner J (1962) Die Morphologie der Wundheilung. Langenbecks Arch Chir 301:39–70
Lindner J (1967) Vitale Reaktionen. Dtsch Z Gerichtl Med 59:312–344
Lindner J (1980) Morphologie und Biochemie der Wundheilung. Langenbecks Arch Chir 358:153–160
Lindner J, Huber P (1973) Biochemische und morphologische Grundlagen der Wundheilung und ihre Beeinflussung. Med Welt 24:897–911
Lorente JA (1996) Cathepsin D as a marker of the vitality of the wounds. In: Oehmichen M, Kirchner H (eds) The wound healing process – forensic pathological aspects, Research in legal medicine, vol 13. Schmidt-Römhild, Lübeck, pp 69–81
Ma WX, Yu TS, Fan YY, Zhang ST, Ren P, Wang SB, Zhao R, Pi JB, Guan DW (2011) Time-dependent expression and distribution of monoacylglycerol lipase during the skin-incised wound healing in mice. Int J Legal Med 125:549–558
MacGregor RR, Safford M, Salit M (1988) Effect of ethanol on function required for delivery of neutrophils to sites of inflammation. J Infect Dis 157:682–689
Mackie EJ, Halfter W, Liverani D (1988) Induction of tenascin in healing wounds. J Cell Biol 107:2757–2767
Mann M, Bednar B (1977) Influence of age and different drugs on the healing process in human skin wounds. Gerontology 23:277–289
Martin P (1997) Wound healing – aiming for perfect skin regeneration. Science 276:75–81
Mauch C, Oono T, Eckes B, Krieg T (1994) Cytokines and wound healing. In: Luger TA, Schwarz T (eds) Epidermal growth factors and cytokines. M. Dekker, New York, pp 325–344
Maxeiner H (1987) Zur lokalen Vitalreaktion nach Angriff gegen den Hals. Z Rechtsmed 99:35–54
Maxeiner H (1994) Zur lokalen Vitalreaktion bei Unterkühlung. Rechtsmed 4:80–84
McKay IA, Leigh IM (1991) Epidermal cytokines and their role in cutaneous wound healing. Br J Dermatol 124:513–518
Müller PK, Brinckmann J (1996) Collagen and wound healing – a summary. In: Oehmichen M, Kirchner H (eds) The wound healing process – forensic pathological aspects, Research in legal medicine, vol 13. Schmidt-Römhild, Lübeck, pp 243–246
Mulligan MS, Till GO, Smith CW, Anderson DC, Miyasaka M, Tamatani T, Todd RF, Issekutz TB, Ward PA (1994) Role of leucocyte adhesion molecules in lung and dermal vascular injury after thermal trauma of skin. Am J Pathol 144:1008–1015
Murakami R, Yamaoka I, Sakakura T (1989) Appearance of tenascin in healing skin of the mouse: possible involvement in seaming of wounded tissue. Int J Dev Biol 33:439–444
Naeve W, Bause HW (1974) Experimentelle postmortale Kopf- und Hirnverletzungen. Z Rechtsmed 74:187
Nakajima T, Hayakawa M, Yajima D, Motani-Saitoh H, Sato Y, Kiuchi M, Ichinose M, Iwase H (2006) Time-course changes in the expression of heme oxygenase-1 in human subcutaneous hemorrhage. Forensic Sci Int 158:157–163
Nerlich ML, Bosch U (1988) Wunde und Wundbehandlung. Tetanusprophylaxe. Orthopade 17:11–16
Ninggou L, Yijiu C, Xiaohua H (2006) Fibronectin EIIIA splicing variant: a useful contribution to forensic wounding interval estimation. Forensic Sci Int 162:178–182
Oehmichen M (1984) Blutabbau in den Lungenalveolen: Zeichen der Vitalität und Bestimmung der Überlebenszeit. Z Rechtsmed 92:47–57
Oehmichen M (1990a) Die Wundheilung. Springer, Heidelberg
Oehmichen M (1990b) Theorie und Praxis der Chronomorphologie von Verletzungen in der forensischen Pathologie. Springer, Berlin
Oehmichen M, Cröpelin A (1995) Temporal course of intravital and post-mortem proliferation of epidermis cells after injury – an immunohistochemical study using bromodeoxyuridine in rats. Int J Legal Med 107:257–262
Oehmichen M, Kirchner H (eds) (1996) The wound healing process – forensic pathological aspects, Research in legal medicine, vol 13. Schmidt-Römhild, Lübeck
Oehmichen M, Raff G (1980) Timing of cortical contusion. Correlation between histomorphologic alterations and post-traumatic interval. Z Rechtsmed 84:79–94
Oehmichen M, Karres-Balting U, Saternus KS (1987) Reaktive Veränderungen bei Weichteilunterblutungen im Kehlkopfinneren. Beir Gerichtl Med 45:73–78
Oehmichen M, Frasunek J, Zilles K (1988a) Cytokinetics of epidermal cells in skin from human cadavers: I. Dependency on sex, age and site. Z Rechtsmed 101:161–171
Oehmichen M, Frasunek J, Zilles K (1988b) Cytokinetics of epidermal cells in skin from human cadavers: II. Dependency on sex, age and site. Z Rechtsmed 101:173–182

Oehmichen M, Schmidt V, Stuka K (1989) Freisetzung von Proteinase-Inhibitoren als vitale Reaktion im frühen posttraumatischen Intervall. Z Rechtsmed 102:461–472

Oehmichen M, Gronki T, Meissner C, Anlauf M, Schwark T (2009) Mast cell reactivity at the margin of human skin wounds: an early cell marker of wound survival? Forensic Sci Int 191:1–5

Ogbuihi S, Müller Z, Zink P (1988) Quantitative polarizing microscopy for the evaluation of collagen types I and III in paraffin-embedded sections. Z Rechtsmed 100:101–111

Ordmann LJ, Gillmann T (1966) Studies in the healing of cutaneous wounds. I. The healing of incisions through the skin of pigs. Arch Surg 93:857–882

Ortonne JP, Löning T, Schmitt D, Thivolet J (1981) Immunomorphological and ultrastructural aspects of keratinocyte migration in epidermal wound healing. Virchows Arch A Pathol Anat Histol 392:217–230

Pechníková M, Mazzarelli D, Poppa P, Gibelli D, Baggi ES, Cattaneo C (2015) Microscopic pattern of bone fractures as an indicator of blast trauma: a pilot study. J Forensic Sci 60:1140–1145

Pierce GF, Yanagihara D, Kopchin K et al (1994) Stimulation of all epithelial elements during skin regeneration by keratinocyte growth factor. J Exp Med 179:831–840

Pinsker JE, Kain C, Keller L, Rooks VJ (2016) Vitamin D deficiency versus non-accidental trauma: comment on "Rickets or abuse? A histologic comparison of rickets and child abuse-related fractures?". Forensic Sci Med Pathol 12:119–120

Pioch W (1969) Epidermale Esterase-Aktivität als Beweis der vitalen Einwirkung von stumpfer Gewalt. Beitr Gerichtl Med 25:136–145

Püschel K, Schulz-Schaeffer WJ, Brück M (1996) Time-dependent morphological alterations of injection marks. In: Oehmichen M, Kirchner H (eds) The wound healing process – forensic pathological aspects, Research in legal medicine, vol 13. Schmidt-Römhild, Lübeck, pp 293–307

Radzun HJ (1996) Pathology of wound healing and repair. In: Oehmichen M, Kirchner H (eds) The wound healing process – forensic pathological aspects, Research in legal medicine, vol 13. Schmidt-Römhild, Lübeck, pp 35–39

Raekallio J (1960) Enzymes histochemically demonstrable in the earliest phase of wound healing. Nature 188:234–235

Raekallio J (1964) Histochemical distinction between antemortem and postmortem skin wounds. J Forensic Sci 9:107–118

Raekallio J (1965a) Die Altersbestimmung mechanisch bedingter Hautwunden mit enzymhistochemischen Methoden. Schmidt-Römhild, Lübeck

Raekallio J (1965b) Histochemical demonstration of enzymatic response to injure in experimental skin wounds. Exp Mol Pathol 4:303–310

Raekallio J (1970) Enzyme histochemistry of wound healing. Fischer, Stuttgart

Raekallio J (1972) Determination of the age of wounds by histochemical and biochemical methods. Forensic Sci 1:3–16

Raekallio J (1973) Estimation of the age of injuries by histochemical and biochemical methods. Z Rechtsmed 73:83–102

Raekallio J (1976) Timing of wounds in forensic medicine. Jpn. J Legal Med 30:125–136

Raekallio J (1980a) Histological estimation of the age of injuries. In: Perper JA, Wecht CH (eds) Microscopic diagnosis in forensic pathology. Springfield, Thomas, pp 3–16

Raekallio J (1980b) Histological and biochemical estimation of the age of injuries. In: Perper JA, Wecht CH (eds) Microscopic diagnosis in forensic pathology. Springfield, Thomas, pp 17–35

Raekallio J, Mäkinen PL (1967) Biochemical and histochemical observations on aminopeptidase activity in early wound healing. Nature 213:1037–1038

Raekallio J, Mäkinen PL (1974) The effect of ageing on enzyme histochemical vital reactions. Z Rechtsmed 75:105–111

Rolvien T, Butscheidt S, Herrmann J, Pueschel K (2016) Methodological approach for the histological comparison between rickets and child abuse. Rechtsmedizin 26:313–315

Ross R (1968) The fibroblast and wound repair. Biol Rev 43:51–96

Schaeffer-Schulz WJ, Brück W, Püschel K (1996) Macrophage subtyping in the determination of age of injection sites. Int J Legal Med 109:29–33

Schollmeyer W (1965) Über die Altersbestimmung von Injektionsstichen. Beitr Gerichtl Med 23:244–249

Singer AJ, Clark RA (1999) Cutaneous wound healing. N Engl J Med 341:738–746

Suárez-Penarada JM, Rodríguez-Calvo MS, Ortiz-Rey JA, Munoz JI, Sánchez-Pintos P, da Silva EA, de la Fuente-Buceta A, Concheiro-Carro L (2002) Demonstration of apoptosis in human skin injuries as an indicator of vital reaction. Int J Legal Med 116:109–112

Sun JH, Wang YY, Zhang L, Gao CR, Zhang LZ, Guo Z (2010) Time-dependent expression of skeletal muscle troponin I mRNA in the contused skeletal muscle of rats: a possible marker for wound age estimation. Int J Legal Med 124:27–33

ten Dijke P, Iwata KK (1989) Growth factors for wound healing. Biotechnology 7:793–798

Thomsen H (1996) Platelets and wound healing – a review. In: Oehmichen M, Kirchner H (eds) The wound healing process – forensic pathological aspects, Research in legal medicine, vol 13. Schmidt-Römhild, Lübeck, pp 151–172

Tian ZL, Jiang SK, Zhang M, Wang M, Li JY, Zhao R, Wang LL, Li SS, Liu M, Zhang MZ, Guan DW (2016) Detection of satellite cells during skeletal muscle wound healing in rats: time-dependent expressions of Pax7 and MyoD in relation to wound age. Int J Legal Med 130:163–172

Tutsch-Bauer E, Baur C, Tröger HD, Liebhardt E (1981) Untersuchungen zur Altersbestimmung an künstlich gesetzten Hämatomen. Beitr Gerichtl Med 39:83–86

van de Goot FRW, Korkmaz HI, Fronczek J, Witte BI, Visser R, Ulrich MMW, Begieneman MPV, Rozendaal L, Krijnen PAJ, Niessen HWM (2014) A new method to determine wound age in early vital skin injuries: a probability scoring system using expression levels of fibronectin, CD62p and factor VIII in wound hemorrhage. Forensic Sci Int 244:128–135

Vieira DN (1996) Application of ions, proteinase, inhibitors and PGF2a in the differential diagnosis between vital and post-mortem skin wounds. In: Oehmichen M, Kirchner H (eds) The wound healing process – forensic pathological aspects, Research in legal medicine, vol 13. Schmidt-Römhild, Lübeck, pp 83–105

Walcher K (1936) Die vitale Reaktion bei der Beurteilung des gewaltsamen Todes. Dtsch Z Ges Gerichtl Med 26:193–211

Weber MA, Risdon RA, Offiah AC, Malone M, Sebire NJ (2009) Rib fractures identified at post-mortem examination in sudden unexpected death in infancy (SUDI). Forensic Sci Int 189:75–81

Willems IEMG, Arends JW, Daemen MJAT (1996) Tenascin and fibronectin expression in healing human myocardial scars. J Pathol 179:321–325

Wyler D (1996) Determining the age and assessing the vitality of wounds by immunohistochemical detection of cell adhesion molecules. In: Oehmichen M, Kirchner H (eds) The wound healing process – forensic pathological aspects, Research in legal medicine, vol 13. Schmidt-Römhild, Lübeck, pp 133–138

Yagi Y, Murase T, Kagawa S, Tsuruya S, Nakahara A, Yamamoto T, Umehara T, Ikematsu K (2016) Immunohistochemical detection of CD14 and combined assessment with CD32B and CD68 for wound age estimation. Forensic Sci Int 262:113–120

Yu TS, Cheng ZH, Li LQ, Zhao R, Fan YY, Du Y, Ma WX, Guan DW (2010) The cannabinoid receptor type 2 is time-dependently expressed during skeletal muscle wound healing in rats. Int J Legal Med 124:397–404

Zarbock A, Ley K (2008) Mechanism and consequences of neutrophil interaction with the endothelium. Am J Pathol 172:1–7

Zhao R, Guan DA, Zhang W, Du Y, Xiong CY, Zhu BL, Zhang JJ (2009) Increased expressions and activation of apoptosis-related factors in cell signaling during incised skin wound healing in mice: a preliminary study for forensic wound age estimation. Legal Med 11:S155–S160

Aspiration and Inhalation

11

While aspiration of objects and coarse material, including gastric contents, can often be diagnosed macroscopically, aspiration of liquids or finer foreign matter, including blood or dust, can often only be proved with microscopy. Aspiration is considered to be evidence of vitality when the aspirated material has reached the peripheral branches of the bronchial tree (small bronchi, pulmonary alveoli). In the case of terminal or agonal aspiration, the aspirated material can at deepest be found in the tracheal lumen and the main bronchi, as well as occasionally in the segmental bronchi. However, the spread of aspirated material to the periphery of the bronchial tree as a result of resuscitation measures must be considered when making a diagnosis. Histological examinations are particularly necessary to demonstrate aspiration as a sign of vitality, which is usually possible histologically but also radiologically prior to autopsy in more severe cases (Yen et al. 2005).

Some authors do not consider the breathing in of soot, aerosols, and airborne particulate substances (e.g., fungal spores) as aspiration in the strict sense (Janssen 1977); the term "inhalation" is more appropriate here.

Aspiration or inhalation may play a significant role in various correlations at forensic autopsy:

- Aspiration of freshwater or salt water during drowning.
- Aspiration of blood after traumatic brain injury including basal skull fracture
- Aspiration of dust, in particular soot dust in fatalities from fire or smoldering fire
- Aspiration of gastric content after vomiting
- Aspiration of amniotic fluid containing or not containing meconium particles in newborns
- Aspiration of other foreign materials (aerosols, water components such as diatoms, plant constituents in water, fine sand, dust such as flour dust, volatile substances, etc.)
- Inhalation of gases and sprays

Substances which allow for a more precise classification of the aspirated foreign matter (e.g., bile components in aspirated gastric content or milk aspiration in infant death cases by immunostaining with antihuman alpha-lactalbumin antibody; Iwadate et al. 2001) can frequently be seen microscopically. Acute suffocation caused by aspiration of foreign material may be the sole cause of death in the case of accidents, as well as in cases where the swallowing and gag reflexes are suppressed. This applies, for example, in cases of serious intoxication and traumatic or nontraumatic brain injury. The aspirated material is often clearly visible in the lumina of the peripheral bronchi after routine staining (H&E, van Gieson, Sudan III), unless only water has been aspirated. Demonstrating aspiration of water, however, is important to clarify the question of vitality and to prove cause of death (Revenstorf 1904).

R. B. Dettmeyer, *Forensic Histopathology*, https://doi.org/10.1007/978-3-319-77997-3_11

11.1 Aspiration of Water

Findings which appear in the case of aspiration of freshwater or salt water are described on the basis of animal experiments: the influx of fluids causes a wide range of reactions from the development of alveolar–interstitial edema in combination with intracellular and intercellular vesiculation and karyolysis with swollen homogenized nuclei of the subendothelial, septal, and epithelial cells to necrosis of all cellular elements. Pronounced microangiopathy with edema of the vascular walls, hydrops of the myocytes containing large vacuoles, and perivascular edema with dilated lymphatic channels may also be found. Alveolar macrophage numbers can be considerably increased. Sporadic rupture of the alveolar walls and microhemorrhage can occur (see also Chap. 3).

In saltwater drowning, alterations in the shape of both erythrocytes (crab-apple form) and alveolar epithelium, in combination with detachment of the pneumocytes from the alveolar walls, as well as villous transformations prevail. In addition, capillary hyperemia and sludge are found. In careful specimen analysis, differentiation of the findings between vital reactions and postmortem effects of fluid may be possible (Brinkmann et al. 1983).

Particularly in the case of freshwater aspiration, diatoms (silica algae), as well as impurities in the aspirated water such as amorphous foreign particles, like soot particles (Fig. 11.1) or plant constituents (Fig. 11.2), are often observed. There is debate as to whether drowning without aspiration should be considered as a possible diagnosis (Modell et al. 1999).

It is possible that the composition of various types of diatoms could be traced back to a particular body of water, but this does not apply to plant constituents. However, such a classification calls for further complex analysis. As a histomorphological correlate of emphysema aquosum, pulmonary alveoli coalesce to form vesicular cavities with flattened interalveolar septa, which may only be visible as stubby sections under the microscope. If this finding is absent in the case of death by drowning, a reflex event should also be considered. The initial aspiration of water may cause an extremely low heart rate and low blood pressure due to reflex vagal inhibition, which can result in even a strong swimmer drowning after loss of consciousness (Suzuki et al. 1985). The temperature of the water may play an important role (Keating and Hayward 1981). Near drowning can predispose a person to a systemic mycotic infection following severe aspiration of muddy water leading to mycotic pneumonia (Ortmann et al. 2010).

The intrapulmonary expression of aquaporin-5 (AQP5) has been examined in an experimental drowning model and forensic autopsy cases in

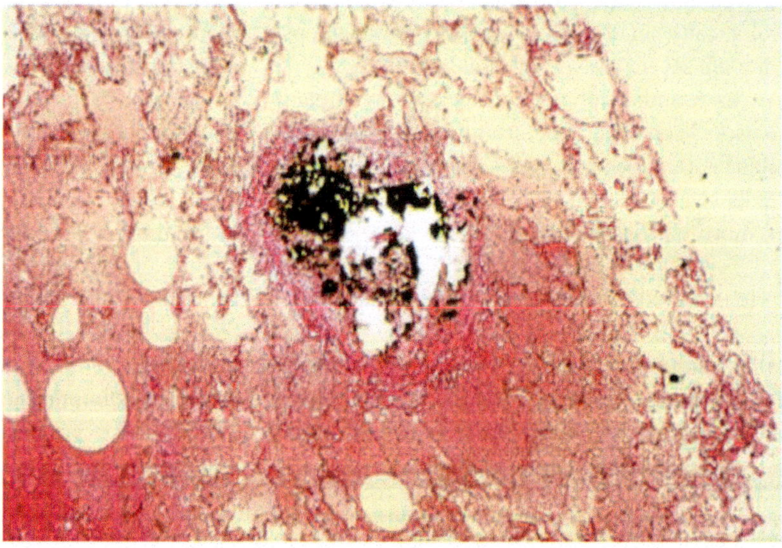

Fig. 11.1 Aspirated water polluted with soot particles in the lumen of a peripheral bronchus in the case of death by drowning (H&E ×125)

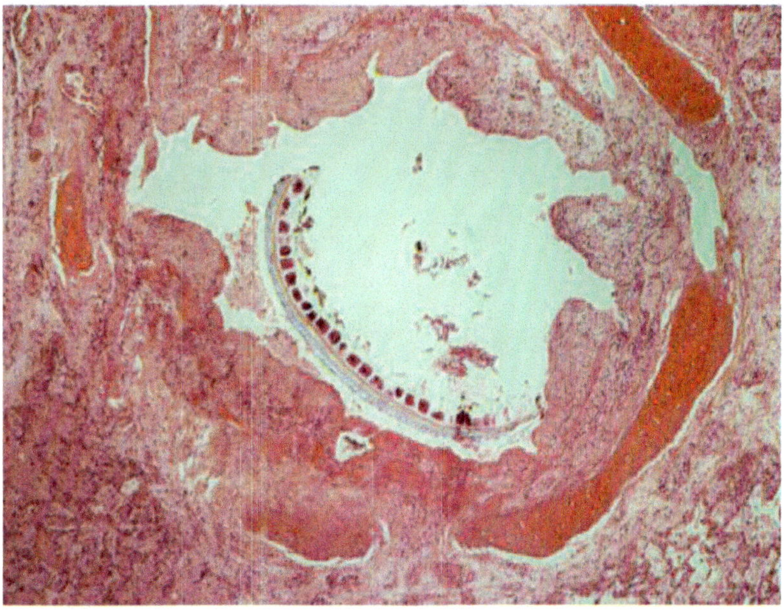

Fig. 11.2 Aspiration of plant constituents in a case of freshwater drowning (H&E ×40)

the hope of differentiating between freshwater drowning (FWD) and saltwater drowning (SWD). The authors reported that AQP5 mRNA could be detected in all lung samples under the experimental conditions employed: the intrapulmonary gene expression of AQP5 in FWD was significantly attenuated, and the observations imply that AQP5 expression in type I alveolar epithelial cells was suppressed by hypotonic water to prevent hemodilution. The authors concluded that analysis of intrapulmonary AQP5 expression would be forensically useful for differentiation between FWD and SWD or between FWD and postmortem immersion (Hayashi et al. 2009).

11.2 Aspiration of Blood

The aspiration of blood may have various causes, including:

- In the case of traumatic brain injury
- Following sharp force injury in homicides or suicides (e.g., deep stab wounds to the throat)
- In the case of preexisting pulmonary disease (malignant diseases, infections such as pulmonary tuberculosis)
- Iatrogenically following pulmonary endoscopic procedures in the course of bronchoscopy (Sato et al. 2009; Strange et al. 1987) or following implantation of a bronchial wall stent (Spendlove et al. 2007)
- Rarely in alcoholics with acute esophageal variceal bleeding, Mallory–Weiss syndrome (see Chap. 6) and alcohol-related impairment of the coughing reflex

Pathological histological results can be found in the lungs in particular, but histological investigations into the underlying disease must also be made. The histological verification of blood in the lumina of peripheral bronchi and pulmonary alveoli needs to be performed with intact alveolo-capillary walls in order to exclude the possibility of bleeding of septal capillaries caused by the rupture of basal membranes (Fig. 11.3).

Traumatic Brain Injury (TBI) In the case of severe traumatic brain injury including basal skull fracture and hemorrhage in the oral cavity, massive aspiration of blood is likely. This may result in peripheral pulmonary emphysema (emphysema hemorrhagicum)—with an identical pathophysiological mechanism to

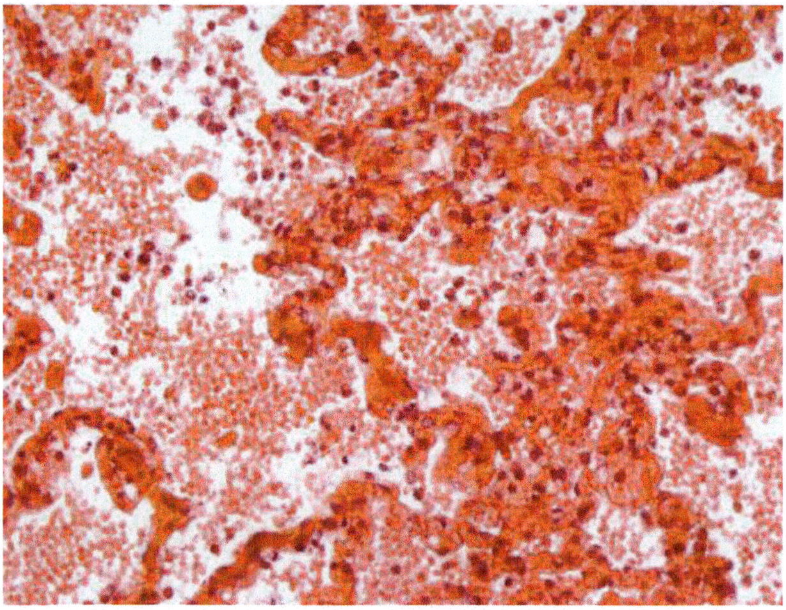

Fig. 11.3 Densely packed erythrocytes in the lumina of the pulmonary alveoli following massive aspiration of blood due to traumatic brain injury and basal skull fracture with simultaneous acute vascular congestion after a traffic accident (H&E ×200)

drowning. Within the lung tissue, alveoli in the periphery will coalesce to small vesicular cavities by rarefaction of the narrow interalveolar septa, such that often only stubby interalveolar septa remain. This histological picture can also be seen in the case of death by drowning (emphysema aquosum), but areas with aspirated blood also appear in the lumina of the alveoli, where densely packed erythrocytes can be observed. Similar blood aspiration may also occur following decapitation (Leopold 1959). In very rare cases, aspiration of brain tissue in addition to blood has been described (Walcher 1930).

Aspiration Following Intrapulmonary Hemorrhage Acute bleeding may occur in the case of a preexisting pulmonary disease, in particular malignant diseases (metastases, primary bronchial carcinomas) or infections such as pulmonary tuberculosis.

To clarify acute intrapulmonary bleeding after endoscopic surgery, a subtle microscopic examination of the endoscopic puncture site is needed in order to find the source of bleeding (Dettmeyer et al. 2003). An example of this is bleeding after bronchoscopic puncture of a suspected pseudopolyp (Fig. 11.4) or preexisting vascular ectasias (Fig. 11.5) (Chajed et al. 2003). Pulmonary hemorrhage caused by insertion of a right heart catheter has also been described (Preuss et al. 2005). In such cases, histological examinations can provide essential findings for the clarification of medical malpractice claims (Eisenmenger et al. 1980).

Examinations have shown that, in case of survival, degradation and resorption of the aspirated blood follow a certain chronology: in addition to H&E staining, siderin was identified with the Prussian blue reaction, and the activities were determined by tartrate-resistant acid phosphatase, as a macrophage marker, and naphthol AS-D chloroacetate esterase, as a granulocyte marker. The first sign of vitality is granulocyte emigration, which was initially observed after a survival period of 5 min. Erythrophages were found after a survival time of at least 30 min and siderophages after at least 17 h (Oehmichen 1984). Depending on the survival time following blood aspiration, one can expect a histologically detectable rapid adhesion of erythrocytes and phagocytes. Within the first 30–90 min, this also leads to adhesion of granulocytes and erythrophages. In the case of adhesion of erythrocytes to the surface of macrophages, a rosette-shaped pattern is visible. With erythrophagocytosis, one can

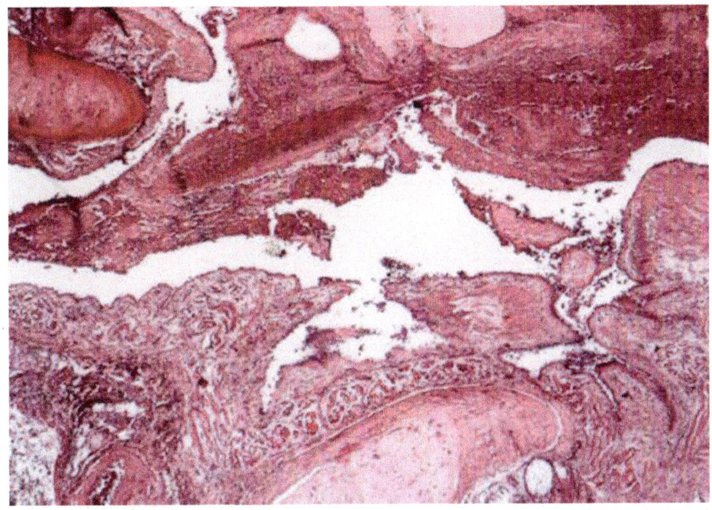

Fig. 11.4 Bronchoscopically punctured fibrous pseudopolyp of the bronchial mucosa followed by intrapulmonary bleeding in a case of suspected cancer (H&E ×40)

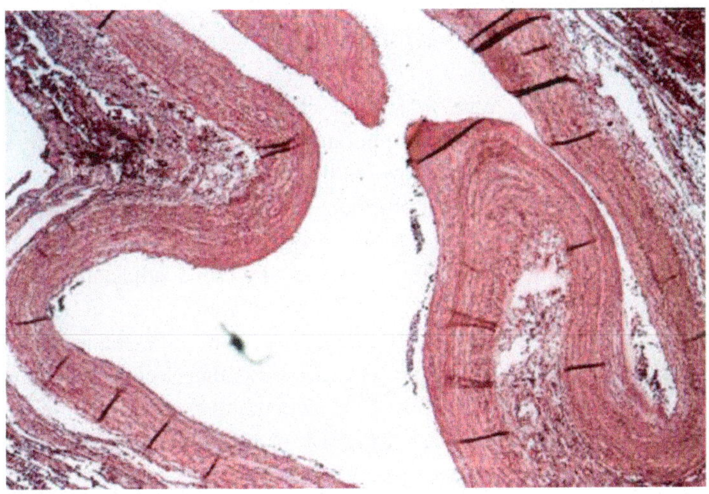

Fig. 11.5 Unusually pronounced angiectasia in the direct vicinity of a fibrous pseudopolyp following bronchoscopic biopsy with acute lethal blood aspiration (H&E ×40)

find an intracytoplasmic inclusion of erythrocytes, which may be recognizable as shadowy forms (Oehmichen 1984). Only after many hours does digestion include hemolysis, fragmentation of the phagocytosed cells, and intracytoplasmic siderin deposition. In contrast to the appearance of granulocytes, the adhesion itself cannot be considered a vital phenomenon in this context.

Animal experiments with rats have shown that, following blood aspiration, hemolyzed blood disappears from the lumina of the alveoli after a few days. Deposits of hemosiderin were shown to be found after 4 days (Mueller et al. 1960), which seems rather early in the case of intra-alveolar bleeding. Similar results have been presented by Graev and Fabroni (1962), although the extrapolation of their findings to humans is not necessarily possible. Blood aspiration that has initially been survived can, at least for a certain period of time after resorption, be proven histologically by detecting hemosiderin pigment-laden macrophages in the lumen of the alveoli (Fig. 11.6).

The differential diagnosis of intrapulmonary hemorrhage must take hemorrhagic lung infarction, hemorrhagic pulmonary edema, and pneumonia, e.g., hemorrhagic influenza pneumonia, into consideration. There are rare cases where lethal bilateral hemoaspiration was not necessarily the result of trauma and where the bleeding site was not situated above the trachea (Tsokos

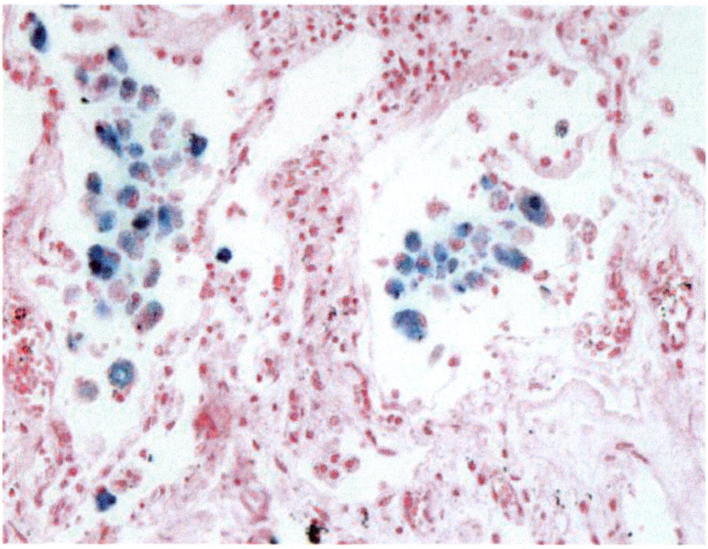

Fig. 11.6 Status following blood aspiration with hemosiderin pigment-laden macrophages remaining in the alveolar space (Prussian blue ×200)

and Byard 2007). With regard to severe iatrogenic endoscopy-induced intrapulmonary bleeding, and irrespective of how well-trained the physician might be, an appropriate emergency protocol should be established to manage severe bleeding complications. Indeed, the use of a balloon catheter to immediately close a vessel wall leak seems to be well suited (Spendlove et al. 2007). Prior to endoscopic surgery and the implantation of a bronchial stent, the patient must be thoroughly informed about the risk of bleeding complications.

11.3 Aspiration of Gastric Content or Chyme

Aspirated gastric content can be identified histologically by providing evidence of bile pigment and food components. To demonstrate aspirated amylum, cellulose, and bilirubin, a modified Stein's reaction was proposed. This reaction stains bilirubin green, cellulose light yellow, and amylum dark blue (Jobba 1971). Gastric acid may lead to initial digestion of the lung tissue (pneumomalacia acida), which cannot easily be differentiated from postmortem autolysis and putrefaction. In specific cases, a local inflammatory reaction with signs of initial digestion of the lung tissue can serve as an indication of at least short-term survival of chyme aspiration. In the case of classification problems, numerous specimens from various localizations need to be evaluated. Aspirated material can be seen in several adjacent alveoli or in one lobule, whereas other sections are not involved.

Aspirated chyme in particular is colonized relatively rapidly by bacteria. Thus, aspirated material interspersed with basophilic bacterial colonies (rod-shaped bacteria and/or cocci) can be verified in the lumina of the peripheral bronchi and pulmonary alveoli (Fig. 11.7).

If chyme aspiration is initially survived, aspiration pneumonia may develop within hours. The histological picture of acute bronchopneumonia with several segmented neutrophil granulocytes and embedded aspirated foreign material is then apparent (Figs. 11.8 and 11.9).

This type of aspiration pneumonia can be found on the one hand in particular in cases of alcohol- or drug-induced intoxications following longer agonal periods or after severe traumatic brain injury. On the basis of an appropriate anamnesis, demonstration of fresh aspiration pneumonia can serve as evidence of initial survival of the aspiration. On the other hand, there have been histological findings in recent aspirations without any tissue reaction (no prediges-

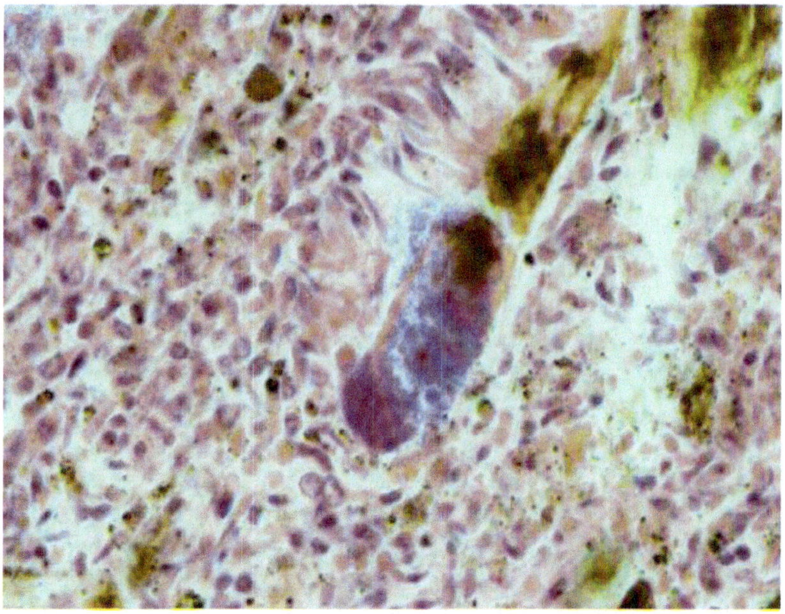

Fig. 11.7 Chyme colonized with bacteria in a peripheral bronchus with basophilic bacteria colonies—cocci—next to cylindrical bronchial epithelium following deep chyme aspiration in an intoxicated alcoholic (H&E ×400)

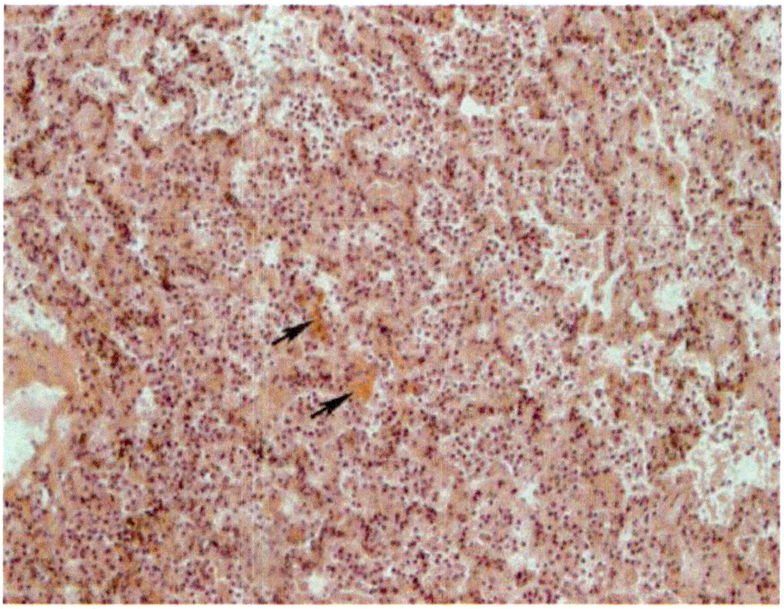

Fig. 11.8 Localized, verifiable foreign material (*arrows*) in the case of acute granulocyte-rich aspiration pneumonia following chyme aspiration in a drug-related death following a prolonged agonal period (29-year-old decedent) (H&E ×100)

tion of the tissue, no hemorrhage, no inflammatory reaction). In these cases, a final or agonal chyme aspiration without any relevance to the cause of death must be taken into consideration. Aspiration exacerbated by resuscitation measures must also be considered. Aspects such as these are also discussed, although not exclusively, in the context of sudden infant death (Bajanowski et al. 1996). If, on the basis of histological results, short-term survival of aspiration can be proven, the aspiration must be considered in each individual case with regard to its significance in a fatal causal chain where the primary cause needs to be determined. Fatal aspiration of the stomach contents is also possible in infants (Schmidt et al. 2003).

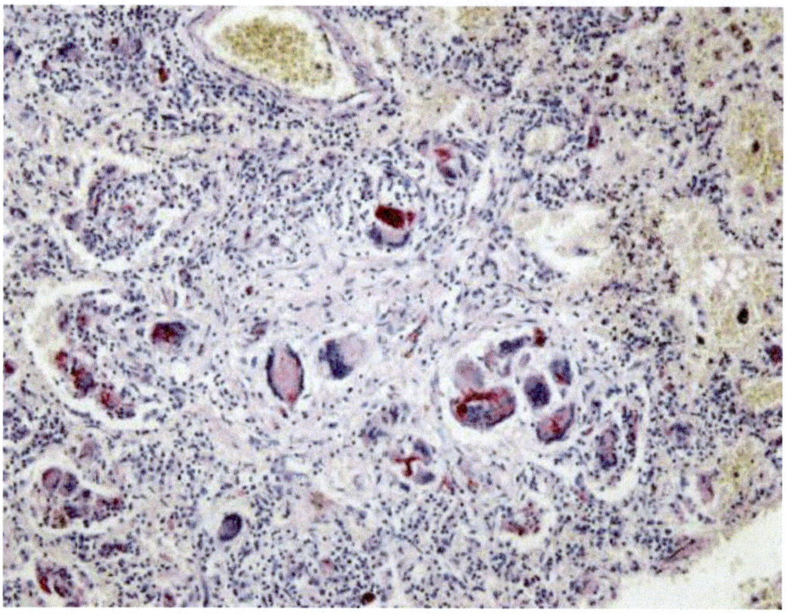

Fig. 11.9 Older aspiration pneumonia after chyme aspiration with embedded foreign material and distinct post-inflammatory fibrosis as well as polynuclear foreign-body giant cells (PAS ×100)

11.4 Amniotic Fluid Aspiration

Microscopic detection of amniotic fluid aspiration is particularly significant when determining the cause of death in stillborns and newborns. Reliable methods are required to quantify the modifications in the bronchi and lung parenchyma that were directly caused by amniotic fluid aspiration (Althoff and Cremer 1989; Sinicina et al. 2009). Amniotic fluid is a solution consisting of 98–99% water and 1–2% soluble and insoluble matter, mainly comprised of proteins, electrolytes, lipids, enzymes, and cellular debris from the fetal skin, urinary tract, respiratory system, and gastrointestinal tract (Fracasso et al. 2010).

Amniotic fluid aspiration during pregnancy is a paraphysiological event occurring to a fetus with intrauterine respiratory movements. Severe respiratory distress syndrome has been described after massive aspiration of uncontaminated amniotic fluid. The aspirated contents of amniotic fluid primarily include:

- Sebum
- Exfoliated epithelial cells of the fetal epidermis
- Lanugo hair
- Meconium (Bransilver 1970)

Aspiration of a small amount of amniotic fluid during birth or immediately after birth is physiologically possible. Thus, unless the cause of death has been determined, diagnosis of fatal amniotic fluid aspiration always requires examination of all pulmonary lobes.

The systematic examination of cases of intrapartal death of various causes has demonstrated that intrapartal aspiration of amniotic fluid only occurs when the function of the umbilical cord is impaired. For the purposes of forensic medicine, this means that death by intrapartal asphyxia can also be assumed when concurrent findings demonstrate that aspiration is absent and hypoxic changes in the organs are present (Dirnhofer and Sigrist 1983).

Due to amniotic fluid aspiration, the affected parts of the lung may show unfolding of the alveoli, which may simulate ventilation of the lung tissue (Janssen 1984 referring to Dell'Erba and Vimercati 1966, Janssen 1977, 1984). A histological examination is indispensable for verifying or excluding amniotic fluid aspiration in cases of alleged stillbirth and unlawful killing of a newborn.

Mild amniotic fluid aspiration not involving meconium aspiration is seldom relevant to the cause of death. However, massive amniotic fluid aspiration with abundant anucleated keratin

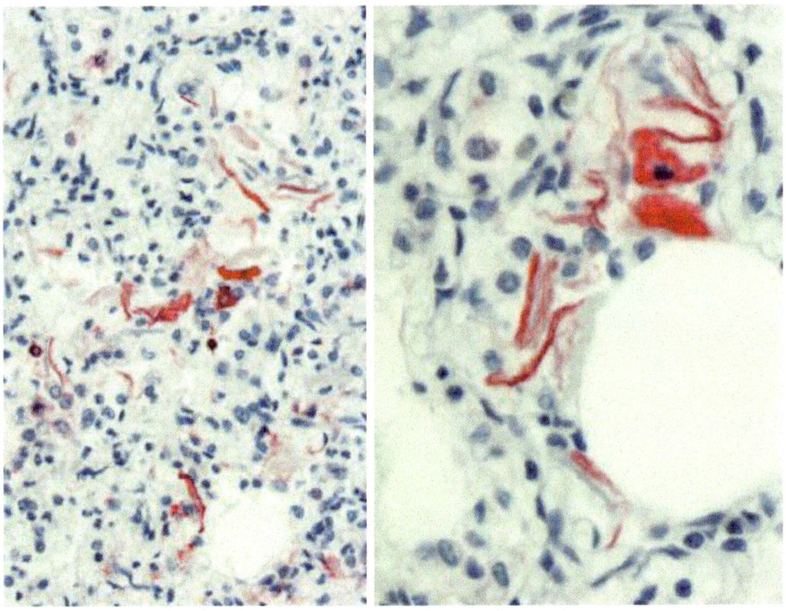

Fig. 11.10 Lung tissue following amniotic aspiration: intra-alveolar, partially anucleated keratin lamellae exfoliated from the fetal epidermis can be seen by immunohistochemistry (anti-cytokeratin ×250; ×400)

lamellae in the pulmonary alveoli has been described in congenital fetal epidermolysis bullosa. In such cases, however, it is important to histologically identify both epidermolysis bullosa and extensive amniotic fluid aspiration (Farkaš et al. 2015; Leslie 2009; Smith et al. 1992).

With some experience in microscopy, amniotic fluid aspiration can be easily diagnosed in most cases by means of conventional histological staining of tissue sections. Immunohistochemical examinations using an antibody against keratin lead to a clear representation of aspirated epidermal cells (Fig. 11.10).

In cases of chronic intrauterine meconium aspiration, distinctive subpleural infarcts of the lungs caused by meconium-induced vasoconstriction of peripheral preacinar arteries are possible, potentially even lung rupture and meconium embolism. The infarcts may contain inspissated meconium with a granulomatous reaction (Kearney 1999).

Inspissated meconium should be sought if anucleated or nucleated keratin lamellae are detected in the lung of neonates or newborns (Fig. 11.11). Meconium is found in amniotic fluid primarily as a result of intrauterine hypoxic stress. Inspissated meconium can cause thickening of the alveolocapillary exchange surface and injury to the surfactant, leading to severe impairment of ventilation. In the case of aspiration of non-sterile meconium, bacterial colonies are sporadically detected. An inflammatory reaction may ensue, involving aspiration pneumonia, atelectasis, and areas of hyperinflation in line with focal pulmonary emphysema. Clinical symptoms may include severe dyspnea, cyanosis, low muscle tone, and symptoms of shock, referred to as meconium aspiration syndrome. In this setting, the radiological work-up (chest X-ray) will be abnormal. In isolated cases, death following amniotic fluid or meconium aspiration can occur days after birth.

Normal infant lungs show atelectatic areas in addition to well-ventilated alveoli. The interstitial space seems thick, and the general impression is that of a cell-rich organ (Fracasso et al. 2010). Clumps of squames can be observed in the alveoli, but identification with simple H&E or PAS staining may be difficult for the less experienced investigator. Better identification is achieved with immunohistochemical techniques. Death related to amniotic fluid is represented by cases of embolism in uterine veins during labor and delivery but also by possible aspiration in the airways of the newborn during delivery (Ikeda et al. 1989).

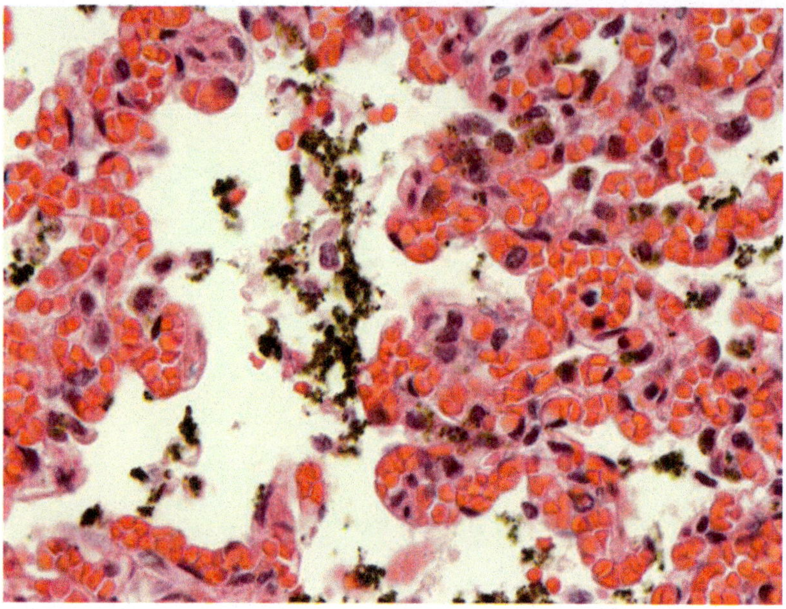

Fig. 11.11 Acute blood stasis in the lungs and massive pulmonary aspiration of meconium in a neonate (H&E ×400) (image kindly provided by Prof. J. Preuß-Wössner, Kiel/Lübeck, Germany)

11.5 Aspiration of Barium Sulfate

Barium sulfate is an insoluble salt and therefore nontoxic when ingested. Nevertheless, it plays a role in rare cases, e.g., suicide (Downs et al. 1995). It is usually used for contrast radiography of the digestive tract. Rare complications related to extravasation of barium sulfate into the peritoneal or retroperitoneal space, or intravasation into the blood stream, have been reported during barium enema examinations (Pelissier-Alicot et al. 1999; Deixonne et al. 1983; Gross and Howard 1972). Barium granuloma of the rectum is described as a benign complication occurring when contrast material is forced through a discontinuity in the rectal mucosa (Lewis et al. 1975). In rare cases, accidental aspiration of barium sulfate may occur (Zhang et al. 2015; Buschmann et al. 2011), causing damage to the lung tissue.

Aspiration pneumonia is expected with acute aspiration of barium sulfate. Histological findings show intra-alveolar rhomboid crystals with early granulocytic demarcation corresponding to the aspirated barium sulfate. In addition, indications of shock lung are found, in particular with hyaline membranes.

Protracted course: In the case of an insufficient reaction of the organism and a more prolonged survival period, a pattern of carnificating pneumonia may develop. Histologically, H&E and Elastica van Gieson stainings show dense collagen fibers in the alveolar lumina, alveolar walls broadened by connective tissue, loose lymphomonocytic inflammatory infiltrates, and possibly fibrin bands. Patients die after aspiration of barium-containing contrast medium as a result of ARDS (adult respiratory distress syndrome) despite intensive medical intervention (Tsokos et al. 1998).

11.6 Aspiration of Textile Material and Fibers

Diagnosis may be very challenging in cases of death due to smothering (Schmeling et al. 2009; Banaschak et al. 2003; Hicks et al. 1990). Histological findings may reveal dystelectasis of the lungs with varying degrees of emphysema, while the alveolar spaces may show hemorrhagic edema. Additionally, the alveolar septa may be stretched, acutely lacerated, and edematous together with activated macrophages (Schmeling et al. 2009). Nevertheless, these histological findings are not specific and do not allow for diagnosis of smothering, although they point to obstructive asphyxia.

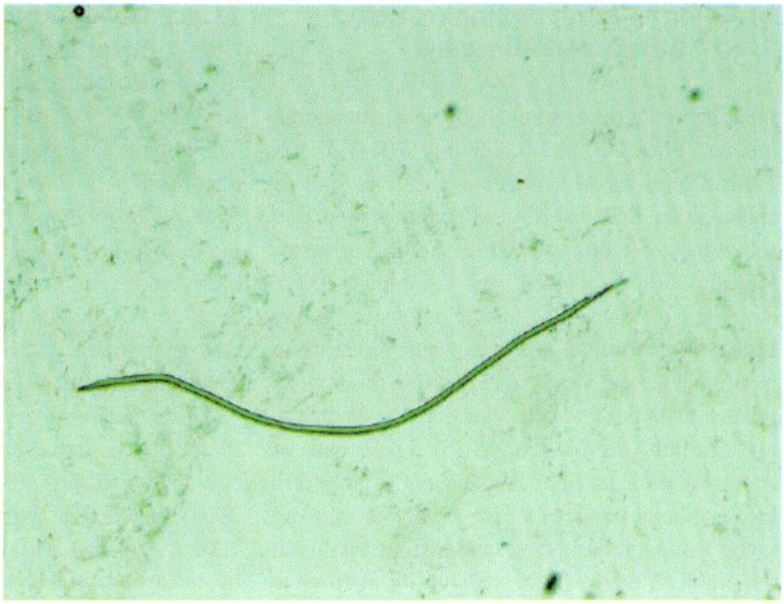

Fig. 11.12 Textile fiber detected in the sediment of a tracheobronchial lavage—consistent with the pillow used as a tool to suffocate by covering nose and mouth (×40)

In such cases, it is important to search for evidence of aspiration of fabric fibers. The preservation of traces around the mouth and nose with scotch tape can demonstrate close contact of, e.g., a pillow with the face. However, it is necessary to find fibers in the trachea to prove the vital obstruction of the airways by textile material and aspiration of fibers. A tracheobronchial lavage with distilled water should be carried out during autopsy. After centrifugation of the liquid, the sediment can be smeared on slides and dried. Microscopy can then reveal fibers aspirated during smothering (Fig. 11.12).

11.7 Aspiration of Other Substances

Particularly in the case of accidents, aspiration of foreign matter such as sand or dirt may occur (Saukko and Knight 2004; Glinjongo et al. 2004; Efron and Beierle 2003; Hanson et al. 2002; Koops et al. 1983; Bergeson et al. 1978). Cases reported to date have been due to external causes such as cave-ins (Wales et al. 1983), near drowning, or burial under sand masses (Kettner et al. 2008). Although extensive deep aspiration of sand, gravel, or dirt is a very rare incident, its consequences may be severe requiring immediate intensive care and possibly leading to death. Its distinction from preliminary suffocation in the case of simple agonal aspiration may be very difficult. If the demonstration of foreign matter in the deeper respiratory tracts is successful, this will allow for the assumption of fatal aspiration. This, however, is rarely the case. Histological findings of vital or lethal aspirations show overinflated lung segments, ruptures of the alveolar walls, dystelectasis, and subpleural petechiae. Fat embolism is possible, as well as microthrombi and degenerative changes such as vacuolizations of endothelial cells and hepatocytes (e.g., Kupffer cells). In order to adequately evaluate air, liquid, and vessel contents, as well as alveolar cells, it is necessary to examine at least five to ten lung samples (Maxeiner and Schneider 1985). Following the aspiration of sand, overinflated lung segments have primarily been described (Kettner et al. 2008). No diffuse alveolar edema and only focally small hemorrhagic alveolar edema have been proven. As a result of overinflation, one sees single, persistently stubby, and flattened or narrow alveolar walls without any vascular congestion in the septal capillaries and with ruptures in the alveolar walls—all well demonstrable using silver staining.

11.8 Inhalation of Smoke, Dust, Gases, and Allergens

Inhaling hot gases or smoke may cause inhalation trauma (Fracasso and Schmeling 2011; Peters 1981; Chap. 7). The inhalation of cigarette or cigar smoke, dust, gases, or allergens may lead to sometimes discrete, sometimes significant histological findings (Linch and Prahlow 2008). However, in many cases, there may not be any histological results. Fatal exposure to carbon monoxide perhaps leads to expression of antigens related to hypoxia, stress, and apoptosis in the myocardium (Morita et al. 2013). In the case of soot inhalation, particles of the soot dust found in the peripheral branches of the bronchial tree and in the lumina of the alveoli demonstrate vitality at the outbreak of the fire. Inhalation of aggressive gases, such as chlorine gas, may cause severe necrosis of lung tissue. Inhalation of allergens may lead to acute allergic shock. Other inhaled volatile substances may also cause death (Wick et al. 2007). In an acute setting, allergic-vasoneurotic laryngeal edema is possible, which is otherwise typically of noninflammatory origin. Fatal acute phlegmonous laryngitis is very rare (Ortmann et al. 2000).

Cigarette and Cigar Smoke An increase in the number of so-called smoker cells in lung tissue has been described in people who smoke. Cytological examinations of lung impression preparations from smokers' lungs revealed that the percentage of smoker cells within lung tissue increases up to a daily consumption of 40 cigarettes. Additional cigarette consumption above 40 per day does not raise the number of smoker cells present. A determination of nuclear content in the smoker cells of patient groups with different consumption rates showed that the number of macrophages with more than two nuclei increases in proportion to the number of cigarettes smoked. If more than 50 cigarettes a day were smoked, many multinucleated giant cells were observed (Reiter 1985).

11.8.1 Histopathological Findings After Inhalation of Volatile Substances

The intentional inhalation of a volatile substance ("sniffing") causing euphoria and hallucinations is an under-recognized form of substance abuse in children and adolescents leading to high morbidity and mortality (Schrot et al. 2009; Pfeiffer et al. 2006). Sudden death can be caused by cardiac arrhythmia, asphyxia, or trauma (Shepherd 1989; Janssen 1984).

The inhalation of volatile substances such as fuel vapors (Byard et al. 2003), isobutane (Pfeiffer et al. 2006; Rohrig 1997), propane (Sugie et al. 2004), or *n*-butane (Ago et al. 2002; Wehner et al. 2002; Segal and Wason 1990) is usually verified by means of toxicologic examinations. Autopsy findings are most often relatively unspecific. There are reports of intra-alveolar edema and activated macrophages, as well as intrapulmonary circulatory disturbances, and, in long-term use of isobutane by inhalation, for example, diffuse myocardial fibrosis has been described. In cases of fatalities after isobutane inhalation, fresh myocardial fiber necrosis demonstrated by intrasarcolemmal accumulation of fibronectin and fresh necrosis of single cardiomyocytes demonstrated by the loss of the cardiac antigen troponin C were found (Pfeiffer et al. 2006; Chap. 13).

Additionally, histopathologic findings may show aspiration of stomach contents, acute occlusive hyperemia (congestion), pulmonary edema, cerebral edema, and acute encephalopathy (Kaelan et al. 1986), as well as chronic neuropathological findings such as gliosis, cerebellar atrophy, and cerebral infarcts. The detection of pigmented foreign material within alveolar macrophages is described in cases of inhalation of dyestuffs which may contain titanium dioxide or solvents such as toluene (Byard et al. 2007). In such cases, the inherent color of the material can be seen using microscopy without staining. Lethal courses following inhalation of volatile substances are rare, generally accidental, and only rarely suicidal (Klitte et al. 2002). In some cases, massive acute myocardial necrosis may occur, as has been reported after inhalation of hydrogen sulfide (Christia-Lotter et al. 2007).

Inhalation of Trichloroethylene Solvents may be inhaled accidentally or with suicidal intent (von Lüpke et al. 1978). This includes the inhalation or "sniffing" of vapors over a prolonged period of time causing damage to the organism. The literature reports at least one attempted homicide by means of inhalation of trichloroethylene (Le Breton et al. 1963). Most other cases usually involve industrial accidents, followed by the aspiration of oil sludge in one case (waste oil sediments) (Fischer et al. 1977). Histologically, fatty degeneration of liver cells with hepatocellular necrosis and an inflammatory reaction in the portal tracts are predominantly seen. A further consequence is severe tubular nephrosis including necrosis of the proximal tubuli, as well as massive proteinuria. Kidneys and lungs show edema, while intrapulmonary hemorrhage will develop. After aspiration of particulate foreign matter, these particles may be demonstrated histologically; oily or greasy substances can only be partially resorbed, depending on the survival period (Fischer et al. 1977).

Inhalation of Hydrogen Sulfide A handful of case studies have reported fatal inhalation of H_2S, a toxic, flammable, and colorless gas. Histologically, superficial necrosis and mucosal desquamation were found most notably in the upper airways. Lung tissue was striking due to confluent hemorrhage and areas of emphysema (Dura et al. 2015; Reedy et al. 2011; Maebashi et al. 2011).

Cadmium Poisoning by Inhalation There have been several reports of acute accidental cadmium poisoning by inhalation (Townshead 1968; Evans 1966; Paterson 1947). The longer the survival time, the more distinct the indications of pulmonary damage caused by inhalation of cadmium-containing vapors (Yamamoto et al. 1983); histologically, alveolar spaces may be occupied by mononuclear cells, which are considered to be pneumocytes. An exudate presents signs of organization with fibroblasts in the interstitium and the intra-alveolar space. Patchy areas of leukocyte infiltration and intra-alveolar hemorrhage can be observed. In the liver, fatty degeneration is present around the central vein. The renal tubular epithelia show degenerative changes. Severe hypoxemia leads to myocardial single-cell necrosis and fibrotic changes.

Inhalation of Fuel Vapors Fatalities following fuel vapor inhalation have been reported as case studies. However, dermotoxic damage by petroleum hydrocarbons must also be considered. A paper-thin detachment of the epidermis is described, which is histologically accompanied by swelling and spongiosis (toxic epidermolysis). In addition, hyperemia and, depending on survival time, a leukocytic reaction may be observed (Rabl et al. 1989; Carnevale et al. 1983).

Inhalation of Propane (C_3H_8) There are rare cases with inhalation of propane or butane (C_4H_{10}) in suicidal intent (Sugie et al. 2004). Lung tissue may present severe congestion, numerous granulocytic infiltrations (Fig. 11.13), and fibrinous membranes. The liver can be found with fresh necroses, inflammatory reactions, and fragments of destroyed cells in the portal triads and also concerning hepatocytes next to the portal triads (Fig. 11.14). In cases of sudden death after isobutane sniffing, sectional total anemia of the microcirculation in the lungs is described as well as multiple intracapillary and endothelial "blebs" with total obstruction of the capillary lumen (Pfeiffer et al. 2006). Additionally, myocardium represents with fresh myocardial necroses demonstrated by intrasarcolemmal accumulation of fibronectin (see Chap. 13), accompanied by intracellular loss of the cardiac antigen troponin C (Pfeiffer et al. 2006).

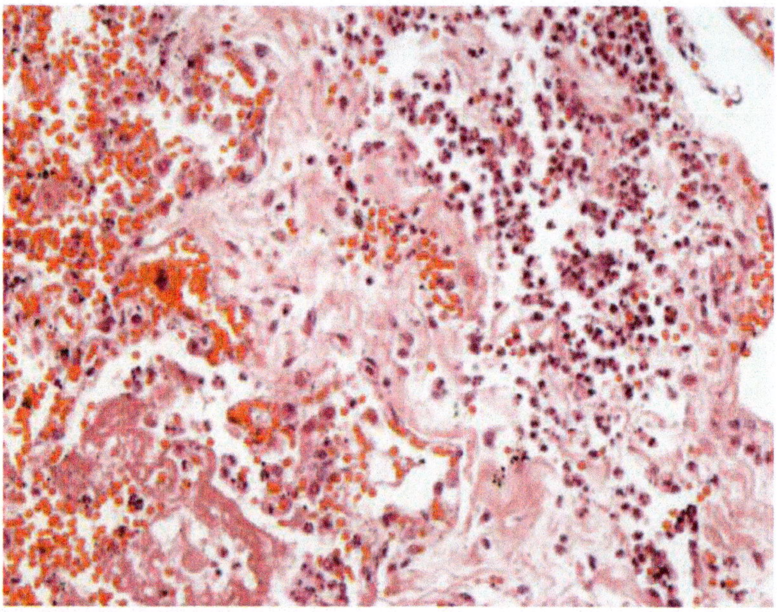

Fig. 11.13 Diffuse granulocytic infiltration in the walls of the bronchial tree and the lung tissue with cellular necrosis and fibrinous membranes—48-year-old man found dead following propane gas inhalation and with unknown survival period (H&E ×200)

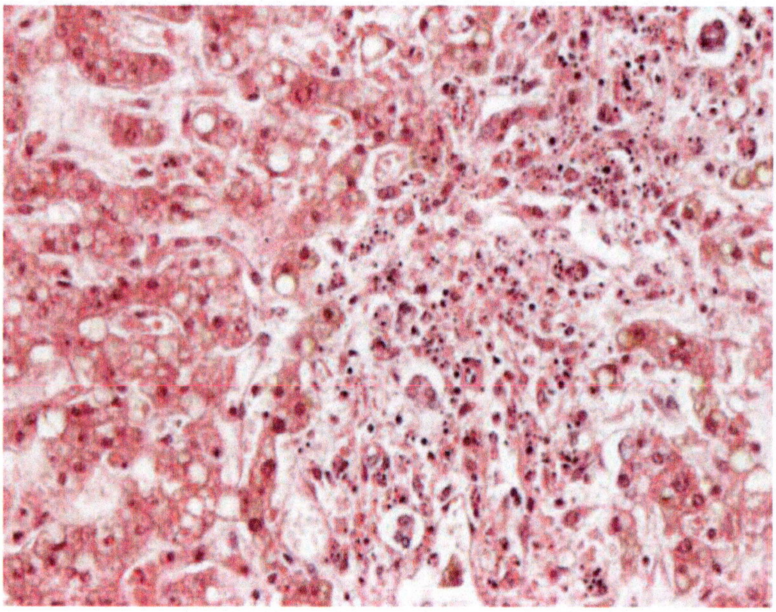

Fig. 11.14 Fresh necroses and multiple cell fragments in the portal fields and of hepatocytes in the liver following propane gas inhalation—same case as Fig. 11.13 (H&E ×200)

Inhalation of 1,1-Difluoroethane (HFC-152a) Mild interstitial edema was diffusely found in the myocardium, intra-alveolar edema with macrophages was observed, the capillary endothelia presented focal vesicularization in the lungs, and capillaries in the alveolar wall were generally congestive (Sakai et al. 2011).

Inhalation of Brake Cleaner Aerosols Brake cleaner liquid is commonly used for cleaning of engines and motor parts and contains volatile hydrocarbons (e.g., acetone, isopropanol, 2-methylpetane, 3-methylpentane, hexane). Inhalation leads to hypoxia-induced brain damage with cerebral edema and severe lung edema. After inhalation, volatile hydrocarbons disrupt the surface tension of the lung thereby impairing lung function. Furthermore the inhaled hydrocarbons enter the bloodstream affecting the central nervous system (CNS). The mechanism of action seems to be dose dependent (Bowen et al. 2006). High doses exert sedative effects; stimulating mechanisms were described for low doses (Howard et al. 2011). A severe congestion and hemorrhagic edema in all parts of the lungs can be found (Figs. 11.15 and 11.16).

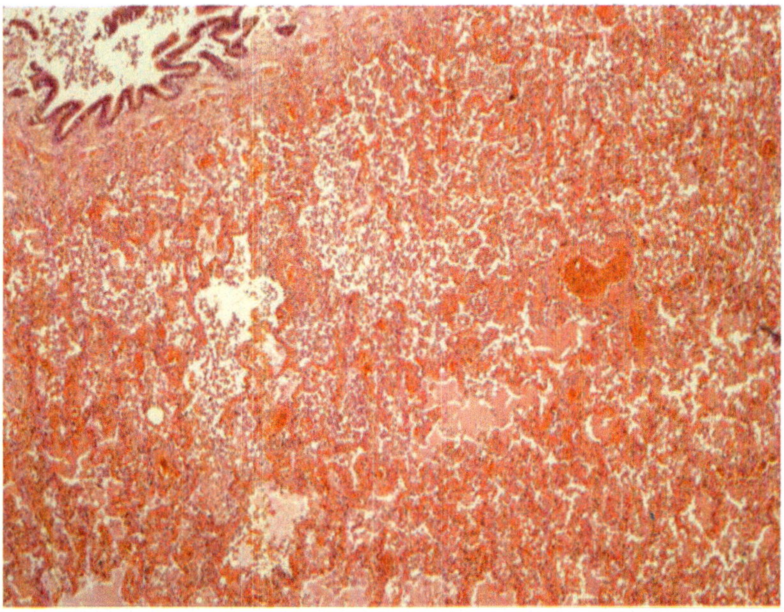

Fig. 11.15 Severe hemorrhagic edema in a case of accidental inhalation of brake cleaner aerosols (H&E ×40)

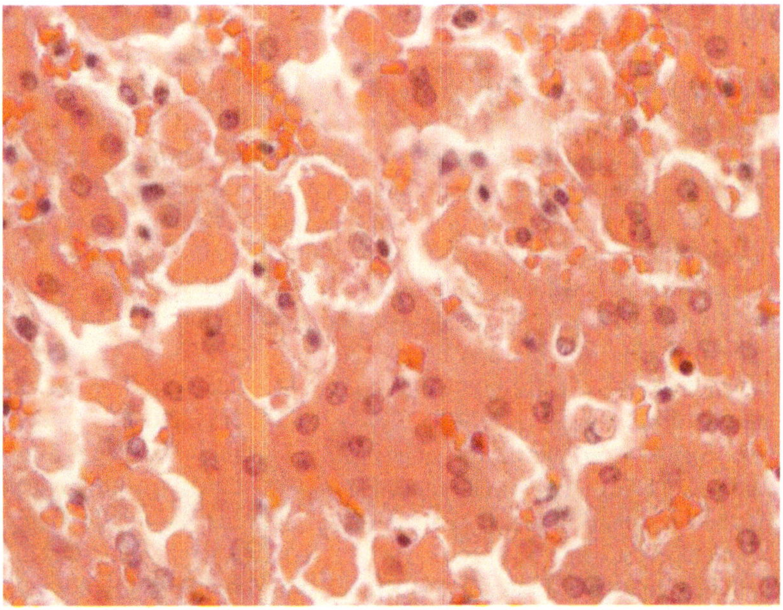

Fig. 11.16 Lethal brake cleaner inhalation with multiple single necroses of hepatocytes in the liver (H&E ×400)

11.8.2 Asthma and Fatal Anaphylaxis

It is well established that infiltration by mast cells, eosinophils, and activated T-lymphocytes plays a central role in anaphylactic reactions and asthmatic airway inflammation (Costa et al. 1997), although differential diagnosis can be difficult (Da Broi and Moreschi 2011; Perskvist and Edston 2007; Rainbow and Browne 2002; Pumphrey and Roberts 2000). Perskvist and Edston (2007) reported on marked differences in cellular composition of the lung between fatal anaphylaxis and asthmatic death. Anaphylactic shock represents the most severe type of anaphylaxis: a rapid release of large quantities of immunological mediators from mast cells takes place as an allergic response, e.g., histamine, serotonin, leukotrienes. Therefore, mast cell degranulation can be found microscopically, but conventional histopathology is nonspecific for anaphylaxis (Heinze et al. 2010). Mast cells appear to be the main cell type involved in IgE-induced passive sensitization, and mast cell-derived tryptase is also involved in the mechanisms of IgE-related hyperresponsiveness in asthmatic patients (Berger et al. 1998; Gerber et al. 1971). Drug-induced fatal anaphylactic shock is well known after administration of antibiotics, nonsteroidal anti-inflammatory drugs, anesthetics, contrast reagents, and extracts of allergen (Lenler-Petersen et al. 1995).

Asthma and Fatal Anaphylaxis Asthma is not a frequent cause of sudden death, but unexpected, unexplained sudden death in young asthmatic subjects is well known (Tsokos and Paulsen 2002; Robin and Lewiston 1989; Preston and Bowen 1987; Balachandra et al. 1987); Pentillä (1980) found only two cases in his series of 799 cases. Other authors had no such cases in their study of 77 sudden deaths (Särkioja and Hirvonen 1984). Asthma is a disorder characterized by increased responsiveness of the airways to various stimuli. It is classically subdivided into extrinsic (atopic) and intrinsic (idiopathic) types. Death from asthma in adults is rare; it is also rare in childhood (Champ and Byard 1994; Morild and Giertsen 1989; Benatar 1986). Often, viral respiratory tract infections were commonly associated findings. Most cases of sudden death due to asthma present with a long history and prolonged medication or hospitalization. In children, there is evidence of growth retardation in the form of height or weight below the third percentile (Champ and Byard 1994).

Most cases show bulky, hyperinflated lungs and mucus plugging of airways on cut sections, although collapsed lung parenchyma can sometimes be noted. Histologically, a variable thickening of bronchial basement membranes can be found together with hypertrophy of bronchiolar and bronchial smooth muscle, mucus gland hyperplasia, and mucus plugging of many of the minor airways (Fig. 11.17).

Eosinophils can be evident within the submucosa and also within mucus plugs; occasionally, Charcot–Leyden crystals are visible as octahedrite crystals. However, there are also focal areas of the lungs that appear relatively normal. Chronic inflammatory cell infiltrates and lymphoid follicular hyperplasia within the wall of the trachea and the major bronchi are suggestive of viral upper respiratory tract infections (Champ and Byard 1994).

Children are usually atopic, with attacks triggered by specific allergens which bind to presensitized IgE-covered mast cells resulting in the release of mediators such as histamine, leukotrienes, prostaglandin, and platelet-activating factors. Some victims experience right cardiac hypertrophy, while emphysema has also been seen (Copeland 1986), although this is not a characteristic finding in asthma patients (Morild and Giertsen 1989).

Death due to anaphylaxis often occurs suddenly and outside a hospital setting (Edston and van Hage-Hamsten 2005). Anaphylaxis is known to result in approximately 18 deaths per year in the USA compared to 2.4 million deaths per year from all causes in the USA (Unkrig et al. 2010). Serological investigations are helpful in the diagnosis of anaphylaxis (Nishio et al. 2005). Anaphylactic deaths do not show emphysema or significant mucous bronchial secretions, whereas all asthmatic deaths do (Table 11.1). Additionally, anaphylactic deaths present with severe pulmonary congestion and edema. The

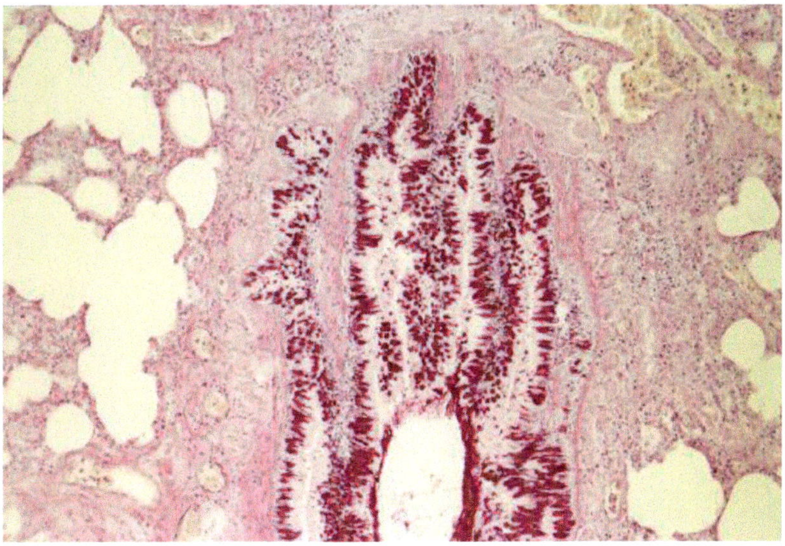

Fig. 11.17 Bronchus wall in asthma with papillar formations of the mucosa, goblet cell hyperplasia, thickening of the subepithelial basement membrane, and smooth muscle cell hyperplasia (PAS ×100)

Table 11.1 Histological and immunohistochemical findings in cases of fatal asthma

Organ	Findings
Internal organs	Acute occlusive hyperemia (congestion); facultative perivascular accumulation of $CD117^+$ mastocytes
Lung	• Acute eosinophilic pulmonary edema
	• Facultative peripheral coalesced pulmonary alveoli after bronchospasm (H&E)
	• Thickening of bronchial basement membranes
	• Hypertrophy of bronchiolar and bronchial smooth muscle
	• Mucus gland hyperplasia
	• Mucus plugging of many of the minor airways
	• Dilated vessels with perivascular inflammatory infiltrates consisting of mast cells, lymphocytes, and eosinophils (Shiang et al. 2009; Tsokos 2006; Carroll et al. 1996)
	• Epithelial desquamation (finding with different interpretations; Holgate and Davies 2001; Ordonez et al. 2000)
Bronchial lumina	Facultatively increased mucous accumulation (PAS)
Pulmonary interstitium	Accumulation of $CD117^+$ mastocytes
Bronchial walls	Possibly increased number of IgE^+ cells, demonstrated by immunohistochemistry

For anaphylactic shock, see also Chap. 15

symptomatology of anaphylaxis with mucosal and parenchymal edema could be explained by the activation of mast cells both centrally and peripherally in the lung parenchyma (Perskvist and Edston 2007). This seems to result in generally increased vascular permeability and, in combination with systemic vasodilatation, also results in severe congestion. In contrast, cases of acute asthma show eosinophils and mast cells mainly located in the bronchial wall (Fig. 11.18) and mucosa leading to the typical symptoms of bronchial smooth muscle constriction and mucous secretion (Tsokos 2006; Hays and Fahy 2003). Postmortem IgE tests can cause a high titer of IgE antibodies as well as serum tryptase. However, to definitively prove an acute rise in the enzyme blood concentration—due to mast cell degranulation and pathognomonic in anaphylaxis—a baseline measurement is necessary. Otherwise, mast cell degranulation can be visualized using immunohistochemistry and specific markers such as CD117 and particularly anti-tryptase antibodies. Mast cells must show a reaction to anti-tryptase in the cells and also around the cells in the extracellular space (Chap. 15). Allergic and asthmatic reactions to heroin and alcoholic drinks are discussed (Vally and Thompson 2003; Krantz et al. 2003; Shaikh

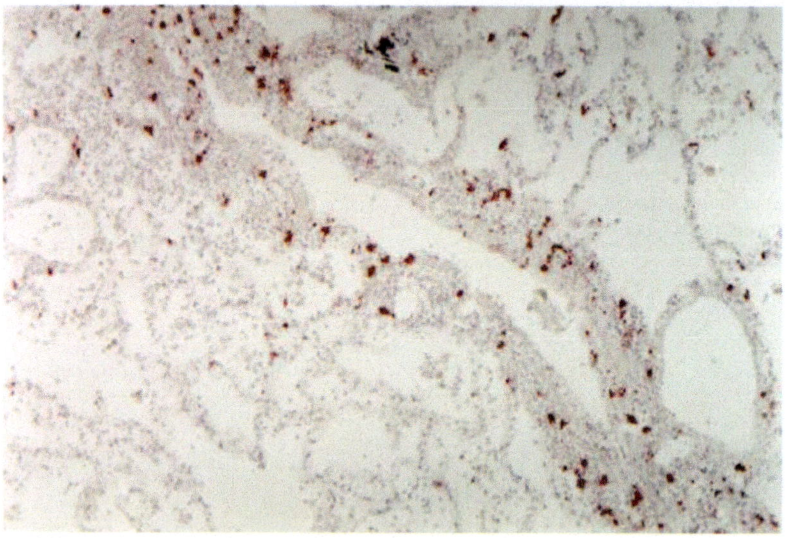

Fig. 11.18 Accumulation of immunohistochemical IgE-positive cells in the bronchial wall in a case of acute allergic asthma (IgE ×100)

1990, Hughes and Caverly 1988). Expression of pulmonary lactoferrin in sudden-onset (death within 1 h of the onset of an asphyctic asthma attack) and slow-onset asthma (time interval between onset of asthma attack and death >2.5 h) with fatal outcome was investigated in comparison to controls (Tsokos and Paulsen 2002).

Eosinophilic Pneumonia The pathology of eosinophilic pneumonia, a rare allergic syndrome, is usually characterized by diffuse eosinophilic granulocyte infiltration in the lungs. The majority of patients affected are middle-aged females (Liang et al. 2010). Only a few clinical and epidemiological studies have been carried out concerning eosinophilic pneumonia. In fatal cases, eosinophilic granulocytes can be found not only in the lungs but also in the lumina of peripheral vessels (Fig. 11.19) at the portal tracts of the liver, in the splenic sinuses, in the mucosa of the gastric fundus, and in the intestinal epithelium (Liang et al. 2010).

11.8.3 Inhalation of Hairspray ("Hairspray Lung")

There are isolated reports in the literature on the primarily histopathological findings in lung tissue following long-term excessive inhalation of hairspray (Lang et al. 2015; Wright and Cockcroft 1981; Gebbers et al. 1979, 1980; Nagata et al. 1997) or of an antiperspirant aerosol (Uchida et al. 2015). Findings from animal tests conducted on rats and hamsters are also available (Kawajiri et al. 2004; Gupta and Drew 1976). Focal deposits of amorphic material in lung tissue (Fig. 11.20), lymphomonocytic alveolitis, sometimes with a granulomatous reaction, multinucleated foreign-body-type giant cells, and increased alveolar macrophages accompanied by fibrosing inflammation ("hairspray lung") have been reported. If hairspray is inhaled from the moist milieu of a plastic box that is repeatedly used, fungal spores may accumulate and be concomitantly inhaled (Fig. 11.21).

In the case of one young woman, perivascular cell defects and lipophage accumulations were seen in brain tissue (Fig. 11.22). Hairspray inhalation as such does not usually cause histopathological findings in lung tissue that can account for death.

Paraphenylenediamine (PPD) or black dye is an aromatic amine derivative of the aniline, which is traditionally used as cosmetic product, particularly in hair dye preparations in the Maghreb countries and India. There are reports of lethal cases of PPD poisoning causing myocarditis associated with rhabdomyolysis (Jedidi et al. 2016, Trikha et al. 2013).

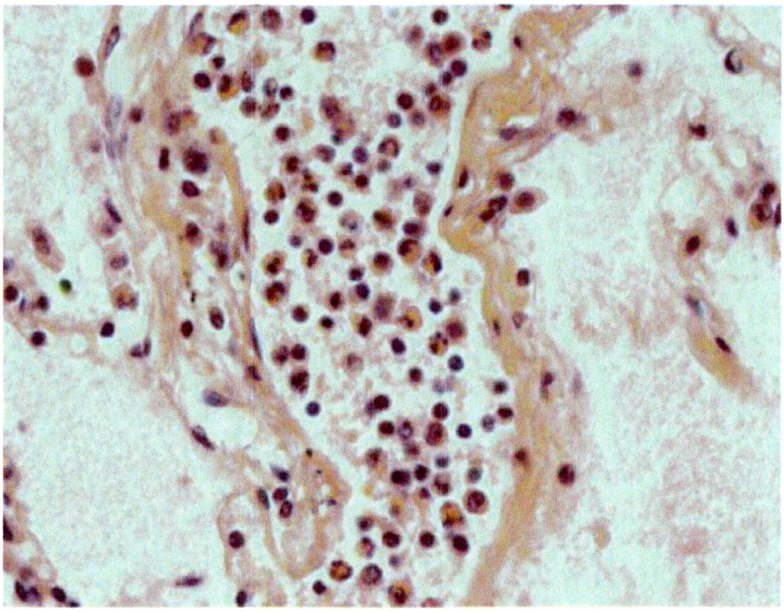

Fig. 11.19 Eosinophilic pneumonia: lung tissue with numerous eosinophilic granulocytes in the lumina of peripheral vessels (H&E ×400)

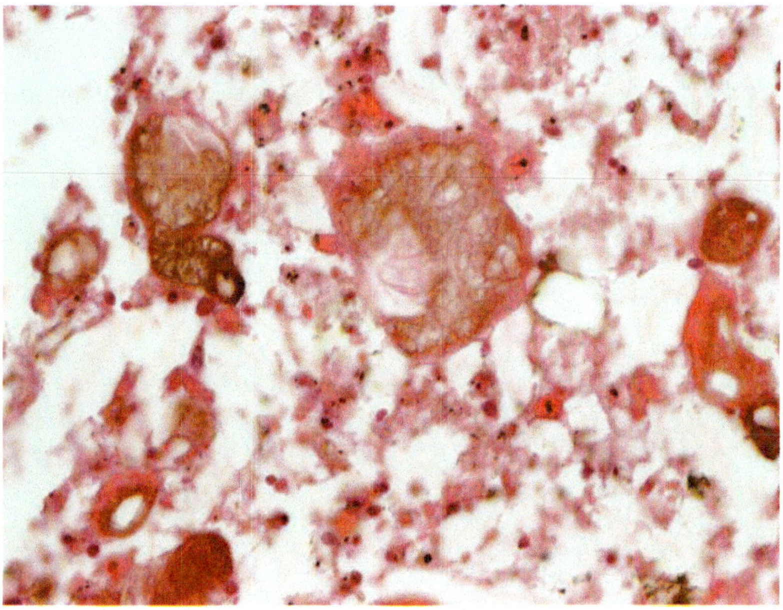

Fig. 11.20 Amorphous foreign material deposits in the lungs following long-term hairspray inhalation (H&E ×400)

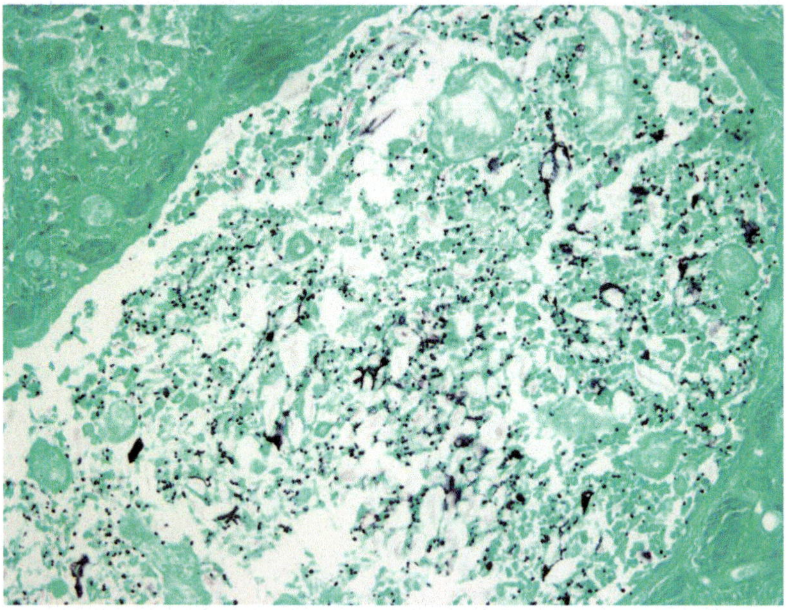

Fig. 11.21 Hairspray lung with abundant intrabronchial fungal hyphae and conidia (Grocott ×100)

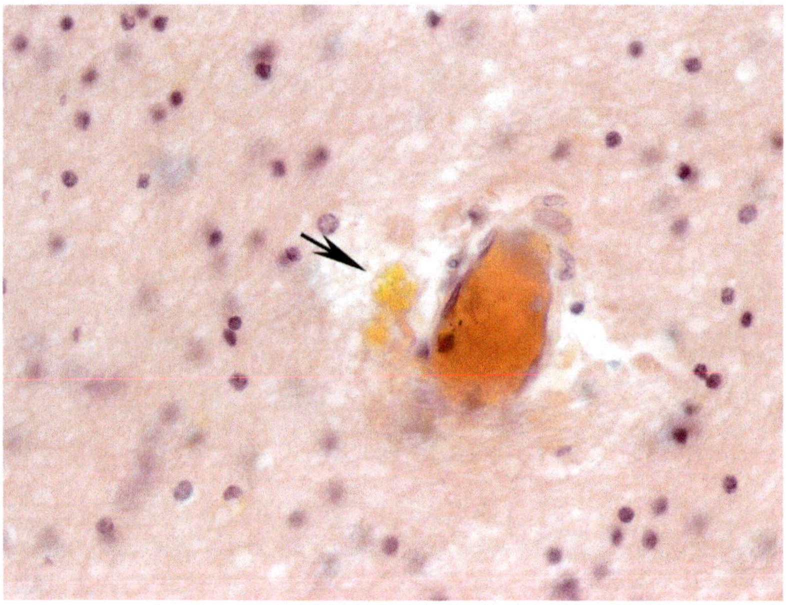

Fig. 11.22 Hairspray inhalation of many years' standing and numerous perivascular accumulations of lipophages in the brain (H&E ×400)

References

Ago M, Ago K, Ogata M (2002) A fatal case of n-butane poisoning after inhaling anti-perspiration aerosol deodorant. Legal Med 4:113–118

Althoff H, Cremer U (1989) Aspects of preliminary proceedings according to criminal law against physicians and morphological requirements for fatal aspiration of amniotic fluid. Z Rechtsmed 102:11–23

Bajanowski T, Ott A, Jorch G, Brinkmann B (1996) Frequency and type of aspiration in cases of sudden infant death (SID) in correlation with the body position at the time of discovery. J SIDS Infant Mortal 1: 271–279

Balachandra AT, O'Connor R, Bowden DH (1987) Sudden unexpected death in asthmatics. J Can Soc Forensic Sci 20:227

Banaschak S, Schmidt P, Madea B (2003) Smothering of children older than one year of age – diagnostic

significance of morphological findings. Forensic Sci Int 134:163–168
Benatar SR (1986) Fatal asthma. N Engl J Med 314: 423–427
Berger P, Walls AF, Marthan R, Tunon-de-Lara JM (1998) Immunoglobulin E-induced passive sensitization of human airways: an immunohistochemical study. Am J Respir Crit Care Med 157:610–616
Bergeson PS, Hinchcliffe WA, Crawford RF, Sorenson MJ, Trump DS (1978) Asphyxia secondary to massive dirt aspiration. J Pediatr 92:506–507
Bowen SE, Batis JC, Paez-Martinez N, Cruz SL (2006) A direct comparison of inhalant effects on locomotor activity and schedule-controlled behavior in mice. Exp Clin Psychopharmacol 6:235–247
Bransilver BR (1970) Massive aspiration in the newborn. Obstet Gynecol 35:608–612
Brinkmann B, Fechner G, Püschel K (1983) Lung histology in aspiration of watery fluids of different osmolarities. Z Rechtsmed 89:267–277
Buschmann C, Schulz F, Tsokos M (2011) Fatal aspiration of barium sulfate. Forensic Sci Med Pathol 7: 63–64
Byard RW, Chivell WC, Gilbert JD (2003) Unusual facial markings and lethal mechanisms in a series of gasoline inhalation deaths. Am J Forensic Med Pathol 24:298–302
Byard RW, Gilbert JD, Terlet J (2007) Death associated with volatile substance inhalation – histologic, scanning electron microscopic and energy dispersive X-ray spectral analyses of lung tissue. Forensic Sci Int 171:118–121
Carnevale A, Chiarotti M, Giovanni ND (1983) Accidental death by gasoline ingestion. Case report and toxicological study. Am J Forensic Med Pathol 4: 153–157
Carroll N, Carello S, Cooke C, James A (1996) Airway structure and inflammatory cells in fatal attacks of asthma. Eur Respir J 9:709–715
Chajed PN, Malouf MA, Glanville AR (2003) Risk of bleeding associated with transbronchial lung biopsy. Chest 123:2162
Champ CS, Byard RW (1994) Sudden death in asthma in childhood. Forensic Sci Int 66:117–127
Christia-Lotter A, Bartoli C, Piercecchi-Marti MD, Demory D, Pelissier-Alicot AL, Sanvoisin A, Leonetti G (2007) Fatal occupational inhalation of hydrogen sulfide. Forensic Sci Int 169:206–209
Copeland AR (1986) Asthmatic deaths in the medical examiner's population. Forensic Sci Int 31: 7–12
Costa JJ, Weller PF, Galli SJ (1997) The cells of the allergic response: mast cells, basophils and eosinophils. JAMA 278:1815–1822
Da Broi U, Moreschi C (2011) Post-mortem diagnosis of anaphylaxis: a difficult task in forensic medicine. Forensic Sci Int 204:1–5
Deixonne B, Baumel H, Mauras Y, Allain P, Robert C, Raffanel C (1983) A case of barium-peritoneum with neurological involvement. Importance of barium determination in biological fluids. J Chir 120:611–613
Dell'Erba A, Vimercati F (1966) Inalacione di liquido amniotico e causa della morte dell prodotto di concedimento. G Med Leg Infortun Tossicol 12:349
Dettmeyer R, Schmidt P, Driever F, Stiel M, Madea B (2003) Letale pulmonale Hämorrhagien als plötzliche und unerwartete Todesursache. 11th Spring Meeting of the German Society of Forensic Medicine, Kiel
Dirnhofer R, Sigrist T (1983) Intra partum death or infanticide? A contribution on intrapartal asphyxia. Z Rechtsmed 91:145–151
Downs JC, Milling D, Nichols CA (1995) Suicidal ingestion of barium-sulfide-containing shaving powder. Am J Forensic Med Pathol 16:56–61
Dura H, Morar S, Cipăian CR (2015) Chemical suicide by inhalation of hydrogen sulfide in Sibiu County, Romania. Case report and literature review. Rom J Leg Med 23:289–292
Edston E, van Hage-Hamsten M (2005) Postmortem diagnosis of anaphylaxis. In: Tsokos M (ed) Forensic pathology reviews, vol 3. Humana, Totowa, pp 267–281
Efron PA, Beierle EA (2003) Pediatric sand aspiration: case report and literature review. Pediatr Surg Int 19: 409–412
Eisenmenger W, Liebhardt E, Tröger HD (1980) Zwischenfälle bei endoskopischen Eingriffen und ihre Beurteilung aus rechtsmedizinischer Sicht. Beitr Gerichtl Med 38:25–28
Evans DM (1966) Cadmium poisoning. Br Med J 1:173–174
Farkaš D, Ŝvajdler MM, Fröhlichová L, Ŝprláková J, Iannaccone SF, Szép Z, Nyitrayová O (2015) Unusual lung finding of massive alveolar filling with foamy macrophages in congenital epidermolysis bullosa after amnion fluid aspiration in 15-day-old newborn without any clinical signs of respiratory impairment. Cesk Patol 51:89–93
Fischer H, Kahler J, Megges G, Steiner R (1977) Zur Kasuistik der Ölschlammaspiration. Z Rechtsmed 79:241–244
Fracasso T, Schmeling A (2011) Delayed asphyxia due to inhalation injury. Int J Legal Med 125:289–292
Fracasso T, Karger B, Vennemann M, Bajanowski T, Golla-Schindler UM, Pfeiffer H (2010) Amniotic fluid aspiration in cases of SIDS. Int J Legal Med 124:113–117
Gebbers O, Tetzner C, Burkhardt A (1979) Alveolitis due to hair-spray. Ultrastructural observations in two patients and the results of experimental investigations. Virchows Arch A Pathol Anat Histol 382:323–338
Gebbers O, Burkhardt A, Tetzner C, Rüdiger HW, von Wichert P (1980) "Hair-spray lung". Clinical and morphological findings. Schweiz Med Wochenschr 110:610–615
Gerber MA, Paronetto F, Kochwa S (1971) Immunohistochemical localization of IgE in asthmatic lungs. Am J Pathol 62:339–348

Glinjongo C, Kiatchaipipat S, Thepcharoenniran S (2004) Severe sand aspiration: a case report with complete recovery. J Med Assoc Thail 87:825–828
Graev M, Fabroni F (1962) Sulla evoluzione dei focolai di aspirazione ematica polmonare. Min Med Leg 82:255
Gross GF, Howard MA (1972) Perforations of the colon from barium enema. Am Surgeon 38:583–585
Gupta BN, Drew RT (1976) The effect of aerosol hair spray inhalation in the hamster. Am Ind Hyg Assoc J 37:357–360
Hanson KA, Gilbert JD, James RA, Byard RW (2002) Upper airway occlusion by soil – an unusual cause of death in vehicle accidents. J Clin Forensic Med 9:96–99
Hayashi T, Ishida Y, Mizunuma S, Kimura A, Kondo T (2009) Differential diagnosis between freshwater drowning and saltwater drowning based on pulmonary aquaporin-5 expression. Int J Legal Med 123:7–13
Hays SR, Fahy JV (2003) The role of mucus in fatal asthma. Am J Med 115:68–69
Heinze S, Erbersdobler A, Tsokos M (2010) Cause of death: anaphylaxis. Autopsy findings and additional investigations. Rechtsmedizin 20:282–284
Hicks LJ, Scanlon M, Bostwick TC, Batten TJ (1990) Death by smothering and its investigation. Am J Forensic Med Pathol 11:291–293
Holgate ST, Davies DE (2001) Epithelia desquamation in asthma. Am J Respir Crit Care Med 164:1997
Howard MO, Bowen SE, Garland EL, Perron BE, Vaughn MG (2011) Inhalant use and inhalant use disorders in the United States. Addict Sci Clin Pract 6:18–31
Hughes S, Caverly PMA (1988) Heroin inhalation and asthma. BMJ 297:1511–1512
Ikeda N, Yamakawa M, Imai Y, Suzuki T (1989) Sudden infant death from atelectasis due to amniotic fluid aspiration. Am J Forensic Med Pathol 10:340–343
Iwadate K, Doy M, Ito Y (2001) Screening of milk aspiration in 105 infant death cases by immunostaining with anti-human alpha-lactalbumin antibody. Forensic Sci Int 122:95–100
Janssen W (1977) Forensische Histologie. Schmidt-Roemhild, Lübeck, pp 207–210
Janssen W (1984) Pregnancy, abortion, aborticide. The problem of the cause of death. In: Janssen W (ed) Forensic histopathology. Springer, Berlin, pp 205–207
Jedidi M, Bel Hadj M, Masmoudi T, Ben Adelkarim S, Mlayeh S, Ben Dhiab M, Souguir MK (2016) Fatal toxic myocarditis induced by paraphenylene diamine. A case report. Rom J Led Med 24:17–20
Jobba G (1971) Nachweis von aspiriertem Amylum und Cellulose mit der modifizierten Steinschen Reaktion. Z Rechtsmed 68:204–206
Kaelan C, Harper C, Vieira BI (1986) Acute encephalopathy and death due to petrol sniffing: neuropathological findings. Aust NZ J Med 16:804–807
Kawajiri T, Nagata N, Morimoto Y, Ishimatsu S, Hori H, Tanaka I, Yatera K, Yoshii C, Kido M (2004) Pathology and mechanism of lung toxicity following inhalation of hair spray in rats. Inhal Toxicol 16:147–153
Kearney MS (1999) Chronic intrauterine meconium aspiration cause fetal lung infarcts, lung rupture, and meconium embolism. Pediatr Dev Pathol 2:544–551
Keating WR, Hayward MG (1981) Sudden death in cold water and ventricular arrhythmia. J Forensic Sci 26: 451–461
Kettner M, Ramsthaler F, Horlebein B, Schmidt PH (2008) Fatal outcome of a sand aspiration. Int J Legal Med 122:499–502
Klitte A, Gilbert JD, Lokan R, Byard RW (2002) Adolescent suicide due to inhalation of insect spray. J Clin Forensic Med 9:22–24
Koops E, Püschel K, Hadjiraftis K, Brinkmann B (1983) Ungewöhnliche Aspirations-Todesfälle. Beitr Berichtl Med 42:47–56
Krantz AJ, Hershow RC, Prachand N, Hayden DM, Franklin C, Hryhorczuk DO (2003) Heroin insufflation as a trigger for patients with life threatening asthma. Chest 1213:510–517
Lang J, Felske-Zech H, Veit F, Lasczkowski G, Dettmeyer R (2015) Chronic abuse of hairspray by inhalation and sudden death of a 20-year-old woman. Rom J Leg Med 23:285–288
Le Breton R, Bourtris L, Garat J (1963) Un cas d' empoisonnement criminel par le trichlorethylene. Ann Med leg 43:281–283
Lenler-Petersen P, Hansen D, Andersen M (1995) Drug-related fatal anaphylactic shock in Denmark 1968–1990. A study based on notifications to the committee on adverse drug reactions. J Clin Epidemiol 48:1185–1188
Leopold D (1959) Blutaspirationen bei Dekapitationen. Zeitschr ärztl Fortb 53:1043–1045
Leslie KO (2009) My approach to interstitial lung disease using clinical, radiological and histopathological patterns. J Clin Pathol 62:387–401
Lewis JW Jr, Kerstein MD, Koss N (1975) Barium granuloma of the rectum: an uncommon complication of barium enema. Ann Surg 181:418–423
Liang M, Sunnassee A, Yan L, Zheng N, Zhuo L, Haidong Z, Liang L (2010) Fatal anaphylaxis in the presence of eosinophilic pneumonia in an asthmatic patient. A case report. Rom J Leg Med 18:193–198
Linch CA, Prahlow JA (2008) Microscopical examination of particles on smoked cigarette filters. Forensic Sci Med Pathol 4:228–233
Maebashi K, Iwadate K, Sakai K, Takatsu A, Fukui K et al (2011) Toxicological analysis of 17 autopsy cases of hydrogen sulfide poisoning resulting from the inhalation of intentionally generated hydrogen sulfide gas. Forensic Sci Int 207:91–95
Maxeiner H, Schneider V (1985) Death by suffocation as a result of occlusion of the respiratory tract by sand. Z Rechtsmed 94:173–189
Modell JH, Bellefleur M, Davis JH (1999) Drowning without aspiration: is this an appropriate diagnosis? J Forensic Sci 44:1119–1123
Morild I, Giertsen JC (1989) Sudden death from asthma. Forensic Sci Int 42:145–150
Morita S, Furukawa S, Wingenfeld L, Nishi K (2013) Expression of antigens related to hypoxia, stress, and

apoptosis in the myocardium after fatal carbon exposure. Rom J Leg Med 21:253–258
Mueller B, Erbach A, Ottmar U (1960) Studien über das Schicksal von Blutaspirationsherden. Riv Med Leg Legislac Sanit 2:7
Nagata N, Kawajiri T, Hayashi T, Nakanishi K, Nikaido Y, Kido M (1997) Interstitial pneumonitis and fibrosis associated with the inhalation of hair spray. Respiration 64:310–312
Nishio H, Takai S, Miyazaki M, Horiuchi H, Osawa M, Uemura K (2005) Usefulness of serum mast cell-specific chymase levels for post-mortem diagnosis of anaphylaxis. Int J Legal Med 119:331–334
Oehmichen M (1984) Blutabbau in den Lungenaleolen: Zeichen der Vitalität und Bestimmung der Überlebenszeit. Z Rechtsmed 92:47–57
Ordonez C, Ferrando R, Hyde DM, Wong HH, Fahy JV (2000) Epithelial desquamation in asthma: artifact or pathology? Am J Respir Crit Care Med 162: 2324–2329
Ortmann C, Fechner G, Schmäl F (2000) Akuter Tod nach Halsschmerzen. 9th Spring Meeting of the German Society of Forensic Medicine. 4–5 May, Leipzig
Ortmann C, Wüllenweber J, Brinkmann B, Fracasso T (2010) Fatal mycotic aneurysm caused by Pseudallescheria boydii after near drowning. Int J Legal Med 124:243–247
Paterson JC (1947) Studies on the toxicity of inhaled cadmium. J Ind Hyg Toxicol 29:294–301
Pelissier-Alicot AL, Leonetti G, Champsaur P, Allain P, Mauras Y, Botta A (1999) Fatal poisoning due to intravasation after oral administration of barium sulfate for contrast radiography. Forensic Sci Int 106:109–113
Pentillä A (1980) Sudden and unexpected natural deaths of adult males. Forensic Sci Int 16:249–259
Perskvist N, Edston E (2007) Differential accumulation of pulmonary and cardiac mast cell-subsets and eosinophils between fatal anaphylaxis and asthma death. A post-mortem comparative study. Forensic Sci Int 169: 43–49
Peters WJ (1981) Inhalation injury caused by the products of combustion. Can Med Assoc J 125:249–252
Pfeiffer H, Al Khaddam M, Brinkmann B, Köhler H, Beike J (2006) Sudden death after isobutene sniffing: a report of two forensic cases. Int J Legal Med 120:168–173
Preston HV, Bowen DAL (1987) Asthma deaths: a review. Med Sci Law 27:89–94
Preuss J, Dettmeyer R, Madea B (2005) Tödliche Blutungskomplikation durch Pulmonalarterienwandruptur bei Rechtsherzkatheter. 84 Annual Meeting of the German Society of Forensic Medicine, 19–24 September, Hamburg
Pumphrey RSH, Roberts ISD (2000) Postmortem findings after anaphylactic reactions. J Clin Pathol 53:273–276
Rabl W, Ambach E, Battista H (1989) Hautschädigung bei tödlicher Benzindampfinhalation. Beitr Gerichtl Med 47:295–300
Rainbow J, Browne GJ (2002) Fatal asthma or anaphylaxis? Emerg Med J 19:415–417
Reedy SJ, Schwarz MD, Morgan BW (2011) Suicide fads: frequency and characteristics of hydrogen sulfide suicides in the United States. West J Emerg Med 12:300–304
Reiter C (1985) Rauchverhalten und Zytologie der Raucherzellen. Z Rechtsmed 95:167–173
Revenstorf V (1904) Der Nachweis der aspirierten Ertrinkungsflüssigkeit als Kriterium des Todes durch Ertrinken. Vjschr Gerichtl Med 27:274
Robin ED, Lewiston N (1989) Unexpected, unexplained sudden death in young asthmatic subjects. Chest 96:790–793
Rohrig T (1997) Sudden death due to butane inhalation. Am J Forensic Med Pathol 18:299–302
Sakai K, Maruyama-Maebashi K, Takatsu A, Fukui K, Nagai T, Aoyagi M, Ochiai E, Iwadate K (2011) Sudden death involving inhalation of 1,1-difluoroethane (HFC-152a) with spray cleaner: three case reports. Forensic Sci Int 206:e58–e61
Särkioja T, Hirvonen J (1984) Causes of sudden unexpected deaths in young and middle-aged persons. Forensic Sci Int 24:247–261
Sato H, Tanaka T, Kasai K, Kita T, Tanaka N (2009) Perforation of the trachea by an endotracheal tube: an autopsy case. Int J Legal Med 123:513–516
Saukko P, Knight B (2004) Immersion deaths. In: Saukko P, Knight B (eds) Knight's forensic pathology. Arnold, London, pp 395–411
Schmeling A, Fracasso T, Pragst F, Tsokos M, Wirth I (2009) Unassisted smothering in a pillow. Int J Legal Med 123:517–519
Schmidt U, Günzel A, Müller L, Thiele K (2003) Plötzlicher Tod eines Kleinkindes durch Mageninhaltsaspiration bei Norwalk-like-Virusinfektion. 82nd Annual Meeting, German Society of Forensic Medicine. 17–20 September, Münster
Schrot M, Schulz F, Andresen H, Püschel K, Römhild W, Szibor R (2009) Forensische Pädopathologie: Tod durch Lösungsmittelinhalation – "Schnüffeltod". Päd 15:35–40
Segal E, Wason S (1990) Sudden death by inhalation of butane and propane. N Engl J Med 323:1638
Shaikh WA (1990) Allergy to heroin. Allergy 45:555–556
Shepherd RT (1989) Mechanism of sudden death associated with volatile substance abuse. Hum Toxicol 8:287–291
Shiang C, Mauad T, Senhorini A, de Araúja BB, Ferreira DS, da Silva LF, Dohlnikoff M, Tsokos M, Rabe KF, Pabst R (2009) Pulmonary periarterial inflammation in fatal asthma. Clin Exp Allergy 39:1450–1452
Sinicina I, Pankratz H, Bise K, Metevossian E (2009) Forensic aspects of post-mortem histological detection of amniotic fluid embolism. Int J Legal Med 124:55–62
Smith LT, Miller AW, Kirz DA, Elias S, Brumbaugh S, Holbrook KA (1992) Separation of noncutaneous epithelia in a fetus diagnosed in utero with junctional epidermolysis bullosa. Pediatr Res 31:561–566
Spendlove D, Trübner K, Bajanowski T (2007) Perforation of the pulmonary artery by a bronchial wall stent. Int J Legal Med 121:204–206
Strange C, Heffner JE, Collins BS, Brown FM, Sahn SA (1987) Pulmonary hemorrhage and air embolism

complicating transbronchial biopsy in pulmonary amyloidosis. Chest 92:367–369
Sugie H, Sasaki C, Hashimoto C, Takeshita H, Nagai T, Nakamura S, Furukawa M, Nishikawa T, Kurihara K (2004) Three cases of sudden death due to butane or propane gas inhalation: analysis of tissues for gas components. Forensic Sci Int 143:211–214
Suzuki T, Ikeda N, Umetsu K, Kashimura S (1985) Swimming and loss of consciousness. Z Rechtsmed 94:121–126
Townshead RH (1968) A case of acute cadmium pneumonitis: lung function tests during a four-year-follow-up. Br J Ind Med 25:68–71
Trikha S, Jatav OP, Rastogi P, Kansal A et al (2013) A case of myocarditis mimicking myocardial infarction in hair dye poisoning. J Ind Coll Cardiol 3:173–176
Tsokos M (2006) Asthma deaths. Phenomenology, pathology and medicolegal aspects. In: Tsokos M (ed) Forensic pathology reviews, vol 4. Humana Press Inc., Totwa, NJ, pp 107–141
Tsokos M, Byard RW (2007) Massive, fatal aspiration of blood: not necessarily a result of trauma. Am J Forensic Med Pathol 28:53–54
Tsokos M, Paulsen F (2002) Expression of pulmonary lactoferrin in sudden-onset and slow-onset asthma with fatal outcome. Virchows Arch 441:494–499
Tsokos M, Schulz F, Vogel H (1998) Barium aspiration with fatal outcome. Aktuelle Radiol 8:201–203
Uchida K, Unuma K, Uemura K (2015) A fatality in a child with severe fatty liver due to n-butane and isopentane poisoning resulting from long-term inhalation of an antiperspirant aerosol. Forensic Sci Med Pathol 11:631–632
Unkrig S, Hagemeier L, Madea B (2010) Postmortem diagnostics of assumed food anaphylaxis in an unexpected death. Forensic Sci Int 198:e1–e4
Vally H, Thompson PJ (2003) Allergic and asthmatic reactions to alcoholic drinks. Addict Biol 8:3–11
von Lüpke H, Gerchow J, Schmidt K (1978) Über zwei Fälle von tödlicher Trichloräthylenvergiftung. Z Rechtsmed 81:237–241
Walcher K (1930) Über Aspiration und Verschlucken von Gehirnstücken als Zeichen intravitaler Entstehung schwerer Verletzungen. Z Rechtsmed 15:398–406
Wales J, Jackimczyk K, Rosen P (1983) Aspiration following a cave-in. Ann Emerg Med 12:99–101
Wehner F, Benz D, Wehner HD (2002) Tödiche Inhalation von Butan-Propan-Gas. Arch Kriminol 209:165–168
Wick R, Gilbert JD, Felgate P, Byard RW (2007) Inhalant deaths in South Australia – a 20-year retrospective autopsy study. Am J Forensic Med Pathol 28:319–322
Wright JL, Cockcroft DW (1981) Lung diseases due to abuse of hairspray. Arch Pathol Lab Med 105:363–366
Yamamoto K, Ueda M, Kikuchi H, Hattori H, Hiraoka Y (1983) An acute fatal occupational cadmium poisoning by inhalation. Z Rechtsmed 91:139–143
Yen K, Plattner T, Dirnhofer R (2005) Retrograde blood aspiration: a vital reaction. Forensic Sci Int 154:13–18
Zhang L, Yang Y, Zhang J, Zhou X, Dong H, Zhou Y (2015) Barium sulfate aspiration: severe chemical pneumonia induced by a massive reflux of contrast medium during small bowel barium enema. Forensic Sci Int 253:e16–e19

12 Forensic–Histological Diagnosis of Species, Gender, Age, and Identity

Histological analysis of tissue samples and organ material contributes only rarely to the identification of a deceased person. However, a range of tests and conclusions are possible by means of microscopic diagnosis, including:

- Species diagnosis: human or nonhuman (e.g., by examining hair or bones).
- Cytological gender determination.
- Assigning biological material to certain tissues or organs.
- Determining blood group.
- Skin type (light- or dark-skinned) may be determined with skin samples.
- Based on histological criteria, the approximate age of a person may be estimated.

In cases where there are specific indications of histologically verifiable findings, e.g., a tattoo which is assumed to have been removed from a certain skin area, these can be proven microscopically to aid in the verification of identity. This is also true for residues of former implantations (Palazzo et al. 2010).

12.1 Species Diagnosis

Based on bone tissue samples, species diagnosis (human or nonhuman) is often possible macroscopically. However, with some bones, macroscopic species diagnosis is difficult or even impossible. In such cases, a histological examination may be helpful (Caccia et al. 2016; Dillon et al. 2016; Brits et al. 2014; Verhoff et al. 2006; Schiwy-Bochat 1993). Ground bone sections are analyzed to determine the number and width of Haversian canals, which are known to show significant differences between humans and animals (Rämsch and Zerndt 1963; Table 12.1).

Other studies investigated primarily cortical bone in a variety of animals [brown rat, *Rattus norvegicus*; hare, *Lepus americanus* (snowshoe hare); *Lepus oryctolagus* (European hare); European badger, *Meles meles*; raccoon dog, *Nyctereutes procyonoides*; cat, *Felis silvestris catus*; dog, *Canis lupus familiaris*; pig, *Sus scrofa domesticus*; goat, *Capra aegagrus hircus*; sheep, *Ovis aries*; cow, *Bos taurus*; deer, *Odocoileus virginianus*; horse, *Equus caballus*; water buffalo, *Bubalus arnee*; chimpanzees, *Pan troglodytes*; Old World monkeys, Cercopithecidae; rhesus macaques, *Macaca mulatta*; New World monkeys, Platyrrhini)], as well as the possibilities of age and gender determination (Hillier and Bell 2007). If a body has been largely dissolved by acids, it may be that, under certain circumstances, only microscopic residues of bone can be detected (Vermeij et al. 2015).

For histological species determination based on bone examination, the use of the proximal femur diaphysis is preferred (Janssen 1977). First, the bone tissue is macerated and decalcified; 10–15 μm thick tissue sections are then stained (e.g., thionin) and analyzed microscopically. Counting 100 visual fields is recommended, as is

R. B. Dettmeyer, *Forensic Histopathology*, https://doi.org/10.1007/978-3-319-77997-3_12

Table 12.1 Histological distinction between human and animal bone tissue on the basis of Haversian canals (Rämsch and Zerndt 1963, according to Dürwald 1987)

Haversian canals	Average diameter (µm)	Average number per visual field	Haversian canals in overview magnification
Human neonate	54.5	2.3	Medium-sized to very large, increasing in size toward the center, round to oval shape
Human, 6 months	60.5	1.7	–
Human, 12 months	71.6	1.6	–
Human, 18 months	56.8	1.7	–
Human, 41 years	52.9	1.7	–
Human, 70 years	70.0	1.5	–
Horse	30.0	2.7	Small to medium-sized, predominantly medium-sized, regularly shaped
Cattle	47.9	1.4	Predominantly medium-sized but also large, regularly shaped
Goat	21.2	2.4	Predominantly medium-sized but also large, becoming smaller toward the center
Sheep	18.2	3.6	Predominantly medium-sized but also large, irregular structure
Pig	32.8	2.1	Predominantly medium-sized but also large, becoming smaller toward the center
Dog	21.2	3.0	Predominantly very small but also medium-sized, regularly shaped
Rabbit	12.6	8.0	Very small, round to oval
Cat	20.3	2.8	Predominantly very small but also medium-sized, irregular structure
Chicken	14.0	7.0	Very small, round
Goose	15.7	14.4	Medium-sized, irregularly shaped

Very small, <10 µm; small, 11–20 µm; medium-sized, 21–40 µm; large, 41–80 µm; very large, >80 µm

exact morphometric measurement of canal diameter (metric histology), which is sometimes possible with newer technologies. Human bones show a random distribution of round, discretely polygonal, almost equi-sized osteons and Haversian canals, whereas numerous domestic animals typically show a plexiform, sometimes linear formation of osteons of various sizes. Ground bone sections may also be examined without previous decalcification (Fig. 12.1).

The distinction between human hair and animal hair may be possible using microscopy. For this purpose, it is necessary to examine the cross section of the hair shaft (Fig. 12.2). In cases where certain animal species are under particular legal protection, a distinction between animal species is required. Microscopic hair analysis can contribute to this differentiation (Tridico et al. 2014; Sato et al. 2010; Sahajpal et al. 2009). It is generally accepted that nuclei degrade in developing hair shafts. The point at which this nuclear degradation occurs was investigated using transmission electron microscopy to investigate when nuclei and mitochondria are no longer visible in the developing hair shaft (Linch 2009).

12.2 Cytological Gender Determination

Nuclear morphological examinations of body tissues or secretions enable the microscopic verification of so-called Barr bodies in females (Michailow 1975; Helmer 1970). It is sometimes necessary to determine the gender of individuals in order to establish their identity. Saliva stains found at the scene of a crime can be highly useful in such cases. Mittal et al. (2008) studied buccal mucosal scrapings from 100 men and 100 women using the Papanicolaou staining method. They examined the

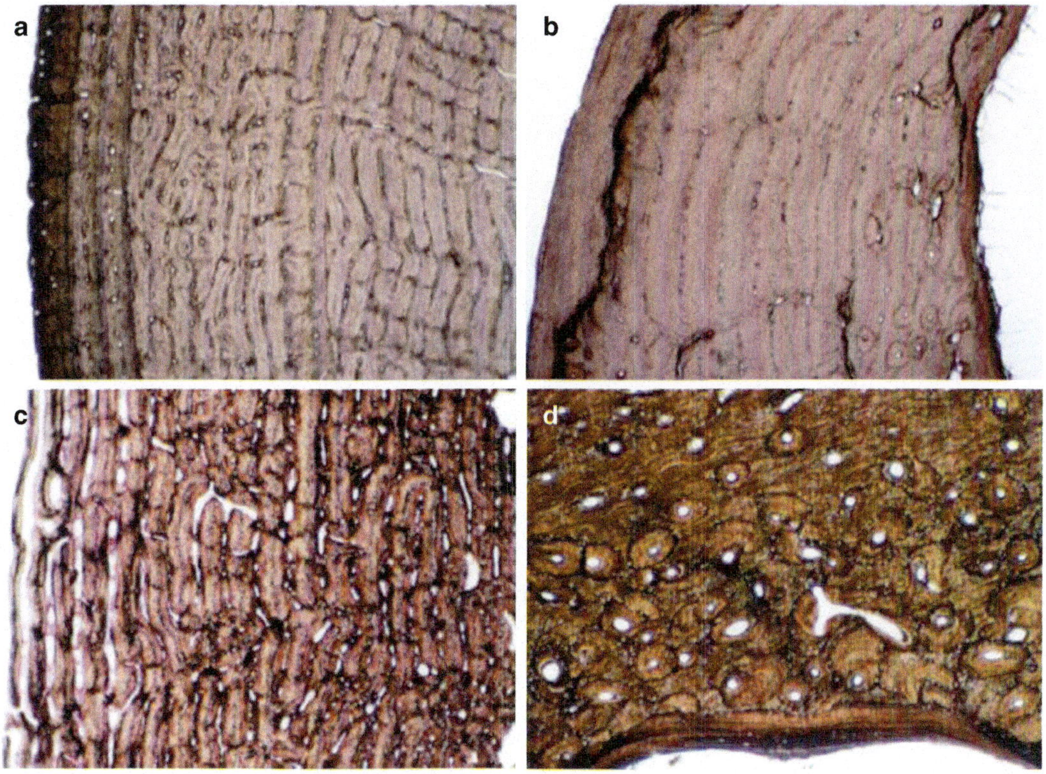

Fig. 12.1 Ground bone sections of mammal bones for species differentiation. Undecalcified ground sections of the compact bone tissue of long tubular bones of different mammals: (**a**) sheep, (**b**) dog, (**c**) pig, (**d**) human (Kossa ×4) (Figures kindly provided by Dr. F. Ramsthaler, Homburg, Germany)

cells for Barr bodies under oil immersion with a compound microscope. It was observed that 1.14% of buccal mucosal cells in men (range 0–4%) and 39.29% of buccal mucosal cells in women (range 20–78%) showed Barr bodies (Rai 2010). Unlike other studies (Anoop et al. 2004; Manjulabai et al. 1997; Aggarwal et al. 1996), the authors here have discussed the influence of ethnic origin on the cytological evidence of Barr bodies. Analogous chromatin densifications were found by other authors, appearing as "drumstick" shapes in polymorphonuclear leukocytes in females.

Verification of the Y chromatin, a typical characteristic of male gender, can be performed by detecting fluorescent bodies (F-bodies) using Atabrine staining. In some syndromes, such as the Klinefelter syndrome, males have Barr bodies (Rai 2010; Pralea and Mihalache 2007). Also, H3K27me3 immunostaining, which has been reported to label the inactivated X chromosome, can predict sex with high accuracy in both neoplastic and nonneoplastic tissues as well as X-inactive specific transcript RNA in situ hybridization (XIST ISH) (Schaefer et al. 2016; Tschui and Hewer 2017; Crotty et al. 2017).

12.3 Tissue and Organ Determination

In the case of body parts, microscopic classification depending on the type of tissue (fatty, muscular, nervous tissue, etc.) or according to a certain organ (liver, lung, kidney, etc.) can be made. This is especially helpful when only tissue or organ remains are found. In uncertain cases, it is possible to use organ-specific immunohistochemical markers where available.

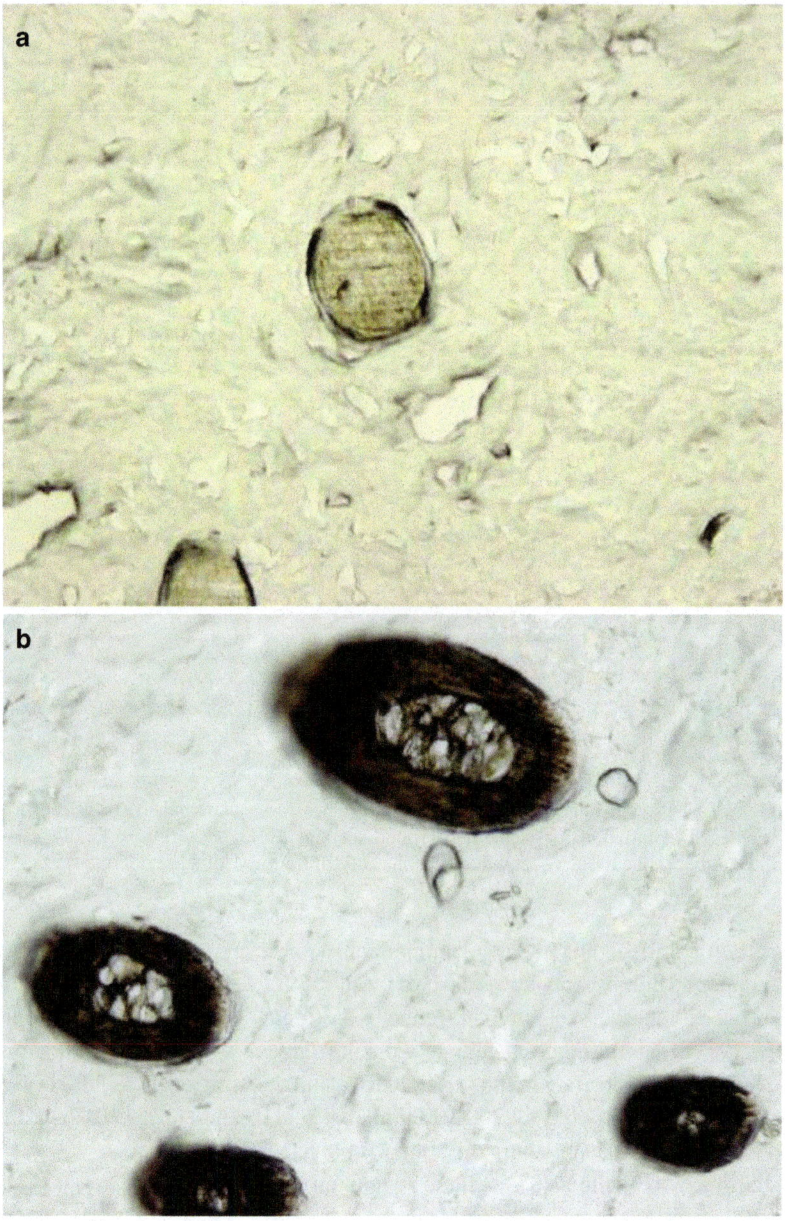

Fig. 12.2 Microscopic image: human (**a**) and dog (**b**) hair in cross section, both ×200

12.4 ABO Blood Type Verification

Determining a person's blood type using histological cross sections is only of theoretical interest and rarely of any practical importance when there is no opportunity to perform forensic DNA analysis. In principle, blood types can be reliably identified with tissue sections of the brain, heart, liver, kidney, or spleen by means of the absorption–elution method (Tröger and Jungwirth 1975; Slavik and Meluzin 1972; Moharrem 1934). It is not essential, however, to use surgically removed tissue; tissue samples retained at autopsy can also be examined successfully. Identifying ABO blood groups has been performed successfully even with samples which were up to 10 years old. Standard anti-A and anti-B serums were used as antiserums. In the case of a positive reaction, clustered agglutinations are observed microscopically; in the case of a negative reaction, a homogeneous distribution of erythrocytes over the entire visual field is seen.

12.5 Histological Age Estimation

The need for accurate techniques of age estimation is great due to an increased number of unidentified cadavers and human remains (Ritz-Timme et al. 2000). The contribution of microscopic examinations to the histological age estimation or identification of an individual, however, is somewhat limited. With experience in microscopy, an attempt can be made to roughly estimate age after examining tissue samples from all inner organs and taking macroscopic evidence into consideration. However, a high-level reliability in microscopic diagnosis cannot be assumed, and significant interobserver variability can be expected (Lynnerup et al. 1998).

12.5.1 Tooth Cementum Annulation for Age Estimation

Accurate age determination from skeletal and dental remains is an important goal for biological anthropologists. One of the techniques deemed promising utilizes tooth cementum annulations (TCA). Recent research indicates that TCA may be used more reliably than other morphological or histological traits of the adult skeleton to estimate age (Roksandic et al. 2009; Wittwer-Backofen et al. 2004). The tooth organ is the hardest organ in the human body, with a loose connective tissue of dental pulp situated within a rigid encasement of mineralized surrounding tissues. Histologically, beneath the dentin, a layer of odontoblasts circumscribes the outermost part of the pulp. The odontoblast is considered to be a fixed postmitotic cell; once it has fully differentiated, it does not appear to undergo further cell division. Counting the number of odontoblasts in samples taken within 24 h after death and determining the average density of odontoblasts per square millimeter can provide an additional parameter for estimating the time since death in the early postmortem period for up to 5 days (Vavpotić et al. 2009).

12.5.2 Age Estimation from Human Bones

There are studies on the estimation of age at death from human bones using histological techniques (Martrille et al. 2009; Crowder and Rosella 2007; Stout et al. 1994; Thompson and Calvin 1983; Watanabe et al. 1998; Stout 1988; Stout and Gehlert 1980; Kerley 1965). For this examination, tissue samples from the ribs (Cannet et al. 2010; Crowder and Rosella 2007; Kim et al. 2007; Paine and Brenton 2006; Stout et al. 1994; Iscan et al. 1984) and femur (Chan et al. 2007; Watanabe et al. 1998) were chosen among other tissues. Histological and histodynamic parameters of bone remodeling of the ribs are well documented. Nevertheless, published data should not be used uncritically for age estimation. Special education, experience, and training are required for the application of all methods (Ritz-Timme et al. 2000). A recent study reported changes in costal cartilage that appear at the microscopic level throughout life, especially during the ossification process: the costochondral junction has the character of a growth plate. Resorbing, calcified, hypertrophic, proliferative, and reserve zones can be identified in this location. Several types of ossification patterns in human costal cartilage seem to exist. Additionally, it was shown that peripheral ossification patterns can be considered as a finding specific to the male sex, while central lingual ossification patterns determine female sex (Rejtarová et al. 2009). Meanwhile, histomorphometric analysis is required. Cannet et al. (2010) presented a study attempting to estimate age at death by using histomorphometric analysis from the fourth left rib adjacent to the costochondral joint in 80 forensic cases. The use of picrosirius dye ensured reliable staining of the decalcified paraffin-embedded ribs. Cannet et al. were able to sufficiently discriminate between three age groups: 20–39 (adulthood), 40–59 (middle age), and above 60 years of age (elderly). One of the methods used in forensic anthropology to estimate age at the time of death may be the histological study of cranial sutures, e.g., the frontosphenoidal suture (Dorandeu et al. 2009). Some studies have used computer-assisted histomorphometry to determine age at death (Martrille et al. 2009). Nevertheless, currently, all recommended methods are represented by several scientific groups, each using their own methodological protocol and different procedures for the evaluation of their method. Therefore, there is a severe limitation in terms of comparability, reproducibility, and verification of results. As stated over a decade ago, there are still no generally accepted guidelines concerning quality assurance in age estimation, particularly for histological and histomorphometric methods (Ritz-Timme et al. 2000).

12.5.3 Age Estimation Using Routine Histology

At least degenerative changes and natural aging processes can be retraced histologically, including the degree of severity of arteriosclerosis or arteriolosclerosis of the kidneys, portal fibrosis in the liver, and the intensity of the lipofuscin deposits (age pigment), e.g., next to the nuclei of cardiomyocytes and in hepatocytes. This can serve as a point of reference to determine whether the tissue sample stems from a very young or a more elderly person. Any possible influencing factors must be considered when interpreting findings. Some authors have examined the thickness of the splenic capsule (Shibata et al. 1963a) and the degree of anthracosis in lung tissue (Shibata et al. 1963b) for the purposes of histological age estimation; the results, however, remain vague und imprecise.

Using the degree of sclerotization of the glomeruli of the kidneys for age estimation (Fukuda et al. 2010), for example, has also been suggested. The authors report that glomerular sclerosis is one of the age-related causes of nephron damage. Histological studies of cadaver kidneys in several ethnic groups have shown that there is a consistent relationship between the percentage of sclerotic glomeruli and age. Immunohistochemical demonstration of amelogenin in order to estimate the age of unidentified bodies has also been examined (Wehner et al. 2007). According to the World Health Organization (WHO), estimating fetal age is essential to assess viability, particularly after 20 weeks. The proposed methods generally use long bone measurements. To determine fetal age more precisely, forensic pathologists should use both histological and anthropometric data as accurately as possible (Piercecchi-Marti et al. 2004).

12.6 Other Histological Age Determinations

When bones are found, not only the question of human specificity and gender arises but also of how old the individual was at the time of death. Investigations to this end may concentrate on individual bones, e.g., the hyoid bone (Fisher et al. 2016), or bone tissue from various regions or localizations of the body may undergo investigation. In this context, histomorphological investigations of bone tissue are of interest in forensic medicine, anthropology, and archeology. Histological investigations of the Haversian canals/osteons are known (Patrascu et al. 2014; Ahlquist and Damsten 1969; Bouvier and Ubelaker 1977; Chan et al. 2007; Cho et al. 2002; Crowder and Rosella 2007; Ericksen 1991; Ericksen and Stix 1991; Kerley 1965; Kerley and Ubelaker 1978; Kim et al. 2007; Maat et al. 2006; Paine and Brenton 2006; Stout 1986; Stout 1988; Stout et al. 1994; Stout and Gehlert 1980; Stout and Paine 1992; Stout et al. 1996; Thompson 1979, 1981; Thompson and Calvin 1983; Watanabe et al. 1998; Yoshino et al. 1994). Here, histomorphometric analysis of bone tissue from defined localizations (femur, clavicle, ribs, etc.) is required. These investigations permit, at least with relatively high probability, the classification of a bone into ranges of adult ages, e.g., 20–39 years, 40–59 years, and over 60 years (Goliath et al. 2016; Cannet et al. 2011). However, attention must be paid to the method of investigation, from the choice of fixative and the number of samples to the type of microscopic analysis and staining method. Decalcified bone samples offer sharper contrast and readily evaluable structures using picrosirius staining (Junqueira et al. 1979; Puchtler et al. 1973). When evaluating histological sections, one needs to bear in mind possible interobserver variability on the one hand and, on the other, the uniformity of sectioning planes, i.e., the distinction between transverse, oblique, and longitudinal sections (Dragoi et al. 2014). To determine age at the time of death, histological and immunohistochemical methods were also used in investigations of frontosphenoidal sutures (Dorandeu et al. 2009). Freezing bone tissue evidently does not have a negative effect on microscopic investigations (Tersigni 2007).

When determining age or pregnancy duration in the case of an embryo or fetus, guidance is taken primarily from body weight, body length (e.g., femur length), and other signs of maturity. However, histological criteria that are believed to permit the determination of gestational age have also been reported (Barbet et al. 1988; Emery and Mithal 1960). Here, one can consider the developmental stage of internal organs, as well as draw conclusions about the duration of pregnancy from placental histology (Vogel 1986).

The development of the nucleus of ossification of Beclard in the distal femoral epiphysis is considered a general sign of maturity (Fig. 12.3). If macroscopic inspection of the section surface shows no clear bone nucleus, histological analysis may be useful.

12.6.1 Age Determination and the Development of Internal Organs in Embryos and Fetuses

When assessing the degree of development of internal organs, quantitative findings, e.g., skin thickness or the number of thymic corpuscles, as well as the degree of differentiation into organ structures, can be helpful. Table 12.2 provides more details in this regard.

Table 12.2 Histological findings to determine the age of embryos or fetuses (modified according to Piercecchi-Marti et al. 2004)

Organ	Finding
Epidermis	Epidermis thickness in various regions, e.g., skin on the abdomen, hand, or foot
Skin	Occurrence of skin appendages (e.g., sebaceous glands, Pacini bodies)
Kidneys	Number of glomeruli in a defined region in the renal cortex
Adrenal gland	Occurrence of neuroblasts in the adrenal medulla
Thymus gland	Increasing number of thymic corpuscles
Lungs	Number of pulmonary alveoli between the last bronchiole and the visceral pleura
Lungs	Developmental stage of pulmonary tissue (a) (Pseudo-) glandular stage (b) Canalicular stage (c) Saccular stage (d) Alveolar stage

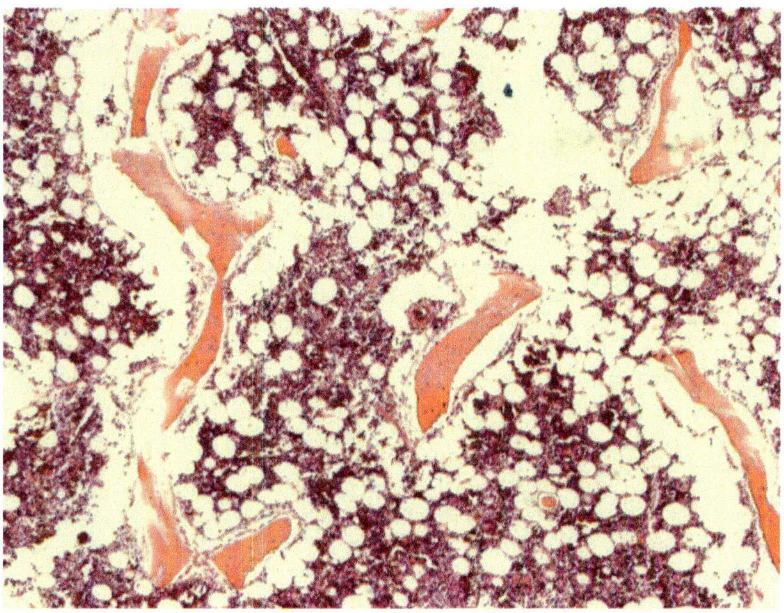

Fig. 12.3 Histological demonstration of the nucleus of ossification of Beclard in the distal femoral epiphysis with fine bone trabeculae and regular hematopoietic bone marrow

Due to relatively early-onset autolysis, brain tissue is less suitable in age determinations.

12.6.2 Developmental Stages of the Human Placenta in the Embryonic and Fetal Periods

The histological criteria when assessing the developmental stage of the human placenta initially include the chorionic plate and its placental villi. In the case of regular growth, both structures—chorionic plate and placental villi—exhibit a maturation process that can be attributed to a defined gestation period (Table 12.3).

The placenta also ages as the pregnancy advances. The following criteria are given for the aging process: increasing formation of vascularized terminal villi, inter- and perivillous microfibrin deposits, increasing concentration of villous stroma, as well as deposits of microcalcification. At the same time, the picture of placental histology becomes less homogeneous in the final trimester of

Table 12.3 Histological stages of development of the placenta from the 5th to the 20th week of gestation (according to Vogel 1986)

Pregnancy duration	Chorionic plate	Placental villi
5th–6th week of gestation	Embryonic connective tissue; separated subamniotic and chorionic tissue space; allantoic vessels exhibit thin walls, only isolated capillaries	Uniformly plump villi; embryonic stroma is coarsely meshed, scant vessels, only red blood cells with nuclei in the vascular lumina; numerous sections of trophoblast columns; broad, invariably two-layered chorion epithelium
7th–8th week of gestation	Subamniotic and chorionic tissue margins coalesce and collagen fiber bands appear	Plump villi; embryonic stroma with Hofbauer cells. Central villous, thin-walled allantoic vessels in stem villi, primarily adjacent to the plate; subepithelial capillaries, as well as two-layered chorionic epithelium, individual syncytiotrophoblast branches
9th–10th week of gestation	Broader vessel walls with early development of a media; denser collagen fibers	Partially plump, partially slender villi, loose collagen fibers along the stem villi vessels, allantoic vessel processes down to basal peripheral stem villi; flat chorionic epithelium that is still two-layered; very rarely, gaps in the cytotrophoblastic shell
11th–12th week of gestation	Stroma made up of collagen fibers; well-developed vascular media in the chorionic plate	Transition from plump to narrow villi diameter; reticular stroma in stem villi; denser collagen fibers adjacent to the allantoic vessels, pronounced media in the vessel walls; peripheral villi with capillaries in cross section; erythrocytes mostly without nuclei; some gaps in the cytotrophoblastic shell, abundant syncytial trophoblast cells in the intervillous space
14th–16th week of gestation	Increasing villi density, collagen fiber tissue along the vessels in stem villi; reticular stroma with subepithelial Hofbauer cells; several capillaries in cross section per villus; chorion frondosum and chorion laeve are distinguishable	
18th–20th week of gestation	Numerous villi with reticular stroma, stem villi with greater cell density; wide-meshed stroma in the intervillous space; subepithelial capillaries with early so-called metabolic membranes, proliferation buds in the nearby area	

pregnancy, such that the histological findings described here can only be used as a guide in the determination of pregnancy duration or age and only if tissue samples are taken from different localizations.

Nevertheless, there is a close relationship between placental growth and maturation in relation to neonate weight. Thus, the weight of the placenta also enables conclusions to be drawn about pregnancy duration; the relevant weights in correlation to the week of gestation are provided in table form in the literature. The relationship between placental weight and the weight of the neonate is expressed by the placental ratio, according to which the weight of the placenta (excluding the umbilical cord and amnion) is divided by the weight of the neonate. If the placental ratio is 10.0:9.3 in the 2nd month of pregnancy, it will already be at 2.5:1.0 in the 4th month of pregnancy and reduces between the 28th and 42nd weeks of gestation from 0.27 to 0.138 (with deviations). Although the placental ratio provides guidance when determining pregnancy duration, it does not enable any conclusions to be drawn on placental function.

Pathological changes to the placenta that are able to explain intrauterine fetal death or stillbirth are not rare and include, e.g., impaired placental maturation in the form of delayed villous maturation, fibrosis of the villous stroma, intervillous thrombus, anemic placental infarction, placentitis and chorioamnionitis, deposits of microfibrin and microcalcification, thromboangiitis obliterans, and chorangiomatosis of the placenta.

12.7 Evidence of Tattoo Remnants in the Identification Process

In histological sections, tattoos appear as aggregates of black material within the interstitium and macrophages within the upper dermis, usually without significant inflammatory reaction (Cains and Byard 2008).

In cases where tattoo removal from a certain location is suspected, a microscopic examination of skin tissue samples can be helpful to identify the deceased. Since complete removal of tattoo pigments is generally not possible, tattoo remnants can be still detected with microscopy, partially surrounded by fibrosis with relatively few cells in the superficial layer of the corium (Fig. 12.4). Adjacent draining regional lymph nodes, often axillary lymph nodes, may also show aggregated black pigment.

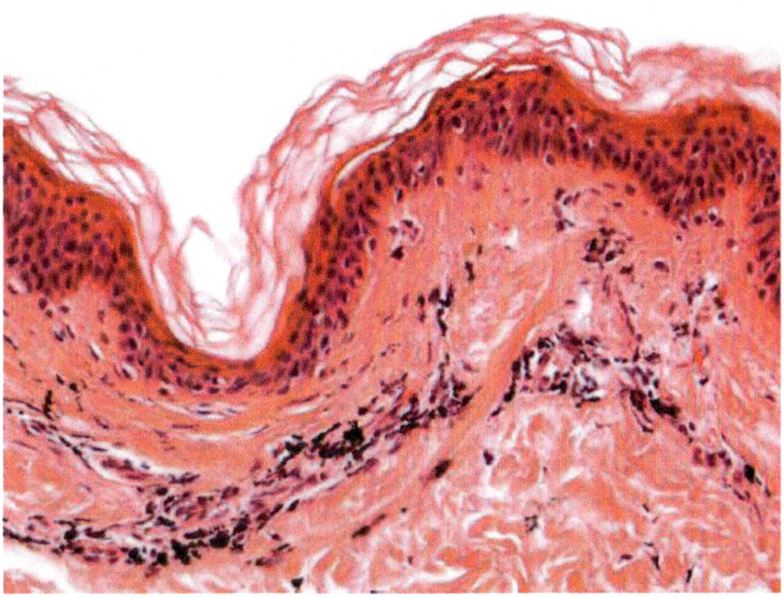

Fig. 12.4 Microscopically demonstrable pigment remnants of a partly removed tattoo in the superficial layer of the corium (H&E ×200)

Additionally, the release of metals from osteosynthesis implants can be used for identification using postmortem histopathological and ultrastructural methods. The discovery of intra-bone metal particles in tissues treated by osteosynthesis is possible even in bone areas where implants have been removed and even if there are no longer any radiological signs of their application (Palazzo et al. 2010).

In some cases, in addition to demonstrating a tattoo, histological examination of the skin can provide information about the degree of skin tanning at the time of death (Fig. 12.5) or about the color of the hair (Fig. 12.6).

Intense blackish, streaky discolorations on the anucleate keratin lamellae of the epidermis or the outer corneal layer of the skin are produced by contamination with rail grease. This finding can usually be observed on body parts after being run over by a rail vehicle. Using Prussian blue staining, the rail grease appears intensely iron-positive (Fig. 12.7).

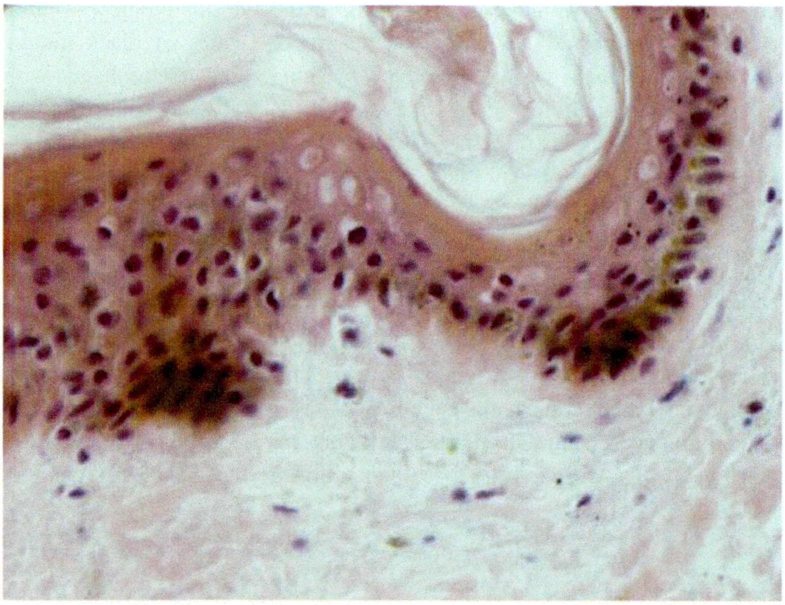

Fig. 12.5 Skin sample of an unidentified deceased person with signs of putrefaction; nevertheless, marked tanning is still detectable by demonstrating melanin pigment in the basal layers of the epidermis (H&E ×200)

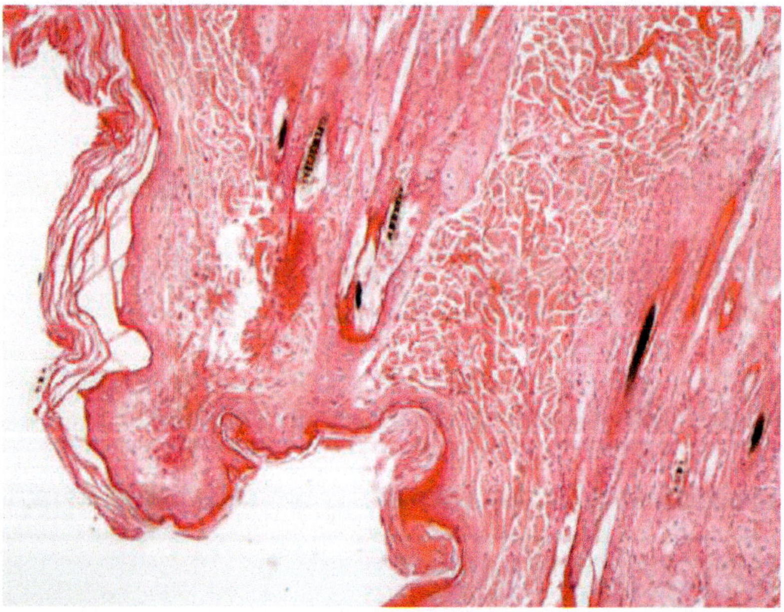

Fig. 12.6 Skin sample of an unidentified deceased person without demonstrating melanin pigment in the basal layers of the epidermis but with black hair (H&E ×100)

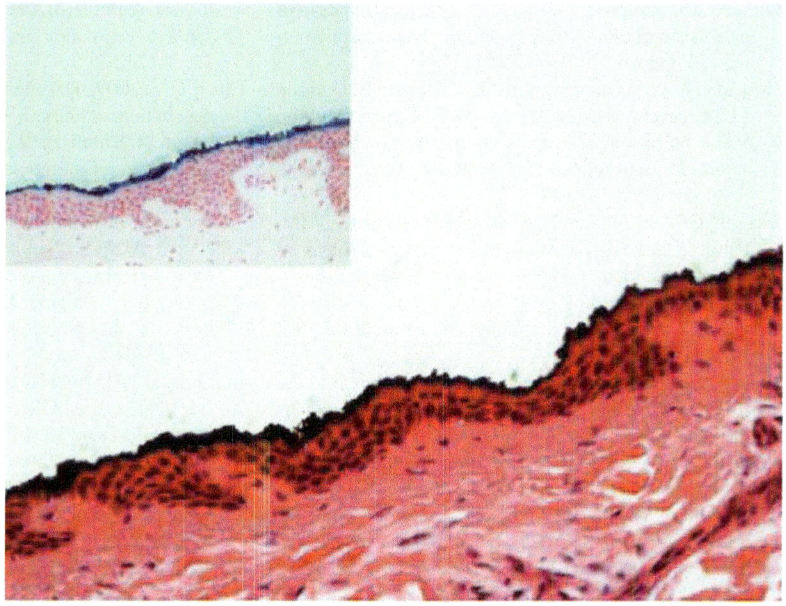

Fig. 12.7 Skin of a body part after the victim was run over by a rail vehicle: intense iron-positive streaky contaminations of rail grease (H&E ×200; Insert: Prussian blue ×200)

12.8 Xenogeneic Tissue

With the exception of bone findings, it is rare in forensic practice to investigate tissue that is of questionable human specificity. A case involving abortion material that actually originated from a dog, with histological findings that could not be attributed to a human embryo, has been reported. It was pointed out in this context that species differentiation may also be possible using placental morphology.

References

Aggarwal NK, Kumar S, Banerjee KK, Agarwal BBL (1996) Sex determination from buccal mucosa. J Forensic Med Toxicol 13:43–44

Ahlquist J, Damsten O (1969) A modification of Kerley's method for the microscopic determination of age in human bone. J Forensic Sci 14:205–212

Anoop UR, Ramesh V, Balamurali PD, Nirima O, Premalatha B, Karthikshree VP (2004) Role of Barr bodies obtained from oral smears in the determination of sex. Indian J Dent Res 15:5–7

Barbet JP, Houette A, Barres D, Durigon M (1988) Histological assessment of gestational age in human embryos and fetuses. Am J Forensic Med Pathol 9:40–44

Bouvier M, Ubelaker DH (1977) A comparison of two methods for the microscopic determination of age of death. Am J Phys Anthropol 46:391–394

Brits D, Steyn M, L'Abbé EN (2014) A histomorphological analysis of human and non-human femora. Int J Legal Med 128:369–377

Caccia G, Magli F, Tagi VM, Porta DGA, Cummaudo M, Márquez-Grant N, Cattaneo C (2016) Histological determination of the human origin from dry bone: a cautionary note for subadults. Int J Legal Med 130: 299–307

Cains GE, Byard RW (2008) The forensic and cultural implications of tattooing. In: Tsokos M (ed) Forensic pathology reviews, vol 5. Humana Press, Totowa, pp 197–220

Cannet C, Baraybar JP, Kolopp M, Meyer M, Ludes B (2010) Histomorphometric estimation of age in paraffin-embedded ribs: a feasibility study. Int J Legal Med 125(4):493–502

Cannet C, Baraybar JP, Kolopp M, Meyer P, Ludes B (2011) Histomorphometric estimation of age in paraffin-embedded ribs: a feasibility study. Int J Legal Med 125:493–502

Chan AHW, Crowder CM, Rogers TL (2007) Variation in cortical bone histology within the human femur and its impact on estimating age at death. Am J Phys Anthropol 132:80–88

Cho H, Stout SD, Madsen RW, Streeter MA (2002) Population-specific histological age-estimating method: a model for known African-American and European-American skeletal remains. J Forensic Sci 47: 12–18

Crotty R, Arora K, Prasad S, Ting DT, Rivera MN, Deshpande V (2017) X-inactive specific transcript RNA in-situ hybridization as a tool for resolving contamination events. Histopathology 71(4):662–665

Crowder C, Rosella L (2007) Assessment of intra- and intercostal variation in rib histomorphometry: its impact on evidentiary examination. J Forensic Sci 52:271–276

Dillon S, Cunningham C, Felts P (2016) Quantification of osteon morphology using geometric histomorphometrics. J Forensic Sci 61:402–408

Dorandeu A, de la Grandmaison GL, Coulibaly B, Durigon M, Piercecchi-Marti MD, Baccino E, Leonetti G (2009) Value of histological study in the fronto-sphenoidal suture for the age estimation at the time of death. Forensic Sci Int 191:64–69

Dragoi GS, Melingte PR, Dinca I, Botoran MM, Patrascu E (2014) Histomorphometric evaluation of osteons inside the compacta of long bones diaphysis. Implication in pathology. Rom J Leg Med 22:109–116

Dürwald W (1987) Gerichtliche Medizin. Barth JA, Leipzig, 3. Aufl., p 75

Emery JL, Mithal A (1960) The number of alveoli in the terminal respiratory unit of man during late intrauterine life and childhood. Arch Dis Child 35:544–547

Ericksen MF (1991) Histologic estimation of age at death using the anterior cortex of the femur. Am J Phys Anthropol 84:171–179

Ericksen MF, Stix AI (1991) Histological examination of age of the first African Baptist church adults. Am J Phys Anthropol 85:247–252

Fisher E, Austin D, Werner HM, Chuang YJ, Bersu E, Vorperian HK (2016) Hyoid bone fusion and bone density across the lifespan: prediction of age and sex. Forensic Sci Med Pathol 12:146–157

Fukuda N, Suzuki Y, Sato K, Yajima D, Hayakawa M, Motani H, Kobayashi K, Otsuka K, Nagasawa S, Iwase H (2010) Estimation of age from sclerotic glomeruli. Forensic Sci Int 197:123.e1–123.e4

Goliath JR, Stewart MC, Stout SD (2016) Variation in osteon histomorphometrics and their impact on age-at-death estimation in older individuals. Forensic Sci Int 262:282.e1–282.e6

Helmer R (1970) Möglichkeiten und Methoden der zellkernmorphologischen Geschlechtserkennung an Körpergeweben und Sekreten. In: Weinig E, Berg S (eds) Arbeitsmethoden der medizinischen und naturwissenschaftlichen Kriminalistik. Bd. 9. Schmidt-Römhild, Lübeck

Hillier ML, Bell LS (2007) Differentiating human bone from animal bone: a review of histological methods. J Forensic Sci 52:249–263

Iscan MY, Loth SR, Wright RK (1984) Age estimation from the rib by phase analysis: white males. J Forensic Sci 29:1094–1104

Janssen W (1977) Forensische histologie. Schmidt-Römhild, Lübeck

Junqueira LC, Bignolas G, Brentani RR (1979) Picrosirius staining plus polarization microscopy, a specific method for collagen detection in tissue sections. Histochem J 11:447–455

Kerley ER (1965) The microscopic determination of age in human bone. Am J Phys Anthropol 23:149–163

Kerley ER, Ubelaker DH (1978) Revisions in the microscopic method of estimating age at death in human bone. Am J Phys Anthropol 49:545–546

Kim YS, Dim KI, Park DK, Lee JH, Chung NE, Lee WT, Han SH (2007) Assessment of histomorphological features of the sternal end of the fourth rib for age estimation in Koreans. J Forensic Sci 52: 1237–1242

Linch CA (2009) Degeneration of nuclei and mitochondria in human hairs. J Forensic Sci 54:346–349

Lynnerup N, Thomsen JL, Frohlich B (1998) Intra- and inter-observer variation in histological criteria used in age-at-death determination based on femoral cortical bone. Forensic Sci Int 91:219–230

Maat GJR, Maes A, Aarents MJ, Nagelkerke NJD (2006) Histological age prediction from the femur in a contemporary dutch sample: the decrease of non-remodeled bone in the anterior cortex. J Forensic Sci 51: 230–237

Manjulabai KH, Yadwad BS, Patil PV (1997) A study of Barr bodies in Indian, Malaysian and Chinese subjects. J Forensic Med Toxicol 14:9–13

Martrille L, Irinopoulou T, Bruneval P, Baccino E, Fornes P (2009) Age at death estimation in adults by computer-assisted histomorphometry of decalcified femur cortex. J Forensic Sci 54:1231–1237

Michailow R (1975) Die Häufigkeit des Geschlechtschromatins in den Zellkernen innerer Organe, untersucht mit der Abstrichmethode. Z Rechtsmed 76: 27–30

Mittal T, Sralaya KM, Kuruvilla A, Achary C (2008) Sex determination from buccal mucosa scrapes. Int J Legal Med 123(5):437–440

Moharrem J (1934) Über den Nachweis von gruppenspezifischen Stoffen in formalinfixierten Organen. Dtsch Z Gesamte Gerichtl Med 23:197–205

Paine PR, Brenton BP (2006) Dietary health does affect histological age assessment: an evaluation of the Stout and Paine (1992) age estimation equation using secondary osteons from the rib. J Forensic Sci 51:489–492

Palazzo E, Andreola S, Battistini A, Gentile G, Zoja R (2010) Release of metals from osteosynthesis implants as a method for identification: post-autopsy histopathological and ultrastructural forensic study. Int J Legal Med 125:21–26

Patrascu E, Melinte PR, Dragoi GS (2014) Optimized morphologic evaluation of biostructures by examination in polarized light and differential interference contrast microscopy. Rom J Leg Med 22:275–282

Piercecchi-Marti MD, Adalian P, Liprandi A, Figarella-Branger D, Dutour O, Leonetti G (2004) Fetal visceral maturation: a useful contribution to gestational age estimation in human fetuses. J Forensic Sci 49: 912–917

Pralea CE, Mihalache G (2007) Importance of Klinefelter syndrome in the pathogenesis of male infertility. Rev Med Chir Soc Med Nat Iasi 111:373–378

Puchtler H, Waldrop FS, Valentine LS (1973) Polarization microscopic studies of connective tissue stained with picro-sirius red F3BA. Beitr Pathol Anat 150:174–187

Rai B (2010) Comments an sex determination from buccal mucosa scrapes. Int J Legal Med 124:261

Rämsch R, Zerndt B (1963) Vergleichende Untersuchungen der Haversschen Kanäle zwischen Menschen und Haustieren. Arch Kriminol 131:74

Rejtarová O, Hejna P, Soukup T, Kuchař M (2009) Age and sexually dimorphic changes in costal cartilages. A preliminary microscopic study. Forensic Sci Int 193:72–78

Ritz-Timme S, Cattaneo C, Collins MJ, Waite ER, Schütz HW, Kaatsch HJ, Borrman HIM (2000) Age estimation: the state of the art in relation to the specific demands of forensic practise. Int J Legal Med 113:129–136

Roksandic M, Vlak D, Schillaci MA, Voicu D (2009) Technical note: applicability of tooth cementum annulation to an archaeological population. Am J Phys Anthropol 140:583–588

Sahajpal V, Goyal SP, Thakar MK, Jayapal R (2009) Microscopic hair characteristics of a few bovid species listed under Schedule-I of Wildlife (Protection) Act 1972 of India. Forensic Sci Int 189:34–45

Sato I, Nakaki S, Murata K, Takeshita H, Mukai T (2010) Forensic hair analysis to identify animal species on a case of pet animal abuse. Int J Legal Med 124:249–256

Schaefer IM, Minkovsky A, Hornick JL (2016) H3K27me3 immunohistochemistry highlights the inactivated X chromosome (Xi) and predicts sex in non-neoplastic tissues. Histopathology 69:702–704

Schiwy-Bochat KH (1993) Automatische Kompaktaanalyse zur Speziesdifferenzierung. In: Pesch HJ (ed) Osteologie aktuell VII. Springer, Berlin, pp 512–514

Shibata M, Hirota A, Tsurozono M, Teranishi N, Uehara M, Yamamoto H, Kita H (1963a) Estimation of age of victims from pieces of their organs. I. The spleen. 1. The thickness of capsule of human spleen. Jpn J Leg Med 17:75

Shibata M, Naripa N, Hirota A, Tsurozono M, Teranishi N, Uehara M, Yamamoto H, Kita H (1963b) Estimation of age of victims from pieces of their organs. II. The lungue. 1. Anthracosis. Jpn J Leg Med 17:83

Slavik V, Meluzin F (1972) Bestimmung der Gruppenzugehörigkeit im system ABO aus histologischem material. Z Rechtsmed 70:79–88

Stout SD (1986) The use of bone histomorphometry in skeletal identification: the case of Francisco Pizarro. J Forensic Sci 31:296–300

Stout SD (1988) The use of histomorphology to estimate age. J Forensic Sci 33:121–125

Stout SD, Dietze WH, Iscan MY, Loth SR (1994) Estimation of age at death using cortical histomorphometry of the sternal end of the fourth rib. J Forensic Sci 39:778–784

Stout SD, Gehlert SJ (1980) The relative accuracy and reliability of histological aging methods. Forensic Sci Int 15:181–190

Stout SD, Paine PR (1992) Brief communication: histological age estimation using rib and clavicle. Am J Phys Anthropol 87:111–115

Stout SD, Porro MA, Perotti B (1996) Brief communication: a test and correction for the clavicle method of Stout and Paine for histological age estimation of skeletal remains. Am J Phys Anthropol 100:139–142

Tersigni MA (2007) Frozen human bone: a microscopic investigation. J Forensic Sci 52:16–20

Thompson DD (1979) The core technique in the determination of age at death in skeletons. J Forensic Sci 24:902–915

Thompson DD (1981) Microscopic determination of age at death in an autopsy series. J Forensic Sci 26: 470–475

Thompson DD, Calvin CA (1983) Estimation of age at death by tibial osteon remodeling in an autopsy series. Forensic Sci Int 22:203–211

Tridico SR, Houck MM, Kirkbride KP, Smith ME, Yates BC (2014) Morphological identification of animal hair: myths and misconceptions, possibilities and pitfalls. Forensic Sci Int 238:101–107

Tröger HD, Jungwirth J (1975) Bestimmung der AB0-Gruppenzugehörigkeit an histologischen Präparaten. Beitr Gerichtl Med 33:326–329

Tschui J, Hewer E (2017) H3K27me3 immunostaining for sex determination in the context of presumed tissue misidentification. Histopathology 72(2):358–359. https://doi.org/10.1111/his.13364

Vavpotić M, Turk T, Martinčič DS, Balažic J (2009) Characteristics of the number of odontoblasts in human dental pulp post-mortem. Forensic Sci Int 193:122–126

Verhoff MA, Kreutz K, Ramsthaler F, Schiwy-Bochat KH (2006) Forensic anthropology and osteology – synopsis and definition. Dtsch Ärztebl 103:A782–A788

Vermeij E, Zoon P, van Wijk M, Gerretsen R (2015) Microscopic residues of bone from dissolving human remains in acids. J Forensic Sci 60:770–776

Vogel M (1986) Histologische Entwickungsstadien der Chorionzotten in der Embryonal- und der frühen Fetalperiode (5. bis 20. SSW). Pathologe 7:59–61

Watanabe Y, Konishi M, Shimada M, Ohara H, Iwamoto S (1998) Estimation of age from the femur of Japanese cadavers. Forensic Sci Int 98:55–65

Wehner F, Secker K, Wehner HD, Gehring K, Schulz MM (2007) Immunhistochemischer Nachweis von Amelogenin an Zähnen – ein Beitrag zur Abschätzung des Lebensalters bei der Identifikation unbekannter Leichen. Arch Kriminol 220:40–50

Wittwer-Backofen U, Gampe J, Vaupel JW (2004) Tooth cementum annulation for age estimation: results from a large known-age validation study. Am J Phys Anthropol 123:119–129

Yoshino M, Imaizumi K, Miyasaka S, Seta S (1994) Histological estimation of age at death using microradiographs of humeral compact bone. Forensic Sci Int 64:191–198

13 Coronary Sclerosis, Myocardial Infarction, Myocarditis, Cardiomyopathy, Coronary Anomalies, and the Cardiac Conduction System

Sudden unexpected deaths occur frequently in forensic autopsy practice. In such cases, pathological findings in the heart can often explain the acuteness of death (Fineschi et al. 2006; Fineschi and Pomara 2004). In addition to ruptured myocardial infarcts, these pathological changes include rare diseases, such as a primary heart tumor (atrial myxoma, rhabdomyosarcoma, *cardiac fibroma*; Ventura et al. 2012; Pusta et al. 2015) or pericardial tamponade in the case of a dissecting aortic aneurysm. Pathological changes also include:

- Acute coronary insufficiency in the case of stenosing coronary sclerosis
- Myocardial infarction
- All forms of myocarditis
- Cardiomyopathies of varying etiology
- Hereditary anomalies of coronary artery development
- Lesions of the cardiac conduction system
- Primary cardiac tumors

Histological and/or immunohistochemical findings of varying severity can be expected in all of the abovementioned pathological changes to the heart, on the one hand, confirming the macroscopically suspected diagnosis and, on the other, only then enabling the crucial differential diagnosis. Primary cardiac tumors are extremely rare as a cause of sudden death (Jiang et al. 2009). Sudden cardiac death (SCD) is one of the most common causes of death, and an important number of sudden deaths, especially in the young, are due to genetic heart disorders, both with structural and arrhythmogenic abnormalities (Rodríguez-Calvo et al. 2008). TUNEL can be a useful screening method in sudden cardiac death (Edston et al. 2002). There are a number of different terms for sudden cardiac death in the absence of coronary atherosclerosis: *Pokkuri death syndrome* (PDS) in Japan, "Lai Tai" in Thailand, "bangungut" in the Philippines, "dream disease" in Hawaii, and "sudden unexpected nocturnal death syndrome" among South Asian immigrants in the USA. Lipid metabolism disorders, for instance, are discussed as a possible cause (Takeichi et al. 2001). In order to document the various diseases underlying the phenomenon of sudden cardiac death, the Association for European Cardiovascular Pathology published their "Guidelines for autopsy investigation of sudden cardiac death" (Basso et al. 2008a, b). Finally, the literature describes comparatively rare findings that are seen in rare diseases or that infrequently occur following medical procedures. For example, calcified myocardial necrosis in pediatric patients following cardiopulmonary reanimation has been reported (Buschmann et al. 2013), as well as a combination of arrhythmogenic right ventricular cardiomyopathy and cystic tumor of the atrioventricular (AV) node (Cavanaugh and Prahlow 2013).

R. B. Dettmeyer, *Forensic Histopathology*, https://doi.org/10.1007/978-3-319-77997-3_13

13.1 Sudden Coronary Death

Autopsy frequently shows a stenosing coronary sclerosis of varying severity in subjects with acute or sudden death, also in defined patient collectives such as adolescents (Weiler and Knieriem 1975; Weiler and Risse 1981; Janssen 1968; Walthard 1942) or young women (Althoff 1983) *or smokers* (Leone 2014). On the one hand, autopsies have shown severe forms of arteriosclerotic stenosing coronary scleroses—partly infected with *Chlamydia pneumoniae* (Dettmeyer et al. 2006a)—in people who, until death, had had sufficient cardiac function. On the other hand, autopsies have also shown partially isolated coronary scleroses with only moderate stenoses of the vascular opening, which are given as the cause of death. In such cases, evidence of acute or protracted ischemia of the myocardium is crucial, either in extensive areas of the myocardium as a myocardial infarction or in the form of fresh and possibly focal myocardial ischemia under stress.

In conventional histology, a morphological equivalent of clinically indicated acute lethal coronary insufficiency is often difficult to identify; at best small scarred areas can be found as an indication of older, preceding local ischemia with circumscribed myocardial necrosis and scarring. Occasionally, single necrosis with homogeneous eosinophilia, myofibrillar degenerations, contraction bands, and thick cytoplasm accompanied by interstitial edema are also found. Acute myocardial ischemia can be displayed immunohistochemically by means of a wide range of primary antibodies (Xiaohong et al. 2002; Xu et al. 2001; Zhang and Riddick 1996; Brinkmann et al. 1993; Greve et al. 1990; Shekhonin et al. 1990; Steenbergen et al. 1987). Unlike circumscribed myocardial infarction, immunohistochemical investigations in cases of subtotal obturating thrombosis and coronary sclerosis show a rather diffuse pattern of damage (Brinkmann et al. 1993). Additionally, there are cases of sudden cardiac death in non-atherosclerotic and noninflammatory intimal cellular proliferations usually affecting small and medium caliber arteries (Dermengiu et al. 2010a, b, c). Fibromuscular dysplasia (FMD) was first described in 1958 by McCormack who reported its histological appearance in four patients with renovascular hypertension. Meanwhile, FMD is defined as an idiopathic, segmentary, noninflammatory, and non-atherosclerotic condition of the arterial walls, leading to stenosis in small and medium arteries (Dermengiu et al. 2010c with definitions for non-atherosclerotic histological alterations of the intima).

Coronary Thrombosis

Occasionally, it is difficult to macroscopically differentiate postmortem blood clots from intravascular thrombosis. Very small thromboses, for example, in a disrupted atheroma bed, may be overlooked. Histological evaluation of coronary thrombosis, which also serves as evidence, is often necessary, especially in the context of a legal expert opinion.

A note on dissection: Opening the coronary arteries longitudinally is not recommended, but rather lamellar cuts should be made perpendicular to the axis of the vessel and their localization from proximal to distal recorded. Postmortem coronary angiography might also be helpful. Tissue cross sections of the coronary vessels should include the arterial adventitia and adjacent soft tissue.

Coronary thrombosis (Fig. 13.1) normally involves white thrombi (see Chap. 9). The histological findings in the coronary arterial wall regularly show pathological arteriosclerotic changes, which are considered to be the cause of the wall-adherent thrombosis and early organization. In individual cases, a primarily inflammatory vascular disease (e.g., coronaritis, Kawasaki disease) might be the cause of coronary thrombosis; in extremely rare cases, the cause may be previous trauma (cardiac contusion). Staining methods recommended for diagnosis are as follows: HE, Elastica van Gieson, PTAH, and Prussian blue. Nuclear

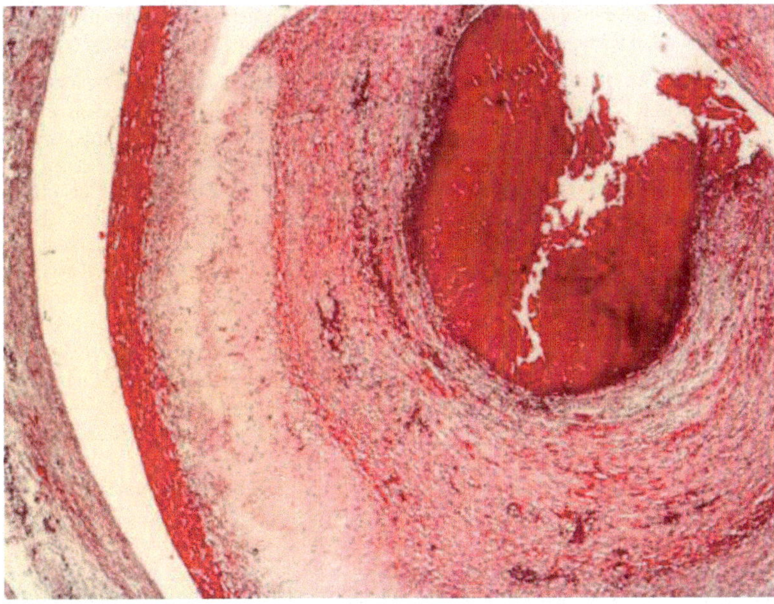

Fig. 13.1 Obturating coronary thrombosis in the setting of coronary sclerosis as a cause of acute myocardial infarction: atherosclerotic stenosis with fresh, central thrombosis (H&E ×40) (see Chap. 9 for determination of thrombus age)

morphometry of the myocardial cells as a diagnostic tool in cases of sudden death due to coronary thrombosis was investigated (Lazaros et al. 1998).

Meanwhile, immunohistochemical techniques have been widely utilized in the study and diagnosis of early myocardial ischemia. Large numbers of experiments indicate that myoglobin or desmin depletion, for example, can be used as morphologic parameters to diagnose early myocardial ischemia. Other authors investigated the immunohistochemical distributions of myocardial hypoxia-inducible factor (HIF)-1-α and its downstream factors, erythropoietin (Epo) and vascular endothelial growth factor (VEGF), in cardiac deaths. HIF-1-α was found weakly positive in cardiomyocytes in the cardiac necrotic region and intensely positive in the nuclei of cardiomyocytes showing eosinophilic change. Epo and VEGF were weakly positive in cardiomyocytes in the necrotic region, but intensely positive in the cytoplasm with eosinophilic change. Additionally, Epo was shown to be positive in macrophages of necrotic areas (Zhu et al. 2008). The diagnostic value of selected histological staining and immunohistochemical markers can be seen in Table 13.1. However, the spectrum of possible immunohistochemical markers to prove fresh myocardial infarction is more extensive, based in part also on animal models. The following markers, although not all adequately supported by studies, have been mentioned: myoglobin, C1, C3, C8, C9, CD59, α-actinin, vinculin, FABP, HIF-1α, PHD2, PHD3, CT-I, dystrophin, SORBS2, S100A1, npCX-43, CX-43, GAL-1, dityrosine, IL-15, MCP-1, GAL-3, CTn1, H-FABP, and Jun B. Here, positive evidence of antigen expression is in some cases significant and in others its loss, and thus the failure to detect it is relevant to diagnosis (Sabatasso et al. 2016).

Contraction band necrosis (*CBN*), *myofibrillary degeneration* (*MFD*). Histologically, this form of myocardial necrosis is characterized by:

- Irreversible hypercontraction of cardiomyocytes
- Markedly thickened Z-lines
- Extremely short sarcomeres
- Breakdown of the whole contractile apparatus
- Irregular pathological and eosinophilic cross-bands consisting of segments with hypercontracted or coagulated sarcomeres
- Total disruption of myofibrils
- A granular aspect of the whole cell without clear-cut pathological bands

Table 13.1 Conventional histological and immunohistochemical staining methods or techniques used to diagnose early myocardial damage in cases of cardiac and noncardiac perfusion damage (selection)

Conventional histological staining	Immunohistochemical markers
H&E and H&E in combination with fluorescence (Saukko and Knight 1989; Badir and Knight 1987; Fechner and Sivaloganathan 1987; Al-Rufaie et al. 1983; Carle 1981) After approximately 30 min first visible contraction bands as a consequence of the collapse of the myofibril apparatus (Amberg 1995)	Complement C5b-$9_{(m)}$: positive reaction in the case of macroscopically visible myocardial infarction and in borderline cases (Thomsen and Held 1995; Thomsen et al. 1990; Schäfer et al. 1986; Knight 1967); also for the detection of group necroses; if C5b-$9_{(m)}$-positive, then also fibrinogen-positive reaction; early necrosis marker with positive reaction especially in desmin-negative areas; detectability may vanish after the acute stage; C5b-$9_{(m)}$ should only be positive if contraction bands can be detected in the chromotrope aniline blue stain (CAB) (Amberg 1995)
Luxol fast blue (LFB) staining (Oehmichen et al. 1990a, b; Pedal and Oehmichen 1990; Arnold et al. 1985)	Fibronectin: positive detection in the case of macroscopically visible myocardial infarction and in borderline cases (Shekhonin et al. 1990); also for the detection of group necroses (Fischbein et al. 1986)
Hematoxylin basic fuchsin picric acid (HBFP staining) (Janssen 1984; Lie et al. 1971; Lie 1968): shows early myocardial ischemia; staining is very sensitive but not very specific (Amberg 1995)	Desmin (structural protein) + myoglobin (functional protein)—in both cases negative reaction, i.e., no desmin and no myoglobin in the acute ischemic area (Chumachenko and Vikkert 1991; Leadbetter et al. 1989, 1990; Ishiyama et al. 1982), possible focal depletions in the case of diffuse myocardial ischemia
Chromotrope aniline blue (CAB) stain (Zollinger 1983): presents visible contraction bands due to the collapse of the myofibril apparatus after approximately 30 min (Amberg 1995)	Troponin I: early negative reaction in the case of myocardial infarction (Hansen and Rossen 1999)
Alizarin complex stain: detection of early hypoxic myocardial damage by determining free oxygen radicals may be possible (Amberg 1995)	Fibrinogen: positive detection in the case of macroscopically visible myocardial infarction and in borderline cases (Shekhonin et al. 1990)
	HIF-1-α (hypoxia-inducible factor 1α)—stains necrotic areas within the first 2 h (Pampín et al. 2006)

Data is based on animal experiments and/or studies on human myocardium

Contraction band necrosis (Fig. 13.2), defined as above, can be observed in many human pathologies (Curca et al. 2011; Oehmichen et al. 1990a, b) and is reproduced experimentally by intravenous infusion of catecholamines. It does not represent an ischemic change (Baroldi et al. 2001; Todd et al. 1985a, b). Conditions associated with contraction band necrosis are (according to Karch 2009 and modified from Karch and Billingham 1986) reperfusion, steroid therapy, electrocution, defibrillation, cardiopulmonary resuscitation (Curca et al. 2011), drowning, cocaine, amphetamine, epinephrine, isoproterenol, norepinephrine, cobalt poisoning, starvation, myocardial infarction, free-radical injuries, brain death, phenylpropanolamine, intracerebral hemorrhage, and MDMA.

The detection of contraction bands or myofibrillar degeneration is carried out by means of H&E and PTAH staining methods, particularly with the modified Luxol fast blue staining method according to Arnold et al. (1985). Corresponding lesions, however, are found in multiple causes of death (e.g., drowning, shock, intoxication, hanging). CBN or MFD are therefore unspecific phenomena, which are indicative of asphyxia and are taken as evidence of an event during life (Oehmichen et al. 1990b).

Frequently, no histomorphological findings (neither macroscopic nor obtained using conventional histological staining) which could have led to heart failure or acute lethal cardiac arrhythmia can be seen to explain, e.g., local myocardial ischemia. Exceptions include findings in the

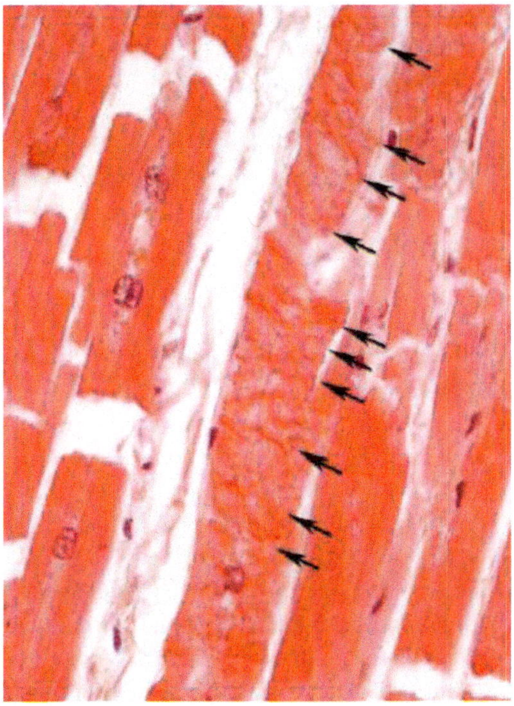

Fig. 13.2 Contraction band necrosis—myofibrillary degeneration (H&E ×400)

cardiac conduction system, for example, at the sinoatrial node; however, the significance of these findings is controversial. What is crucial in many cases is that a limit has been exceeded (e.g., physical and/or emotional stress, postprandial myocardial ischemia in the case of a full stomach), resulting in localized or diffuse myocardial ischemia. These diagnostic problems have resulted in a range of immunohistochemically usable myocardial ischemia markers now being recommended (Brinkmann et al. 1993).

If these immunohistochemical findings, along with anamnesis and macroscopic findings in the coronary arteries and myocardium, reveal a similar pattern, a diagnosis of acute lethal coronary insufficiency in the setting of stenosing coronary sclerosis is indicated. The degree of severity is less meaningful, however, in some cases. This applies to all cases where competing causes of death need to be excluded.

The conventional histological and immunohistochemical ischemia markers which have been recommended in the literature can also be used in cases of perfusion disturbance of noncardiac origin. Some immunohistochemical markers for the diagnosis of myocardial ischemia are explained here in more detail.

C5b-9$_{(m)}$. This is activated complement C5 with one C6–C8 molecule and six C9 molecules. Ischemically damaged cell membranes cause C5 activation. Complete myocardial necrosis can be clearly differentiated using an antibody against activated C5b-9$_{(m)}$.

C5b-9$_{(m)}$ forms transmembrane channels that accelerate the effect of calcium ions and thus lead to a direct toxic effect on myofibrils, or they trigger damaging secondary reactions. Thomsen and Held (1995) reported that they were unable to demonstrate C5b-9$_{(m)}$ in the myocardium of any of their cases of myocardial injury not caused by infarction. This means that C5b-9$_{(m)}$ was negative in cases with direct myocardial lesions, especially those caused by external trauma and with diseases directly affecting the myocardium. Additionally, C5b-9$_{(m)}$ seems to also be negative in indirect myocardial lesions due to systemic factors affecting the entire organism. For the early diagnosis of myocardial infarction, reference is made to the immunohistochemical identification of complement C9 (Piercecchi-Marti et al. 2001).

A note on microscopic analysis: Deeper wall portions of arteries show positive detection of C5b-9$_{(m)}$ in non-ischemic or non-necrotic areas, such that this reaction can be used as an "internal positive control" (Thomsen and Held 1995; Thomsen et al. 1990).

Creatine Kinase MM

Creatine kinase-type MM (CK-MM) for fast energy supply is predominantly found in the myocardium. In animal experiments, a significant decrease in creatine phosphate was detected as early as 30 s after ligating a coronary artery (Osuna et al. 1990). Immunohistochemically, CK-MM is normally represented homogeneously. Detection may be patchy or completely absent, depending on the duration of ischemia; this also applies to circumscribed perfusion disturbances. Parallel to this, the detectability of desmin drops off (Amberg 1995).

Desmin

Desmin is a structural protein which is topographically associated with Z-lines of the muscle cell. Hypoxia-based activations of proteases are said to change the structure of desmin in such a way that the immunohistochemically used antibody no longer recognizes the antigen, while desmin can be well represented immunohistochemically in normally perfused heart muscle tissue (Wick and Siegal 1988). The result is that desmin is no longer identifiable in ischemically damaged myocardium (Fig. 13.3).

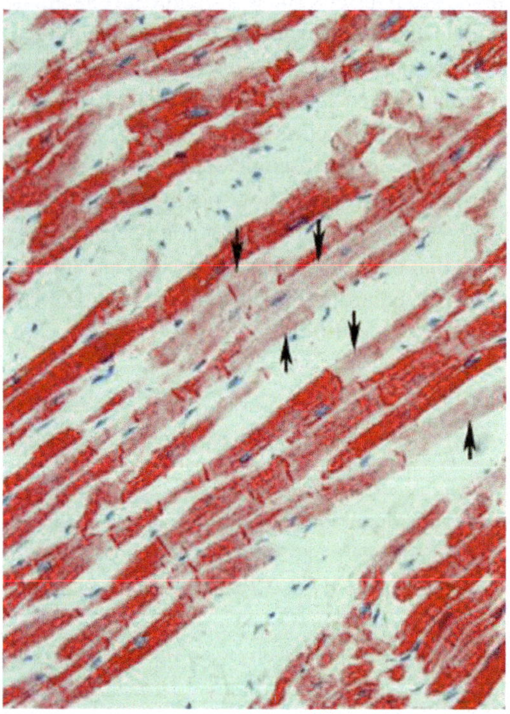

Fig. 13.3 Ischemically damaged cardiomyocytes—immunohistochemically detectable loss of desmin (*arrows*) (×400)

Fibrinogen

In an experimental rat model, fibrinogen seemed to increase 30 min after coronary artery ligation (Xiaohong et al. 2002), while fibrinogen staining extended in accordance with changes in myoglobin depletion 2–3 h after ligation.

Fibronectin

Fibronectin is a protein situated at the cell surface, also appearing in the serum. It is produced in fibroblasts, monocytes, and epithelial cells and apparently plays a role in fibrillogenesis in heart muscle cells. Fibronectin cannot be detected immunohistochemically in the normally oxygenated adult myocardium (Casscells et al. 1990) and is currently considered to be the earliest immunohistochemical necrosis marker, which, in terms of time, is identifiable even before $C5b\text{-}9_{(m)}$ (Hu et al. 2002).

Myoglobin

Myoglobin is a myocardial cytoplasmic component, and local and incomplete myoglobin depletion occurred in the subendocardial cells in front of the left ventricle after 30 min of myocardial ischemia (animal experiment; Xiaohong et al. 2002).

Troponin I

Cardiac troponin I is like myoglobin, myosin, and other muscle protein components of normal myocardial cells and appears elevated in serum after acute myocardial infarction due to leakage from the damaged myocardial cells (Adams et al. 1993).

Troponin I is specific for heart muscle cells and not found in other tissues. Cases of definite myocardial infarction show a well-defined area with loss of troponin I (Hansen and Rossen 1999; Leadbetter et al. 1989). Autolytic areas show a diffuse reduction in troponin I.

In cases of acute diffuse perfusion disturbance of the myocardium, there is no localized ischemia in terms of myocardial infarction. The abovementioned conventional histological stainings and immunohistochemical markers can show findings or absence of findings in all areas of the myocardium. This supports the assumption of acute coronary insufficiency. However, conclusions on the chronology of acute cardiac death must be drawn very cautiously.

For further information on the abovementioned and other immunohistochemical ischemia markers, please refer to the appropriate literature. There are several animal models and studies on autopsy tissue performed in order to determine the age of ischemia in cases of myocardial findings. However, to date, no reliable and generally accepted spectrum of reproducible immunohistochemical markers has been found. This also applies to age determination of myocardial infarction, even if in this case a concentration on certain immunohistochemical examinations is apparent.

Small Vessel Disease. This remains an umbrella term for various disorders of the small arteries in the heart (myocardial atherosclerosis). Sclerosis of the arterioles and small arteries are likely to be the most common forms; having said that, hereditary medial necrosis, fibromuscular dysplasia, amyloid deposits, and vasculitis have also been described. There is no proven correlation between small vessel disease and hypertension. A narrow vessel lumen in myocardial samples taken at autopsy does not reflect antemortem vessel width, but rather an artifact arising from the fact that the arteries were not fixated under physiological pressure (Hort 2000). In terms of histological changes, focal or diffuse loss of smooth muscle cells in the arterial media and their replacement by a fibrous tissue have been described in addition to narrowing of the vessel lumen. Hyperelastosis of the vessel wall and degenerative changes are also seen (Rahlf 1980). It is only with great caution that a diagnosis of small vessel disease as the cause of death should be made on the basis of lesions of this kind and only if an alternative cause of death has been ruled out and if the circumstances of death tally with the patient history.

13.2 Myocardial Infarction

Acute myocardial ischemia leads to myocardial necrosis which will be reabsorbed and fibrously organized if the patient survives. Since ischemia is normally considered to be the consequence of an incident such as coronary sclerosis with insufficient blood supply to the myocardium, smaller ischemic areas (up to 1 cm) are also called coronary insufficiency scars. Such coronary insufficiency scars may coalesce to larger scar zones. If the diameter of the ischemia-based myocardial necrosis is more than 1 cm, this can be considered a myocardial infarction. If the coronary arteries are narrowed, relative anemia following blood loss due to injury can lead to myocardial ischemia or myocardial infarction.

Conventional Histology

The hemorrhagic halo which occurs in fresh myocardial infarction and which is macroscopically visible, as well as the leukocytic demarcation which develops later, can be detected histologically.

In cases of coronary insufficiency calluses or myocardial infarctions, the age of the lesion can be determined histologically. In this context, conventional histology with various stainings and methods is still relied upon (Mihatsch 1988; Sahai 1976; Bouchardy and Majno 1974; McVie 1970; Knight 1967), but immunohistochemical techniques are increasingly used (Piercecchi-Marti et al. 2001; Brinkmann et al. 1993; Leadbetter et al. 1989, 1990). However, the detection of very fresh myocardial infarction is sometimes impossible, both macroscopically and using conventional histology. In such cases, improved diagnosis was initially achieved in the past using enzyme-histochemical methods.

Enzyme Histochemistry

Over 40 years ago, it was demonstrated that myocardial infarction can be detected with enzyme-histochemical methods in cases where there are no pathological findings in conventional histology. It was found that cytochrome oxidase activity is an early indicator of fresh myocardial infarction, showing a marked reduction even before the reduction of succinate dehydrogenase activity (Jääskeläinen 1968). Enzyme-histochemical methods have only been partially accepted in histological practice, while immunohistochemical techniques are now widespread.

Immunohistochemistry

By means of immunohistochemical control of structural and repair proteins, it is possible to provide evidence of a myocardial infarction even before it is visible macroscopically or detectable histologically. Primary antibodies have proven to be effective as infarction markers against the repair proteins fibronectin, $C5b\text{-}9_{(m)}$, and fibrinogen, as well as against the structural protein myoglobin, all of which can also display diffuse myocardial ischemia (see Table 13.1). Positive findings in repair proteins can in part also be seen in traumatic myocardial damage and in the case of fibrinogen in other organs (Raza-Ahmad 1994). Along with immunohistochemical detection of repair proteins, the loss of structural proteins is evidence of myocardial ischemia also in cases of myocardial infarction, such as the loss of troponin I (Hansen and Rossen 1999) and desmin. On the other hand, immunohistochemical analysis in animal models showed increased expression of *dityrosine*, a protein product in oxidative stress, in the affected ischemic and infarcted myocardial areas after only a very short ischemia time (approximately 5 min; Mayer et al. 2014, 2016). The angiotensin type 2 receptor was proposed as a marker of acute myocardial infarction with positive detection in the peripheral region of the infarcted myocardium after 12–24 h (Rentea et al. 2016; Mondello et al. 2017).

Coagulative necrosis and contraction band necrosis are microscopically visible using H&E/autofluorescence staining, diffuse myofibrillar degeneration is visible using Luxol fast blue staining (LFB) (Arnold et al. 1985), and contraction bands are also visible using chromotrope aniline blue staining (Zollinger 1983). Details on the chronology of myocardial infarction or on age determination of an infarction can be seen in Table 13.2 (see also Figs. 13.4, 13.5, 13.6, 13.7, 13.8, 13.9, and 13.10).

Table 13.2 Chronology of microscopic findings of myocardial infarction

Time	Microscopic findings
From 15 min	Measuring distances between horizontal stripes in myocardial fibers in unstained sections: several myocardial sections are compared using an eyepiece micrometer on a phase contrast microscope; extension is evidence of myocardial infarction (Hort 1965)
Up to 30 min	Electron microscopic changes to the mitochondria with swelling and dissolution of the cristae mitochondriales (Büchner and Onishi 1968)
30–60 min	Edema of the myocardial fibers; decrease in glycogen; in animal studies immunohistochemical loss of myoglobin and early detection of fibrinogen (Xiaohong et al. 2002); in cases of ischemia of at least 30 min, contraction bands can be seen in the chromotrope aniline blue staining (CAB) as an expression of collapse of the myofibril apparatus (Amberg 1995)
From 60 min	Positive tartaric acid cresyl violet inclusion staining: preserved musculature, blue-violet to red-violet; damaged musculature, pale blue to sky blue (Holczabek 1970, 1973)
2–3 h	First homogeneous eosin red hyalinized myocardial fibers (Fig. 13.4) in peripheral areas of myocardial infarction (Janssen 1977); the stain according to Lie: dark red ischemic myocardial fibers (Tausch 1974)
	Unfixed tissue sections: Fluorochromization with acridine orange can represent damaged myocardium by means of bright green fluorescence (Korb and Knorr 1962)
3–4 h	First agglutinated sarcolemma tubes, discrete fatty degeneration of the myocardial fibers; possible hemorrhagic demarcation of the infarction with hyperemic edges (can also be present at an earlier stage), first tamping cell nuclei of the cardiomyocytes
4–5 h	Immunohistochemical representation of the infarct area with the early necrosis markers fibronectin and C5b-9(m) (Fig. 13.6); fibrinogen is also positive; visible loss of desmin and myoglobin
4–7 h	Necrosis in the infarct area, first peripheral leukocyte reaction, gradual general eosinophilia of the myocardial fibers, and shrinkage of the heart muscle cells in the infarct area, nuclear dyeability (Fig. 13.5) (Janssen 1977)
9 h	Pronounced necrosis in the infarct area, strong leukocyte reaction—now also in the infarct area, nuclear dyeability of the cardiomyocytes no longer possible, cell nuclei of the interstitial connective tissue can be dyed for somewhat longer (Fig. 13.7)
18–24 h	Pronounced necrosis, further leukocyte penetration of the infarct area
5–6 days	Continued leukocyte penetration of the infarct area, abscess-like dissolutions are possible with myocytolysis and rupture of the heart chamber wall (Fig. 13.8) (Janssen 1977)
2–3 weeks	More pronounced peripheral granulation tissue with sprouted capillary blood vessels, fibrocytes, fibroblasts, lymphocytes, few plasma cells, macrophages, possibly siderophages, few granulocytes
5 weeks to 2–3 months	Collagen fiber or scar tissue with endothelially coated capillary blood vessels of varying density (Mallory et al. 1939), siderophages still possible, loose infiltration with lymphocytes, few plasma cells, scant granulocytes (Fig. 13.9)
3–6 months	Scar tissue with fewer cells, few capillary blood vessels, scant siderophages
6–12 months	Scar tissue with few cells (DiMaio and Dana 2007), dystrophic calcification with basophilic calcium salt deposits is possible later (Fig. 13.10)

Summary according to the literature, own experience, and in line with Sandritter and Thomas (1977)

13.3 Acute and Chronic Viral Myocarditis

Myocarditis of varying etiology is often the explanation for sudden and unexpected death (Kiryakova et al. 2016; Kittulwatte et al. 2010; Dettmeyer et al. 2002a). A variety of causes may trigger myocarditises, from infection to the involvement of the myocardium in cases of systemic diseases (Table 13.3).

The most frequent and frequently unrecognized myocarditis is viral myocarditis (Fairley et al. 1996; Friman et al. 1995; Friman and Fohlman 1993; Karjalainen et al. 1980). Bacterial purulent myocarditises, tuberculous or rheumatoid myocarditis, fungal myocarditis, as well as

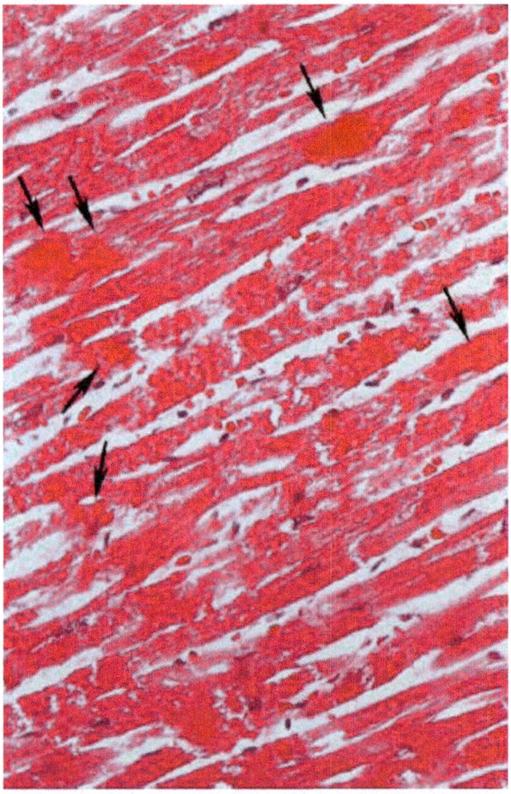

Fig. 13.4 Fresh myocardial infarction with homogeneous eosin red hyalinized myocardial fibers (*arrows*), fiber breaks, intensive myocardial decay, tamping cell nuclei, and interstitial edema—infarct age, approximately 2–4 h (H&E ×400)

inflammatory myocardium involvement in cases of systemic diseases or sarcoidosis are all very rare. Other rare diagnoses include myocarditises which respond well to medication (see Chap. 5), which frequently show pronounced infiltration with eosinophil leukocytes (Aoki et al. 1996), and giant-cell myocarditis.

It is remarkable that viral myocarditis can present clinically as ischemic heart disease (IHE), the ECG-mimicking myocardial infarction (Bültmann et al. 2003a; Kühl et al. 2003; Lauer et al. 1998; Tyson et al. 1989; Miller et al. 1973). The (viral) inflammation is said to act as an arrhythmia trigger, such that sudden and unexpected death in the case of viral myocarditis can be explained by acute cardiac arrhythmia with only discrete histological and immunohistochemical findings (Klein et al. 1995, 2000). Viral myocarditis should be considered in the case of sudden unexpected death when taking exercise or without any known physical strain (Bux et al. 2002; Byard 2002; Karjalainen and Heikkila 1999; McCaffrey et al. 1991; Drory and Hiss 1991; Philips et al. 1986).

Improved immunohistochemical methods in connection with the molecular pathological evidence of viruses in the myocardium allow a

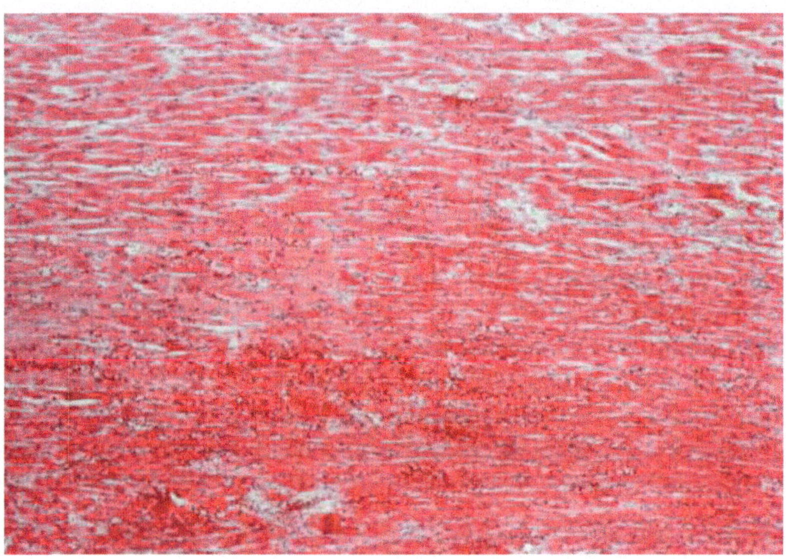

Fig. 13.5 Fresh myocardial infarction with hemorrhagic edges (*bottom*) and largely preserved nuclear dyeability of the cardiomyocytes—infarct age <7 h (H&E ×40)

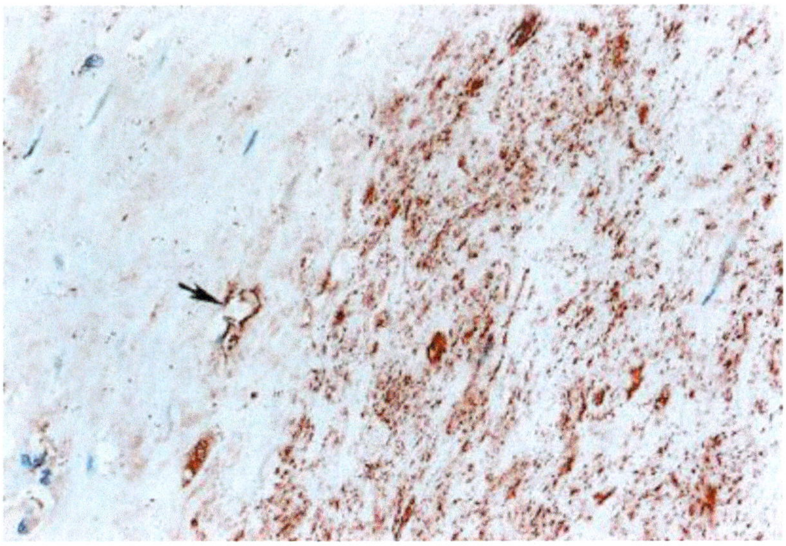

Fig. 13.6 Fresh myocardial infarction with evidence of the early ischemia marker C5b-$9_{(m)}$. Note: C5b-$9_{(m)}$ expression in the wall of a neighboring artery as "internal positive control" (*arrow*) (×200)

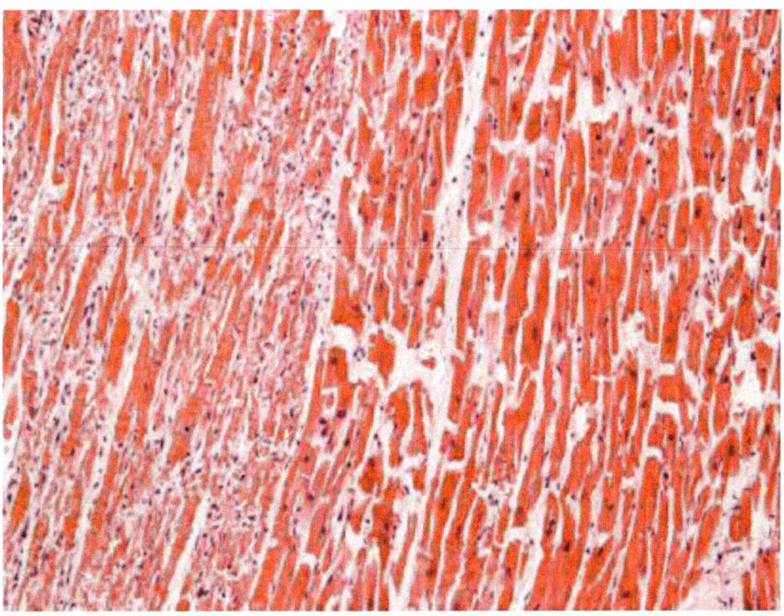

Fig. 13.7 Peripheral region of a myocardial infarction with lost heart muscle fibers, diffuse leukocyte infiltration, absent or almost completely tamped cell nuclei (*left*) adjacent to unaffected myocardium (*right*)—infarct age at least 7–9 h (H&E ×100)

better understanding of pathophysiological mechanisms in the case of acute and chronic myocarditis, even if a lot of questions remain unanswered (Liu and Mason 2001). Immunohistochemical staining first enabled the quantification of interstitial inflammatory cells in the myocardium (Klages and Gerken 1972) and more recently enabled the qualification of individual cell types (Noutsias et al. 2002; Kühl et al. 1994, 1997). Despite advances in the diagnosis of myocarditis, there is still controversy about how to judge small, focal inflammatory infiltrates in the myocardium in terms of their significance to the cause of death. Focal

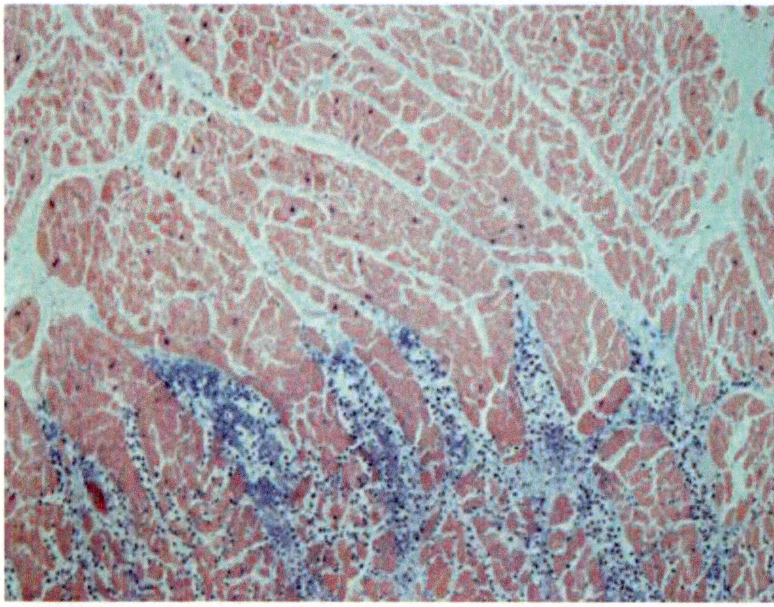

Fig. 13.8 Myocardial infarction, abscess-like leukocyte penetration of the infarct area—infarct age, approximately 24–48 h, few days (H&E ×100)

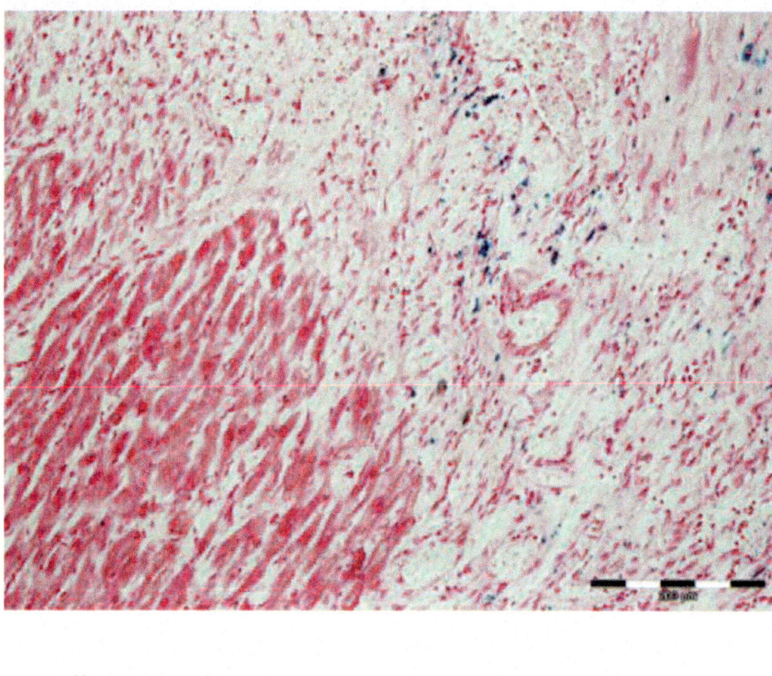

Fig. 13.9 Myocardial infarction which is no longer fresh with substituting granulation tissue: collagen fiber tissue with fibroblasts and fibrocytes, sprouted capillary blood vessels, a large number of siderophages as residuals of intramyocardial bleeding (Prussian blue ×200)—infarct age, approximately 3 weeks or older

infiltrates with inflammatory cells are occasionally seen in the myocardium in adults, evidently more frequently as a reactive event following the use of a wide variety of drugs, e.g., antibiotics (Zhang et al. 2013). Findings of this kind cannot necessarily be deemed relevant to death. Myocardial inflammatory infiltrates in the infant heart are of greater significance in terms of cause of death (see Chap. 17).

13.3.1 Acute Viral Myocarditis

The diagnosis of acute, subacute, or abating myocarditis is made partly with the help of conventional histological methods, as well as by using immunohistochemical myocarditis diagnostics established in the 1990s. This is currently supplemented by molecular pathological detection of viruses in the myocardium.

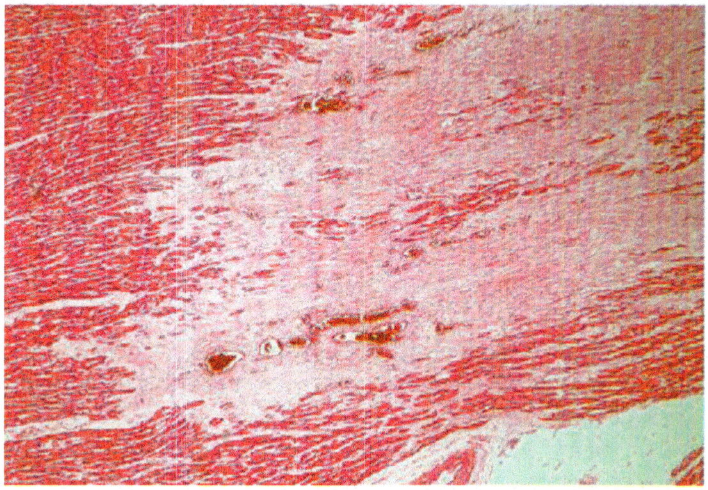

Fig. 13.10 Old myocardial infarction scar with dense collagen fiber tissue, partially revascularized with capillary blood vessels, and no inflammatory infiltrates (H&E×100)—infarct age, at least 6 months

Table 13.3 Classification of the etiology of myocarditis

Etiology	Triggering agent (selection)
Infection	Viruses (in particular enteroviruses, coxsackieviruses B1–B5, coxsackieviruses A4 and A16, echoviruses 9 and 22, polioviruses, parvovirus B19, adenoviruses, human herpes virus 6, Epstein–Barr virus, human cytomegaly virus, influenza viruses, mumps virus, herpes simplex virus, varicella-zoster virus, respiratory syncytial virus, measles virus, rubella virus, human immunodeficiency virus)
	Bacteria [staphylococci, *Pseudomonas*, *Proteus*, *Klebsiella*, pneumococci, mycobacteria (Tbc), meningococci, mycoplasma pneumoniae, *Borrelia burgdorferi* (Lyme carditis)]
	Fungi (candida, aspergilla)
	Protozoans (*Trypanosoma cruzi*–Chagas disease, *Toxoplasma gondii*)
Allergic/autoimmune	Immune reaction (autoimmune or eosinophilic myocarditis, rheumatic carditis, myocarditis which responds well to medication, e.g., antibiotics, diuretics, anticonvulsives, neuroleptics)
Pharmacological/toxic	Anthracyclines, amphetamines, catecholamines, cocaine, *Corynebacterium diphtheriae* (exotoxin), drugs
Systemic diseases	For example, lupus erythematodes (LE)
Physical	For example, radiotherapy
Rare forms	Giant-cell myocarditis, sarcoidosis, hypereosinophilic syndrome, Kawasaki disease with myocardium involvement, transplant rejection

Conventional Histological Myocarditis Diagnostics

With the exception of more rare forms of myocarditis, microscopic diagnosis was and still is performed using conventional histological staining methods (in particular H&E, LFB, Elastica van Gieson, Mallory's stain, Giemsa stain), according to the Dallas criteria in the first instance (Aretz 1987; Aretz et al. 1987; Table 13.4). Descriptions of histological findings include, e.g., inflammatory infiltrates and fibrosis:

Table 13.4 Conventional histological diagnosis of myocarditis according to the Dallas criteria (Aretz 1987)

First myocardial biopsy	Findings
Active myocarditis	Myocytolysis, lymphomonocytic interstitial inflammatory infiltrate in the myocardium, interstitial edema (Fig. 13.11)
Borderline myocarditis	Sparse accumulation of lymphocytes, subsequent control biopsy
Control biopsy	Findings
Persistent myocarditis	Unchanged evidence of a myocarditis
Healing myocarditis	Decrease in lymphomonocytic infiltration
Healed myocarditis	No myocytolysis, no necrosis, no increase in lymphomonocytic cells

1. Inflammatory infiltrates
   (a) Focal, confluent, and diffuse
   (b) Mild, moderate, and severe
   (c) Lymphocytic, eosinophilic, granulomatous, giant cells, neutrophilic, and mixed
2. Fibrosis
   (a) Endocardial
   (b) Mild, moderate
   (c) Perivascular and replacement

The complete picture of viral myocarditis shows dense, diffuse lymphomonocytic interstitial infiltrates, necrosis of single cardiomyocytes, more extensive group necrosis, interstitial edema, empty sarcolemma tubes, and leukocytes adhering to the vascular endothelium in the vascular space (Fig. 13.11). A 2013 consensus statement emphasized the diagnostic value of *endomyocardial biopsy (EMB)* in the diagnosis of myocarditis and highlighted the diagnostic possibilities presented by immunohistochemistry and molecular pathology testing for viruses (Thiene et al. 2013).

In the case of purulent myocarditis, granulocyte infiltration may lead to microabscesses, or a focal abscess may be induced by embolic spread of bacterial colonies. In cases of myocarditis responsive to drug treatment, relatively well-demarcated focal lymphomonocytic infiltrates with plasma cells and eosinophil granulocytes may appear (see Chap. 5). Within the scope of a removal reaction, macrophages may occur en masse; fibrocytes and fibroblasts will then drive the replacement of eliminated cardiomyocytes with collagenous connective tissue. However, with regard to myocarditis, the tissue is rather diffuse and not within a well-demarcated area as seen with myocardial infarct. It is possible that myocarditis is followed to some extent by circular perivascular fibrosis.

Two disadvantages of myocarditis diagnostics according to the Dallas criteria were already highlighted early on:

1. Questionable representativeness of the myocardial samples examined, hence the sampling error (Hauck et al. 1989)
2. Significantly different diagnoses from individual observers, hence the "interobserver variability" (Shanes et al. 1987)

Nevertheless, clarification of myocarditis according to the Dallas criteria is the first step in myocarditis diagnosis. If the findings for myocarditis according to the Dallas criteria listed in Table 13.4 are absent, viral infection of the myocardium is not in any way excluded, and

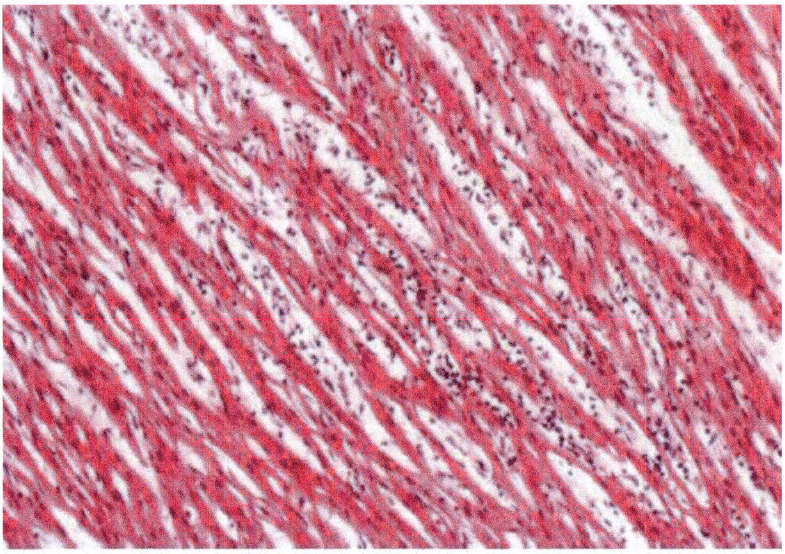

Fig. 13.11 Acute lymphomonocytic viral myocarditis according to the Dallas criteria with myocardial necrosis, myocytolyses, leukocyte infiltration, and interstitial edema (H&E ×100)

immunohistochemical examinations may be needed. Investigations to differentiate fatal myocarditis from incidental myocarditis show that myocardial necrosis is not necessarily required to establish the diagnosis of myocarditis (Casali et al. 2012). The molecular genetic detection of viral genomes in myocardial samples taken at autopsy remains methodologically complex, and conflicting results have been presented. Especially retrospective studies in old myocardial samples stored for long periods of time seem to yield more virus-negative findings (Nielsen et al. 2014a, b).

In the case of acute death and macroscopically normal findings at autopsy, conventional histological examinations may largely show normal findings despite myocarditis. Since viral myocarditis only offers a circumscribed focal interstitial lymphomonocytic inflammatory infiltrate, a sufficiently high number of tissue samples are needed for microscopic diagnosis to ensure detectability of these focal infiltrates.

According to personal experience, a minimum of eight myocardial samples from a defined area should be examined (localization of the specimens; see Chap. 17) concerning babies. For adults, other authors ask for eight samples from the right and eight samples from the left myocardium, additionally samples from the cardiac conduction system, a reasonable proposal (Janssen 1977). If indications of myocarditis are found, e.g., a focal inflammatory infiltrate, step sections of all tissue samples may lead to the detection of additional focal leukocyte infiltrates, thus supporting the diagnosis of myocarditis.

The anamnesis of patients with myocarditis often reveals a viral infection of the respiratory system or gastrointestinal tract which may have been perceived as insignificant in the preceding weeks. At forensic autopsy and particularly in the case of sudden death in relatively young subjects due to physical stress, myocarditis should be considered once other cardiac diseases have been excluded. This includes death while participating in sports (e.g., soccer), swimming, military duty, or in cases of sudden cardiac death.

The chronology of acute myocarditis corresponds to electron-microscopic, immunohistochemical, and conventional histological findings. The conventional histological diagnosis, however, is no longer reliable during the early phase and while the myocarditis is subsiding. Thus, with no virus detected in the myocardium, only a histomorphologically justified suspected diagnosis remains (Table 13.5).

Table 13.5 Diagnostic phases of acute viral myocarditis: postinfection findings

Phase	Findings
Early phase (hours following infection)	Ultrastructural and molecular pathological diagnosis: evidence of ultrastructural changes (electron microscopy); molecular pathological evidence of a virus
From approx. 24–48 h	Immunohistochemical diagnosis: growing immunohistochemically provable findings with expression of proinflammatory molecules; adhesion molecules, cytokines, leukocyte infiltration, expression of non-cellular proinflammatory molecules
From approx. 24–48 h	Conventional histological diagnosis: possible development of myocarditis according to the Dallas criteria

Note: When the immune system is intact, possible early elimination of the virus in the myocardium may be considered, such that the myocardium may be affected only temporarily and in a confined area

According to Feldmann and McNamara (2000) and Mall (1995)

Finally, it is not clear to what extent viral infections impact the myocardium, but cardiotropic viruses, including certain enteroviruses, may have a greater impact than other viruses. Currently, there is no research into the interplay between rapid elimination of the viral genome and the organism's immune defense, the intensity and duration of the viral infection and a possible genetic variation, or into whether chronic myocarditis with viral persistence often develops when the number of viral copies is extremely low. A reduction in interstitial and especially perivascular fibroses is occasionally proposed as an indication of healed, viral myocarditis. If there are zones of fibrosis with a discrete lymphomonocytic inflammatory infiltrate and myocardial single-cell necrosis, a transition to chronic myocarditis or inflammatory cardiomyopathy should be considered.

Immunohistochemical Diagnosis of Myocarditis

One improvement in the diagnosis of myocarditis was based on immunohistochemical methods (Noutsias et al. 2002; Yazaki et al. 1998; Kühl et al. 1996, 1997; Maisch et al. 1995; Mall 1995; Schwartzkopff et al. 1995; Maisch 1994, among others). Due to significant interobserver variability (Shanes et al. 1987) and also because the examined myocardial samples are not sufficiently representative with low sample counts when myocardium particles are very small, immunohistochemical methods were established to demonstrate inflammatory processes in the myocardium. In this context, interstitial leukocytes, T-lymphocytes, and macrophages are qualified and quantified, proinflammatory molecules are immunohistochemically expressed, and the degree of expression is semiquantitatively determined. This process, which has been an established part of the diagnostic work-up in adult myocarditis since the 1990s, has since been transferred to cases of sudden infant death (Dettmeyer and Kandolf 2009, Dettmeyer et al. 2004a, 2006c; Dettmeyer and Madea 2004; see Chap. 17).

According to personal experience, it is remarkable that with expression of proinflammatory MHC class II molecules, the myocardium apparently reacts as a whole; relatively even expression of this proinflammatory marker can also be found when cellular infiltration is only detectable focally.

A larger spectrum of immunohistochemical markers has meanwhile been proposed for the diagnosis of myocarditis. However, the focus remains on the extent of cellular infiltration of the myocardial interstitium, oriented to empirically derived limit values for adults and cases of sudden infant death. Thus for adults, a T-lymphocyte number (marker CD3; Figs. 13.12 and 13.13) of >2.0 cells/visual field (high power field; ×400) or >7.0 cells/mm^2 is regarded as a pathological finding, as well as <14 T-lymphocytes and macrophages (CD68; Fig. 13.14) per mm^2, marked expression of MHC class I and II molecules (Fig. 13.15), or adhesion molecules (CD18, CD54, VLA-4) on cells and the vascular endothelium (Fig. 13.16) (Kühl et al. 1997). Other studies propose a threshold value of 11–16 T-lymphocytes/mm^2, whereas the quantification of intramyocardial macrophages using the CD68 macrophage marker is deemed infeasible (Nielsen et al. 2014a, b).

If these limit values are exceeded, the diagnosis of myocarditis is definite or highly probable,

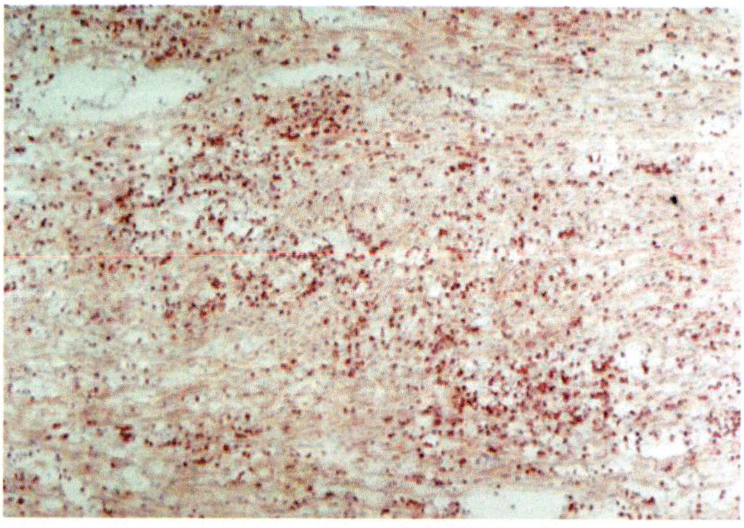

Fig. 13.12 Myocarditis with diffusely increased infiltration by CD3$^+$-T-lymphocytes (×100)

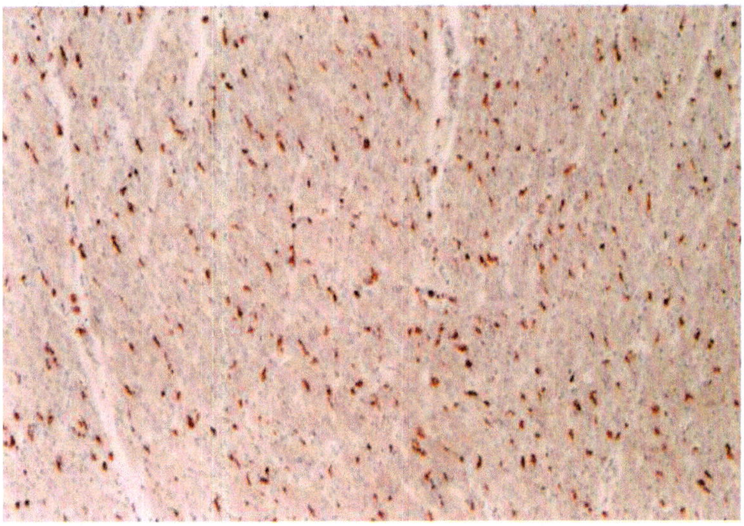

Fig. 13.13 Myocarditis with diffusely increased infiltration by CD45R0⁺-T-lymphocytes (×100)

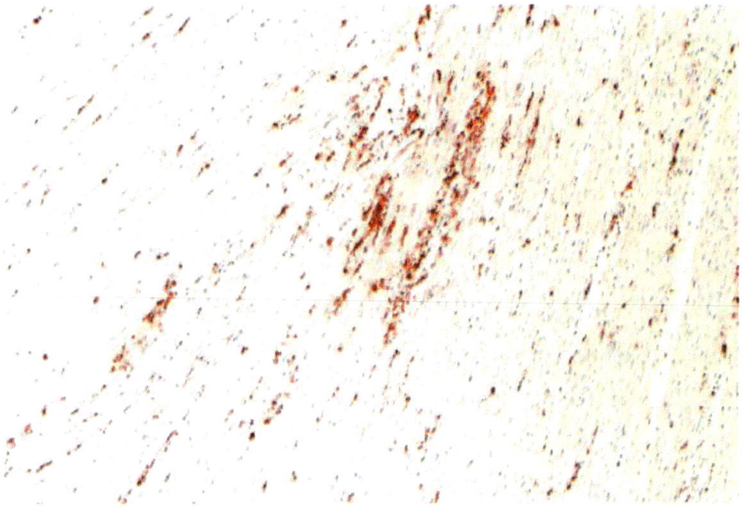

Fig. 13.14 Focally dense infiltration by CD68⁺ macrophages in the posterior wall of the left ventricular myocardium (×100)

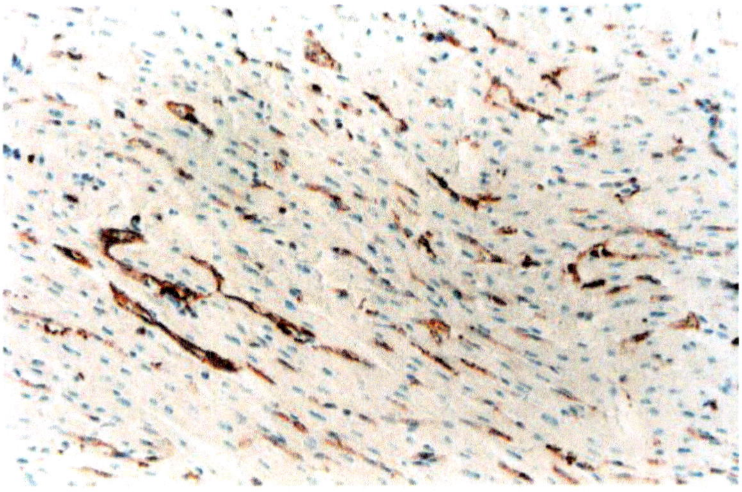

Fig. 13.15 Diffusely marked expression of the MHC class II molecules (+++) in the presence of viral myocarditis in myocardial samples taken from various locations (×100)

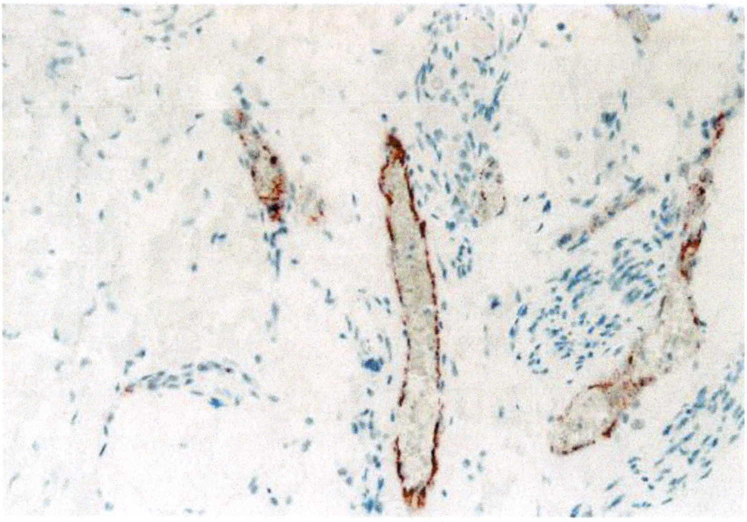

Fig. 13.16 Marked endothelial expression of E-selectin in peripheral arterial branches of the myocardium in the presence of myocarditis (×200)

Table 13.6 The spectrum of cellular and non-cellular inflammatory markers in immunohistochemical diagnosis of myocarditis (selection)

Marker	Antigen
Leukocytes	Leukocyte common antigen (LCA)
T-lymphocytes	CD2, CD3
B-lymphocytes	CD19-CD22
Macrophages	CD68
Natural killer cells	CD57
Lymphocyte subpopulations	
Helper-inducer cells	CD4
Suppressor-cytotoxic cells	CD8
Activated cells	
Lymphocytes	CD25, CD71, CD45R0 (Fig. 13.13)
Macrophages	27E10, RM3/1, 25 F9
Vascular endothelial cells	HLA-I/DR, CD54
Other inflammatory molecules	
Major histocompatibility complex	MHC-I (A,B,C), MHC-II (DP,DQ,DR)
Adhesion molecules, cytokines, etc.	CD18, CD54, VLA-4, E-selectin, etc.

According to Dettmeyer et al. (2006b)

but as with suspicious cases, molecular genetic evidence of a viral presence in the myocardium is desirable to support the diagnosis. In addition, the literature mentions a spectrum of immunohistochemical markers which are used within the scope of myocarditis diagnosis (Table 13.6). Other immunohistochemical antigens were tested, e.g., ICAM-1 (Wojnicz et al. 1998); the increase in number of T-lymphocytes in the myocardial interstitium is of the greatest diagnostic importance.

Given that the quality of immunohistochemical diagnosis depends to a large extent on the methodical approach, the guidelines given in Table 13.7 should be followed for the diagnosis of myocarditis. This method refers in particular to the selection of the fixative and the duration of fixation, while some flexibility remains in the selection of immunohistochemical markers, in addition to the antibodies needed for the qualification and quantification of interstitial leukocytes; new proinflammatory antibodies are being tested.

The immunohistochemical diagnosis of myocarditis is initially based on the qualification and quantification of interstitial leukocytes, T-lymphocytes, and macrophages within the scope of empirically determined standard values for adults (Kühl et al. 1997; Azzawi et al. 1997; Milei et al. 1990; Chow et al. 1989; Schnitt et al. 1987; Steenbergen et al. 1986; Cassling et al. 1985; Linder et al. 1985; Edwards et al. 1982). For the expression of proinflammatory endothelial markers and non-cellular molecules, a semi-quantitative evaluation (0, +, ++, +++) is recommended, also against the background of empirically determined levels of expression, e.g., for MHC class I and II molecules (Daar et al. 1984a, b) and other proinflammatory markers

Table 13.7 Method of recommended conventional histological, immunohistochemical, and molecular genetic investigations for the diagnosis of myocarditis

Method	Important points requiring attention
Fixative	Neutrally buffered formaldehyde (pH-control) or an acceptable alternative fixative
Duration of fixation	Up to 36–48 h
Routine histology	Hemalaun–eosin staining of representative samples for all internal organs
Conventional histology of the myocardium	Hemalaun–eosin staining, additionally Mallory, LFB, and EvG staining; taking at least eight myocardial samples from defined locations is recommended for postmortem diagnosis
Immunohistochemistry	Qualification and quantification of interstitial leukocytes, T-lymphocytes, and macrophages (marker: e.g., LCA, CD45R0, CD68, CD3): count 20 high power fields (hpf) at ×400 or per mm^2; then determine average value
Immunohistochemistry	Detection and semiquantitative evaluation of proinflammatory, e.g., endothelial proteins or molecules (e.g., MHC class I and II, selectin, cytokine, necrosis marker-like fibronectin and C5b-9(m), ICAM-1, etc.)
Molecular genetic agent diagnosis	The myocardial samples with more pronounced lymphomonocytic infiltrates are preferred: PCR and rt-PCR on DNA and RNA viruses [especially enteroviruses (EV), coxsackieviruses, belonging in particular to Group B (CVB; especially CVB3), adenoviruses (AV), Epstein–Barr virus (EBV), parvovirus B19 (PVB19), Herpes simplex viruses, especially Type 6 (HHSV-6), cytomegaly viruses (CMV), etc.]

(Noutsias et al. 1999; Hufnagel and Maisch 1991). In addition, the significance of such markers is partially proven in animal experiments, especially in connection with Group B coxsackievirus infection (Seko et al. 1990).

An immunohistochemical antibody against the enterovirus envelope protein VP1 can provide immediate microscopic evidence of enteroviruses in the myocardium (Li et al. 2000). According to personal experience with these antibodies, the findings could not be reliably reproduced and led to incorrect positive results, as shown by a molecular pathological control.

Molecular and Pathological Evidence of a Viral Presence in the Myocardium

In tissue samples adequately treated with formalin and embedded in paraffin, virus genomes can be found in connection with conventional, histological, and immunohistochemical diagnosis of myocarditis including RNA viruses like the enteroviruses and DNA viruses such as adenoviruses, Epstein–Barr viruses, parvovirus B19, etc. (Dettmeyer et al. 2003, 2004a, b, 2006b, c; Baasner et al. 2003a, b; Chia and Jackson 1996; Zell et al. 1995; Cassinotti et al. 1993; Jin et al. 1990). According to personal experience, evidence of viruses in the myocardium is possible, even when histological and immunohistochemical findings show rather discrete deviations from the standard.

Enteroviruses are common pathogens of myocarditis, particularly cardiotropic Group B coxsackievirus (Gaaloul et al. 2011; Dettmeyer et al. 2006c; Bendig et al. 2001; Huber et al. 1999; Lau 1994; Kandolf et al. 1993; Muir 1993; Jin et al. 1990; Bowles et al. 1986; Lau 1983), but also cytomegaly virus (Kytö et al. 2005; Maisch et al. 1993), Epstein–Barr virus (Lentini et al. 2001; Hebert et al. 1995), adenovirus (Lozinski et al. 1994), influenza virus (Drescher et al. 1987), and parvovirus B19 (Klingel and Kandolf 2009; Bültmann et al. 2003a, b; Dettmeyer et al. 2003; Murry et al. 2001; Enders et al. 1998; Orth et al. 1997). Especially in cases of drug addicts with known hepatitis B or C, myocarditis caused by hepatitis virus should be taken into consideration. Coinfections with two or more pathogens of a myocarditis exist but are relatively rare (Rohayem et al. 2001). The most common pathogens of acute and chronic myocarditis or inflammatory cardiomyopathy are various types of the enterovirus, whereby the Group B coxsackieviruses, specifically CVB3, are considered as particularly cardiotropic (Lang et al. 2008; Klingel et al. 2000; Klump et al. 1990; Pauschinger et al. 1994, 1998; Martino et al. 1995; Kandolf 1995; Klingel et al. 1992a, b; Kandolf et al. 1987).

Enteroviruses (EV)

To determine the importance of detecting enteroviruses in the human myocardium, both pathophysiological aspects and epidemiological findings should be taken into consideration. Based on epidemiological investigations, enteroviruses are recognized as the most common pathogens of viral myocarditis; the coxsackieviruses B1–B5 (CVB), of which the CVB3 is recognized to be particularly cardiotropic (Chrysohoou et al. 2009; Priemer et al. 1999; Klump et al. 1990). Enteroviral infections show seasonal variability (Moral et al. 1993), appearing more often in the summer (Druyts-Voets et al. 1993; Grady and Costanzo-Nordin 1989), while occasional epidemics are reported (Braun et al. 2002; Dettmeyer and Madea 2002; Mounts et al. 2001; Philipps et al. 1980). Human pathogenic enteroviruses are one of the most examined virus systems (Kandolf 1995). Genetic factors not yet identified are assumed to be responsible; for most people, spontaneous elimination of the virus from the myocardium is possible. This effective virus elimination is supposedly associated with an adequate, natural killer cell response, elimination of the virus-infected cell with the help of T-cells, as well as suppression of histocompatible antigens (MHC class). In addition, cytokine-mediated activation of phagocytic macrophages and the induction of apoptotic cell death of virus-infected cells (Ventéo et al. 2010; Schaper et al. 1999; Narula et al. 1996; Kawano et al. 1994) are assumed. Meanwhile, a coxsackievirus and adenovirus receptor (CAR) has been isolated, suggesting a molecular basis for the particular cardiotropic nature of certain viruses (Bergelson et al. 1997; Noutsias et al. 2001). Although a rare exception, enteroviral myocarditis that follows a fulminant course with severe clinical symptoms and rapid death has been described (Oka et al. 2005).

In the early phase of enteroviral myocarditis, endocytic invasion of cardiomyocytes is followed by virus replication with only electron microscopically detectable intracytoplasmic vesicle formation (Klingel et al. 2000; Kandolf 1993, 1995). As part of this process, the number of virus components inside the infected cell may rapidly replicate. If the cell has viral proteins and RNA genomes in sufficient numbers, these components are assembled into infectious viruses (self-assembly). Viral proteins include, for example, envelope proteins of the enteroviruses and capsid proteins 1–4 (VP1–4). The enteroviral proteinase 2A destroys the dystrophin-glycoprotein complex, an extra-sarcomeric protein of the cardiomyocyte cytoskeleton, and thus attacks the contractile apparatus of the host cell. Molecular biological investigations led to the exact breakpoint, and the “Hinge 3” region could be localized (Noutsias et al. 2002; Badorff et al. 1999, 2000a, b).

Increased expression of proinflammatory cytokines, however, should already have a pro-arrhythmogenic effect (Klein et al. 1995). Within the scope of comprehensive observation and based on current knowledge, it is assumed that detection of enteroviruses in the myocardium should be seen as a pathological diagnosis in its own right.

Parvovirus B19 (PVB19)

According to current investigations, parvovirus B19 in the myocardium should not necessarily be regarded as a less significant finding and irrelevant in terms of cause of death. PVB19 preferentially affects the endothelial cells of peripheral arterioles and capillaries and may lead to acute endothelial dysfunction (Bock et al. 2010; Klingel and Kandolf 2009; Bültmann et al. 2003a, b; Schwartzkopff et al. 1998). According to personal experience, histologically and immunohistochemically diagnosed chronic myocarditis may be caused by PVB19 infection (Dettmeyer and Madea 2003; Dettmeyer et al. 2003). In an older study, a PVB19 variant led to the sudden death of young dogs as a result of myocarditis (Hayes et al. 1979).

Epstein–Barr Virus (EBV)

Epstein–Barr viruses are known as potential pathogens of viral myocarditis; in the context of infectious mononucleosis (Pfeifer's mononucleosis, "kissing disease"), sudden unexpected death may occur (Ishikawa et al. 2005; Byard 2002). EVB-induced myocarditis and pericarditis are rarely observed in the clinical setting, despite the fact that the incidence of EBV infection increases with age and is high in adults. However, death in infancy can occur (Hebert et al. 1995). Knowledge of molecular EBV pathology is limited. According to individual cases, EBV-induced myocarditis may clinically and echocardiographically simulate acute myocardial infarction with cardiogenic shock (Lentini et al. 2001; Tyson et al. 1989; Miller et al. 1973), but the exact mechanism of damage remains unknown.

Adenoviruses (AV)

Of the pathogens of viral myocarditis, adenoviruses are often mentioned second to enteroviruses, in particular adenoviruses 2 and 5 (Oyer et al. 2000; Bergelson et al. 1997; Lozinski et al. 1994; Martin et al. 1994). Meanwhile, common membrane-linked receptors for coxsackie- and adenoviruses (Liu and Mason 2001; Bergelson et al. 1997) have been successfully identified. This coxsackievirus and adenovirus receptor (CAR) belongs to the immunoglobulin superfamily and is able to react with other viruses of the enteroviruses group (Liu and Mason 2001). CAR is an embryonic gene product with high expression levels during embryonic development, as well as early downregulation already in the neonatal phase. Under physiological conditions, the receptor is absent on adult cardiomyocytes (Noutsias et al. 2002; Bergelson et al. 1997). At least in immature newborns and preterm infants, postnatal, initially persistent, and relatively high expression levels of the CAR gene could represent a molecular basis for the increased cardiotropic nature of coxsackie- and adenoviruses, but possibly also of enteroviruses.

Cytomegalovirus (CMV)

Cytomegaloviruses are regarded as relatively rare pathogens of myocarditis; they are occasionally found in babies and children in the glandular epithelia of the salivary glands, particularly the parotid gland (Cecchi et al. 1995; Cremer and Althoff 1991). More recent investigations suggest a greater role for cytomegalovirus-induced myocarditis in the case of fatal outcome (Dettmeyer et al. 2006d; Kytö et al. 2005).

Influenza A H1N1-Associated Myocarditis

During the 2009/2010 A/H1N1 influenza pandemic, fatal cases were seen showing molecular pathological evidence of infection and interstitial myocarditis accompanied by myocardial necrosis in the absence of significant respiratory tract and pulmonary infection (Gdynia et al. 2011).

Autoimmune Myocarditis. This involves an immune reaction to endogenous cardiac myosin producing the histological picture of lymphocytic myocarditis. It is not uncommon for this entity to be preceded by viral myocarditis, with the immune reaction developing in a delayed manner once the virus has already been eliminated. Therefore, in such cases of postviral myocarditis, the viral genome is no longer detectable in myocardial samples. However, our knowledge of the basics of immunopathology is still patchy. Autoimmune myocarditis is challenging to differentiate from chronic myocarditis with at least partial but often undetectable viral persistence. For this reason, chronic myocarditis is sometimes also referred to as autoimmune myocarditis.

13.3.2 Chronic Myocarditis

Acute myocarditis may either heal or become chronic. In particular, immunohistochemical and molecular pathological investigations over the past 20 years have shown that most of the macroscopically diagnosed dilative cardiomyopathies are the result of chronic myocarditis; evidence of virus persistence is only possible in some cases. It is clear that, despite successful elimination of the virus, the result may be an autoimmune response with persistent myocardial inflammation (autoimmune myocarditis). In some cases, diagnostic differentiation from concomitant myocarditis may be difficult following microscopic diagnosis, but this is usually still possible within the scope of a comprehensive histological examination of all internal organs.

Conventional staining will result in diagnostic findings which already indicate a chronic inflammatory process; if necessary, further immunohistochemical diagnostic tests should follow (see Table 13.8). Following death of a heart muscle cell, there is increased cellular infiltration in the myocardial interstitium, accompanied by partially interstitial, partially perivascular fibrosis, as well as some streaky fibrosis (Fig. 13.17). Studies to date have focused on myocarditis and its transition to a chronic inflammatory process (D'Ambrosio et al. 2001; Strauer et al. 2001; Maisch et al. 2000; Kawai 1999; Noutsias et al. 1996; Martino et al. 1994; Schultheiß 1993; Klingel et al. 1992a, b; Herzum and Maisch 1988; Kawai et al. 1987).

Table 13.8 Histological and immunohistochemical diagnosis of chronic myocarditis, dilated myocarditis, or dilated cardiomyopathy, inflammatory type (DCMi)

Histology	Immunohistochemistry/molecular pathology
Focal, interstitial edema, fiber structures with partially and somewhat irregular appearance	Often only a moderate increase in leukocytes, T-lymphocytes, and macrophages
Interstitial fibrosis, caliber deviation of the cardiomyocytes, differences in size of nuclei	Somewhat increased expression of MHC class I and II molecules
Pronounced perivascular fibrosis (EvG stains)	Sign of progressive restructuring with expression of tenascin at the margin of microscopically small zones of fibrosis
Myocardial single-cell necrosis	Focal loss of desmin detectability
Single, empty sarcolemma tubes	Myocardial single-cell necrosis, seldom group necrosis (fibronectin, $C5b\text{-}9_{(m)}$)
Potential microscopically small zones of scarring	Expression of additional proinflammatory markers (see Table 13.6)
Circumscribed endocardial fibroses	Molecular pathology (PCR, rt-PCR), possible detection of viral genome with typically small number of viral copies (Bowles et al. 1989; Arola et al. 1998)

The differentiation between chronic myocarditis and inflammatory cardiomyopathy has been discussed in the literature (Kühl et al. 1992)

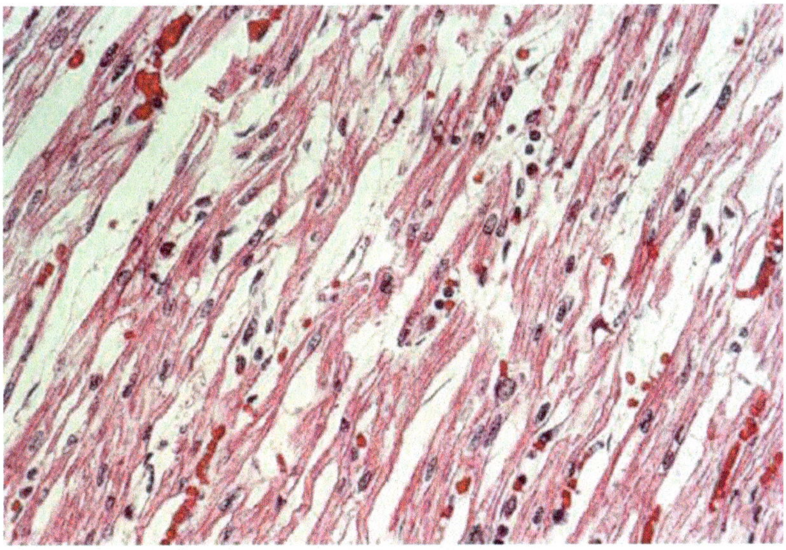

Fig. 13.17 Chronic myocarditis with somewhat increased cellular infiltration, interstitial edema, and degeneration of heart muscle fibers (H&E ×400)

The term "chronic myocarditis" is appropriate for a macroscopically normal heart with the microscopic diagnosis of a chronic inflammatory process. If dilated cardiomyopathy is present macroscopically, in addition to a histologically or immunohistochemically observed inflammatory process, the term "dilated cardiomyopathy, inflammatory type (DCMi)" may be used. The spectrum of possible viruses responsible remains unknown, although according to more recent tests, the virus PVB19, for example, is being considered (Bock et al. 2005; Klingel et al. 2004).

Apoptosis

Apoptosis is a form of programmed cell death with cell shrinkage and dismantling of the DNA into defined fragments by endonucleases, which may be detected with the help of the TUNEL method (Chap. 2). From the histological perspective, the affected cell separates from the cell environment and becomes increasingly eosinophilic and smaller. The cell nucleus becomes small and compact. Effector caspases, primarily caspases 3, 6, and 7, lead to apoptotic cell death. Investigations into apoptosis from a forensic perspective are currently being undertaken in only a few studies. Nevertheless, cardiomyocyte apoptosis, a key pathologic feature of heart failure, may play a critical role in patients with acute myocarditis (Abbate et al. 2009; Kawano et al. 1994) and in cases of dilated cardiomyopathy (Schaper et al. 1999).

13.4 Non-virus-Based Myocarditis

Rare forms of non-virus-based myocarditis sometimes appear at autopsy. For example, *Chagas disease*, a disorder widespread in some areas of South America and involving an intracellular parasite (*Trypanosoma cruzi*), can cause chronic lymphocytic myocarditis (de Lourdes Higuchi et al. 1993). Since these findings often explain sudden death due to natural causes and are histologically characteristic, brief explanations should be sufficient here to cover the different forms.

13.4.1 Bacterial Myocarditis

In the context of bacterial infection, which usually involves sepsis accompanying bacteremia, partially diffuse and partially granulocytic infiltrates with focal emphasis can be found in the myocardium (Figs. 13.18 and 13.19). At the same time, some cases may show basophilic colonies of bacteria (cocci, coccoid rods) which are more effectively detected using specialized stains. In addition, histological findings, such as septic shock, are made on a regular basis. Particularly in cases of focal infection with purulent abscess and central bacterial colonies, embolic spread of pathogens should be taken into consideration.

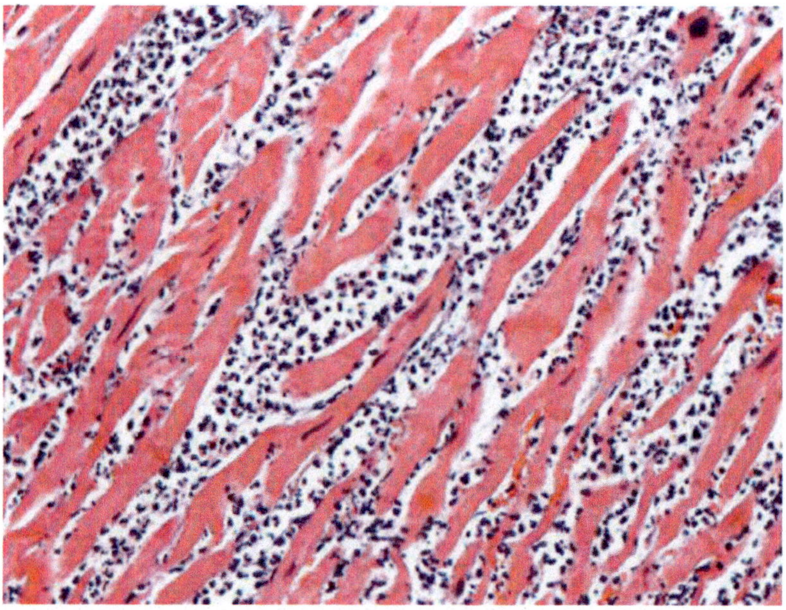

Fig. 13.18 Acute purulent myocarditis with multiple granulocytes (H&E ×200)

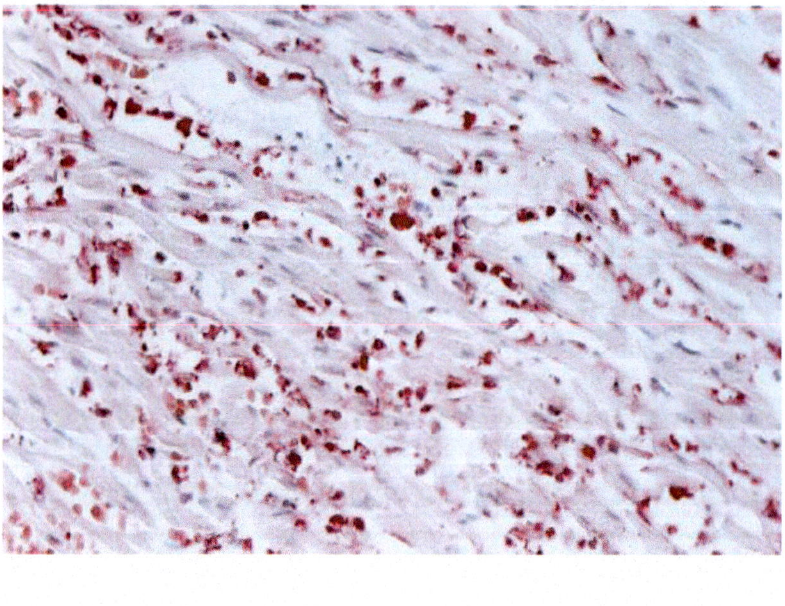

Fig. 13.19 Acute purulent myocarditis with enzyme-histochemical detection of granulocytes (*red*) in the interventricular septal myocardium and bulky degeneration of individual cardiomyocytes, interstitial edema, and drifting apart of heart muscle fibers (ASD ×400)

13.4.2 Tuberculous Myocarditis

Tuberculosis rarely involves the myocardium (Dada et al. 2000). At autopsy, decedents with a weakened immune system (e.g., chronic alcoholics) should be examined for the possibility of cardiac tuberculosis, followed by investigations to establish whether other organs are affected (particularly the lung). Tuberculosis pathogens can be seen using Ziehl–Neelsen staining (oil immersion microscopy ×1000); however, this method is frequently unsuccessful. Tuberculous bacteria are often found in the peripheral region of caseous necrosis, adjacent to the lymphocyte wall and Langerhans giant cells. However, diagnosis may easily be based on classic histological diagnosis with no detection of agents: Necrotic zone with a lymphocytic border, peripheral fibrosis, multinucleated Langhans giant cells, and the cores of these giant cells are frequently arranged in a horseshoe form.

13.4.3 Fungal Myocarditis

When using conventional stains under microscopy, an experienced pathologist may recognize fungal components in the myocardium, often with marked surrounding inflammation. Grocott stains (Fig. 13.20) are usually used to show fungal spores and hyphae. The entry site often remains undetected, as with other myocarditis pathogens. However, sources of infection can regularly be observed in other organs (lungs, liver, kidney).

13.4.4 Rheumatoid Myocarditis

Diagnosis of rheumatoid myocarditis as the cause of premature sudden death is extremely rare. Map-like necrotic zones with dense, raised margins full of inflammatory cells with no multinucleated Langhans giant cells appear next to Aschoff nodules (Fig. 13.21) (Fraser et al. 1995). There have also been reports of seasonal variations in myocardial involvement in rheumatism (Metze et al. 1993). Sudden death in the setting of rheumatic heart disease in children is seen in extremely rare cases (Rérolle et al. 2016).

13.4.5 Giant-Cell Myocarditis

Giant-cell myocarditis (Fig. 13.22) is a special form of myocarditis, which has been described

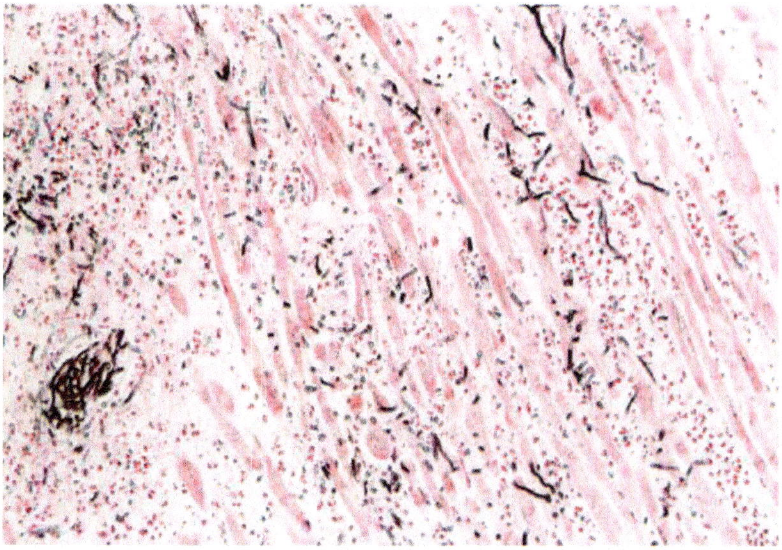

Fig. 13.20 Fungal hyphae demarcated by inflammatory cells in the myocardium in the presence of fungal myocarditis (Grocott ×200)

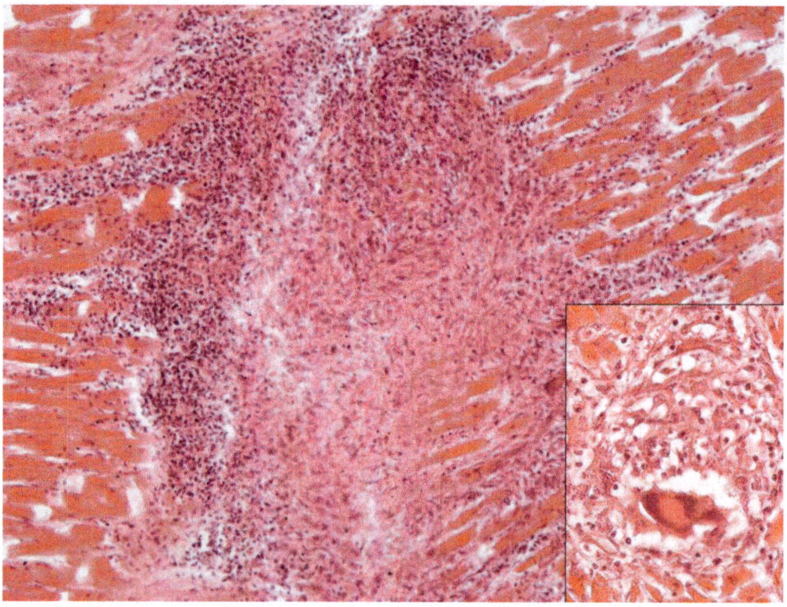

Fig. 13.21 Rheumatoid myocarditis with central necrosis and a dense wall of inflammatory cells as the cause of unexpected sudden death (H&E ×100; ×400)

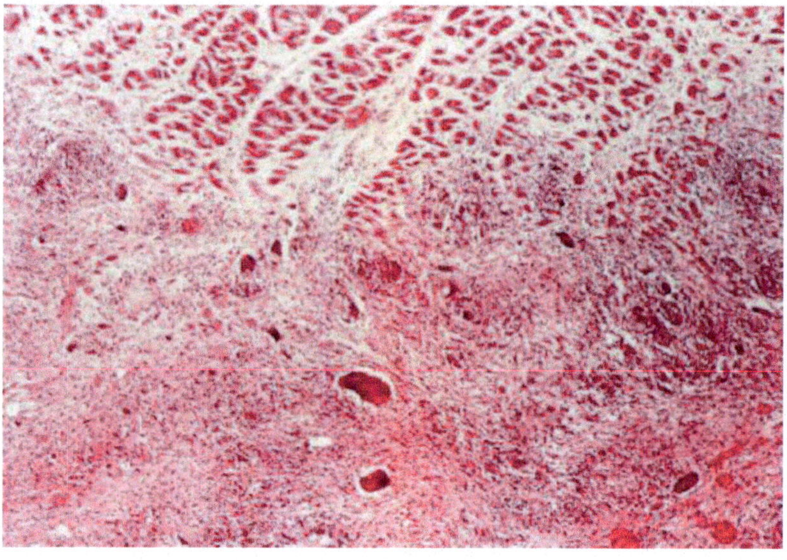

Fig. 13.22 Acute giant-cell myocarditis with significant fibrous components (H&E ×100)

as a cause of sudden death (Martinez et al. 2013; Matejic et al. 2010; Blauwet and Cooper 2010; Langlois 2009; Murty 2008; Hamilton et al. 2007). Microscopically, the myocardium is frequently replaced by extensive collagen connective tissue with a lymphohistiocytic inflammatory infiltrate, which often includes numerous multinucleated giant cells with no characteristic alignment of cell nuclei. Epithelioid and granulomatous structures are absent, and other organs are not involved. Healed, fibrous areas occur alongside reparative processes. Young adults are particularly affected by giant-cell myocarditis. An autoimmune process as a possible cause is under investigation.

13.4.6 Myocardial Involvement in Sarcoidosis

Sarcoidosis may affect internal organs (Bernstein et al. 1929), and systemic sarcoidosis may cause myocardial inflammation. In this case, sarcoidosis is often detectable in other organs, particularly in the lungs. The forensic literature reports undetected myocardial involvement in sarcoidosis, which remained undiagnosed up to the point of autopsy, as the cause of sudden death (Ginellinová et al.; Bagwan et al. 2011; Riezzo et al. 2009; Byard et al. 2008; Riße et al. 2008; Veinot and Johnston 1998; Ogbuihi et al. 1993).

With the help of microscopic investigations, scattered foci of granulomatous inflammation with epithelioid giant cells, lymphocytes, mononuclear cells, and foci of myocytic necrosis can be found (Fig. 13.23). Specific stains for fungi and acid fast bacilli are always negative. In addition to multinucleated giant cells and noncaseating epithelioid granulomas, there have been occasional reports of intracytoplasmic inclusions in sarcoidosis: so-called Hamazaki-Wesenberg bodies, Schaumann bodies (as laminated proteinaceous concretions), birefringent calcium oxalate crystals under polarized light microscopy, and asteroid bodies (as stellate-shaped inclusions within giant cells) (Ginellinová et al. 2016). The diagnostic differentiation from idiopathic giant-cell myocarditis can be challenging. Myocardial necrosis and increased eosinophilic granulocytes suggest giant-cell myocarditis.

13.4.7 Eosinophilic Myocarditis

The literature mentions idiopathic eosinophilic endocarditis and myocarditis (Janík and Hejna 2017; Fragkouli et al. 2011); however, in individual cases, allergic myocarditis, in particular myocarditis responsive to drug therapy, should also be considered when histological accumulations of eosinophilic granulocytes can be detected in the myocardium (Fineschi et al. 2004; Burke et al. 1991; Löffler 1936; see Chap. 5, Fig. 4.13).

In certain cases, immunohistochemical stains may provide additional evidence of IgE and an allergic-responsive cause, for example, in increased mast cells in lung tissue. If possible, evidence of the trigger allergen should be provided. Eosinophilic myocarditis can be part of "drug-induced hypersensitivity syndrome (DIHS)," also called "drug rash with eosinophilia and systemic symptoms (DRESS)," and is a

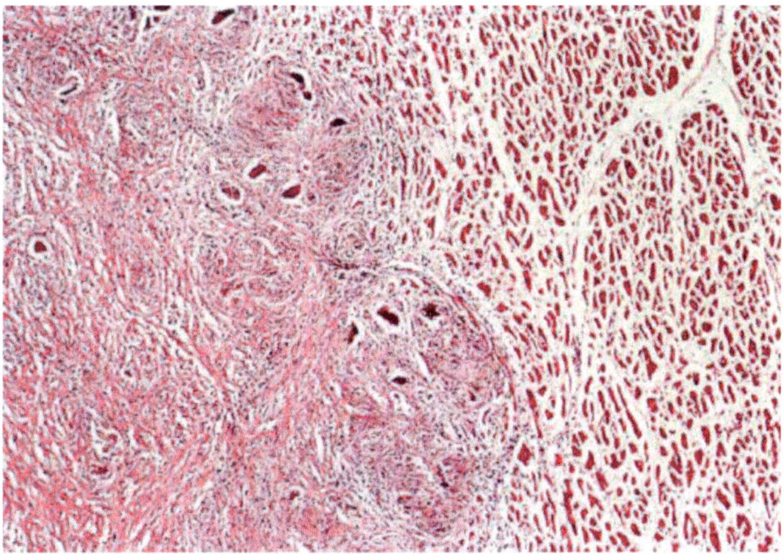

Fig. 13.23 Myocardial involvement in sarcoidosis (H&E ×100)

severe reaction usually characterized by fever, rash, and multiorgan failure, occurring 1–8 weeks after drug introduction. It is an immune-mediated reaction involving macrophage and T-lymphocyte activation and cytokine release, although no consensus has been reached as to its etiology (Ben m'rad et al. 2009).

13.5 Cardiomyopathy

The term cardiomyopathy includes various diseases of the heart muscle, with a distinction between primary and secondary cardiomyopathies. The expert consensus panel proposes a definition (Maron et al. 2006):

> Cardiomyopathies are a heterogenous group of diseases of the myocardium associated with mechanical and/or electrical dysfunction that usually (but not invariably) exhibit inappropriate ventricular hypertrophy or dilatation and are due to a variety of causes that frequently are genetic. Cardiomyopathies either are confined to the heart or are part of generalized systemic disorders, often leading to cardiovascular death or progressive heart failure-relatively disability.

Cardiomyopathy is a disease of the heart muscle which has not been caused by coronary artery disease, mechanical stress through congenital heart disease, a coronary anomaly, or hypertension in the large and small circulation.

Primary cardiopathy types are classified according to the revised version (Maron et al. 2006) of the 1996 American Heart Association (AHA) definitions (Richardson et al. 1996). In addition, the European Society of Cardiology Working Group produced a statement on myocardial and pericardial types (Elliott et al. 2008). Hypertrophic cardiomyopathy and other forms of cardiomyopathy which may become symptomatic in infants have a genetic cause (Schwartz et al. 1996; Seidman et al. 1992; Takahashi et al. 2008). A modified classification of cardiomyopathy is given in Table 13.9 (for additional details, please refer to the relevant literature).

As with nonviral myocarditis, only the classic histology of the most important forms of cardiomyopathy in forensics will be discussed here. Microscopic diagnosis is suitable for the investigation of a suspicious macroscopic diagnosis; in some cases, immunohistochemical findings may provide additional diagnostic confirmation.

13.5.1 Hypertrophic Cardiomyopathy

Evidence of hypertrophic cardiomyopathy can be detected at autopsy in both children and adults; however, this condition may also affect children with less conspicuous macroscopic findings (Bryant 1999). In this case, myocardial samples should be specifically taken from

Table 13.9 Modified classification of cardiomyopathy types

Genetic forms	Mixed forms	Acquired forms
Hypertrophic cardiomyopathy (HCM), e.g., as idiopathic, hypertrophic subaortic stenosis (IHSS)	Dilative cardiomyopathy (DCM)	Inflammatory dilative cardiomyopathy (DCMi)
Arrhythmogenic right ventricular cardiomyopathy (ARVCM)	Restrictive cardiomyopathy	Stress-induced cardiomyopathy
		Takotsubo cardiomyopathy
Glycogen reservoir diseases		Periportal cardiomyopathy
Transition defects		Tachycardia-induced cardiomyopathy
Mitochondrial cardiomyopathy		Acquired in children with insulin-dependent diabetic mothers
Ion channel defects		Thyrogenic cardiomyopathy
Isolated noncompaction cardiomyopathy (NCCM)		Drug-induced forms, e.g., cocaine cardiomyopathy

There are other rare forms of acquired cardiomyopathy

the affected area for investigation (primarily H&E, van Gieson staining). For example, samples should be taken from the portion of the interventricular septum below the aortic valve, as well as the left ventricular wall in cases of idiopathic hypertrophic subaortic stenosis (IHSS).

The histological picture varies between children and adults (Wigle et al. 1985; Frenzel et al. 1987; Maron 2002), whereby the following are frequent:

- Manifest disturbance of the texture of the left ventricular myocardial tissue partially with storiform patterns (disarray) (Fig. 13.24)
- Circumscribed hypertrophic cardiomyocytes (myofiber hypertrophy) with partially bizarre cell nuclei (Fig. 13.25)

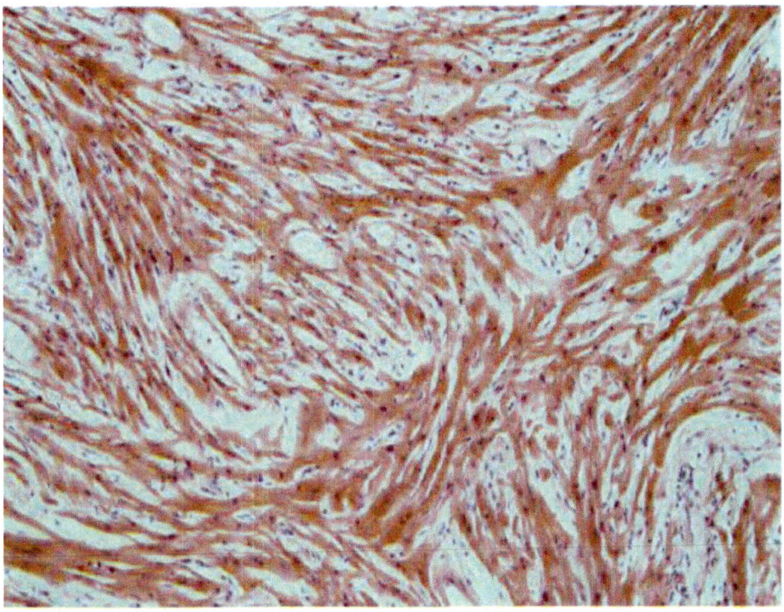

Fig. 13.24 Histologically irregular dendritic texture of heart muscle fibers with a denoted storiform basic pattern in hypertrophic cardiomyopathy (Elastica van Gieson ×100)

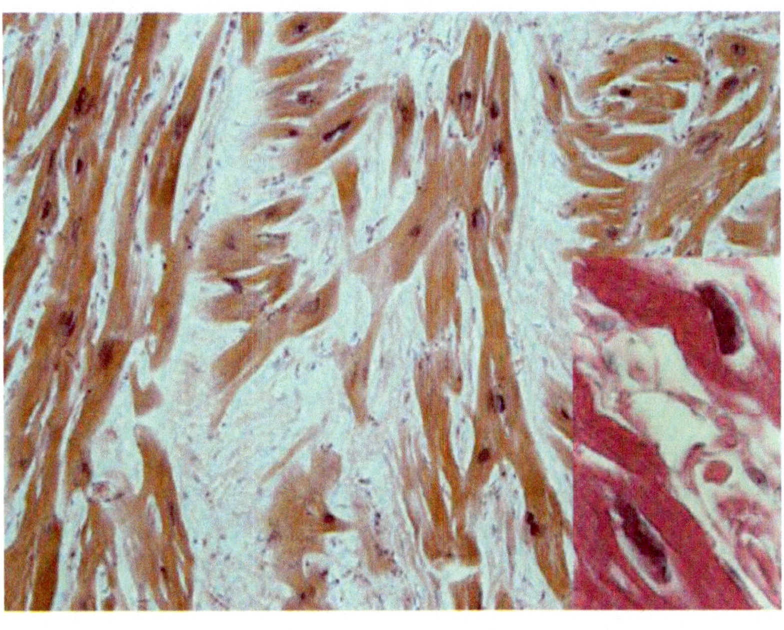

Fig. 13.25 Irregular dendritic heart muscle fibers in hypertrophic cardiomyopathy with enlarged cell nuclei (van Gieson ×100; Insert: H&E ×1000)

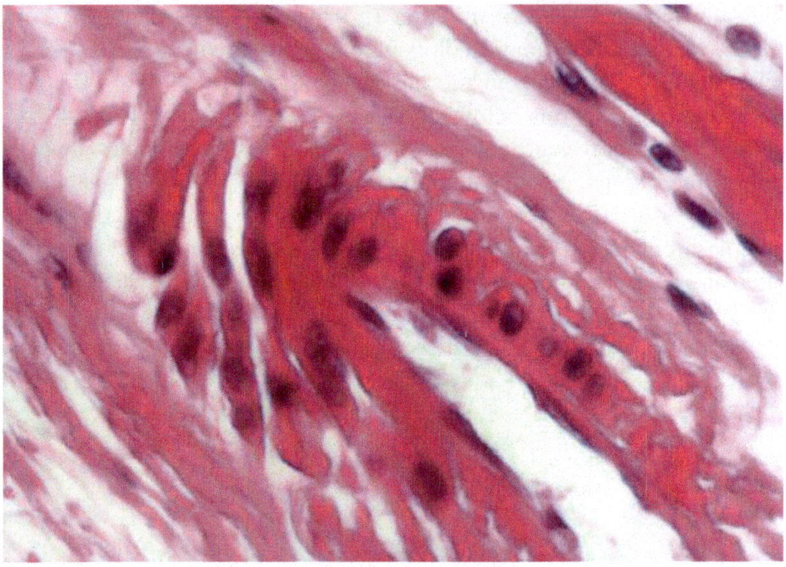

Fig. 13.26 Hypertrophic cardiomyopathy: dysplastic vessels with increased thickness of the wall and enlarged hyperchromatic nuclei of vascular smooth muscle cells (H&E ×400)

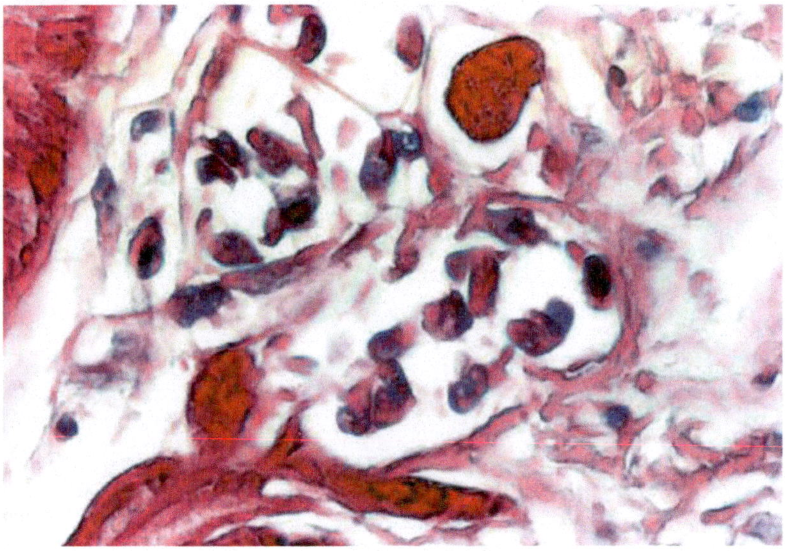

Fig. 13.27 Hypertrophic cardiomyopathy with empty sarcolemma tubes in which accumulations of enlarged hyperchromatic heart muscle cell nuclei are found (H&E ×1000)

- Cardiomyocytes with irregular myofibril structure
- Peripheral vessels with thickened walls and smooth muscle cells showing enlarged and hyperchromatic nuclei (Fig. 13.26)
- Occasional focal accumulation of $CD68^+$ macrophages
- In isolated cases, empty sarcolemma tubes can be present in which accumulated cell nuclei can be seen (Fig. 13.27)
- Interstitial fibrosis may appear in places

In the case of confirmed hypertrophic cardiomyopathy, a genetic diagnosis is recommended in cases where this could be of therapeutic significance for relatives and where such an examination is desired (Maron et al. 1997). After an often longer course, hypertrophic cardiomyopathy may appear macroscopically as dilative cardiomyopathy (Riedel et al. 1997; Lin et al. 1998) and in some cases may be difficult to differentiate from inflammatory cardiomyopathy (Dettmeyer et al. 2004b).

13.5.2 Dilative Cardiomyopathy (DCM)

Dilative cardiomyopathy is characterized by dilation and enlargement of the left ventricle with a partially thickened, partially normal, and partially thinning ventricle wall which shows reduced motility. Histopathologically, degeneratively modified cardiomyocytes as well as hypertrophic heart muscle fibers with enlarged, and occasionally abnormally shaped, cell nuclei are found. Additionally, there are zones of interstitial fibrosis which can be found particularly in subendocardial sections. The extracellular matrix contains collagen, proteoglycan, and glycoprotein, which may be involved in fibrotic restructuring. Components of the extracellular matrix also include glycoprotein tenascin, for example, which is more significantly expressed at the margin of relatively discrete zones of fibrosis, but also in enlarged cardiomyocytes and next to necrotic heart muscle cells (see alcoholic cardiomyopathy; Chap. 6). Tenascin expression is seen as a continuous, progressive restructuring process in the myocardium (Tamura et al. 1996), connexin (Cx), especially the relationship between Cx43, and sudden death in patients with dilated cardiomyopathy was examined (Chen and Zhang 2006).

Both primary obstructive hypertrophic cardiomyopathy and the resulting secondary dilative cardiomyopathy show a similar histological picture. If dilative cardiomyopathy is a chronic inflammatory process (termed dilative inflammatory cardiomyopathy), chronic myocarditis is involved, often of viral genesis (Figulla 2004; Kühl et al. 1994, 1996; see also above). Attention should be paid to perivascular fibrosis (Fig. 13.28) in addition to moderately increased cellular infiltration. Increased mRNA expression of *coxsackievirus and adenovirus receptor (CAR)*, whose pathophysiological role remains the subject of discussion, has been observed in both dilated and ischemic cardiomyopathy (Tatrai et al. 2011). CAR can perhaps be regarded as a novel modifier of ventricular conduction and arrhythmia vulnerability in the setting of myocardial ischemia. Genetic determinants of arrhythmia susceptibility, such as CAR, may constitute future targets for risk stratification of potentially lethal ventricular arrhythmias in patients with coronary artery disease (Marsman et al. 2014).

13.5.3 Arrhythmogenic Right Ventricular Cardiomyopathy/Dysplasia (ARVCM)

Arrhythmogenic right ventricular cardiomyopathy/dysplasia (ARVCM) may be the cause of sudden unexpected death, for example, under

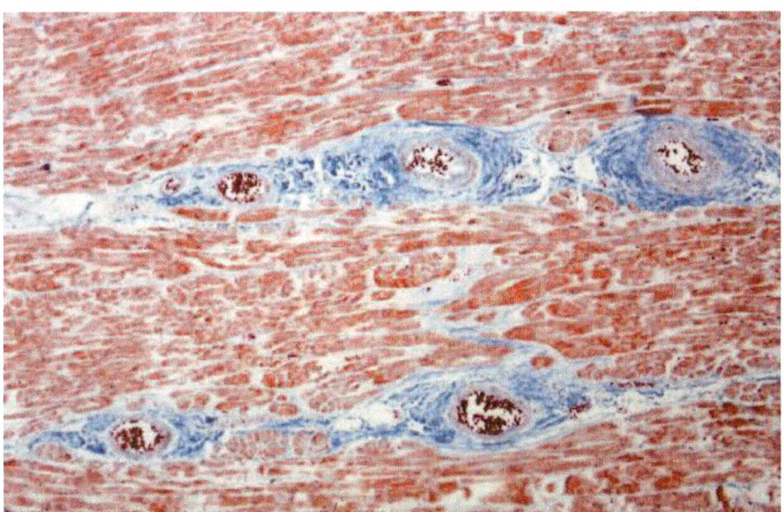

Fig. 13.28 Dilative cardiomyopathy with multifocal, perivascular fibrosis—most likely inflammatory dilative cardiomyopathy (DCMi) (Mallory ×125)

physical stress (Wingenfeld et al. 2010; Mund et al. 2002). A prevalence of 1:2500 to 1:5000 has been indicated for ARVCM (Basso et al. 2009), but considerable regional variation has been described. It is inherited in a predominantly autosomal dominant manner; 11 different genotypes are currently known. In the case of ARVCM, progressive adiposis of mainly the right ventricular myocardium is present; heart muscle fibers are replaced by adipose and connective tissue (Fig. 13.29) (Basso et al. 2008a, b; Angelini et al. 1996; Angelini et al. 1993). The remaining myocardium often is partially hypertrophied but may appear atrophic as well. Cardiomyocytes can appear vacuolated or may show coagulation necroses. Sometimes they are surrounded by inflammatory, mostly lymphocytic infiltrates (Huckenbeck and Papadomanolakis 2005). Although there are a number of reports concerning histologically detectable adipose and fibrous infiltrations of the left ventricular myocardium with left ventricular functional disorders, in all these cases, a concomitant infiltration of the right ventricle was present. The literature contains criteria for diagnosis which also include clinical data and family anamnesis (McKenna et al. 1994). Evidence of transmural replacement of myocardium by fat and connective tissue with fat cell nests reaching as far as under the right ventricular endocardium is histologically significant (Lobo et al. 1992). These changes, however, can only be detected in localized areas of the right ventricular wall and, alone, are not sufficiently specific (Basso et al. 2008a, b; Angelini et al. 1993). Similar findings can also be seen in older hearts (Basso and Thiene 2005; Tansey et al. 2005). For this reason, a histomorphometric method was suggested to determine the percentage of fat and connective tissue in seven visual fields at a 400× magnification using a diagram analysis system (Angelini et al. 1993). Diagnosis of ARVCM requires a minimum of 3% fat tissue on average and more than 40% fibrotic tissue. Other investigators regard 5–20% fat tissue as suspicious (Hort 2000; Dalal et al. 1994). In 2010, a modified method was introduced to evaluate digital microphotographs treating five myocardial regions, each with seven fields of view, together with Elastica van Gieson staining and Sudan III staining (Hagemeier et al. 2010). Patients with ARVCM may suffer from a myocardial viral infection, which may at least in part explain interstitial fibrosis and accompanying inflammatory infiltrates (Bowles et al. 2002). It was shown that ARVCM in children coexists with chronic myocarditis, as was shown with the aid of immunocytochemical staining for markers for T-lymphocytes (CD3, CD4, CD8)

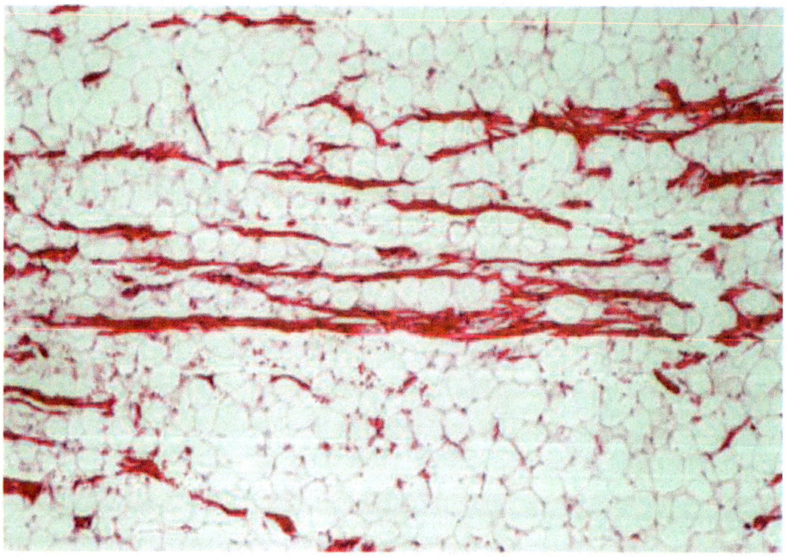

Fig. 13.29 Arrhythmogenic right ventricular cardiomyopathy/dysplasia (ARVCM) with a fatty replacement of cardiac muscle in the right ventricular myocardium. Adipose tissue infiltration is associated with atrophic heart muscle cells (H&E ×40)

B-lymphocytes (CD22), and macrophages (CD68) and for adhesion molecules (ICAM-1, VCAM, ELAM) and endothelial marker (CD31/PECAM-1) (Woźniewicz et al. 1998). Clinically, the arrythmogenic right ventricular cardiomyopathy may lead to cardial arrhythmias. However, the disease is often asymptomatic until the diagnosis is made by an autopsy performed for the analysis of a sudden unexpected death. Recent investigations propose mutations believed to occur more frequently in patients with ARVCM, despite the fact that histological findings in the cases investigated were not typical for ARVCM (Sato et al. 2015). Plakoglobin is believed to be a suitable immunohistochemical diagnostic marker for ARVCM (Munkholm et al. 2015).

13.5.4 Isolated Noncompaction Cardiomyopathy

Isolated noncompaction cardiomyopathy (NCCM) was first described in 1984 (Engberding and Bender 1984). Fatal cases are usually seen in the pediatric population (Handlos et al. 2017; Lim and Langlois 2016; Buschmann et al. 2006). The term "isolated noncompaction of left ventricular myocardium" was suggested later (Chin et al. 1990). The clinical picture of NCCM varies greatly. In addition to heart insufficiency, intraventricular thrombosis and thromboembolic events occur (Binz et al. 2003; Bleyl et al. 1997a, b), including microcirculation imbalance (Jenni et al. 2002). It is reported to be the third most frequent form in children, after dilative cardiomyopathy (DCM) and hypertrophic cardiomyopathy (HCM) (Andrews et al. 2008; Arola et al. 1997), and carries a serious prognosis (Oechslin et al. 2000).

There are sporadic cases as well as cases showing familial prevalence (Ichida et al. 2001). Meanwhile, a genetic basis for the disease has been identified (Rodríguez-Calvo et al. 2008; Hermido-Prieto et al. 2004; Kenton et al. 2004; Sasse-Klaassen et al. 2003, 2004; Ichida et al. 2001; Bleyl et al. 1997a, b).

Histologically, there are sinusoidal recesses with an immunohistochemically CD34-positive endothelial or endocardial lining in the affected myocardial area which run deep into the left ventricular myocardium (Fig. 13.30) (Chin et al. 1990; Burke et al. 2005). In the right ventricle, it is almost impossible to distinguish this type of change from the regular trabecula system; thus NCCM is considered as localized, pathological left ventricular trabeculation. The corresponding endocardium may show subendocardial fibrosis (Jenni et al. 2002). In sudden infant death, NCCM may be considered in the differential diagnosis; it is possible that some cases of sudden infant death can be explained in this way (Dettmeyer and Kandolf 2009).

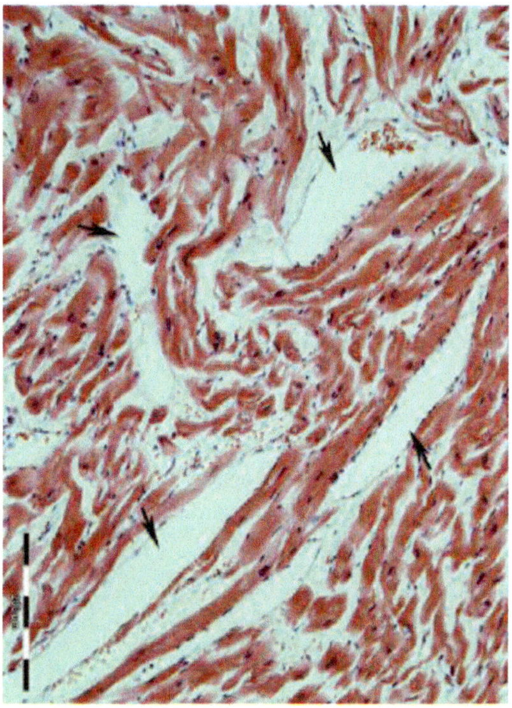

Fig. 13.30 Noncompaction cardiomyopathy: cross section of trabeculations (*arrows*) focally reaching far into the myocardium (H&E ×200)

13.5.5 Alcoholic Cardiomyopathy

Alcoholic cardiomyopathy belongs to the group of toxic cardiomyopathies (Bulloch et al. 1972). In addition to alcohol consumption reported during anamnesis, alcoholic cardiomyopathy appears macroscopically as dilative cardiomyopathy. It is under discussion whether at least some cases of presumed alcoholic cardiomyopathy should actually be categorized as inflammatory dilative cardiomyopathy (DCMi) (Dettmeyer et al. 2002b). For more information, see Chap. 6.

13.5.6 Rare Forms of Cardiomyopathy

Rare forms of cardiomyopathy include:

- Thyrogenic cardiomyopathy
- Histiocytoid/oncocytic cardiomyopathy
- Takotsubo cardiomyopathy

Thyrogenic Cardiomyopathy
Hyperthyreosis may lead to cardiomyopathy with an eccentric myocardial hypertrophy, including necrosis, focal fibroses, and fine adiposis of the heart muscle fibers. Thyrotoxicosis of long standing may lead to the diagnosis of dilative cardiomyopathy (Santer 2004). Diagnosis always requires evidence of hyperthyreosis that has existed over a longer period of time (see Chap. 16).

Histiocytic/Oncocytic Cardiomyopathy
This rare childhood disease affects girls more often than boys. Microscopically, transformed muscle cells can be detected with partially vacuolized, partially eosinophilic and granular cytoplasm. Necrosis and an inflammatory response are absent (Stahl et al. 1997; Ruszkiewicz and Vernon-Roberts 1993; Ferrans et al. 1976). Eston and Perskvist (2009) reported on the association between histiocytoid cardiomyopathy and left ventricular hypertrabeculation in the death of a female infant. Histiocytoid cardiomyopathy and noncompaction cardiomyopathy are occasionally associated with mitochondrial disease (Finsterer and Stöllberger 2009; Finsterer 2008; Finsterer et al. 2007; Vallance et al. 2004).

Takotsubo Cardiomyopathy. Stress-Induced Cardiomyopathy (SICM)
Takotsubo cardiomyopathy (also called transient apical ballooning and stress cardiomyopathy; Angelini 2016; Indorato and Bartolini 2016; Indorato et al. 2015; Prasad et al. 2008; Cebelin and Hirsch 1980) is characterized by transient left ventricular dysfunction, electrocardiographic changes, and minimal release of myocardial enzymes (modest elevation of cardiac troponin), which mimic acute myocardial infarction. Patients do not present with coronary artery disease, and the pathomechanism is unknown. Takotsubo cardiomyopathy occurs primarily in postmenopausal women (Stöllberger et al. 2010; Fineschi et al. 2010; Bybee and Prasad 2008; Hansen 2007). Currently, there is no consensus on the diagnostic criteria for Takotsubo cardiomyopathy; some investigators proposed diagnostic criteria in 2004, which included the absence of pheochromocytoma and myocarditis (Akashi et al. 2008). The expert consensus panel (Maron et al. 2006) proposes a definition about stress cardiomyopathy:

> … a recently described clinical entity characterized by acute but rapidly reversible LV systolic dysfunction in the absence of atherosclerotic coronary artery disease, triggered by profound psychological stress. This distinctive form of ventricular stunning typically affects older women and preferentially involves the distal portion of the LV chamber ("atypical ballooning"), with the basal LV hypercontractile. Although presentation often mimics ST-segment-elevation myocardial infarction, outcome is favorable with an appropriate medical therapy.

There is no known specific histomorphologic correlate for Takotsubo cardiomyopathy, and a more precise histological documentation is needed for all cases with different kinds of behavior who suddenly died following emotional stress. Of the patients who underwent endomyocardial biopsy, interstitial infiltrates consisting primarily of mononuclear lymphocytes and macrophages and contraction bands without myocyte necrosis were observed (Wittstein et al. 2005). Myocardial contraction band necrosis is the pathognomonic lesion of myocardial catecholamine damage linked with peroxidation (Fineschi et al. 2010). Other investigations revealed intensely increased expression of β_1-adrenergic receptors in subendocardial as well as deeper layers of the cardiac musculature. At the same time, areas of myocardial damage and cellular apoptosis (TUNEL assay) were found (D'Errico et al. 2011). Other authors describe lymphocytic infiltrates, macrophages, contraction band necrosis, as well as endocardial myoelastofibrosis, smaller myocardial infarctions, hypereosinophilia, and myocardial fibrosis (Angelini 2016; Indorato and Bartolini 2016; Kammal et al. 2015).

Toxic Cardiomyopathies

Numerous toxins are essentially capable of causing cardiomyopathies, including drugs, poisons, and narcotic drugs, such as cocaine (see Chap. 5) or amphetamines (Karch 2011). Cobalt-beer cardiomyopathy became known after cobalt chloride started being added to beer.

13.6 Coronary Anomalies

Anomalies of the coronary arteries that have been classified and studied at autopsy and by clinical angiography can be divided into minor and major forms (Lipsett et al. 1994; Pedal and Teufel 1993; Taylor et al. 1992; Roberts 1986; Pedal 1976; Alexander and Griffith 1956). Descriptions of the various forms cover a wide range of entirely asymptomatic courses up to cases with sudden cardiac death. The incidence of the entire group of coronary anomalies is 0.036–6.5% (Thierauf et al. 2007; Yamanaka and Hobbs 1990). The most common anomaly is an aberrant course of the circumflex artery with an incidence of 0.16–0.35% (Barriales et al. 2001). The most common anomalous origin is the aberrant origin of the circumflex artery (Cx) from the right aortic sinus (RSV) with normal origin of the left anterior descending branch (LAD) (Cohle et al. 1986). Unexpected stimulation can work as a trigger of sudden cardiac death in the presence of a coronary abnormality (Kurosu et al. 2016).

A single coronary artery is rare in hearts without other congenital malformations (McConnell and Collins 1998). In about 0.4% of adults undergoing angiography, single coronary arteries are present (Thierauf et al. 2007). Clinical symptoms occur in 11–41% of patients with coronary anomalies (Eber et al. 1991). Angina pectoris, myocardial infarction, cardiac dysrhythmia, and acute cardiac death have all been reported as possible manifestations of coronary anomalies (Joswig et al. 1978). Major coronary anomalies often result in cardiac dysfunction and may cause cardiac failure and death. Minor anomalies tend to have no pathophysiological significance and include alterations in the number and location of coronary ostia. The anomalous origin of the left main coronary artery can be divided into four subtypes: intertruncal course, anterior free wall course before the right ventricular outflow, posterior course with the left coronary artery or one of the great branches passing behind the aorta, and an intertruncal–septal course through the crista supraventricularis (Aoki et al. 1999; Roberts and Shirami 1992).

In the case of insufficient perfusion of areas of the myocardium as a result of a coronary anomaly, there will often be areas of fibrosis of varying sizes replacing the myocardium, a finding highlighted by a Masson's trichrome stain. Surrounding myocytes exhibit hypertrophic changes with large hyperchromatic nuclei. At times, several foci of dystrophic calcifications with fibrosis may be noted, and often intimal proliferations of intramyocardial vessels are evident (McConnell and Collins 1998). Additionally, sections of the cerebrum can reveal neuronal subacute hypoxic changes, and siderophages can be found within pulmonary alveoli.

There are rare cases where the right coronary artery departs from a Valsalva sinus aneurysm (Albalooshi et al. 2008) or cases with an initial anomaly of this artery with Roemheld syndrome (Hagemeier and Madea 2009). Radiological examinations are helpful to detect various forms of coronary anomaly (McConnell et al. 1995), including hypoplastic coronary arteries (McConnell and Collins 1998; Zugibe et al. 1993). The forensic literature contains various descriptions of coronary anomalies which lead to death (Hagemeier and Madea 2009; Albalooshi et al. 2008; Iino et al. 2007; Madea and Dettmeyer 1998); when young athletes die suddenly, a coronary anomaly should be considered (Tsung et al. 1982). Myocardial ischemia is also described in connection with abnormal continuous forms between the aorta and the departure of the pulmonary trunk (Roynard et al. 1994). In cases of abnormal origin of the left coronary artery (LCA) from the right sinus, the clinical significance is determined by the course of the artery. Cases of sudden death, especially in young people during exercise, are mainly reported in connection with an intertruncal course of the artery (Madea and Dettmeyer 1998; Janssen 1975). There have been individual cases which reported the presence of multiple coronary anomalies together with a borderline hypertrophic cardiomyopathy (Dermengiu et al. 2010a).

The following is valid in histological evaluation: Myocardial samples must be removed from the outer range of the supply areas of the coronary arteries. Confluent coronary insufficiency scars can be observed even macroscopically. Older collagen scar tissue can be seen which replaces the preexisting myocardium on the one hand, while partially fresh myocardial necrosis is detectable in an acute or subacute course on the other; this is partially a sign of organizing myocardial necrosis with alternating dense collagen connective tissue, macrophages, lymphocytes, fibrocytes, fibroblasts, and branched capillary blood vessels in the form of granulation tissue.

Myocardial Bridging

Myocardial bridging is a common coronary anomaly characterized by the presence of a muscle bridge above an epicardial artery (Srettabunjong 2016; Sunnassee et al. 2011; Weiler and Risse 1994; Ferreira et al. 1991). According to the literature, interstitial fibrosis (Brodsky et al. 2008), interstitial edema, and hypoxia-induced changes, particularly inside the left ventricular front wall (Dermengiu et al. 2010b), are often found in myocardial bridging (Riße and Weiler 1985). Individual studies report myocardial infarction in connection with myocardial bridging (Baldassarre et al. 1996; Bestetti et al. 1987; Bezerra et al. 1987). Nevertheless, controversy exists over whether myocardial bridging can actually cause sudden cardiac death (Biggs et al. 2008; Möhlenkamp et al. 2002).

13.7 Cardiac Conduction System (CCS)

When the cause of death remains unclear, and in those cases where the cause of death cannot be explained even after the case history and autopsy findings have been examined, one should also consider lesions of the cardiac conduction system, particularly of the sinoatrial node (Ogbuihi 1989; Doerr 1980; Smith and Davis 1997). However, up to now histological examinations of the cardiac conduction system are carried out too rarely in cases of sudden cardiac death caused by conduction disturbances (Zack and Wegener 1994). This is also valid for cases which do not demonstrate relevant microscopic myocardial or coronary findings. In this case, samples should be taken from various areas of the heart, which may lead to pathologic findings, as has been frequently the case. In addition, while histological examination of the cardiac conduction system is useful, the findings require interpretation (Suarez-Mier and Aguilera 1998; Suarez-Mier et al. 1995) and are sometimes regarded as inconclusive (Pedersen 1980). Cystic tumors of the atrioventricular nodal region are a rare cause of sudden death (Patel and Sheppard 2011).

13.7.1 Examining the CCS

Earlier studies suggested methods to examine the cardiac conduction system, many of which required differentiated tissue work-up with between hundreds and thousands of tissue sections per case (Bharati and Lev 1995; Song et al. 1991; Okada and Kawai 1983; Hudson 1963; Lenègre and Chevalier 1951). Currently, there are suggestions for a modified and simplified method to examine the conduction system (Michaud et al. 2002; Sigrist and Germann 1998; Song et al. 1997; Charlton and Williams 1990; Chandrasiri 1985). Song et al. (1997, 1991) described a revised technique in which the sinoatrial node, the AV node, the distal part of the His bundle, and the bundle branches of the CCS are demonstrated in longitudinal sections by cutting between four and five blocks. This method reduces workload and can make examination of the CCS a routine procedure to some extent.

Sigrist and Germann (1998) described a further possible dissection approach:

1. Firstly, the coronary arteries are dissected, including the sinoatrial node and AV node arteries (Haas' artery).
2. Secondly, the coronary ventricles are opened either by cutting with scissors alongside the blood flow or by cutting with a knife vertically to the heart axis. The upper third of the interventricular septum must not be damaged.
3. Thirdly, starting at the left ventricular chamber, one can easily observe the membranous portion. Four radical incisions with the scalpel are made in this region:
   (a) Firstly, through the attachment of the frontal valvula mitralis at the septum interventriculare
   (b) Secondly, parallel to the first incision, approximately 1.5 cm before the membranous part
   (c) Thirdly, 1 cm above the membranous portion vertically through the vestibule septum
   (d) Fourthly, parallel to the third incision 2 cm below the membranous portion

With these four incisions, a tissue sample almost rectangular in shape has been removed which may be sliced into 2–3-mm-thick slices after formaldehyde fixation. These tissue slices can be used to prepare tissue sections suitable for histological examination. Occasionally, the cross section of the His bundle can be recognized as a light brown point structure inside the membranous portion. Other investigators have described a similar examination technique, in particular Michaud et al. (2002), Davies et al. (1975), and Hudson (1963).

13.7.2 Histopathologic Findings in the CCS

Histopathological changes such as a fibromuscular dysplasia (James and Marshall 1976), modular wall thickening, or thrombosis of the sinoatrial node artery are described in numerous publications (Zack et al. 2011). However, for some of these findings, there are no systematic investigations into their frequency or their relevance in terms of the cause of death. Some of the histological changes in the cardiac conduction system evidently occur more frequently than previously assumed and cannot necessarily be considered as pathological findings. For example, it was found that fibromuscular proliferation of the AV node artery is also seen relatively frequently in individuals free of cardiac disease (Zack et al. 2016). Fat cell nests, moderate lumen-narrowing proliferations in the wall of the sinus node artery, and discrete inflammatory infiltrates in the sinus node or surrounding area are found more commonly in individuals that died of a nonnatural cause of death (Zack et al. 2016). Therefore, findings of this type should at most—if at all—only be considered in the diagnosis of cause of death once other causes of death have been ruled out. In this context, any coincidence of arrhythmogenic or cardiotoxic drugs and histopathological findings in the cardiac conduction system should prompt consideration of a cumulative cause of death, for instance, in pronounced lipomatosis of the atrioventricular node and simultaneous sertindole and pipamperone use (Zack et al. 2014a). Traumatic damage is possible in addition to degenerative changes and inflammatory infiltrates. Local fibrosis with degeneration of the specific musculature is also reported (Ogbuihi 1989). This fibrosis may explain sick sinus syndrome. However, previous studies have not proven that there is increased fibrosis of the sinoatrial node with increasing age (Hudson 1960; Doerr 1959), nor which degree of fibrosis can be regarded as a pathological finding at all (Song et al. 1999). However, examination of the conduction system in 150 Finnish subjects led to the result that an increase in fibrosis and adiposis of the cardiac conduction system (CCS) could be observed with increasing age (Song et al. 2001). In about half of the subjects examined, there were calcium deposits in the central fibrous body, membranous portion, and the top of the musculature in the interventricular septum. In seven cases, the AV node, His bundle, or bundle branches (right bundle branch, left bundle branch) were compressed by the calcium deposits. Hemorrhage, inflammation, amyloidosis, tumor, fatty infiltration, and development malformations were observed in 31 cases. Although 28 cases died of myocardial infarction, no involvement of the CCS was observed in these subjects (Song et al. 2001).

Arteriosclerotic changes, especially those of the sinoatrial node artery, can certainly lead to even fatal cardiac arrhythmia (Lev et al. 1970), including surgical and other trauma to the region of the conduction system (Cohle and Lie 1998; Titus et al. 1963). There is one case of elective fatty degeneration of the specific heart muscle cells in connection with digitoxin intoxication described in the literature (Doerr 1969).

Histological findings on the CCS after acute hypoxia such as perinuclear vacuoles and cavities next to the cell nuclei with fish bone-like deformation have been known for a long time. These findings include "tubular myopathy" with tube-shaped cavity formation and peripheral displacement of the cytoplasm, whereby the cross-sectional fibers retain a ring-like appearance (Büchner 1975; Pichotka 1942). These findings could also be proven at autopsy. A loss of specific heart muscle fibers is the result of chronic lack of oxygen (Sigrist and Germann 1998).

Pathologic changes in the cardiac conduction system may already be found intrauterine. Piercecchi-Marti et al. (2003) provide the description of a fetus in the 29th gestational week with histologically proven alterations of the AV node and the His bundle with fibrosis, calcification, endocardial fibroelastosis, and mononuclear inflammatory infiltration. Embolism caused by adiposis of the CCS is also described (Schwartz et al. 1988).

A correlation between histopathological changes and clinically diagnosed cardiac arrhythmias should be considered first, including fatal arrhythmias (Lev et al. 1979; Doerr 1975). Nevertheless, in individual cases, histopathologic findings in relation to their importance in terms of the time of death are often difficult to interpret, and other causes of death must be excluded first (Nishida et al. 2002; Zack and Wegener 1994; Ogbuihi 1989; Voigt 1976).

Sinus Node Fibrosis

In addition to histopathological lesions in the region of the AV node and bundle of His, findings made in the sinus node could explain death, assuming other causes have been excluded. Sinus node fibrosis is of particular relevance in this regard. As part of this process, the specific muscle fibers may be largely destroyed (Zack et al. 1996; Ogbuihi 1989). Individual fat cell nests have been reported, as have occasional lymphocytic infiltrates (Knieriem et al. 1979) (Fig. 13.31).

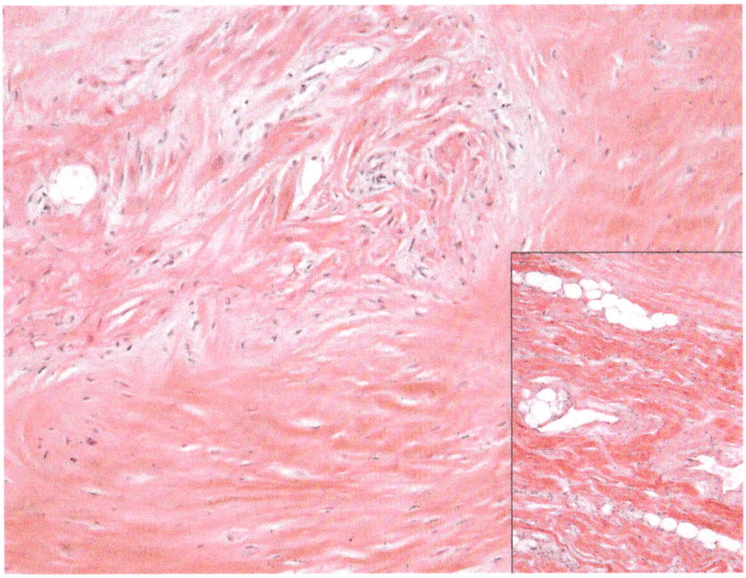

Fig. 13.31 Largely fibrosed sinus node region with peripheral fibrosis, scant lymphocytic infiltration, and tiny individual fat cell nests (H&E ×100)

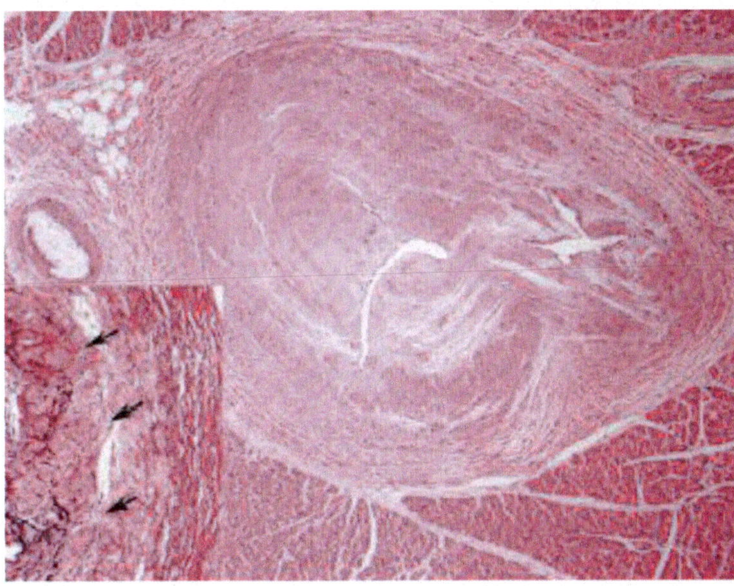

Fig. 13.32 AV node artery (AVNA) of the heart with strong thickening of the arterial wall, narrowing of the lumen (H&E ×100), and destruction of the internal elastic lamina (*arrows*; Elastica van Gieson ×400)

Fibromuscular Dysplasia

Intramyocardial small vessel anomalies are not commonly recognized. Small vessel disease has been reported as an isolated cardiac anomaly in individuals with sudden death. The best known anomaly is fibromuscular dysplasia (Fig. 13.32), involving the sinoatrial or AV nodal artery. Histological findings include prominent vascular dilatation, interstitial edema, and marked vascular narrowing of intramyocardial arterioles due to fibromuscular dysplasia. The vessel presents a thick media which is disorganized, causing narrowing of the vessel (Veinot et al. 2002).

Finally, in the case of sudden death with no histomorphological correlation to a plausible cause of death, rare genetic defects should be considered (e.g., ion channel defects). In order to clarify these defects, molecular genetic investigations are necessary (Michaud et al. 2011; Kauferstein et al. 2009). Doubts about the pathophysiological significance of fibromuscular dysplasia have been expressed, since this entity is not infrequently an incidental finding in the context of thorough investigations (Zack et al. 2014b, 2016). Evidently, the vessel lumen stenosis associated with fibromuscular dysplasia does not necessarily cause acute ischemia under strain; one assumes sufficient formation of collateral vessels. In the case of negative histopathological findings and assumed sudden cardiac death, molecular genetic testing is able to determine cardiac ion channel defects as the cause of death in some cases (Kauferstein et al. 2013; Campuzano et al. 2014).

References

Abbate A, Sinagra G, Bussani R, Hoke NN, Merlo M, Varma A, Toldo S, Salloum FN, Biondi-Zoccai GG, Vetrovec GW, Crea F, Silvestri F, Baldi A (2009) Apoptosis in patients with acute myocarditis. Am J Cardiol 104:995–1000

Adams JE, Bodor GS, Dávila-Román VG et al (1993) Cardiac troponin I: a marker with high specificity for cardiac injury. Circulation 88:101–106

Akashi YJ, Goldstein DS, Barbaro G, Ueyama T (2008) Takotsubo cardiomyopathy. A new form of acute, reversible heart failure. Circulation 118:2754–2762

Albalooshi Y, Hagemeier L, Doberentz E et al (2008) Abgang der rechten Herzkranzarterie aus einem Aneurysma des Sinus Valsalvae. Rechtsmedizin 18:437–440

Alexander RW, Griffith GC (1956) Anomalies of the coronary arteries and their clinical significance. Circulation 14:800–805

Al-Rufaie HK, Elorio RA, Olsen EGJ (1983) Comparison of the haematoxylin basic fuchsin picric acid method and the fluorescence of haematoxylin and eosin stained sections for the identification of early myocardial infarction. J Clin Pathol 36:646–649

Althoff H (1983) Zur morphologie des akuten koronartodes jüngerer frauen. Z Rechtsmed 91:85–99

Amberg R (1995) Immunmorphologische Reaktionsmuster des Myokard bei kardialen und nicht-kardialen Perfusionsstörungen. In: Bratzke H, Schröter A (eds) Immunhistochemie in der Rechtsmedizin. Hänsel-Hohenhausen, Egelsbach, pp 101–116

Andrews RE, Fenton MJ, Ridout DA, Burch M (2008) British congenital cardiac association. New onset heart failure due to heart muscle disease in childhood: a prospective study in the United Kingdom and Ireland. Circulation 117:79–84

Angelini A, Thiene G, Boffa GM et al (1993) Endomyocardial biopsy in right ventricular cardiomyopathy. Int J Cardiol 40:273–282

Angelini A, Basso C, Nava A, Thiene G (1996) Endomyocardial biopsy in arrhythmogenic right ventricular cardiomyopathy. Am Heart J 132:203–206

Angelini P (2016) Do pathologists agree on how to diagnose takotsubo cardiomyopathy? Forensic Sci Med Pathol 12:226

Aoki Y, Nata M, Hashiyada M, Sagisaka K (1996) Sudden unexpected death in childhood due to eosinophilic myocarditis. Int J Legal Med 108:221–224

Aoki Y, Saigusa K, Nakayama Y (1999) Sudden infant death with anomalous origin of the left coronary artery from the pulmonary artery. Legal Med 1:250–253

Aretz HT (1987) Myocarditis: the Dallas criteria. Hum Pathol 18:619–624

Aretz HT, Billingham ME, Edwards W, Factor SM, Falllon JT, Fenoglio JJ et al (1987) Myocarditis: a histopathologic definition and classification. Am J Cardiovasc Pathol 1:5–14

Arnold G, Kaiser C, Fischer R (1985) Myofibrilläre degeneration – a common type of myocardial lesion and its selective identification by a modified Luxol fast blue stain. Pathol Res Pract 180:405–415

Arola A, Jokinen E, Ruuskanen O, Saraste M, Pesonen E, Kuusela AL, Tikanojja T, Paavilainen T, Simell O (1997) Epidemiology of idiopathic cardiomyopathies in children and adolescents. A nationwide study in Finland. Am J Epidemiol 146:385–393

Arola A, Kallajoki M, Ruuskanen O, Hyypia T (1998) Detection of enteroviral RNA in end-stage dilated cardiomyopathy in children and adolescents. J Med Virol 56:364–371

Azzawi M, Hasleton PS, Kann SW, Hillier VF, Quigley A, Hutchinson IV (1997) Distribution of myocardial macrophages in the normal human heart. J Anat 191:417–423

Baasner A, Dettmeyer R, Graebe M, Madea B (2003a) PCR-based diagnosis of enterovirus and parvovirus B19 in paraffin-embedded heart tissue. In: Brinkmann B, Carracedo A (Hrsg.) Progress in Forensic Genetics 9, 19th International ISFG Congress, 28.08–01.09.2001, Münster, Germany; International Congress Series 1239, p. 715–717

Baasner A, Dettmeyer R, Graebe M, Rissland J, Madea B (2003b) PCR-based diagnosis of Enterovirus and Parvovirus B19 in paraffin embedded heart tissue of children with suspected sudden infant death syndrome. Lab Investig 83:1451–1455

Badir B, Knight B (1987) Fluorescence microscopy in the detection of early myocardial infarction. Forensic Sci Int 34:99–102

Badorff C, Lee GH, Lamphear BJ, Martone ME, Campbell KP, Rhoads RE, Knowlton KU (1999) Enteroviral protease 2A cleaves dystrophin: evidence of cytoskeletal disruption in an acquired cardiomyopathy. Nat Med 5:320–326

Badorff C, Berkeley N, Mehrotrar S, Talhouk JW, Rhoads RE, Knowlton KU (2000a) Enteroviral protease 2A directly cleaves dystrophin and is inhibited by a dystrophin-based analogue. J Biol Chem 275:1191–1197

Badorff C, Lee GH, Knowlton KU (2000b) Enteroviral cardiomyopathy: bad news for the dystrophin-glycoprotein-complex. Herz 25:227–232

Bagwan IN, Hooper LVB, Sheppard MN (2011) Cardiac sarcoidosis and sudden death. The heart may look normal or mimic other cardiomyopathies. Virchows Arch 458:671–678

Baldassarre S, Unger P, Renard M (1996) Acute myocardial infarction and myocardial bridging: a case report. Acta Cardiol 51:461–465

Baroldi G, Mittleman RE, Parolini M, Silver MD, Fineschi V (2001) Myocardial contraction bands. Definition, quantification and significance in forensic pathology. Int J Legal Med 115:142–151

Barriales R, Moris C, Lopz Muniz A, Hernandez LC, San Roman L, Barriales Alvarez V, Testa A, de la Hara J, Sammartin JC, Cortina A (2001) Anomalías congénitas de las arterias coronarias del adulto descritas en 31 años de estudios coronariográficos en el Principado de Asturias: principales características angiográficas y clínicas. Rev Esp Cardiol 54:269–281

Basso C, Thiene G (2005) Adipositas cordis, fatty infiltration of the right ventricle, and arrhythmogenic right ventricular cardiomyopathy. Just a matter of fat? Cardiovasc Pathol 14:37–41

Basso C, Burke M, Fornes P, Gallagher PJ, Henriques de Gouveia R, Sheppard M, Thiene G, van der Wal A (2008a) Guidelines for autopsy investigation of sudden cardiac death. Virchows Arch 452:11–18

Basso C, Ronco F, Marcus F et al (2008b) Quantitative assessment of endomyocardial biopsy in arrhythmogenic right ventricular cardiomyopathy/dysplasia: an in vitro validation of diagnostic criteria. Eur Heart J 29:2760–2771

Basso C, Corrado D, Marcus F et al (2009) Arrhythmogenic right ventricle cardiomyopathy. Lancet 373:1289–1300

Ben m'rad M, Leclerc-Mercier S, Blanche P, Franck N, Rozenberg F, Fulla Y, Guesmi M, Rollot F, Dehoux M, Guillevin L, Moachon L (2009) Drug-induced hypersensitivity syndrome: clinical and biologic disease patterns in 24 patients. Medicine 88:131–140

Bendig JWA, O'Brien PS, Muir P, Porter HJ, Caul EO (2001) Enterovirus sequences resembling coxsackievirus A2 detected in stool and spleen from a girl with fatal myocarditis. J Med Virol 64:482–486

Bergelson JM, Cunningham JA, Droguett G, Kurt-Jones EA, Krithivas A, Hong JS et al (1997) Isolation of a common receptor for coxsackie B viruses and adenoviruses 2 and 5. Science 275:1320–1323

Bernstein M, Konzelman FW, Sidlick DM (1929) Boeck's sarcoid: a report of a case with visceral involvement. Arch Intern Med 4:721–734

Bestetti RB, Finzi LA, Amaral FTV (1987) Myocardial bridging of coronary arteries associated with an impending acute myocardial infarction. Clin Cardiol 10:129–131

Bezerra AJC, Prates JC, DiDio LJA (1987) Incidence and clinical significance of bridges of myocardium over the coronary arteries and their branches. Surg Radiol Anat 9:273–280

Bharati S, Lev M (1995) Cardiac conduction system involvement in sudden death of obese young people. Am Heart J 129:273–281

Biggs MJ, Swift B, Sheppard MN (2008) Myocardial bridging: is it really a cause of sudden cardiac death? In: Tsokos M (ed) Forensic pathology reviews, vol 5. Humana, Totawa, pp 115–127

Binz G, Knirsch W, Lewin MA, Haas NA, Koch W, Kandolf R, Uhlemann F (2003) Isolated myocardial noncompaction in childhood – case report and review of the literature. Z Kardiol 92:1039–1044

Blauwet LA, Cooper LT (2010) Myocarditis. Prog Cardiovasc Dis 52:274–288

Bleyl SB, Mumford BR, Brown-Harrison MC, Pagotto LT, Carey JC, Pysher TJ, Ward K, Chin TK (1997a) Xq28-linked noncompaction of the left ventricular myocardium: prenatal diagnosis and pathologic analysis of affected individuals. Am J Med Genet 72:257–265

Bleyl SB, Mumford BR, Thompson V, Carey JC, Pysher JT, Chin TK, Ward K (1997b) Neonatal, lethal noncompaction of the left ventricular myocardium is allelic with Barth syndrome. Am J Hum Genet 61:868–872

Bock CT, Klingel K, Aberle S, Duechting A, Lupescu A, Lang F, Kandolf R (2005) Human parvovirus B19: a new emerging pathogen of inflammatory cardiomyopathy. J Vet Med B Infect Dis Vet Public Health 52:340–343

Bock CT, Klingel K, Kandolf R (2010) Human parvovirus B19-associated myocarditis. N Engl J Med 362:1248–1249

Bouchardy B, Majno G (1974) Histopathology of early myocardial infarcts. A new approach. Am J Pathol 74:301–330

Bowles NE, Richardson PJ, Olsen EGJ, Archard LC (1986) Detection of coxsackie-B-virus-specific RNA sequences in myocardial biopsy samples from patients with myocarditis and dilated cardiomyopathy. Lancet 17:1120–1122

Bowles NE, Rose ML, Taylor P, Banner NR, Morgan-Capner P, Cunningham L et al (1989) End-stage dilated cardiomyopathy. Persistence of enterovirus RNA in myocardium at cardiac transplantation and lack of immune response. Circulation 80:1128–1136

Bowles NE, Ni J, Marcus F, Towbin JA (2002) The detection of cardiotropic viruses in the myocardium of patients with arrhythmogenic right ventricu-

lar dysplasia/cardiomyopathy. J Am Coll Cardiol 39:892–895
Braun R, Hassler D, Kimmig P (2002) Myokarditis durch Enteroviren in Griechenland – und bei uns? Dtsch Med Wochenschr 127:1364
Brinkmann B, Sepulchre MA, Fechner G (1993) The application of selected histochemical and immunohistochemical markers and procedures to the diagnosis of early myocardial damage. Int J Legal Med 106:135–141
Brodsky SV, Roh L, Ashar K, Braun A, Ramaswamy G (2008) Myocardial bridging of coronary arteries: a risk factor for myocardial fibrosis? Int J Cardiol 124:391–392
Bryant RM (1999) Hypertrophic cardiomyopathy in children. Cardiol Rev 7:92–100
Büchner F (1975) Strukturveränderungen durch allgemeinen Sauerstoffmangel, insbesondere bei der Höhenkrankheit. In: Grundmann E (ed) Hypoxie. Springer, Berlin
Büchner F, Onishi S (1968) Der Herzmuskel bei akuter Coronarinsuffizienz im elektronenmikroskopischen Bild. Urban & Schwarzenberg, München
Bulloch RT, Pearce MB, Murphy ML, Jenkins BJ, Davis JL (1972) Myocardial lesions in idiopathic and alcoholic cardiomyopathy. Study by ventricular septal biopsy. Am J Cardiol 29:15
Bültmann BD, Klingel K, Sotlar K, Bock CT, Baba HA, Sauter M, Kandolf R (2003a) Fatal parvovirus B19-associated myocarditis clinically mimicking ischemic heart disease: an endothelial cell-mediated disease. Hum Pathol 34:92–95
Bültmann BD, Klingel K, Sotlar K, Bock CT, Kandolf R (2003b) Parvovirus B19: a pathogen responsible for more than hematologic disorders. Virchows Arch 442:8–17
Burke AP, Saenger J, Mulick F, Virmani R (1991) Hypersensitivity myocarditis. Arch Pathol Lab Med 115:764–769
Burke A, Mont E, Kutys R, Virmani R (2005) Left ventricular noncompaction: a pathological study of 14 cases. Hum Pathol 36:403–411
Buschmann C, Stenzel W, Martin H, Heppner FL, Guddat SS, Tsokos M (2013) Calcified myocardial necrosis in pediatric patients after cardiopulmonary resuscitation. Forensic Sci Med Pathol 9:543–550
Buschmann C, Schäfer HJ, Püschel K, Schulz F (2006) Innate heart deformation as a cause of sudden death in a 7-year-old girl. Rechtsmedizin 16:64–68
Bux R, Bratzke H, Rothschild MA, Lutz FU (2002) Plötzlicher Tod einer 12-Jährigen mit klinisch inapparenter Myokarditis unter psychischer und physischer Belastung. Rechtsmedizin 12:229–232
Byard RW (2002) Unexpected death due to infectious mononucleosis. J Forensic Sci 47:202–204
Byard RW, Manton N, Tsokos M (2008) Sarcoidosis and mechanism of unexpected death. J Forensic Sci 53:460–464
Bybee KA, Prasad A (2008) Stress-related cardiomyopathy syndromes. Circulation 118:397–409
Campuzano O, Allegue C, Partemi S, Iglesias A, Oliva A, Brugada R (2014) Negative autopsy and sudden cardiac death. Int J Legal Med 128:599–606
Carle BN (1981) Autofluorescence in the identification of myocardial infarcts. Hum Pathol 12:643–646
Casali MB, Lazzaro A, Gentile G, Blandino A, Ronchi E, Zoja R (2012) Forensic grading of myocarditis: an experimental contribution to the distinction between lethal myocarditis and incidental myocarditis. Forensic Sci Int 223:78–86
Casscells W, Kimura H, Sanchez J, Yu Z, Ferrans VJ (1990) Immunohistochemical study of fibronectin in experimental myocardial infarction. Am J Pathol 137:801–810
Cassinotti P, Weitz M, Siegl G (1993) Human parvovirus B 19 infections: routine diagnosis by a new nested polymerase chain reaction assay. J Med Virol 40:228–234
Cassling RS, Linder J, Sears TD, Waller BF, Rogler WC, Wilson JE, Kugler JD, Kay DH, Dillon JC, Slack JD et al (1985) Quantitative evaluation of inflammation in biopsy specimen from idiopathically failing or irritable hearts: experience in 80 pediatric and adult patients. Am Heart J 110:713–720
Cavanaugh J, Prahlow JA (2013) Sudden cardiac death due to arrythmogenic right ventricular cardiomyopathy and cystic tumor of the AV node. Forensic Sci Med Pathol 9:407–412
Cebelin MS, Hirsch CS (1980) Human stress cardiomyopathy. Myocardial lesions in victims of homicidal assaults without internal injuries. Hum Pathol 11:123–132
Cecchi R, Bajanowski T, Kahl B, Wiegand P (1995) CMV-DNA detection in parenchymatous organs in cases of SIDS. Int J Legal Med 107:291–295
Chandrasiri N (1985) Histopathological re-study of the human cardiac conduction system. Med Sci Law 25:29–43
Charlton I, Williams R (1990) Cardiac conducting tissue: a simplified technique for examination of the SA and AV nodes. Am J Forensic Med Pathol 11:213–218
Chen X, Zhang Y (2006) Myocardial Cx43 expression in the cases of sudden death due to dilated cardiomyopathy. Forensic Sci Int 162:170–173
Chia JKS, Jackson B (1996) Myopericarditis due to parvovirus B19 in an adult. Clin Infect Dis 23:200–201
Chin TK, Perloff JK, Vuillemin M, Thompson RP, Anderson RH (1990) Isolated noncompaction of left ventricular myocardium. A study of eight cases. Circulation 82:507–513
Chow LH, Ye Y, Linder J, McManus BM (1989) Phenotypic analysis of infiltrating cells in human myocarditis. Arch Pathol Lab Med 113:1357–1362
Chrysohoou C, Tsiamis E, Brili S, Barbetseas J, Stefanadis C (2009) Acute myocarditis from coxsackie infection, mimicking subendocardial ischaemia. Hell J Cardiol 50:147–150
Chumachenko PV, Vikkert AM (1991) Immunomorphologic diagnosis of early myocardial

necrosis using monoclonal antibodies to desmin and vimentin. Arkh Patol 53:16–19
Cohle SD, Lie JT (1998) Histopathologic spectrum of the cardiac tissue in traumatic and noncardiac sudden death patients under 30 years of age: an analysis of 100 cases. Anat Pathol 3:53–76
Cohle SD, Graham MA, Pounder DJ (1986) Nonatherosclerotic sudden coronary death. Pathol Annu 21:217–249
Cremer U, Althoff H (1991) Nachweis und Inzidenz von Zytomegalievirusinfektionen bei plötzlichen Kindstodesfällen (SIDS). Rechtsmedizin 1:25–28
Curca GC, Dermengiu D, Ceausu M, Francisc A, Rusu MC, Hostiuc S (2011) Cardiac lesions associated with cardiopulmonary resuscitation. Rom J Legal Med 19:1–6
D'Ambrosio A, Patti G, Manzoli A, Sinagra G, Di Lenarda A, Silvestri F, Di Sciascio G (2001) The fate of acute myocarditis between spontaneous improvement and evolution to dilated cardiomyopathy: a review. Heart 85:499–504
Daar AS, Fuggle SV, Fabre JW, Ting A, Morris J (1984a) The detailed distribution of HLA-A, B, C antigens in normal human organs. Transplantation 38:287–292
Daar AS, Fuggle SV, Fabre JW, Ting A, Morris PJ (1984b) The detailed distribution of MHC class II antigens in normal human organs. Transplantation 38:293–298
Dada MA, Lazarus NG, Kharsany ABM, Sturm AW (2000) Sudden death caused by myocardial tuberculosis. Am J Forensic Med Pathol 21:385–388
Dalal P, Fujisic K, Hupart P, Schweizer P (1994) Arrhythmogenic right ventricular dysplasia: a review. Cardiology 85:361–369
Davies JM, Pomerance A, Lamb D (1975) Techniques in examination and anatomy of the heart. In: Pomerance A, Davies MJ (eds) The pathology of the heart. Blackwell, Oxford
de Lourdes Higuchi M, Guitierrez PS, Demarchi Aiello V, Palomino S, Bocchi E, Kalil J, Bellotti G, Pileggi F (1993) Immunohistochemical characterization of infiltrating cells in human chronic Chagas myocarditis: comparison with myocardial rejection process. Virch Arch A Pathol Anat 423:157–160
D'Errico S, Neri M, Nieddu A, Mazzeo E, Riezzo I, Turillazi E, Fineschi V (2011) Cardiac $ß_1$-adrenoceptor expression in two stress-induced cardiomyopathy-related deaths. Forensic Sci Int 207:e8-e11
Dermengiu D, Ceausu M, Rusu MC, Dermengiu S, Curca GC, Hostiuc S (2010a) Sudden death with borderline hypertrophic cardiomyopathy and multiple coronary anomalies. Case report and literature review. Rom J Legal Med 18:3–12
Dermengiu D, Vovolis I, Hostiuc S, Curca GC, Rusu MC, Luca L (2010b) Morphological features in myocardial bridging. Rom J Legal Med 18:163–170
Dermengiu D, Curcă GC, Sărbu N, Hostiuc S, Ceauşu M (2010c) Sudden cardiac death in non-atherosclerotic and non-inflammatory intimal cellular proliferations. A case report. Rom J Legal Med 18:183–188
Dettmeyer R, Kandolf R (2009) Cardiomyopathies – misdiagnosed as sudden infant death syndrome (SIDS). Forensic Sci Int 194:e21–e24
Dettmeyer R, Madea B (2002) Myokarditis durch Enteroviren in Griechenland – und bei uns? Leserbrief zum Beitrag aus Dtsch Med Wochenschr 127:1364 (2002). Dtsch Med Wochenschr 27:2467–2468
Dettmeyer R, Madea B (2003) Commentary to the letter of Arya SC and Agarval N to our report "Fatal parvovirus B19 myocarditis in an 8-year-old boy", J Forensic Sci 2003; 48:183–186 – authors response. J Forensic Sci 48:1205
Dettmeyer R, Madea B (2004) Sudden, unexpected death related to viral myocarditis. A survey of histological, immunohistochemical, and molecular pathological methods for the postmortem diagnosis. In: Tsokos M (ed) Forensic pathology reviews, vol 2. Humana Press, Totowa, pp 169–186
Dettmeyer R, Haag C, Madea B (2002a) Leserbrief zum Beitrag "Plötzlicher Tod einer 12-jährigen mit klinisch inapparenter Myokarditis unter psychischer und physischer Belastung". Rechtsmedizin 12:229–232 (2002). Rechtsmedizin 12:395–396
Dettmeyer R, Reith K, Madea B (2002b) Alcoholic cardiomyopathy versus chronic myocarditis – immunohistological investigations with LCA, CD3, CD68 and tenascin. Forensic Sci Int 126:57–62
Dettmeyer R, Kandolf R, Baasner A, Banaschak S, Eis-Hübinger AM, Madea B (2003) Fatal parvovirus B19 myocarditis in an 8-year-old boy. J Forensic Sci 48:183–186
Dettmeyer R, Padosch SA, Baasner A, Madea B (2004a) PCR-based diagnosis of adenovirus and Epstein-Barr virus in paraffin-embedded heart tissue. In: Doutremépuich C, Morling N (eds.) Progress in Forensic Genetics 10. Proceedings of the 20th International ISFG Congress, Arcachon, 9.-13. September 2003, France. Int Congr Ser 1261:605–607
Dettmeyer R, Schmidt P, Kandolf R, Madea B (2004b) Evolution of dilated cardiomyopathy (DCM) from idiopathic hypertrophic cardiomyopathy (IHCM) vs. inflammatory dilated cardiomyopathy (DCMi): a rare case of sudden death in an 8-year-old boy. Pathol Res Pract 200:411–415
Dettmeyer R, Stiel M, Madea B (2006a) Heat shock protein 60 (cHSP60) as a marker for chronic infection with Chlamydia pneumoniae in atherosclerosis – investigation of atherosclerotic coronary arteries by immunocytochemistry. Forensic Sci Med Pathol 2:173–178
Dettmeyer R, Strehler M, Winkelmann S, Madea B (2006b) Myokarditis. Rechtsmedizin 16:138–142
Dettmeyer R, Padosch SA, Madea B (2006c) Lethal enterovirus-induced myocarditis and pancreatitis in a 4-month-old boy. Forensic Sci Int 156:51–54
Dettmeyer R, Müller J, Poster S, Madea B (2006d) PCR-based diagnosis of cytomegaloviruses in paraffin-embedded heart tissue in cases of suspected sudden infant death syndrome (SIDS). In: Progress in Forensic Genetics11. Proceedings of the 21st international

ISFG congress, 13–16 Sept 2005, Portugal. Int Congr Ser 1288:771–773

DiMaio VJM, Dana SE (2007) Handbook of forensic pathology. CRC Taylor & Francis, Boca Raton

Doerr W (1959) Histopathologie des Reizbildungs- und Reizleitungssystems des Herzens. Verh Dtsch Ges Inn Med 65:459–495

Doerr W (1969) Normale und pathologische Anatomie des reizbildenden und erregungsleitenden Gewebes. Verh Dtsch Ges Herz Kreislaufforsch 35:1–36

Doerr W (1975) Morphologische Äquivalente bei Rhythmusstörungen des Herzens. Verh Dtsch Ges Inn Med 81:36–69

Doerr W (1980) Sekundenherztod. Beitr Gerichtl Med 39:1–25

Drescher JZP, Verhagen W, Flik J, Milbradt H (1987) Recent influenza virus A infections in forensic cases of sudden unexplained death. Arch Virol 92:63–76

Drory TY, Hiss Y (1991) Sudden unexpected death in persons less than 40 years of age. Am J Cardiol 68:1388–1392

Druyts-Voets E, van Renterghem L, Gerniers S (1993) Epidemiology. Coxsackie B virus epidemiology and neonatal infection in Belgium. J Infect 27:311–316

Eber B, Kilzer K, Luha O, Schumacher M, Fruhwald FM, Gasser R, Klein W (1991) Coronary artery anomalies in adulthood. Wien Med Wochenschr 141:406–411

Edston E, Perskvist N (2009) Histiocytoid cardiomyopathy and ventricular non-compaction in a case of sudden death in a female infant. Int J Legal Med 123:47–53

Edston E, Grontoft L, Johnsson J (2002) TUNEL: a useful screening method in sudden cardiac death. Int J Legal Med 116:22–26

Edwards WD, Holmes DR Jr, Reeder GS (1982) Diagnosis of active lymphocytic myocarditis by endomyocardial biopsy. Quantitative criteria for light microscopy. Mayo Clin Proc 57:419–425

Elliott P, Andersson B, Arbustini E, Bilinska Z, Cecchi F, Charron P, Dubourg O, Kühl U, Maisch B, McKenna WJ, Montserrat L, Pankuweit S, Rapezzi C, Seferovic P, Tavazzi L, Keren A (2008) Classification of the cardiomyopathies; a position statement from the European Society of Cardiology Working Group on myocardial and pericardial diseases. Eur Heart J 29:270–277

Enders G, Dotsch J, Bauer J et al (1998) Life-threatening parvovirus B19-associated myocarditis and cardiac transplantation as possible therapy: two case reports. Clin Infect Dis 26:355–358

Engberding S, Bender F (1984) Identification of a rare congenital anomaly of the myocardium by two dimensional echocardiography: persistence of isolated myocardial sinusoids. Am J Cardiol 53:1733–1734

Fairley CK, Ryan M, Wall PG, Weinberg J (1996) The organisms reported to cause infective myocarditis and pericarditis in England and Wales. J Infect 32:223–225

Fechner GG, Sivaloganathan S (1987) Demonstration of myocardial infarction in putrefying bodies. J Clin Pathol 40:922–929

Feldmann AM, McNamara D (2000) Myocarditis. N Engl J Med 343:1388–1398

Ferrans VJ, McAllister HA, Haese WH (1976) Infantile cardiomyopathy with histiocytoid change in cardiac muscle cells. Report of six patients. Circulation 53:708–719

Ferreira AG, Trotter SE, König B, Décourt LV, Fox K, Olsen EG (1991) Myocardial bridges: morphological and functional aspects. Br Heart J 66:364–367

Figulla HR (2004) Transformation of myocarditis and inflammatory cardiomyopathy to idiopathic dilated cardiomyopathy: facts and fiction. Med Microbiol Immunol 193:61–64

Fineschi V, Pomara C (2004) A forensic pathological approach to sudden cardiac death. In: Tsokos M (ed) Forensic pathology reviews, vol 5. Humana, Totawa, pp 139–168

Fineschi V, Neri M, Riezzo I, Turillazzi E (2004) Sudden cardiac death due to hypersensitivity myocarditis during clozapine treatment. Int J Legal Med 118:307–309

Fineschi V, Baroldi G, Silver MA (2006) Pathology of the heart and sudden death in forensic medicine. CRC Press, Boca Raton

Fineschi V, Michalodimitrakis M, D'Errico S, Neri M, Pomara C, Turillazzi E (2010) Insight into stress-induced cardiomyopathy and sudden cardiac death due to stress. A forensic cardio-pathologist point of view. Forensic Sci Int 194:1–8

Finsterer J (2008) Histiocytoid cardiomyopathy: a mitochondrial disorder. Clin Cardiol 31:225–227

Finsterer J, Stöllberger C (2009) Is mitochondrial disease the common cause of histocytoid cardiomyopathy and non-compaction? Int J Legal Med 123:507–508

Finsterer J, Stöllberger C, Karner J, Keller H, Feichtinger F (2007) Left ventricular hypertrabeculation (noncompaction) with prominent calcifications in a patient with mannose-binding lectin deficiency and unclassified myopathy. Cardiovasc Pathol 16:310–312

Fischbein MC, Kulber D, Stancl M, Edwalds G (1986) Distribution of fibrinogen and albumin in normal, ischaemic, and necrotic myocardium during the evolution of myocardial infarction: an immunohistochemical study. Cardiovasc Res 20:36–41

Fragkouli K, Mitselou A, Boumba V, Michalis L, Vougiouklakis T (2011) An autopsy case of necrotizing eosinophilic myocarditis causing left ventricular wall rupture. Forensic Sci Med Pathol 7:350–354

Fraser WJ, Haffejee Z, Cooper K (1995) Rheumatic Aschoff nodules revisited: an immunohistological reappraisal of the cellular component. Histopathology 27:457–461

Frenzel H, Schwartzkopff B, Reinecke P, Kamino K, Lösse B (1987) Evidence for muscle fiber hyperplasia in the septum of patients with hypertrophic obstructive cardiomyopathy (HOCM). Quantitative examination of endomyocardial biopsies (EMCB) and myectomy specimens. Z Kardiol 76(suppl 3):14–19

Friman G, Fohlman J (1993) The epidemiology of viral heart disease. Scand J Infect Dis 88(suppl):7–10

Friman G, Wesslen L, Fohlman J, Karjalainen J, Rolf C (1995) The epidemiology of infectious myocarditis, lymphocytic myocarditis and dilated cardiomyopathy. Eur Heart J 16(suppl O):36–41

Gaaloul I, Riabi S, Harrath R, Evans M, Huber S, Aouni M (2011) Coxsackie B3 myocarditis in a case of sudden unexpected death in young athlete: histopathological, immunohistochemical and molecularpathological for diagnosis. Forensic Sci Int 208:e10–e14

Gdynia G, Schnitzler P, Brunner E, Kandolf R, Bläker H, Daum E, Schnabel P, Schirmacher P, Roth W (2011) Sudden death of an immunocompetent young adult caused by novel (swine origin) influenza A/H1N1-associated myocarditis. Virchows Arch 458:371–376

Ginellinová A, Farkaš D, Farkašová Iannaccone S, Vyhnálkova V (2016) Sudden unexpected death due to severe pulmonary and cardiac sarcoidosis. Forensic Sci Med Pathol 12:319–323

Grady KL, Costanzo-Nordin MR (1989) Myocarditis: review of a clinical enigma. Heart Lung 18:347–354

Greve G, Rotevath S, Svendby K, Grong K (1990) Early morphologic changes in cat heart muscles cells after acute coronary artery occlusion. Am J Pathol 136:273–283

Hagemeier L, Madea B (2009) Ursprungsanomalie der rechten Koronararterie und Roemhild-Syndrom – Ursache eines plötzlichen Todes. Rechtsmedizin 19:30–33

Hagemeier L, Mohr C, Schyma C et al (2010) Diagnose der arrythmogenen rechtsventrikulären Kardiomyopathie. Histomorphometrisches Verfahren zum postmortalen Nachweis. Rechtsmedizin 20:13–18

Hamilton RA, Sullivan L, Wolf BC (2007) Sudden cardiac death due to giant cell inflammatory processes. J Forensic Sci 52:943–948

Handlos P, Gruszka T, Staňková M, Marecová K, Joukal M (2017) Biventricular noncompaction cardiomyopathy with malignant arrhythmia as a cause of sudden death. Forensic Sci Med Pathol 13. https://doi.org/10.1007/s12024-017-9889-y

Hansen PR (2007) Takotsubo cardiomyopathy: an underrecognized myocardial syndrome. Eur J Intern Med 18:561–565

Hansen SH, Rossen K (1999) Evaluation of cardiac troponin I immunoreaction in autopsy hearts: a possible marker of early myocardial infarction. Forensic Sci Int 99:189–196

Hauck AJ, Kearney DL, Edwards W (1989) Evaluation of postmortem endomyocardial biopsy specimens from 38 patients with lymphocytic myocarditis: implications for role of sampling error. Mayo Clin Proc 64:1235–1245

Hayes MA, Russell RG, Babiuk LA (1979) Sudden death in young dogs with myocarditis caused by parvovirus. J Am Vet Med Assoc 174:1197–1203

Hebert MM, Yu C, Towbin JA, Rogers BB (1995) Fatal Epstein-Barr virus myocarditis in a child with repetitive myocarditis. Pediatr Pathol Lab Med 15:805–812

Hermido-Prieto M, Montserrat L, Castro-Beiras A, Laredo R, Soler R, Peteiro J, Rodriguez E, Bouzasa B, Alvarez N, Muniz J et al (2004) Familial dilated cardiomyopathy and isolated left ventricular noncompaction associated with lamin A/C gene mutations. Am J Cardiol 94:50–54

Herzum M, Maisch B (1988) Humoral and cellular immune response in human myocarditis and dilated cardiomyopathy. Pathol Immunopathol Res 7:240–250

Holczabek W (1970) Über das histologische Bild der ischämischen Schädigung des Herzfleisches bei Anwendung der Weinsteinsäure-Kresylechtviolett-Einschlußfärbung. Beitr Gerichtl Med 27:275

Holczabek W (1973) Nachweis von Isoproterenol-bedingten Herzmuskelschäden an der Ratte mittels der Weinsteinsäure-Kresylechtviolett-Einschlußfärbung. Beitr Gerichtl Med 30:175

Hort W (1965) Ventrikeldilatation und Muskelfaserdehnung als früheste morphologische Befunde beim Herzinfarkt. Virchows Arch 339:72

Hort W (ed) (2000) Pathologische Anatomie des Herzens und seiner Hüllen II. Pathologie des Endokard, der Kranzarterien und des Myokard. Springer, Berlin

Hu BJ, Chen YC, Zhu JZ (2002) Study on the specificity of fibronectin for post-mortem diagnosis of early myocardial infarction. Med Sci Law 42:195–199

Huber SA, Gauntt CJ, Sakkinen P (1999) Enteroviruses and myocarditis: viral pathogenesis through replication, cytokine induction, and immunopathogenicity. Adv Virus Res 51:35

Huckenbeck W, Papadomanolakis A (2005) Right and left ventricular arrythmogenic dysplasia. Pathological features and medicolegal significance. In: Tsokos M (ed) Forensic pathology reviews, vol 3. Humana Press, Totowa, pp 253–165

Hudson REB (1960) The human pacemaker and its pathology. Br Heart J 22:153–167

Hudson REB (1963) The human conducting-system and its examination. J Clin Pathol 16:492–499

Hufnagel G, Maisch B (1991) Expression of MHC class I and II antigens and the IL-2 receptor in rejection, myocarditis and dilated cardiomyopathy. Eur Heart J 12(suppl D):137–140

Ichida F, Tsubata S, Bowles KR, Haneda N, Uese K, Miyawaki T, Dreyer WJ, Messina J, Li H, Bowles NE et al (2001) Novel gene mutations in patients with left ventricular noncompaction or Barth syndrome. Circulation 103:1256–1263

Iino M, Kimura T, Abiru H, Kaszynski RH, Yuan QH, Tsuruyama T, Tamaki K (2007) Unexpected sudden death resulting from anomalous origin of the right coronary artery from the left sinus of Valsalva: a case report involving identical twins. Legal Med 9:25–29

Indorato F, Akashi YJ, Rossitto C, Raffino C, Bartoloni G (2015) Takotsubo cardiomyopathy associated with rupture of the left ventricular apex: assessment of histopathological features of a fatal case and literature review. Forensic Sci Med Pathol 11:577–583

Indorato F, Bartolini G (2016) Post-mortem Takotsubo cardiomyopathy diagnosis: the challenge is open! Forensic Sci Med Pathol 12:227–228

Ishikawa T, Zhu BL, Li DR, Zhao D, Maeda H (2005) Epstein-Barr virus myocarditis as a cause of sudden death: two autopsy cases. Int J Legal Med 119:231–235

Ishiyama I, Kamiya M, Rose M, Komuro E, Takatsu A (1982) Fulminant deletion of myoglobin from myocardial fibers in state of acute cardiac failure including sudden cardiac arrest. Lancet 2:1468–1469

Jääskeläinen AJ (1968) Enzymhistochemischer Nachweis des frischen Myokardinfarkts bei Fällen von vermutetem gewaltsamem Tod. Dtsch Z Gerichtl Med 64:1–8

James TN, Marshall TK (1976) Multifocal stenosis due to fibromuscular dysplasia of the sinus node artery. Circulation 53:736–742

Janík M, Hejna P (2017) Necrotizing eosinophilic myocarditis. Forensic Sci Med Pathol 13:255–258

Janssen W (1968) Zur Arteriosklerose der Coronararterien jugendlicher Menschen. Morphologische und forensische Bedeutung. Dsch Zschr Gerichtl Med 62:39–50

Janssen W (1975) Todesfälle im Rahmen emotionaler Belastung. Beitr Gerichtl Med 33:97–102

Janssen W (1977) Forensische histologie. Schmidt-Römhild, Lübeck

Janssen W (1984) Forensic histopathology. Springer, Berlin, pp 187–190

Jenni R, Wyss CA, Eochslin EN, Kaufmann PA (2002) Isolated ventricular noncompaction is associated with coronary microcirculatory dysfunction. J Am Coll Cardiol 39:450–454

Jiang WX, Gao C, Sun J, Bunai Y (2009) Sudden cardiac death caused by a primary intimal sarcoma of the left coronary artery. Int J Legal Med 123:503–506

Jin O, Sole M, Butany JW, Chia WK, McLaughlin PR, Liu P et al (1990) Detection of enterovirus RNA in myocardial biopsies from patients with myocarditis and cardiomyopathy using gene amplification by polymerase chain reaction. Circulation 82:8–16

Joswig BC, Warren SE, Vieweg WV, Hagan AD (1978) Transmural myocardial infarction in the absence of coronary arterial luminal narrowing in a young man with single coronary arterial anomaly. Catheter Cardiovasc Diagn 4:297–304

Kammal AL, Püschel K, Tsokos M (2015) Takotsubo cardiomyopathy. Pathomorphological and medicolegal aspects of a rare syndrome. Rechtsmedizin 25:474–480

Kandolf R (1995) Molekulare Pathogenese der Enterovirusmyokarditits. Viruspersistenz und chronische Entzündung. Internist 36:430–438

Kandolf R, Ameis D, Kirschner P, Canu A, Hofschneider PH (1987) In situ detection of enteroviral genomes in myocardial cells by nucleic acid hybridization: an approach to the diagnosis of viral heart disease. Proc Natl Acad Sci U S A 84:6272–6276

Kandolf R, Klingel K, Zell R, Canu A, Fortmuller U, Hohenadl C et al (1993) Molecular mechanisms in the pathogenesis of enteroviral heart disease: acute and persistent infections. Clin Immunol Immunopathol 68:153–158

Karch SB (2009) Karch's pathology of drug abuse, 4th edn. CRC Press, Boca Raton, p 101

Karch SB, Billingham ME (1986) Myocardial contraction band revisited. Hum Pathol 17:9–13

Karch SB (2011) The unique histology of methamphetamine cardiomyopathy: a case report. Forensic Sci Int 212:e1–e4

Karjalainen J, Heikkila J (1999) Incidence of three presentations of acute myocarditis in young men in military service. A 20-year experience. Eur Heart J 20:1120–1125

Karjalainen J, Nieminen M, Heikkila J (1980) Influenza A1 myocarditis in conscripts. Acta Med Scand 207:27–30

Kauferstein S, Kiehne N, Neumann T, Pitschner HF, Bratzke H (2009) Cardiac gene defects can cause sudden cardiac death in young people. Dtsch Arztebl Int 106:41–47

Kauferstein S, Kiehne N, Peigneur S, Tytgat J, Bratzke H (2013) Cardiac channelopathy causing sudden death as revealed by molecular autopsy. Int J Legal Med 127:145–151

Kawai C (1999) From myocarditis to cardiomyopathy: mechanisms of inflammation and cell death. Circulation 99:1091–1100

Kawai C, Matsumori A, Fujiwara H (1987) Myocarditis and dilated cardiomyopathy. Annu Rev Med 38:221–239

Kawano H, Okada R, Kawano Y, Sueyoshi N, Shirai T (1994) Apoptosis in acute and chronic myocarditis. Jpn Heart J 35:745–750

Kenton AB, Sanchez X, Coveler KJ, Kavar KA, Jiminez S, Ichida F, Murphy RT, Elliott PM, McKenna W, Bowles NE et al (2004) Isolated left ventricular noncompaction is rarely caused by mutations in G4.5, alpha-dystrobrevin and FK Binding Protein-12. Mol Genet Metab 82:162–166

Kiryakova T, Nikolov D, Alexandrov A (2016) Sudden death due to asymptomatic myocarditis – a forensic case report. Rom J Leg Med 24:281–283

Kittulwatte ID, Kim PJH, Pollanen MS (2010) Sudden death related myocarditis: a study of 56 cases. Forensic Sci Med Pathol 6:13–19

Klages U, Gerken F (1972) Eine Methode zur Objektivierung fraglicher entzündlicher Zellvermehrung im Interstitium des Herzmuskels. Beitr Z Gerichtl Med 14:429

Klein RM, Vester EG, Perings C, Strauer BE (1995) Arrhythmien bei Myokarditis. Internist 36:458–468

Klein RM, Vester EG, Brehm MU et al (2000) Entzündung des Myokards als Arrhythmietrigger. Z Kardiol 89(suppl 3):24–35

Klingel K, Kandolf R (2009) Virale Myokarditis im Kindesalter. Stellenwert der modernen kardiopathologischen Diagnostik. Rechtsmedizin 18:349–358

Klingel K, Albrecht M, Canu A, Hofschneider PH, Kandolf R (1992a) Molekulare Pathogenese der Myokarditis: Viruspersistenz und chronische Herzmuskelentzündung. Verh Dtsch Ges Pathol 76:394

Klingel K, Hohenadl C, Canu A et al (1992b) Ongoing enterovirus-induced myocarditis is associated with persistent heart muscle infection: quantitative analysis of virus replication, tissue damage and inflammation. Proc Natl Acad Sci U S A 89:314–318

Klingel K, Selinka HC, Huber M, Sauer M, Leube M, Kandolf R (2000) Molecular pathology and structural features of enteroviral replication. Towards understanding the pathogenesis of viral heart disease. Heart 25:216–220

Klingel K, Sauer M, Bock CT, Szalay G, Schnorr JJ, Kandolf R (2004) Molecular pathology of inflammatory cardiomyopathy. Med Microbiol Immunol 193:101–107

Klump WM, Bergmann I, Muller BC, Ameis D, Kandolf R (1990) Complete nucleotide sequence of infectious Coxsackievirus B3 cDNA: two initial 5′ uridine residues are regained during plus-strand RNA syntheses. J Virol 64:1573–1583

KnieriemHJ,MeckingD,SeipelL(1979)Pathomorphologie des Sinusknotens beim Sinusknotensyndrom und anderen Herzrhythmusstörungen. Pathologie 1:233

Knight B (1967) Early myocardial infarction: practical methods for its postmortem demonstration. J Forensic Med 14:101–107

Korb G, Knorr G (1962) Vergleichende licht- und fluoreszenzmikroskopische Untersuchungen frischer Herzmuskelschäden beim Menschen. Virchows Arch 335:159

Kurosu A, Kuroyanagi K, Yamauchi S, Omura K, Saito K (2016) Sudden death caused by anomalous origin on the coronary artery during exercise. J Forensic Sci 61:548–550

Kühl U, Daun B, Seeberg B, Schultheiss HP, Strauer BE (1992) Dilatative kardiomyopathie – eine chronische myokarditits? Herz 17:97–106

Kühl U, Noutsias M, Seeberg B, Schannwell M, Welp LB, Schultheiss HP (1994) Chronic inflammation in the myocardium of patients with clinically suspected dilated cardiomyopathy. J Card Fail 1:13–25

Kühl U, Noutsias M, Seeberg B, Schultheiß HP (1996) Immunohistochemical analysis of the chronic inflammatory process in dilated cardiomyopathy. Heart 75:295–300

Kühl U, Pauschinger M, Schultheiss HP (1997) Neue konzepte zur diagnostik der entzündlichen herzmuskelerkrankung. Dtsch Med Wochenschr 122:690–698

Kühl U, Pauschinger M, Bock T, Klingel K, Schwimmbeck CPL, Seeberg B, Krautwurm L, Poller W, Schultheiss HP, Kandolf R (2003) Parvovirus B19 infection mimicking acute myocardial infarction. Circulation 108:945–950

Kytö V, Vuorinen T, Saukko P, Lautenschlager I, Lignitz E, Saraste A, Voipio-Pulkki LM (2005) Cytomegalovirus infection of the heart is common in patients with fatal myocarditis. Clin Infect Dis 40:683–688

Lang C, Sauter M, Szalay G, Racchi G, Grassi G, Rainaldi G, Mercantanti A, Lang F, Kandolf R, Klingel K (2008) Connective tissue growth factor: a crucial cytokine-mediating cardiac fibrosis in ongoing enterovirus myocarditis. J Mol Med 86:49–60

Langlois NE (2009) Sudden adult death. Forensic Sci Med Pathol 5:210–232

Lau RCH (1983) Coxsackie B virus infections in New Zealand patients with cardiac and non-cardiac diseases. J Med Virol 11:131–137

Lau G (1994) Acute fulminant fatal coxsackie B virus infection: a report of two cases. Ann Acad Med 23:917–920

Lauer B, Schulze K, Kühl U, Pauschinger M, Schwimmbeck PL, Strauer BE, Schultheiss HP (1998) Biphasischer Verlauf der linksventrikulären Funktion bei einer 22 jährigen Patientin mit akuter Myokarditis. Dtsch Med Wochenschr 123:74–80

Lazaros GA, Stefanaki KS, Panayiotides IG, Tzardi MN, Vlachonikolis IG, Kanavaros PE, Delides GS (1998) Nuclear morphometry of the myocardial cells as a diagnostic tool in cases of sudden death due to coronary thrombosis. Forensic Sci Int 96:173–180

Leadbetter S, Wawman HM, Jasani B (1989) Immunocytochemical diagnosis of early myocardial ischaemic/hypoxic damage. Forensic Sci Int 40:171–180

Leadbetter S, Wawman HM, Jasani B (1990) Further evaluation of immunocytochemical staining in the diagnosis of early myocardial ischaemic/hypoxic damage. Forensic Sci Int 45:135–141

Lenègre J, Chevalier H (1951) Note technique préliminaire concernant l'étude histologique de la cloison du cœur. Arch Mal Coeur 44:512–524

Lentini S, Klingel K, Skowasch R, Kandolf R, Bauriedel G (2001) Epstein-Barr virus assoziierte perikarditis. Dtsch Med Wochenshr 126:1043–1046

Leone A (2014) Relation between coronary lesions and cigarette smoking of subjects deceased from acute myocardial infarction. A histopathological study. J Cardiobiol 2:1–5

Lev M, Kinave SG, Pick A (1970) The pathogenesis of atrioventricular block in coronary disease. Circulation 42:409–426

Lev M, Nordenberg A, Carvalho AG, Bharati S, Rosen K, Varghese JP, Bauernfeind RA (1979) The anatomic substrate for the sick sinus syndrome in adolescence. Circulation 59(suppl II):437

Li Y, Bourlet T, Andreoletti L, Mosnier JF, Peng T, Yang Y, Archard LC, Pozzetto B, Zhang H (2000) Enteroviral capsid protein is present in myocardial tissues from some patients with myocarditis or dilated cardiomyopathy. Circulation 101:231–234

Lie JT (1968) Detection of early myocardial infarction by the acid fuchsin staining technic. Am J Clin Pathol 50:317–319

Lie JT, Holley KE, Kampa WR, Titus IL (1971) New histochemical method for morphologic diagnosis of early stages of myocardial ischemia. Mayo Clin Proc 46:319–327

Lim A, Langlois N (2016) Non-compaction cardiomyopathy. Forensic Sci Med Pathol 12:104–107

Lin YT, Chen CH, Ding PY (1998) Evolution of dilated cardiomyopathy from hypertrophic obstructive cardiomyopathy in a child. J Formos Med Assoc 97:416–419

Linder J, Cassling RS, Rogler WC, Wilson JE, Markin RS, Sears TD, McManus BM (1985) Immunohistochemical characterization of lymphocytes in uninflamed ventricular myocardium. Arch Pathol Lab Med 109:917–920
Lipsett J, Cohle SD, Berry PJ, Russell G, Byard RW (1994) Anomalous coronary arteries: a multicenter pediatric autopsy study. Pediatr Pathol 14:287–300
Liu PP, Mason JW (2001) Advances in the understanding of myocarditis. Circulation 104:1076–1082
Lobo FV, Ha H, Butany J et al (1992) Right ventricular dysplasia: morphological findings in 13 cases. Can J Cardiol 8:261–268
Löffler W (1936) Endocarditis parietalis fibroplastica mit Bluteosinophilie. Ein eigenartiges Krankheitsbild. Schweiz Med Wochenschr 66:817
Lozinski GM, Davis GG, Krous HF, Billman GF, Shimizu H, Burns JC (1994) Adenovirus myocarditis: retrospective diagnosis by gene amplification from formalin-fixed, paraffin-embedded tissues. Hum Pathol 25:831–834
Madea B, Dettmeyer R (1998) Sudden death in cases with anomalous origin of the left coronary artery. Forensic Sci Int 96:91–100
Maisch B (1994) Myokarditis. Internist 35:91–93
Maisch B, Schönian U, Crombach M, Wendl I, Bethge C, Herzum M et al (1993) Cytomegalovirus associated inflammatory heart muscle disease. Scand J Infect Dis Suppl 88:135–148
Maisch B, Schönian U, Herzum M, Hufnagel G (1995) Immunserologische und immunhistologische Untersuchungen bei Myokarditis und Perikarditis. Internist 36:448–457
Maisch B, Portig I, Ristic A, Hufnagel G, Pankuweit S (2000) Definition of inflammatory cardiomyopathy (myocarditis): on the way to consensus. Herz 25:200–209
Mall G (1995) Morphologie der myokarditis. Internist 36:426–429
Mallory GK, White PD, Salcedo Salgar J (1939) The speed of healing of myocardial infarction. A study of the pathologic anatomy in seventy-two cases. Am Heart J 18:647
Maron BJ (2002) Hypertrophic cardiomyopathy: a systemic review. JAMA 287:1308–1320
Maron BJ, Bonow RO, Cannon RO, Leon MB, Epstein SE (1997) Hypertrophic cardiomyopathy: interrelations of clinical manifestations, pathophysiology, and therapy: parts 1 and 2. N Engl J Med 316:780–789. 844–852
Maron BJ, Towbin JA, Thiene G, Antzelevith C, Corrado D, Arnett D, Moss AJ, Seidman CE, Young JB (2006) Contemporary definitions and classifications of the cardiomyopathies: an American heart association scientific statement from the council on clinical cardiology, heart failure and transplantation committee; quality of care and outcomes research and functional genomics and translational biology interdisciplinary working group; and council on epidemiology and prevention. Circulation 113:1807–1816
Marsman RFJ, Bezzina CR, Freiberg F, Verkerk AO, Adriaens ME, Podliesna S, Chen C, Purfürst B, Spallek B, Koopmann TT, Baczko I, dos Remedios CG, George AL, Bishopric NH, Lodder EM, de Bakker JMT, Fischer R, Coronel R, Wilde AAM, Gotthardt M, Remme CA (2014) Coxsackie and adenovirus receptor is a modifier of cardiac conduction and arrhythmia vulnerability in the setting of myocardial ischemia. J Am Coll Cardiol 63:549–559
Martin AB, Webber S, Fricker FJ, Jaffe R, Demmler G, Kearney D et al (1994) Acute myocarditis: rapid diagnosis by PCR in children. Circulation 90:330–339
Martinez S, Miranda E, Kim P, Pollanen MS (2013) Giant cell myocarditis associated with amoxicillin hypersensitivity. Forensic Sci Med Pathol 9:403–406
Martino TA, Liu P, Sole MJ (1994) Viral infection and the pathogenesis of dilated cardiomyopathy. Circ Res 74:182–188
Martino TA, Liui P, Petric M, Sole MJ (1995) Enteroviral myocarditis and dilated cardiomyopathy: a review of clinical and experimental studies. In: Rothbard HA (ed) Human enterovirus infections. American Society for Microbiology, Washington DC, pp 291–350
Matejic D, Schönfeld C, Tsokos M (2010) Plötzlicher Tod bei akuter idiopathischer Riesenzellmyokarditis. Rechtsmedizin 20:275–277
Mayer F, Pröpper S, Ritz-Timme S (2014) Dityrosine, a protein product of oxidative stress, as a possible marker of acute myocardial infarctions. Int J Legal Med 128:787–794
Mayer F, Falk M, Huhn R, Behmenburg F, Ritz-Timme S (2016) Dityrosine as a marker of acute myocardial infarction? Experiments with the isolated Langendorff heart. Int J Legal Med 130:1053–1060
McCaffrey FM, Braden DS, Strong WB (1991) Sudden cardiac death in young athletes. Am J Dis Child 145:177–183
McConnell SE, Collins KA (1998) Sudden unexpected death from an anomalous hypoplastic left coronary artery. J Forensic Sci 43:708–711
McConnell MV, Ganz P, Selwyn AP, Li W, Edelmann RR, Manning WJ (1995) Identification of anomalous coronary arteries and their anatomic course by magnetic resonance coronary angiography. Circulation 92:3158–3162
McKenna WJ, Thiene G, Nava A et al (1994) Diagnosis of arrhythmogenic right ventricular dysplasia/cardiomyopathy. Br Heart J 71:215–218
McVie JG (1970) Postmortem detection of inapparent myocardial infarction. J Clin Pathol 23:203–209
Metze K, Meves R, Moreira PRS (1993) Seasonal variation in rheumatic heart disease – letter to the editor. Int J Cardiol 38:01–102
Michaud K, Romain N, Taroni F, Horisberger B, Mangin P (2002) Evaluation of a simplified method of the conduction system analysis in 110 forensic cases. Forensic Sci Int 130:13–24
Michaud K, Mangin P, Elger BS (2011) Genetic analysis of sudden cardiac death victims: a survey of

current forensic autopsy practices. Int J Legal Med 125:359–366

Mihatsch MJ (1988) Die morphologie des myokardinfarkts. Schweiz Med Wochenschr 118:1688–1691

Milei J, Bortman G, Fernandez-Alonso G, Grancelli H, Beigelman R (1990) Immunohistochemical staining of lymphocytes for the reliable diagnosis of myocarditis in endomyocardial biopsies. Cardiology 77:77–85

Miller R, Ward C, Amsterdam E (1973) Focal mononucleosis myocarditis simulating myocardial infarction. Chest 63:102–105

Möhlenkamp S, Wort W, Ge J, Erbel R (2002) Update on myocardial bridging. Circulation 106:2616–2622

Mondello C, Cardia L, Ventura-Spagnolo E (2017) Immunohistochemical detection of early myocardial infarction: a systematic review. Int J Leg Med 131:411–421

Moral GL, Rubio-Calduch EM, Broto-Escapa P, Caballero-Requero E, Calico-Bosch I, Bertran-Sangues JM (1993) Enteroviral infections in children: clinical and epidemiological findings in 530 patients (1984–1991). An Esp Pediatr 39:521–527

Mounts AW, Amr S, Jamshidi R, Graves C, Dwyer D, Guarner J et al (2001) A cluster of fulminant myocarditis cases in children, Baltimore, Maryland, 1997. Pediatr Cardiol 22:34–39

Muir P (1993) Enteroviruses and heart disease. Br J Biomed Sci 50:258–271

Mund MT, Hailemariam S, Gathomas G (2002) Die arrhythmogene rechtsventrikuläre Kardiomyopathie als Ursache des plötzlichen Herztodes. Rechtsmedizin 12:371–374

Munkholm J, Andersen CB, Ottesen GL (2015) Plakkoglobin: a diagnostic marker of arrhythmogenic right ventricular cardiomyopathy in forensic pathology? Forensic Sci Med Pathol 11:47–52

Murry CE, Jerome KR, Reichenbach DD (2001) Fatal parvovirus myocarditis in an 5-year-old girl. Hum Pathol 32:342–345

Murty OP (2008) Giant cell myocarditis with cardiac tamponade. Am J Forensic Med Pathol 29:245–248

Narula J, Haider N, Virmani R, DiSalvo TG, Kolodgie FD, Hajjar RJ et al (1996) Apoptosis in myocytes in end-stage heart failure. N Engl J Med 335:1182–1189

Nielsen TS, Nyengaard JR, Møller J, Banner J, Nielsen LP, Baandrup UT (2014a) Quantitative diagnosis of lymphocytic myocarditis in forensic medicine. Forensic Sci Int 238:9–15

Nielsen TS, Hansen J, Nielsen LP, Baandrup UT, Banner J (2014b) The presence of enterovirus, adenovirus, and parvovirus B19 in myocardial tissue samples from autopsies: an evaluation of their frequencies in deceased individuals with myocarditis and in non-inflamed control hearts. Forensic Sci Med Pathol 10:433–350

Nishida N, Ikeda N, Kudo K, Tsuji A, Kiyoshima A (2002) Forensic significance of conduction system abnormalities as a precise cause of accidental death. Int J Legal Med 116:344–349

Noutsias M, Seeberg B, Schultheiss HP, Kühl U (1999) Expression of cell adhesion molecules in dilated cardiomyopathy. Evidence for endothelial activation in inflammatory cardiomyopathy. Circulation 99:2124–2131

Noutsias M, Fechner H, de Jonge H, Wand X, Dekkers D, Houtsmuller AB, Pauschinger M, Bergelson JM, Warraich R, Yacoub M et al (2001) Human coxsackie-adenoviruses receptor is colocalized with integrins alpha(v)beta(3) and alpha(v)beta(5) on the cardiomyocyte sarcolemma and upregulated in dilated cardiomyopathy: implications for cardiotropic viral infections. Circulation 104:275–280

Noutsias M, Pauschinger M, Kühl U, Schultheiss HP (2002) Myokarditis und dilatative Kardiomyopathie. Neue Wege in Diagnostik und Therapie. Münch Med Wochenschr 144:36–40

Oechslin EN, Attenhofer JCH, Rojas JR, Kaufmann PA, Jenni R (2000) Long-term follow-up of 34 adults with isolated left ventricular noncompaction: a distinct cardiomyopathy with poor prognosis. J Am Coll Cardiol 36:493–500

Oehmichen M, Pedal I, Hofmann P (1990a) Diagnostic significance of myofibrillar degeneration of cardiocytes in forensic pathology. Forensic Sci Int 48:163–173

Oehmichen M, Pedal I, Hohmann P (1990b) Myofibrilläre degeneration der herzmuskulatur: diagnostische wertigkeit am ausgesuchten forensisch-pathologischen fallmaterial. Beitr Gerichtl Med 48:245–249

Ogbuihi S (1989) On the forensic significance of sinuatrial node lesions in sudden death. Z Rechtsmed 102:315–322

Ogbuihi S, Fechner G, Brinkmann B (1993) Sudden death due to cardiac sarcoidosis in a case of suspected homicide. Int J Legal Med 106:99–102

Oka K, Oohira K, Yatabe Y, Tanaka T, Kurano K, Kosugi R, Murata M, Hakozaki H, Nishikawa T, Tsutsumi Y (2005) Fulminant myocarditis demonstrating uncommon morphology – a report of two cases. Virchows Arch 446:259–264

Okada R, Kawai S (1983) Histopathology of the conduction system in sudden cardiac death. Jpn Circ J 47:573–580

Orth T, Herr W, Spahn T et al (1997) Human parvovirus B19 infection associated with severe acute perimyocarditis in an 34-year-old man [letter]. Eur Heart J 18:524–525

Osuna E, Perez Carceles MD, Jakobson SW, Luna A (1990) Biochemical and morphological markers in the post mortem diagnosis of ischemic heart distress. Acta Med Leg Soc 40:275–283

Oyer CE, Ongeapin EH, Ni J, Bowles NE, Towbin JA (2000) Fatal intrauterine adenoviral endomyocarditis with aortic and pulmonary valve stenosis: diagnosis by polymerase chain reaction. Hum Pathol 31:1433–1435

Pampín JB, Aranzazu García Rivero S, Cepeda JLO, Vázquez Boquete A, Forteza Vila J, Fonseca RH (2006) Immunohistochemical expression of HIF-1-alpha in response to early myocardial ischemia. J Forensic Sci 51:120–124

Patel J, Sheppard MN (2011) Cystic tumour of the atrioventricular node: three cases of sudden death. Int J Legal Med 125:139–142

Pauschinger M, Meissner G, Preis S, Kühl U, Kandolf R, Schultheiss HP et al (1994) Detection of enteroviral RNA by polymerase chain reaction in patients with myocarditis and dilated cardiomyopathy. JACC 1994:880

Pauschinger M, Kühl U, Dörner A, Schieferecke K, Petschauer S, Rauch U, Schwimmbeck PL, Kandolf R, Schultheiss HP (1998) Nachweis enteroviraler RNA in endomyokardialen Biopsien bei inflammatorischer Kardiomyopathie und idiopathischer dilatativer Kardiomyopathie. Z Kardiol 87:443–452

Pedal I (1976) Ursprungsanomalie einer Koronararterie. Dtsch Med Wochenschr 101:1601–1604

Pedal I, Oehmichen M (1990) Myofibrilläre Degeneration der Herzmuskulatur: Histologisches Bild und pathophysiologische Bedeutung. Beitr Gerichtl Med 48:237–244

Pedal I, Teufel M (1993) Plötzlicher Herztod im Kindesalter durch eine Ursprungsanomalie der Koronararterie. Dtsch Med Wochenschr 118:861–866

Pedersen PK (1980) Poor results in attempting to demonstrate the cause of death by examination of the conduction system of the heart in cases of sudden death. Forensic Sci Int 16:281–282

Philipps CA, Aronson MD, Tomkow J, Philipps ME (1980) Enteroviruses in Vermont, 1969–1978: an important cause of illness throughout the year. J Infect Dis 141:162–164

Philips M, Robiniwitz M, Higgins JR, Boran KJ, Reed T, Virmani R (1986) Sudden cardiac death in air force recruits. JAMA 256:2696–2699

Pichotka J (1942) Tierexperimentelle Untersuchungen zur pathologischen Histologie des akuten Höhentodes. Beitr Pathol Anat 197:117

Piercecchi-Marti MD, Lepidi H, Leonetti G, Vire O, Cianfarani F, Pellissier JF (2001) Immunostaining by complement C9: a tool for early diagnosis of myocardial infarction and application in forensic medicine. J Forensic Sci 46:328–334

Piercecchi-Marti MD, Mohamed H, Chau C, Liprandi A, Fredouille C (2003) Congenital atrioventricular block: histological aspects. Forensic Sci Int 136:12–15

Prasad A, Lerman A, Rihal CS (2008) Apical ballooning syndrome (Tako-Tsubo or stress cardiomyopathy): a mimic of acute myocardial infarction. Am Heart J 155:408–417

Priemer F, Keil W, Kandolf R (1999) Hydrocution in a case of Coxsackie virus infection. Int J Legal Med 112:368–371

Pusta CT, Mihalache G, Buhas C, Pop O (2015) A rare case of cardiac fibroma in a dead truck driver. Rom J Leg Med 23:247–250

Rahlf G (1980) Intramyocardial microarteriopathy. Virch Arch A Path Anat Histol 388:289–311

Raza-Ahmad A (1994) Fibrinogen: a diagnostic marker for early ischemia. Biotech Histochem 69:268–272

Rentea I, Voinea OC, Hostiuc S, Iancu CB, Petre N, Ceausu M (2016) Usefulness of angiotensin type 2 receptor in establishing the histological age of myocardial infarction. Rom J Leg Med 24:100–105

Rérolle C, Faisant M, Lefrancq T, Saint-Martin P (2016) Sudden death due to undiagnosed rheumatic heart disease in a child. J Forensic Sci 61:848–850

Richardson P, McKenna W, Bristow M, Maisch B, Mautner B, O'Connell J, Olsen E, Thiene G, Goodwin J, Gyarfas I, Martin I, Nordet P (1996) Report on the 1995 world health organization/international society and federation of cardiology task force on the definition and classification of cardiomyopathies. Circulation 93:841–842

Riedel J, Neudorf U, Schmaltz AA (1997) Rasche Progredienz einer hypertrophen Kardiomyopathie in eine dilatative Form – Ungewöhnlicher Verlauf bei einem jugendlichen Patienten. Eine Fallbeschreibung. Z Kardiol 88:427–432

Riezzo I, Ventura F, D'Errico S, Neri M, Turillazzi E, Fineschi V (2009) Arrhythmogenesis and diagnosis of cardiac sarcoidosis. An immunohistochemical study in a sudden cardiac death. Forensic Sci Int 183:e1–e5

Riße M, Weiler G (1985) Die koronare Muskelbrücke und ihre Beziehungen zu lokaler Koronarsklerose, regionaler Myokardischämie und Koronarspasmus. Eine morphometrische Studie. Z Kardiol 74:700–705

Riße M, Verhoff MA, Dettmeyer R (2008) Kardiale sarkoidose. Rechtsmedizin 18:267–268

Roberts WC (1986) Major anomalies of coronary arterial origin seen in adulthood. Am Heart J 111:941–963

Roberts WC, Shirami J (1992) The four subtypes of anomalous origin of the left main coronary artery from the right aortic sinus (or from the right coronary artery). Am J Cardiol 70:119–123

Rodríguez-Calvo MS, Brion M, Alleque C, Concheiro L, Carracedo A (2008) Molecular genetics of sudden cardiac death. Forensic Sci Int 182:1–12

Rohayem J, Dinger J, Fischer R et al (2001) Fatal myocarditis associated with acute parvovirus B19 and human herpesvirus 6 coinfection. J Clin Microbiol 39:4585–4587

Roynard JL, Cattan S, Artigou JY (1994) Anomalous course of the left anterior descending coronary artery between the aorta and pulmonary trunk: a rare cause of myocardial ischaemia at rest. Br Heart J 72:397–399

Ruszkiewicz AR, Vernon-Roberts E (1993) Sudden death in an infant due to histiocytoid cardiomyopathy. A light-microscopic, ultrastructural and immunohistochemical study. Am J Forensic Med Pathol 16:74–80

Sabatasso S, Mangin P, Fracasso T, Moretti M, Docquier M, Djonov V (2016) Early markers for myocardial ischemia and sudden cardiac death. Int J Legal Med 130:1265–1280

Sahai VB (1976) The post-mortem detection of early myocardial infarction by a simple fluorescent method. Med Sci Law 16:17–20

Sandritter W, Thomas C (eds) (1977) Histopathologie. F.K. Schattauer, Stuttgart

Santer R (2004) Metabolische kardiomyopathien. Monatsschr Kinderheilkd 152:639–648

Sasse-Klaassen S, Gerull B, Oechslin E, Jenni R, Thierfelder L (2003) Isolated noncompaction of the left ventricular myocardium in the adult is an autosomal dominant disorder in the majority of patients. Am J Med Genet A 119:162–167

Sasse-Klaassen S, Probst S, Gerull B, Oechslin E, Nurnberg P, Heuser A, Jenni R, Hennies HC, Thierfelder L (2004) Novel gene locus for autosomal dominant left ventricular noncompaction maps to chromosome 11p15. Circulation 109:2720–2723

Sato T, Nishio H, Suzuki K (2015) Identification of arrhythmogenic right ventricular cardiomyopathy-causing gene mutations in young sudden unexpected death autopsy cases. J Forensic Sci 60:457–461

Saukko P, Knight B (1989) Evaluation of eosin-fluorescence in the diagnosis of sudden cardiac death. Forensic Sci Int 40:285–290

Schäfer H, Mathey D, Hugo F, Bhakdi S (1986) Deposition of the terminal C5b-9 complement complex in infarcted areas of human myocardium. J Immunol 137:1945–1949

Schaper J, Lorenz-Meyer S, Suzuku K (1999) The role of apoptosis in dilated cardiomyopathy. Herz 24:219–224

Schnitt SJ, Ciano PS, Schoen FJ (1987) Quantitation of lymphocytes in endomyocardial biopsies: use and limitations of antibodies to leukocyte common antigen. Hum Pathol 18:796–800

Schultheiß HP (1993) Die dilatative Kardiomyopathie – eine chronische Myokarditis? Neue Aspekte zur Diagnostik und Therapie. Z Kardiol 82(suppl 4):25–33

Schwartz DA, Finkelstein SD, Lumb GD (1988) Fat embolism to the cardiac conduction system associated with sudden death. Hum Pathol 19:116–119

Schwartz ML, Cox GF, Lin AE, Korson MS, Perez-Atayde A, Lacro RV, Lishultz SE (1996) Clinical approach to genetic cardiomyopathy in children. Circulation 94:2021–2038

Schwartzkopff B, Klein RM, Strauer BE (1995) Diagnostik und therapie der myokarditis. Internist 36:469–483

Schwartzkopff B, Klein RM, Strauer BE (1998) Evidence of endothelial dysfunction of epicardial coronary arteries in patients with immunohistochemically proven myocarditis. Am Heart J 136:389–397

Seidman CD, McKenna WJ, Watkins HC, Seidman JG (1992) Molecular genetic approaches to diagnosis and management of hypertrophic cardiomyopathy. In: Braunwald E (ed) Heart disease. A textbook of cardiovascular medicine. W.B. Saunders Co, New York, pp 77–83

Seko Y, Tsuchimochi H, Nakamura T, Okumura K, Naito S, Imatako K (1990) Expression of major histocompatibility complex class I antigen in murine ventricular myocytes infected with Coxsackievirus B3. Circ Res 67:360–367

Shanes JG, Ghali J, Billingham ME, Ferrans VJ, Fenoglio JJ, Edwards WD, Tsai CC, Saffitz JE, Isner J, Furner S (1987) Interobserver variability in the pathologic interpretation of endomyocardial biopsy results. Circulation 75:401–405

Shekhonin BV, Guriev SB, Irgashev SB, Koteliansky VE (1990) Immunofluorescent identification of fibronectin and fibrinogen/fibrin in experimental myocardial infarction. J Mol Cell Cardiol 22:533–541

Sigrist T, Germann U (1998) Morphological alterations in the conducting system for the diagnosis of sudden cardiac death. Rechtsmedizin 8:69–72

Smith ET, Davis G (1997) Sudden cardiac death associated with hypoplasia of the coronary arteries and conduction system alteration. Am J Forensic Med Pathol 18:189–193

Song Y, Yao Q, Luo B, Zhu J, Liang S (1991) A simplified method for examining the human cardiac conduction system. Chin. J Forensic Med 6:92–93

Song Y, Zhu J, Laaksonen H, Saukko P (1997) A modified method for examining the cardiac conduction system. Forensic Sci Int 86:135–138

Song Y, Yao Q, Zhu J, Bin L, Shangyon L (1999) Age-related variation in the interstitial tissues of the cardiac conduction system; an autopsy study of 230 Han Chinese. Forensic Sci Int 104:133–142

Song Y, Laaksonen H, Saukko P, Toivonen S, Zhu J (2001) Histopathological findings of cardiac conduction system of 150 Finns. Forensic Sci Int 119:310–317

Srettabunjong S (2016) Myocardial bridging of coronary arteries: sudden unexpected deaths in a 24-year-old man. Rom. J Leg Med 24:83–86

Stahl J, Couper RTL, Byard RW (1997) Oncocytic cardiomyopathy: a rare cause of early childhood death associated with fitting. Med Sci Law 37:84–87

Steenbergen C, Kolbeck PC, Wolfe JA, Anthony RM, Sanfilippo FP, Jennings RB (1986) Detection of lymphocytes in endomyocardium using immunohistochemical techniques. Relevance to evaluation of endomyocardial biopsies in suspected cases of lymphocytic myocarditis. J Appl Cardiol 1:63–73

Steenbergen C, Hill ML, Jennings RB (1987) Cytoskeletal damage during myocardial ischemia: changes in vinculin immunofluorescence staining during total in vitro ischemia in canine heart. Circ Res 60:478–486

Stöllberger C, Sporn R, Skala K, Schneider B, Finsterer J (2010) Assault-induced Takotsubo cardiomyopathy associated with persisting anterograde amnesia and myopathy. Int J Legal Med 124:467–470

Strauer B, Kandolf R, Mall G, Maisch B, Mertens T, Figulla HR et al (2001) Myokarditis – kardiomyopathie. Update 2001. Med Klin 96:608–625

Suarez-Mier MP, Aguilera B (1998) Histopathology of the conduction system in sudden infant death. Forensic Sci Int 93:143–154

Suarez-Mier MP, Fernandez-Simón L, Gawallo C (1995) Pathologic changes of the cardiac conduction tissue in sudden cardiac death. Am J Forensic Med Pathol 16:193–202

Sunnassee A, Shaohua Z, Liang R, Liang L (2011) Unexpected death of a young woman: is myocardial bridging significant? A case report and review of the literature. Forensic Sci Med Pathol 7:42–46

Takahashi S, Kanetake J, Moriya T, Funayama M (2008) Sudden infant death from dilated cardiomyopathy with endocardial fibroelastosis. Legal Med 10:277–280

Takeichi S, Nakajima Y, Yukawa N, Saito T, Seto Y, Huang XL, Kusakabe T, Jin ZB, Hasegawa I, Nakano T, Saniabadi R, Adachi M, Ohara N, Wang T, Nakajima K (2001) Association of plasma triglyceride-rich lipoprotein remnants with "Pokkuri disease". Legal Med 3:84–94

Tamura A, Kusachi S, Nogami K, Yamanishi A, Kajikawa Y, Hirohata S, Tsuji T (1996) Tenascin expression in endomyocardial biopsy specimens in patients with dilated cardiomyopathy: distribution along margin of fibrotic lesions. Heart 75:291–294

Tansey DK, Aly Z, Sheppard MN (2005) Fat in the right ventricle of the normal heart. Histopathology 46:98–104

Tatrai E, Bedi K, Kovalszky I, Hartyanszky I, Laszik A, Acsady G, Sotonyi P, Hubay M (2011) No mutation but high mRNA expression of Coxsackie-Adenovirus receptor was observed in both dilated and ischemic cardiomyopathy. Forensic Sci Int 212:47–50

Tausch D (1974) Experimentelle Untersuchungen über den histologischen Nachweis frischer ischämischer Herzmuskelschädigungen mit der Methode nach Lie und Mitarb. Beitr Gerichtl Med 32:274–278

Taylor AJ, Rogan KM, Virman R (1992) Sudden cardiac death associated with isolated congenital coronary anomalies. J Am Coll Cardiol 20:640–647

Thiene G, Bruneval P, Veinot J, Leone O (2013) Diagnostic use of the endomyocardial biopsy: a consensus statement. Virchows Arch 463:1–5

Thierauf A, Dettmeyer R, Wollersen H, Madea B (2007) Aplastic right coronary artery and left coronary artery with a separate origin of the circumflex branch in a 31-year-old man. Forensic Sci Int 173:178–181

Thomsen H, Held H (1995) Immunohistochemical detection of C5b-9 (m) in myocardium: an aid in distinguishing infarction-induced ischemic heart muscle necrosis from other forms of lethal myocardial injury. Forensic Sci Int 71:87–95

Thomsen H, Schulz A, Bhakdi S (1990) Immunohistochemische C5b-9-Komplement-Komplex-Darstellung in Frühstadien der Herzmuskelnekrosen am Paraffinschnitt. Z Rechtsmed 103:199–206

Titus JL, Daugherty GW, Kirklin JW, Edwards JE (1963) Lesions of the atrio-ventricular conduction system after repair of ventricular septal defect. Relation to heart block. Circulation 28:82–88

Todd GL, Baroldi G, Pieper GM, Clayton F, Eliot RS (1985a) Experimental catecholamine-induced myocardial necrosis. I Morphology, quantification and regional distribution of acute contraction band lesions. J Mol Cell Cardiol 17:317–338

Todd GL, Baroldi G, Pieper GM, Clayton F, Eliot RS (1985b) Experimental catecholamine-induced myocardial necrosis. II Temporal development of isoproterenol-induced contraction band lesions correlated with ECG, hemodynamic and biochemical changes. J Mol Cell Cardiol 17:647–656

Tsung SH, Huang TY, Chang HH (1982) Sudden death in young athletes. Arch Pathol Lab Med 106:168–170

Tyson AA, Hackshaw BT, Kutcher MA (1989) Acute Epstein-Barr virus myocarditis simulating myocardial infarction with cardiogenic shock. South Med J 82:1184–1187

Vallance HD, Jeven G, Wallace DC, Brown MD (2004) A case of sporadic infantile histiocytoid cardiomyopathy caused by the A8344G (MERRF) mitochondrial DNA mutation. Pediatr Cardiol 25:538–540

Veinot JP, Johnston B (1998) Cardiac sarcoidosis – an occult cause of sudden death: a case report and literature review. J Forensic Sci 43:715–717

Veinot JP, Johnston B, Acharya V, Healey J (2002) The spectrum of intramyocardial small vessel disease associated with sudden death. J Forensic Sci 47:384–388

Ventéo L, Bourlet T, Renois F, Douche-Aourik F, Mosnier JF, Maison GL, Pluot M, Pozzetto B, Andreoletti L (2010) Enterovirus-related activation of the cardiomyocyte mitochondrial apoptotic pathway in patients with acute myocarditis. Eur Heart J 31:728–736

Ventura F, Landolfa MC, Leoncini A, Gentile R, Gaggero G, Bonsignore A, de Stefano F (2012) Sudden death due to primary atrial neoplasms: report of two cases and review of the literature. Forensic Sci Int 214:e30–e33

Voigt J (1976) Reflections on the value of histological examination of the cardiac conduction system in cases of natural unexpected death. Forensic Sci Int 8:29–31

Walthard B (1942) Die Koronarsklerose der Jugendlichen. Schweiz Med Wochenschr 72:1261

Weiler G, Knieriem HJ (1975) Beitrag zur Morphometrie der Coronarsklerose. Z Rechtsmed 75:241–254

Weiler G, Risse M (1981) Morphological examinations in cases of stenosing coronary sclerosis and their importance for evaluation of competing causes of death. Forensic Sci Int 18:131–139

Weiler G, Risse M (1994) New aspects concerning the morphology and significance of coronary muscle bridges. Cardiovasc Pathol 3:51–55

Wick MR, Siegal GP (1988) Antibodies to desmin in diagnostic pathology. In: Wick MR (ed) Monoclonal antibodies in diagnostic immunohistochemistry. Marcel Dekker, New York, pp 93–114

Wigle ED, Sasson Z, Henderson MA, Ruddy TD, Fulop J, Rakoski H, Williams WG (1985) Hypertrophic cardiomyopathy: the importance of the site and the extent of hypertrophy: a review. Prog Cardiovasc Dis 28:1–83

Wingenfeld L, Freislederer A, Schulze-Bahr E, Paul M, Bajanowski T (2010) Life-threatening hobbies in the youth? Two autoptic cases suggesting arrhythmogenic right ventricular cardiomyopathy. Forensic Sci Int 171:e1–e4

Wittstein IS, Thiemann DR, Lima JA, Baughman KL, Schulman SP, Gerstenblith G, Wu KC, Rade JJ, Bivalacqua TJ, Champion HC (2005) Neurohumoral features of myocardial stunning due to sudden emotional stress. N Engl J Med 352:539–548

Wojnicz R, Nowalany-Kozielska E, Wodniecki J, Szczurek-Katanski K, Nożyński J, Zembala M, Rozek MM (1998) Immunohistological diagnosis of myocarditis – potential role of sarcolemmal induction of the MHC and ICAM-1 in the detection of autoimmune mediated myocyte injury. Eur Heart J 19:1564–1572

Woźniewicz B, Czarnowska E, Kubicka K, Ziółkowska L, Cielecka-Kuszyk J, Zaleska T (1998) Coexistence of arrhythmogenic right ventricular cardiomyopathy and chronic myocarditis in children. Ann Diagn Paediatr Pathol 2:13–17

Xiaohong Z, Xiaorui C, Jun H, Qisheng Q (2002) The contrast of immunohistochemical studies of myocardial fibrinogen and myoglobin in early myocardial ischemia in rats. Legal Med 4:47–51

Xu XH, Chen JG, Zhu JZ (2001) Primary study of vascular endothelial growth factor immunohistochemical staining in the diagnosis of early acute myocardial ischemia. Forensic Sci Int 118:11–14

Yamanaka O, Hobbs RE (1990) Coronary artery anomalies in 126,595 patients undergoing coronary angiography. Catheter Cardiovasc Diagn 21:28–40

Yazaki Y, Isobe M, Yamazaki S, Sekiguchi M, Usuda N (1998) Ultrastructural and immunohistochemical analysis of biopsy-proven chronic active myocarditis with numerous clusters of lymphocytes. Virchows Arch 433:161–166

Zack F, Rummel J, Büttner A (2011) Fibromuscular dysplasia and sudden cardiac death. Brief review. Rechtsmedizin 21:513–517

Zack F, Manhart J, Rentsch D, Büttner A (2014a) Rare cause of death due to treatment of schizophrenia and alcohol abuse. Rechtsmedizin 24:22–25

Zack F, Kutter G, Blaas V, Rodewald AK, Büttner A (2014b) Fibromuscular dysplasia of cardiac conduction system arteries in traumatic and non-natural sudden death victims aged 0 to 40 years: a histological analysis of 100 cases. Cardiovasc Pathol 23:12–16

Zack F, Rummel J, Wegener R (1996) Hochgradige Sinusknotenfibrose als Ursache eines plötzlichen Herztodes. Rechtsmedizin 6:133–136

Zack F, Wegener R (1994) Zur Problematik der Diagnose "rhythmogener Herztod" durch histologische Untersuchungen des Erregungsbildungs- und -leitungssystems. Rechtsmedizin 5:1–5

Zack F, Rodewald AK, Blaas V, Büttner A (2016) Histologic spectrum of the cardiac conducting tissue in non-natural deaths under 30 years of age: an analysis of 43 cases with special implications for sudden cardiac death. Int J Legal Med 130:173–178

Zell R, Klingel K, Bültmann B, Kandolf R (1995) Nachweis enteroviraler RNA aus Formalin-fixiertem Paraffin-eingebettetem Myokardgewebe durch nested RT-PCR. Verh Dtsch Ges Pathol 79:359

Zhang JM, Riddick L (1996) Cytoskeleton immunohistochemical study of early ischemic myocardium. Forensic Sci Int 80:229–238

Zhang M, Tavora F, Zhang Y, Ripple M, Fowler D, Li L, Zhao Z, Burke A (2013) The role of focal myocardial inflammation in sudden unexpected cardiac death and noncardiac deaths – a clinicopathological study. Int J Legal Med 127:131–138

Zhu BL, Tanaka S, Ishikawa T, Zhao D, Li DR, Michiue T, Quan L, Maeda H (2008) Forensic pathological investigation of myocardial hypoxia-induced factor-1a, erythropoietin and vascular endothelial growth factor in cardiac death. Legal Med 10:11–19

Zollinger U (1983) Die Chromotrop-Anilinblau-Färbung zur besseren Darstellung frischer Herzmuskelfaserschädigungen. Z Rechtsmed 90:269–275

Zugibe FT, Zugibe FT Jr, Costello JT, Breithaupt MK (1993) Hypoplastic coronary artery disease within the spectrum of sudden unexpected death in young and middle age adults. Am J Forensic Med Pathol 14:276–283

14 Vascular, Cardiac Valve, and Metabolic Diseases

Sudden death prompting a judicial postmortem can be attributed to natural causes arising from a spectrum of vascular, cardiac valve, and metabolic diseases. The diseases most frequently reported in the forensic literature can only be diagnosed in part using macroscopic methods; however, cardiac valve disease in particular often demonstrates macroscopic findings. Suspected diagnoses require microscopic confirmation. In this context, almost all vascular, cardiac valve, and metabolic diseases demonstrate a histological and partly also immunohistochemical correlation. Occasionally, congenital vascular and cardiac valve diseases, as well as metabolic diseases undetected until postmortem, are the cause of sudden death, e.g., congenital heart defects, endocarditis, or aortic coarctation (Lynch et al. 2008; Karayel et al. 2006); endocardial fibroelastosis is rarely reported in the literature.

Undetected lethal cardiac valve disease primarily affects children and relatively young people with congenital cardiac valve defects, acquired cardiac valve stenosis, or cardiac valve insufficiency. Macroscopically detectable anomalies in coronary arteries in particular are also rare (Schmitt 1973). In contrast, arteriosclerotic aneurysms are unproblematic; however, their distinction from primary vasculitides is occasionally challenging (Desinan et al. 2010; Dettmeyer et al. 2006, 1998a).

Congenital and, more rarely, iatrogenic vascular anomalies can lead to lethal complications; primary among these are gross congenital malformations of the heart and vascular system. Severe malformations quickly become clinically symptomatic, while less life-threatening malformations can long remain undetected. Cases of sudden death associated with intracerebral hemangioma and arteriovenous malformations have also been reported (see Chap. 20). In the case of hemangioma, cavernous hemangioma needs to be differentiated from capillary hemangioma.

14.1 Vascular Diseases

The following potentially lethal vascular diseases are particularly noteworthy:

- General atherosclerosis (very common), including cerebral sclerosis, carotid and renal artery sclerosis, etc.
- Coronary sclerosis (see Chap. 13)
- Various forms of aneurysm which are either congenital or which develop in the setting of atherosclerosis
- Special forms of dissecting aneurysm in the setting of, e.g., idiopathic cystic medial necrosis (Erdheim–Gsell), Marfan syndrome, Ehlers–Danlos syndrome, and, rarely, syphilis (lues)

R. B. Dettmeyer, *Forensic Histopathology*, https://doi.org/10.1007/978-3-319-77997-3_14

- Arteritides and/or angitides as isolated or system disease (Wang et al. 2002)
- Congenital vascular anomalies such as capillary or cavernous hemangioma or arteriovenous tumors
- Rare syndromes with vascular involvement which, in individual cases, can be the cause of sudden death, e.g., Osler–Weber–Rendu syndrome (Byard et al. 2001)

A comprehensive list of all possible vascular diseases and their potentially lethal variants is beyond the scope of this work. Atherosclerotic lesions and their complications are the most common. In a number of cases, vascular disease has been proven as the cause of pregnancy-related sudden death (Risse et al. 2010; Risse and Weiler 1987). In addition, there are very rare findings of, e.g., coronary artery fibromuscular dysplasia as a cause of death (Zack et al. 1996). Also, cases of lethal complications of arteriovenous malformations, e.g., rupture and spontaneous hemothorax (Ishikawa et al. 2010), have been reported.

Posttraumatic arterial rupture may also be significant in terms of insurance law, particularly in cases where a two-stage event is suspected; in this case, a histomorphological correlation should be provided where possible. Thus, in initially incomplete rupture of the aorta, thrombosed ruptured fissure, partially necrotic vascular wall, and focal linear necrosis of the aortic muscle, for example, have all been described. In addition to the detection of micromorphologic signs of trauma, histological investigation also serves to exclude/include preexisting vascular diseases (trauma-related degenerative lesions in elastic fibers, acidic mucopolysaccharide deposition, microcystic lesions, and inflammatory processes). The final rupture of the remaining layers is mainly thought to be due to posttraumatic necrosis. A significant degree of atherosclerosis partly favors the onset of rupture, a fact that should be considered when giving an opinion in civil litigation (Brinkmann 1974). The same problem associated with expert opinions is also valid, e.g., for two-stage ruptures or dissecting aneurysms of the carotid or vertebral arteries following trauma or chiropractic intervention.

14.1.1 General, Coronary, and Cerebral Sclerosis

Sudden or unexpected death from natural causes may be the result of a wide range of sometimes extraordinary disorders. Although atherosclerotic coronary artery disease is by far the most frequent cause of sudden death, there are a number of differential diagnoses to consider:

Severe forms of general atherosclerosis with stenosing coronary sclerosis and cerebral sclerosis are diseases which, as a result of long-standing hypertension, nicotine abuse, metabolic disorders, or diabetes, among others, can lead to vascular wall rupture, stenosis, thrombosis, etc., with lethal hemorrhage, as in the case of massive intracerebral hypertonic hemorrhage. Severe atherosclerotic findings are often observed histologically:

- Rarefaction of the arterial media with elastic fiber fragmentation
- Intimal fibrosis, cholesterol crystal deposition
- Basophilic, partly tubular wall calcification
- High-grade atherosclerotic vascular narrowing

However, sudden cardiac death in relatively young men with no coronary atherosclerosis has also been reported. This type of sudden unexplained death has been known as "Pokkuri death syndrome" (PDS) in Japan, "Lai Tai" in Thailand, "bangungut" in the Philippines, "dream disease" in Hawaii, and "sudden unexpected nocturnal death syndrome" among South Asian immigrants in the USA (Nakajima et al. 2010).

14.1.2 Aneurysms

Aneurysms which can lead to lethal complications, generally hemorrhage following rupture, include:

- Atherosclerotic aneurysms, in particular infrarenal aortic aneurysms
- Congenital, occasionally multiple, aneurysms, e.g., of aortic, coronary, or cerebral arteries
- Aneurysms of the heart wall, generally following previous myocardial infarct

- Dissecting aneurysms, generally of the aorta, but rarely also of other arteries (splenic or coronary arteries, etc. (D'Ovidio et al. 2015)
- Iatrogenic aneurysms (Lau 2002)
- Ductal aneurysm

All forms of aneurysm can thrombose as a secondary event or even demonstrate accompanying inflammatory reactions. These inflammatory infiltrates are often encountered only focally and need to be distinguished from primary inflammatory vascular disease, which could itself be the cause of the aneurysm. Unusual localizations of aneurysms have also been described in the recent forensic literature (Desinan et al. 2010; Kodikara and Sivasubramanium 2009). In some cases, histological investigations can reveal, e.g., vasculitis or fibromuscular dysplasia as the cause of (dissecting) aneurysm or provide evidence of thrombosis and fungal colonization (Ortmann et al. 2010; Hagemeier et al. 2009).

14.1.3 Dissecting Aortic Aneurysm in Idiopathic Cystic Medial Necrosis

Aortic dissection is defined as follows: penetration of blood into the vessel wall through a tear in the intima, forming a split between coats or medial laminae that may be complicated by rupture; it is due to degeneration of connective or elastic fibers of the media, and the main predisposing factors include hypertension, Marfan syndrome, idiopathic cystic medial necrosis, pregnancy, some congenital cardiovascular diseases, as well as damage due to arterial catheterization or aortic valve surgery (Desinan et al. 2010; Dermengiu et al. 2009). In individual cases, consideration should be given to whether aortic dissection could have occurred in the setting of resuscitation measures (Patterson et al. 1974; Nelson and Ashley 1965). Erdheim–Gsell medial necrosis is a significant cause of aortic dissection and aortic rupture, and there is only a short time window available between onset of symptoms and administration of the necessary treatment (Maeso Madronero et al. 2000).

An acute dissection of the ascending aorta must be treated surgically as soon as possible, since the mortality rate in untreated dissections increases by 1–2% hourly. A higher frequency of medial degeneration associated with hypertension is well known (Carlson et al. 1970; Gore 1953; Rottino 1939). A long history of hypertension is reported in nearly 90% of all cases of aortic dissection (Stegmann 1987).

Dissecting aortic aneurysm is known as a cause of sudden unexpected death; however, clinical symptoms may be confused with those of myocardial infarction (Stegmann 1987). Dissection extending to the pericardium leads to acute pericardial tamponade; ruptures in the (usually left) pleural cavity or free abdominal cavity are less common. Entry and exit sites of aortic dissection are often in the ascending aorta (type A); aneurysms not involving the aorta are classified as type B (Li et al. 2015). Whether a genetic component is a causal factor in aortic dissection is currently the subject of discussion (Robertson et al. 2016). When reaching the origin of the ascending aorta, a dissecting aneurysm can lead to luminal compression in the large branching coronary arteries resulting in acute death. Cases where hemorrhage is absent are known as "bloodless aortic dissection" (Dettmeyer et al. 1998b; Dickens and Khoo 1993; Cambria et al. 1988).

In cases of "bloodless aortic dissection," an alternative pathophysiological mechanism must be discussed: increasing hypertension during progressive extension of the dissection, followed by sudden disruption of the subendothelially localized cardiac conduction system. The aortic dissection may also cause variations in blood pressure due to the undulating surface of the intimal layer, which may be enhanced by simultaneously increasing blood levels of catecholamines due to intensive chest pain. A comparative mechanism of sudden heart failure has been proposed in cases of aortic stenosis and coarctation of the aorta, which are known to cause sudden death (Frank et al. 1973).

Idiopathic medial necrosis is a frequent cause of dissecting aneurysm (Fig. 14.1) (Maeso Madronero et al. 2000; Leu and Leu 1988).

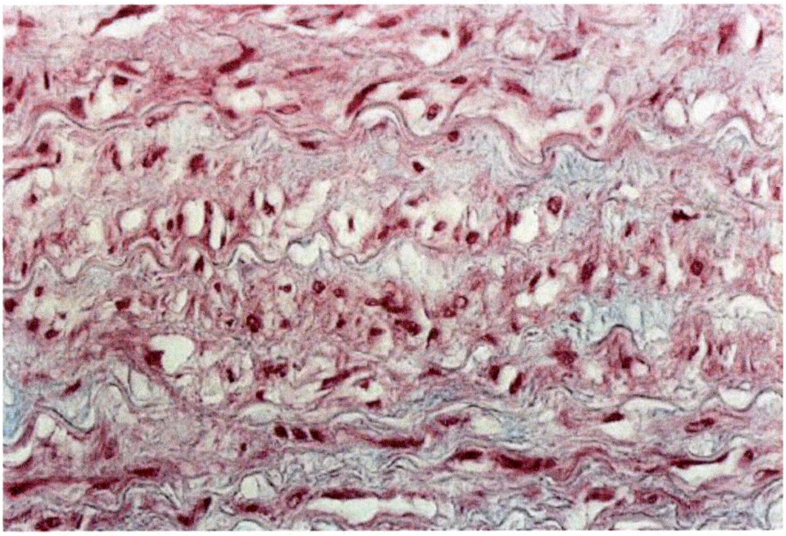

Fig. 14.1 Idiopathic microcystic medial necrosis as the cause of a dissecting aneurysm (H&E ×400)

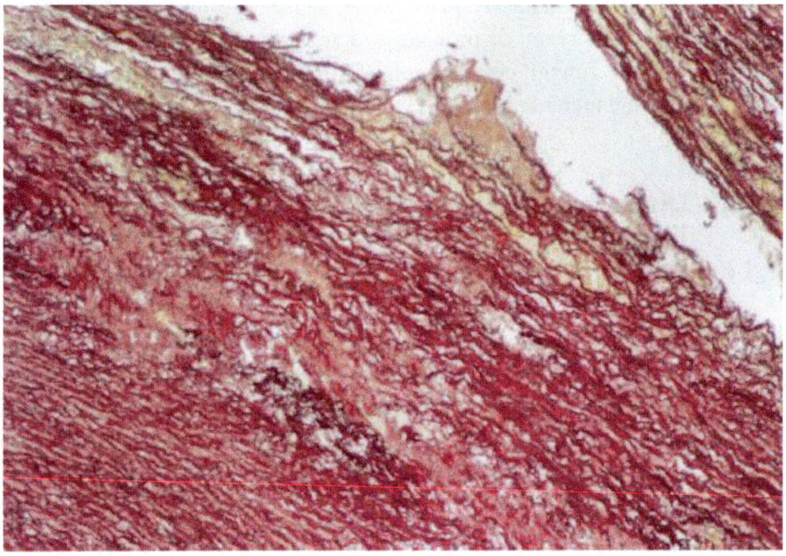

Fig. 14.2 Dissecting aneurysm of the descending aorta with longitudinal splitting of the vascular wall and fragmentation of elastic fibers in idiopathic medial necrosis (Elastica van Gieson ×40)

It was first described by Gsell (1928) and Erdheim (1929a, b) as a disease entity of the aortic vascular wall (Guitierrez et al. 1991; Hirst and Gore 1976). Pathogenetically, it leads to destruction of the aortic or arterial media with destruction of smooth muscle fibers, mesenchyme, and elastic fibers (Fig. 14.2). The degree of severity can vary greatly. Histologically, noninflammatory mucoid degeneration in the arterial media with only scant rarefaction and splitting of elastic fibers is seen; this can be easily detected using Elastica van Gieson staining. Necrosis and microcysts can only be detected in some cases; the extracellular matrix contains Alcian Blue-positive mucopolysaccharides (chondroitin sulfuric acid), starting most likely in the inner third of the arterial media (Fig. 14.3). In the case of extensive findings, muscular, collagen, and elastic fibers which have been forced apart can be seen, even in the absence of light microscopic confirmation of necrosis of elastic elements (Bode-Jänisch et al. 2012; Jungmann et al. 2010; Schmidt et al. 1996; Nashima et al. 1990; Schnapka et al. 1983; Schlatman and

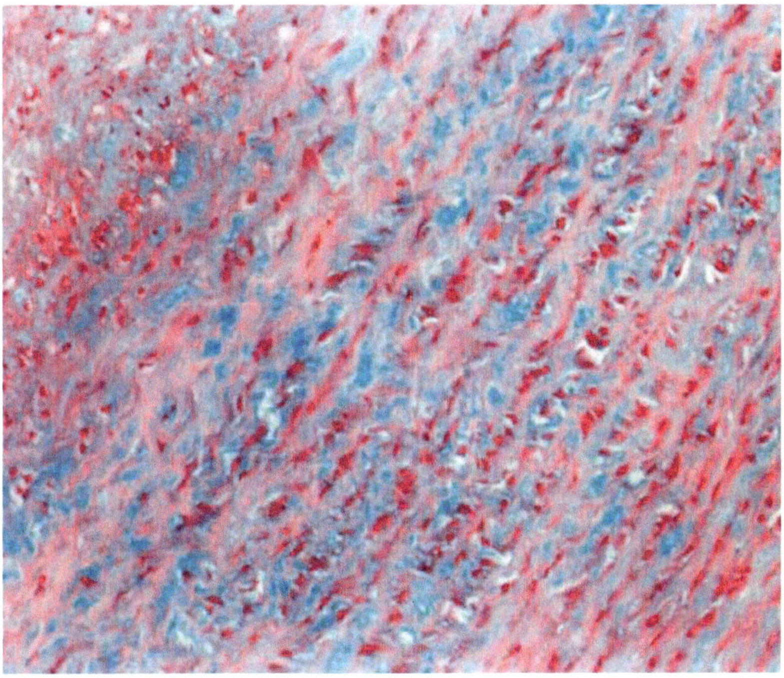

Fig. 14.3 Extensive Alcian Blue-positive mucopolysaccharides in the wall of the descending aorta in dissecting aortic aneurysm in the setting of idiopathic medial necrosis (×100)

Becker 1977; Brinkmann 1974; Anagnostopoulos et al. 1972; Burman 1960).

The severity of shrinkage and fragmentation of elastic fibers correlates with the extent of arterial intimal sclerosis, atrophy, and fibrosis of the muscular media. The vasa vasorum also demonstrates changes (Sorger 1968):

- Muscle hyperplasia
- Vascular ectasia
- Hyaline fusion of the vascular wall
- Endothelial swelling
- Intimal proliferation
- Intravascular thrombosis formation

Scant mucoid deposits can occur at any age and have no pathological relevance.

The term "segmental mediolytic arteritis"—often encountered in Anglo-Saxon countries—is ambiguous since no inflammatory vascular process is present (Lie 1992). Dissecting aneurysms are more rarely found in other arteries, such as the temporal, internal carotid, medial cerebral, basilar, coronary, splenic, femoral, anterior tibial, and vertebral arteries (Leu 1993). In such cases, histological investigation of vascular wall specimens can help clarify the cause. Cases of aortic dissection following cocaine consumption have been described (Palmiere et al. 2004).

14.1.4 Marfan Syndrome

Marfan syndrome is one of the most frequent genetic connective tissue disorders with a prevalence of 1 in 5000 Europeans (Wang et al. 2016; Hugar et al. 2014; von Kodolitsch and Robinson 2007; Byard 2006). It is an inherited connective tissue disorder with mutation on the fibrillin-1 gene (more than 500 identified mutations) (Klintschar et al. 2009; Byard 2006). Family clustering has been described (Hirani et al. 2008) and an autosomal dominant trait with complete penetrance but with phenotypic expression that varies considerably, both between and within families. Affected individuals develop varying patterns of organ involvement including the cardiovascular, ocular, skeletal, and pulmonary systems, as well as the skin and dura (Judge and Dietz 2005). Undiagnosed Marfan patients usually die from acute aortic dissection or rupture and thus have an average life expectancy of about 32 years (Klintschar et al. 2009; Hirani et al. 2008; Hugar et al. 2014).

In Marfan syndrome, the aortic arch is particularly affected, demonstrating aneurysmal bulging which forms the point of origin of a dissecting aneurysm, as well as dilation of the aortic valve ring. Sudden, unexpected, and spontaneous rupture is possible (Bratzke and Wojahn 1977; Melsen 1973). If specimens are taken from the appropriate site, localized destruction of elastic fibers can be seen histologically (Elastica van Gieson staining).

The differential diagnosis between idiopathic cystic medial necrosis (Erdheim–Gsell) and changes seen in Marfan syndrome cannot be reliably made using histology, since both demonstrate loss and fragmentation of elastic fibers as well as pseudocystic areas in the aortic media with deposits of Alcian Blue-positive mucoid substances (Sariola et al. 1986; Saruk and Eisenstein 1977). However, in contrast to Marfan syndrome, there is no history of extravascular findings in idiopathic cystic medial necrosis, either in the deceased or their relatives. The differential diagnosis should take Ehlers–Danlos syndrome (Banaschak et al. 2002) or Loeys–Dietz syndrome into consideration; Marchesani syndrome also belongs to this group of diseases. Cases of familial dissecting aortic aneurysm have been reported (Schürch 1970). Even in younger people, a dissecting aneurysm should be considered (Gore 1953), whereby it is in precisely such cases that a genetic disposition is possible (Rippberger et al. 2009). In the case of death as a result of a ruptured dissecting aneurysm while performing an insured activity, issues relating to expert opinions may be raised, in some cases even medicolegal problems (Schmidt et al. 1996; Vock and Schulz 1986; Brinkmann 1974; Naeve and Brinkmann 1971). Distinction must be made in the differential diagnosis of dissecting aneurysm in the setting of atherosclerosis.

14.1.5 Ehlers–Danlos Syndrome

Ehlers–Danlos syndrome (EDS) is a connective tissue disorder characterized by the inability to produce sufficient amounts of collagen or a defect in the structure of collagen (Banaschak et al. 2002). EDS type IV, the vascular type, is marked by four clinical characteristics:

- Thin skin with visible veins
- Distinctive facial features
- Rupture of vessels and/or viscera
- Easy bruising/hematomas

While representing only 4% of the EDS cases, type IV poses the risk of premature death from spontaneous arterial, intestinal, or uterine rupture and may remain undiagnosed until postmortem examination (Shields et al. 2010; Prahlow and Wagner 2005; Wimmer et al. 1996). The median survival is approximately 48 years (Shields et al. 2010). Most deaths are caused by arterial dissection or rupture, involving a thoracic or abdominal vessel; cases with incidental myocardial infarction are rare (Gilchrist and Duflou 2005). There are also rare cases with type IV EDS presenting as sudden infant death (Byard et al. 1990) or leading to fatal hemoptysis (Yost et al. 1995). Additionally, there are reports where the cause of death was hemorrhage of the central nervous system. Histology and electron microscopy may demonstrate the findings of arterial wall thinning, decreased collagen content, and distorted collagen fibril structure. In routine histology (H&E, Elastica van Gieson), there are often no diagnostic microscopic pathological findings. Immunohistochemical detection of collagen type III reveals a significant reduction in the aortic media and adventitia, within the renal interstitium and the intrarenal vascular walls, as well as in the alveolar capillary regions of the lungs in particular (Banaschak et al. 2002). EDS can lead to myocardial infarction due to coronary artery dissection (Adés et al. 1995), to rupture of the coronary, thoracic, and other arteries (Aru et al. 1999; Collins et al. 1999; Evans and Fraser 1996; Nerlich et al. 1994), as well as to aneurysms of varying sizes (Eriksen et al. 1992). Nontraumatic vascular or bowel ruptures may cause sudden death even in children or adolescents (Aru et al. 1999; Kinnane et al. 1995; Soucy et al. 1990). The postmortem diagnosis can be supported by fibroblast cultures or by immunohistochemical examination of organ tissue (Reis et al. 1998). In rare cases, EDS may simulate child abuse (Saulsbury and Hayden 1985; Owen and Durst 1984; Roberts et al. 1984). EDS can also cause sudden death in an infant in extremely rare cases (Byard et al. 1990).

14.1.6 Aneurysms in Other Arteries

In addition to atherosclerotic aneurysms of varying forms, other vascular wall changes can infrequently lead to dissecting aneurysms; primary vasculitides should be borne in mind in particular as the cause of secondary aneurysms. While aortic dissection frequently extends into its branches, isolated dissections of peripheral arteries, such as renal, coronary, pulmonary, and carotid vessels, are exceptional (Byard et al. 2017). In contrast, aneurysms of the visceral arteries are not a rare feature with the splenic artery being the most common site (Desinan et al. 2010; Thierauf et al. 2007; Saukko and Knight 2004; Merrell and Gloviczki 1992; Cosgrave et al. 1947). Ductal aneurysms are very rare. A primary defect in the internal elastic lamina of the ductal wall is assumed to be causal. A distinction is made between true ductal aneurysms, which can occur either as fusiform or dissecting variants, and so-called traction aneurysms, in which indentations in the aortic wall are drawn into the insertion of the ductus arteriosus (Früchtnicht and Albrecht 1998). Although atherosclerotic aortic aneurysms predominate in the majority of cases, there are reports on dissecting, as well as other, aneurysms, e.g., of the subclavian artery, the vertebral artery, the renal artery, the coronary artery (Makino et al. 2015; Jung et al. 2013; Erbersdobler and Tsokos 2006), or the splenic artery, sometimes in the setting of vasculitis (Desinan et al. 2010); isolated cases during pregnancy have also been reported (Srettabunjong 2013; Barbesier et al. 2013; Jung et al. 2013). For vertebral artery dissections, there are more reports on a traumatic cause of rupture (Kaiser et al. 2008; Galtés et al. 2012; Kristoffersen et al. 2012). As in basilar artery and coronary artery aneurysms, there is evidence of a genetic predisposition also in aortic dissection (Rippberger et al. 2009). In the case of traumatic aneurysm, histological tests should be performed to rule out primary vasculitis as a competing explanation for the aneurysm (Kaiser et al. 2008). The detection of hemorrhage at a survival time of approximately 3 days and longer, as well as the detection of siderophages, supports the assumption of a traumatic etiology of the aneurysm in the absence of primary vascular disease (Galtés et al. 2012; Kristoffersen et al. 2012; Kaiser et al. 2008) (Fig. 14.4).

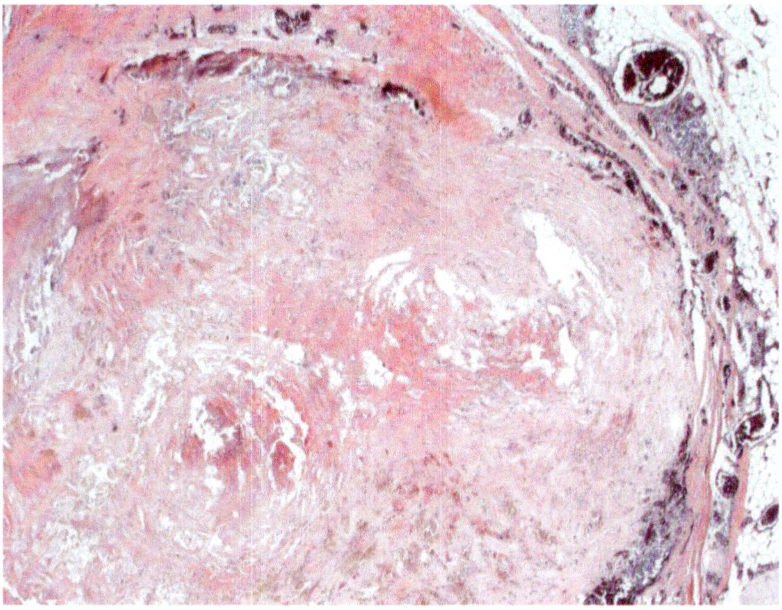

Fig. 14.4 Peripheral region of a thrombosed left circumflex artery aneurysm (H&E ×40)

14.1.6.1 Osler–Weber–Rendu Syndrome

Osler–Weber–Rendu syndrome, also known as *hereditary hemorrhagic telangiectasia (HHT)*, is a genetically inherited disease (Byard et al. 2001). Pulmonary arteriovenous malformations are predominantly found (Fig. 14.5); in the case of rupture or fistula formation, these can lead to hemothorax and death due to bleeding. More than half of all pulmonary arteriovenous malformations are seen in patients with Osler–Weber–Rendu syndrome (Ishikawa et al. 2010). If the pulmonary malformation is located in the subpleural region, rupture can rapidly result in hemothorax. If localized elsewhere in the lung, bleeding in peripheral branches of the bronchial tree and death due to blood aspiration are conceivable. From a differential diagnostic perspective, primary lung cancer, tumor metastasis, other vascular tumors (hemangiomas), and—as a rarity—extrauterine endometriosis in lung tissue (Morcos et al. 2006) should be considered.

In the differential diagnosis of Osler–Weber–Rendu syndrome, the *Klippel–Trenaunay syndrome*, a congenital angiodysplasia of venous vessels characterized by three main symptoms, cutaneous vascular nevi, hypertrophy of a limb, and varicosis or venous malformations, has to be pointed out (Pourhassan et al. 2007).

14.2 Arteritis

Of the underlying diseases with possible involvement of the coronary arteries, panarteritis nodosa, thromboangiitis obliterans, giant-cell arteritis (Shields et al. 2012; Pery et al. 1983), luetic arteritis (Frank et al. 1999; Glenewinkel et al. 1996), Takayasu's arteritis, Churg–Strauss syndrome (Schön et al. 2005), and rheumatic disease are mentioned in the literature.

14.2.1 Syphilitic Mesaortitis

Syphilitic aortitis is a complication of tertiary stage syphilis; histologically, up to 80% of patients show involvement of the cardiovascular system. Between 10 and 20 years may elapse from the time of infection to the clinical picture of syphilitic aortitis, although a faster disease course is possible. In addition to uncomplicated syphilitic aortitis, syphilitic aortic aneurysm, syphilitic endocarditis of aortic valve in particular with aortic insufficiency, as well as syphilitic

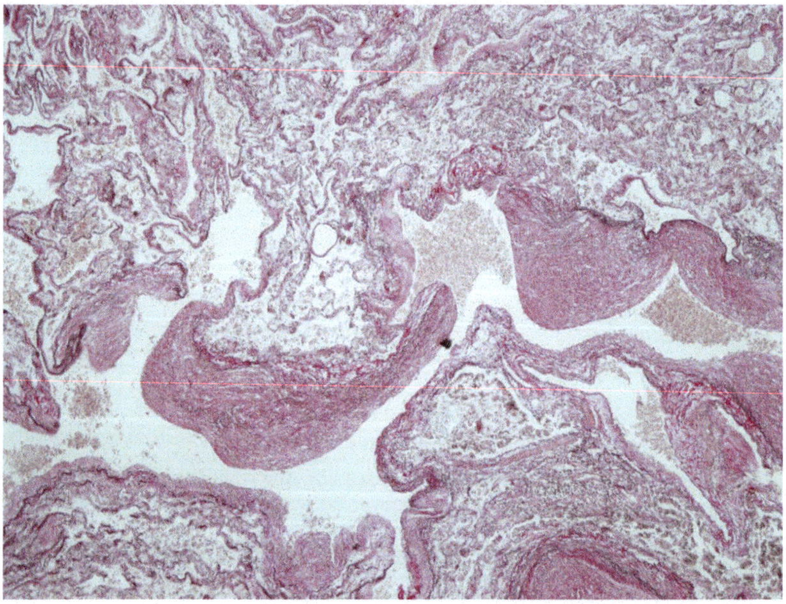

Fig. 14.5 Pulmonary *arteriovenous malformation* in Osler–Weber–Rendu syndrome with fatal blood aspiration following malformation rupture (Elastica van Gieson ×40)

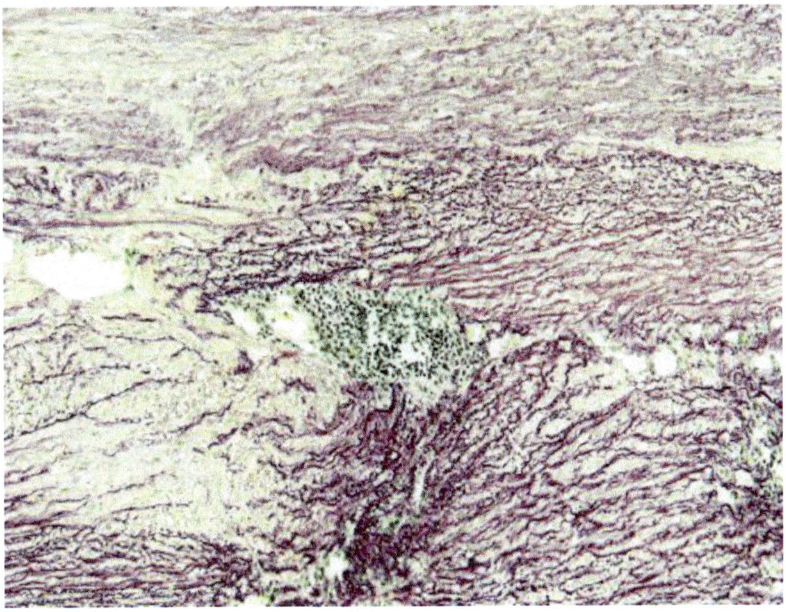

Fig. 14.6 Syphilitic aortitis with focal loss of fiber structures in the aortic media, as well as focal inflammatory infiltration with lymphocytes and plasma cells (Elastica van Gieson ×100)

coronary artery ostial stenosis may develop (Glenewinkel et al. 1996; Scharfman et al. 1950). The histological picture includes marked fibrous thickening of the aortic wall with lymphocytic and plasma cell infiltrates at the border between intima and media, in the media, and in the adventitial connective tissue (Fig. 14.6). These infiltrates may be more pronounced around the vasa vasorum. The elastic fibers of the aortic or arterial media are rarefied and fragmented and partially replaced by collagenous scar tissue. The histological picture described here, however, requires serological confirmation prior to a definitive diagnosis (Gormsen 1984).

14.2.2 Suppurative Aortitis in Atherosclerosis

The spectrum of rare primary inflammatory vascular diseases also includes suppurative arteritis, more rarely primary coronaritis (Dettmeyer et al. 1998a), and hypersensitivity angiitis. These vascular diseases can have a fatal outcome as a result of acute obturating thrombosis, vascular stenosis, or rupture. Histopathologically, granulomatous, giant-cell containing, and lymphoplasma cellular arteritis can be found (Cassling et al. 1985; Hushang et al. 1984). Only few cases describe inflammatory aneurysm of the abdominal aorta in the setting of existing coronaritis (Cohle and Lie 1988; Pereira et al. 1981).

The severity of the inflammatory process can vary greatly: on the one hand, findings may reveal scant inflammatory infiltration of the vascular wall and perivascular tissue, while on the other, dense lymphocytic infiltrates may be present accompanied by germinal center formation in longer disease courses. Hypersensitivity angiitis should be considered in the differential diagnosis if eosinophilic granulocytes are present. Nonspecific angiitis is frequently found, while suppurative aortitis in the setting of infected aortic atherosclerosis (Fig. 14.7), which can lead to vascular wall rupture, is rare (Eplinius and Hädrich 2014). Aortitis as the cause of death in infants is extremely rare (Schäfer and Püschel 1996).

14.2.3 Giant-Cell Arteritis

Intramyocardial vascular involvement in the context of systemic vascular wall inflammation is occasionally seen in the form of uncharacteristic and nonspecific vasculitis (Fig. 14.8; Table 14.1).

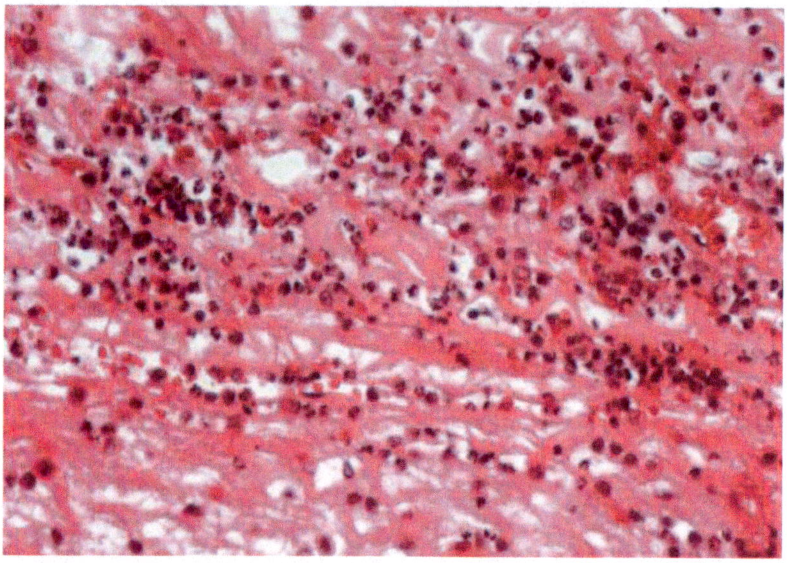

Fig. 14.7 Acute rupture of suppurative aortitis in severe atherosclerosis (H&E ×200)

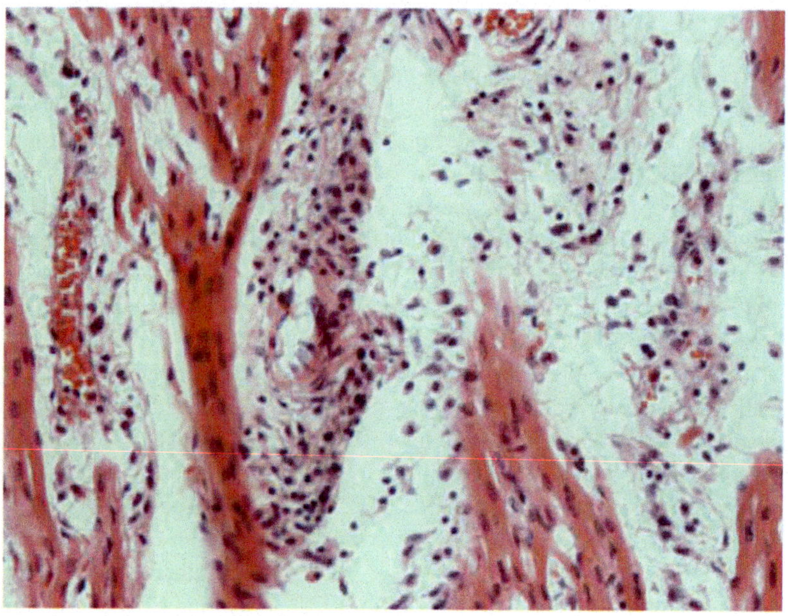

Fig. 14.8 Nonspecific vasculitis of peripheral intramyocardial arterial branches (H&E ×200)

Giant-cell arteritis occurs as temporal arteritis; the aorta is less frequently affected, as are the coronary arteries. Thus, giant-cell arteritis could be proven histologically as the cause of aortic rupture (Pery et al. 1983; Ainsworth and Gresham 1961); coronary artery involvement is also possible in giant-cell arteritis (Fig. 14.9) (Karger and Fechner 2006; Kumar et al. 2002). Giant-cell arteritis is an arterial disease of unclear etiology seen in the elderly, in the form of temporal arteritis and rheumatic polymyalgia (Salvarani et al. 2002). Appearing in almost all arteries, it was first described in 1932 (Horton et al. 1932). In the case of coronary artery involvement, myocardial infarction (Karger and Fechner 2006; Martin et al. 1980) or dissecting aneurysm (Magarey 1950) may result, both with fatal outcomes (Cohle et al. 1982).

Immunohistochemically, the giant cells react positively to the macrophage-specific antibody CD68 (Wagner et al. 1994) and are negative for the antibodies MRP 8 and 14 (Karger and

Table 14.1 Differential diagnosis of giant-cell arteritis

Term	Characteristic histological findings	Preferential localization
Syphilitic mesaortitis (mesaortitis syphilitica, lues)	Focal necrosis of the aortic media; lymphoplasma cellular infiltrate perivascularly around the vasa vasorum	Ascending aorta
Takayasu's arteritis	Granulation tissue with polynuclear giant cells, fibrosis of the aortic intima, elastic fiber degeneration, and fragmentation	Aortic arch, aortic arch arteries
Giant-cell arteritis	Giant cells (CD68+) in granulation tissue, intimal fibrosis, "skip" lesions, degeneration, and fragmentation of elastic fibers	Aorta, primarily large and medium arteries, rarely coronary arteries
Panarteritis nodosa	Fibrinoid necrosis, followed by scarred granulation tissue, and sectorial lesions	Medium and small muscle-like arteries
Coronaritis	As giant-cell arteritis; primary isolated coronaritis without giant cells, with thick lymphocytic infiltrate, and germinal centers	As giant-cell arteritis, usually involvement of all coronary artery; as primary arteritis, segmental involvement

Modified from Pery et al. (1983)

Fechner 2006). The cores of the giant cells are frequently arranged in a horseshoe or circular form. The giant cells are localized in close association to fragmented fibers of the internal elastic lamina (Kimmelstiel et al. 1952) and are often accompanied by a dense lymphocyte-rich inflammatory infiltrate of all three wall layers. Additionally, neutrophil granulocytes and macrophages can be observed. The arterial wall is thickened, and a concentric narrowing of the lumen by intimal hyperplasia may be present (Karger and Fechner 2006).

Churg–Strauss syndrome (CSS). This rare syndrome with an incidence of 1–3 cases per 1 million individuals per year is characterized by systemic eosinophilic granulomatous vasculitis, in later stages with involvement of all internal organs including life-threatening eosinophilic myocarditis. Inflammatory eosinophilic infiltrates can show granuloma-like arrangement and necrosis. Without histological examination of tissue samples, it is not possible to correctly diagnose eosinophilic myocarditis and/or perimyocarditis. The presence of extravascular eosinophilic blood cells appears to be the most relevant diagnostic criterium for Churg–Strauss syndrome. Most important differential diagnoses include rheumatologic diseases and allergic asthma (Schön et al. 2005; Noth et al. 2003).

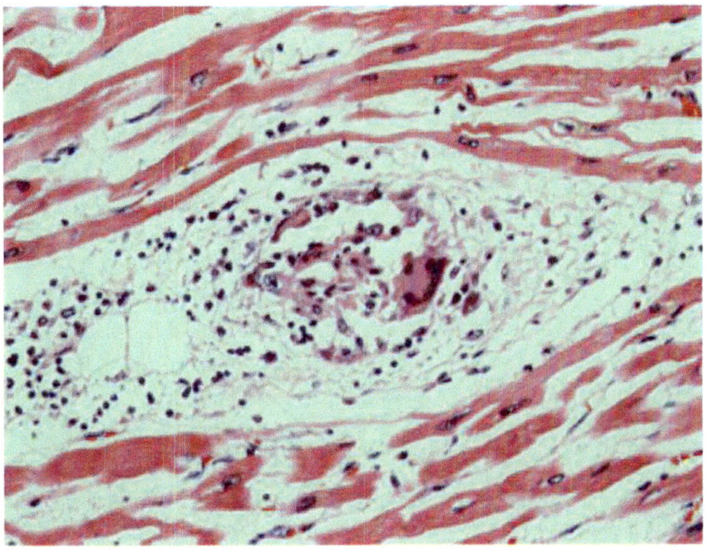

Fig. 14.9 Intramyocardial giant-cell arteritis in peripheral coronary artery branches (H&E ×200)

14.2.4 Isolated Coronary Arteritis

There are numerous case reports in the literature on inflammatory changes in the coronary arteries as a cause of sudden cardiac death (Inokuchi et al. 2014; Norita et al. 2012; Dettmeyer et al. 1998a; August and Holzhausen 1992; Fujita et al. 1992; Paul et al. 1990; Tanaka et al. 1988; Lie 1987; Mitchinson et al. 1984). Isolated coronaritis, however, is very rare. Macroscopically, marked thickening of the segmentally involved coronary wall is conspicuous, with clear luminal narrowing. Inflammatory changes can be seen in a circular pattern. Histologically, giant-cell arteritis of the coronary arteries or granulomatous arteritis may be present (Aufderheide et al. 1981). In the absence of evidence of polynuclear giant cells, and in the case of isolated, segmental involvement of the coronary arteries, coronaritis demonstrates a dense, primarily lymphocytic inflammatory infiltrate, in addition to which germinal centers may be present (Fig. 14.10), while densely aggregated hemosiderin deposits may be found in granulation tissue (Fig. 14.11). Pronounced coronaritis can be a plausible cause of death. Neutrophil granulocytes are barely detectable, while eosinophil granulocytes may be present in only scant numbers (Kajihara et al. 2013).

14.2.5 Takayasu's Arteritis

Takayasu's arteritis is a very rare, special form of arteritis, affecting women more commonly than men (Johnston et al. 2002; Gravanis 2000; Amano and Suzuki 1991; Lupi-Herrera et al. 1977; Rosen and Gaton 1972). Typically, segmental involvement of one artery is seen, while vascular occlusion is possible in smaller arteries. Coronary artery involvement can be the cause of sudden death (Krompecher et al.

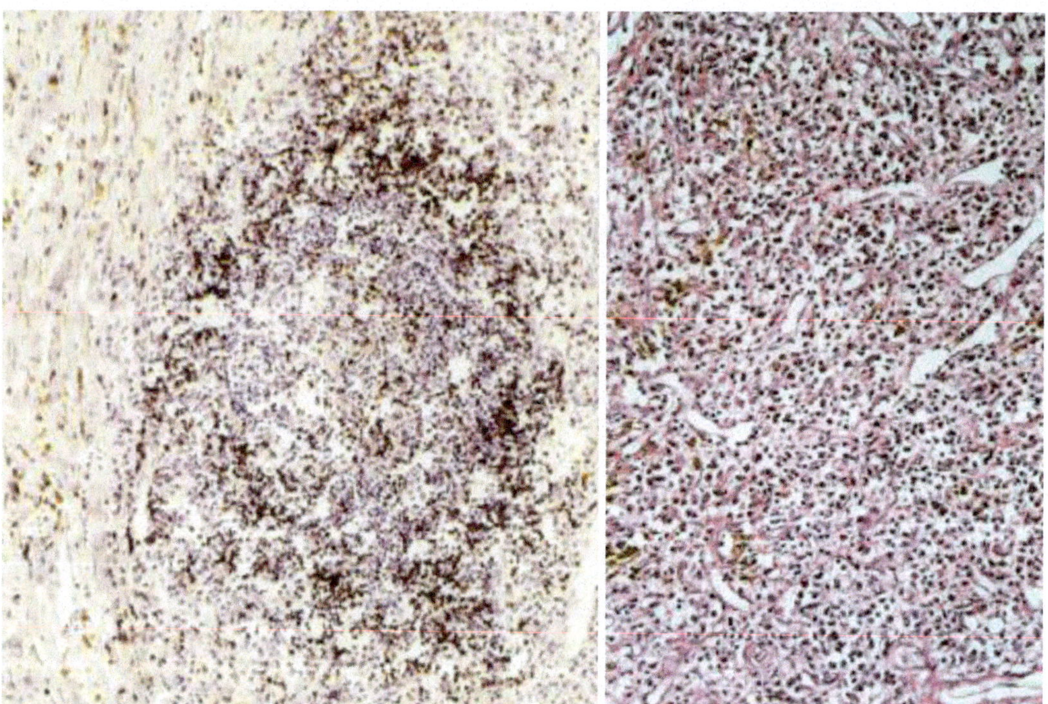

Fig. 14.10 Lethal coronaritis: pronounced stenosing coronaritis with germinal center formation in the circular, stenosing lymphoplasma cellular infiltrates within the vascular wall and in perivascular tissue; immunohistochemical detection of CD3+ T-lymphocytes (CD3 ×100; left); section of the left coronary artery wall with dense lymphoplasma cellular infiltration in loose granulation tissue (H&E ×200; right)

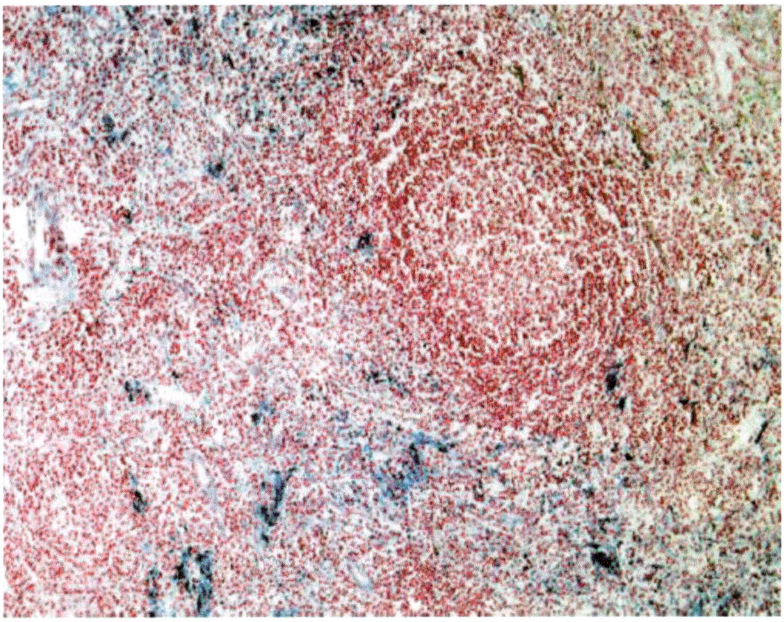

Fig. 14.11 Lethal coronaritis: inflammatory granulation tissue with densely aggregated lymphocytes, plasma cells, scant eosinophil granulocytes, and siderophages (Prussian blue ×200)

1984). Histologically, segmental lymphoplasma cellular inflammation of an artery wall section can be seen at acute and subacute stages; the arterial intima and adventitia in particular may be severely affected. Inflammatory cells may be embedded in a well-vascularized, fine connective tissue. Depending on stage, areas of fibrosis may already be found, while inflammatory cells can infiltrate the arterial media, which generally remains clearly discernible. Necrosis and granulomas are rare; single polynuclear isolated giant cells have been described. Approximately 30% of cases of Takayasu's arteritis show coronary artery involvement, the proximal sections being those mostly commonly affected. Isolated involvement of a cardiac artery is very rare (Seguchi et al. 1990; Rosen and Gaton 1972; Krompecher et al. 1984). Occasionally, the disease can involve the aortic base, with extension into the aortic valve, coronary arteries, and interventricular septum, causing sudden death. Segmental involvement of the abdominal aorta produces aneurysms. Newly formed lesions may be found in the splenic and renal arteries (Aufderheide et al. 1981).

14.2.6 Kawasaki Disease

Kawasaki disease (mucocutaneous lymph node syndrome, MLNS), first identified in 1967 by Tomisaku Kawasaki, is an acute systemic but self-limiting vasculitis of childhood that can result in coronary artery aneurysms, myocardial infarction, and sudden death in previously healthy children (Rowley and Shulman 2010; Wood and Tulloh 2009; Suzuki et al. 2000; Bayer Kristensen and Østergaard Kristensen 1994; Althoff 1990; Landing and Larson 1987; Tanaka et al. 1986; Missliwetz et al. 1981; Yutani et al. 1981; Kawasaki et al. 1974). In more than 20% of patients, severe inflammation of the vasa vasorum led to coronary arteritis with aneurysm formation, thrombosis, and severe fibrous stenosis (Fineschi et al. 1999). Morbidity and mortality are mainly associated with the development of coronary aneurysms (Canino-Rodriguez and Cox 2008; Murai et al. 1989; Schultz 1989). Of unknown etiology, it is the most common cause of acquired heart disease in young children (Ashrafi et al. 2007). The intense inflammatory process has a predilection for the coronary arteries, resulting in the development of aneurysmal lesions, arterial thrombotic occlusion, or, potentially, sudden death. Giant aneurysms due to Kawasaki disease can rupture, presenting histological findings with aggregations of neutrophils containing myeloperoxidase and neutrophil elastase scattered in chains over the aneurysm wall. These findings suggest that destruction of the wall by an enzyme may cause aneurysm rupture (Sunagawa et al. 2008). Cases with late sudden death from obliteration of the lumen of the full length of the left anterior descending coronary artery are reported (McConnell et al. 1998). The clinical picture of Kawasaki disease varies greatly, and even extensive myocardial damage may be asymptomatic for many years (Kristensen and Kristensen 1994). Long-term follow-up of coronary artery lesions has revealed several characteristic features, including progressive localized stenosis, extensive recanalizations, and development of collateral arteries. Saccular aneurysms can be large with calcified, thin walls, composed of an internal fibrocalcified layer and an external thin tunica media (Fineschi et al. 1999). Late stages present without any signs of active inflammation. Usually, individuals affected were completely healthy, often asymptomatic, and without an identifiable risk factor for cardiovascular disease prior to the fatal event (Rozin et al. 2003). With regard to histological examinations, it is important to note that myocarditis also frequently occurs in the acute phase of Kawasaki syndrome, even in the case of prior normal echocardiography (Yoshikawa et al. 2006; Yonesaka et al. 1992). Juvenile periarteritis should be considered in the differential diagnosis (Missliwetz et al. 1981).

14.2.7 Drug-Associated Vasculitis

There are reports in the literature on necrotizing angiitis associated with drug abuse (Halpern and Citron 1971) and heroin-associated cerebral arteritis (King et al. 1978), as well on neurosurgical complications of heroin addiction including brain abscess and mycotic aneurysm (Amine 1997).

14.3 Heart Valve Defect: Endocarditis

Acute, frequently polypoid and occasionally bacterially infected inflammation of a heart valve (ulcerative polypoid endocarditis) is found primarily at the mitral and aortic valves. Macroscopic diagnosis can be confirmed histologically by evidence of partially fibrin-covered granulation tissue at the surface (Fig. 14.12), capillarization of valve tissue, and pos-

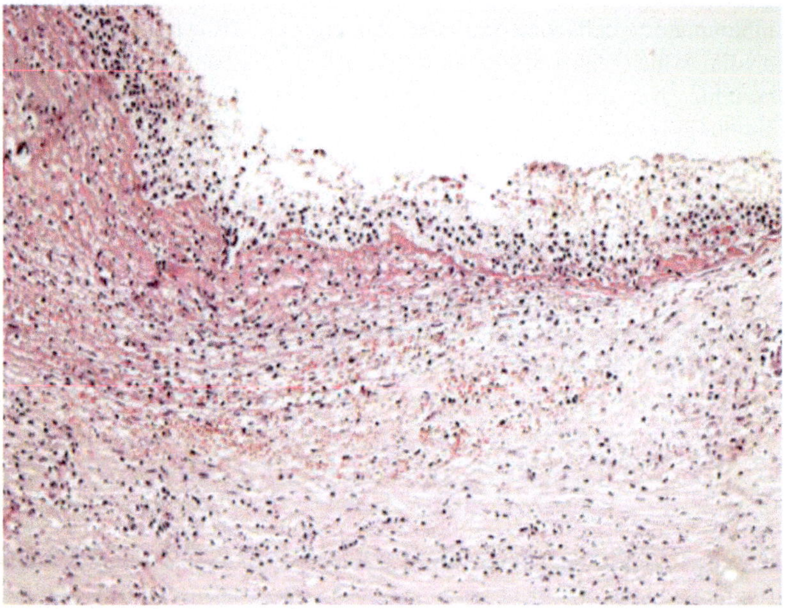

Fig. 14.12 Acute recurrent fibrinous endocarditis of the mitral valve: flat fibrin layer, infiltrated by a mixed-cell inflammatory infiltrate, edematous fibrous cardiac valve tissue (H&E ×100)

sible detection of an adherent thrombosis, in addition to which basophilic bacterial colonies can be seen in infective endocarditis. Inflammatory processes of longer standing may fibrose and reveal basophil calcium salt deposits (Fig. 14.13). Aortic bicuspid valve, infective endocarditis, and subaortic aneurysm appear to be associated (Saint-Martin et al. 2009). Post-inflammatory mitral valve stenosis can lead to hemosiderin-laden macrophages in the lungs (Fig. 14.14).

14.4 Amyloidosis

The spectrum of potentially lethal metabolic diseases relevant in forensic practice covers a multitude of diseases. In addition to congenital metabolic diseases or mitochondrial diseases [e.g., medium-chain acyl-CoA dehydrogenase deficiency (MCAD) in neonates and infants], diabetes (see Chap. 16), and mucoviscidosis, sudden unexpected death also occurs in various forms of

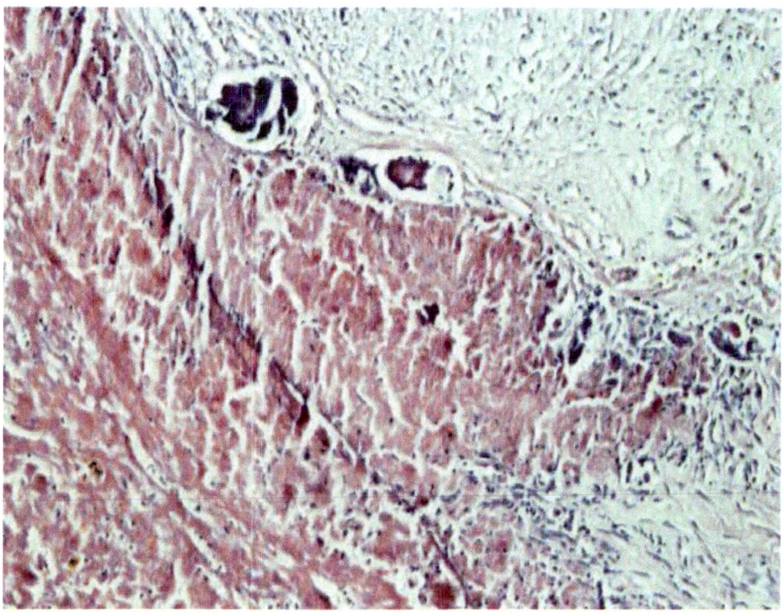

Fig. 14.13 Endocarditis of the aortic valve with dystrophic basophil calcification of the valve ring (H&E ×100)

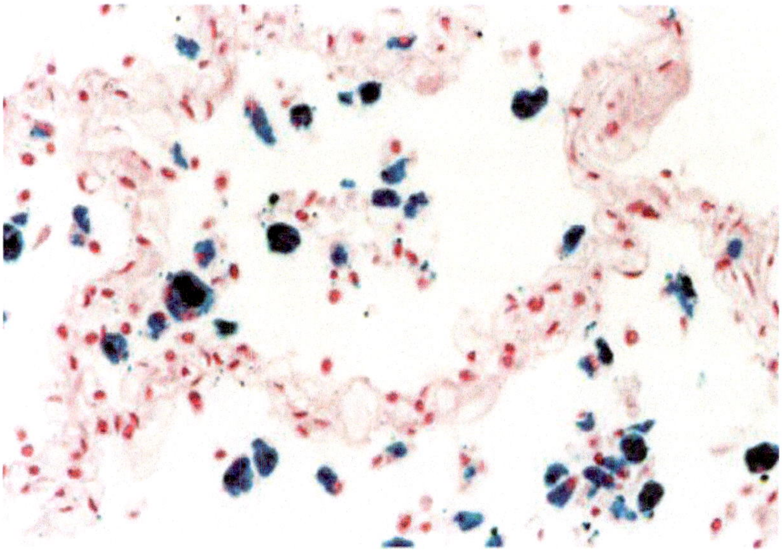

Fig. 14.14 Multiple hemosiderin-laden macrophages in the lungs following post-inflammatory mitral valve stenosis (Prussian blue ×400)

amyloidosis, Addison's disease (see Chap. 16), undetected pheochromocytoma (see Chap. 16), or cases of sudden death due to Fabry disease, which is regarded as an underdiagnosed disease (Hoffmann and Mayatepek 2009).

Amyloidosis. Amyloidosis is a multisystem disease. Amyloid deposits are found in various organs or organ systems. Amyloids are proteins of varying chemical structure, which forms the basis for the amyloid classification (Röcken 2009). In this context, a letter code is used, whereby, e.g., "A" represents amyloid fibril protein and the abbreviation "TTR" represents the precursor protein transthyretin (formerly prealbumin). Approximately 75 amyloid TTR variants have been identified to date (Merlini 2003).

Amyloidosis is a chronic disease which can long remain symptom-free and undetected; hereditary forms are also known (Gertz 1992). The distribution and extent of amyloid deposits determines the disease course, occasionally also the acuteness of death, particularly in the case of cardiac involvement (Röcken 2008). Amyloidosis is only macroscopically suspected in severe forms; here the conspicuously light red tissue has a markedly hardened consistency, in particular the spleen (so-called ham spleen), and the myocardium has a rubbery consistency.

Amyloid deposits can be detected in all organs and organ systems as homogeneous eosin red glycoprotein complexes using conventional amyloid staining or Congo red staining. Characteristic apple-green deposits are seen when visualized through crossed polarimetric filters; in fluorescence microscopy, amyloid deposits have a yellowish-orange color. The distribution pattern of the amyloid deposits in the organism enables typing as, e.g., cardiovascular-type amyloidosis (Kieninger et al. 2010). Amyloidosis can exhibit different protein structures and, likewise, can be classified on this basis, e.g., AA amyloidosis or ATTR amyloidosis. The most common systemic variant is an immunoglobulin-derived light chain (AL) amyloidosis (Morgenthal et al. 2016). A classification of myocardial amyloidosis based on the intensity of amyloid deposits has been proposed, whereby the degree of deposition was evaluated on the basis of visual judgment. At grade I, less than 25% of the myocardial area consisted of amyloid; at grade II, 25–50%; and at grade III, more than 50% (Kieninger et al. 2010). A distinction is made between various amyloid types depending on distribution patterns. In cardiovascular amyloidosis, primarily arteries have thickened vascular walls, containing striped, semicircular Congo red-positive amyloid deposits in the vascular wall media (Figs. 14.15 and 14.16); massive

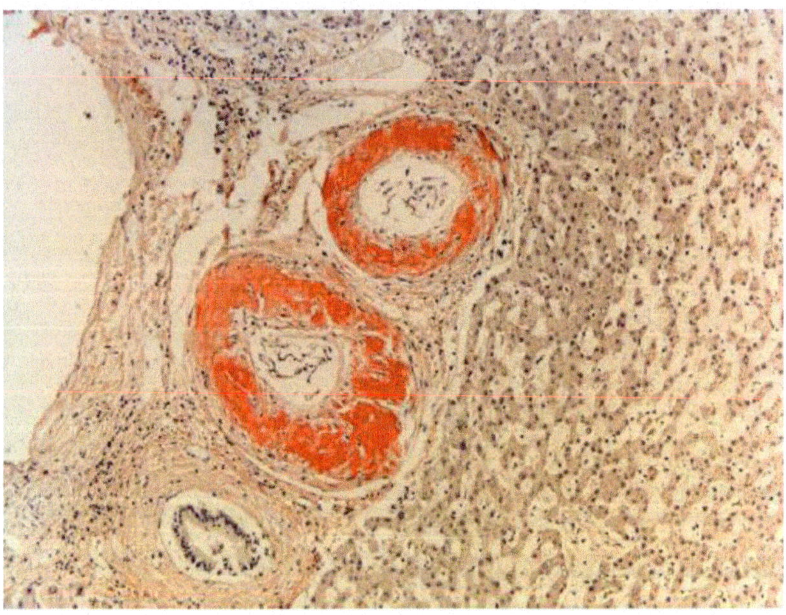

Fig. 14.15 Vascular amyloidosis with striped, Congo red-positive amyloid deposits in intrahepatic vascular branches (Congo red ×200)

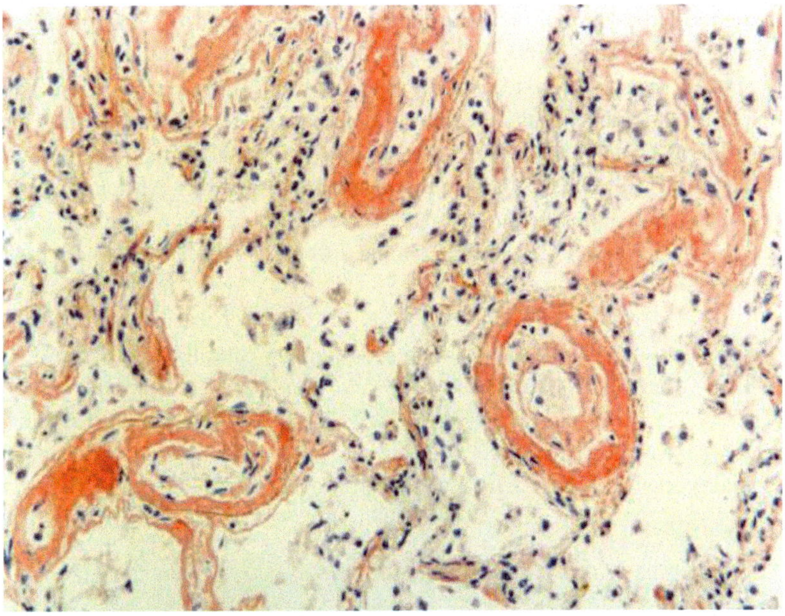

Fig. 14.16 Intra pulmonary vascular amyloidosis (Congo red ×200)

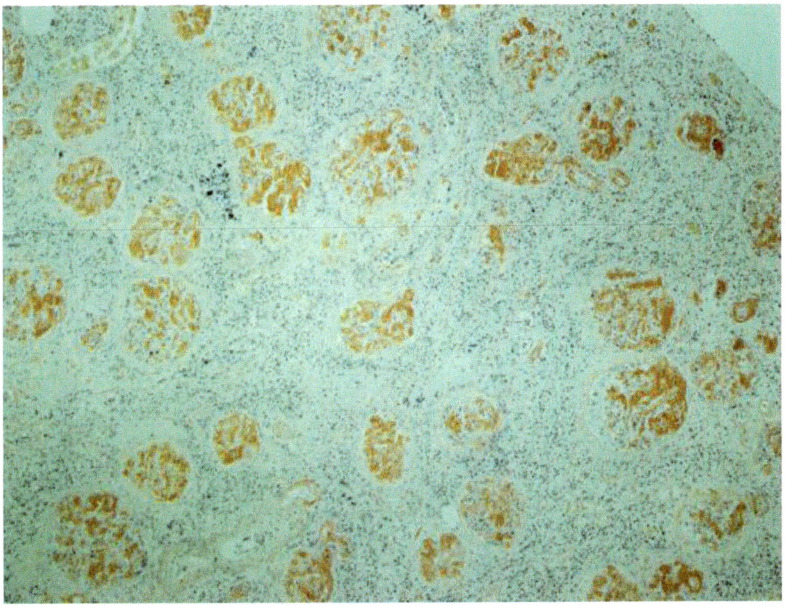

Fig. 14.17 Intrarenal amyloidosis with involvement of the glomeruli (Congo red ×40)

involvement of renal glomeruli also is possible (Fig. 14.17). In the myocardium, these deposits can be detected in the interstitium, leading to restrictive cardiomyopathy. In this context, the contractile function of cardiomyocytes is impaired to the same extent as the cardiac conduction system and cardiac microcirculation. Distinct amyloid deposits could represent a plausible explanation for acute rhythmic cardiac death (see Chap. 1, Fig. 1.3) (Gertz 1992; Hassan et al. 2005; Dröber et al. 2010).

The prognosis of cardiac amyloidosis depends on the nature and origin of the amyloid protein deposited (Kieninger et al. 2010). Patients with cardiac amyloidosis can show persistent elevated troponin levels. Therefore, it is important to consider cardiac amyloidosis in patients with troponin elevation and heart failure (Kraemer et al. 2009).

Other vascular and metabolic diseases can explain sudden unexpected death (e.g., mucoviscidosis, etc.). In this respect, diseases are also encountered in forensic practice for which a histological and immunohistochemical correlation can be found in the relevant general and specialized forensic literature.

14.5 Hemochromatosis

Hereditary hemochromatosis is a frequent autosomal recessive disease which causes iron overload of various organs. Symptoms and organs involved can vary, and only a minority develops liver cirrhosis and pancreatic fibrosis. However, the life expectancy of persons with moderate or subclinical symptoms is reduced (Niederau et al. 1985). Although there are cases with myocardial damage leading to cardiomyopathy with an increased risk of sudden cardiac death, there are only single case reports in the forensic literature (Klintschar and Stiller 2004). Microscopically, the liver will show micronodular cirrhosis with portal fibrosis containing slight inflammatory infiltration. Prussian blue and therefore iron-positive granules may be abundant in phagocytes and bile duct epithelia (Fig. 14.18). Iron may also

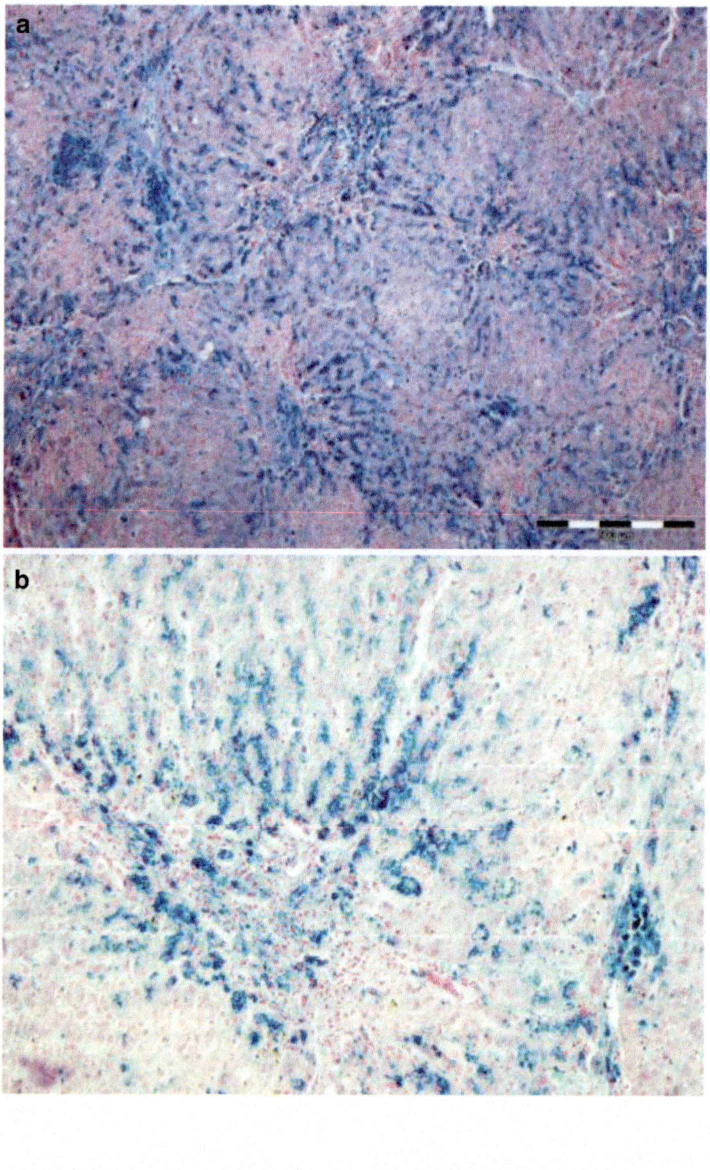

Fig. 14.18 Hemochromatosis with (**a**) iron overload and beginning liver cirrhosis (Prussian blue ×100) and (**b**) multiple iron-positive granules in hepatocytes, phagocytes, and bile duct epithelia (Prussian blue ×200)

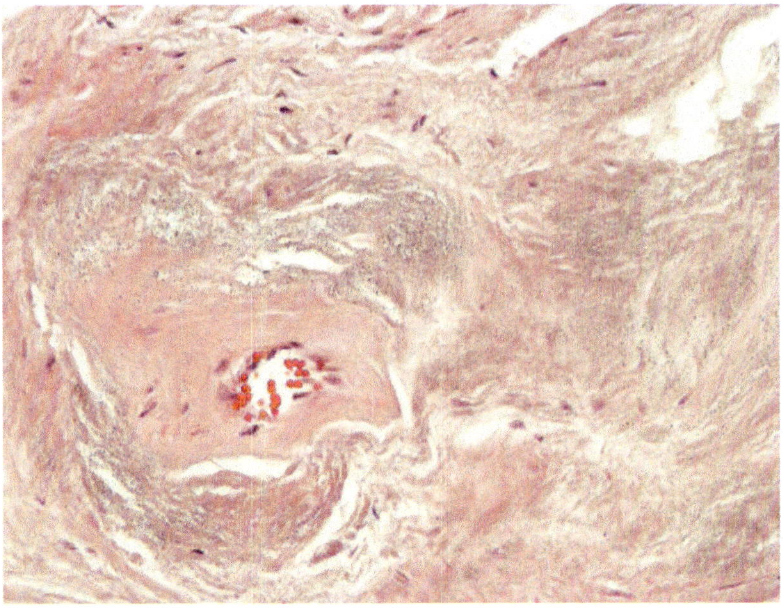

Fig. 14.19 Ochronosis with fine, dustlike blackish-brown deposits in collagenous scar tissue within the myocardium (H&E ×400)

be present in all other parenchymal organs. Iron-containing granules in the myocardium, combined with marked dilation and disconnection of the muscle fibers accompanied by microfocal necrosis, may explain sudden cardiac death (Klintschar and Stiller 2004; Passen et al. 1996).

14.6 Ochronosis

Ochronosis is a rare, congenital, autosomal recessive metabolic disease with an incidence of between 1:250,000 and 1:1,000,000. It is characterized by an accumulation of homogentisic acids in the body and their excretion in urine (*alkaptonuria*). When polymerized homogentisic acids are deposited in collagen-containing tissue (sclera, skin, hyaline cartilage, blood vessel intima, intervertebral discs), these tissues take on a blackish-brown color—a finding that is macroscopically patent at autopsy in advanced cases (Breer et al. 2012). From a histopathological perspective, dust-like blackish-brown deposits are seen particularly in intervertebral disc tissue and joint capsules. Deposits in thyroid tissue in the setting of ochronosis can cause the clinical picture of "black thyroid," as also described in minocycline use (see Chap. 16). In individual cases, deposits are found even in small areas of fibrotic scarring within the myocardium (Fig. 14.19). Other manifestation sites of ochronosis can include, e.g., the coronary arteries, the aortic wall, and the dura mater.

References

Adés LC, Waltham RD, Chiodo AA, Baterman JF (1995) Myocardial infarction resulting from coronary artery dissection in an adolescent with Ehlers-Danlos syndrome type IV due to a type III collagen mutation. Br Heart J 74:112–116

Ainsworth RW, Gresham GA (1961) Giant cell aortitis with rupture of the aorta. J Pathol Bacteriol 82:203–205

Althoff H (1990) Zur Ätiopathogenese der infantilen Koronarsklerose beim sog. Kawasaki-Syndrom. Pathologe 11:41–47

Amano J, Suzuki A (1991) Coronary artery involvement in Takayasu's arteritis. J Thorac Cardiovasc Surg 102:554–560

Amine ARC (1997) Neurosurgical complications of heroin addiction: brain abscess and mycotic aneurysm. Surg Neurol 7:385–386

Anagnostopoulos CE, Manakavalan JS, Kittle CF (1972) Aortic dissections and dissecting aneurysms. Am J Cardiol 30:263–273

Aru GM, English WP, Netherland D, Heath BJ (1999) Internal thoracic artery rupture in a child with type IV Ehlers-Danlos syndrome. J Thorac Cardiovasc Surg 117:1021–1022

Ashrafi AH, Wang J, Stockwell CA, Lloyd D, McAlvin JB, Russo P, Shehata BM (2007) Kawasaki disease: four case reports of cardiopathy with an institutional and literature review. Pediatr Dev Pathol 10: 491–499

Aufderheide A, Henke B, Parker E (1981) Granulomatous coronary arteritis (Takayasu disease). Arch Pathol Lab Med 105:647–649
August C, Holzhausen HJ (1992) Isolierte Koronararteriitis – Fallbericht und Nomenklaturdiskussion. Pathologe 13:280–285
Banaschak S, Driever F, Nerlich A, Madea B (2002) Aortenruptur bei einem 18-jährigen Mann. Postmortale Diagnose eines Ehlers-Danlos-Syndroms Typ IV. Rechtsmedizin 12:153–158
Barbesier M, Duncanson ER, Mackey-Bojack SM, Roe SJ, Thomas LC (2013) Sudden death due to spontaneous acute dissection of the left subclavian artery with rupture during postpartum period: a case report. Int J Legal Med 127:453–457
Bayer Kristensen I, Østergaard Kristensen B (1994) Sudden death caused by thrombosed coronary artery aneurysm. Two unusual cases of Kawasaki disease. Int J Legal Med 106:277–280
Bode-Jänisch S, Schmidt A, Günther D, Stuhrmann M, Fieguth A (2012) Aortic dissection aneurysm – histopathological findings. Forensic Sci Int 214:13–17
Bratzke H, Wojahn H (1977) Spontane Aortenrupturen aus gerichtsmedizinischer Sicht. Z Rechtsmed 79:159–182
Breer S, Amling M, Püschel K, Klein A, Schulz F, Zustin J (2012) Ochronose. Rechtsmedizin 22:49–53
Brinkmann B (1974) Zur Histomorphologie und Begutachtung zweizeitiger Aortenrupturen. Z Rechtsmed 74:235–243
Burman JO (1960) Medial degeneration and its relation to dissecting aneurysm. Int Abstr Surg 110:1–8
Byard RW (2006) Sudden death in Marfan syndrome. In: Tsokos M (ed) Forensic pathology reviews, vol 4. Humana Press, Totowa, pp 93–106
Byard RW, Keeley FW, Smith CR (1990) Type IV Ehlers-Danlos syndrome presenting as sudden infant death. Am J Clin Pathol 93:579–582
Byard RW, Schliebs J, Koszyca BA (2001) Osler-Weber-Rendu syndrome – pathological manifestations and autopsy considerations. J Forensic Sci 46:698–701
Byard RW, Gilbert JD, Langlois NEI (2017) Spontaneous coronary artery dissection. Forensic Sci Med Pathol 13:248–251
Cambria RP, Brewster DC, Gertler J, Moncure AC, Gusberg R, Tilson MD, Darling RC, Hammond G, Mergerman J, Abbott WM (1988) Vascular complications associated with spontaneous aortic dissection. J Vasc Surg 7:199–209
Canino-Rodriguez A, Cox RA (2008) Giant coronary aneurysms in a young adult patient with Kawasaki disease. P R Health Sci J 27:382–386
Carlson RG, Lillehei CW, Edwards JE (1970) Cystic medial necrosis of the ascending aorta in relation to age and hypertension. Am J Cardiol 25:411–415
Cassling RS, Lortz JB, Olson DR, Hubbard TF, McManus BM (1985) Fatal vasculitis (periarteritis nodosa) of the coronary arteries: angiographic ambiguities and absence of aneurysms at autopsy. J Am Coll Cardiol 6:707–714
Cohle SD, Lie JT (1988) Inflammatory aneurysm of the abdominal aorta with coronary arteritis. Arch Pathol Lab Med 112:1121–1125
Cohle SD, Titus JL, Espinola A, Hachimczyk A (1982) Sudden unexpected death due to coronary giant cell arteritis. Arch Pathol Lab Med 106:171–172
Collins MH, Schwarze U, Carpentieri DF, Kaplan P, Nathanson K, Meyer JS, Byers PH (1999) Multiple vascular and bowel ruptures in an adolescent male with sporadic Ehlers-Danlos syndrome type IV. Pediatr Dev Pathol 2:86–93
Cosgrave GE Jr, Watts JC, Kaump DH (1947) Spontaneous rupture of splenic arterial aneurysms: report of three cases. Am J Clin Pathol 17:372–382
D'Ovidio C, Sablone S, Carnevale A (2015) Spontaneous coronary artery dissection: case report and literature review. J Forensic Sci 60:801–806
Dermengiu S, Ceausu M, Hostiuc S, Curca GC, Dermengiu D, Turculet C (2009) Spontaneous aortic dissection due to cystic medial degeneration. Report of a sudden death and review of the literature. Rom J Leg Med 17:89–96
Desinan L, Scott CA, Piai I, Mazzolo GM (2010) Sudden death due to spontaneous rupture in splenic artery atypical dissection with features of vasculitis: case report and review of the literature. Forensic Sci Int 200:e1–e5
Dettmeyer R, Amberg R, Varchmin-Schultheiß K, Madea B (1998a) Sudden cardiac death due to atypical isolated coronary arteritis? Forensic Sci Int 95:193–200
Dettmeyer R, Schmidt P, Madea B (1998b) Two cases of unexpected sudden death due to cystic medianecrosis of the aorta associated with bloodless aortic dissection. Forensic Sci Int 94:161–166
Dettmeyer R, Stiel M, Madea B (2006) Chlamydial heat-shock protein 60. A marker for chronic infection with chlamydia pneumoniae in atherosclerosis: investigation of atherosclerotic coronary arteries by immunocytochemistry. Forensic Sci Med Pathol 2:173–178
Dickens P, Khoo US (1993) Sudden death associated with bloodless aortic dissection. Forensic Sci Int 59:149–155
Dröber J, Buschmann CT, Blechschmidt C, Martin H, Tsokos M (2010) Kardiale Amyloidose als Ursache eines plötzlichen Todes. Rechtsmedizin 20:278–281
Eplinius F, Hädrich C (2014) Acute aortic dissection caused by *Clostridium septicum* aortitis. Forensic Sci Int 244:e38–e41
Erbersdobler A, Tsokos M (2006) Sudden, unexpected death resulting from a giant coronary artery aneurysm. Forensic Sci Med Pathol 2:199–201
Erdheim J (1929a) Medianecrosis aortae idiopathica. Virchows Arch Pathol Anat Physiol 273:454–479
Erdheim J (1929b) Medionecrosis aortae indiopathica cystica. Virchows Arch A Pathol Anat Histopathol 276:187–229
Eriksen UH, Aunsholt NA, Nielsen TT (1992) Enormous right coronary artery aneurysm in a patient with type IV Ehlers-Danlos syndrome. Int J Cardiol 35: 259–261

Evans RH, Fraser AG (1996) Spontaneous coronary artery rupture and cardiac tamponade in Ehlers-Danlos syndrome type IV. Int J Cardiol 54:283–286
Fineschi V, Paglicci Reatelli L, Baroldi G (1999) Coronary artery aneurysms in a young adult: a case of sudden death. A late sequelae of Kawasaki disease? Int J Legal Med 112:120–123
Frank S, Johnson A, Ross J Jr (1973) Natural history of valvular aortic stenosis. Br Heart J 35:41–46
Frank MW, Mehlman DJ, Tsai F, Lomasney JW, Joob AW (1999) Syphilitic aortitis. Circulation 100:1582–1583
Früchtnicht W, Albrecht R (1998) Aneurysma des Ductus Botalli bei einem 6 Wochen alt gewordenen Säugling. In: 7th spring meeting of the German Society of Forensic Medicine, Bonn, 5–6 June 1998
Fujita M, Abe A, Itoh T, Saitoh K, Noguchi M, Sano K, Fujiioka Y, Nagashima K (1992) Nonarthritic rheumatoid valvulitis with coronary arteritis causing myocardial infarction. Virchows Arch A Pathol Anat Histopathol 420:109–112
Galtés I, Borondo JC, Cos M, Subirana M, Martín C, Castellà J, Medallo J (2012) Traumatic bilateral vertebral artery dissection. Forensic Sci Int 214:e12–e15
Gertz MA (1992) Familial amyloidosis and the heart. Arch Intern Med 166:1805–1813
Gilchrist ER, Duflou JA (2005) Incidental myocardial infarction in Ehlers-Danlos syndrome type IV? J Forensic Sci 50:461–464
Glenewinkel F, Schmidt P, Arnold G, Henßge C (1996) Plötzlicher Tod beim subtotalen Verschluß des rechten Koronarostiums durch eine Mesaortitis luica. Rechtsmedizin 6:49–52
Gore I (1953) Dissecting aneurysm of the aorta in persons under forty years of age. Arch Pathol 5:1–3
Gormsen H (1984) Postmortem diagnosis of syphilitic aortitis, including serological verification on postmortem blood. Forensic Sci Int 24:51–56
Gravanis MB (2000) Giant cell arteritis and Takayasu aortitis: morphologic, pathogenic and etiologic factors. Int J Cardiol 75(Suppl):S21–S33
Gsell O (1928) Wandnekrosen der Aorta als selbständige Erkrankung und ihre Beziehung zur Spontanruptur. Virchows Arch A Pathol Anat Histopathol 276: 1–36
Guitierrez PS, Correia de Almeida I, Nader HB, de Lourdes HM, Stolf N, Dietrich CP (1991) Decrease in sulphated glycosaminoglycans in aortic dissection – possible role in the pathogenesis. Cardiovasc Res 25:742–748
Hagemeier L, Unkrig S, Madea B (2009) Dissezierendes Milzarterienaneurysma bei fibromuskulärer Dysplasie. Rechtsmedizin 19:21–24
Halpern M, Citron BP (1971) Necrotizing angiitis associated with drug abuse. Am J Roentgenol 111:663–671
Hassan W, Al-Sergani MW et al (2005) Amyloid heart disease. New frontiers and insights in pathophysiology, diagnosis, and management. Tex Heart Inst J 32:178–184
Hirani R, Koszyca B, Byard RW (2008) Marfan syndrome and sudden death within a family – aetiologic, molecular and diagnostic issues at autopsy. J Forensic Legal Med 15:205–209
Hirst AE, Gore J (1976) Is cystic medianecrosis the cause of dissecting aorta aneurysms? Circulation 53:915–916
Hoffmann B, Mayatepek E (2009) Fabry disease – often seen, rarely diagnosed. Dtsch Arztebl Int 106: 440–447
Horton BT, Magath TB, Browne GE (1932) An undescribed form of arteritis of the temporal vessels. Proc Staff Meet Mayo Clin 7:700–701
Hugar BS, Praveen S, Kainoor SK, Shetty ARS (2014) Sudden death in Marfan Syndrome. J Forensic Sci 59:1126–1128
Hushang M, Payan MD, Enid F, Gilbert MD (1984) Granulomatous coronary arteritis. Arch Pathol Lab Med 108:136–137
Inokuchi G, Hayakawa M, Kishimoto T, Makino Y, Iwase H (2014) A suspected case of coronary periarteritis due to IgG4-related disease as a cause of ischemic heart disease. Forensic Sci Med Pathol 10:103–108
Ishikawa T, Pollak S, Pflugradt R, Bohnert M, Große Perdekamp M, Thierauf A, Maeda H (2010) Pulmonary arteriovenous malformation causing sudden death due to spontaneous hemothorax. Int J Legal Med 124:459–465
Johnston SL, Lock RJ, Gompels MM (2002) Takayasu arteritis: a review. J Clin Pathol 55:481–486
Judge DP, Dietz HC (2005) Marfan's syndrome. Lancet 366:1965–1976
Jung H, Lostun A, Matei DB (2013) Coronary artery dissection as cause of sudden death. Rom J Leg Med 21:85–90
Jungmann L, Bohnert M, Schmidt U, Pollak S (2010) Plötzlicher Tod durch spontane Aortenruptur: zwei ungewöhnliche Manifestationensformen. Arch Kriminol 226:55–65
Kaiser C, Schnabel A, Berkefeld J, Bratzke H (2008) Traumatic rupture of the intracranial vertebral artery due to rotational acceleration. Forensic Sci Int 182:e15–e17
Kajihara H, Tachiyama Y, Hirose T, Takata A, Saito K, Murai T, Yasui W (2013) Eosinophilic coronary periarteritis (vasospastic angina and sudden death), a new type of coronary arteritis: report of seven autopsy cases and a review of the literature. Virchows Arch 462:239–248
Karayel F, Ozaslan A, Turan AA, Pakis I, Ketenc C, Eroglu AG (2006) Sudden death in infancy due to bicuspid aortic valve. J Forensic Sci 51:1147–1150
Karger B, Fechner G (2006) Sudden death due to giant cell coronary arteritis. Int J Legal Med 120:377–379
Kawasaki T, Kosaki F, Okawa S, Shigematsu I, Yanagawa H (1974) A new infantile acute febrile mucocutaneous lymph node syndrome (MLNS) prevailing in Japan. Pediatrics 54:271–276
Kieninger B, Eriksson M, Kandolf R, Schnabel PA, Schönland S, Kristen AV, Hegenbart U, Lohse P, Röcken C (2010) Amyloid in endomyocardial biopsies. Virchows Arch 456:523–532

Kimmelstiel P, Gilmour MT, Hodges HH (1952) Degeneration of elastic fibers in granulomatous giant cell arteritis (temporal arteritis). Arch Pathol 54:157–168

King J, Richards M, Tress B (1978) Cerebral arteritis associated with heroin abuse. Med J Aust 2:444–445

Kinnane J, Priebe C, Caty M, Kuppermann N (1995) Perforation of the colon in an adolescent girl. Pediatr Emerg Care 11:230–232

Klintschar M, Stiller D (2004) Sudden cardiac death in hereditary hemochromatosis: an underestimated cause of death? Int J Legal Med 118:174–177

Klintschar M, Bilkenroth U, Arslan-Kirchner M, Schmidke J, Stiller D (2009) Marfan syndrome: clinical consequences resulting from a medicolegal autopsy of a case of sudden death due to aortic rupture. Int J Legal Med 123:55–58

Kodikara S, Sivasubramanium M (2009) Bilateral pulmonary artery aneurysms. Legal Med 11:S496–S497

Kraemer BF, Seizer P, Geisler T, Klingel K, Kandolf R, Lindemann S, Gawaz M (2009) Persistent troponin elevation in a patient with cardiac amyloidosis. Clin Cardiol 32:E39–E42

Kristoffersen S, Vetti N, Morild I (2012) Traumatic dissection of the vertebral artery in a toddler following a short fall. Forensic Sci Int 221:e34–e38

Krompecher T, Saraga EP, Gardiol G (1984) Plötzlicher Tod aus natürlicher Ursache: Isolierter Befall eines Herzkranzgefäßes durch eine Arteriitis vom Typ Takayasu. Beitr Gerichtl Med 42:155–163

Kumar P, Velissaris T, Sheppard MN, Pepper JR (2002) Giant cell arteritis confined to intramural coronary arteries. Unforeseen hazards myocardial protection. Cardiovasc Surg 43:647–649

Landing BH, Larson EJ (1987) Pathological features of Kawasaki disease (mucocutaneous lymph node syndrome). Am J Cardiovasc Pathol 1:218–229

Lau G (2002) Fatal pulmonary haemorrhage from a perforated and possibly iatrogenic thoracic aortic aneurysm. Forensic Sci Int 126:167–170

Leu HJ (1993) Spontane dissezierende Aneurysmen von Arterien des muskulären Bautyps infolge mukoider Mediadegeneration (mediolytische Arteriopathie). Pathologe 14:325–329

Leu AJ, Leu HJ (1988) Eigenartige bandförmige Degeneration der Aortenmedia als Ursache multipler Aneurysmata der Aorta thoracalis und abdominalis. Pathologe 9:366–369

Li Y, Li L, Mu HS, Fan SL, He FG, Wang ZY (2015) Aortic dissection and sudden unexpected deaths: a retrospective study of 31 forensic autopsy cases. J Forensic Sci 60:1206–1211

Lie JT (1987) Coronary vasculitis. Arch Pathol Lab Med 111:224–233

Lie JT (1992) Segmental mediolytic arteritis. Not an arteritis but a variant of arterial fibromuscular dysplasia. Arch Pathol Lab Med 116:238–241

Lupi-Herrera E, Sanchez-Torres G, Marcushamer J, Mispireta J, Horwitz S, Vela JE (1977) Takayasu's arteritis: clinical study of 107 cases. Am Heart J 93:94–103

Lynch MJ, Woodford NWF, Dodd MJ (2008) Sudden death due to aortic rupture complicating undiagnosed coarctation of the aorta in a teenager – a case report and review of the literature. J Forensic Legal Med 15:443–446

Maeso Madronero JL, Aretz S, Theis U, Morgenroth K, Bergbauer M (2000) Aortenruptur bei idiopathischer Medianekrose Gsell-Erdheim. Dtsch Med Wschr 125:1195–1198

Magarey FR (1950) Aneurysm in giant-cell aortitis. Dissecting aneurysm due to giant-cell aortitis. J Pathol Bact 62:445–447

Makino Y, Inokuchi G, Yokota H, Hayakawa M, Yajima D, Motomura A, Chiba F, Torimitsu S, Nakatani Y, Iwase H (2015) Sudden death due to coronary artery dissection associated with fibromuscular dysplasia revealed by postmortem selective computed tomography coronary angiography: a case report. Forensic Sci Int 253:e10–e15

Martin JF, Kittas C, Triger DR (1980) Giant cell arteritis of coronary arteries causing myocardial infarction. Br Heart J 43:487–489

McConnell ME, Hannon DW, Steed RD, Gilliland MG (1998) Fatal obliterative coronary vasculitis in Kawasaki disease. J Pediatr 133:259–261

Melsen F (1973) Spontaneous rupture of the aorta in the Marfan's syndrome. Z Rechtsmed 73:53–60

Merlini G (2003) Molecular mechanism of amyloidosis. N Engl J Med 349:583–596

Merrell SW, Gloviczki P (1992) Splenic artery dissection: a case report and review of the literature. J Vasc Surg 15:221–225

Missliwetz J, Reiter C, Winter RE (1981) Differential diagnosis of Kawasaki syndrome. Beitr Gerichtl Med 39:307–316

Mitchinson MJ, Wight DJD, Arno J (1984) Chronic coronary periarteritis in two patients with coronary periaortitis. J Clin Pathol 37:32–36

Murai T, Kuroda N, Shinozuka T, Kurihara K, Yanagida J, Watanabe H, Saito K, Maurai N, Imai M (1989) Coronary aneurysms in a young adult: report of a case suspected of Kawasaki's disease. Med Sci Law 29:59–63

Morcos M, Alfiano M, Gompel A, Regnard J (2006) Life-threatening endometriosis-related hemopneumothorax. Ann Thorac Surg 82:726–729

Morgenthal S, Bayer R, Schneider E, Zachäus M, Röcken C, Dreßler J, Ondruschka B (2016) Nodular pulmonary amyloidosis with spontaneous fatal blood aspiration. Forensic Sci Int 262:e1–e4

Naeve W, Brinkmann B (1971) Zur Begutachtung der Medianecrosis aortae idiopathica als Todesursache beim Sport. Z Rechtsmed 68:101–104

Nakajima K, Takeichi S, Nakajima Y, Fujita MQ (2010) Pokkuri death syndrome: sudden cardiac death cases without coronary atherosclerosis in South Asian young males. Forensic Sci Int 207(1–3):6–13

Nashima Y, Kurozumi T, Sueishi K, Tanaka K (1990) Dissecting aneurysms: a clinicopathologic and histopathologic study of 111 autopsied cases. Hum Pathol 21:291–296
Nelson DA, Ashley PF (1965) Rupture of the aorta during closed-chest cardiac massage. JAMA 193:681–683
Nerlich AG, Stöss H, Lehmann H, Krieg T, Müller PK (1994) Pathomorphological and biochemical alterations in Ehlers-Danlos-syndrome type IV. Pathol Res Pract 190:697–706
Niederau C, Fischer R, Sonnenberg A, Stremmel W, Trampisch HJ, Strohmeyer G (1985) Survival and causes of death in cirrhotic and noncirrhotic patients with primary hemochromatosis. N Engl J Med 313:1256–1262
Norita K, de Noronha SV, Sheppard MN (2012) Sudden cardiac death caused by coronary vasculitis. Virchows Arch 460:309–318
Noth I, Strek ME, Leff AR (2003) Churg-Strauss-syndrome. Lancet 361:587–594
Ortmann C, Wüllenweber J, Brinkmann B, Fracasso T (2010) Fatal mycotic aneurysm caused by *Pseudallescheria boydii* after near drowning. Int J Legal Med 124:243–247
Owen SM, Durst RD (1984) Ehlers-Danlos syndrome simulating child abuse. Arch Dermatol 120:97–101
Palmiere C, Burkhardt S, Staub C, Hallenbarter M, Pizzolato G, Dettmeyer R, La Harpe R (2004) Thoracic aortic dissection associated with cocaine abuse. Forensic Sci Int 141:137–142
Passen EL, Rodriguez R, Neumann A, Tan CD, Parillo JE (1996) Cardiac hemochromatosis. Circulation 94:2302
Patterson RH, Burns WA, Jannotta FS (1974) Complications of external cardiac resuscitation: a retrospective review and survey of the literature. Med Ann Dist Columbia 43:389–394
Paul RA, Helle MJ, Tarssanen LT (1990) Sudden death as sole symptom of coronary arteritis. Ann Med 22:161–162
Pereira MC, Filho AA, Lastoria S (1981) Inflammatory aneurysm of the abdominal aorta with coronary arteritis. Arch Pathol Lab Med 105:678–679
Pery C, Frenzel H, Schindler P (1983) Aortenruptur als seltene Komplikation der Riesenzell-Arteriitis. Pathologe 4:204–211
Pourhassan S, Grotemeyer D, Klar V, Sandmann W (2007) Klippel-Trenaunay syndrome associated with multiple visceral arteries aneurysm. Vasa 36:124–129
Prahlow JA, Wagner SA (2005) Death due to Ehlers-Danlos syndrome type IV. Am J Forensic Med Pathol 26:78–82
Reis ED, Martinet OD, Mosimann F (1998) Spontaneous rupture of the oesophagus in an adolescent with type IV Ehlers-Danlos syndrome. Eur J Surg 164:313–316
Rippberger T, Tröger HD, Schmidtke J (2009) The genetic message of sudden unexpected death due to thoracic aortic dissection. Forensic Sci Int 187:1–5
Risse M, Weiler G (1987) Spontanes Aneurysma dissecans einer Kranzschlagader als seltene Ursache eines postpartalen Todes der Kindesmutter. Z Rechtsmed 99:143–150
Risse M, Lasczkowski G, Dettmeyer R, Verhoff MA (2010) Spontane Aortenruptur ohne Dissektion. Plötzlicher Tod während der Schwangerschaft. Rechtsmedizin 20:34–35
Roberts DL, Pope FM, Nicholls AC, Narcisi P (1984) Ehlers-Danlos syndrome type IV mimicking non-accidental injury in a child. Br J Dermatol 111:341–345
Robertson EN, Hambly BD, Jeremy RW (2016) Thoracic aortic dissection and heritability: forensic implications. Forensic Sci Med Pathol 12:366–368
Röcken C (2008) Pathologie der Amyloidose. Nephrologe 3:275–284
Röcken C (2009) Update immunhistologischer Klassifikation der Amyloidose. Pathologe 30(suppl 2):121–123
Rosen N, Gaton E (1972) Takayasu's arteritis of coronary arteries. Arch Pathol 94:225–229
Rottino A (1939) Medial degeneration of the aorta. A study of two hundred and ten routine autopsy specimens by a serial block method. Arch Pathol 28:377–385
Rowley AH, Shulman ST (2010) Pathogenesis and management of Kawasaki disease. Expert Rev Anti-Infect Ther 8:197–203
Rozin L, Koehler SA, Shakir A, Ladham S, Wecht CH (2003) Kawasaki disease: a review of pathologic features of stage IV disease and two cases of sudden death among asymptomatic young adults. Am J Forensic Med Pathol 24:45–50
Saint-Martin P, Rogers C, Carpenter E, Fishbein MC, Lau S, Sathyavagiswaran L (2009) Subaortic pseudoaneurysm of the left ventricle complicating staphylococcal endocarditis. J Forensic Sci 54:930–932
Salvarani C, Cantini F, Boiardi L, Hunder GG (2002) Polymyalgia rheumatica and giant cell arteritis. N Engl J Med 347:261–271
Sariola H, Viljanen T, Luosto R (1986) Histological pattern and changes in extracellular matrix in aortic dissections. J Clin Pathol 39:1074–1081
Saruk M, Eisenstein R (1977) Aortic lesion in Marfan syndrome. The ultrastructure of cystic medial degeneration. Arch Pathol Lab Med 101:74–77
Saukko P, Knight B (2004) Knight's forensic pathology, 3rd edn. Arnold, London, pp 492–526
Saulsbury FT, Hayden GF (1985) Skin conditions simulating child abuse. Pediatr Emerg Care 1:147–150
Schäfer H, Püschel K (1996) Proximale Aortitis als Ursache eines unerwarteten plötzlichen Herztodes bei einem Kleinkind. Pathologe 17:324
Scharfman WB, Wallach JB, Angrist A (1950) Myocardial infarction due to syphilitic coronary ostial stenosis. Am Heart J 40:603–613
Schlatman TJM, Becker AE (1977) Pathogenesis of dissecting aneurysma of aorta. Comparative histopathologic study of significance of medial changes. Am J Cardiol 39:21–26
Schmidt P, Madea B, Oehmichen M, Gerling I (1996) Plötzlicher Tod bei idiopathischer cystischer Medianekrose – Analyse von 6 Fällen

unter Berücksichtigung arztrechtlicher Fragen. Rechtsmedizin 6:39–44
Schmitt HP (1973) Die Bedeutung von Varianten im Bereich der Arteriae vertebrales und der Arteria basilaris für die forensische Medizin. Z Rechtsmed 73:23–28
Schnapka G, Dietze O, Propst A (1983) Morphometrische Untersuchungen bei idiopathischer Medianekrose. Pathologe 4:303–306
Schön C, Ramaswamy A, Barth PJ (2005) Churg-Strauss-Syndrom. Rechtsmedizin 15:173–176
Schultz TC (1989) Coronary artery aneurysms in a young adult. Am J Forensic Med Pathol 10:63–66
Schürch W (1970) Familäre dissezierende Aneurysmen der Aorta. Arch Kreislaufforsch 63:288–319
Seguchi M, Hino Y, Aiba S, Yasukohchi S, Momma K, Takao A, Endo M (1990) Ostial stenosis of the left coronary artery as a sole clinical manifestation of Takayasu's arteritis: a possible cause of unexpected sudden death. Heart Vessel 5:188–191
Shields LBE, Rolf CM, Davis GJ, Hunsaker JC (2010) Sudden and unexpected death in three cases of Ehlers-Danlos Syndrome type IV. J Forensic Sci 55:1641–1645
Shields LBE, Burge M, Hunsaker JC (2012) Sudden death due to polyarteritis nodosa. Forensic Sci Med Pathol 8:290–295
Sorger K (1968) Über Veränderungen der Vasa vasorum bei Medianecrosis aortae. Virchows Arch Abt A Path Anat 345:107–120
Soucy P, Eidus L, Keeley F (1990) Perforation of the colon in an 15-year-old girl with Ehlers-Danlos syndrome type IV. J Pediatr Surg 25:1180–1182
Stegmann T (1987) Aortendissektion: Nicht mit dem Herzinfarkt verwechseln. Dtsch Ärztebl 84:282–285
Srettabunjong S (2013) Spontaneous rupture of acute ascending aortic dissection in a young pregnant woman: a sudden unexpected death. Forensic Sci Int 232:e5–e8
Sunagawa K, Mitsumata M, Ayusawa M, Kusumi Y (2008) Ruptured giant aneurysm of the left anterior descending coronary artery in Kawasaki disease. Pediatr Cardiol 29:1115–1119
Suzuki A, Miyagawa-Tomita S, Nakazawa M, Yutani C (2000) Remodeling of coronary artery lesions due to Kawasaki disease: comparison of arteriographic and immunohistochemical findings. Jpn Heart J 41:245–256
Tanaka N, Naoe S, Masuda H, Ueno T (1986) Pathological study of sequelae of Kawasaki disease (MCLS). With special reference to the heart and coronary arterial lesions. Acta Pathol Jpn 36:1513–1527
Tanaka A, Fukajama M, Funata N, Koike M, Saito K (1988) Coronary arteritis and aortoarteritis in the elderly males. Virchows Arch A Path Anat Histopathol 414:9–14
Thierauf A, Preuss J, Dettmeyer R, Madea B (2007) Fatal rupture of an undiagnosed aneurysm of the splenic artery – medico-legal implications. Forensic Sci Int 171:133–136
Vock R, Schulz E (1986) Marfan syndrome. A case report. Z Rechtsmed 96:67–78
von Kodolitsch Y, Robinson PN (2007) Marfan syndrome: an update of genetics, medical and surgical management. Heart 93:755–760
Wagner AD, Goronzy JJ, Weyand CM (1994) Functional profile of tissue-infiltrating and circulating CD68+ cells in giant cell arteritis: evidence for two components of the disease. J Clin Invest 94:1134–1140
Wang L, Thelmo WL, Axiotis CA (2002) Microscopic polyangiitis with massive myocardial necrosis and diffuse pulmonary hemorrhage. Virchows Arch 441:202–204
Wang Y, Chen S, Wang R, Huang S, Yyang M, Liu L, Liu Q (2016) Postmortem diagnosis of Marfan syndrome in a case of sudden death due to aortic rupture: detection of a novel FBN1 frameshift mutation. Forensic Sci Int 261:e1–e4
Wimmer PJ, Howes DS, Rumoro DP, Carbone M (1996) Fatal vascular catastrophe in Ehlers-Danlos syndrome: a case report and review. J Emerg Med 14:25–31
Wood LE, Tulloh RM (2009) Kawasaki disease in children. Heart 95:787–792
Yonesaka S, Takahashi T, Furukawa H, Matubara T, Tomimoto K, Oura H, Nakada T, Sunagawa Y (1992) Histopathological analysis of myocardial damages following Kawasaki disease with repeated endomyocardial biopsy. Kokyu To Junkan 40:375–381
Yoshikawa H, Nomura Y, Masuda K, Hazeki D, Yotsumoto K, Arata M, Kamenosono A, Yanagi S, Yoshinaga M, Kawano Y (2006) Four cases of Kawasaki syndrome complicated with myocarditis. Circ J 70:202–205
Yost BA, Vogelsang JP, Lie JT (1995) Fatal hemoptysis in Ehlers-Danlos syndrome. Chest 107:1465–1467
Yutani C, Go S, Kamiya T, Hirose O, Misava H, Maeda H, Kozuka T, Onishi S (1981) Cardiac biopsy of Kawasaki disease. Arch Pathol Lab Med 105:470–474
Zack F, Terpe H, Hammer U, Wegener R (1996) Fibromuscular dysplasia of coronary arteries as a rare cause of death. Int J Legal Med 108:215–218

15 Lethal Infections, Sepsis, and Shock

Infections are a common cause of death, with the highest mortality rates seen with various types of viral (e.g., Landi and Coleman 2008) and bacterial infection, such as pneumonias, myocarditises (Chap. 13), and secondary infections (e.g., gastrointestinal infections such as salmonellae or ascending infections). Sudden unexpected death may also occur due to infection with rare pathogens which would otherwise follow a non-fatal course, e.g., leptospirosis (Luchini et al. 2008), influenza A infection (Tsokos et al. 2005), or meningoencephalitis caused by *Bartonella henselae* bacteria (Gerber et al. 2002). Especially cases of sudden unexpected death due to infection are found frequently in the forensic literature, e.g., fatal *necrotizing fasciitis* (Heinze et al. 2011), fatal human ehrlichiosis caused by obligate intracellular bacteria (Pavelites and Prahlow 2011), ruptured aortic aneurysm in syphilis (Tsokos 2012), and fatal gastric wall rupture (De-Georgia et al. 2015). Fatalities due to *Corynebacterium diphtheriae* infection (Beh and Byard 2015), as well as tuberculosis (Thu et al. 2014), have been described.

Meningitides that remained undetected prior to death are also seen (Chap. 20). In addition, infections following medical treatment can occur, such as postoperative wound infection, phlegmon and abscesses, ascending cholangitises following endoscopic retrograde cholangiopancreatography (ERCP), and lethal sepsis due to decubitus or liposuction (Preuss et al. 2006a). In the case of sudden death unrelated to medical treatment, the infection is often unknown at the time of autopsy. In other cases, characteristic symptoms have been described, and only a suspected diagnosis could be provided. Rare infections undetected prior to death, such as malaria or lethal measles infection, can also be found in forensic medical practice (Dettmeyer 2006; Risse et al. 2008). Obligations to report infections such as tuberculosis or meningitis must be considered insofar as this is required by law.

Typical findings from a wide range of lethal infections are highlighted below; for more detailed information relating to some cases, the reader is referred to the pathology literature. In addition, selected forms of infection considered to be significant are mentioned, such as malaria and overwhelming postsplenectomy infection (OPSI) syndrome.

The diagnosis of an infection can be established either directly by detecting the pathogen or indirectly by detecting the corresponding signs of an inflammatory process using microscopy. Viral infections primarily cause lymphocytic infiltration, bacterial infection, or granulocytic (purulent) infiltration, as well as phlegmonous-purulent inflammation and abscess. Other pathogens, e.g., fungi, parasites, etc., can cause mixed-cell infections. Sepsis arises if an infection site develops within the body from which pathogenic bacteria spread constantly or periodically into the bloodstream. This happens in such a way that this invasion triggers subjective and objective symptoms. Sepsis can also be triggered by fungi (fungal

R. B. Dettmeyer, *Forensic Histopathology*, https://doi.org/10.1007/978-3-319-77997-3_15

sepsis), for instance. There are numerous publications in the literature on immunohistochemical findings in sepsis. All cases of sepsis result in a strain on the entire organism, meaning that the organism's ubiquitous reaction in the form of the expression of numerous markers that can be demonstrated immunohistochemically is not surprising. Many of these markers (E-selectin = CD62E; VLA-4 = CD49d/CD29; ICAM-1 = CD54; VEGF; lactoferrin, lectins, etc.) react in part acutely, in part in a delayed manner not only in sepsis but also in the setting of other causes of shock, be these prolonged hemorrhagic shock or allergic shock. Thus, the reliability of the relevant immunohistochemical investigations may be limited; however, in combination with conventional histological findings, they may be able to provide guidance in terms of the age of the process (fresh, no longer fresh, older). Therefore, whether immunohistochemical diagnostic methods always yield additional information compared with the combined evaluation of macroscopic and conventional histological findings must still be deemed unclear at present. The forms of inflammation most frequently encountered in forensic practice, as well as a number of rarer inflammatory diseases and their characteristic findings, are discussed below. Information on other forms of inflammation relevant to cause of death, in particular myocarditis, can be found in other chapters of this book.

15.1 Pneumonias

Various forms of pneumonia are differentiated conceptually and morphologically:

- Bronchopneumonia (bacterial and purulent)
- Interstitial pneumonia (viral)
- Caseous pneumonia (tuberculous)
- Lobar pneumonia (staged disease course)
- Carnificating pneumonia (pneumonia with impaired healing)
- Aspiration pneumonia (pneumonia following aspiration of, e.g., stomach contents)
- Hypostatic pneumonia (pneumonia due to immobility)
- Hemorrhagic pneumonia (pneumonia with clear intraparenchymal hemorrhage)
- Atypical pneumonias (viral, fungal, or parasitic)

In the case of unequivocal histological or immunohistochemical findings, pneumonias are named after the triggering pathogen, e.g., cytomegalovirus-induced pneumonia (CMV pneumonia), measles pneumonia, or infection with *Mycoplasma pneumoniae* (Tsokos 2004).

Since conventional histological diagnosis of viral and in particular bacterial pneumonias typically provides adequate results, immunohistochemical diagnosis of pneumonia is only needed in certain cases. Occasionally, methodological problems are encountered when choosing an adequate pretreatment or contradictory findings are obtained. For example, proinflammatory P-selectin can be found in cases of pneumonia, but, according to Ortmann and Brinkmann (1997), P-selectin is also detected in megakaryocytes, platelets, and both activated and non-activated endothelium.

15.1.1 Purulent Bronchopneumonia

The most common pneumonias are bacterial purulent bronchopneumonias (Figs. 15.1 and 15.2) with multiple polymorphonuclear neutrophil granulocytes in the pulmonary alveoli, originating from an accompanying purulent bronchitis (Fig. 15.1). In advanced cases with a weakened immune system and in the absence of antibiotic therapy, a purulent lung-melting pneumonia with abscesses may develop. Isolated cases of infection-triggered *hemophagocytic syndrome (HPS)* in pneumococcal pneumonia have been reported. Histologically, one finds diplococci, neutrophil granulocytes, macrophages, and fibrin-filled alveoli. Elevated granulopoiesis, megakaryocytes in a typical distribution, and diffuse increased histiocytes or CD-68-positive macrophages, and erythrocyte ingestion consistent with HPS were detected in bone marrow (Ondruschka et al. 2015).

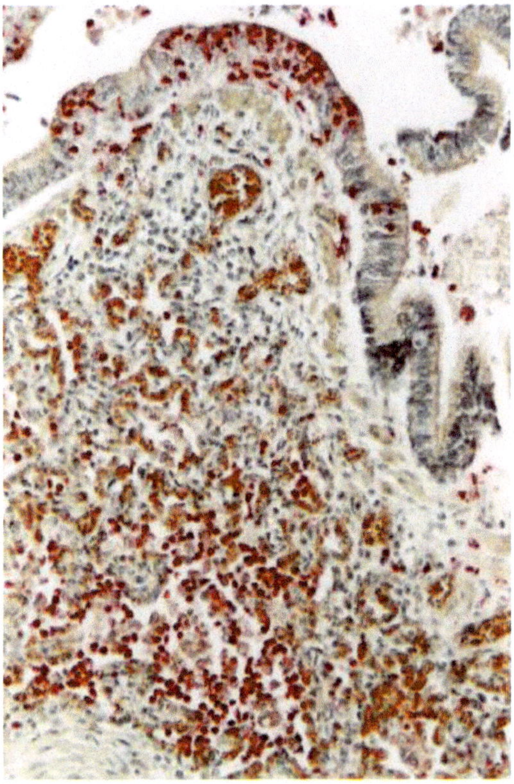

Fig. 15.1 Purulent bronchitis with polymorphonuclear neutrophil granulocytes in the bronchial wall (ASD ×200)

15.1.2 Lobar Pneumonia and Carnificating Pneumonia

Lobar pneumonia (Fig. 15.3) is a specific form of pneumonia in which one or more pulmonary lobes are affected; the disease occurs in stages. A chronology can be assigned to the stages, and thus conclusions can be drawn with respect to the age of lobar pneumonia (Table 15.1).

In the case of impaired or insufficient healing of the pneumonia, the affected lung tissue develops a meat-like consistency (carnificating pneumonia) (Fig. 15.4). Histologically, fibrously spread alveolar septa can be seen with striated pulmonary hyaline membranes, some fibrously organized and some in the repair process. The pathological changes increase right heart overload and can lead to right ventricular hypertrophy and acute heart failure.

Uremic pneumonitis (in dialysis patients), contrast medium aspiration, or toxin inhalation, e.g., chloric gas, should be considered in the differential diagnosis of carnificating pneumonia.

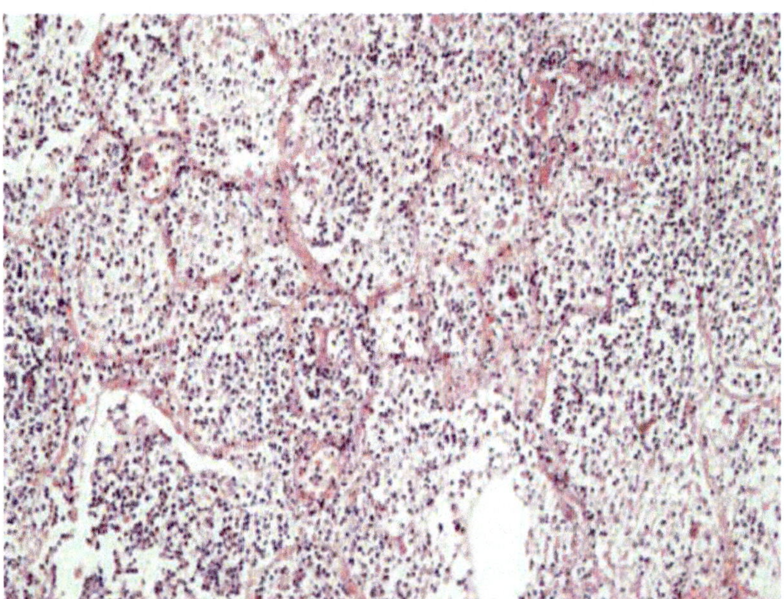

Fig. 15.2 Purulent bronchopneumonia with multiple polymorphonuclear neutrophil granulocytes in the pulmonary alveoli (H&E ×200)

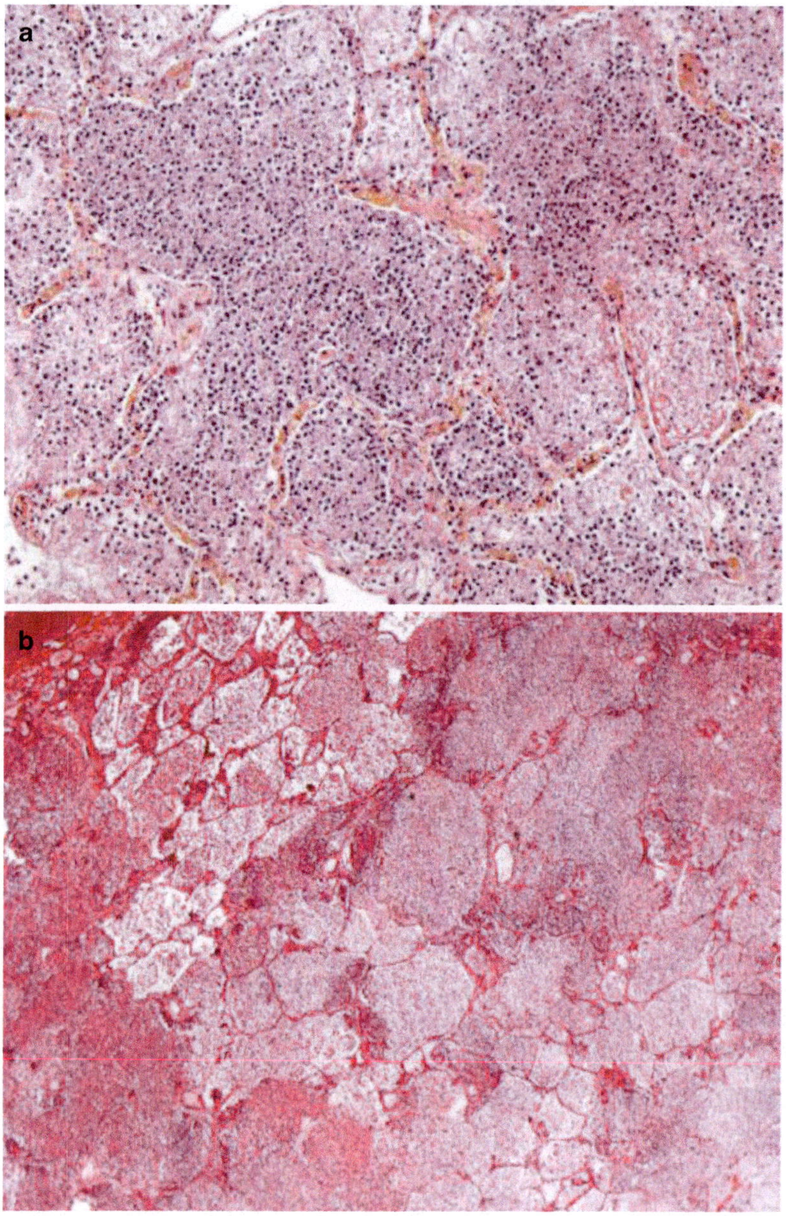

Fig. 15.3 Lobar pneumonia (**a**) in the macroscopically gray hepatization stage (H&E ×100) and (**b**) in the macroscopically yellow hepatization stage (H&E ×20)

15.1.3 Fungal Pneumonia

A fungal lung infection can often only be detected microscopically (Brandt 1980). In the case of simultaneous granulocytic infiltration, it is sometimes difficult to say whether the culprit is a primary fungal pneumonia or a secondary fungal infection following a preexisting purulent bronchopneumonia. Fungal spores, conidia, or hyphae can be seen with H&E staining by an experienced examiner but can also be well detected with Grocott staining (Fig. 15.5). Overstaining should be avoided, however, since connective tissue fibrils, mucus, mucous glands, erythrocytes, granulocytes, and bacteria will start to stain positive. Grocott staining is a nonspecific stain; detection of the fungal structure is important. This applies in particular to unusual fungal infections, e.g., *Aspergillus* infection of the aortic wall (Shintaku et al. 2001). Aspergillosis is often

Table 15.1 Stages of lobar pneumonia

Stage	Microscopy
1. Engorgement (1st–2nd day) Macroscopic: red section rich in blood; moist foamy fluid which can be collected	Inflammatory exudate in the pulmonary alveoli, shed alveolar epithelia, homogeneous protein complexes, few granulocytes and erythrocytes; rarely determined histologically since death typically occurs later
2. Red hepatization (3rd–4th day) Macroscopic: red, solid brittle section	Abundant erythrocytes, fibrin in the form of a dense network of fine strands, few granulocytes and alveolar epithelia. Fibrin can also be made visible by dimming the condenser. Hyperemia in the septal capillaries, increased fibrin thrombi
3. Gray hepatization (5th–6th day) Macroscopic: gray, brittle-dry section, finely grained (fibrin thrombi)	Exudation of fibrinogen in the alveoli, red fibers (blue in the fibrin staining according to Weigert), fibrin fibers are connected with adjacent alveoli via the pores of Cohn (Fig. 15.3a)
4. Yellow hepatization (6th–9th day) Macroscopic: yellow, soft section due to dissolution of fibrinous exudate (lysis); tissue is easily torn	Homogenous overview, abundant leukocytes in the alveoli, no abscesses, but many granulocytes (Fig. 15.3b)
5. Chronic (carnificating) pneumonia (as of day 10) Macroscopy: meat-like consistency (carnification), red followed by gray-white; lung shrinkage	Since cell lysis does not occur, organization of the fibrinous exudate by means of granulation tissue (van Gieson stain). Young yellow and older red collagen fibers, angioblasts, capillaries, fibroblasts, lymphohistiocytic infiltrates in the alveolar septa, hyperplasia of smooth muscles (muscular cirrhosis)

found in immunosuppressed patients. Pulmonary aspergillosis is the most common form, usually triggered by *Aspergillus fumigatus* (Figs. 15.6 and 15.7). In addition to local dissemination, hematogenic spread to various organs is seen (Young et al. 1970).

In addition to aspergillosis, there are diseases (including fungal sepsis) that can essentially be caused by other fungi. According to own experience, immunosuppressed patients, as well as diabetics with poor blood sugar control, appear to be at higher risk for infection. *Pneumocystis jirovecii* infection belongs to the group of rarer infections (Fig. 15.8).

15.1.4 Pulmonary Tuberculosis

Tuberculosis—usually restricted to the lung—can sometimes be detected in chronically ill, undernourished, or drug-/alcohol-addicted decedents. In rare cases, tuberculosis that remained undiagnosed antemortem is found to be the cause of sudden infant death (Dempers et al. 2011). In addition to miliary tuberculosis of the lung that may be macroscopically unrecognized or misdiagnosed as bronchopneumonia, active and inactive pulmonary tuberculosis occurs, in severe cases with cavern formation.

Histologically, pulmonary tuberculosis typically shows a sufficiently characteristic diagnostic picture: central necrosis of varying extent is surrounded by a seam of connective tissue in which polynuclear giant cells (Langerhans giant cells) and a dense collection of inflammatory cells (primarily lymphocytes and histiocytes) can be found (Fig. 15.9). Only in certain cases may it be possible to microscopically determine tubercle bacilli using Ziehl–Neelsen staining (1000× magnification with oil immersion). Generally, tubercle bacilli can be detected at the periphery of caseous necrosis as reddish, acid-resistant rods using Ziehl–Neelsen staining.

If histological findings are characteristic, diagnosis can also be confirmed without pathogen detection.

In the case of miliary tuberculosis of the lung (Fig. 15.10), small dispersed grains (milium = grain) can be seen in the pulmonary parenchyma. Histologically, the grains show no or only mild central necrosis; however, Langerhans giant cells, fibrosis, and lymphocyte accumulation can be seen. In terms of a differential diagnosis, pulmonary sarcoidosis may be considered in some cases.

Extrapulmonary tuberculosis occurs more rarely; urogenital tuberculosis is a possible consideration, while tuberculous myocarditis is extremely

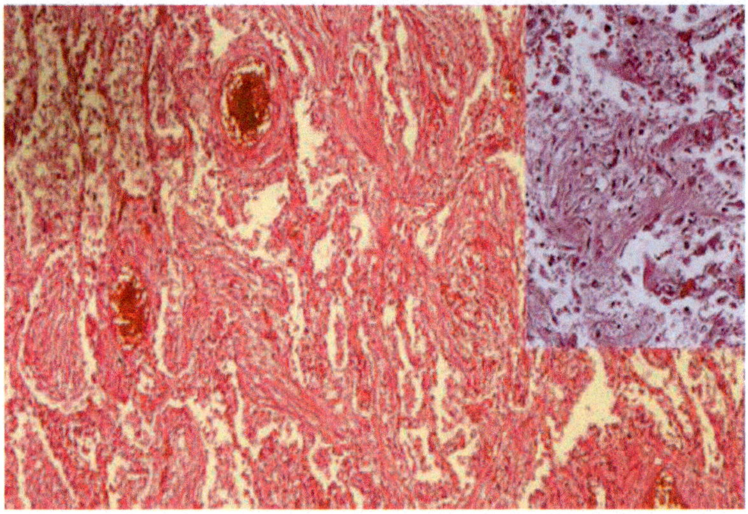

Fig. 15.4 Post-inflammatory carnificating pneumonia (H&E ×125; Insert: H&E ×500)

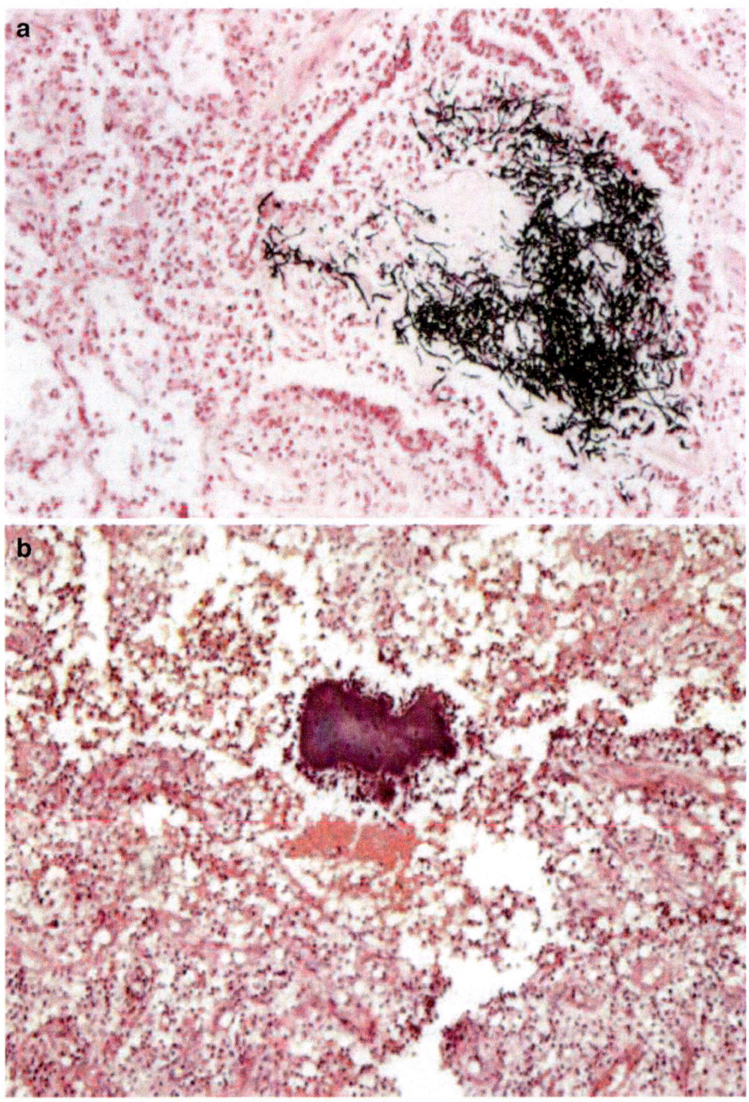

Fig. 15.5 Pronounced fungal pneumonia with numerous fungal fibers (candida type) (**a**) in the bronchial lumen (Grocott ×200) and abscesses with actinomyces (**b**) (H&E ×100)

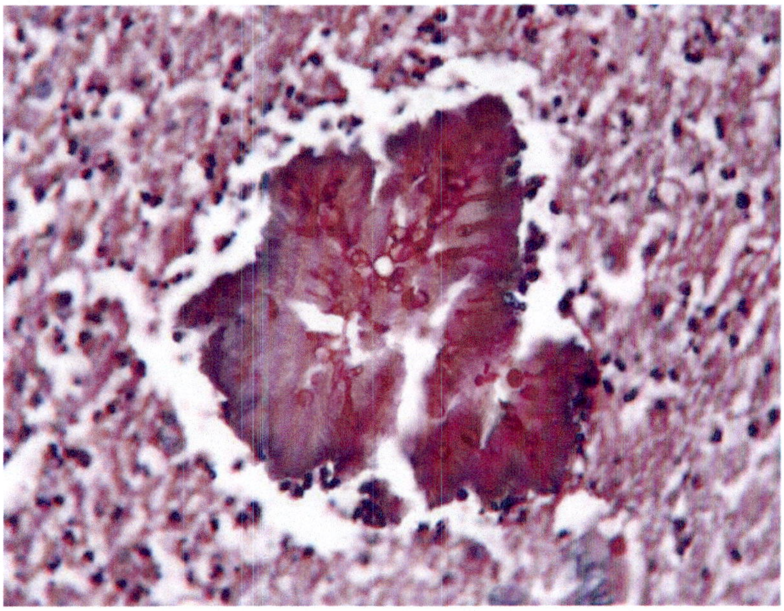

Fig. 15.6 *Aspergillus* infection (image kindly provided by Dr. D. Farkas, Kosice, Slovakia)

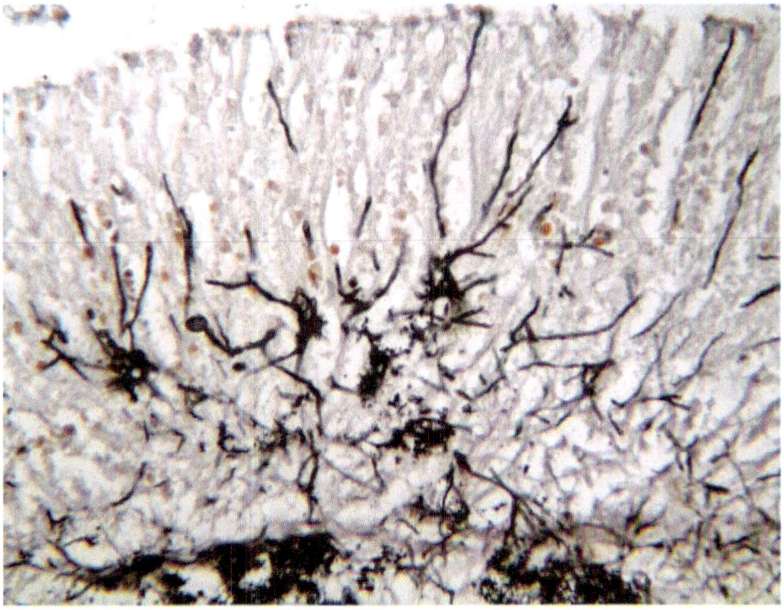

Fig. 15.7 *Aspergillus fumigatus* in Grocott staining (image kindly provided by Dr. D. Farkas, Kosice, Slovakia)

rare. In severe cases, a generalized infection with a lethal course following intracutaneous BCG vaccination may occur (Molz et al. 1986).

15.1.5 Viral Pneumonia

Virus-induced pneumonias are interstitial pneumonias with lymphomonocytic infiltration of the pulmonary interstitium of varying density (Fig. 15.11). Accumulations of alveolar macrophages with polymorphic hyperchromatic cell nuclei can be seen, sometimes in the alveolar lumen. Binuclear and sometimes polynuclear cells can be found. Severe forms of virus-induced pneumonia can lead to microscopically small necrosis. Since the respiratory epithelium is frequently affected, primary viral and secondary bacterial bronchitis and pneumonia are not unusual. Typically, histological findings do not enable any conclusions as to the triggering virus.

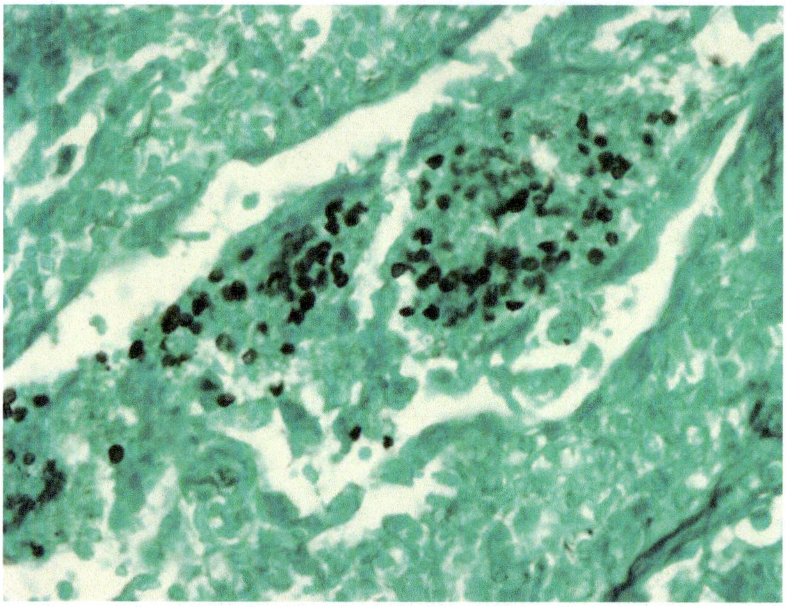

Fig. 15.8 *Pneumocystis jirovecii* infection (Grocott ×400—image kindly provided by Dr. K. Varchmin-Schultheiss, Münster, Germany)

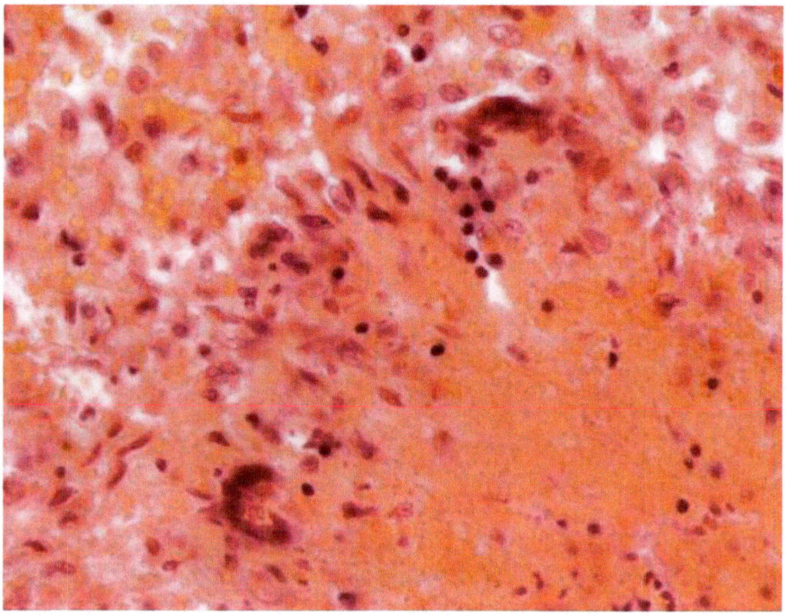

Fig. 15.9 Pulmonary tuberculosis with central caseous necrosis, fibrosis, polynuclear giant cells, lymphocytes, and histiocytes (H&E ×500)

Cytomegalovirus (CMV) pneumonia. Histolo gically, characteristic inflammatory infiltrates indicate CMV pneumonia if so-called owl's eye cells can be determined, i.e., enlarged cells in the alveoli with polymorphic cell nuclei surrounded by an optically blank circle. If doubts remain, diagnosis can be reliably confirmed immunohistochemically with a marker for CMV. Based on personal experience, CMV-infected cells typically show immunohistochemical evidence of E-selectin. Thus, CMV-positive cells can be clearly determined immunohistochemically (Fig. 15.12).

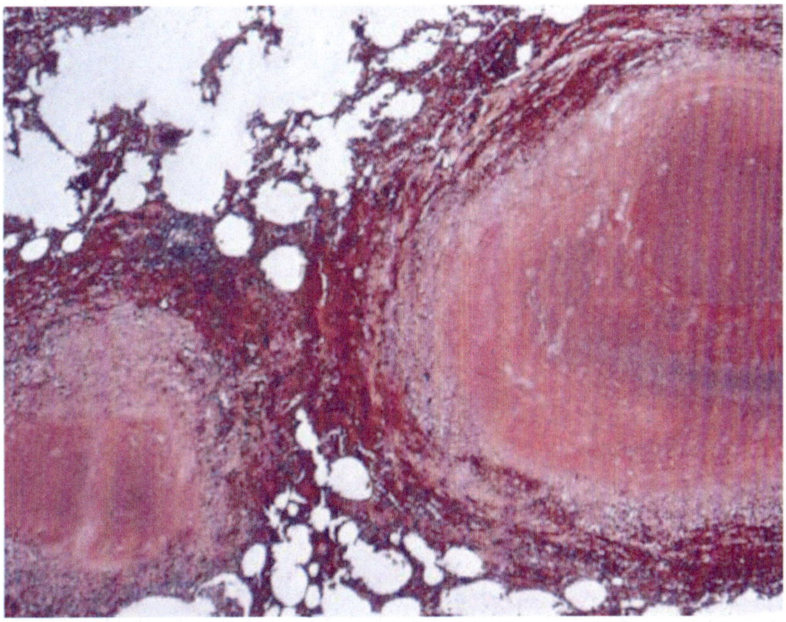

Fig. 15.10 Miliary tuberculosis of the lung (bronchopneumonia suspected macroscopically), incidental finding in a dialysis patient (H&E ×100)

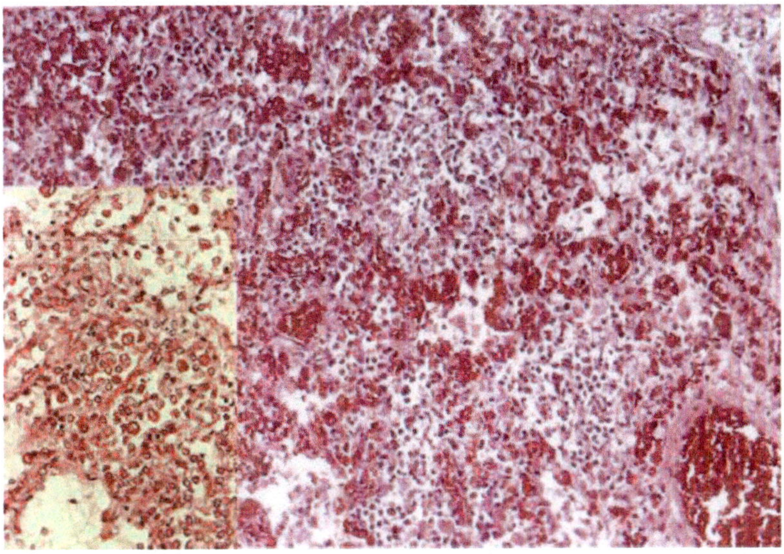

Fig. 15.11 Pronounced interstitial lymphomonocytic viral pneumonia with dense lymphomonocytic inflammatory infiltrate (H&E ×200) and cell engorgement in the alveolar lumina. Alveolar macrophages (pneumocytes) with polymorphic hyperchromatic cell nuclei in a case of viral pneumonia (H&E ×400)

15.1.6 Acute Interstitial Pneumonitis (*Hamman–Rich Syndrome*)

Acute interstitial pneumonitis, also known as Hamman–Rich syndrome and first described in 1935 and then 1944, is a distinct type of idiopathic interstitial pneumonia affecting patients of both genders without preexisting lung diseases (Buris et al. 1963; Diamond 1958; White and Craighead 1957; Peabody et al. 1955). The disease culminates in acute respiratory failure and often in death. In fact, the mortality rate of Hamman–Rich syndrome is approximately 50%, despite mechanical ventilation. Histological lung examination shows diffuse alveolar damage with alveolar septa mildly thickened by edema and capillary

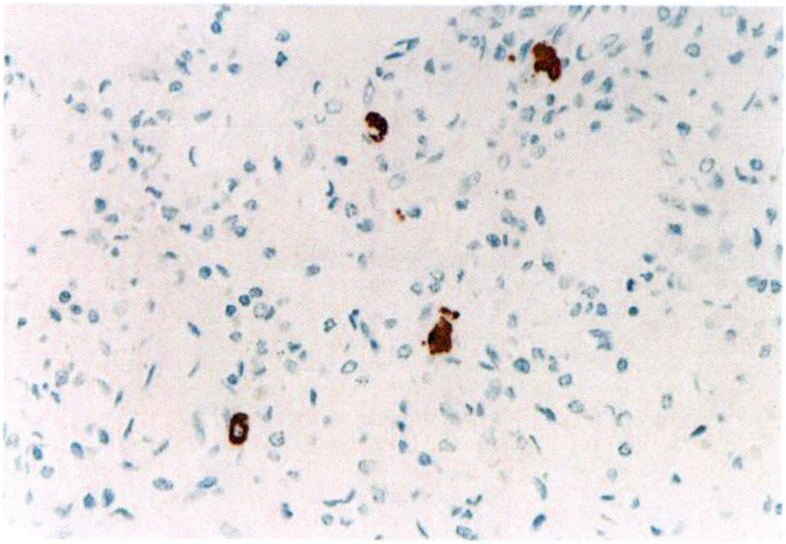

Fig. 15.12 Immunohi stochemical detection of CMV-positive cells in a case of viral pneumonia (CMV ×400)

congestion, alveolar edema, hyaline membranes lining the denuded alveolar walls, hyperplastic type-II pneumocytes, alveolar infiltrates of polymorphonuclear neutrophilic leukocytes, macrophages, monocytes, and plasma cells. In addition, fibrin thrombi can be found in small arteries, and numerous endoalveolar erythrocytes may be observed. Bronchial walls show epithelial denudation, while inside the lumen infiltrates of leukocytes, primarily neutrophils, may be present, as well as a moderate quantity of eosinophilic amorphous material (Turillazzi et al. 2007). Currently, there are only single reports concerning acute interstitial pneumonitis in the forensic literature. Desquamative interstitial pneumonia, one of the rarer forms of pneumonia, can cause death in isolated cases if undiagnosed (Plenzig et al. 2016).

15.2 Pancreatitis

Acute pancreatitis can lead to sudden death and represents a spectrum of diseases ranging from a mild, transitory illness to a severe, rapidly progressive hemorrhagic form, accompanied by massive necrosis and mortality rates of up to 24% (Tsokos and Braun 2007; Tümer and Dener 2007). Typically, only fulminant, mostly hemorrhagic pancreatitides have a lethal course. Macroscopic findings predominate, while histological findings can contribute to the detection or exclusion of preexisting damaged pancreatic tissue. Causes of pancreatitis include:

- Acute relapse caused by inflammation (Fig. 15.13) in the setting of a preexisting chronic fibrotic and frequently alcoholic pancreatitis (Chap. 6)
- Cholangio-pancreatitis, possibly with accompanying and mostly purulent cholangitis, cholangiolithiasis, and obstruction of the junction of the common bile duct and pancreatic duct
- Post-endoscopic retrograde cholangiopancreatography (ERCP) pancreatitis
- Postoperative pancreatitis with post-inflammatory adhesions
- Tumor-related pancreatitis
- Other rare forms

While gall stones represent the main etiologic factor in numerous extensive clinical studies, biliary etiology seems to play only a minor role in outpatient deaths subject to medicolegal autopsies (Tsokos and Braun 2007). Complications due to acute pancreatitis include lung edema, acute respiratory distress syndrome, peritonitis, disseminated intravascular coagulation, and sepsis.

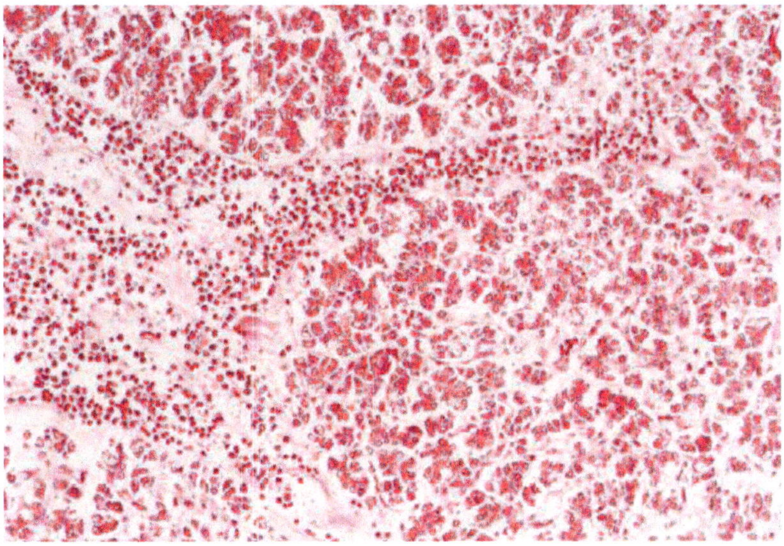

Fig. 15.13 Acute purulent pancreatitis (ASD ×100)

Histologically, necrosis of the parenchyma, necrosis of adipose tissue islets inside and outside pancreatic tissue, and hemorrhage can frequently be seen. Instead of adipose tissue, it is possible that only slightly homogeneous eosin red or bluish material can be detected, as well as fatty acid crystals or diffuse hematogenous deposits. In the acute stage, necrosis is demarcated by granulocytes, while granulation tissue and fibrosis can be seen later. Postmortem fatty tissue necrosis due to autolysis does not show vital reactions in the form of leukocytic demarcation. Pancreatitides occur more frequently in the case of alcohol abuse with inflammatory fatty liver (termed fatty liver hepatitis). Chronic pancreatitides show a marked increase in collagen fibers with lymphocytes, plasma cells, and histiocytes. The progressive inflammatory process can have an intermittent course. Pseudocysts, duct ectasia with secretion retention (dyschylia), and basophilic concretion can develop following inflammation. The islets of Langerhans are long spared and will only decay in the final phase which leads to diabetes mellitus. In the case of acute relapsing, focal hemorrhagic, and chronic fibrotic pancreatitis, the histological findings mentioned in Table 15.2 can be seen.

Table 15.2 Histological findings in the case of acute relapsing, hemorrhagic, and predominantly chronic fibrotic pancreatitis

Localization	Findings
Pancreatic lobules	Partly diffuse, partly netlike post-inflammatory fibrosis with embedded lymphocytes and monocytes
Glandular ducts	Duct ectasias; glandular epithelium with cellular and nuclear polymorphism, potential cell dysplasias (differential diagnosis: highly differentiated adenocarcinoma of the pancreas)
Glandular lumina	Accumulation of chyle, in part amorphous basophilic calcification (dyschylia)
Islets of Langerhans	These are not necessarily affected but are frequently rarefied
Peripancreatic adipose tissue	Finely spotted, tryptic fatty tissue necrosis that may have fibrous scarring and calcification (basophil calcium salt sediments)
Acute inflammatory episode	Focal pancreatic necrosis with accompanying hemorrhage

In the case of cholangio-pancreatitis, retained bile pigment may appear in adjacent glandular excretory ducts of the pancreas in addition to extrahepatic cholestasis in the liver tissue and potentially accompanying icterus. With a subacute course, cholemic nephrosis might be determined histologically, i.e., resorbed bile pigment in the epithelia of the renal tubes (Chap. 6). Acute rupture of the arteria pancreatica magna can be a complication of an immature pseudocyst in chronic pancreatitis (Lunetta et al. 2002).

15.3 Malaria

Malaria is one of the most common infectious diseases worldwide. In Europe, malaria belongs to the group of acute lethal diseases that rarely go unrecognized, in particular tropical malaria (Yagmur et al. 2015; Dettmeyer 2006; Siveke et al. 2001; Püschel et al. 1998; Albert et al. 1995). Previous history, including arrival or return from a malaria region, corresponding symptoms, and an enlarged spleen at autopsy with a black-red section are highly indicative of malaria (Rauch et al. 1999). Histological evidence of malaria pigment (hemozoin pigment) is possible in all vascularized internal organs including the brain, kidney, lung, heart, and liver, even in the presence of putrefactive changes (Naeve 1971). This pigment is characteristic of the disease and leads to the diagnosis of malaria (Figs. 15.14 and 15.15). Typical capillary blockades with parasite-infested erythrocytes or schizonts positive for malaria pigment can sometimes be determined in brain tissue. Alveolar macrophages, liver, and spleen may be positive for the malaria pigment. Under magnification, merozoites arranged in rosette patterns can be seen in the schizonts and under higher magnification (up to ×1000); trophozoites and possibly disintegrated pathogens (schizonts) can be determined in postmortem blood smears. Polymerase chain reaction can be used for the postmortem diagnosis of malaria (Becker et al. 1999).

15.4 Clostridia

Fatal cases of clostridial gas gangrene are rare (Jänisch et al. 2010; Hausmann et al. 2004; Sasaki et al. 2000; Burke and Opeskin 1999; Soper 1986; Ruf et al. 1986; Andes 1982; Metter and Schulz 1977). The causative agent is primarily *Clostridium perfringens* but may also be, e.g., *Clostridium sordellii*. Clostridial infection is often related to trauma and more rarely to intravenous injection (Mahfoud et al. 2002). Characterized by extensive tissue necrosis and a complete absence of an accompanying leukocyte infiltration or tissue inflammatory response, the histopathological picture of clostridial gas gangrene is distinctly different from other bacterial infections. Occasionally, in cases without trauma, it may be impossible to verify the portal of entry of the responsible pathogen (Tsokos et al. 2008).

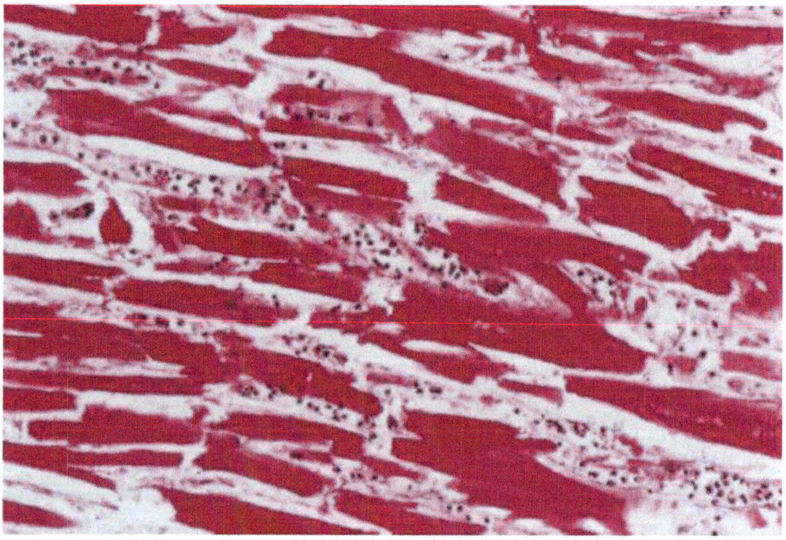

Fig. 15.14 Abundant malaria pigment in intramyocardial capillary blood vessels (H&E ×200)

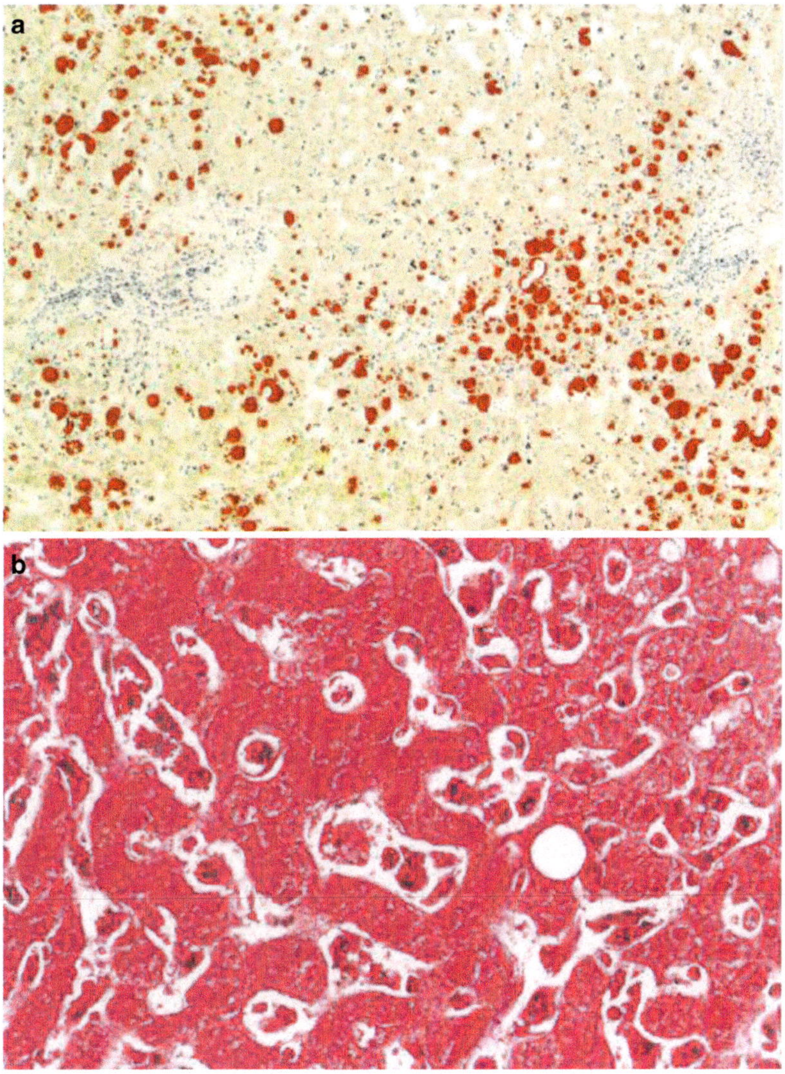

Fig. 15.15 (**a**) Steatosis hepatis (Sudan III ×100) and (**b**) abundant malaria pigment in liver sinusoids (H&E ×400)

Histological examination of the affected skel etal musculature may demonstrate separation of myofibers by abundant gram-positive, rod-shaped bacteria without an associated inflammatory reaction. In the brain, liver, and kidneys, empty cystic spaces can be seen lined by bacteria corresponding to clostridia (Figs. 15.16 and 15.17). Additionally, an accumulation of clostridia within alveolar capillaries as well as an accumulation of phagocytosed clostridia in Kupffer cells in the liver seem to be typical histopathological features. The combination of extensive tissue necrosis and the absence of an inflammatory response are distinct from other bacterial infections. Otherwise, clostridia are often found in the heart, blood, and organs of corpses showing putrefactive changes, and it can sometimes be difficult to distinguish between an antemortem infection caused by gram-positive, anaerobic, spore-forming bacteria and postmortem putrefactive changes (Jänisch et al. 2010; Kernbach-Wighton et al. 2003).

Necrotizing infection caused by *Clostridium perfringens* (gram-positive, spore-forming, obligate anaerobic rods) is occasionally seen (so-called gas gangrene). Other possible causes of gas gangrene include *Clostridium histolyticum*, *Clostridium septicum*, *Clostridium novyi*, and

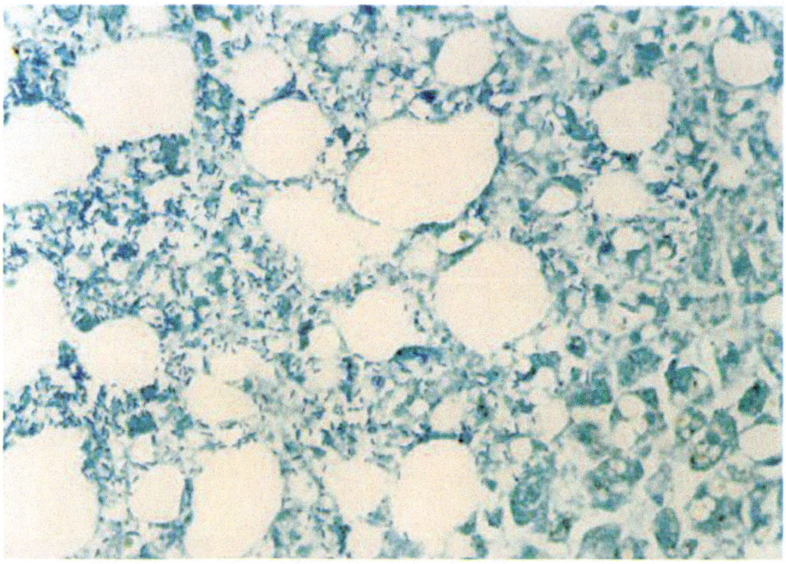

Fig. 15.16 Accumulation of bacteria corresponding to clostridia located near empty cystic spaces in the partly necrotic liver (methylene blue ×40)

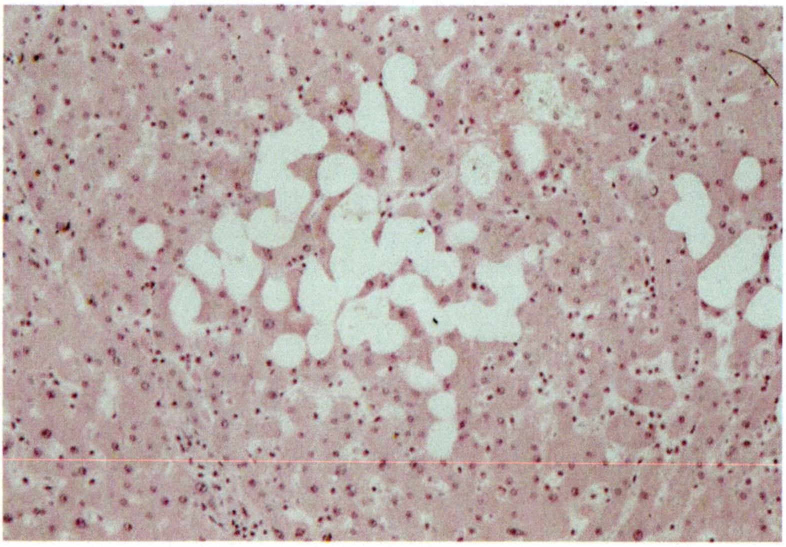

Fig. 15.17 Empty cystic spaces in the liver in a case of clostridial gas gangrene (H&E ×100—image kindly provided by Dr. R. Amberg, Freiburg, Germany)

Clostridium fallax. Histologically, one sees extensive necrosis in the affected areas, and sepsis with acute kidney failure develops rapidly. Areas of focal spread can appear blown-up like a balloon, at times with microscopically tiny bubble-like cavities and adjacent gram-positive rods (Fig. 15.18). A posttraumatic infective subcutaneous emphysema is possible, classically including *Clostridia* sp. or *Streptococcus* sp., but may also involve coliform and anaerobic bacteria (Byard 2016).

15.5 Measles

Fatal measles infection is relatively rare in Western countries with high immunization rates but does sometimes occur in areas where too few children

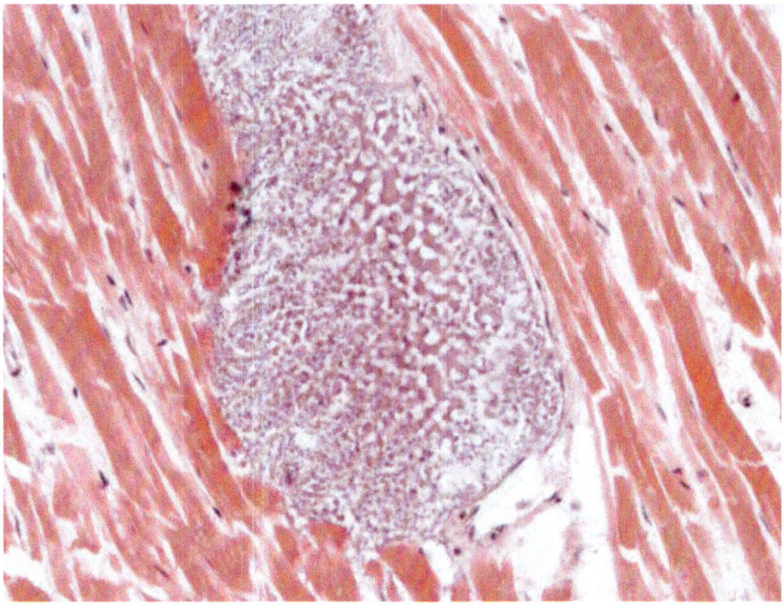

Fig. 15.18 Histological gram-positive rods, areas blown-up like a balloon, and microscopically small, round cavities with a honeycomb-like pattern in the setting of fatal *Clostridium septicum* infection of the myocardium following partial colon resection and wound infection in an adipose female patient (H&E ×400)

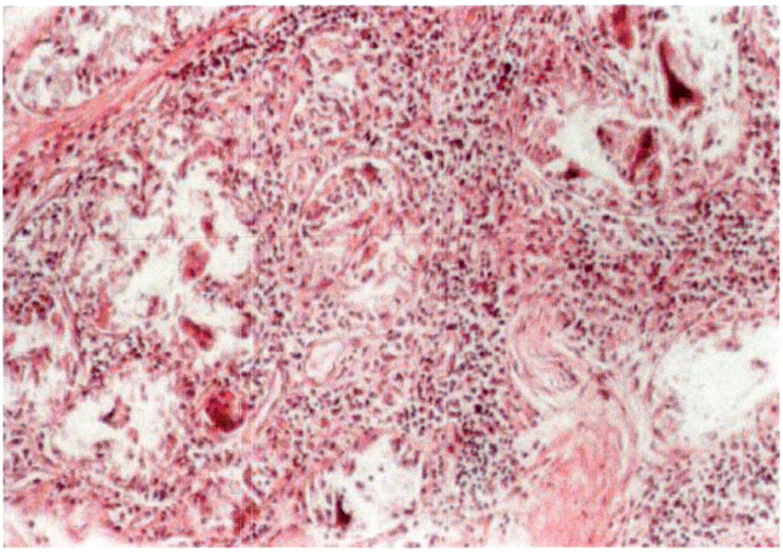

Fig. 15.19 Pronounced lymphadenitis of paratracheal lymph nodes with reactive sinus histiocytosis, multiple polynuclear giant cells, and substantial cell and nuclear polymorphism in a case of measles infection (H&E ×100)

are vaccinated over a prolonged period to prevent spread of the highly infectious measles viruses (Risse et al. 2008). In lethal courses or in the case of measles infections causing permanent neurological deficits (e.g., measles-induced meningitis, measles encephalitis), an allegation of parental negligence should be considered on the basis of parental failure to vaccinate children. Without explicit legal vaccination requirements, however, it is unlikely that the allegation can be prosecuted. In the acute stage, pronounced lymphadenitis (Fig. 15.19) with polynuclear giant cells can be seen histologically. These giant cells can also be determined in the bronchial epithelium as well as in the case of measles

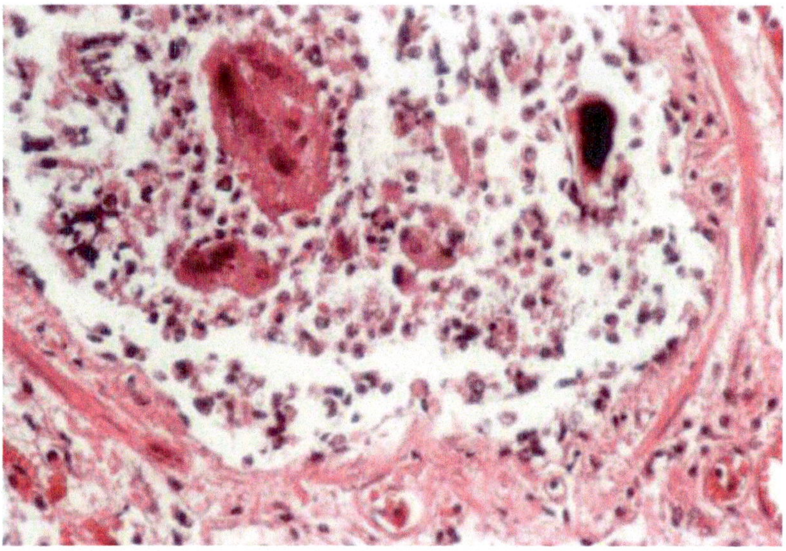

Fig. 15.20 The lumen of a bronchiolus with epithelial cells, polymorphonuclear leukocytes, and giant cells with multiple and in part bizarrely configured hyperchromatic cell nuclei in a case of measles infection (H&E ×200)

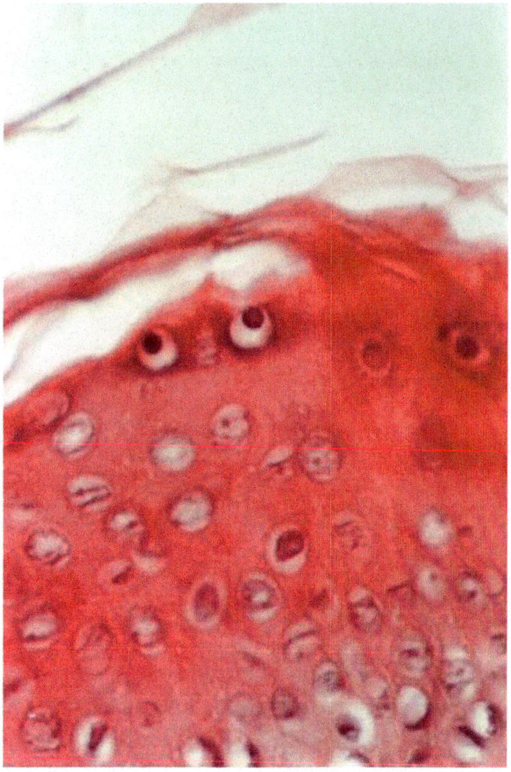

Fig. 15.21 Skin findings in a case of measles with virus-infected squamous epithelial cells, so-called koilocytes (H&E ×400)

pneumonia (Fig. 15.20). Virus-infested squamous epithelial cells, termed koilocytes, can be seen in the infected parts of the epidermis (Fig. 15.21).

15.6 Hydatid Disease (Echinococcosis)

Echinococcosis is endemic in some parts of the world, e.g., in sheep-raising areas. Most cases of hydatid disease in human populations are due to *Echinococcus granulosus* (Byard 2009). The dog is the usual host of *Echinococcus granulosus*, but humans may serve as an intermediate host upon ingestion of tapeworm ova. Although hydatid disease may remain asymptomatic, occasional cases of sudden and unexpected death do present at autopsy. Hydatid disease is a dangerous condition due to the risk of complications, and some authors suggest that human alveolar echinococcosis is underreported (Jorgensen et al. 2008).

The liver is involved in particular, whereas cardiac involvement with hydatid cysts is rare but may cause sudden unexpected death (Butcovan et al. 2010; Bennis et al. 2000; Murphy et al. 1971). Microscopically, an internal layer containing daughter cysts, an external laminated layer, and a cystic fibrotic wall can be detected (Fig. 15.22). This structure is surrounded by a moderate inflammatory cellular infiltration (eosinophils, lymphocytes, and plasma cells). If such intravascular findings are detectable, the cause of death can be deemed to be anaphylactic shock due to intravascular spread of the hydatid cyst content. Intracavitary expansion is also

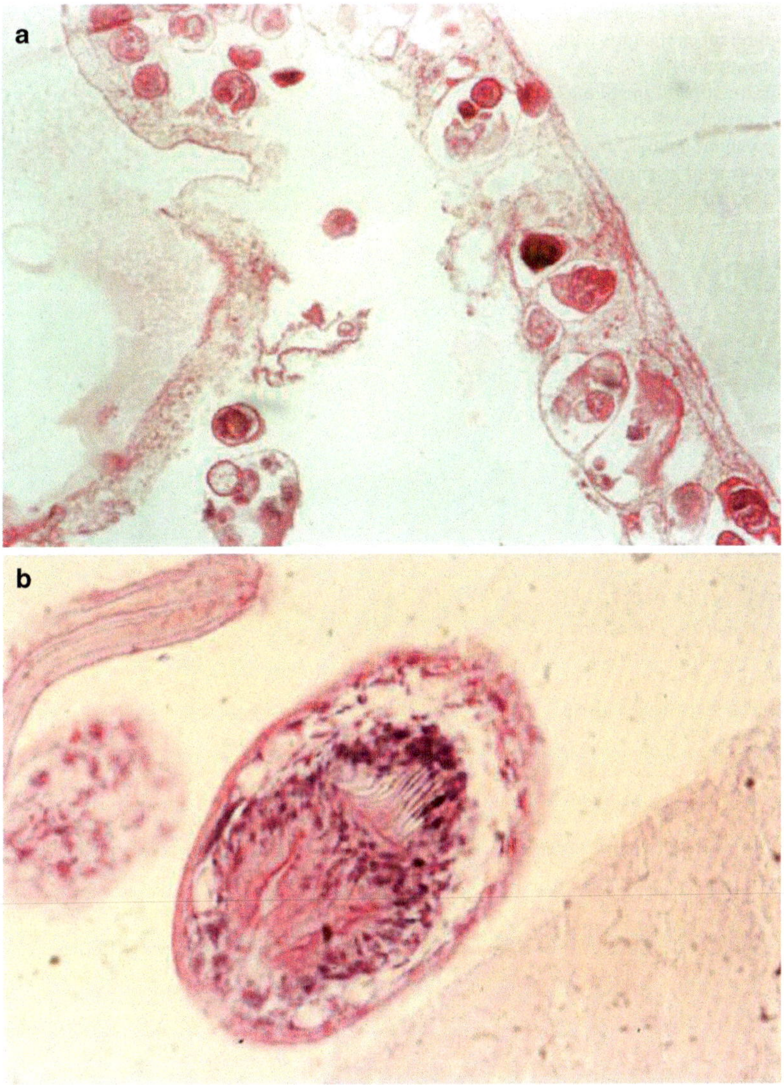

Fig. 15.22 (**a**) Internal germinal layer with daughter cysts in a case of *Echinococcus granulosus* (H&E ×40) and (**b**) characteristic scolices (H&E ×100)

possible (Kaplan et al. 2001). Cardiac echinococcosis is mostly symptomatic including angina due to pressure effects of the cyst on the coronary arteries, dyspnea, and palpitation (Telli and Durgut 2001) but may also be asymptomatic (Kucukarslan et al. 2005).

15.7 Ascending Cholangitis

Ascending cholangitis typically occurs as bacterial purulent cholangitis but also as fungal cholangitis in rare cases. If cholangitis spreads to liver tissue, an inflamed cellular infiltration of the bile duct walls can be seen (Figs. 15.23 and 15.24). In cases of fungal infection, periductal fungal infection can also be found.

15.8 Ascending Urinary Tract Infections

These are ascending canalicular or lymphogenic urinary tract infections (often *Escherichia coli*) due to congestion, urethral stenosis, prostatic hypertrophy, etc. Histologically, polymorphonuclear leukocytes can be found in the interstitium and renal tubules. The infiltrates are typically arranged in a striated manner; abscesses in particular develop in the cortical

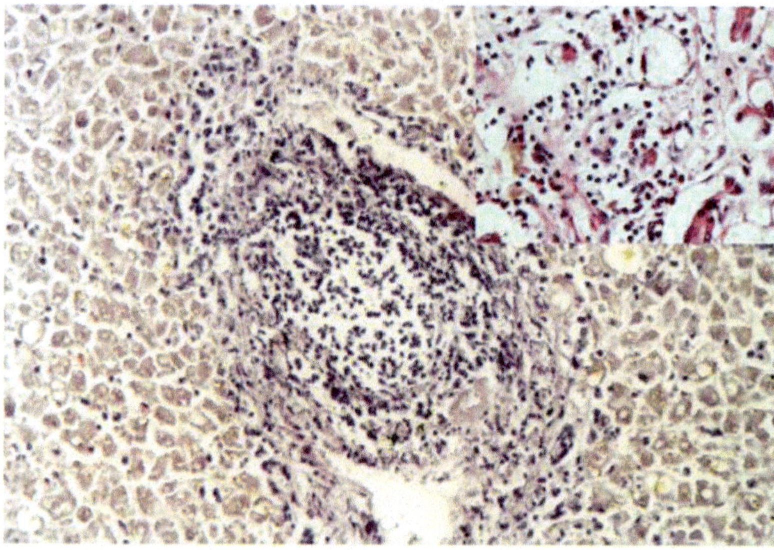

Fig. 15.23 Ascending purulent cholangitis with inflammatory destruction of the bile duct wall and polymorphonuclear neutrophil granulocytes (methylene blue ×200)

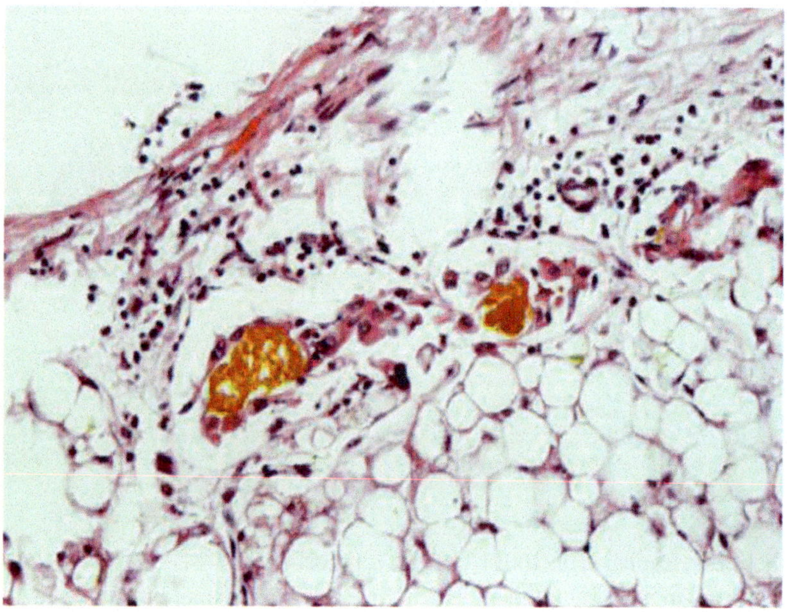

Fig. 15.24 Pronounced extrahepatic cholestasis in a case of ascending purulent cholangitis with severe hepatic steatosis (H&E ×200)

region. Hyaline obliteration of glomeruli and interstitial fibrosis with lymphocytic infiltration can be seen after healing. Inflammation remains focally restricted in contrast to hematogenic renal abscesses. Occasionally, ascending fungal infections in the efferent urinary tract system are present (Fig. 15.25).

15.9 Glomerulonephritis

Cases of unrecognized glomerulonephritis are very rare in forensic practice. Goodpasture's syndrome, which must be considered in any differential diagnosis (Goodpasture 1919;

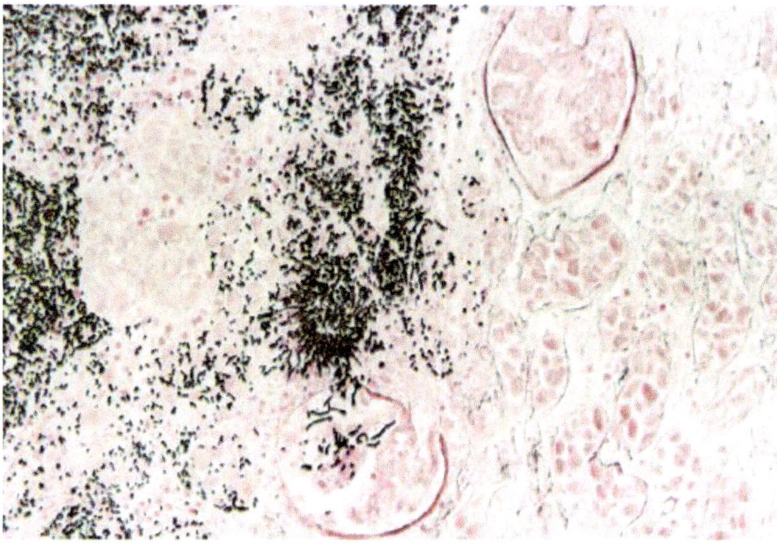

Fig. 15.25 Ascending fungal infection with detectable fungal conidia and fungal fibers in the renal parenchyma (Grocott ×200)

McCaughey and Thomas 1962; Clausnitzer and Müntefering 1975), should always be considered as a possible cause of sudden natural death in young adults if merely unusual; disseminated pulmonary hemorrhage represents the essential finding at autopsy. The final diagnosis is made by microscopic evidence of additional diffuse hemosiderosis of the lungs and proliferative glomerulonephritis. In addition, fibrinoid necrosis of lung capillaries and loss of elastic fibers in the lung can be observed. Nevertheless, glomerulonephritis can be observed as acute postinfection endocapillary glomerulonephritis, affecting mainly children and adolescents.

Classic poststreptococcal glomerulonephritis can begin 1–2 weeks after streptococcal infection and show macro- and microhematuria, proteinuria, and edema formation. Microscopically, glomeruli with numerous neutrophil granulocytes in capillary lumina, a swollen endothelium, and an increased number of cells in the mesangium can be seen (Fig. 15.26). Immunohistochemically, coarse particle deposition of complement C3 can be detected on the glomerular capillary walls.

15.10 OPSI Syndrome

Overwhelming postsplenectomy infection (OPSI) syndrome is characterized by an acute lethal course in splenectomy patients following commonplace injuries that become infected (Rizzo et al. 2004; Kanthan et al. 1999; Locker et al. 1995; Lindblad and Lindblad 1990; Curti et al. 1985; Ramsay and Bouskill 1973). The syndrome was first described in children (Schumaker Jr 1952) and is characterized by severe clinical symptoms, very rapid progression, and a frequently dismal prognosis (Dickerman 1979; Kribben et al. 1995; Bisno 1971; Grinblat and Gilboa 1975; Diamond 1969; Holdsworth et al. 1991). Although more rarely, adults are also affected. Typically, the syndrome is observed within the first 2 years following posttraumatic splenectomy (Kühn et al. 1983; Seufert and Böttcher 1982). Even leaving spleen tissue in the abdomen posttraumatically—termed peritoneal splenosis—is insufficient to prevent postsplenectomy sepsis (Seufert and Böttcher 1982; van Wyck et al. 1980). Frequently, the fulminant course does not leave time for the diagnosis of sepsis (Reavy and Nakonechny 1979; Locker

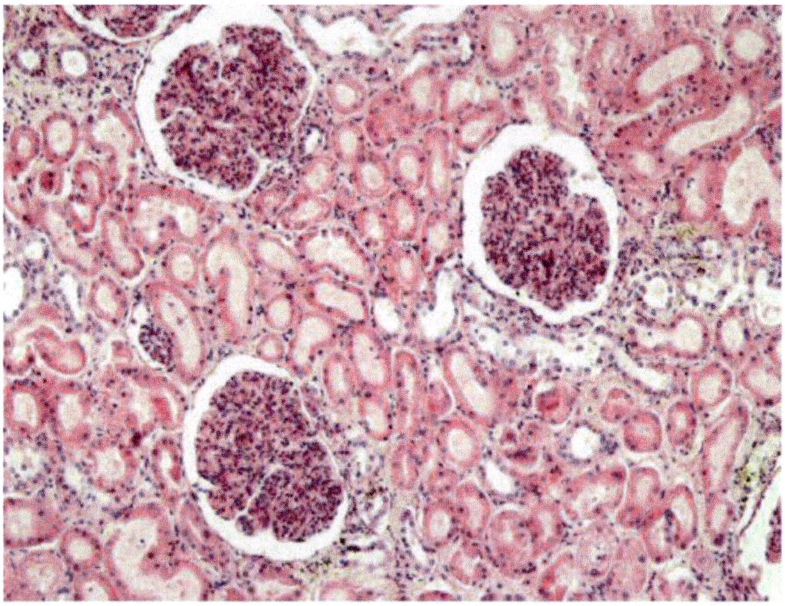

Fig. 15.26 Acute glomerulonephritis (H&E ×100)

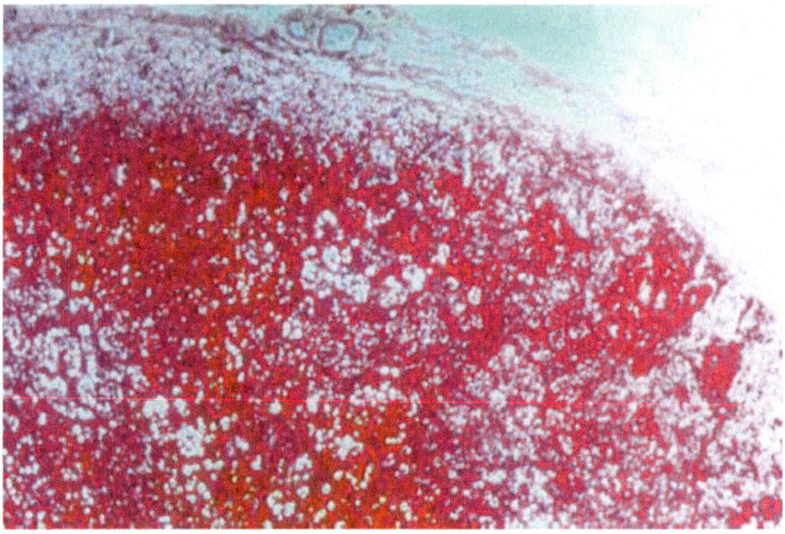

Fig. 15.27 Hemorrhagic necrosis in the adrenal glands in a case of OPSI syndrome (H&E ×200)

et al. 1995; Rodriguez Gomez et al. 1997). Lethal OPSI syndrome may even occur many years after splenectomy has been performed (Grinblat and Gilboa 1975; Kühn et al. 1983; Urata et al. 1997). Even patients who have been vaccinated against the most frequent agent, *Streptococcus pneumoniae*, can be affected (Lindblad and Lindblad 1990). Autopsy findings including hemorrhagic necrosis of the adrenal glands (Fig. 15.27) are similar to those of Waterhouse–Friderichsen syndrome or Sanarelli–Shwartzman phenomenon, both of which have also been rarely observed in adults. Pregnancy-related OPSI syndrome is rarely seen (Dettmeyer et al. 1999).

The mortality rate for OPSI syndrome ranges from 24 to 75% (Kühn et al. 1983). Most cases of mortality occur within the first year following splenectomy; the risk for splenectomy patients to develop OPSI is said to lie between 0.4 and 2.5% (Kribben et al. 1995). In the majority of cases

(50–70%), *Streptococcus pneumoniae* often is the causative agent, followed by *Haemophilus influenzae* (Kribben et al. 1995; Locker et al. 1995). Some authors require an obligatory vaccination following splenectomy and prior to hospital discharge to lower the risk of OPSI syndrome. As a prophylactic measure, spleen-preserving surgery or peritoneal splenosis has been promoted by leaving spleen tissue in the abdomen (Kribben et al. 1995; Seufert and Böttcher 1982). In the case of body temperatures above 37 °C, 1 g of amoxicillin should be given immediately. The shock event due to the distribution of bacterial endotoxins is mostly irreversible and, within a few hours, develops into sepsis with disseminated intravascular coagulation and microcirculatory disturbance.

15.11 Shock

The term "shock" refers to various pathophysiological processes that lead to a state which can result in death due to multiorgan failure. However, only in some cases does the cause of shock offer different histological findings. The literature on pathophysiology, clinical picture, and morphology of shock is very comprehensive.

In the literature, the term "shock" is known in the following forms:

- Hemorrhagic-hypovolemic shock (bleeding to death)
- Septic shock, e.g., due to very rare infectious agents such as pneumatosis cystoides intestinales (Suzuki et al. 2009) or fungi (Thierauf et al. 2007; Tsokos 2006a, b)
- Anaphylactic shock (anaphylaxis)
- Shock due to metabolism irregularity, e.g., Addison's disease, Sheehan's syndrome, or thyrogenic shock (Chap. 16)
- Pancreatogenic shock
- So-called burn shock
- Symptomatic shock
- Toxic shock

The histological distinctness of the findings in a shock event depends considerably on patient survival time. If death occurs rapidly, less pronounced findings are usually detectable. In a shock event, the regulation systems of the organism will not only be activated but will also decompensate. For this reason, a certain homogeneity of histological and immunohistochemical findings in types of shock of different origins is not surprising (see, e.g., shock lung, Fig. 15.28). There are numerous

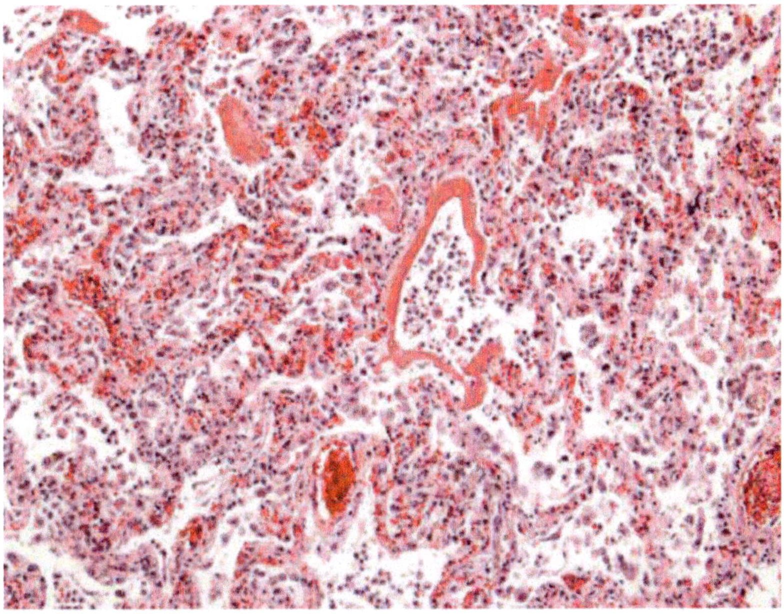

Fig. 15.28 Shock lung with widespread hyaline membranes and megakaryocyte embolism (H&E ×100)

comparative investigations of various types of shock that demonstrate, with the present state of knowledge, that histological and immunohistochemical findings alone do not allow for a determination of shock origin without knowing patient medical history (Weis and Bohnert 2008).

Septic shock. Sepsis is a systemic inflammatory disease with a high mortality rate.

> Sepsis arises if an infection site develops within the body from which pathogenic bacteria spread constantly or periodically into the bloodstream. This happens in such a way that this invasion triggers subjective and objective symptoms.

Human sepsis refers to a spectrum of pathophysiological changes in the host system resulting from a generalized activation and systemic expression of the host's inflammatory pathways in response to infection (Levy et al. 2003).

Often, autopsy findings and routine histology in cases of suspected fatal sepsis are nonspecific and unconvincing. Various immunohistochemical markers have been investigated in cases of sepsis, especially with regard to changes in the lungs (Müller et al. 2008; Tsokos 2003, 2005; Tsokos et al. 2001, 2002, 2003; Tsokos and Fehlauer 2001). Immunohistochemical evidence of E-selectin on endothelial cells of the interstitial pre- and postcapillary vascular system and of lactoferrin on intravascular, interstitial, and intra-alveolar leukocytes, as well as the biochemical parameter procalcitonin, are typically included in sepsis diagnosis (Müller and Tsokos 2006). However, immunohistochemical staining of tissue showing putrefactive changes can only be analyzed to a certain extent (Ortiz-Rey et al. 2008; Ortmann et al. 2000).

The vascular endothelium controls leukocyte extravasation into tissue by induction and modulation of endothelial cell adhesion molecules, such as E-selectin (CD62E). E-selectin is not expressed by non-stimulated endothelium but expressed due to the release of cytokines. E-selection on activated endothelium initiates neutrophil recruitment in sepsis-induced lung injury. Immunohistochemical detection of an intense expression of E-selectin in lung tissue may prove to be a valuable diagnostic tool in the forensic postmortem elucidation of death due to sepsis (Tsokos et al. 2000). Immunohistochemical detection of CCR2 and CX3CR1 expression in the lungs should also be considered a valuable diagnostic tool for the postmortem diagnosis of sepsis (An et al. 2009). ICAM-1 was upregulated in endothelium and in leukocytes within the lungs as well as lactoferrin and VLA-4 in pulmonary leukocytes, while vascular endothelial growth factor (VEGF) is downregulated in sepsis-induced lung injury (Lau and Lai 2008).

Regardless of the cause of shock, histological and immunohistochemical findings of varying distinctness can be found in internal organs, whereby preexisting diseases may also be of prognostic significance in the case of sepsis, e.g., previous ischemic damage in the right ventricular myocardium, which can be demonstrated using the immunohistochemical marker fibronectin (Fracasso et al. 2016). Currently, however, immunohistochemical findings do not allow for a reliable differentiation with respect to the cause of shock or for a reliable conclusion as to the chronology of the shock; thus the reader is referred to the relevant literature. A short overview of the various types of shock with details or examples as to etiology, pathophysiology, and histology is provided in Table 15.3.

In summary, histological findings in the lung, liver, and kidneys typically allow for the diagnosis of a shock event. Immunohistochemical studies on sepsis-induced findings in lung tissue are available, e.g., on the expression of tumor necrosis factor-α (Miyashita et al. 2006).

However, etiology of the shock event must be derived from differential autopsy findings (myocardial infarction, pulmonary embolism, etc.) in association with the patient's history. Even if there are significant variations as to the chronology of shock events, in particular in the case of simultaneous intensive medical therapy, it is possible to provide an approximate timeline for the stages of shock (Table 15.4).

The intravascular microthrombi that occur during shock can be eliminated by fibrinolysis. With prolonged postmortem intervals, postmortem fibrinolysis must be considered (Janssen 1977). In order to detect microthrombi and hyaline membranes, PAS reaction (Fig. 15.29),

Table 15.3 Overview of the types of shock with etiology, pathogenesis, and histology

Type of shock	Etiology or pathophysiology	Histological findings
Cardiogenic shock	Myocardial infarction, myocarditis, mechanical trauma, arrhythmias, rupture of the papillary muscle, thrombosis, myxoma, heart valve defect	According to etiology
Circulatory shock	Pulmonary embolism, pneumothorax, pleural effusions, dissecting aneurysm, diaphragmatic hernias, mediastinal emphysema; always resulting in right heart failure	Thrombosis and embolism (Chap. 9), aneurysms (Chap. 14)
Septic shock (endotoxin or exotoxin shock)	Endotoxin formation, in particular in the case of pleural empyema and peritonitis, urogenital infections, pyoderma, possibly endocarditis	Shock organs: megakaryocyte embolism in the lung, pulmonary hyaline membranes (Fig. 15.23), centrilobular necrosis in the liver, hyperemia in the renal medulla
Intoxication (toxic shock)	Barbiturates, anesthetics, antihypertensives, etc.	Possibly substance-specific findings (Chap. 5), nonspecific signs of intoxication, such as hepatocellular vacuolization
Anaphylactic shock (e.g., after colloid plasma solutions) or neurogenic shock (e.g., craniocerebral trauma, meningoencephalitis, intracranial bleeding, spinal marrow injury)	Antigen–antibody reaction with release of IgE, histamine, tryptase, etc.	According to etiology, presentation of eosinophil granulocytes, degranulated mast cells, IgE
Hemorrhagic-hypovolemic shock	Exsiccosis, severe diuresis, vomiting, diarrhea, exudation (cholera, burnings), acute edemas and effusions, bleeding to death	Signs of blood loss, more frequently subendocardial hemorrhages
Symptomatic shock; primary pulmonary edema	Respiratory insufficiency with hypoxidosis	Evidence of aspirated material, aqueous emphysema, histological signs of hypothermia or hyperthermia
Aspiration		
Drowning		
Hypothermia		
Hyperthermia		
Endocrine shock (Chap. 16)	Specific dysregulation	Findings according to the cause of endocrine shock
Addisonian crisis		
Diabetic coma		
Pheochromocytoma		
Hypothyreotic coma		
Thyrotoxicosis		
Parathyrotoxicosis		

The various causes of shock have a combined effect in the terminal vascular system: varying degrees of enlargement of artery, capillary, and venule lumina, stasis phenomena, damage to endothelial cells, microthrombi in the terminal vascular system, edemas, and peripheral hypoxia with necrosis

trichrome staining according to Goldner, PTAH, and Ladewig stains have been recommended as staining methods. Ladewig stains fibrin bright red, erythrocytes orange, and thrombocytes blue. In the case of postmortem hemolysis with hyalinization of the vascular content, precipitation of fibrin that typically interfuses the complete microthrombus is lacking. The intravital formation of fibrin clots shows long fibers that run parallel to the vascular wall. If such fibrin thrombi are fibrously organized, so-called Siegmund's nodes may remain.

In some cases, there may be alternate explanations for histological findings with respect to shock events. Thus in the liver, for example, it might be difficult to differentiate between

Table 15.4 Stages of shock

Stage	Conventional histological findings
Early stage (minutes up to 1 h)	*Lung*: interstitial and alveolar edema rich in proteins, dilated lymphatic vessels, aggregation of erythrocytes in the terminal vascular system, sometimes with accumulation of thrombocytes (termed sludge phenomenon), first microthrombi
	Kidneys: microthrombi in the glomeruli, major parts of the renal tubules with wide lumina (approximately 70%), intratubular protein cylinders (approximately 40–50%)
	Liver: acute venous hyperemia (particularly in the case of cardiogenic shock), homogeneous blood columns in the sinusoids of the liver (in the differential diagnosis, differentiation from postmortem intravascular homogenization is facilitated by azan or Lepehne's staining) (Janssen 1977)
	Brain: pronounced perivascular edema
Mid stage I (1–24 h)	*Lung*: damage and swelling of endothelial cells with adhesion of granulocytes and monocytes, microthrombi (obstruction of pulmonary circulation with sudden death is possible), necrosis of the alveolar epithelium, erythrocyte extravasation, focal atelectases, initial discharge of fibrin into the interstitium, then into the alveolar lumina, and formation of hyaline membranes up into the terminal bronchioli and hyaline membranes coating the surface of the alveoli, hemorrhage—particularly in the case of septic shock, megakaryocyte embolism
	Kidneys: focal tubular necrosis, major parts are initially swollen, then flattened epithelial cells, frequently enlarged nuclei
	Liver: disseminated hepatocellular single and group necrosis or necrosis with bright zonal demarcation in a centroacinar or annular arrangement around the central nerves (Müller et al. 1970)
	In general: numerous microthrombi in all body regions, intravascular "shock-bodies" in round to oval formations up to 200 µm in diameter (in the context of disseminated intravascular coagulation, DIC)—in particular in the case of endotoxin shock, liver and kidneys are less affected than the lungs
Mid stage II (>24 h to 1 week)	*Lung*: early proliferation of connective tissue into the protein-rich exudate
	Kidneys: inflammatory infiltration, particularly lymphocytes, development of interstitial fibrosis; development of mostly double-sided cortex necrosis is possible (renal cortex ischemia)
	Liver: microthrombi, nonspecific reaction of Kupffer stellate cells (phagocytic activity), centrilobular dissociation of hepatocytes, loss of cytoplasmic basophilia, reduced dyeability with eosin; confluence of centrilobular necrosis with interlobular bridge formation is possible; histiocytic reaction starts after approximately 48 h (Janssen 1977)
Late stage (>1 week)	*Lung*: regeneration of the vascular and alveolar epithelium, fibrous thickening of interalveolar septa, development of pulmonary fibrosis with chronic respiratory insufficiency
	Kidneys: lymphocytic inflammation and tubular atrophy; in the case of bilateral necrosis of the renal cortex or with so-called crush kidney, dialysis treatment might be required
	Liver: centrilobular necrosis, pronounced hypoxic steatosis of hepatocytes possible

Hemorrhagic erosions of the mucosa can be found as a sign of shock in the gastrointestinal tract with necrosis of the intestinal epithelium (after 4–5 h) and bleeding complications. The heart is not typically directly affected by a shock event. However, hypoxic myocardial damage cannot be excluded, such as fibrillar necrosis (contraction band necrosis) of the myocardium, subendocardial hemorrhage, or intimal and medial necrosis of the coronary arteries

a preexisting chronic congested liver and focal autolytic areas. In the case of purulent-inflammatory processes, an inflammatory reaction in the spleen (Fig. 15.30) may develop. In the case of abdominal inflammation, this reaction typically occurs faster than with intrathoracic or intracranial inflammation. During septic shock, microabscesses can be determined in all body regions, for example, in the renal tubules (Fig. 15.31, particularly with purulent urinary tract infections, but also in the heart muscle (Fig. 15.32). If fungal conidia or fungal fibers can be determined in

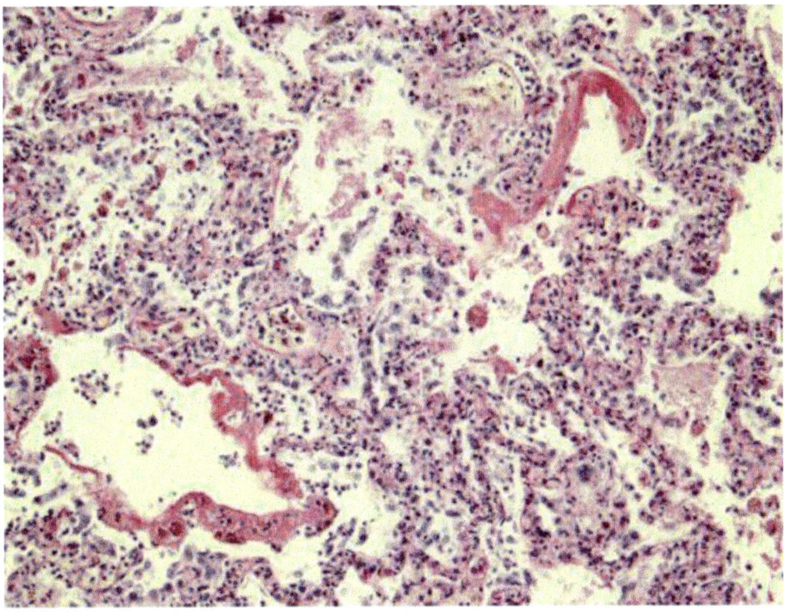

Fig. 15.29 Shock lung with widespread hyaline membranes, pulmonary necrosis, mixed inflammatory cell reaction, and single megakaryocyte embolisms (PAS ×100)

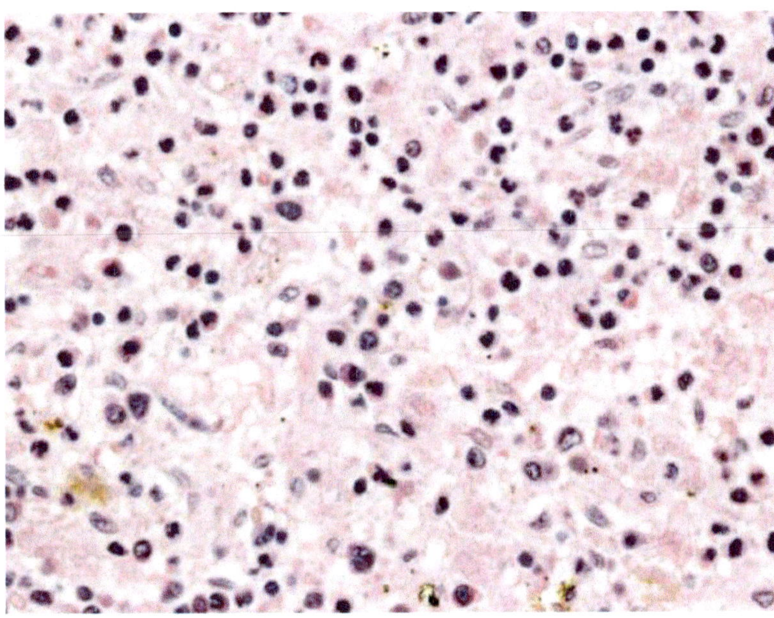

Fig. 15.30 Septic shock with inflammatory spleen reaction: numerous polymorphonuclear neutrophil granulocytes in the splenic sinuses (H&E ×400)

connection with an inflammatory reaction, this is referred to as fungal sepsis (Fig. 15.33).

15.12 Iatrogenic Infections

Hospital and iatrogenically acquired infections are not uncommon, especially in surgical patients. Severely ill patients who require intensive care or who are diabetic and/or immunocompromised appear to be particularly vulnerable to nosocomial infections. Methicillin-resistant *Staphylococcus aureus* (MRSA) may be responsible for a large number of these infections. MRSA, as well as *Pseudomonas aeruginosa*, are implicated in

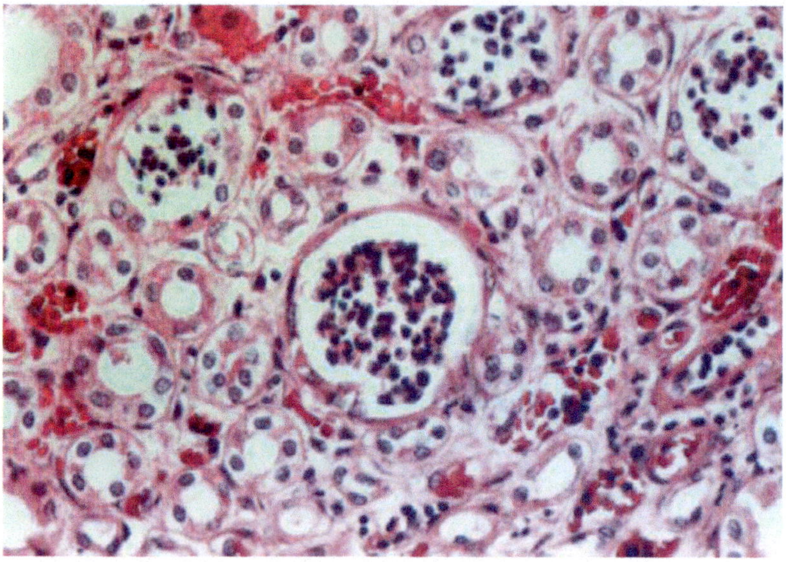

Fig. 15.31 Ascending purulent urinary tract infection with microabscesses in the renal tubules and septic shock (H&E ×400)

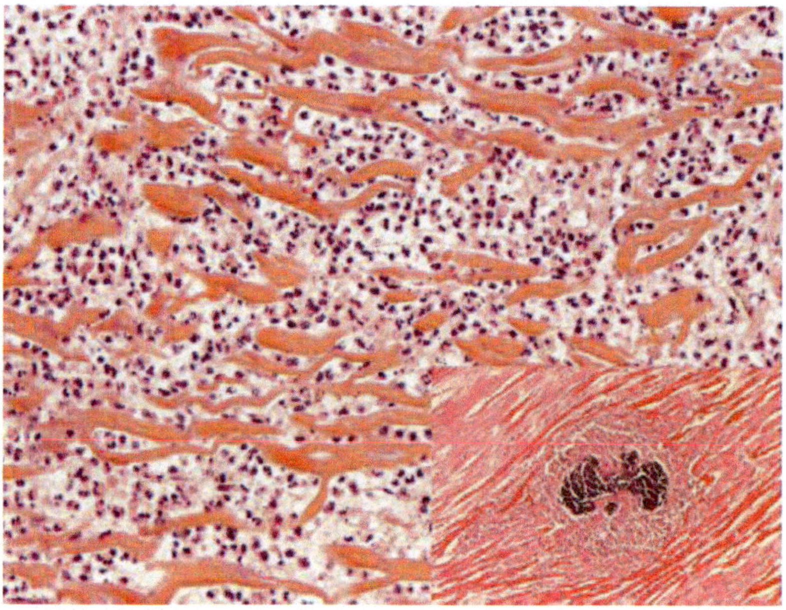

Fig. 15.32 Sepsis with purulent heart muscle necrosis, numerous polymorphonuclear neutrophil granulocytes, and cardiomyocytes with almost no nuclear dyeability (H&E ×200), as well as focal basophilic bacterial colonies (H&E ×400)

postoperative respiratory infections; potentially 40% of patient–nurse interactions in intensive care may result in the transmission of *Klebsiella* species and *Clostridium difficile*, even after only minimal contact (Lau 2005).

In addition to infections resulting from hospital pathogens, lethal infections that can have consequences under criminal law are known in forensic practice. Examples of such iatrogenically acquired infections include:

- Postoperative infections due to prolonged immobilization (urinary tract infection, bronchopneumonia, decubitus, and sepsis)
- Phlegmon and sepsis after liposuction (Simini 1999) (Chap. 1)
- Infected electrode probe for a cardiac pacemaker
- Ascending canalicular cholangitis or pancreatitis following ERCP
- Sepsis due to care errors in third- to fourth-degree decubitus, sometimes with osteomyelitis

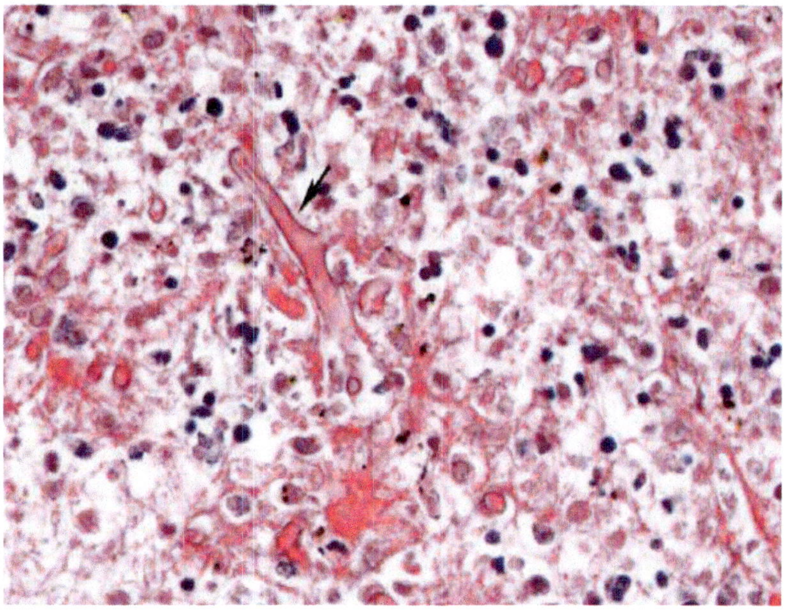

Fig. 15.33 Fungal sepsis with fungal fibers that can already be recognized in H&E staining (*arrow*) (H&E ×400)

- Peritonitis and septicemia resulting from biliary leaks induced by laparoscopic cholecystectomy
- Endoscopically or intraoperatively induced perforations resulting in peritonitis (Preuss et al. 2006b)
- Leptomeningitis and epidural abscesses after laminectomy and decompression
- Osteomyelitis after surgical stabilization
- Meningitis after neurosurgery (e.g., open resection of a meningioma)
- Septicemia following intravenous and intramuscular injection

The forensic diagnosis of *Staphylococcus aureus* septicemia following iatrogenic injections, for example, should be critically evaluated. This diagnosis can be established routinely in cases with delayed autopsy only when no other cause of death is revealed, no apparent source of infection other than the insertion site can be detected, and careful attention is paid to histological and bacteriological findings (Tsokos and Püschel 1999).

15.13 Allergies, Insect Bites, and Anaphylactic Shock

Sudden anaphylactic death occurring outside a hospital setting, in an emergency room, or in a medical treatment setting is usually subject to forensic autopsy. The forensic literature on anaphylactic deaths includes numerous case reports and a few population-based studies (Edston and van Hage-Hamsten 2005). The actual incidence of anaphylaxis ranges from 10 to 20/100,000 people per year (Da Broi and Moreschi 2011).

There are numerous triggers for allergic hypersensitive shock reactions, including foodstuffs (Unkrig et al. 2010; Sampson 2000), cat-hair allergy, insect bites (Prahlow and Barnard 1998; Barnard 1967), dust mite allergy (Edston and van Hage-Hamsten 2003), contrast agent allergy in connection with radiological diagnostics (Fineschi et al. 1999), or anaphylactic latex reaction, e.g., during anesthesia (Turillazzi et al. 2008). Allergic anaphylactic reactions to antibiotics, such as penicillins or cephalosporins, are relatively common and occasionally cause sudden death. Metamizole can also trigger allergic anaphylactic shock (Sterzig et al. 2016). In cases of sudden death such as these, marked splenic eosinophilia using pagoda red stain has been described (Reggiani Bonetti et al. 2015; Trani et al. 2008). Rarer triggers of anaphylactic shock have been described, e.g., injury by a crown-of-thorns starfish (Ihama et al. 2014). Nevertheless it is in doubt, whether death in anaphylactic shock can be diagnosed by autopsy alone.

Table 15.5 Response phases of the *allergic anaphylactic reaction*

Phase	Response
Phase I: sensitization	The immune system identifies foreign substances as allergens. Plasma cells then synthesize IgE-type antibodies and IgG4-type immunoglobulins as antibodies to the allergen. These antibodies bind with high affinity to Fc receptors on the membranes of mast cells and basophils. The affinity to Fc receptors on the surface membranes of eosinophilic and neutrophilic granulocytes, thrombocytes, as well as monocytes or macrophages is believed to be much lower
Phase II: immediate response	Only once (previous) sensitization has taken place does a second exposure occur with binding to IgE on the cell membranes from around 15–30 days following initial exposure. This triggers the degranulation of mast cells and basophils with the release of mediators (histamine, adenosine, chymase, tryptase, heparin) within 5–30 min following exposure These mediators cause the clinical symptoms: urticaria, conjunctivitis, rhinitis, bronchial asthma, angioedema with laryngospasm, anaphylactic shock
Phase III: delayed response	Several hours following (renewed) exposure to the allergen, secondary mediators that have been newly synthesized in the proinflammatory cells are released: noteworthy among these are, e.g., major basic protein (MBP) and eosinophil cationic protein (ECP). These mediators cause cell and tissue damage

Morphological diagnosis of anaphylactic by counting mast cells in the lung and airways has failed to gibe consistent results (Edston 2013).

The phases described in Table 15.5 for immediate-type anaphylactic reactions are distinct from an immunological allergic reaction, which affects the entire organism (Roncati et al. 2013). By using an anti-IgE antibody, it is possible to detect increased expression immunohistochemically. While eosinophils can be identified by hematoxylin and eosin staining, mast cells are better seen with the Giemsa stain; the membrane of mast cells can be demonstrated immunohistochemically using CD117 (c-kit) (Kounis et al. 2013). The number of CD117 (c-kit)-positive mast cells was observed higher in subjects who had died of asphyxia than in controls, particularly in the proximity of vessels in pulmonary samples (Muciaccia et al. 2016).

A distinction is often made between granulated and non-granulated mast cells, whereby degranulation likely takes place in the context of an acute allergic anaphylactic reaction. Only at higher magnifications is it possible to assess whether mast cells are still granulated or already degranulated. At 400× magnification, it is possible to demonstrate mast cells with granules immunohistochemically (Fig. 15.34).

Kounis syndrome is described as a hypersensitive reaction of the coronary arteries involving coronary spasms and cardiogenic heart failure (Kounis 2013; Kounis et al. 2013, 2014).

Postmortem determination of *tryptase*, *histamine*, and *diamine oxidase* in serum has yielded varying results. Accordingly, blood or serum should ideally be taken within 24 h postmortem for histamine determination, since levels can be expected to rise thereafter. Elevated levels in samples taken earlier support the diagnosis of anaphylactic shock, as do elevated tryptase levels. The value of serum diamine oxidase (DAO) determination is questionable (Mayer et al. 2011). However, elevated tryptase levels have also been described in other causes of death, such as trauma, asphyxia, myocardial infarction, heroin intoxication, hypereosinophilic *parasitosis*, and systemic *mastocytosis*, and these need to be ruled out in individual cases (Da Broi and Moreschi 2011). As a general rule, a number of adhesion molecules and their ligands are expressed in the context of allergic reactions, as has been shown, for instance, in allergic lung diseases (Popper et al. 2002).

Since anaphylaxis represents classical IgE-mediated hypersensitivity, both type E immunoglobulins (IgE) and tryptase can be mentioned as indicators (Osawa et al. 2008; Ansari et al. 1993; Yunginger et al. 1991; Edston and van Hage-Hamsten 1998), although there are reports of increased tryptase levels without anaphylaxis (Randall et al. 1995). In addition to findings on the skin, respiratory, cardiovascular, and

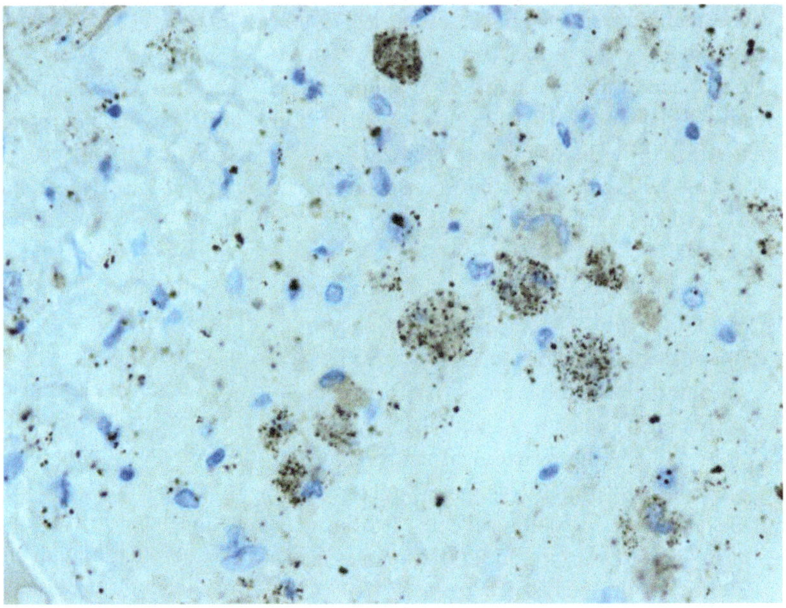

Fig. 15.34 Granulated *mast cells* demonstrated immunohistochemically using CD117 (×400)

gastrointestinal symptoms have also been described. Frequently, biphasic reactions can be observed with symptom improvement that ranges from temporary to complete recovery with recurring health problems after 8–12 h, often with bronchospasm. Apart from the clinical and chemical evidence of increased levels of IgE and tryptase, nonspecific findings should be present in a lethal course, such as acute stasis hyperemia of internal organs and pulmonary edema (Heinze et al. 2010), or increased mucus accumulation in the branches of the bronchial tree (Carson and Cook 2009). Immunohistochemically, degranulating perivascular mast cells can be determined via an anti-CD117 antibody. These mast cells can also be detected in the pulmonary interstitium (Shen et al. 2009; Heinze et al. 2010). Although antibodies do not address a specific epitope, they can identify mast cells using immunohistochemistry (Rimmer et al. 1984). Antibodies against histamine were also found to be effective (Johansson et al. 1992), but postmortem histamine is unstable. Meanwhile, the identification of neutral proteases as constituents of mast cell granules and new monoclonal antibodies against mast cell tryptase and chymase has facilitated the accurate identification of mast cells in histological sections (Perskvist and Edston 2007; Edston and van Hage-Hamsten 2005; Walls et al. 1990a, b; Glenner and Cohen 1960). In the case of a final event of acute bronchospasm, pulmonary alveoli that have coalesced peripherally to form small blisters can be detected microscopically. Examination with an anti-IgE antibody may lead to the detection of increased IgE-positive cells in the bronchial wall, which also supports the diagnosis of anaphylactic shock (Chap. 11).

Insect bites. Examinations of anaphylactic shock following a single insect bite revealed that the bite extended to the corium. Histologically, single microhemorrhages could be seen in the corium, as well as a sting canal and focal necrosis that could sporadically be traced back into the subcutaneous fat tissue. The tissue surrounding the sting canal has a loosened, edematous appearance, is penetrated by leukocytes, and shows significantly enlarged capillaries. Some studies showed that no particular inflammatory cells were seen histologically in airway edema or at the site of the sting (Barnard 1967), while others showed pronounced eosinophilia in the upper airway edema and inflammation with epithelial sloughing in cases of mucous plugging (Pumphrey and Roberts 2000). Some authors also reported an increased number of eosinophils in the splenic red pulp (Delage and Irey 1972;

Vance and Strassmann 1941; Dean 1922) and myocardial lesions in the form of discrete myocyte damage in 80% of 30 cases of anaphylactic deaths (Delage et al. 1973). Removal of the skin area affected by the insect bite is always necessary. This will then be cut into consecutive sections to reliably analyze the tissue layer with the sting canal.

Anaphylactic Reactions to Latex

Various patient groups are at risk for potentially life-threatening anaphylactic reactions to latex during surgical and medical procedures, primarily those receiving obstetric and gynecological care (Turillazzi et al. 2008; Draisci et al. 2007; Diaz et al. 1996).

15.14 H1N1 Infection

The first known infections with the new H1N1 virus (swine flu) were reported in April 2009. Sudden and unexpected deaths can occur in connection with H1N1 infections, whereby women are primarily affected. In two postmortem examinations carried out by the author, prominent lymph nodes, which showed pronounced nonspecific lymphadenitis histologically, were evident macroscopically (Fig. 15.37). Wide lymph sinuses with reactive sinus histiocytosis and an increased mitotic index can be seen. Others reported on lymphomonocytic pneumonia with granulocyte involvement, florid myocarditis, and extensive hemorrhage in the lung tissue and airways (trachea, bronchia) with an accompanying inflammatory reaction (Edler et al. 2011), which may also be observed in spleen tissue. The key histopatho-

Food Allergies

Allergic reactions to foodstuffs occur frequently but rarely lead to death. In the USA, 125–150 deaths per year are reported (Unkrig et al. 2010; Heinze et al. 2010; Sampson 2000). In the case of severe, typically acute, and potentially lethal forms that develop immediately (minutes to several hours) after food intake, this is termed anaphylactic shock. One possible trigger is a peanut allergy (Fig. 15.35). In the case of food allergies, increased numbers of eosinophil granulocytes can be detected in the gastric mucosa (Fig. 15.36). An analysis of more than 4000 cases of anaphylaxis in Germany, Switzerland, and Austria revealed insect venom to be the trigger in around 50% of cases, followed by food (ca. 25%) and medications (ca. 15%). The following foods were reported: peanut, hazelnut, wheat, cow's milk, hen's egg, fish, celery, shellfish/crustaceans, and walnut (Worm et al. 2014).

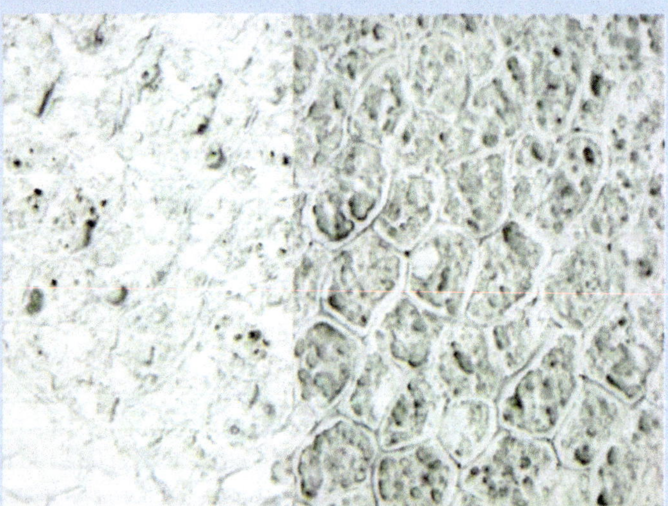

Fig. 15.35 Micro scopically detectable structures in the stomach content (*left*) consistent with a known peanut sample (*right*) (H&E ×400)

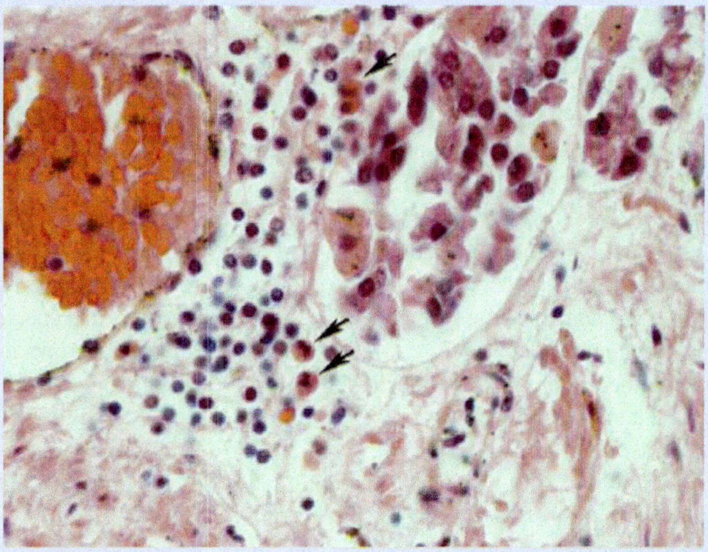

Fig. 15.36 Same case as in Fig. 15.29 with microscopically detectable eosinophil granulocytes (*arrows*) in the gastric mucosa (H&E ×400)

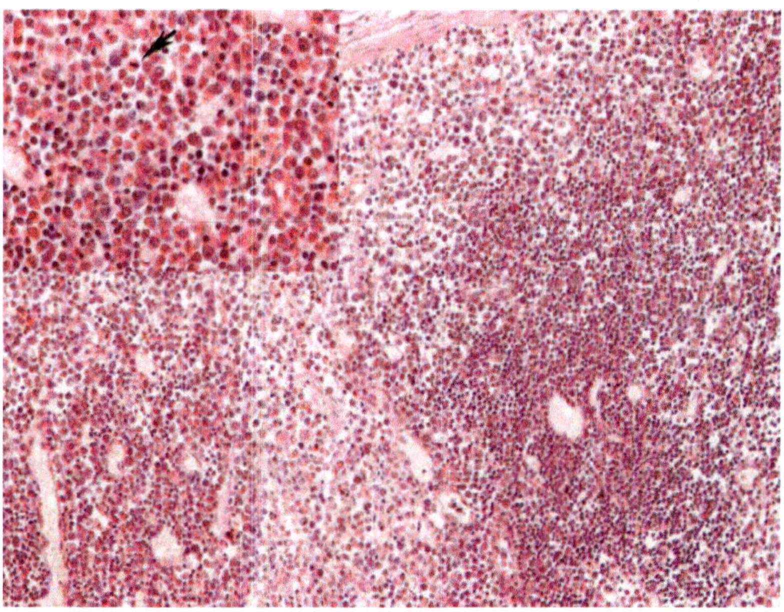

Fig. 15.37 Pronounced nonspecific lymphadenitis with reactive sinus histiocytosis and an increased mitotic index (*arrow*) in the case of lethal H1N1 infection (H&E ×100, Insert: H&E ×400)

logical features include acute lung injury (diffuse alveolar damage), lymphopenia in lymph nodes and spleen, and hemophagocytosis in lymphoid organs and bone marrow. The sites where the virus can be identified by immunohistochemistry—although not widely available at present—and virological molecular diagnostics are the lung, intestines, lymph node lymphocytes, and blood. The fresh tissue samples taken by autopsy for the microbiology departments include lower airways and lung tissue, lymph node (not spleen), distal small bowel, and blood. The blood should ideally include both whole blood from a peripheral vein and serum from centrifugation of whole blood. The whole blood should be placed in an EDTA tube, the serum in an untreated sample bottle. Additionally for histopathology with formalin fixation and according to the Royal College of Pathologists, a standard set of samples should comprise all the major organs including intestine and must include the lung, trachea, and bronchus. Recommended minimum samples:

- Central (hilar) lung with segmental bronchi
- Right and left primary bronchi
- Trachea (proximal and distal)
- Pulmonary parenchyma from right and left lung
- Vertebral bone marrow
- Hilar lymph nodes
- Any other organ that indicates a possibly relevant comorbidity

In summary, the histological findings are somewhat nonspecific, e.g., lymphadenitis, (hemorrhagic) pneumonia, lung edema, and signs of respiratory tract inflammation. The lungs are primarily affected. There are guidelines for personal protection during autopsy, and an appropriate mask (FFP3) should be worn (Ramsthaler et al. 2010). For details please see:

The Royal College of Pathologists: Advice for pathologists and anatomical pathology technologists for autopsy of cadavers with known or suspected new/virulent strains of influenza A (2nd edition, 2009)—Website: www.rcpath.org.

15.15 *Leptospirosis*

Leptospirosis (*Weil's disease*, *canicola fever*) is caused by *Leptospira spirochetes* and transmitted by animals. The disease is on the whole rare in Europe; the species most commonly found in Western Europe is *Leptospira interrogans.* The incubation period is 7–13 days and follows a biphasic course: sudden high fever, nonspecific symptoms such as headache and limb pain, and in some cases mild flu-like infections. Particularly in the case of infection with the serotype *Leptospira icterohaemorrhagiae*, severe organ disease (e.g., meningitis, myocarditis, and/or nephritis) may be seen shortly after the resolution of fever (Fig. 15.38). The mortality rate is as high as 10%, and the pathogen can be detected using molecular pathology (Luchini et al. 2008). *Leptospira* may persist in the kidneys and be excreted in urine for long periods of time.

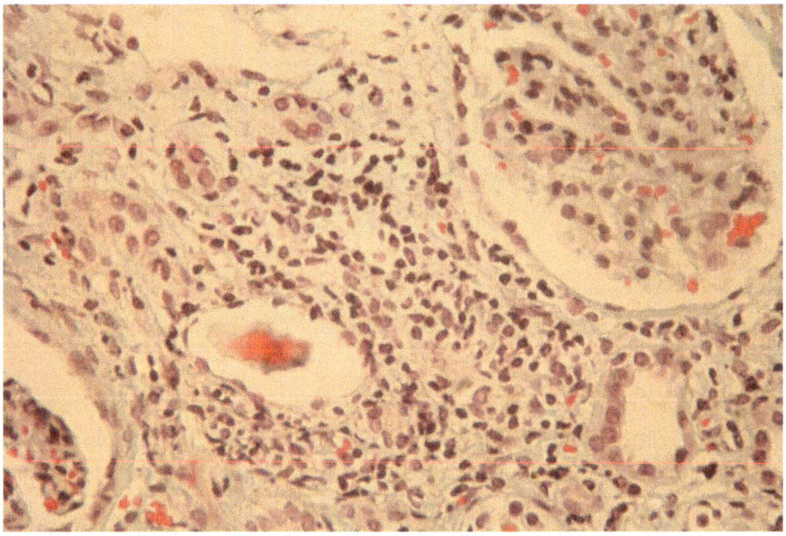

Fig. 15.38 Lymphocytic *interstitial nephritis* in leptospirosis (H&E ×400)

15.16 *Schistosomiasis (Bilharzia)*

Schistosomiasis is a disease caused by trematodes (flukes) that occurs in East Asia, Egypt, and Central and South America. Infection is caused by exposure to cercaria in standing or slow-moving water. The sexually mature *Schistosoma japonicum* or *Schistosoma mansoni* females lay their eggs in peripheral branches of the mesenteric veins, from where the eggs spread to fine branches of the hepatic portal vein, reaching as far as the liver sinusoids. Granulomas with multinucleated giant cells, partially surrounding epithelioid cells, and a connective tissue capsule that may exhibit inflammatory infiltrates can develop in the liver (Figs. 15.39 and 15.40). One also sees prominent macrophages that store schistosoma pigment, the natural color of which is grayish-brown. Severe complicated chronic schistosomiasis involving the development of liver cirrhosis is rare. In the absence of giant-cell detection, granulomas can be confused with a granulomatous drug reaction.

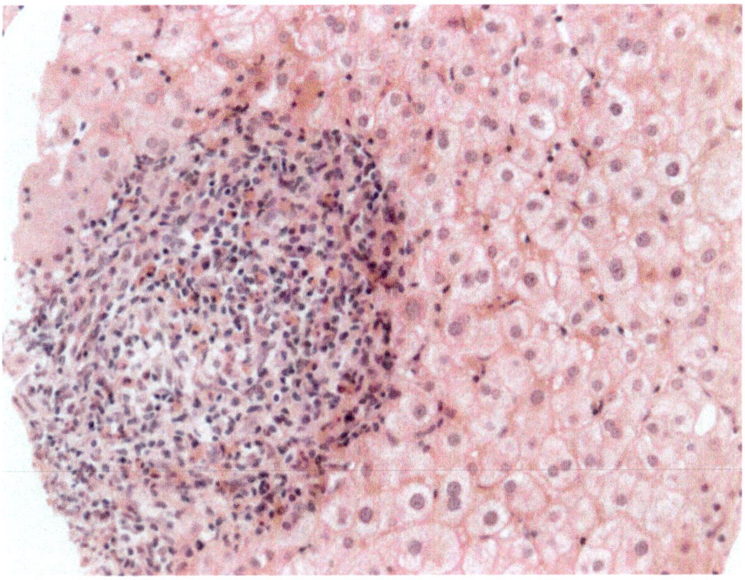

Fig. 15.39 A hepatic granuloma in schistosomiasis (H&E ×200)

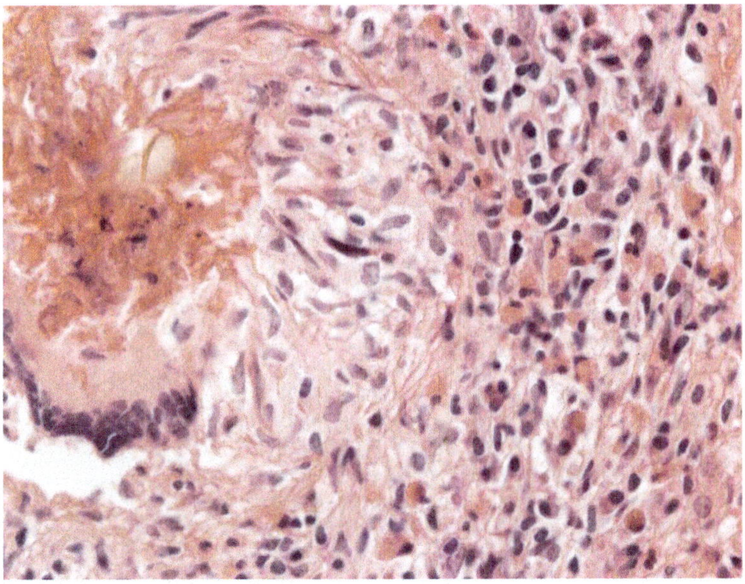

Fig. 15.40 Schistosomiasis with granulomatous inflammation of the liver, epithelioid cells, and a multinucleated giant cell (H&E ×400)

References

Albert S, Schröter A, Bratzke H, Brade V (1995) Postmortem diagnosis of falciparum malaria. Dtsch Med Wochenschr 120:18–22

An JL, Ishida Y, Kimura A, Tsokos M, Kondo T (2009) Immunohistochemical detection of CCR2 and CX3CR1 in sepsis-induced lung injury. Forensic Sci Int 192:e21–e25

Andes WA (1982) Spontaneous clostridial sepsis and sudden death. South Med J 75:378–379

Ansari MQ, Zamora JL, Lipscomb MF (1993) Postmortem diagnosis of acute anaphylaxis by serum tryptase analysis. Am J Clin Pathol 99:101–103

Barnard JH (1967) Allergic and pathologic findings in fifty insect-sting fatalities. J Allergy 40:107–114

Becker K, Ortmann C, Bajanowski T, Brinkmann B, Peters G (1999) Use of polymerase chain reaction for post-mortem diagnosis of malaria. Diagn Mol Pathol 8:211–215

Beh P, Byard RW (2015) Diptheria and lethal upper airway obstruction. Forensic Sci Med Pathol 11: 133–135

Bennis A, Darif A, Mehadji BE, Chraibi N (2000) Cardiac hydatid cyst revealed by the complete heart block. Heart Vessel 15:46–48

Bisno AL (1971) Hyposplenism and overwhelming pneumococcal infection, a reappraisal. Am J Med Sci 262:101

Brandt G (1980) Pathohistologische Diagnostik der Gewebsformen einheimischer Mykosen. Pathologe 1:100–105

Buris L, Szabó M, Kelemen J (1963) Hamman-Rich-Syndrom beim plötzlichen Tod. Dtsch Z Gesamte Gerichtl Med 54:211–216

Burke MP, Opeskin K (1999) Nontraumatic clostridial myonecrosis. Am J Forensic Med Pathol 20:158–162

Butcovan D, Grigoriu C, Astărăstoae V (2010) Cardiac echinococcosis causing unexpected death. A case report. Rom J Leg Med 18:189–192

Byard RW (2009) An analysis of possible mechanisms of unexpected death occurring in hydatid disease (Echinococcosis). J Forensic Sci 54:919–922

Byard RW (2016) Gross and microscopic features of extensive subcutaneous emphysema. Forensic Sci Med Pathol 12:372–375

Carson HJ, Cook BA (2009) Mast cell tryptase in a case of anaphylaxis due to repeat antibiotic exposure. Legal Med 11:234–236

Clausnitzer H, Müntefering H (1975) Ein Fall von Goodpasture-Syndrom in der gerichtsärztlichen Praxis. Z Rechtsmed 76:245–251

Curti AJ, Lin JH, Szabo K (1985) Overwhelming post-splenectomy infection with Plesiomonas shigelloides in a patient cured of Hodgkin's disease. Am J Clin Pathol 83:522–524

Da Broi U, Moreschi C (2011) Post-mortem diagnosis of anaphylaxis: a difficult task in forensic medizince. Forensic Sci Int 204:1–5

Dean HR (1922) Histology of a case of anaphylactic shock. J Pathol Bacteriol 25:305–315

De-Georgia F, Lodise M, Pascali VL, Spagnolo AG, d'Aloja E, Arena V (2015) An unusual case showing fatal rupture of a gastric ulcer or gastromalacia acida? The importance/role of histology for differential diagnosis. J Forensic Sci 60:240–242

Delage C, Irey NS (1972) Anaphylactic deaths. A clinicopathologic study of 43 cases. J Forensic Sci 17:525–540

Delage C, Mullick FG, Irey NS (1973) Myocardial lesions in anaphylaxis. A histochemical study. Arch Pathol 95:185–189

Dempers J, Sens MA, Wadee SA, Kinney HC, Odendaal HJ, Wright CA (2011) Progressive primary pulmonary tuberculosis presenting as the sudden unexpected death in infancy: a case report. Forensic Sci Int 206:e27–e30

Dettmeyer R (2006) Malaria tropica: Bericht zu einer Erkrankung mit tödlichem Ausgang. Robert Koch Institut. Epidemiologisches Bulletin, p 51

Dettmeyer R, Varchmin-Schultheiß K, Madea B (1999) Postpartales letales OPSI-Syndrom bei posttraumatischer Splenosis peritonei. In: 8th spring-meeting of the German society of forensic medicine – northern region, Hamburg, 7–8 May 1999

Diamond I (1958) The Hamman-Rich syndrome in childhood. Pediatrics 22:27

Diamond LK (1969) Splenectomy in childhood and the hazard of overwhelming infection. Pediatrics 43:886–889

Diaz T, Martinez T, Antepara I, Usandizaga JM, Lopez Valverde M, Jaurequi I (1996) Latex allergy as a risk during delivery. Br J Obstet Gynaecol 103:173–175

Dickerman JD (1979) Splenectomy and sepsis. Pediatrics 63:938–941

Draisci G, Nucera E, Pollastrini E, Forte E, Zanfini B, Pinto R, Patriarca G, Schiavino D, Pietrini D (2007) Anaphylactic reactions during cesarean section. Int J Obstet Anesth 16:63–67

Edler C, Klein A, Gehl A, Ilchman C, Scherpe S, Schrot M (2011) The new influenza A (H1N1/09): symptoms, diagnostics, and autopsy results. Int J Legal Med 125:157–161

Edston E, van Hage-Hamsten M (1998) ß-Tryptase measurements post-mortem in anaphylactic deaths and in controls. Forensic Sci Int 93:135–142

Edston E, van Hage-Hamsten M (2003) Death in anaphylaxis in a man with house dust mite allergy. Int J Legal Med 117:299–301

Edston E, van Hage-Hamsten M (2005) Postmortem diagnosis of anaphylaxis. In: Tsokos M (ed) Forensic pathology reviews, vol 3. Humana Press, Totowa, pp 267–281

Edston E (2013) Accumulation of eosinophils, mast cells, and basophils in the spleen in anaphylactic deaths. Forensic Sci Med Pathol 9:496–500

Fineschi V, Monasterolo G, Rosi R, Turillazzi E (1999) Fatal anaphylactic shock during a fluorescein angiography. Forensic Sci Int 100:137–142

Fracasso T, Jentgens L, Pfeiffer H, Sauerland C, Mangin P, Schmeling A (2016) Right heart ischemia in cases of sepsis. Forensic Sci Int 259:106–109

Gerber JE, Johnson JE, Scott MA, Madhusudhan KT (2002) Fatal meningitis and encephalitis due to bartonella henselae bacteria. J Forensic Sci 47:640–644

Glenner GG, Cohen LA (1960) Histochemical demonstration of species-specific trypsin-like enzyme in mast cells. Nature 105:846–847

Goodpasture EW (1919) The significance of certain pulmonary lesions in relation to the etiology of influenza. Am J Med Sci 158:863

Grinblat J, Gilboa A (1975) Overwhelming pneumococcal sepsis 25 years after splenectomy. Am J Med Sci 270:523

Hausmann R, Albert F, Geißdörfer W, Betz P (2004) Clostridium fallax associated with sudden death in a 16-year-old boy. J Med Microbiol 53:581–583

Heinze S, Erbersdobler A, Tsokos M (2010) Todesursache: anaphylaxie. Rechtsmedizin 20:282–284

Heinze S, Püschel K, Tsokos M (2011) Necrotizing fasciitis with fatal outcome: a report of two cases. Forensic Sci Med Pathol 7:278–282

Holdsworth RJ, Irving AD, Cuschieri A (1991) Postsplenectomy sepsis and its mortality rate. Actual versus perceived risks. Br J Surg 78:1031–1038

Ihama Y, Fukasawa M, Ninomiya K, Kawakami Y, Nagai T, Fuke C, Miyazaki T (2014) Anaphylactic shock caused by sting of crown-of-thorns starfish (*Acanthaster planci*). Forensic Sci Int 236:e5–e8

Jänisch S, Günther D, Fieguth A, Bange FC, Schmidt A, Debertin AS (2010) Postmortal detection of clostridia – putrefaction or infection? Arch Kriminol 225:99–108

Janssen W (1977) Forensische histologie. Schmidt-Römhild, Lübeck, pp 189–216

Johansson O, Virtanen M, Hilliges M, Yang Q (1992) Histamine immunohistochemistry: a new and highly sensitive method for studying cutaneous mast cells. Histochem J 24:283–287

Jorgensen P, Heiden M, Kern P, Schöneberg I, Krause G, Alpers K (2008) Underreporting of human alveolar echinococcosis, Germany. Emerg Infect Dis 14:935–937

Kanthan R, Moyana T, Nyssen J (1999) Asplenia as a cause of sudden unexpected death in childhood. Am J Forensic Med Pathol 20:57–59

Kaplan M, Demirtas M, Cimen S, Ozler A (2001) Cardiac hydatid cyst with intracavitary expansion. Ann Thorac Surg 71:2034–2035

Kernbach-Wighton G, Böhnel H, Saternus KS (2003) Zur Phänomenologie beim positiven Clostridien-Nachweis. Rechtsmedizin 13:86–90

Kounis NG, Soufras GD, Kounis GN, Hahalis G (2013) Suicidal anaphylactic death: is Kounis anaphylaxis associated syndrome the cause? Forensic Sci Int 232:e42–e43

Kounis NG (2013) Coronary hypersensitivity disorder: the Kounis syndrome. Clin Ther 35:563–571

Kounis NG, Soufras GD, Hahalis G (2014) Accumulation of eosinophils, mast cells, and basophils in the spleen and the coronary arteries in anaphylactic deaths: is the Kounis hypersensitivity associated syndrome present? Forensic Sci Med Pathol 10:150–151

Kribben A, Uppenkamp A, Heeman U, Höffkes HG, Meusers P (1995) Postsplenektomie-sepsis (OPSI-Syndrom). Dtsch Med Wochenschr 120:771–775

Kucukarslan N, Savas Oz B, Demirkilic U, Tatar H (2005) An asymptomatic cardiac echinococcus cyst case. Int J Thor Cardiovasc Surg 74:37–42

Kühn H, Kleinfeld F, Pfeifer B (1983) Über das Opsi-Syndrom. Pathologe 4:112–116

Landi KK, Coleman T (2008) Sudden death in toddlers caused by influenza B infection: a report of two cases and a review of the literature. J Forensic Sci 53:213–215

Lau G (2005) Iatrogenic injury. A forensic perspective. In: Tsokos M (ed) Forensic pathology reviews, vol 3. Humana Press, Totowa, pp 351–439

Lau G, Lai SH (2008) Forensic histopathology. In: Tsokos M (ed) Forensic pathology reviews, vol 5. Humana Press, Totowa, pp 239–265

Levy MM, Fink MP, Marshall JC, Abraham E, Angus D, Cook D, Cohen J, Opal SM, Vincent JL, Ramsay G (2003) 2001 SCCM/ESICM/ACCP/ATS/SIS international sepsis definition conference. Crit Care Med 31:1250–1256

Lindblad BE, Lindblad LN (1990) Fatal pneumococcal bacteremia with disseminated intravascular coagulation and Waterhouse-Friderichsen syndrome in a vaccinated, splenectomized adult. Case report. Acta Chir Scand 156:487–488

Locker GJ, Wagner A, Peter A, Staudinger T, Marosi C, Rintelen C, Knapp S, Malzer K, Weiss K, Metnitz P (1995) Lethal Waterhouse-Friderichsen syndrome in post-traumatic asplenia. J Trauma 39:784–786

Luchini D, Meacci F, Oggioni MR, Morabito G, D'Amato V, Gabrielli M, Pozzi G (2008) Molecular detection of Leptospira interrogans in human tissues and environmental samples in a lethal case of leptospirosis. Int J Legal Med 122:229–233

Lunetta P, Penttila A, Salovaara R, Sajantila A (2002) Sudden death due to rupture of the arteria pancreatica magna: a complication of an immature pseudocyst in chronic pancreatitis. Int J Legal Med 116:43–46

Mahfoud B, Heinemann A, Püschel K (2002) Nekrotisierende Myositis durch Clostridium perfringens nach intravenöser Heroinapplikation. Rechtsmedizin 12:109–111

Mayer DE, Krauskopf A, Hemmer W, Moritz K, Jarisch R, Reiter C (2011) Usefulness of post mortem determination of serum tryptase, histamine and diamine oxidase in the diagnosis of fatal anaphylaxis. Forensic Sci Int 212:96–101

McCaughey WTE, Thomas BJ (1962) Pulmonary hemorrhage and glomerulonephritis. The relation of pulmonary hemorrhage to certain types of glomerular lesions. Am J Clin Pathol 38:577

Metter D, Schulz E (1977) Die forensische Begutachtung iatrogener Gasbrandinfektionen. Beitr Gerichtl Med 35:47–54

Miyashita T, Kakimoto N, Ishida Y, Hayashi T, Kimura A, Tsokos M, Kondo T (2006) Immunohistochemical expression of tumor necrosis factor-α in sepsis-induced lung injury. Forensic Sci Med Pathol 2:103–108

Molz G, Hartmann HP, Griesser HR (1986) Generalisierte BCG-Infektion bei einem 7 Wochen alten, plötzlich verstorbenen Säugling. Pathologe 7:216–221

Muciaccia B, Sestili C, de Grossi S, Vestri A, Cipolloni L, Cecchi R (2016) Are mast cells implicated in asphyxia? Int J Legal Med 130:153–161

Müller AM, Tsokos M (2006) Pathology of human endothelium in septic organ failure. In: Tsokos M (ed) Forensic pathology reviews, vol 4. Humana Press, Totowa, pp 161–192

Müller R, Korb G, Gedigk P (1970) Über zentrale Nekrosen in der Leber nach einem Schock. Verh Dtsch Ges Pathol 54:511

Müller AM, Gruhn KM, Herwig MC, Tsokos M (2008) VE-cadherin and ACE: markers for sepsis in post mortem examination? Legal Med 10:257–263

Murphy TE, Kean BH, Venturini A, Lillehei CW (1971) Echinococcus cyst of the left ventricle: report of a case with review of the pertinent literature. J Thorac Cardiovasc Surg 61:443–450

Naeve W (1971) Zum histologischen Nachweis einer akuten Malaria tropica an fäulnisveränderten Organen. Z Rechtsmed 69:210–216

Ondruschka B, Habeck JO, Hädrich C, Dreßler J, Bayer R (2015) Rare cause of natural death in forensic setting: hemophagocytic syndrome. Int J Legal Med 130:777–781. https://doi.org/10.1007/s00414-015-1305-0

Ortiz-Rey JA, Suárez-Peñaranda JM, San Miguel P, Muñoz JI, Rodríguez-Calvo MS, Concheiro L (2008) Immunohistochemical analysis of P-Selectin as a possible marker of vitality in human cutaneous wounds. J Forensic Legal Med 15:368–372

Ortmann C, Brinkmann B (1997) The expression of P-selectin in inflammatory and non-inflammatory lung tissue. Int J Legal Med 110:155–158

Ortmann C, Pfeiffer H, Brinkmann B (2000) Demonstration of myocardial necrosis in the presence of advanced putrefaction. Int J Legal Med 114: 50–55

Osawa M, Satoh F, Horiuchi H et al (2008) Postmortem diagnosis of fatal anaphylaxis during intravenous administration of therapeutic and diagnostic agents: evaluation of clinical laboratory parameters and immunohistochemistry in three cases. Legal Med 10:143–147

Pavelites JJ, Prahlow JA (2011) Fatal human monocytic ehrlichiosis: a case study. Forensic Sci Med Pathol 7:287–293

Peabody JW, Buechner HH, Anderson HE (1955) Hamman-Rich syndrome. Arch Intern Med 43:1127

Perskvist N, Edston E (2007) Differential accumulation of pulmonary and cardiac mast-cell-subsets and eosinophils between fatal anaphylaxis and asthma death: a postmortem comparative study. Forensic Sci Int 169:43–49

Plenzig S, Döring C, Held H, Verhoff MA (2016) On the wrong track. Death of a drug abuser in a penitentiary due to desquamative interstitial pneumonia. Rechtsmedizin 26:440–443

Popper HH, Pailer S, Wurzinger G, Feldner H, Hesse C, Eber E (2002) Expression of adhesion molecules in allergic lung diseases. Virchows Arch 440:172–180

Prahlow JA, Barnard JJ (1998) Fatal anaphylaxis due to fire and stings. Am J Forensic Med Pathol 19: 137–142

Preuss J, Dettmeyer R, Strehler M, Madea B (2006a) Unerkannt akut-letale Infektionen. Ursachen plötzlicher Todesfälle im Erwachsenenalter. Rechtsmedizin 16:165–171

Preuss J, Dettmeyer R, Madea B (2006b) Tödlich verlaufende, postoperative Peritonitiden. Rechtsmedizinische Begutachtung. Rechtsmedizin 16:383–388

Pumphrey RSH, Roberts ISD (2000) Postmortem findings after fatal anaphylactic reactions. J Clin Pathol 53:273–276

Püschel K, Lockemann U, Dietrich M (1998) Recurrent fatal outcome of malaria infections due to late diagnosis. Dtsch Ärztebl 95:2697–2700

Ramsay LE, Bouskill KC (1973) Fatal pneumococcal meningitis in adults following splenectomy: two case reports and a review of the literature. J R Nav Med Serv 59:102–114

Ramsthaler F, Verhoff MA, Gehl A, Kettner M (2010) The novel H1N1/swine-origin influenza virus and its implications for autopsy practice. Int J Legal Med 124:171–173

Randall B, Butts J, Halsey JF (1995) Elevated postmortem tryptase in the absence of anaphylaxis. J Forensic Sci 40:208–211

Rauch E, Tutsch-Bauer E, Penning R (1999) Malaria tropica – a problem in forensic medicine? Rechtsmedizin 10:1–6

Reavy DT, Nakonechny D (1979) Sudden death and sepsis after splenectomy. J Forensic Sci 24:757–761

Reggiani Bonetti L, Maccio L, Trani N, Radheshi E, Palmiere C (2015) Splenic hypereosinophilia in anaphylaxis-related death: different assessments depending on different types of allergens? Int J Legal Med 129:97–103

Rimmer EF, Turberville C, Horton MA (1984) Human mast cells detected by monoclonal antibodies. J Clin Pathol 37:1249–1255

Risse M, Verhoff MA, Lehmann H, Dettmeyer R (2008) Unerkannte letale Maserninfektion bei einem 14-jährigen Mädchen mit Trisomie 21. Rechtsmedizin 18:383–386

Rizzo M, Magro G, Castaldo P (2004) OPSI (overwhelming postsplenectomy infection) syndrome: a case report. Forensic Sci Int 164S:S55–S56

Rodriguez Gomez M, Oehler U, Helpap B (1997) Foudroyant verlaufende Sepsis nach Splenektomie. Pathologe 18:257–260

Roncati L, Barbolini G, Scacchetti AT, Busani S, Maiorana A (2013) Unexpected death: anaphylactic intraoperative death due to Thymoglobulin carbohydrate excipient. Forensic Sci Int 228:e28–e32

Ruf G, Kirchner R, Lausen M, Pelz K (1986) Die Clostridieninfektion der Galle. Chir Praxis 36:13–22

Sampson HA (2000) Food anaphylaxis. Br Med Bull 56:925–935

Sasaki T, Nanjo H, Takahashi M, Sugijama T, Ono I, Masuda H (2000) Non-traumatic gas gangrene in the abdomen: report of six autopsy cases. Gastroenterology 35:382–390

Schumaker B Jr (1952) Splenic studies: I. Susceptibility to infection after splenectomy performed in infancy. Am Surg 136:239

Seufert RM, Böttcher W (1982) Organerhaltende Behandlung von Milzverletzungen. Dtsch Med Wochenschr 107:523–526

Shen Y, Li L, Grant J et al (2009) Anaphylactic deaths in Maryland (United States) and Shanghai (China): a review of forensic autopsy cases from 2004 to 2006. Forensic Sci Int 186:1–5

Shintaku M, Sangawa A, Yonezawa A, Nasu K (2001) Aortic lesions in aspergillosis: histopathological study of two autopsy cases. Virchows Arch 439:640–644

Simini B (1999) Liposuction surgery in Italy leads to Streptococcus pyogenes sepsis. Lancet 353:1164

Siveke J, Caselitz J, Püschel K (2001) Clinical and morphologic features of fatal falciparum malaria. Rechtsmedizin 11:82–88

Soper DE (1986) Clostridial myonecrosis arising from an episiotomy. Obstet Gynecol 68(3 Suppl):26S–28S

Sterzig V, Wild V, Weishaupt J, Tatschner T, Babel B, Bohnert M (2016) Tod beim Hausarzt. Arch Kriminol 238:120–127

Suzuki H, Murata K, Sakamoto A (2009) An autopsy case of fulminant sepsis due to pneumatosis cystoides intestinalis. Legal Med 11:S528–S530

Telli HH, Durgut K (2001) Ruptured cardiac hydatid cyst masquerading as acute coronary syndrome: report of a case. Surg Today 31:908–911

Thierauf A, Dettmeyer R, Wollersen H, Musshoff F, Madea B (2007) Fatal Candida tropicalis infection in an 8-month-old infant with an aplasia of the thymus as a rare cause of death in infancy. Forensic Sci Int 169:228–233

Thu M, Winskong C, Byard RW (2014) Tuberculosis and sudden death. Forensic Sci Med Pathol 10:266–268

Trani N, Reggiani Bonetti LR, Gualandri G, Barbolini G (2008) Immediate anaphylactic death following antibiotics injection: splenic eosinophilia easily revealed by pagoda red stain. Forensic Sci Int 181:21–25

Tsokos M (2012) Syphilitic aortic aneurysm rupture as cause of sudden death. Forensic Sci Med Pathol 8:325–326

Tsokos M (2003) Immunohistochemical detection of sepsis-induced lung injury in human autopsy material. Legal Med 5:73–86

Tsokos M (2004) Fatal respiratory tract infections with Mycoplasma pneumoniae. Histopathological features, aspects of post-mortem diagnosis and medicolegal implications. In: Tsokos M (ed) Forensic pathology reviews, vol 1. Humana Press, Totowa, pp 201–218

Tsokos M (2005) Pathology of sepsis. In: Rutty GN (ed) Essentials of autopsy practice, vol 3. Springer, London, pp 39–85

Tsokos M (2006a) Postmortale Sepsisdiagnostik. Teil 1: Pathomorphologie. Rechtsmedizin 16:231–246

Tsokos M (2006b) Postmortale Sepsisdiagnostik. Teil 2: Immunhistochemie und biochemische Diagnostik. Rechtsmedizin 16:333–342

Tsokos M, Braun C (2007) Acute pancreatitis presenting as sudden, unexpected death: an autopsy-based study of 27 cases. Am J Forensic Med Pathol 28:267–270

Tsokos M, Fehlauer F (2001) Post-mortem markers of sepsis: an immunohistochemical study using VLA-4 (CD49d/CD29) and ICAM-1 (CD54) for the detection of sepsis-induced lung injury. Int J Legal Med 114:291–294

Tsokos M, Püschel K (1999) Iatrogenic staphylococcus aureus septicaemia following intravenous and intramuscular injections: clinical course and pathomorphological findings. Int J Legal Med 112:303–308

Tsokos M, Fehlauer F, Püschel K (2000) Immunohistochemical expression of E-selectin in sepsis-induced lung injury. Int J Legal Med 113: 338–342

Tsokos M, Reichelt U, Jung R, Nierhaus A, Püschel K (2001) Interleukin-6 and C-reactive protein serum levels in sepsis-related fatalities during the early postmortem period. Forensic Sci Int 119:47–56

Tsokos M, Anders S, Paulsen F (2002) Lectin binding patterns of alveolar epithelium and subepithelial seromucous glands of the bronchi in sepsis and controls – an approach to characterize the non-specific immunological response of the human lung to sepsis. Virchows Arch 440:181–186

Tsokos M, Pufe T, Paulsen F, Anders S, Mentlein R (2003) Pulmonary expression of vascular endothelial growth factor in sepsis. Arch Pathol Lab Med 127:331–335

Tsokos M, Zöllner B, Feucht HH (2005) Fatal influenza A infection with Staphylococcus aureus superinfection in a 49-year-old woman presenting as sudden death. Int J Legal Med 119:40–43

Tsokos M, Schalinski S, Paulsen F, Sperhake JP, Püschel K, Sobottka I (2008) Pathology of fatal traumatic and nontraumatic clostridial gas gangrene: a histopathological, immunohistochemical, and ultrastructural study of six autopsy cases. Int J Legal Med 122: 35–41

Tümer AR, Dener C (2007) Diagnostic dilemma of sudden deaths due to acute hemorrhagic pancreatitis. J Forensic Sci 52:180–182

Turillazzi E, Di Donato S, Neri M, Riezzo I, Fineschi V (2007) An immunohistochemical study in a fatal case of acute interstitial pneumonitis (Hamman-Rich syndrome) in a 15-year-old boy presenting as sudden death. Forensic Sci Int 173:73–77

Turillazzi E, Greco P, Neri M, Pomara C, Riezo I, Fineschi V (2008) Anaphylactic latex reaction during anaesthesia: the silent culprit in a fatal case. Forensic Sci Int 179:e5–e8

Unkrig S, Hagemeier L, Madea B (2010) Postmortem diagnosis of assumed food anaphylaxis in an unexpected death. Forensic Sci Int 198:e1–e4

Urata Y, Hasegawa M, Hasegawa H, Shikano M, Kawashima S, Imoto M (1997) A fatal case of overwhelming postsplenectomy infection syndrome developing 10 years after splenectomy. Nihon Rinsho Meneki Gakkai Kaishi 20:184–190

van Wyck DB, Witte MH, Witte CL, Thies AC (1980) Critical splenic mass for survival from experimental pneumococcemia. J Surg Res 28:14–17

Vance BM, Strassmann G (1941) Sudden death following injection of foreign protein. Arch Pathol 34:849–865

Walls AF, Bennett AR, McBride HM, Glennie MJ, Holgate ST, Church MK (1990a) Production and characterization of monoclonal antibodies specific for human mast cell tryptase. Clin Exp Allergy 20:581–589

Walls AF, Jones DB, Williams JH, Church MK, Holgate ST (1990b) Immunohistochemical identification of mast cells in formaldehyde-fixed tissue using monoclonal antibodies specific for tryptase. J Pathol 162:119–126

Weis A, Bohnert M (2008) Expression patterns of adhesion molecules P-selectin, von Willebrand factor and PECAM-1 in lungs: a comparative study in cases of burn shock and hemorrhagic shock. Forensic Sci Int 175:102–106

White RB, Craighead JT (1957) Hamman-Rich syndrome. Dis Chest 31:335

Worm M, Eckermann O, Dölle S, Aberer W, Beyer K, Hawranek T, Hompes S, Koehli A, Mahler V, Nemat K, Niggemann B, Pföhler C, Rabe U, Reissig A, Rietschel E, Scherer K, Treudler R, Ruëff F (2014) Triggers and treatment of anaphylaxis: an analysis of 4000 cases from Germany, Austria and Switzerland. Dtsch Ärztebl Int 111:367–375

Yagmur G, Kara E, Yildirim M, Gurler AS, Eken AE, Babur C (2015) Two cases of malaria due to Plasmodium falciparum resulting in death: postmortem identification. Rom J Leg Med 23:33–36

Young RC, Bennett JE, Vogel CL, Carbone PP, DeVita VT (1970) Aspergillosis. The spectrum of the disease in 98 patients. Medicine 49:147–173

Yunginger JW, Nelson DR, Squillace DL et al (1991) Laboratory investigation of deaths due to anaphylaxis. J Forensic Sci 36:857–865

16 Endocrine Organs

Endocrine organ dysfunction can explain sudden and unexpected death, although this is rarely the case in forensic practice (Püschel 2004). Nevertheless, there is a wide range of possible endocrine diseases which may be relevant at forensic autopsy (Table 16.1).

Examples of findings include:

- Type 1 and type 2 diabetes: lethal hypoglycemia and diabetic coma
- Addison's disease: acute adrenocortical insufficiency
- Lethal and often clinically unrecognized pheochromocytoma
- Thyroid and parathyroid dysfunctions
- Acute hypophyseal dysfunction or necrosis (e.g., Sheehan's syndrome)

Distinct histopathological findings cannot be seen in all cases of endocrine dysfunction; however, less pronounced findings can also be included in forensic evaluation and may explain clinical symptoms.

16.1 Diabetes

Sudden and unexpected death as a result of diabetic metabolism disturbances occurs occasionally due to infection, acute pancreatitis, in cases of islet cell involvement, sometimes accidentally in cases of incorrect dosage of antidiabetics or insulin, in rare cases as homicide with insulin administration, and also rarely as suicide (Banaschak et al. 2000; Kernbach-Wighton and Püschel 1998; Valenzuela 1988; DiMaio et al. 1977). In the case of insulin injection, the dermal and subepidermal injection site should be investigated immunohistochemically using an antibody against insulin (Wehner et al. 1997). In all cases, a rapid urine glucose test at autopsy can provide the crucial hint. Thereafter, postmortem biochemical findings are of prime importance (Osuna et al. 1999, 2005; Karlovsek

Table 16.1 Lethal endocrine dysfunctions

Organ or organ structure	Dysfunction
Hypophysis	Hypopituitarism/Sheehan's syndrome
Parathyroid gland	Hypo- and hyperparathyroidism (adenomas, carcinomas)
Thyroid gland	Underactive thyroid (e.g., thyroiditis)
	Thyrotoxicosis (e.g., Graves' disease, autonomous adenoma, rarely struma ovarii)
Adrenal malfunction	Acute and chronic organic destruction
Adrenal cortex	Hyperfunction: endocrinologically active tumors/Addison's disease
Adrenal medulla	Endocrinologically active tumors (pheochromocytoma)
Pancreatic islet cells	Insulitis, diabetic coma, hypoglycemic coma
Thymus	Myasthenia gravis
Endocrinologically active tumors	For example, serotonin-producing carcinoid

R. B. Dettmeyer, *Forensic Histopathology*, https://doi.org/10.1007/978-3-319-77997-3_16

2004; Kernbach and Brinkmann 1983). The combined findings of glucose and lactate in the cerebrospinal fluid and vitreous humor of the eyes are particularly significant, as are the findings of blood sugar and HbA1c concentration in the blood (Sippel and Möttönen 1992; Ritz and Kaatsch 1990).

Histologically, a hyperglycemic metabolic disturbance can lead to glycogen nephrosis; the correlation of which with biochemical postmortem parameters has been investigated (Lasczkowski and Püschel 1991). After diabetes of long-standing, accompanying diseases (e.g., arterio-arteriolosclerosis) and sometimes even the clinical picture of diabetic glomerulosclerosis (Kimmelstiel–Wilson type) (Fig. 16.1) can be seen histopathologically. This disease must be differentiated from lobular forms of glomerulonephritis in any differential diagnostics (Wehner and Haag 1980).

While acute hypoglycemia will not necessarily show diagnostically relevant findings, a long-lasting hyperglycemia with lethal diabetic coma leads to a resorption of glycogen via epithelial cells, primarily in the main parts of the renal tubules. Vacuolated epithelial cells of the renal tubules can be seen histologically (Fig. 16.2). However, vacuoles do not necessarily contain glycogen, and lipid determination is also

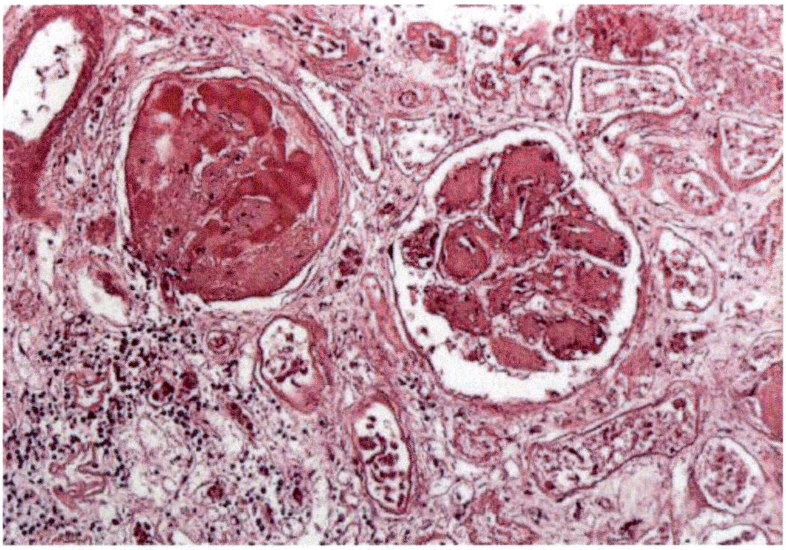

Fig. 16.1 Known dialysis-dependent renal failure in a case of diabetic glomerulosclerosis of Kimmelstiel–Wilson type in a 53-year-old woman with lethal diabetic coma (Elastica van Gieson ×400)

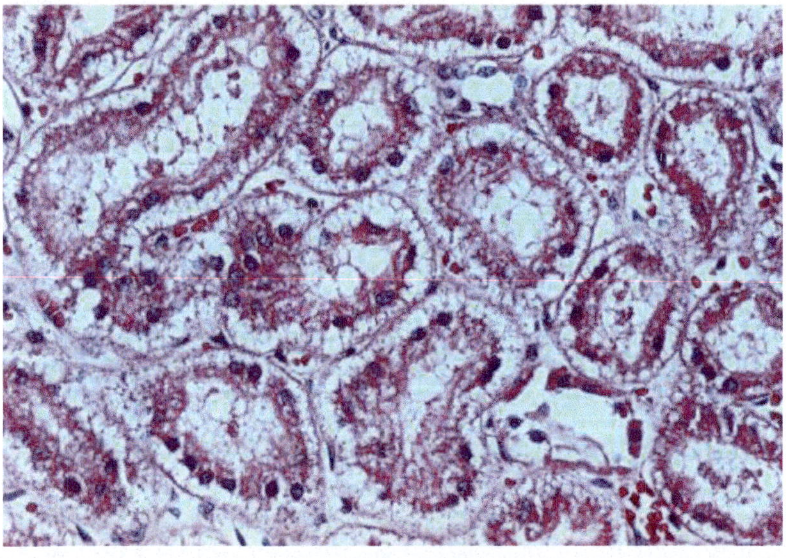

Fig. 16.2 Lethal diabetic coma (postmortem blood sugar level 869 mg/dl) with vacuolated epithelial cells of the renal tubules (H&E ×200)

positive in cases of death due to diabetic coma (Zhou et al. 2015; Thomsen et al. 2006).

If glycogen sediments of this sort are found in epithelial cells of the renal tubules, these cells are then called Armanni–Ebstein cells (Zhou et al. 2010; Ritchie and Waugh 1957). The Armanni–Ebstein lesion was first reported in 1877 and has been associated with deaths due to diabetic ketoacidosis. Meanwhile Armanni–Ebstein cells were also found in cases of nondiabetic individuals who died due to starvation (Milroy and Parai 2011). The glycogen sediments in Armanni–Ebstein cells can be determined in comparatively autolytic kidney tissue (Fig. 16.3), and glycogen drops can be seen in PAS staining (Fig. 16.3). Conventional hematoxylin and eosin staining initially reveals only Armanni–Ebstein cells; however, in addition to glycogen, these can also contain lipids and are found in cases of death due to hypothermia (Byard and Zhou 2010; Zhou and Byard 2011).

In rare cases, impaired sugar metabolism can be caused by an acute dysfunction in insulin production, such as insulitis (Fig. 16.4).

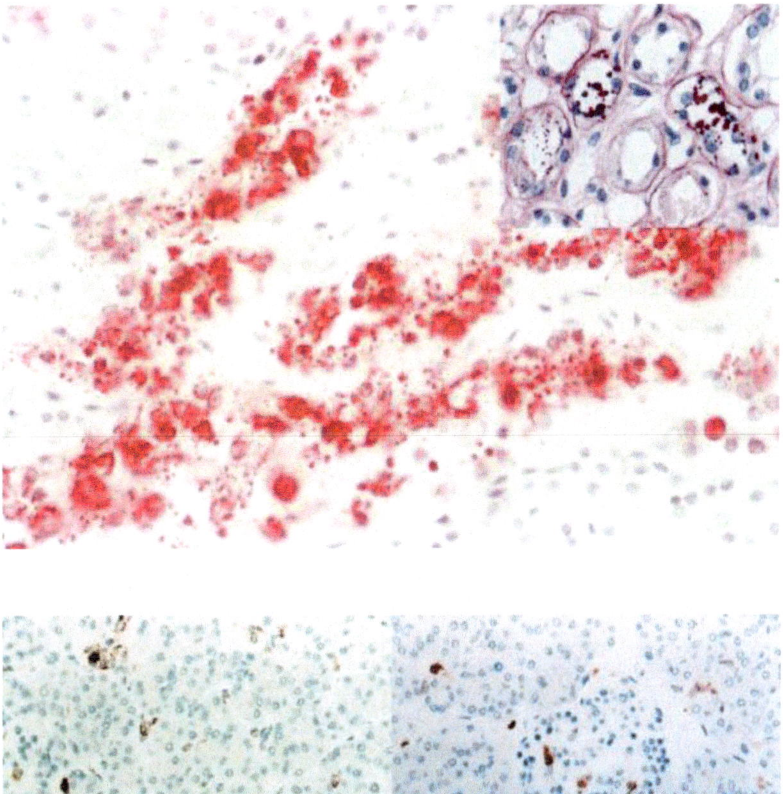

Fig. 16.3 Lethal diabetic coma with glycogenic vacuoles in the cytoplasm of epithelial cells of the renal tubules, referred to as Armanni–Ebstein cells (Best's carmine ×200), and glycogen drops in the lumen of the renal tubules (PAS v200)

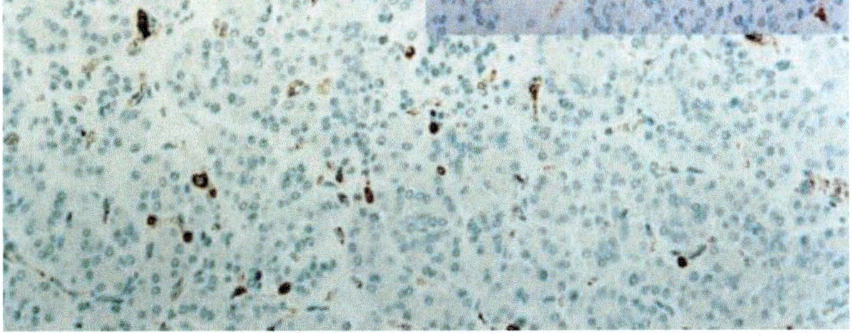

Fig. 16.4 Pancreatic tissue with acute lymphocytic insulitis and an increase in the number of leukocytes in pancreatic islet cells (both LCA ×400)

In cases of hyperglycemia with lethal diabetic coma, extensive infections can often be seen, in particular in the respiratory and genitourinary tract and in rare cases, such as fungal infections, in several organ systems. Vacuoles with a ground-glass appearance in the cell nuclei of hepatocytes are said to indicate a diabetic metabolic state. However, additional causes should be considered, and intoxication should be excluded.

If blood sugar levels remain inadequately controlled in insulin-dependent diabetes over a prolonged period of time, abnormally pronounced *nonalcoholic hepatic steatosis* may develop. As part of this process, mostly small to at most medium-sized vacuoles predominate in the hepatocytes, presenting a relatively uniform picture (Fig. 16.5).

While diabetic metabolic disturbances can only be diagnosed chemically as hypoglycemia or hyperglycemia (determination of glucose concentration and HbA1c value, particularly in blood, serum, liquor, and vitreous humor), indications of underlying diseases can be seen histomorphologically (Table 16.2).

Table 16.2 Histomorphological indications of long-term diabetes mellitus

Organ or organ system	Histomorphological findings
Arterial vascular system	Atherosclerosis at an advanced stage compared to the age of the patient, also arteriolosclerosis
Liver	Microvesicular steatosis of the liver with optically empty vacuoles in the cell nuclei of hepatocytes—nonspecific
Kidneys: glomeruli	Diabetic glomerulosclerosis (Kimmelstiel–Wilson type) of varying severity
Kidneys: arterioles	Relatively pronounced arteriosclerosis
Kidneys: tubules	Vacuolar brightening of the distal tubular cells with Armanni–Ebstein cells, PAS-positive cytoplasm (alternatively, Best's carmine stain)
Pancreas	No pathological findings with conventional histological methods; in some cases, possible insulitis
Infections	Chronic and acute exacerbated infections, including mycoses (pneumonias, infections of the genitourinary tract, etc.)

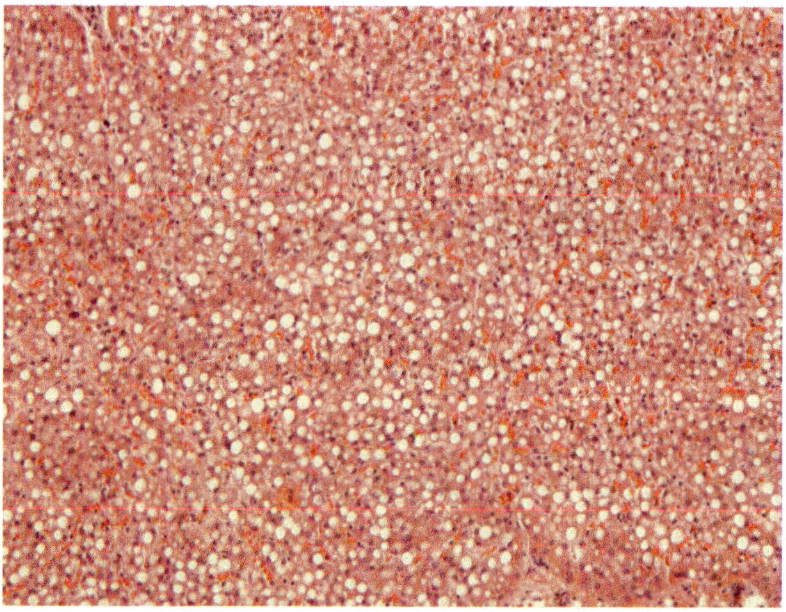

Fig. 16.5 Pronounced nonalcoholic hepatic steatosis in insulin-dependent type 1 diabetes inadequately controlled over a prolonged period of time (H&E ×100)

Hypoglycemia

In cases of hypoglycemia (blood sugar <50 mg%), only scant histological findings can be seen. Nerve cell damage with pyknotic nuclei in nerve and glial cells is described in particular in the central nervous system. Extensive elective parenchymal necrosis occurs, frequently along the sulcal depths. Granular cell necrosis and homogenization of Purkinje cells can occur, in particular in cases of a sudden change from diabetic coma to hypoglycemic coma (Roggendorf 1995). In a case of insulin suicide or homicide, insulin is detectable in routinely formalin-fixed and paraffin-embedded subcutaneous injection marks, in spite of a postmortem interval of day up to weeks. Around birefringent crystalline material, probably zinc phosphate, immunohistochemistry can reveal granular insulin depots as well as an insulin staining along the lipocyte membranes (Lutz et al. 1997).

16.2 Loss of Adrenocortical Lipids

Some authors report that morphological changes in the adrenal cortex are completely absent in acute deaths (Uotila and Pekkarinen 1951). It is only after a prolonged survival time that loss of adrenocortical lipids can be seen (Fig. 16.6; Symington et al. 1956; Spann 1954). Investigations on acute lipid mobilization in cases of very short posttraumatic survival times have been conducted. In these investigations, lipid accumulation in the sinusoids of the adrenal cortex has been found in cases in which death did not occur suddenly, in particular in the middle cortical layer (the fasciculate zone). Scarlet red staining was performed; other staining methods (Nile blue sulfate, Sudan III, osmium IV) did not lead to better differentiation. However, findings were not equally distributed within the fasciculate zone of the adrenal cortex (Heinrichs et al. 1969). The authors interpreted this lipid mobilization as a vital reaction that would also allow for a conclusion as to how rapidly death occurred. However, histological findings should be interpreted with

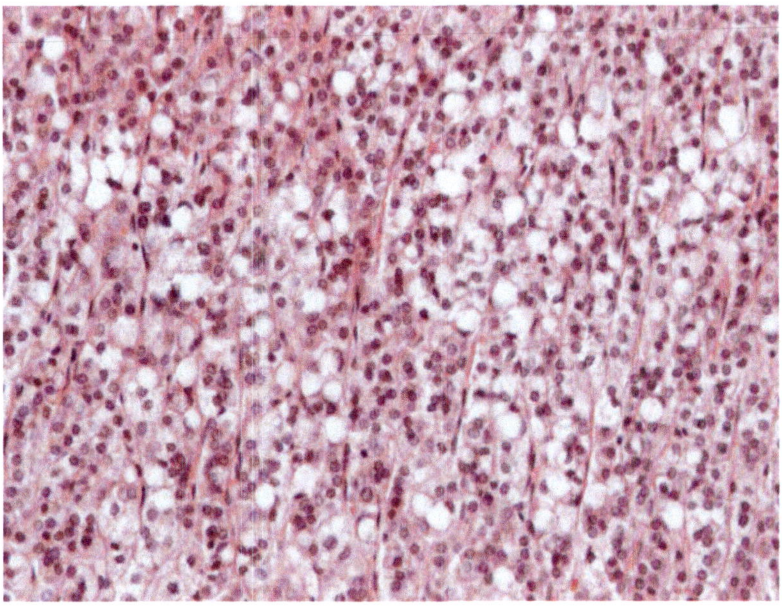

Fig. 16.6 Partial lipid depletion of cells in the zona fasciculata of the adrenal cortex (H&E ×200)

caution. On the one hand, a single histological tissue section cannot be sufficiently representative of the entire adrenal cortex, while on the other there can be various causes for vacuolated lipid depletion in the cells of the zona fasciculata of the adrenal cortex.

16.3 Acute Primary Adrenal Insufficiency (Addison's Disease)

Circulatory lesions, inflammation, and tumors of the adrenal glands can affect the secretion of hormones and may cause lethal metabolic crises (Palmiere et al. 2014; Hecht et al. 2009b; Burke and Opeskin 1999; Al Sabri et al. 1997). Only in very rare cases does adrenocortical carcinoma cause sudden death (Marshall et al. 2007). Even if such cases are quite rare, the primary and secondary morphological findings and symptoms of an acute disease should be known by all forensic medical examiners. Addison's disease is primary adrenal insufficiency due to bilateral destruction of, or damage to, the adrenal cortex, for example, in the setting of tuberculosis (Ward and Evans 1985), due to malignant disease, or in the case of autoimmune adrenalitis. In addition to advanced myasthenia, cachexia and brownish pigmentation of the skin and mucosa (bronze skin disease) can be seen.

An infection (Woenkhaus et al. 2005) or Waterhouse–Friderichsen syndrome can trigger acute adrenal insufficiency with a lethal course. This results in a shock-like condition due to electrolyte deficit with acidosis, vomiting, diarrhea, hemorrhage, and numbness. The disease peaks at between 40 and 50 years of age. In 80% of cases, an autoimmune adrenalitis can be assumed (Fig.16.7), which occurs in isolation in approximately 40% of cases and in connection with an autoimmune polyendocrine process in approximately 60% of cases (Woenkhaus et al. 2005).

Decedents are typically very slim and cachectic, such that anorexia nervosa may also be considered (Arlt and Allolio 2003; Adams et al. 1998). Atrophied adrenal glands are frequently difficult to differentiate during autopsy, and thyroid glands are frequently reduced in size. Histologically, adrenal glands show a significant reduction of the parenchyma in the cortical region and lymphocytic infiltration (almost exclusively in the cortical region), which can be seen as a consequence of an autoimmune process (Palmiere 2015; Govi et al. 2015; Martín Martorell et al. 2002). Inflammation is accompanied by a tendency toward fibrosis of varying degrees. Increased corticotropin (ACTH)-releasing cells

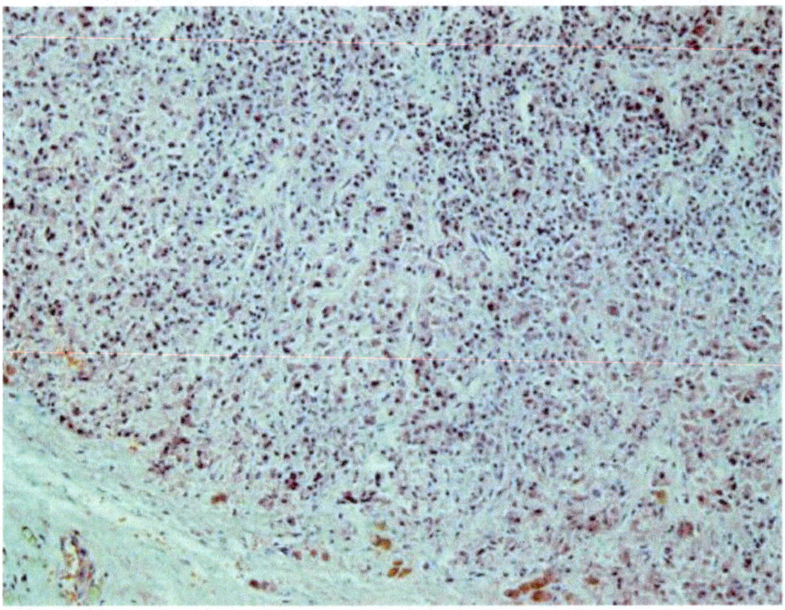

Fig. 16.7 Lymphocytic adrenalitis with clinical symptoms of Addison's disease (H&E ×100)

in the adenohypophysis (apparently reactive) have been reported (Schröder et al. 2009). Medical examinations of the thyroid gland sometimes show chronic thyroiditis with atrophic thyroid follicles.

16.4 Fatal Pheochromocytoma

Pheochromocytomas, tumors of the adrenal gland marrow, are well known as rare causes of sudden death, although they often result in a confusing array of clinical symptoms (Cardesi et al. 1994; Kniseley et al. 1988; James 1976). Pheochromocytomas occur both hereditarily and sporadically (Primhak et al. 1986; Vallance 1957). The biochemical hallmark and characteristic clinical sign of this tumor are secretion of catecholamines, causing dramatic elevations in blood pressure (Badui et al. 1982).

Only a few individual cases describe pheochromocytomas as a cause of sudden death (D'Errico et al. 2009; Preuß et al. 2006; Türk et al. 2004; Vallance 1957). Some authors suggest that pheochromocytomas have been misdiagnosed more often than previously assumed (Lo et al. 2000). Earlier studies showed that <50% of pheochromocytomas found at autopsy were already diagnosed, while the patient was still alive (Benowitz 1990).

Pheochromocytomas are generally found unilaterally (80%) and seldom bilaterally (10%) in the adrenal glands; about 10% are found outside the adrenal glands, but less than 10% are malignant (Preuß et al. 2006). They present as well-circumscribed encapsulated tumors of varying size and show a bright brown carnose color. Relicts of the yellow cortex of the suprarenal gland may be visible at the margin of the tumor. In addition, these tumors have large eosinophilic cells with granular cytoplasm as well as prominent and partly bizarre nuclei with PAS-positive small inclusions (Fig. 16.8). If there is any doubt as to the diagnosis, immunohistochemical investigations using antibodies against neuroendocrine-specific enolase (NSE) will help to demonstrate neuroendocrine granules such as chromogranin A and synaptophysin (Fig. 16.9). Additionally, the so-called sustentacular cells surrounding the tumor can be positive for S-100, a neuroectodermal marker (Preuß et al. 2006). In cases of acute cardiac failure, coagulative myocytolysis or contraction band necrosis can be found, termed catecholamine necrosis. Using confocal laser scanning microscopy, myocardial cells with ruptured myofibrils

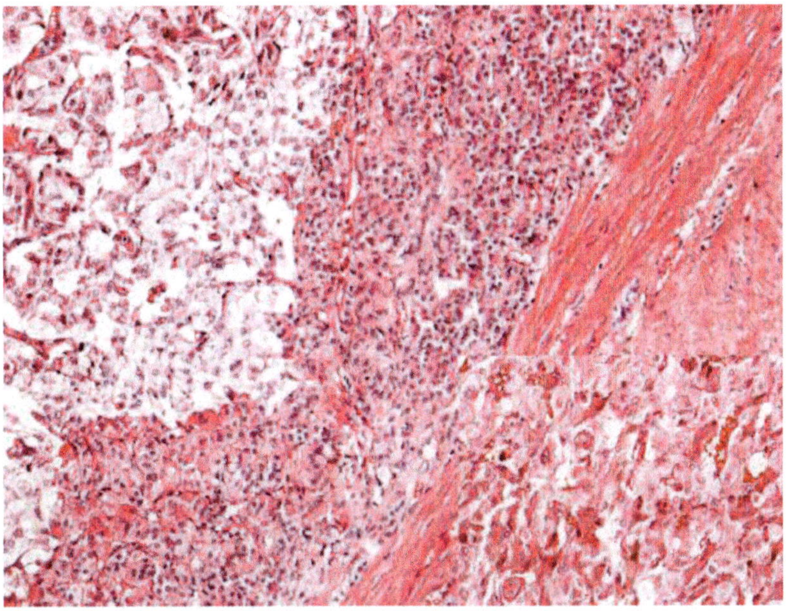

Fig. 16.8 Pheochromocytoma with tumor cells presenting nuclear pleomorphism, round or oval but also some polymorph nuclei, and rare mitoses (H&E ×100, Insert: H&E ×200)

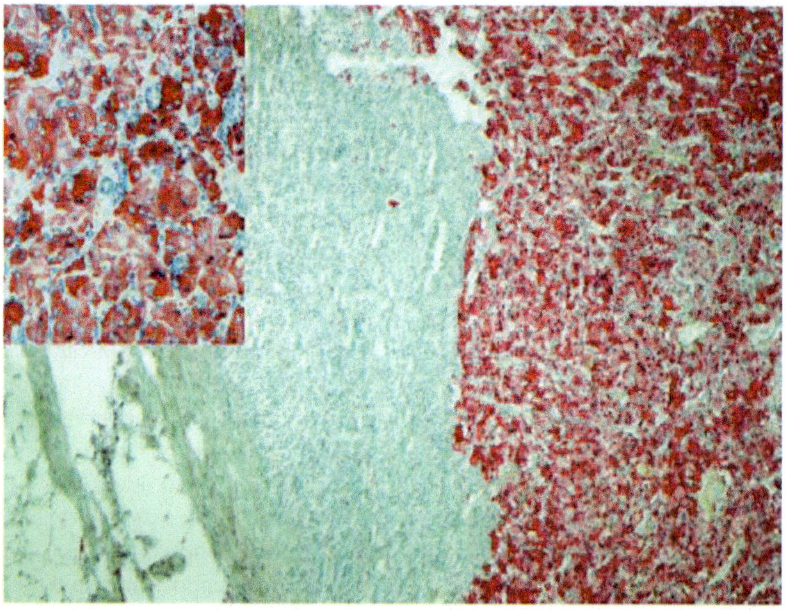

Fig. 16.9 Pheochromocytoma with positive immunohistochemical evidence of expression of synaptophysin (×40) and chromogranin A (Insert: ×200)

are described, characterized by hypereosinophilic bands of hypercontracted sarcomeres demonstrated by granular cytoplasm (D'Errico et al. 2009).

Extra-adrenal Paraganglioma

These tumors seldom occur in adult patients and resemble pheochromocytomas in morphology, functional behavior, and symptoms. They can be found in the region of the para-aortic paraganglia (organ of Zuckerkandl), duodenum, and bladder wall. They predominantly secrete noradrenaline and show a malignant degeneration more frequently than pheochromocytomas. Only a few cases of sudden death due to paragangliomas have been reported (Sperry and Smialek 1986; Isaacson et al. 1960). Causes of death in cases of pheochromocytoma or extra-adrenal paraganglioma are often the result of severe paroxysmal hypertension, such as cerebral vascular accidents, abrupt hemorrhage into the tumor, or acute left ventricular failure (Preuß et al. 2006; James 1976).

16.5 Thyroid and Parathyroid Dysfunction

Sudden death in association with metabolic crises due to dysfunction of the thyroid and parathyroid glands, e.g., thyrotoxicosis, parathyrotoxic crisis, myxedema, and acute hypoparathyroidism, is rarely seen in forensic practice (Hostiuc et al. 2015). Dysfunction can be seen in inflammatory, hyperplastic, and neoplastic processes. Inflammation of the thyroid gland accounts for approximately 20% of all thyroid diseases. According to its clinical course, thyroiditis has been subdivided into acute, subacute, and chronic forms. Classifications are based on the fact that the majority of thyroiditis cases have an autoimmune background. The most common form of this disease is autoimmune thyroiditis, with or without subclinical or manifest hypothyroidism. Thyroiditis is both clinically and morphologically distinct from thyroid tumors. Therefore, a careful examination of organs can provide useful information.

Thyroid and parathyroid dysfunctions do not necessarily show macroscopic findings.

However, appropriate histological findings can often be seen, sometimes in connection with the determination of laboratory parameters (hormone level, calcium level, etc.). Frequently, thyroid dysfunction remains undiscovered without histological controls (Liu and Lin 2015; Edston et al. 2001; Edston 1996). In particular, chronic inflammatory thyroiditises with a reduction in hormone-producing parenchyma can lead to severe dysfunction and may explain sudden death in some cases.

Less common forms of autoimmune thyroiditis include subacute granulomatous (de Quervain's) thyroiditis, postpartum thyroiditis, silent ("painless") thyroiditis, and invasive-sclerosing thyroiditis (Riedel's thyroiditis). Non-autoimmune thyroiditis is very rare (e.g., acute suppurative thyroiditis, radiation thyroiditis).

The following histological diagnoses can only be considered as indications of sudden endocrine-related death, rather than definitive evidence. Comparison with additional findings and hormone analysis to confirm the histomorphological diagnosis are both necessary. If possible, hormone analysis should be performed in the early postmortem interval (Edston et al. 2001; de Letter et al. 2000; Risse et al. 1986).

16.5.1 The Thyroid Gland

Inflammation and, in particular, hyperthyroidism can cause sudden death (Lynch and Woodford 2014; Siegler 1998; Edston 1996). Histological findings may be seen in thyroid tissue, such as papillary formations of the follicular epithelium and increased intracolloidal resorption vacuoles, which can be interpreted as a morphological sign of increased functional activity. Histomorphological findings alone can sometimes indicate that functional disorders are likely but do not provide definitive evidence. In addition, medication can affect the histological picture of the thyroid gland. A goiter develops in 5–15% of patients with chronic lithium intake. Histologically, diffuse hyperplasia can be seen. Anticonvulsants (e.g., phenytoin, carbamazepine) can also cause unspecific thyroiditis (Sheu and Schmid 2003).

Lymphomatous Goiter (Hashimoto's Goiter)
This autoimmune thyroiditis mainly affects women between 40 and 60 years of age. It is a chronic lymphatic thyroiditis with gradual formation of a goiter and hyperthyreosis. Histological findings show destructive inflammation of the thyroid parenchyma. In addition to lymphatic tissue with pronounced germinal centers, a lymphoplasmacellular inflammatory infiltrate can be seen, which moves between the cells of the follicular epithelium (Fig. 16.10). Giant cells can also occur (Schmid and Böcker 1997b), as well as oxyphil metaplasia with eosinophil follicular epithelia.

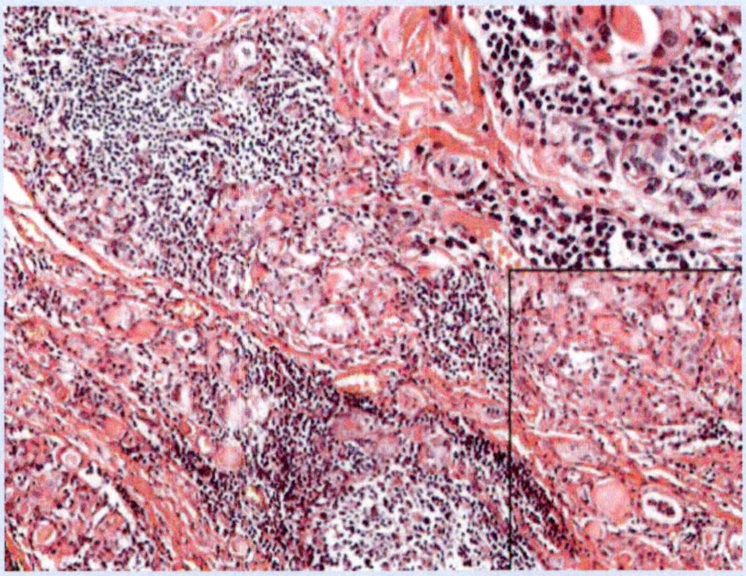

Fig. 16.10 **(a, b)** Hashimoto's goiter with lymphatic germinal centers and a lymphoplasmacellular inflammatory infiltrate invading and partly destroying the follicular epithelium (insert) (H&E ×100, ×400)

Atrophic Autoimmune Thyroiditis

In the case of atrophic autoimmune thyroiditis, clinical signs of hypothyroidism can be seen. Histologically, pronounced fibrosis with macroscopically diminished thyroid glands is evident, while functionally active thyroid tissue is rare, and a loose lymphoplasmacellular inflammatory infiltrate can be seen. Infrequently, dense fibrosis (Riedel's thyroiditis) can be seen, typically in connection with euthyreosis.

De Quervain's Thyroiditis

This is a granulomatous thyroiditis that does not usually lead to severe dysfunction in hormone production. Histologically, both lymphoplasmacellular inflammation and polynuclear giant cells can be seen (Fig. 16.11).

Diffuse Hyperthyroid Goiter (Graves' Disease)

This form of thyroid dysfunction is also an autoimmune disease, typically occurring between 30 and 40 years of age; females are more frequently affected than males. The thyroid gland is enlarged and appears dark red macroscopically. Histologically, a cubic to highly prismatic follicular epithelium can be seen. This epithelium is situated on papillary cell buds which protrude into the follicular epithelium (Fig. 16.12). Adjacent intracolloidal resorption vacuoles can be seen when thyroid colloid is present. A certain fibrotization can be observed subepithelially, along with loosely spread lymphocytes. Autoimmune diseases of the thyroid gland can be accompanied by a myxomatous mitral valve prolapse; the embedded hydrophilic glycosaminoglycans can be detected with Alcian Blue staining. In the case of a thickened mitral valve, valve insufficiency may occur (Kahaly et al. 1995). Cases of sudden unexpected death in undiagnosed Graves' disease have been described (Lynch and Woodford 2014).

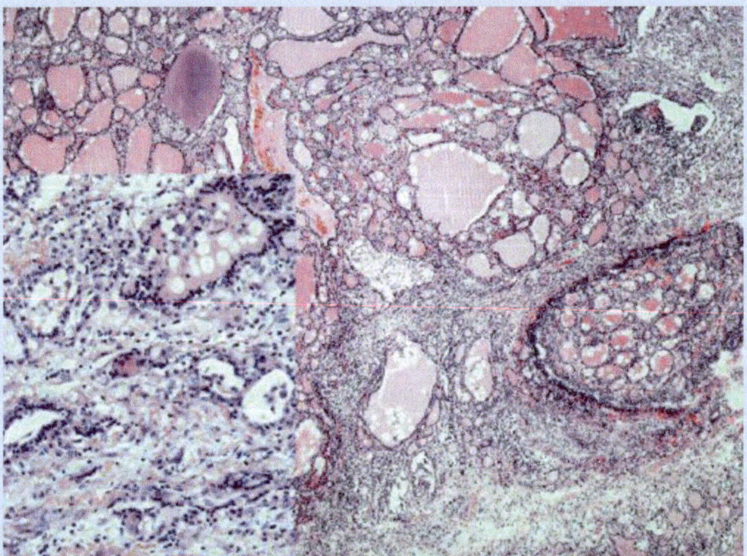

Fig. 16.11 (**a**, **b**) Granulomatous de Quervain's thyroiditis with lymphocytic inflammatory infiltrate, slight interstitial fibrosis, and increased intracolloidal resorption vacuoles as a histological sign of increased functional activity; hyperthyroid phase (H&E ×40, Insert: H&E ×200)

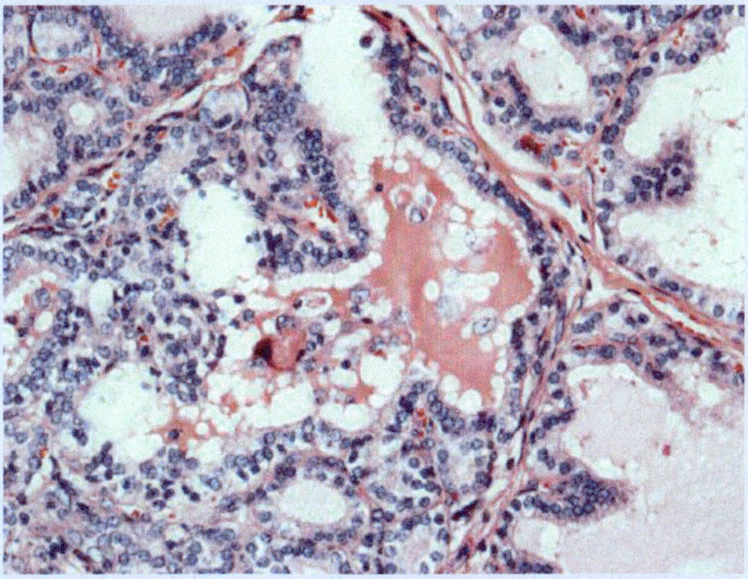

Fig. 16.12 Graves' disease: hyperthyroid goiter with micropapillary formations of the follicular epithelium and intracolloidal resorption vacuoles as a sign of increased functional activity of the thyroid gland (H&E ×200)

Amiodarone-Induced Thyroiditis

Long-term medication with amiodarone or propylthiouracil can promote both hypothyroidism and a thyrotoxic crisis (Sheu et al. 2006; Gough and Gough 2002; Mulligan et al. 1993; Smyrk et al. 1987). Amiodarone, an iodine-containing antiarrhythmic, can lead to severe thyroid dysfunction. Histologically, destructive chronic inflammation with lymphocytes and formation of foam cells from macrophages can be seen; intracolloidal resorption vacuoles as a sign of increased functional activity may also occur. The follicular epithelium will be gradually destroyed, and post-inflammatory fibrosis forms.

Autonomous Thyroid Adenoma

Autonomous or toxic thyroid adenoma is said to be responsible for approximately one third of cases of hyperthyroidism (Hecht et al. 2009b). Histologically, the adenoma is completely surrounded by a modest fibrous fiber capsule. The follicular epithelium shows, as in Graves' disease, micropapillary formations and is relatively bright and high. Abundant intracolloidal resorption vacuoles are visible. Frequently, regressive changes, as can be seen in a goiter, occur, including fibrosis, hemorrhage, calcium deposits, and siderophages. In the case of autonomous adenoma, the remaining thyroid tissue might be atrophic (Schmid and Böcker 1997b). Multiple toxic or autonomous adenoma with a similar histological picture is referred to as toxic multinodular goiter (Plummer's disease). In cases of autonomous adenoma or toxic multinodular goiter, a thyrotoxic crisis may occur on administration of iodine-containing contrast agents (Sheu et al. 2003). The development of thyrogenic cardiomyopathy may be considered, depending on the duration of hyperthyreosis.

Thyrotoxic Crisis

A thyrotoxic crisis is a rare endocrinological emergency with a mortality rate of up to 50% (Burch and Wartofsky 1993). The main clinical symptoms include tachycardia, hyperthermia, and central nervous system disorders. Psychotic states and cramping, as in epileptic seizures, occur (Hecht et al. 2009a; Safe et al. 1990). At autopsy, signs of right heart failure with upper venous congestion, peripheral edemas, and vascular congestion in the internal organs can be seen (Safe et al. 1990; Zierhut and Girlich 2004). Despite inconspicuous findings in the coronary arteries, cardiac arrhythmias and acute myocardial infarctions have been described (Cheah et al. 1971; Kotler et al. 1973), as well as cardiac arrhythmias attributed to coronary spasms (Wei et al. 1979). Typically, a preexisting hyperthyreosis is assumed that may lead to a thyrotoxic crisis when triggering factors occur, such as iodine ingestion or discontinuing thyrostatic therapy (Reschke and Lehnert 2003). In rare cases, accidental or suicidal administration of thyroid hormones should be considered (Hartung et al. 2010; Bhasin et al. 1981). Uncontrolled intake of liothyronine can cause lethal thyroid storm in an euthyroid patient without manifest cardiac disease. Histological findings in such cases include a thyroid gland with plump follicles and a flattened epithelial layer, while the myocardium may present multiple fresh cell necroses (Hartung et al. 2010). Evident uncontrolled intake of liothyronine can cause thyrotoxic crisis and even lethal thyroid storm. In principle, trauma or surgery can also trigger a thyrotoxic crisis.

Hypothyroidism

In the case of a severely underactive thyroid, myxedema and additional symptoms may occur, including ptosis, macroglossia, pasty swelling in the face, cool and dry skin, bradycardia, hypotonia, and even shock (Wall 2000). Hypothyroidism has a mortality rate of up to 20% (Hecht et al. 2009a). There is no morphological correlate for the clinical diagnosis of hypothyroidism.

Radiation-Induced Thyroiditis

External radiation and radioiodide therapy leads to a destruction of thyroid follicles with inflammatory infiltrates, proliferation of fibroblasts, and subsequent fibrosis. Cell nuclei of follicular epithelia may show pronounced pleomorphism and hyperchromasia.

Black Thyroid

A distinctive but very rare side effect of exposure to minocycline, a tetracycline derivate, is black pigmentation of the thyroid gland. Histology findings present clumps of black-brown pigment, visible in epithelial cells and in the colloid (Bell et al. 2001). Also, a granular precipitate of black-brown pigment has been noted in the apical portions of follicular epithelial cells (Tsokos and Schröder 2006). These pigments are also PAS-, Ziehl–Neelsen-, and Sudan IV-positive. Hypothyroidism is occasionally associated with minocycline-related black thyroid, and the development of depressive disorders is possible. No definitive correlation can be drawn between sudden death and black thyroid, which can develop due to chronic intake of high doses of minocycline. The macroscopic picture of "black thyroid" can also form in the setting of *ochronosis* (*alkaptonuria*). Again in this clinical picture, one sees microscopic (partially dustlike, partially fine-grained) deposits of blackish pigment in the thyroid follicles, particularly in the follicular epithelial cells (Fig. 16.13). These deposits are homogentisic acid, which also accumulates especially in bradytrophic tissue (cartilage, intervertebral discs, scar tissue), as well as in the vessel intima of larger vessels. Microscopic analysis reveals partially dustlike blackish pigment. Disorders such as hematochromatosis, chronic arsenic poisoning, porphyrinuria, Addison's disease, and argyrosis need to be considered in the differential diagnosis. Ochronotic changes have been observed following long-term treatment with antimalarial medications (quinacrine, hydroquinone), antibiotic use (tetracyclines such as minocycline), as well as phenothiazine and phenacetin abuse (Klein et al. 2008).

In the event of protracted stress, the thyroid can react to activation, e.g., in gradual hypothermia or malignant hyperthermia (Fig. 16.14). Several thyroid samples need to be analyzed in order to diagnose this type of thyroid function activation; each sample should show increased intracolloidal resorption vacuoles as a sign of increased functional activity.

In the case of severe trauma involving fractures, chest compression, and marked blood congestion in the head and neck area, it is also possible to detect ruptured vessels and hemorrhage in the thyroid follicles (Byard 2013).

Table 16.3 summarizes the histological criteria for the various thyroid disorders (modified from Hostiuc et al. 2015)

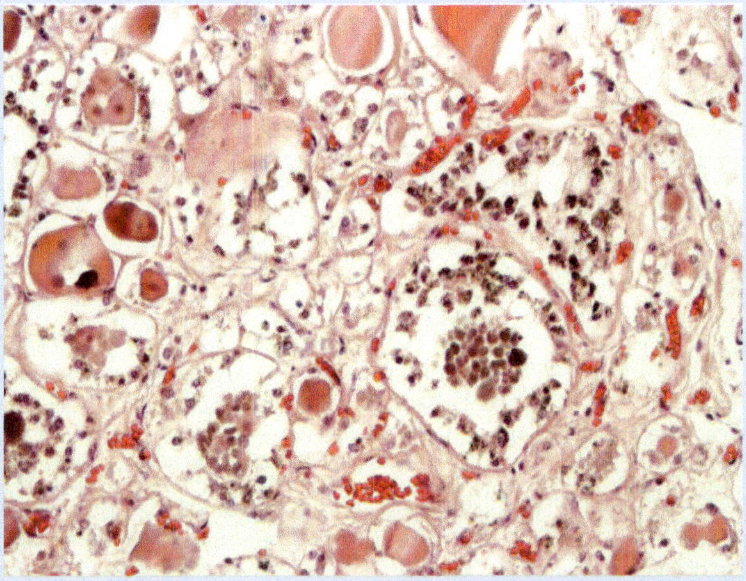

Fig. 16.13 Marked colloid depletion in the thyroid follicles with blackish pigment in the follicular epithelium and follicular spaces, occasionally also in the apical region of the follicular epithelium; "black thyroid" in ochronosis (H&E ×100)

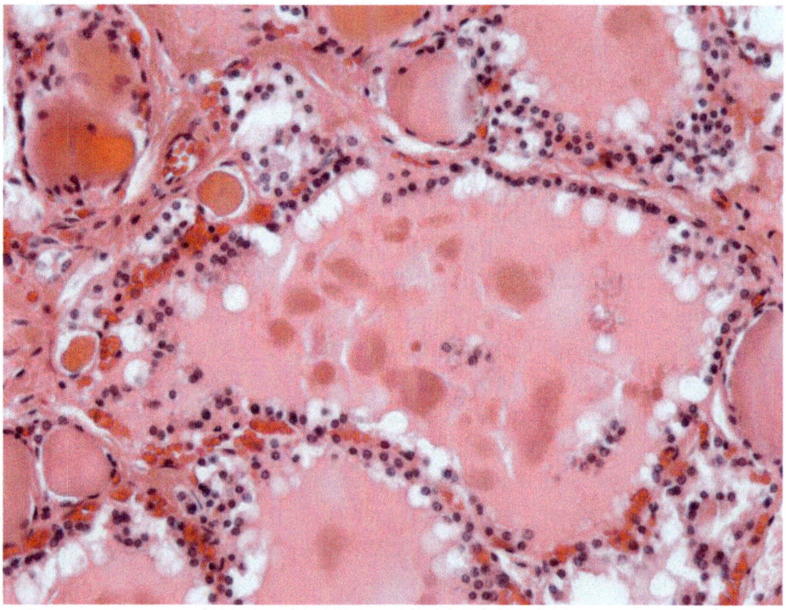

Fig. 16.14 Increased intracolloidal resorption vacuoles as a sign of increased functional thyroid activity (H&E ×200)

Table 16.3 Histological findings in the various thyroid disorders

Diagnosis	Histology
Partially diffuse, partially nodular colloid goiter	Varying thyroid follicle size with a flat, cubic epithelium, no loss of colloid, no inflammation, and no increase in intracolloidal resorption vacuoles Nodular structures, microhemorrhages, interstitial fibrosis with calcifications, ossification, and necrosis are possible
Graves' disease	To some degree small, but also larger thyroid follicles with a high, prominent, and partially pseudopapillary epithelium, lymphocytic infiltrates (generally $CD4^+$-T-lymphocytes), and abundant intracolloidal resorption vacuoles (Fig. 16.12)
Subacute thyroiditis (de Quervain) (Fig. 16.10)	*Hyperthyroid phase:* thyroid colloid depletion, follicle wall rupture, multinucleated giant cells, signs of acute inflammation *Hypothyroid phase:* loss of follicular epithelium, mixed inflammatory cell infiltrates, granulomas surrounding the ruptured follicle *Regenerative phase:* increasing fibrosis and regenerating follicles
Chronic thyroiditis	Buildup of lymphocytic cells in thyroid tissue, some with fully formed germinal centers between the thyroid follicles No histological criteria for increased thyroid function
Riedel's thyroiditis	Cell-poor, strongly fibrosed tissue involving adjacent thyroid tissue, small atrophic residual thyroid follicles with flat epithelium, scant thyroid colloid
Amiodarone thyroiditis	Partially fibrosed, partially chronic inflammatory areas in thyroid tissue as well as tissue that has undergone degenerative change, to an extent involving foam cells in irregularly and diffusely enlarged follicles
"Black thyroid"	Deposits of blackish pigment in apical areas of the follicular epithelium and in the thyroid colloid, e.g., due to tetracycline treatment (ochronosis should be considered in the differential diagnosis; Fig. 16.13)
Autoimmune (Hashimoto) thyroiditis	Atrophic thyroid follicles and oncocytic metaplasia of the follicular epithelium (Hurthle cells), differently sized nuclei, nodular areas, lymphocytic infiltrates with T-cells ($CD4^+$, $CD8^+$) and B-cells of varying density and composition infiltrating the follicular epithelium in places. Frequently enlarged lymph nodes and reactive follicular hyperplasia in adjacent areas (Fig. 16.10)
Increased intracolloidal resorption vacuoles	Uncharacteristic signs of elevated functional activity of varying etiology (Fig. 16.14)
Traumatic crush asphyxia	Congestion-related vessel wall rupture and hemorrhage in thyroid tissue, as well as in thyroid follicles

16.5.2 Parathyroid Glands

As a rule, four parathyroid glands can be seen at autopsy. They lie in pairs and should not normally weigh more than 60 mg. The parathyroid glands in children are somewhat red-brown, while in older people, due to fatty tissue deposits, they appear yellowish-brown. Histologically, a distinction is drawn between clear parathyroid principal cells rich in glycogen (PAS staining) and oxyphil cells. Parathyroid principal cells are solid and situated in small groups, in part with small colloid-containing follicles. Parathyroid dysfunction with increased activity is divided into primary, secondary, and tertiary hyperparathyroidism. These various dysfunctions can result in a hypercalcemic crisis. Reduced activity may lead to lethal hypocalcemia. Here too, histological findings alone cannot verify hyper- or hypocalcemia. However, if further secondary changes are present, particularly in the bones, blood vessels, and soft tissues, it is very likely that chronic hypercalcemia can be verified.

Hyperparathyroidism

The various forms of hyperparathyroidism can lead to a lethal hypercalcemic crisis. In some cases, the underlying cause is a malignant tumor disease with symptoms such as vomiting, renal failure, and coma (Edelson and Kleerekoper 1995). Chronic hyperparathyroidism can lead to calcifications in internal organs, such as the myocardium (Fig. 16.15), kidneys (Fig. 16.16), and lungs (Fig. 16.17), as well as osteomalacia and further vessel and soft tissue calcifications (Schmid and Böcker 1997a).

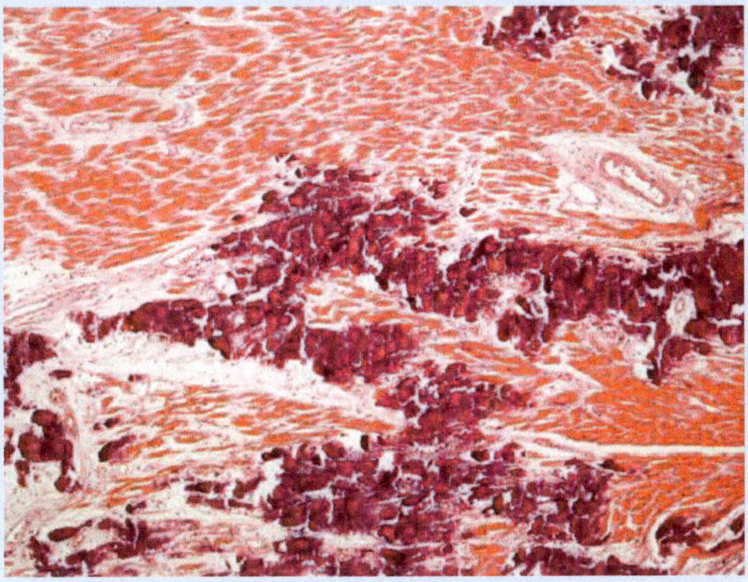

Fig. 16.15 Secondary hyperparathyroidism with severe basophilic calcium salt deposits in the myocardium (H&E ×100)

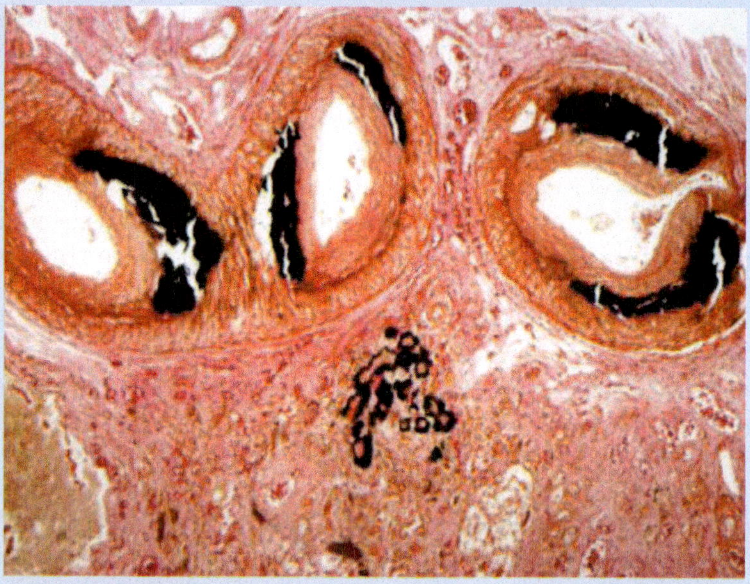

Fig. 16.16 Pronounced nephrocalcinosis with severe calcium deposits in peripheral vascular walls in the case of secondary hyperparathyroidism in a 58-year-old patient with dialysis-dependent renal failure found dead in his home (Kossa ×40)

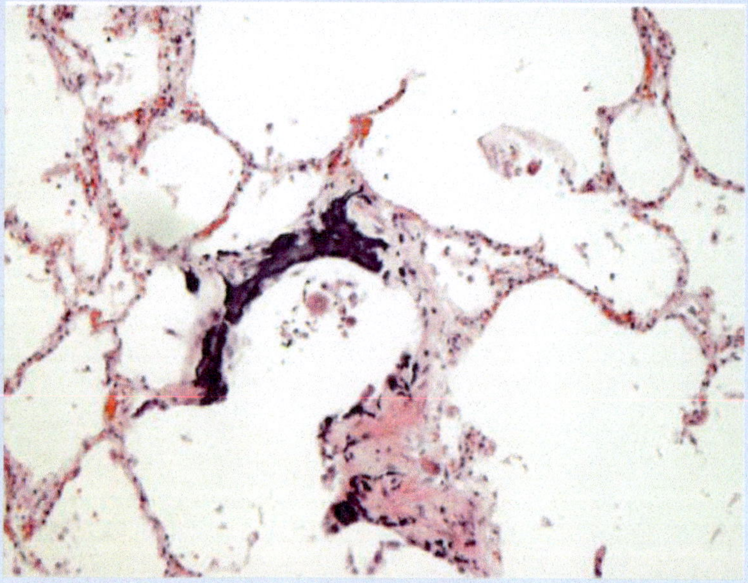

Fig. 16.17 Semicircular streaky basophilic calcifications of a bronchiolar wall in the lung tissue in a case of secondary hyperparathyroidism (H&E ×100)

Hyperplasia of the parathyroid principal cells can be the cause of hyperparathyroidism (Sheu et al. 2003), although not in all parathyroid glands. Histologically, densely situated parathyroid principal cells with fine fibrous septa can usually be found; adipose cells are rarely seen. A complete connective tissue capsule does not need to be present (Hecht et al. 2009b). Additional causes for hyperparathyroidism include parathyroid adenomas (>80% of cases) or parathyroid carcinomas (<3% of cases). In adenoma, a capsule of connective tissue can typically be seen (Sheu et al. 2003). Parathyroid carcinoma mostly affects patients of at least 50 years of age with particularly high calcium levels in their serum. Macroscopically, parathyroid carcinomas are gray-white; histologically, infiltrative growth, regressive changes, and atypical cells can be found.

Hypoparathyroidism/Hypocalcemia

Clinically, acute tetany is known to occur in cases of inadvertent total parathyroidectomy following parathyroid surgery; hypocalcemia can lead to death. Other causes may include autoimmune processes with involvement of parathyroid glands (Schmid and Böcker 1997a, b). Cases of acute heart failure due to hypocalcemia following sodium EDTA therapy for lead poisoning have also been described (Brown et al. 2006).

16.6 Pituitary Gland and Hypophyseal Dysfunction

Pituitary Gland

The pituitary gland (anterior pituitary) contains different cell populations: acidophils, containing prolactin (PRL) and growth hormone (GH), and basophils, containing *luteinizing hormone* (*LH*), *thyroid-stimulating hormone* (*TSH*), and *adrenocorticotropic hormone* (*ACTH*). It should be possible to detect these pituitary hormones immunohistochemically for up to 15 days postmortem—not, however, after longer than 20 days (Ishikawa et al. 2006a). The neurohypophysis (posterior pituitary) is primarily made up of glial cells and nerve fibers, with no glandular structures. During pregnancy, it is possible to visualize the activation of hormone production in the anterior pituitary (Fig. 16.18).

An increased number of vacuoles in the hormone-producing cells of the anterior pituitary have been reported in fatal hypothermia (Ishikawa et al. 2004). Individual studies report increased expression of *clusterin* in the anterior pituitary depending on age (Ishikawa et al. 2006b). Partial or complete hypopituitarism may progress to pituitary coma, resulting in secondary hypothyrosis and/or secondary adrenal insufficiency (Matschke et al. 2000). Hypophyseal dysfunction can lead to sudden death (Bauer et al. 2001; Blisard et al. 1992). Hypophyseal necrosis is typically seen with circulatory shock.

Simmonds' syndrome describes insufficiency of the anterior pituitary gland, i.e., hypopituitarism due to a variety of causes, for example, hypophyseal tumor, hypophysitis, or Sheehan's

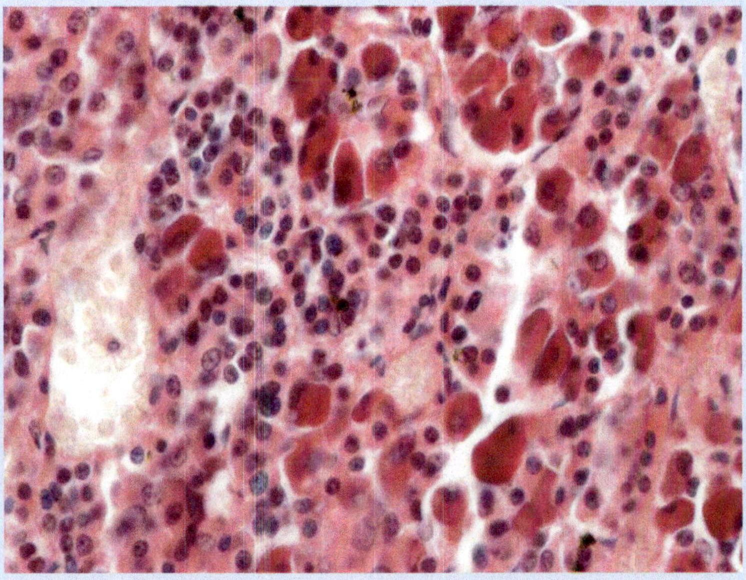

Fig. 16.18 Activated hormone production in the anterior pituitary during pregnancy (H&E ×400)

syndrome. However, these are rare diseases. The lymphocytic type of Simmonds' syndrome with diffusely spread lymphocytes is predominant among primary hypophyseal inflammations, with the possible formation of germinal centers (Hecht et al. 2009b). Inflammation can spread to the neurohypophysis. An autoimmune process is considered to be the underlying disease. Death as a direct result of primary hypophysitis is very rare (Blisard et al. 1992; Gal et al. 1986).

Sheehan's Syndrome

Sheehan's syndrome is accompanied by post-puerperal blood loss with shock symptoms and anterior pituitary insufficiency (Sheehan 1965). Its prevalence has been given in the past as 100–200 cases per 1 million women (Sheehan 1937, 1965). Progression and severity of this disease vary from partial hypopituitarism to panhypopituitarism. Clinical symptoms are variable and can occur at between 1 and 33 years postpartum (Schröder et al. 2009; Huang et al. 2002). Histologically, pronounced fibrosis or scar formation in the adenohypophysis can be found. Small tissue islets with a preserved residual parenchyma can be detected immunohistochemically as follicle-stimulating hormone (FSH) and as prolactin-secreting cells (Schröder et al. 2009; Saeger and Kühn 1984).

Hypophyseal Apoplexy

Hypophyseal adenomas are slow-growing benign tumors that may present with very few symptoms despite suprasellar growth. In some cases, this may lead to hemorrhagic infarction of tumor tissue which, in turn, may lead to the clinical picture of hypophyseal apoplexy. In rare cases, this leads to sudden and unexpected death. Histologically, tumor tissue with widespread hemorrhage and signs of infarction can be seen (Bauer et al. 2000, 2001).

References

Adams R, Hinkebein MK, McQuillen M et al (1998) Prompt differentiation of Addison's disease from anorexia nervosa during weight loss and vomiting. South Med J 91:208–211

Al Sabri AM, Smith N, Busuttil A (1997) Sudden death due to auto-immune Addison's disease in a 12-year-old girl. Int J Legal Med 110:278–280

Arlt W, Allolio B (2003) Adrenal insufficiency. Lancet 31:1881–1893

Badui E, Mancilla R, Szymanski JJ, Gardia-Rubi D, Estanol B (1982) Diverse clinical manifestations of pheochromocytomas. Angiology 33:173–182

Banaschak S, Bajanowski T, Brinkmann B (2000) Suicide of a diabetic by inducing hyperglycemic coma. Int J Legal Med 113:162–163

Bauer M, Lang C, Patzelt D (2000) Hypophysenapoplexie als Ursache eines plötzlichen unerwarteten Todeseintritts. In: 9th spring meeting of the German society of forensic medicine, Leipzig, 4–5 May 2000

Bauer M, Lang C, Patzelt D (2001) Sudden death due to pituitary apoplexy. Legal Med 3:183–186

Bell CD, Kovacs K, Horvath E, Rotondo F (2001) Histologic, immunohistochemical and ultrastructural findings in a case of minocycline-associated black thyroid. Endocr Pathol 12:443–451

Benowitz NL (1990) Pheochromocytoma. Adv Intern Med 35:195–200

Bhasin S, Wallace W, Lawrence JB, Lesch M (1981) Sudden death associated with thyroid hormone abuse. Am J Med 71:887–890

Blisard KS, Pfalzgraf RR, Balko MG (1992) Sudden death due to lymphoplasmatic hypophysitis. Am J Forensic Med Pathol 13:207–210

Brown MJ, Willis T, Omalu B, Leiker R (2006) Deaths resulting from hypocalcemia after administration of edetate disodium: 2003-2005. Pediatrics 118:534–536

Burch HB, Wartofsky L (1993) Life-threatening thyrotoxicosis. Thyroid storm. Endocrinol Metab Clin N Am 22:263–277

Burke MP, Opeskin K (1999) Adrenocortical insufficieny. Am J Forensic Med Pathol 20:60–65

Byard RW (2013) Pathological changes in the thyroid gland in crush asphyxia. Forensic Sci Med Pathol 9:568–572

Byard RW, Zhou C (2010) Erosive gastritis, Armanni-Ebstein phenomenon and diabetic ketoacidosis. Forensic Sci Med Pathol 6:304–306

Cardesi E, Cera G, Gassia A (1994) Pheochromocytoma and sudden death: a case of hyperacute myocardial ischemia. Pathologica 86:670–672

Cheah JS, Lee GS, Chew LS (1971) Myocardial infarction in thyrotoxicosis. Med J Aust 1:393–395

D'Errico S, Pomara C, Riezzo I, Neri M, Turillazzi E, Fineschi V (2009) Cardiac failure due to epinephrine-secreting pheochromocytoma: clinical, laboratory and pathological findings in a sudden death. Forensic Sci Int 187:e13–e17

De Letter EA, Piette MH, Lambert WE, De Leenheer AP (2000) Medico-legal implications of hidden thyroid dysfunction: a study of two cases. Med Sci Law 40:251–257

DiMaio VJM, Sturner WQ, Coe JI (1977) Sudden and unexpected deaths after the acute onset of diabetes mellitus. J Forensic Sci 22:147–151

Edelson GW, Kleerekoper M (1995) Hypercalcemic crisis. Med Clin North Am 79:79–92

Edston E (1996) Three sudden deaths in men associated with undiagnosed chronic thyroiditis. Int J Legal Med 109:94–97

Edston E, Druid H, Holmgren P, Öström M (2001) Postmortem measurements of thyroid hormones in blood and vitreous humor combined with histology. Am J Forensic Med Pathol 22:78–83

Gal R, Schwartz A, Gukovsky-Oren S et al (1986) Lymphoid hypophysitis associated with sudden maternal death: report of a case and review of the literature. Obstet Gynecol Surv 41:619–621

Gough IR, Gough J (2002) Surgical management of amiodarone-associated thyrotoxicosis. Med J Aust 176:128–129

Govi A, Fersini F, Tsokos M (2015) Sudden death due to acute adrenal crisis. Forensic Sci Med Pathol 11:445–447

Hartung B, Schott M, Daldrup T, Ritz-Timme S (2010) Lethal thyroid storm after uncontrolled intake of liothyronine in order to lose weight. Int J Legal Med 124:637–640

Hecht L, Saeger W, Püschel K (2009a) Plötzlicher Tod bei Erkrankungen der Schilddrüse und der Nebenschilddrüsen. Rechtsmedizin 19:11–16

Hecht L, Saeger W, Püschel K (2009b) Plötzlicher Tod bei Erkrankungen der Hypophyse und der Nebennieren. Rechtsmedizin 19:5–10

Heinrichs L, Schulz E, Schwerd W (1969) Morphologischer Nachweis akuter Lipoidmobilisation in der Nebennierenrinde bei sehr kurzen posttraumatischen Überlebenszeiten. Arch Kriminol 143:199–203

Hostiuc S, Luca L, Iliescu DB, Dascălu MI, Drima E, Renţea I, Moldoveanu A, Ceauşu M, Pirici D (2015) Sudden thyroid death. A systematic review. Rom J Leg Med 23:233–242

Huang YY, Ting MK, Hsu BR, Tsai JS (2002) Demonstration of reserved anterior pituitary function among patients with amenorrhea after postpartum hemorrhage. Gynecol Endocrinol 14:99–104

Isaacson C, Rosenzweig D, Seftel HC (1960) Malignant pheochromocytoma of the organs of Zuckerkandl. Arch Pathol 70:725–729

Ishikawa T, Miyaishi S, Tachibana T, Ishizu H, Zhu BL, Maeda H (2004) Fatal hypothermia related vacuolization of hormone-producing cells in the anterior pituitary. Legal Med 6:157–163

Ishikawa T, Zhu BL, Li DR, Zhao D, Michiue T, Maeda H (2006a) Postmortem stability of pituitary hormones in the human adenohypophysis. Legal Med 8:34–38

Ishikawa T, Zhu BL, Li DR, Zhao D, Michiue T, Maeda H (2006b) Age-dependent increase of clusterin in the human pituitary gland. Legal Med 8:28–33

James TN (1976) On the cause of sudden death in pheochromocytoma with special reference to the pulmonary arteries, the cardiac conduction system and the aggregation of platelets. Circulation 54:348–356

Kahaly G, Mohr-Kahaly S, Beyer J, Meyer J (1995) Prevalence of myxomatous mitral valve prolaps in patients with lymphocytic thyroiditis. Am J Cardiol 76:1309–1310

Karlovsek MZ (2004) Diagnostic values of combined glucose and lactate values in cerebrospinal fluid and vitreous humour – our experiences. Forensic Sci Int 146:19–23

Kernbach G, Brinkmann B (1983) Postmortale Pathochemie für die Feststellung der Todesursache Coma diabeticum. Pathologe 4:235–240

Kernbach-Wighton G, Püschel K (1998) On the phenomenology of lethal applications of insulin. Forensic Sci Int 93:61–73

Klein A, Theile A, Körner HW, Schulz F (2008) Ochronose. Seltene Stoffwechselerkrankung mit außergewöhnlichem Sektionsbefund. Rechtsmedizin 19:25–29

Kniseley AS, Sweeney K, Ambler MW (1988) Pheochromocytoma and sudden death as a result of cerebral infarction in Turner's syndrome: report of a case. J Forensic Sci 3:1497–1502

Kotler MN, Michaelides KM, Bouchard RJ, Warbasse JE (1973) Myocardial infarction associated with thyrotoxicosis. Arch Intern Med 132:723–728

Lasczkowski GE, Püschel K (1991) Hyperglykämische Stoffwechselentgleisung: Relation zwischen Glykogennephrose und postmortalen biochemischen Parametern des Glukosestoffwechsels. Rechtsmedizin 1:41–45

Liu H, Lin F (2015) Application of immunohistochemistry in thyroid pathology. Arch Pathol Lab Med 139:67–82

Lo CY, Lam KY, Wat MS (2000) Adrenal pheochromocytoma remains a frequently overlooked diagnosis. Am J Surg 179:212–215

Lutz R, Pedal I, Wetzel C, Mattern R (1997) Insulin injection sites: morphology and immunohistochemistry. Forensic Sci Int 90:93–101

Lynch MJ, Woodford NWF (2014) Sudden unexpected death in the setting of undiagnosed Graves' disease. Forensic Sci Med Pathol 10:452–456

Marshall DT, Gilbert JD, Byard RW (2007) Adrenocortical carcinoma and sudden death. Forensic Sci Med Pathol 3:53–55

Martín Martorell P, Roep BO, Smith JW (2002) Autoimmunity in Addison's disease. Neth J Med 60:269–275

Matschke J, Sperhake J, Saeger W et al (2000) Forensische Pädopathologie – Tödliche Addison-Krise bei idiopathischem Panhypopituitarismus. Päd 6:16–20

Milroy CM, Parai JL (2011) Armanni-Ebstein lesion, ketoacidosis and starvation in a child. Forensic Sci Med Pathol 7:213–216

Mulligan DC, McHenry CR, Kinney W, Esselstyn CB Jr (1993) Amiodarone-induced thyrotoxicosis: clinical presentation and expanded indications for thyroidectomy. Surgery 114:1114–1119

Osuna E, Garcia-Villora A, Pérez-Cárceles MD, Conejero J, Abenza JM, Martinez P, Luna A (1999) Vitreous

humor fructosamine concentrations in the autopsy diagnosis of diabetes mellitus. Int J Legal Med 112:275–279
Osuna E, Vivero G, Conejero J, Abenza JM, Martinez P, Luna A, Pérez-Cáceles MD (2005) Postmortem vitreous humor β-hydroxybutyrate: its utility for the postmortem interpretation of diabetes mellitus. Forensic Sci Int 153:189–195
Palmiere C (2015) Sudden death due to acute adrenal crisis. Forensic Sci Med Pathol 11:629
Palmiere C, de Froidmont S, Mangin P, Werner D, Lobrinus A (2014) Ketoacidosis and adrenocortical insufficiency. J Forensic Sci 59:1146–1152
Preuß J, Woenkhaus C, Schwesinger G, Madea B (2006) Non-diagnosed pheochromocytoma as a cause of sudden death in a 49-year-old man. A case report with medico-legal implications. Forensic Sci Int 156:223–228
Primhak RA, Spicer RS, Variend S (1986) Sudden death after minor abdominal trauma: an unusual presentation of phaeochromocytoma. Br Med J 292:95–96
Püschel K (2004) Plötzlicher Tod im Erwachsenenalter. In: Brinkmann B, Madea B (eds) Handbuch gerichtliche Medizin, vol 1. Springer, Berlin, pp 1020–1021
Reschke K, Lehnert H (2003) Die thyreotoxische Krise. Internist 4:1221–1230
Risse M, Weiler G, Benker G (1986) Comparative histologic and hormonal studies of the thyroid gland with spezial reference to sudden infant death (SIDS). Z Rechtsmed 96:31–38
Ritchie S, Waugh D (1957) The pathology of Armanni-Ebstein-diabetic nephropathie. Am J Pathol 33:1035–1057
Ritz S, Kaatsch HJ (1990) Postmortale Diagnostik von tödlichen diabetischen Stoffwechselentgleisungen: welchen Stellenwert haben Liquor- und Glaskörperflüssigkeitssummenwerte sowie der HbA1-Wert? Pathologe 11:158–165
Roggendorf W (1995) Kreislaufstörungen des zentralen Nervensystems. In: Remmele W, Peiffer J, Schröder JM (eds) Pathologie 6 – Neuropathologie, Skelettmuskulatur, Sinnesorgane, 2nd edn. Springer, Berlin, pp 62–106
Saeger W, Kühn H (1984) Sheehan-Syndrom mit letalem Ausgang. Morphologische und immunhistochemische Untersuchungen eines Falles. Pathologe 5:231–234
Safe AF, Griffiths KD, Maxwell RT (1990) Thyreotoxic crisis presenting as status epilepticus. Postgrad Med J 66:150–152
Schmid KW, Böcker W (1997a) Nebenschilddrüse. In: Remmele W (ed) Pathologie, vol 4, 2nd edn. Springer, Berlin, pp 617–628
Schmid KW, Böcker W (1997b) Schilddrüse. In: Remmele W (ed) Pathologie, vol 4, 2nd edn. Springer, Berlin, pp 579–616
Schröder AS, Hecht L, Sperhake JP, Püschel K, Saeger W (2009) Plötzlicher Tod aus endokriner Ursache. Rechtsmedizin 19:17–20
Sheehan HL (1937) Post-partum necrosis of the anterior pituitary. J Pathol Bacteriol 45:189–214
Sheehan HL (1965) The frequency of post-partum hypopituitarism. J Obstet Gynaecol Br Commonw 72:103–111
Sheu SJ, Schmid KW (2003) Entzündliche Schilddrüsenerkrankungen. Epidemiologie, Klinik und Morphologie. Pathologe 24:339–347
Sheu SY, Otterbach F, Frilling A, Schmid KW (2003) Hyperplasia and tumors of the parathyroid glands. Pathologe 24:373–381
Sheu SJ, Levin S, Schmid KW (2006) Therapy related alterations to the thyroid gland. Pathologe 27:13–18
Siegler RW (1998) Fatal heatstroke in a young woman with undiagnosed chronic thyreoiditis. J Forensic Sci 43:1237–1240
Sippel H, Möttönen M (1992) Combined Glucose and lactate values in vitreous humour for postmortem diagnosis of diabetes mellitus. Forensic Sci Int 19:217–222
Smyrk TC, Goellner JR, Brennan MD, Carney JA (1987) Pathology of the thyroid in amiodarone-associated thyrotoxicosis. Am J Surg Pathol 11:197–204
Spann W (1954) Nebennieren und Unfall. Dtsch Z Gesamte Gerichtl Med 43:103
Sperry K, Smialek JE (1986) Sudden death due to a paraganglioma of the organs of Zuckerkandl. Am J Forensic Med Pathol 7:23–29
Symington T, Duguid WP, Davidson JN (1956) Effect of exogenous corticotropin on the histochemical pattern of the human adrenal cortex and a comparison with the changes during stress. J Clin Endocrinol Metab 16:580–598
Thomsen JL, Bayer Kristensen I, Pottosen PD (2006) The histological demonstration of lipids in the proximal renal tubules of patients with diabetic coma. Forensic Sci Med Pathol 2:249252
Tsokos M, Schröder S (2006) Black thyroid: report of an autopsy case. Int J Legal Med 120:157–159
Türk EE, Sperhake JP, Saeger W, Tsokos M (2004) Phäochromozytom als Ursache des plötzlichen Todes. Z Rechtsmed 14:409–411
Uotila U, Pekkarinen A (1951) The relation of human adrenal glands to the pathological changes produced by intense continuous stress ending in death. Acta Endocrinol 6:23–50
Valenzuela A (1988) Postmortem diagnosis of diabetes mellitus. Quantitation of fructosamine and glycolated haemoglobin. Forensic Sci Int 38:202–208
Vallance WB (1957) Sudden death from an asymptomatic phaeochromocytoma. Br Med J 292:95–96
Wall CR (2000) Myxedema coma: diagnosis and treatment. Am Fam Physician 62:2485–2490
Ward S, Evans CC (1985) Sudden death due to isolated adrenal tuberculosis. Postgrad Med J 61:635–636
Wehner H, Haag G (1980) Morphologische Differentialdiagnose zwischen der nodulären diabetischen Glomerulosklerose und lobulären Glomerulonephritisformen. Pathologe 1:197–205
Wehner F, Schieffer MC, Wehner HD (1997) Immunhistochemischer Insulinnachweis an der Injektionsstelle. In: 76th Annual meeting of the German Society of Forensic Medicine, Jena, 1997

Wei JY, Genecin A, Greene HL, Achuff SC (1979) Coronary spasms with ventricular fibrillation during thyrotoxicosis: response to attaining euthyroid state. Am J Cardiol 43:335–339

Woenkhaus U, Vasold A, Bollheimer LC (2005) Akute Nebenniereninsuffizienz ("Addison-Krise"). Intensivmed 42:345–354

Zhou C, Byard RW (2011) Armanni-Ebstein phenomenon and hypothermia. Forensic Sci Int 206:e82–e84

Zhou C, Gilbert JD, Byard RW (2010) Early diagnosis of Armanni-Ebstein phenomenon at autopsy. Forensic Sci Med Pathol 6:133–134

Zhou C, Moore L, Yool A, Jaunzems A, Byard R (2015) Renal tubular epithelial vacuoles – a marker for both hyperlipidemia and ketoacidosis at autopsy. J Forensic Sci 60:638–641

Zierhut S, Girlich C (2004) Thyrotoxic crisis and myxedema. Intensivmed 41:573–582

Pregnancy-Related Death, Death in Newborns, and Sudden Infant Death Syndrome

17

Sudden natural deaths in pregnant women are very rare in western countries. The cause of death can usually be determined at autopsy and by means of forensic toxicological, microbiological, or histological and immunohistochemical investigations described below. Diagnostic problems may be encountered with newborn deaths, either live or stillbirths—both need to be investigated forensically (Sarioglu and Turowski 2015). Histological and immunohistochemical investigations make considerable contributions toward determining the cause of death and clarifying whether the fetus was alive outside the uterus. Natural and unnatural deaths in infants after the neonatal period and later, i.e., from the 8th to 365th day, need to be clarified histologically in order to determine the cause of death, in relation to findings that could correlate with acts of violence on the one hand, and to exclude competing causes of death on the other. There are numerous publications on the phenomenon of sudden infant death syndrome (SIDS) with histomorphological findings, in particular in the heart and lungs. Accordingly, there are numerous hypotheses on the cause of death in sudden unexpected death in the first year of life as well as in early childhood (Garstang et al. 2015; Kinney et al. 2012; Randall et al. 2012; Opdal and Rognum 2011). Many of these studies suggest an infectious genesis in some cases of sudden infant death, in particular pneumonias and myocarditises with a wider spectrum of pathogens (Dettmeyer 2004; Dettmeyer et al. 2004a, b, 2009a, b; Bajanowski et al. 1996, 2003b; Rambaud et al. 1992).

17.1 Pregnancy-Related Maternal Deaths

Pregnancy-related death is defined as the death of a woman from any cause during pregnancy or in the year after delivery (Herbst et al. 2010; Christiansen and Collins 2006; Carter and Rutty 2004). The WHO classifies pregnancy-associated fatalities as such from the time of nidation of the fertilized egg to 42 days postpartum. The definitions are very broad in terms of their content, since fatal diseases unrelated to pregnancy can occur during pregnancy. For example, there are reports of arterial rupture during pregnancy or shortly following birth (Barbesier et al. 2013). Causes of sudden death during pregnancy or pregnancy-related deaths are primarily internal diseases, infections, intoxications, and accidents (Christiansen and Collins 2006; Shinagawa et al. 1983). In addition to pulmonary thromboembolisms, amniotic fluid embolisms, air embolisms (Banaschak et al. 2014; Baker et al. 2000; Lunetta and Penttilä 1996; Lau 1994; Mirchandani et al. 1988), and ruptured aneurysms (Barbesier et al. 2013; Srettabunjong 2013; Stojanovic et al. 2013; Ventura et al. 2011; Risse and Weiler 1987b), the following diseases should also be considered:

- Unnoticed acute and chronic cardiovascular diseases (acute myocardial infarction, myocarditis, peripartum cardiomyopathy, valvular

R. B. Dettmeyer, *Forensic Histopathology*, https://doi.org/10.1007/978-3-319-77997-3_17

heart disease, endocarditis, arrhythmias, including the long QT syndrome)
- Acute ruptured ectopic pregnancy causing the woman to bleed to death (Strehler et al. 2006; Andersen et al. 2004; Bickell et al. 2004)
- Spontaneous rupture of unscarred gravid uterus (very rare, Gurudut et al. 2011)
- Lethal intoxication, in particular, in drug-addicted pregnant women
- Postnatal bleeding, for example, in cases of unnoticed secondary bleeding due to insufficient medical supervision
- Unnoticed uterine rupture causing the woman to bleed to death
- Lethal HELLP (hemolysis, elevated liver enzymes, low platelet count) syndrome (Tsokos et al. 2002)
- Rare pregnancy-related complications (e.g., acute Sheehan syndrome; Chap. 16)
- Severe infection and sepsis, e.g., amniotic infection syndrome (AIS) (Jänisch et al. 2009)

If no findings relevant to the cause of death can be determined macroscopically, histopathological findings may be able to contribute. This applies to the determination or exclusion of acute or chronic myocarditis and amniotic fluid embolism. In the case of massive hemorrhage following uterine rupture, the cause can be clarified, for example, by detecting granulation and scar tissue at the place of rupture after a Caesarean section. Histologically, siderin deposits can frequently be found in the scar tissue using Prussian blue staining. In individual cases, a postpartum coronary thrombosis following bromocriptine medication is described (Loewe and Dragovic 1998).

17.1.1 Extrauterine Pregnancy or Ruptured Tubal/Ectopic Pregnancy

With timely medical treatment, death due to extrauterine pregnancy can be prevented, although the condition is associated with mortality in rare cases (Strehler et al. 2006; Andersen et al. 2004). The most frequent extrauterine pregnancy is ectopic tubal pregnancy. Extrauterine pregnancy leading to sudden and unexpected death in a pregnant woman occurs early on in pregnancy (Bickell et al. 2004). The autopsy will show massive bleeding in the small pelvis or abdomen in the case of hemato-sactosalpinx and ruptured tubal/ectopic pregnancy (Fig. 17.1). If doubts remain macroscopically as to the origin of hemorrhage because, for example, no fetus can

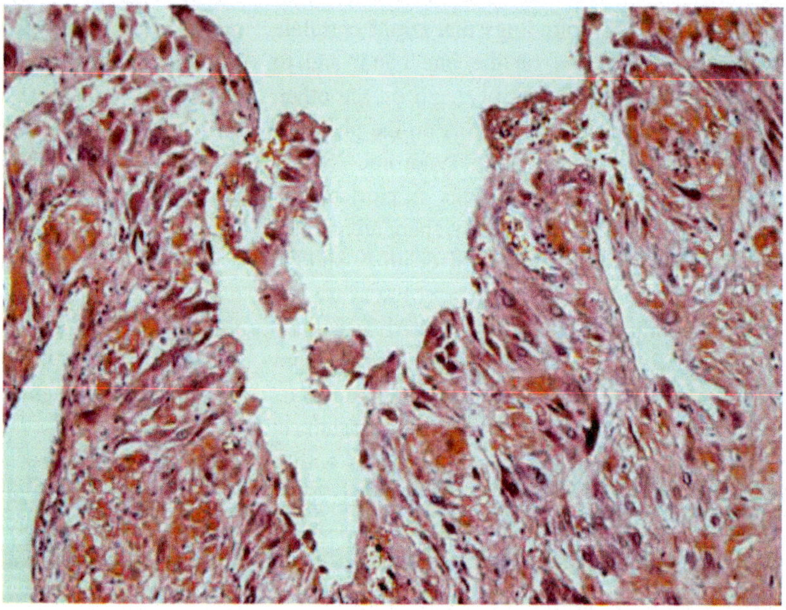

Fig. 17.1 Portions of decidua 24 h after birth without rests of placental tissue (H&E ×100)

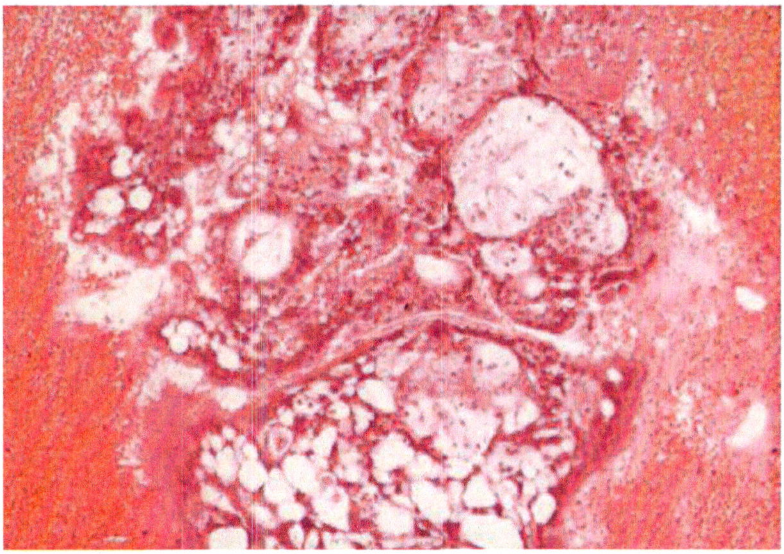

Fig. 17.2 Placental villi with delayed maturation in a case of ruptured extrauterine pregnancy (H&E ×125)

be detected due to an anomaly of the pregnancy, tissue of the suspected extrauterine pregnancy must then be histologically investigated. In the case of a ruptured tubal pregnancy, portions of decidua can be found in the swollen lumen of the uterine tubes, accompanied by hemorrhage in the adjacent fallopian tube. Existing placental villi frequently show delayed maturation (Strehler et al. 2006); in addition to an endometrium highly transformed by secretions with a large-cell decidual stromal reaction (Fig. 17.2), endometrioid glands can show an Arias-Stella phenomenon (Fig. 17.14), a finding which also applies in the case of intrauterine abortion.

17.1.2 HELLP Syndrome

Maternal death from HELLP syndrome, a complication of preeclampsia during pregnancy, is very rare (Tsokos 2004; Tsokos et al. 2002). Petechial hemorrhage and suffusions were found in skin, mucous surfaces, serous coats of internal organs, brain purpura, and the conjunctivae. The histopathological alterations reported relate primarily to the liver and kidneys. The liver presents periportal hepatocellular coagulative necrosis and hemorrhage. This hemorrhage is described as sharply demarcated by an extended fibrin network. Additionally, focal leukocyte sticking in liver sinusoids is evident, as well as swelling of Kupffer cells and bile stasis. An inflammatory reaction is absent, and no fatty vacuolization within the cytoplasm of hepatocytes is seen. The kidneys present bloodless glomeruli with swollen and vacuolated intracapillary cells. Further findings include elongated and obstructed (cigar-shaped) capillary loops or enlarged glomerular tufts, filling Bowman's space with herniation of capillary loops into the proximal convoluted tubules. Swelling of mesangial cells is possible, as is thrombus formation in glomerular capillaries and the vasa recta in cases of severe disseminated intravascular coagulation (DIC). These findings are considered sufficiently characteristic to permit the definitive postmortem diagnosis of HELPP syndrome (Tsokos et al. 2002).

17.1.3 Amniotic Fluid Embolism

Components of amniotic fluid in the arterioles and capillaries of the lungs indicate acute lethal amniotic fluid embolism, for example, cytokeratin-positive skin cells of the fetus or trophoblast cells and mucinous components—see Chap. 9 (Baker et al. 2000; Lunetta and Penttilä 1996). In addition, histopathological findings, in particular in the right ventricular myocardium, may be an indication of an acute rise in pressure in the small circulation (see Chap. 9). Cases of pregnancy-related air embolism are extremely rare (Banaschak et al. 2014).

17.1.4 Histology of the "Soap Abortion"

In countries were the termination of pregnancy is largely prohibited, illegal abortions may be performed by introducing various solutions into the vagina or uterus to cause the embryo to be expelled. For example, there are case studies on the introduction of potassium permanganate solution, formol, zinc chloride, acetic acid, ammonia solution, detergent solutions, and water. The soap solution has become particularly established as a way of inducing the "soap abortion." Side effects primarily include infections (endometritis, parametritis, adnexitis, peritonitis), which can lead to septic shock. One should predominantly consider gram-negative pathogens, but possibly also *Clostridia* as gram-negative pathogens. Histologically, it should be possible to detect abundant fat deposits in the blood and lymph vessels of the endometrium. Curettage material investigated in conjunction with a soap abortion showed largely normal placental tissue, but focal, centrally unreactive, and homogeneous necrosis in the endometrium that had undergone decidual transformation (so-called pregnancy decidua) with low peripheral leukocytic response. In addition to this, small and large hemorrhages in the stroma and microthrombi in the adjacent blood vessels were present. Pronounced sudanophilia should be striking in the areas of necrosis. Depending on the time lapse, regenerative processes may be detectable. The detection of fat in the vessel walls and vascular lumen is considered typical. Also depending on the time of tissue sample collection, extensive inflammation consistent with placentitis and chorioamnionitis may have developed. Septic states following illegal abortion are also seen in conjunction with the use of medications; misoprostol in particular, a prostaglandin E1 analog, is used as an abortive agent (Cittadini et al. 2014).

17.2 Perinatal Fatalities

Forensically, deaths shortly before, during, or after birth raise relevant questions, for example, in connection with suspected medical malpractice. In cases of live births outside maternity units or in cases of live newborns found dead, it must be established whether natural causes of death can be excluded and traces indicating homicide must be secured. As part of this process, it is important to also consider relatively rare congenital diseases, in particular of the cardiovascular system and lungs, e.g., an intrapulmonary vessel malformation that can cause death shortly following birth (Pucci et al. 2003) or primary placental mesenchymal dysplasia (Ventura et al. 2013). Altogether, the spectrum of possible fatal diseases particularly in neonates is relatively broad: disorders worthy of note, for example, include neonatal respiratory distress syndrome, hyaline membrane disease (HMD), pulmonary hemorrhage, acute pulmonary interstitial emphysema, bronchopulmonary dysplasia (BPD), patent ductus arteriosus, myocardial ischemia, thrombosis and embolism, intracranial bleeding, and cystic fibrosis-related disorders (Amann 2000).

17.2.1 Death Shortly Before or During Birth

In addition to potentially life-threatening obstetric complications (shoulder dystocia, unnoticed macrosomia of the fetus, placenta praevia with intrauterine bleeding, true knots in the umbilical cord, umbilical cord around the neck, velamentous insertion of the umbilical cord, uterine rupture, etc.), which may give rise to medical malpractice charges relating to the late induction of Caesarean section, intrauterine causes of death need to be analyzed. The following applies:

Important: Every autopsy of a newborn involves the macroscopic and microscopic examination of the respective placenta.

If serious fetal dysplasias, in particular of the cardiovascular system, are excluded, placental insufficiency and infection must be taken into consideration. There are a number of possible histological findings in the placenta (Melinte et al. 2015; Freitag et al. 2014; Stallmach und Hebisch 2004).

Depending on gestational week at the time of birth, immature lung tissue with insufficient surfactant formation may also be considered. Pulmonary surfactant can be detected immunohistochemically (Zhu et al. 1996).

Histomorphological signs of placental insufficiency include:

- Placental infarctions of various ages (Figs. 17.3 and 17.4)
- Delayed placental maturation

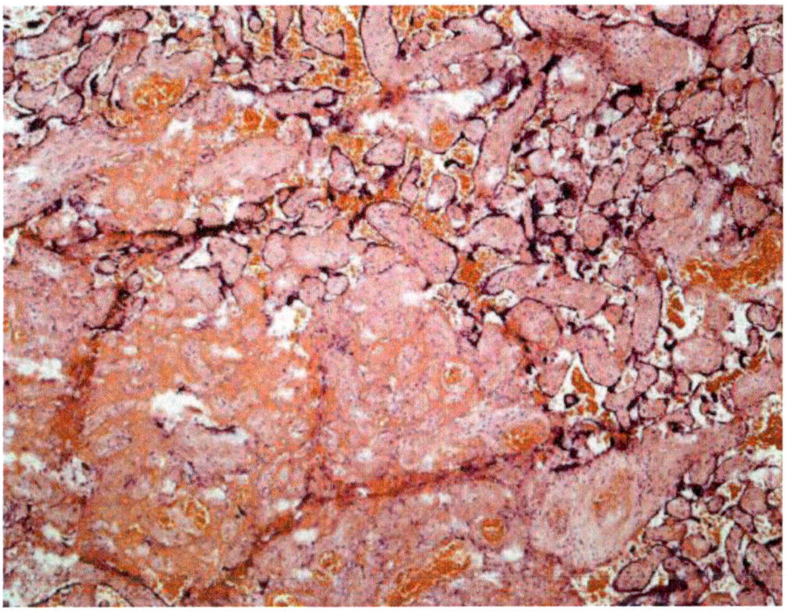

Fig. 17.3 Placental infarction with mostly extinguished cell nuclei (on the *right side*) with scant vascularized terminal villi (H&E ×100)

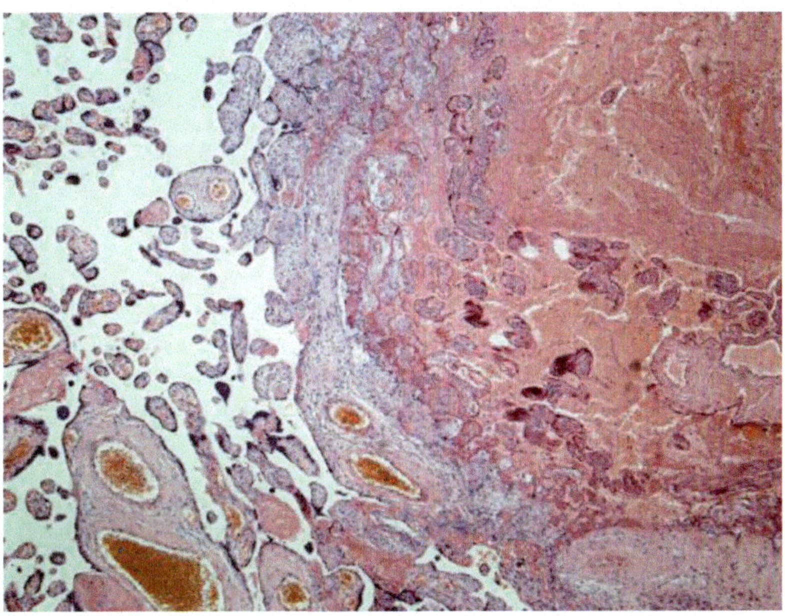

Fig. 17.4 Placental infarction (*right*) next to coarse, poorly vascularized villi (*left*) (H&E ×40)

- Retroplacental hematomas, not only in the case of placenta praevia
- Amniotic infection syndrome (chorioamnionitis, funisitis, placentitis)

In the forensic postmortem examination of perinatal fatalities, it is often difficult to obtain a precise case history, and circumstantial evidence is usually very weak.

Without intensive medical treatment, the viability of a newborn can be assumed from the 22nd to 24th week of pregnancy onward. From approximately the 20th to 22nd week of pregnancy onward, numerous villi of mean diameter can be expected histologically in the case of a normally developed placenta. The reticular stroma has denser cells in the stem villi and is more wide-meshed in the intermediate villi. In the subepithelial layer, capillaries showing formation of nucleus-free epithelial plates can be found (termed metabolic membrane or syncytio-capillary membrane), while proliferation buds can be found in the vicinity (Vogel 1986). Nucleated erythrocyte precursors can also be seen intravascularly. Subsequently, maturation of villi takes place up to maximally reduced vascularized terminal villi containing only scant reticular stroma next to broad capillaries with a noticeable decrease in villus diameter (Fig. 17.5). In the case of immature placental villi, the fiber cuff around the properly produced allantoic vessels may be absent; considerable differences in size between the placental villi are occasionally apparent (Fig. 17.6) (Jänisch et al. 2010).

In cases where an infant survives birth and then dies, delayed pulmonary maturation with incomplete or absent development of the lungs, in particular in preterm infants, must be considered. Histologically, extensive fetal pulmonary atelectasis can be seen in such cases (Fig. 17.7).

In the case of a negative pulmonary floating test (note: positive reaction in the case of putrefaction, sometimes histologically reexpanded lung tissue after amniotic fluid aspiration), fetal pulmonary atelectasis can almost exclusively be expected histologically; ventilated areas of the lung may be due to previous resuscitation measures. The surfactant protein A is essential for the development of lung tissue; the absence or insufficiency of this protein leads to death (De Mello

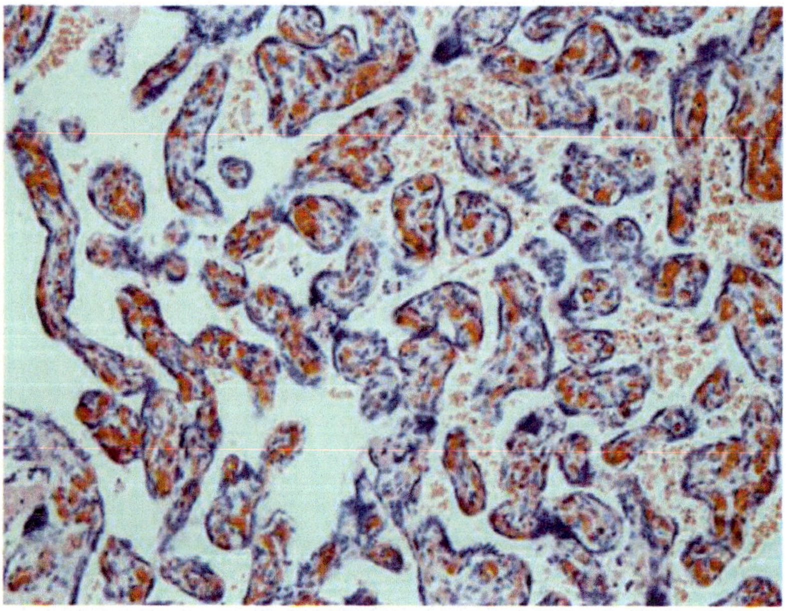

Fig. 17.5 Normal placenta with largely matured and vascularized terminal villi (H&E ×100)

et al. 1993). A further characteristic feature in the differential diagnosis of whether a newborn was alive postpartum is pulmonary interstitial emphysema. However, the utility of pulmonary interstitial emphysema in live-birth determination is not well established. Pulmonary interstitial emphysema is not a sensitive finding in live-born infants but a reliable indicator of live birth, best interpreted in combination with the more sensitive finding of uneven or full aeration of the lung parenchyma (Lavezzi et al. 2004). A causal relationship between florid pulmonary interstitial emphysema and sudden death could not be proven.

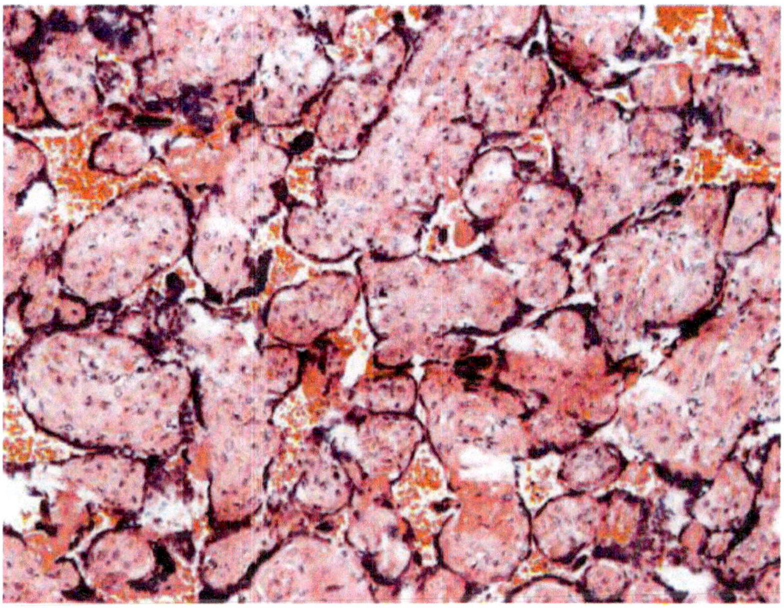

Fig. 17.6 Delayed placental maturation with coarse, poorly vascularized villi rich in connective tissue and covered with a double-rowed trophoblast shell (H&E ×100)

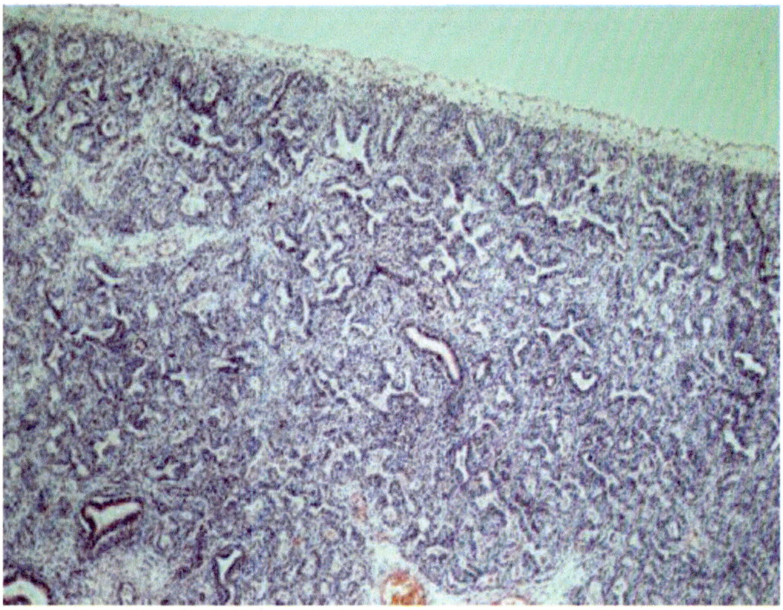

Fig. 17.7 Stillborn infant with extensive fetal pulmonary atelectasis (H&E ×40)

Pulmonary Surfactant
Pulmonary surfactant appears in the late fetal period. Its congenital deficiency is considered to be a fundamental cause of infantile respiratory distress syndrome leading to hyaline membrane disease (Zhu et al. 1996; Kuroki et al. 1986). It has been reported that surfactant production and secretion were enhanced in asphyxia and that immunohistochemical examination was useful to clarify the cause of death in newborns and infants (Funayama et al. 1994; Morita et al. 1985). Surfactant was found to be totally negative until the 24th gestational week, but gradually increased until the 32nd gestational week (Zhu et al. 1996). In an immunohistochemical study, all cases of asphyxia over 36 weeks' gestation showed diffuse, intense staining using antihuman pulmonary surfactant apoprotein A, and maximal staining was observed in the still preserved tissue structure of decomposing lungs (Zhu et al. 1996).

Because of the postmortem stability of the surfactant apoprotein A, it can be assumed that in cases of tissue immunohistochemically positive for surfactant, a newborn found lifeless has at least reached the 36th week of pregnancy (Zhu et al. 1996).

17.2.2 Amniotic Infection Syndrome (AIS) and Sepsis Puerperalis

Amniotic infection syndrome can lead to fetal death and occasionally also to maternal death in cases of severe unnoticed and untreated courses of the disease (Jänisch et al. 2009). After the amniotic sac breaks, there is the risk of an ascending purulent infection of the amnion, umbilical cord, and placenta. Histologically, alternating dense striated granulocytic infiltrates can be seen on the amnion (Fig. 17.8), along the umbilical cord vessels (Fig. 17.9), on the chorionic plate of the placenta (Fig. 17.10), as well as on the placental tissue.

In the case of preexisting *chorioamnionitis*, but also independent of this, purulent endomyometritis may develop and advance to fatal puerperal sepsis in the postpartum period. Group A

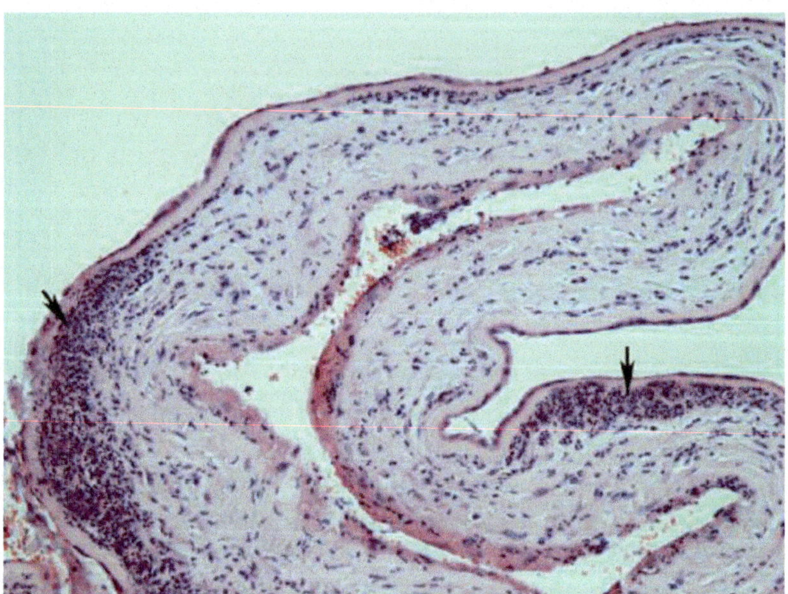

Fig. 17.8 Multiple granulocytes (*arrows*) in a case of pronounced purulent amnionitis (H&E ×100) (Photo courtesy of Dr. F. Driever, Gießen, Germany)

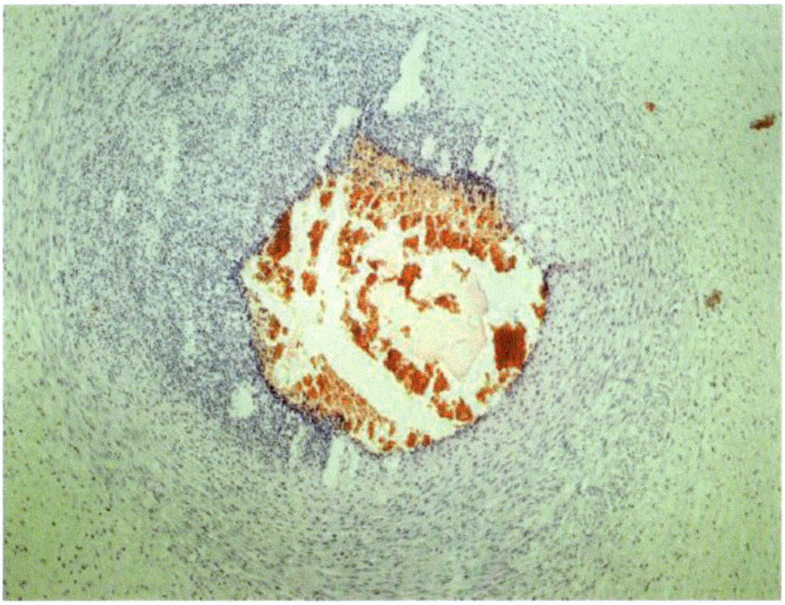

Fig. 17.9 Purulent funisitis following amniotic infection syndrome (H&E ×100) (Photo courtesy of Dr. F. Driever, Gießen, Germany)

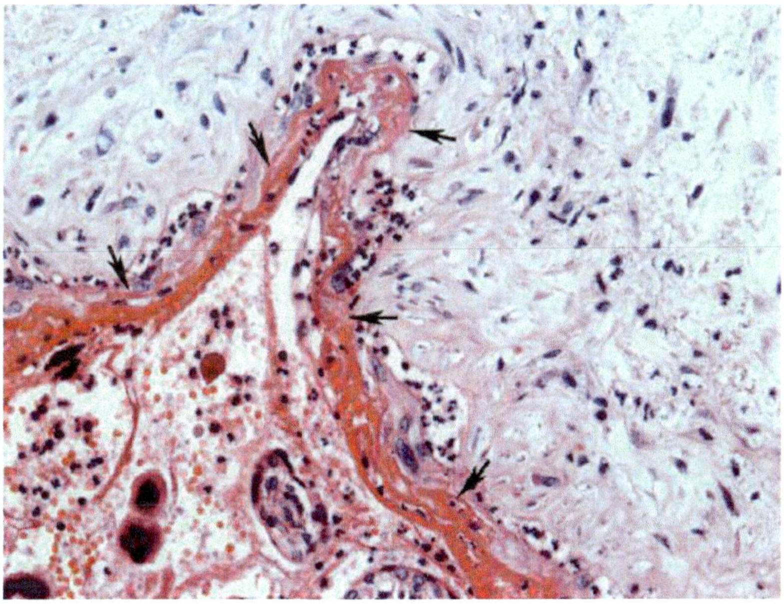

Fig. 17.10 Purulent chorioamnionitis with chorionic plate, granulocytes, striated microfibrin (*arrows*), granulocytes, and coarse placental villi following amniotic infection syndrome (H&E ×200) (Photo courtesy of Dr. C. Haag, Solingen, Germany)

streptococci as superantigen producers should primarily be born in mind in terms of the pathogen (Jänisch et al. 2009).

17.2.3 Endangiitis Obliterans of the Placental Vessels

Depending on the degree of severity, endangiitis obliterans (Fig. 17.11) of the placental vessels can explain sudden intrauterine death or stillbirth. In such cases, obliterated allantoic vessels with partly thrombosed vascular openings, which are difficult to identify, can be seen. The thrombosed material may be in the repair process.

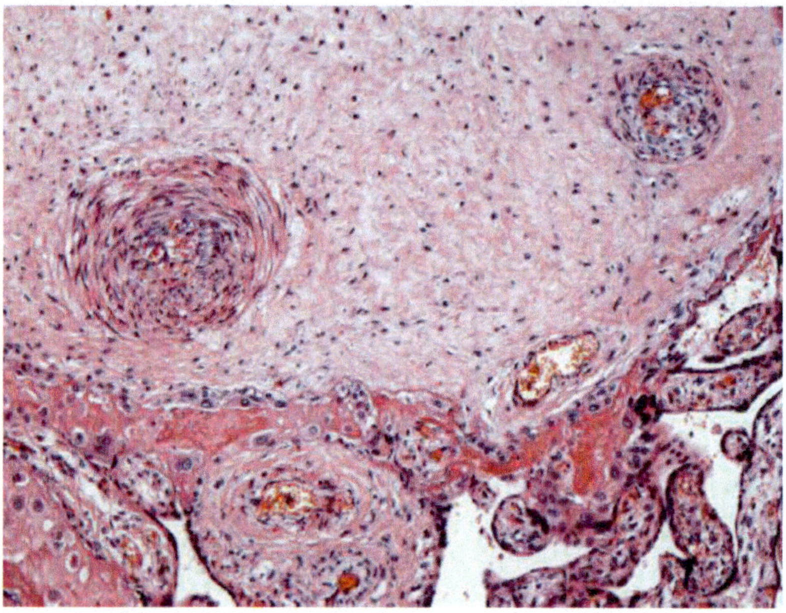

Fig. 17.11 Endangiitis obliterans of placental vessels in the case of intrauterine death (H&E ×100) (Photo courtesy of Dr. C. Haag, Solingen, Germany)

17.3 Newborns Found Lifeless

In the case of newborns found lifeless, several points require clarification:

- Was the baby still alive after it left the womb?
- Signs of maturity which show that the newborn was viable
- Evidence of a disease that could explain the cause of death
- In the case of a stillbirth, an intrauterine cause of death
- An indication of an act of violence that could explain the cause of death
- Evidence of amnionitis, funisitis, chorioamnionitis, placentitis, or placental infarction
- Evidence of amniotic fluid aspiration

This means that the placenta should also be investigated in the case of a newborn found lifeless.

17.3.1 Histological Pulmonary Findings

The histological correlation of the positive pulmonary floating test is properly reexpanded lung tissue with medium pulmonary alveoli (Fig. 17.12).

If all sections of lung tissue are atelectatic, the newborn was not alive after it left the womb. If the lung tissue is partly developed, amniotic fluid aspiration during birth may be considered. Under the microscope, intra-alveolar cells can be seen using conventional stainings, while elongated flat cells with or without a nucleus can be seen in the bronchioles. Immunohistochemically, these cells are shed keratin-positive epithelial cells of fetal skin (Chap. 11; Fig. 11.10). Minor amniotic fluid aspiration is not necessarily an indication of the cause of death.

17.3.2 Pregnancy Decidua and the Arias-Stella Phenomenon

Postnatal evidence of pregnancy can be obtained with histological findings from curettage of residues from partly necrotic and inflamed cellular infiltrated decidua (Fig. 17.13). In addition, endometrial glands can be seen, the epithelial cells of which show shapeless enhancement of cell nuclei with a strong accumulation of chromatin and surrounding brightened cytoplasm (the Arias-Stella phenomenon; Fig. 17.14).

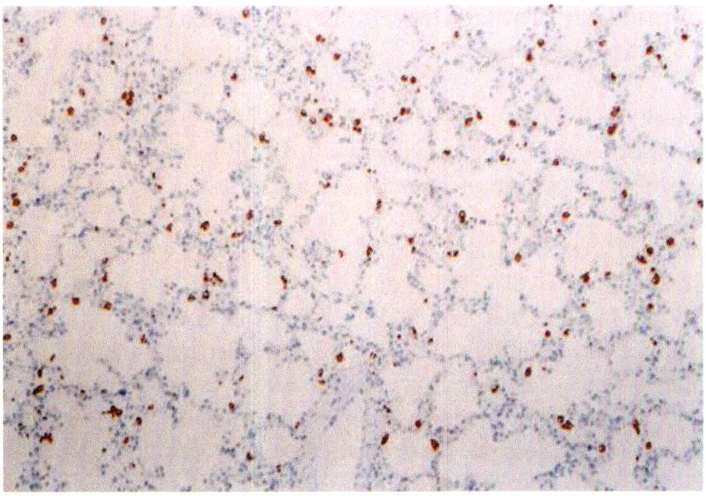

Fig. 17.12 Properly developed lung tissue in a newborn with immunohistochemical detection of CD68+ alveolar macrophages (CD68 ×40)

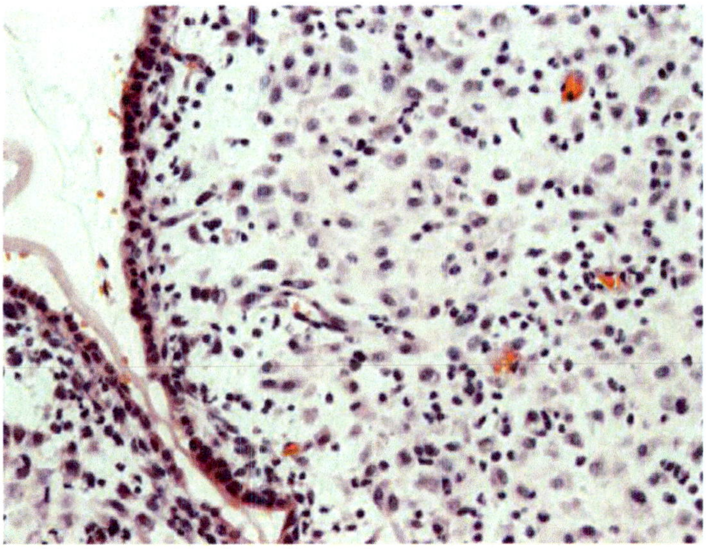

Fig. 17.13 Decidual transformation of pregnancy decidua with inflamed cellular infiltration (H&E ×200)

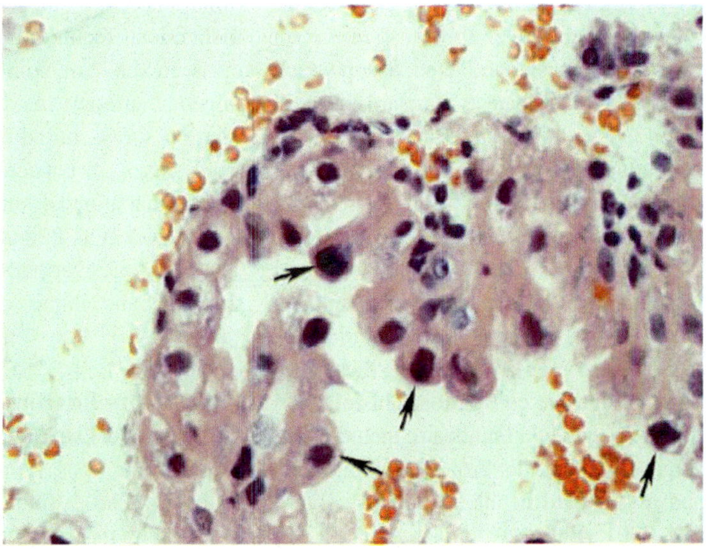

Fig. 17.14 Arias-Stella phenomenon in pregnancy decidua (*arrows*) curettage 1 day post abortion (H&E ×400)

17.4 Sudden Infant Death Syndrome (SIDS)

Sudden infant death syndrome (SIDS) is the most common cause of death in infancy in industrialized countries with an incidence of between 0.3 and 1.5/1000 live births, including seasonal fluctuations (Fitzgerald 2001; Douglas et al. 1997, 1998a, b; Hoppenbrouwers et al. 1981; Adelson and Kinney 1956). In 1969, the term sudden infant death syndrome was defined as "the sudden death of any infant or young child, which is unexplained by history and in which thorough postmortem examination fails to demonstrate an adequate cause of death" (Beckwith 1970; Beckwith et al. 1970). More recently, the upper age limit was defined as 1 year at the time of death, and an extensive investigation of the scene of death was included in the definition (Guntheroth et al. 1994; Willinger et al. 1991). A further classification dating back to 2004 (Krous et al. 2004) involves particular criteria with which the SIDS phenomenon can be excluded as a cause of death (Moon et al. 2007; Rognum 2004; Rognum et al. 2003; Rajs and Hammarquist 1988). The practicability of this classification has been questioned (Bajanowski et al. 2006). A reclassification with minor modifications has also been proposed (Jensen et al. 2012).

Excluding the newborn period, cases of sudden unexpected death at the age of 8–365 days can be assigned to the SIDS phenomenon in cases where no other cause of death can be determined. Since SIDS is a diagnosis of exclusion, this phenomenon should not be considered until histological examinations of organ samples of the most important internal organs have been completed, a step which has not yet been established as standard protocol (Bajanowski and Verhoff 2008; Bajanowski et al. 2007). A routine histological examination of all internal organs and tissues is necessary, including conventional staining (H&E, van Gieson, Alcian blue, PAS, Prussian blue, Sudan III) of the central nervous system (Sawaguchi et al. 2005; Oehmichen et al. 1989, 1998), endocrine organs, muscular system, and lymphatic organs. Meanwhile, there have been cases of extensive conventional histological investigations of sudden infant death, including all internal organs without this protocol having been established as standard in all institutions (Byard and Krous 2001; Rasten-Almqvist et al. 2000; Beech et al. 2000; Castro and Peres 1999; Parham et al. 1998; Becroft et al. 1998; Pattison and Marshall 1997; Baxendine and Moore 1995; Byard and Krous 1995; Thomsen and Saternus 1994; Busuttil and Burchell 1992; Kopp et al. 1993; Stoltenberg et al. 1992; Stramba-Badiale et al. 1992; Berry 1992; Ogbuihi and Zink 1987, 1988, 1989; Wigglesworth et al. 1987; Missliwetz et al. 1986; Stewart et al. 1985; Wilske 1984; Takahashi et al. 1983; Sudnerland 1981; Uren et al. 1980; Berg and Kijewski 1978; Noren et al. 1975).

Some studies suggest an infectious genesis in certain cases of sudden infant death (Wu and Parsons 2017; Vennemann et al. 2007; Debertin et al. 2006; Vege et al. 1995, 1998, 1999; Harrison et al. 1999; Forsyth 1999; Blackwell et al. 1999 Blackwell and Weir 1999; Vege and Rognum 1999; Cubie et al. 1997; Kleemann et al. 1996; Cecchi et al. 1995; Blackwell et al. 1995; Cremer and Althoff 1991; Kleemann et al. 1988; Zink et al. 1987; Williams et al. 1984; Ray et al. 1970; Johnstone and Lawy 1966; Gold et al. 1961).

Autopsy shows findings typical to sudden infant death which, however, are not relevant to the cause of death (Beckwith 1989; Jones and Weston 1976). The following histological and immunohistochemical investigations have shown some distinctive findings; the relevance of which in terms of the cause of death is under discussion. Microscopic findings often suggest an infectious genesis, at least in some cases of sudden infant death. Meanwhile, all organs and organ systems have been intensively examined with conventional histology and some also with immunohistochemical techniques. Unilateral or bilateral otitis media can sometimes already be determined at autopsy. In addition, microscopic investigation shows inflammatory processes in some SIDS cases, in particular in the lungs and submandibular glands, but also in the heart muscle (Dettmeyer et al. 2004a; Bajanowski et al. 1996). The entry sites for pathogens are the gastrointestinal tract and, in particular, the respiratory tract.

17.4.1 The Respiratory Tract and Lungs

Frequently, no distinctive histopathological findings in lung tissue can be seen in suspected SIDS cases, only agonal changes, such as acute congestive hyperemia (Fig. 17.15) and pulmonary edema (Fig. 17.16).

Inflammatory changes can sometimes be found in the lungs (Doi et al. 2000; Dettmeyer et al. 2006d; Entrup and Brinkmann 1990a; Forsyth et al. 1989), or amniotic fluid aspiration can be observed in newborns or within the first few weeks of life (Fracasso et al. 2010; Chap. 11). There are numerous histological examinations of lung tissue in suspected SIDS cases (Bajanowski 2008; de la Grandmaison et al. 1999; Hiller et al. 1997).

Morphological changes typical for viral pneumonia were found significantly more frequently in SIDS cases than in control cases (Entrup and Brinkmann 1990a, b). Immunohistochemically, a mostly loose distribution of CD68-positive alveolar macrophages can be seen. Artificially compressed lung tissue can falsely show a higher macrophage density, particularly in atelectatic areas.

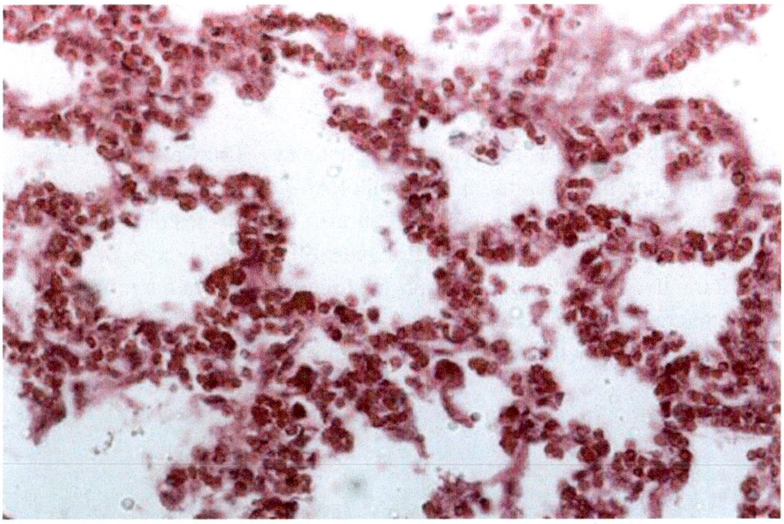

Fig. 17.15 Acute congestive hyperemia in the septal capillaries of the pulmonary alveoli in a 4-month-old male (H&E ×200)

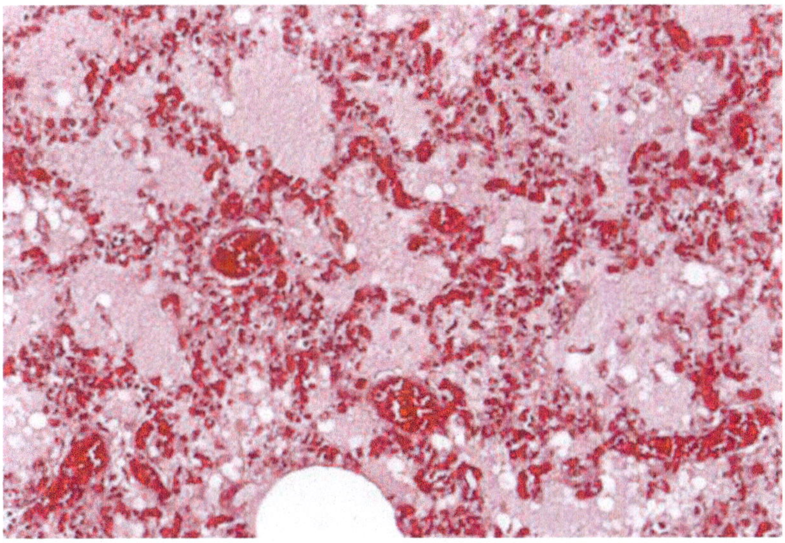

Fig. 17.16 Acute vascular congestion and pronounced eosin pulmonary edema without hemorrhage, desquamated alveolar macrophages, or evidence of inflammation in a 7-month-old female (H&E ×200). Note: In relation to the size of the infant lung, it is necessary in autopsy cases to histologically examination at least one tissue sample per pulmonary lobe that represents the pulmonary parenchyma. Further tissue samples may be preserved

In addition, there are reports of inflammatory changes in lung tissue, including the detection of viral agents of bronchitis and pneumonia (Bajanowski et al. 2003a; Bajanowski and Brinkmann 1995). The investigators found bronchiolitis with peribronchial interstitial inflammatory infiltrates and interstitial pneumonia with lymphomonocytic infiltrates in the alveolar septa, but also purulent bronchitises and bronchopneumonias (Zink 1986; Valdes-Dapena 1982, 1986; Aherne et al. 1970). Ferris et al. (1973) found that in one third of cases of sudden infant death, histological virus-typical changes in the lungs and bronchia were seen. However, bronchiolitis in infancy is not unusual; the mortality rate is given as 2–5% (Berg and Kijewski 1978).

Mast cells in lung tissue of SIDS victims can be detected well in tissue extracted during autopsy using toluidine blue staining and naphthol AS-D chloroacetate. This staining method can also be used for cytological differentiation of interstitial and intra-alveolar cells. In addition to granulocytes, the non-segmented early stages of the neutrophilic line, which are typically difficult to differentiate from other cells, can also be stained. Mast cell degranulation in the lung tissue of SIDS victims has been described, as well as discharged mast cells in the case of inflammatory processes in the lung tissue (Berg and Kijewski 1978). However, another study showed that there were no quantitative differences in the frequency and distribution of mast cells in SIDS victims compared to control cases (Ogbuihi and Zink 1989). The role of noninflammatory cells in lung tissue has been discussed. Although focal proliferation of cells was frequently observed in the vicinity of distended lymphatics in SIDS cases, an inflammatory origin, as in cases of interstitial pneumonia, could not be confirmed (Ogbuihi and Zink 1989).

Some investigations report frequently detectable interstitial and subpleural siderin deposits (Stewart et al. 1985), which are regarded as an indication of preceding intrauterine microhemorrhages or a perinatal near-miss event.

In cases of suspected SIDS, only histological pulmonary findings, including inflammation or prominent bronchus-associated lymphoid tissue (Figs. 17.17 and 17.18), of a certain extent may

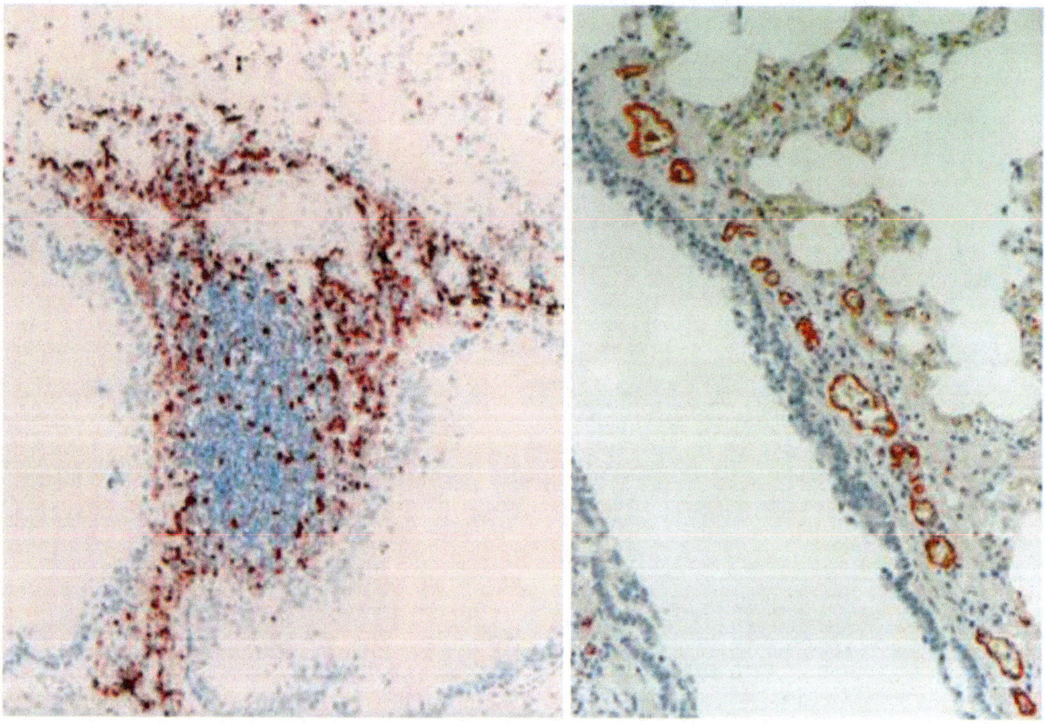

Fig. 17.17 Mildly prominent but nevertheless well-demarcated bronchus-associated lymphoid tissue (BALT) without germinal center formation (*left*; LCA ×200) and peribronchial endothelial expression of P-selectin in a 6-month-old male (*right*; ×200)

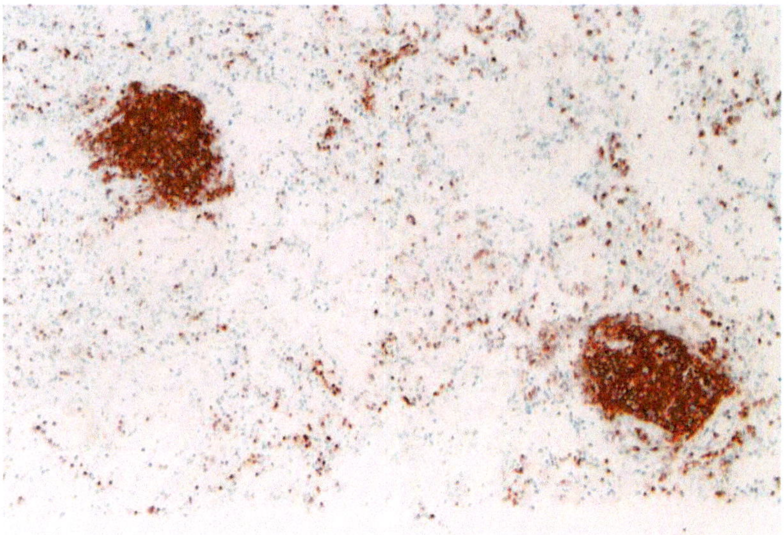

Fig. 17.18 Immunohistochemically detected and well-demarcated bronchus-associated lymphoid tissue (BALT) in a 6-month-old male (LCA ×400)

be an indication of the cause of death. However, pulmonary findings are only relevant for the cause of death after other findings have been excluded (Althoff 1968).

Infections of the Respiratory Tract and Lungs in Infancy

Fatal infections play an important role as a cause of death in infants and children. Infections of the central nervous system, respiratory tract, and circulatory system, including the heart and intestines, can be found. Infections of the respiratory tract cause 0.8% of all deaths within the first year of life, as well as approximately 3% of deaths in children aged between 2 and 15 years (Bajanowski 2008). Important diseases include epiglottitis and various types of pneumonia, mainly bronchopneumonia and interstitial pneumonia, including bronchiolitis and peribronchiolitis (Quan et al. 2000). Cases of suspected SIDS are often associated with inflammatory diseases of the respiratory tract, which are usually insufficient to explain the cause of death.

Unsurprisingly, histopathological findings in the respiratory tract may already show sinusitises of varying degrees, tracheitis, bronchitis, and sometimes interstitial lymphomonocytic pneumonias in routine stains. These latter cases are associated with an expansion of the air–blood barrier in the lung, which may affect disposition to sudden death following hypoxemia (Bajanowski and Brinkmann 2000). The Reid index, an instrument for the evaluation of chronic bronchitis, serves as a reference. The thicknesses of the mucosa and its gland layer are measured, and the relationship is expressed as a gland-wall ratio. Examination of tissue samples taken at autopsy of suspected SIDS cases showed no difference between SIDS cases with and without signs of inflammation in the respiratory tract compared to a control group (Karger et al. 2004).

The most important histopathological findings in the lungs of suspected SIDS cases according to the literature (e.g., Aoki 1994) and personal experience (Dettmeyer et al. 2005) include:

- Pulmonary edema
- Congestion
- Alveolar hemorrhage
- Pulmonary emphysema
- Atelectasis (Fig. 17.19)

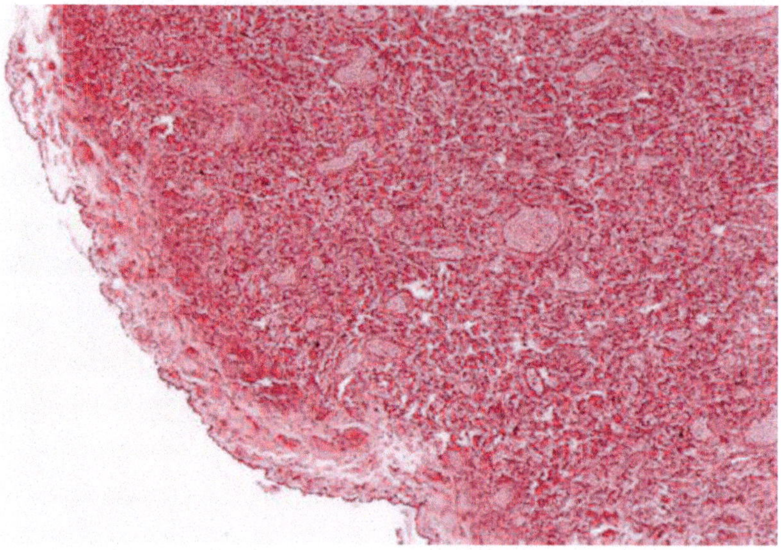

Fig. 17.19 Subpleural pulmonary atelectasis with no inflammation (H&E ×40)

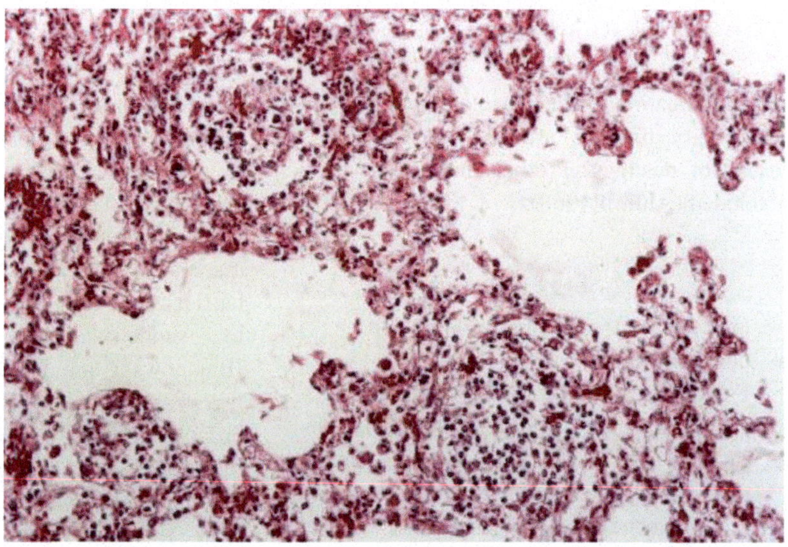

Fig. 17.20 Unsharply outlined prominent BALT with slightly increased cellular infiltration in the interalveolar septa in a 7-month-old male (H&E ×100)

- Increase in alveolar macrophages
- Eminent bronchus-associated lymphoid tissue (BALT)
- Acute and/or chronic inflammation of the trachea
- Bronchitis
- Pneumonia

Some authors classified the severity of the lesions mentioned into four degrees from minimum (1+) to marked (4+) (Aoki 1994). Aoki reported that 12% of SIDS cases had pulmonary emphysema with expanded air spaces and often involvement of the subpleura and alveolar septa. Frequently, atelectasis and pulmonary emphysema were also found; both findings were considered to be caused by cardiopulmonary resuscitation (12 of 13 cases). A mild to marked increase in alveolar macrophages was found in 38% of SIDS cases, whereas BALT was eminent in 17% of cases (Fig. 17.20). Increased macrophages and eminent BALT were also observed in 32% and 12% of explained deaths, respectively. Findings suggesting respiratory infection were noted in 31 (30%) SIDS cases and 27 (54%) explained deaths (Aoki 1994). Bronchitis and

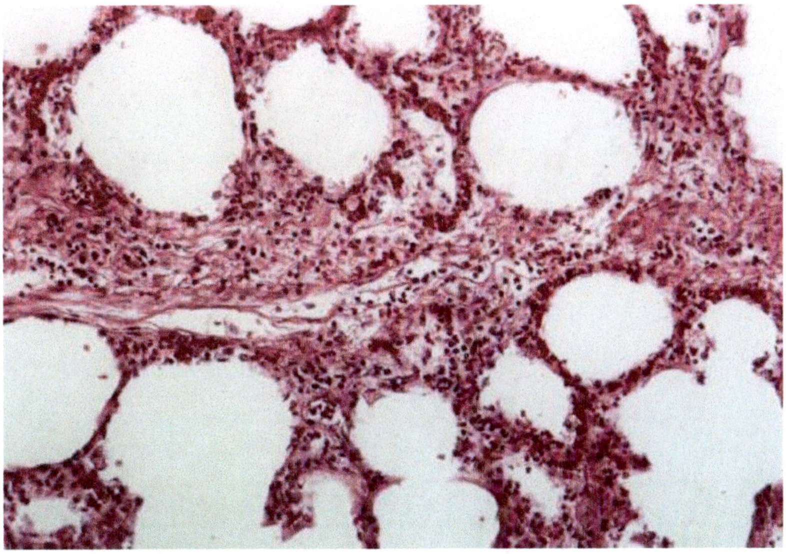

Fig. 17.21 Mild focal interstitial lymphomonocytic infiltration in a 7-month-old male (H&E ×400)

pneumonia were present in 8% and 7% of SIDS cases, respectively (out of 105 SIDS cases) (Aoki 1994). Most histopathological changes were regarded as mild focal lesions and were not considered to alter the SIDS diagnosis (Fig. 17.21)

Evaluation of pneumonia severity is indeed problematic in terms of diagnosing sudden infant death. In 1994 Aoki wrote:

> It would be somewhat subjective and there is no pathological standard to classify whether the lesion is morbid enough to be a cause of death.

According to personal experience, the findings described can be seen in the lung tissue of more than 50% of SIDS victims (Table 17.1). There were, however, differing histopathological diagnoses that showed relatively pronounced inflammation of the respiratory tract and/or lung tissue. As in the heart muscle, lymphomonocytic inflammatory infiltrates and cellular changes if present are dominant and enable the conclusion of a viral infection.

Prominent but no longer well-demarcated BALT enables the conclusion of (early) pneumonia.

The detection of BALT and evaluation of the boundaries of lymphatic tissue, as well as possible lymphatic hyperplasia, can be better performed using immunohistochemical techniques that identify leukocytes and T-lymphocytes.

Table 17.1 Uncharacteristic findings and findings indicating inflammation in lung tissue of suspected SIDS victims

Uncharacteristic findings	Findings indicating inflammation
Pulmonary edema	Lymphomonocytic interstitial infiltrates in the pulmonary interstitium
Acute congestive hyperemia	Prominent bronchus-associated lymphoid tissue (BALT)
Circumscribed intrapulmonary hemorrhage	Lymphomonocytic tracheitis and bronchitis, rarely granulocytic (bacterial)
Atelectatic lung areas	Polymorphonuclear alveolar macrophages with hyperchromasia, binuclear, and polynuclear alveolar macrophages (giant cells)
Megakaryocyte embolism	Strong endothelial expression of P-selectin in arterioles of the bronchial walls
Desquamation of alveolar macrophages into the alveolar space	Evidence of pathogens (e.g., cytomegaloviruses) in the lung tissue along with histopathological signs of inflammation

Regardless of BALT, changes such as considerable cell nucleus polymorphism, hyperchromasia, as well as binuclear and polynuclear giant cells are reminiscent of a viral infection (Fig. 17.22).

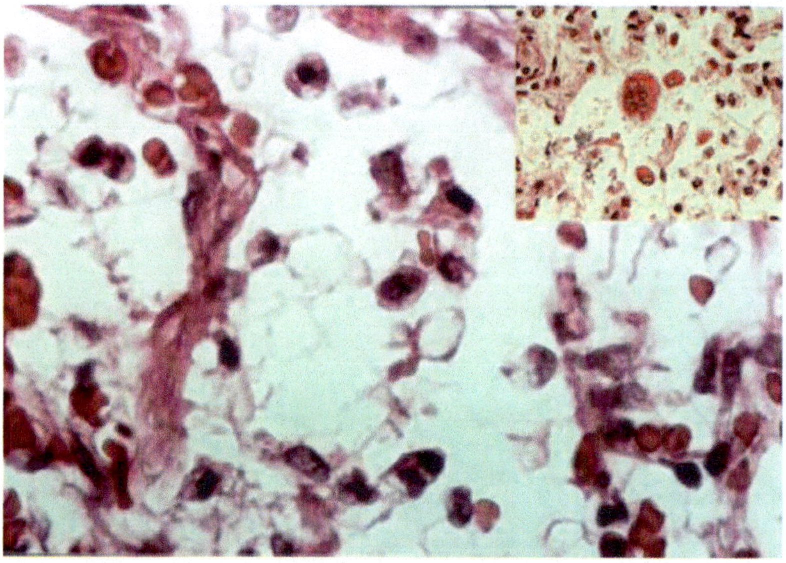

Fig. 17.22 Partially desquamated alveolar macrophages with polymorphic cell nuclei and hyperchromasia, single binuclear cells indicating a viral affection and an alveolar macrophage transformed to a polynuclear giant cell (H&E ×400)

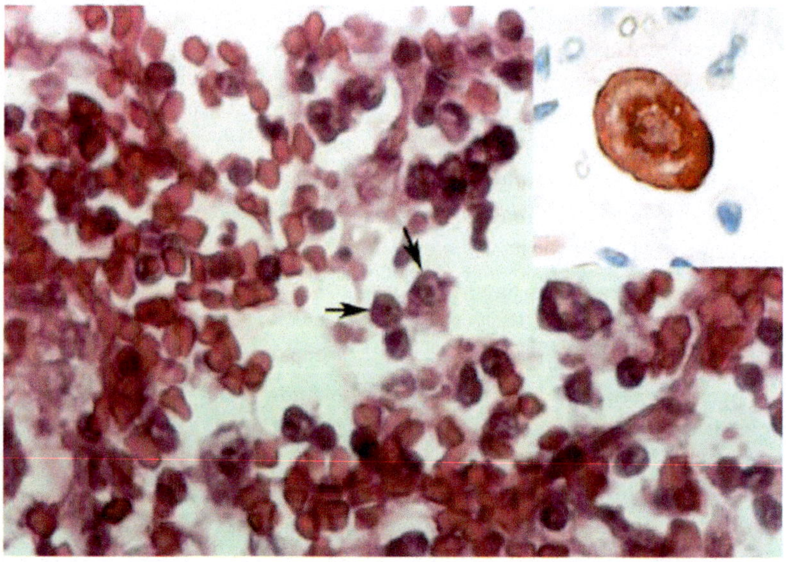

Fig. 17.23 Owl's eye cells with prominent cell nuclei (*arrows*) and a bright perinuclear circle in the case of cytomegaly (H&E ×400) and immunohistochemically a single cytomegalovirus-positive cell in the lung with no inflammatory reaction (insert: ×400)

Occasionally, owl's eye cells can be found, which are morphological signs of cytomegalovirus (CMV) infection (Fig. 17.23). Polynuclear giant cells are also possible with viral infections. If appropriate immunohistochemical antibodies and probes are available for in situ hybridization, these examinations may be extremely useful for correct diagnosis (An et al. 1993).

With an adequate cytological image, detection of CMV may be possible. The viruses can be detected immunohistochemically by means of in situ hybridization (ISH) and by means of molecular pathology (polymerase chain reaction, PCR). According to personal experience, E-selectin can be detected immunohistochemically on CMV-positive cells. If CMV-positive cells have been detected in the lung, samples of the salivary glands should also be examined. Pronounced histopathological findings in the lung tissue with evidence of pneumonia cannot be excluded as a cause of death (Fig. 17.24).

In the case of detection of lymphomonocytic viral tracheitis, bronchitis, and/or pneumonia, performing myocardial diagnosis is recommended, as well as examination of other internal organs for inflammatory processes. However, histological and immunohistochemical findings may

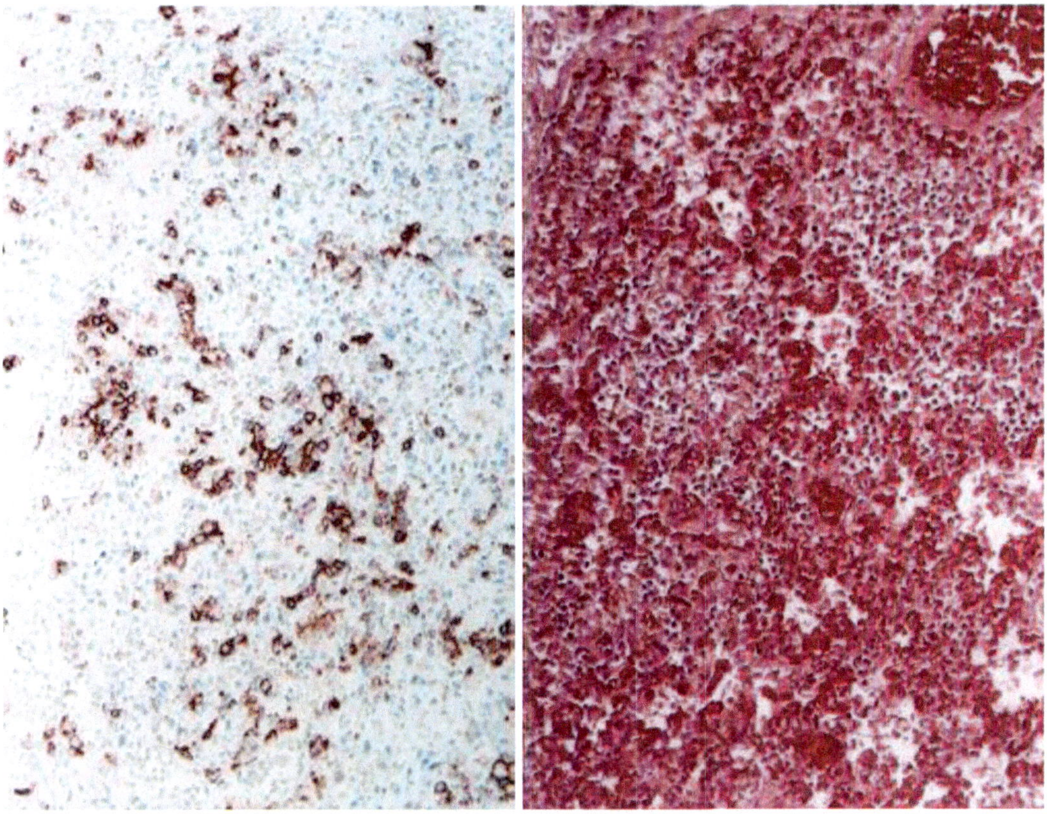

Fig. 17.24 Pronounced lymphomonocytic viral pneumonia (*right*; H&E ×200) and immunohistochemically numerous CD45R0+-T-lymphocytes (*left*; ×200) in a 4-month-old male

be less pronounced, even though an infection is present with postmortem pathogen identification.

Quan et al. (2000) reported on two male infants who died aged 5 months and showed different pulmonary findings. The first case demonstrated strongly congested lungs with marked intra-alveolar hemorrhage, partial emphysema, interstitial edema, mild lymphocytic infiltration, numerous macrophages, and polynuclear giant cells with inclusions. The second case showed highly congested and atelectatic lungs with marked intra-alveolar hemorrhage, focal necrosis of alveolar walls with neutrophil infiltration, numerous macrophages containing gram-positive cocci, and necrotic bronchiolar cells with gram-positive cocci in the alveoli. Microbiological investigations revealed adenovirus DNA in the first case, while *Staphylococcus aureus* was identified in venous blood culture in the second case (Quan et al. 2000).

Such cases clearly show that histological and potentially immunohistochemical examinations are necessary in infants where the cause of death cannot be explained macroscopically before death can be attributed to SIDS.

Further investigations dealt with the cell density of pulmonary neuroendocrine cells (PNECs) in fetal lungs and in the lung tissue of infants, also in relation to maternal smoking (Cutz et al. 1996; Aita et al. 2000). The percentage of PNEC-positive airways reached nearly 100% by term and did not change significantly until 12 months of age in both the SIDS cases and the controls. Nevertheless, the density of PNECs was higher in SIDS cases than in controls, and the authors concluded that the uneven distribution of PNECs may affect respiratory control in SIDS victims (Aita et al. 2000). Alveolar hemosiderin-laden macrophages in histological sections of the lung using Prussian blue staining demonstrate evidence of previous pulmonary hemorrhage and may be associated with features of non-accidental injury (NAI) in infants (Weber et al. 2009).

Basement Membrane Thickness of the Vocal Cord

In 1991 and 1994, Shatz et al. reported on a specific and pathognomonic basement membrane (BM) thickening of the vocal cords in SIDS. Some authors observed fibrinoid vocal cord lesions (Risse et al. 1997), while other authors found no statistically significant difference between a SIDS group and a control group; specific thickening of the basement membrane of the vocal cords in cases of suspected SIDS could not be confirmed (Shatz et al. 1991, 1994; Risse et al. 1997; Van Landeghem et al. 1999).

Mucosa-Associated Lymphoid Tissue (MALT)

The respiratory tract of children in the first 2 years of life, unlike that of adults, contains BALT (Gould and Isaacson 1993) and larynx-associated lymphoid tissue (LALT) with no differences in frequency between SIDS and control children (Tschernig et al. 1995; Hiller et al. 1997). Investigating the distribution of B-, T-, CD4, and CD8 lymphocytes, HLA-D cells, CD68 macrophages, and proliferating cells reveals no differences in the cellular composition of BALT and LALT. The lymphoid follicles contain mainly B-lymphocytes with some CD4 lymphocytes in the germinal centers, and B-lymphocytes were observed in equal numbers in the parafollicular areas (Hiller et al. 1997). Histochemically, it is possible to detect immunoglobulins in SIDS victims (Lemke and Schäfer 1992). The endothelial expression of proinflammatory molecules precedes leukocyte infiltration in the lung or myocardial tissue. These molecules first bring about the invasion of leukocytes in the pulmonary or cardiac interstitium. This also applies to the early phase of pneumonia or myocarditis. However, proinflammatory molecules have also been detected in the endothelium of peribronchial vessels in control cases of nonnatural death in infancy (Fig. 17.25). This raises the question of whether one can assume a generally more pronounced basal expression of this type of molecule in infancy.

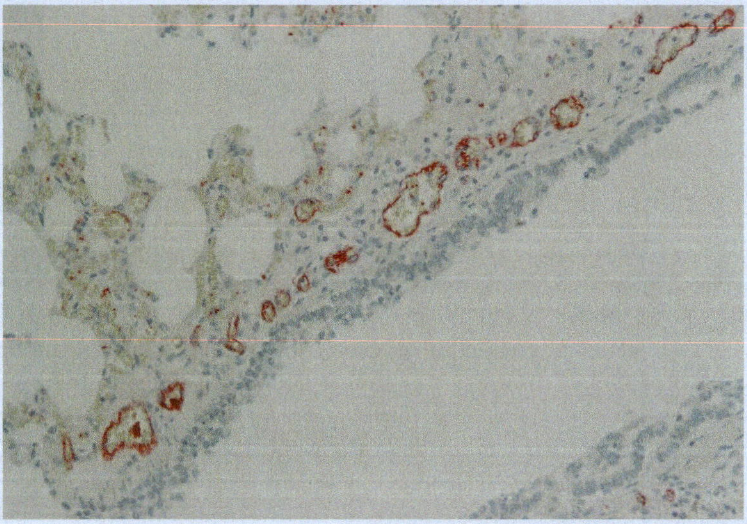

Fig. 17.25 Pronounced basal endothelial expression of proinflammatory P-selectin in peribronchial vessels in the otherwise inflammation-free infant lung; a control case of nonnatural death (×200)

17.4.2 Myocarditis and SIDS

The heart of suspected SIDS cases can show pathological findings (Bajanowski et al. 2003a), including previously undetected malformations (Burkhardt et al. 2005), cardiomyopathies (Dettmeyer and Kandolf 2010; Fried et al. 1979), or expressed endocardial fibroelastosis (Williams and Emery 1987), all of which could explain sudden death. Other findings result from residues of physiological development during the first year of life (Maron and Fisher 1977) or can be coincidental, e.g., intimal thickening of nodal arteries (Kozakewich et al. 1982). Cardiac tumors are extremely rare. Histological examinations to quantify mast cells in the myocardium of infants and toddlers showed an increased number of cells depending on age. This age-dependent increase is interpreted as a physiological process. Considerable quantitative variations may allow for differential diagnostic conclusions with regard to different myocardial alterations (Risse and Weiler 1997). In addition to morphological examinations, studies have been available for many years to prove a link between viruses and infant myocarditis (Bültmann 1992; Berkovich et al. 1968).

There are also symptom-free or symptom-weak myocarditises in infancy (Bux et al. 2002; Forcada et al. 1996). When myocarditis is demonstrated, one should consider arrhythmogenic cardiac death as a diagnosis, especially when relatively moderate histological findings are involved (Klein et al. 1995; Guilleminault 1988). In addition, primary, genetically related disruption of the cardiac conduction system may occur (Bajanowski et al. 2001).

Regardless of genetic heart defects and coronary anomalies undetected prior to autopsy, examinations of the heart muscle show some clues of myocarditis, but in some cases may also show clues of primary cardiomyopathy. The literature also includes references on findings which mention hypoxia as a cause (Fig. 17.26).

With myocarditis, conventional histological diagnosis should be differentiated from the more recently used immunohistochemical diagnosis, which is linked to the detection of molecular pathological agents in the myocardium. Different diagnostic methods are used for several reasons:

- Histological detection of cellular infiltration and necrosis of myocytes
- Immunohistochemical investigations to demonstrate an inflammation-related immunoreaction
- The detection of responsible microorganisms, primarily viruses, by molecular pathological methods

Neonatal Myocarditis

Neonatal myocarditis is well known; in most cases the pathogenic agents have been shown to be enteroviruses (EV) (Freund et al. 2010; Al Senaidi et al. 2009; Gray et al. 2001; Daley et al. 1998; Haddad et al. 1993; Druyts-Voets et al. 1993), which are generally known as the most frequent pathogens of myocarditis (Fairley et al. 1996). Severe EV disease can lead to febrile courses in neonates (Jordán et al. 2009). Parvovirus B19, coxsackieviruses, and echoviruses seem to play an important role (Verboon-Maciolek et al. 2008; Morey et al. 1992; Modlin 1988; Kaplan 1983). Enteroviral infection may cause sepsis and ischemic cardiomyopathy (Nathan et al. 2008); intrauterine adenoviral endomyocarditis has been reported with aortic and pulmonary valve stenosis (Oyer et al. 2000).

Myocarditis: Conventional Histological Diagnosis

The Dallas criteria were introduced for the diagnosis of myocarditis in endomyocardial biopsies and can also be used to estimate autopsy samples. Myocarditis is defined as a non-ischemic process, characterized by cellular infiltration, myolysis, and/or degenerative changes to the myocardium (Aretz et al. 1987).

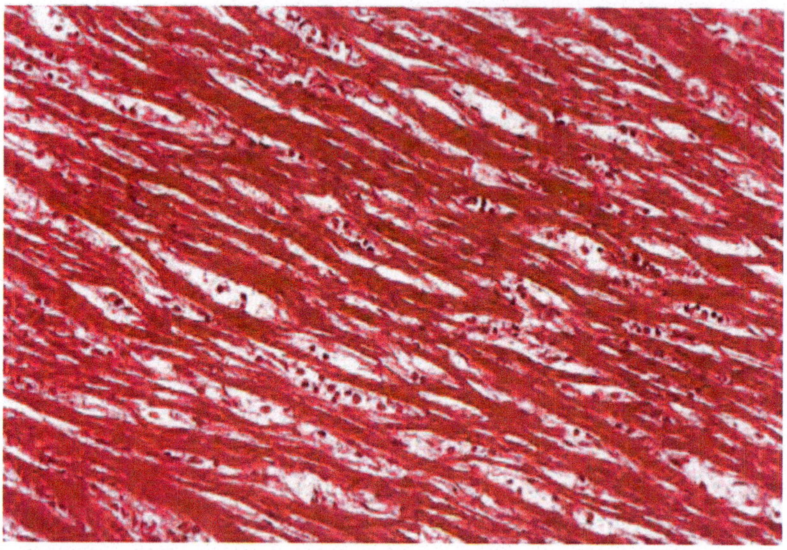

Fig. 17.26 Myocarditis with denser lymphomonocytic infiltration in the left anterior ventricle wall and in other parts of the myocardium in a 7-month-old female (H&E ×400)

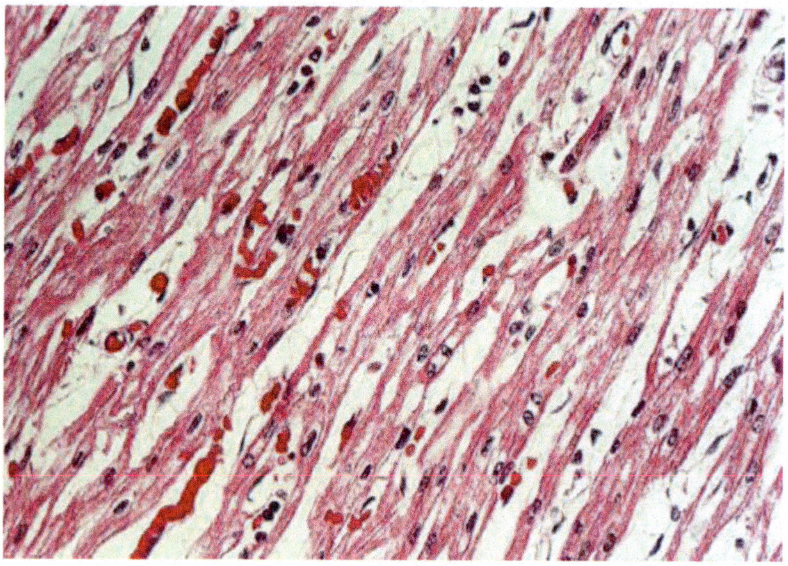

Fig. 17.27 Edematous loosened myocardium with slightly increased cellular infiltration; left posterior ventricle wall, classified as borderline myocarditis in a 4-month-old male (H&E ×400)

Even prior to the establishment of immunohistochemical myocarditis diagnostics, distinct myocarditises have been detected in conventional histological preparations in suspected SIDS cases, or at least a justified suspicion of a myocardial inflammatory process in subtle microscopic diagnostics (Dettmeyer 2008; Dettmeyer and Madea 2002, 2003, 2004; Rasten-Almqvist et al. 2002; Shatz et al. 1997; Rambaud et al. 1992; Kariks 1988, 1992; deSa 1986; Windorfer and Sitzmann 1971; Burgmeister 1963; Müller 1963).

Due to lymphomonocytic infiltrates, findings typically lead to the suspicion of a viral infection in the myocardium; several decades ago, primarily enteroviruses and more specifically coxsackieviruses were considered (Seifert 1961). Bacterial myocarditises with granulocytic infiltration and necrosis of cardiomyocytes are increasingly rare; other myocarditises are a very rare occurrence. Clear lymphomonocytic interstitial infiltrates in the myocardium generally enable an unequivocal diagnosis of viral myocarditis (Fig. 17.25); borderline findings tend to lead to diagnostic ambiguity (Fig. 17.27).

Normally, the myocardial interstitium in infants, including perivascular regions, is only slightly filled with collagen fibers. Clear interstitial and perivascular fibrosis primarily leads to the consideration of a post-inflammatory process (Figs. 17.28 and 17.29).

If persistent inflammatory infiltrates can be demonstrated in a very loose distribution, an intrauterine infection with transition to chronic myocarditis may also be considered in very young infants.

In SIDS victims as in adults, myocarditis can only be demonstrated focally (Dettmeyer 2016). While compact cell groups of lymphomonocytic cells are generally readily identified, the early phase of leukocyte invasion may be more challenging to visualize. Immunohistochemical detection of proinflammatory molecules expressed in the endothelium can help here. Occasionally, edematous areas with leukocytes adhering to the capillary endothelium in an almost "string-of-bead"-like manner can already be seen in H&E staining in the infant myocardium (Fig. 17.30). Without additional immuno-

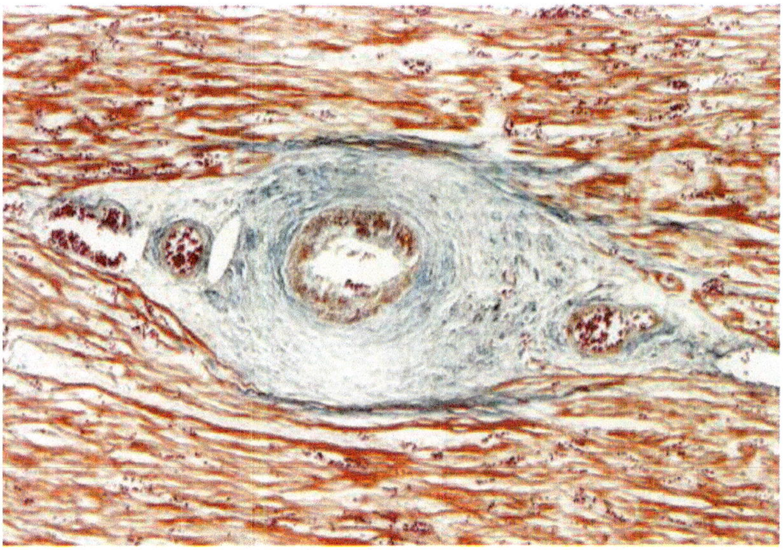

Fig. 17.28 Marked perivascular fibrosis, chronic myocarditis with demonstration of coxsackievirus B3 in a 3-month-old male (Elastica van Gieson ×400)

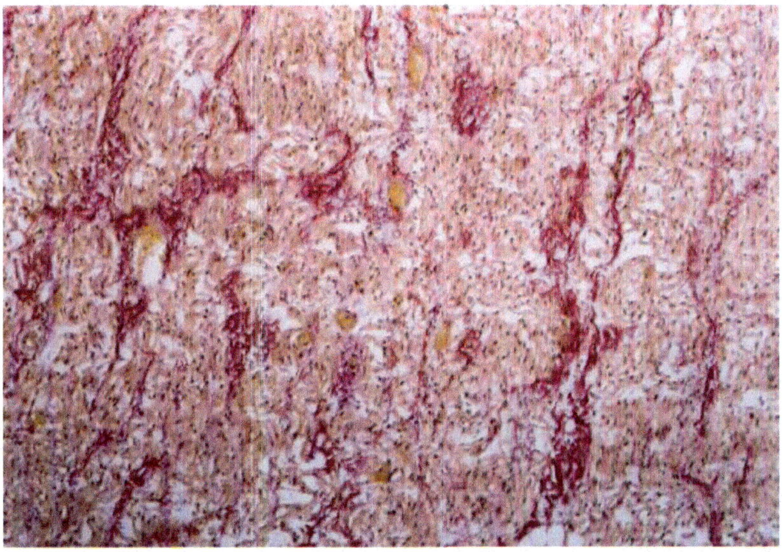

Fig. 17.29 Focal diffuse interstitial fibrosis in the myocardium, suspicion of chronic myocarditis, no virus detection, in a 5-month-old male (Elastica van Gieson ×100)

histochemical investigations, it would be virtually impossible to make findings of this kind using conventional diagnostic tests for myocarditis according to the Dallas criteria.

Weaknesses in myocarditis diagnostics with conventional histological staining (H&E, EvG, etc.) described in the literature have been highlighted (Table 17.2; Chap. 13).

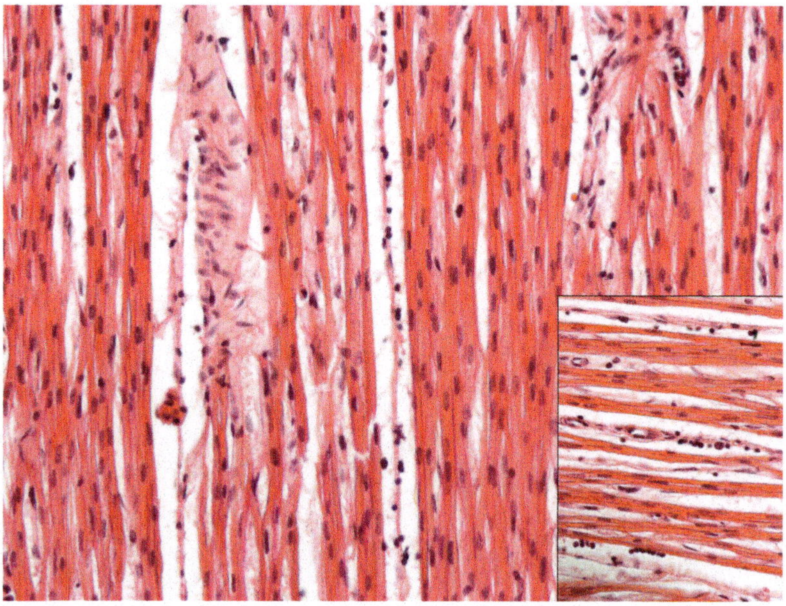

Fig. 17.30 Leukocytes adhering to the capillary endothelium in an almost "string-of-bead"-like manner in the myocardial interstitium as a sign of early-phase myocarditis (H&E ×200; Insert: H&E ×400)

Table 17.2 Disadvantages of conventional histological myocarditis diagnostics according to the Dallas criteria (Aretz et al. 1987)

Problem	Disadvantage
Number of samples	If the number of samples taken from the myocardium is insufficient, a more focally marked inflammation is not detectable; this "sampling error" leads to a false-negative finding
Microscopic finding	When only conventional histological examinations are performed, as per the Dallas criteria, there is significant interobserver variability (Shanes et al. 1987) that may also lead to a false-negative finding
Process monitoring	Biopsy process monitoring is not feasible in victims of suspected SIDS who have undergone autopsy
Early phase of myocarditis	Conventional histological examinations do not detect early phases of myocarditis; at best, these are classified as "borderline myocarditis" or "accompanying myocarditis" in cases of infection localized elsewhere. Here, attention should be paid to the fact that the expression of proinflammatory markers in the myocardium is a prerequisite for cellular invasion of the myocardial interstitium (Feldman and McNamara 2000)
Late phases of myocarditis	The detection of late phases of myocarditis is not reliable, and classification as "healing myocarditis" is possible
Minimum focal infiltrates	Smaller and frequently focal interstitial infiltrates in the myocardium are not regarded as a sign of early- or late-phase myocarditis, but as an accompanying reaction that is not relevant to the cause of death involving an externally localized inflammatory process (Bajanowski et al. 2003a, b). Thus, a minimum inflammatory reaction in the myocardium may be interpreted, for example, as associated with viral interstitial pneumonia, sialoadenitis, or otitis media. However, findings effecting the cardiac conduction system remain feasible

Immunohistochemical Diagnosis of Myocarditis

Following the diagnosis of myocarditis according to the Dallas criteria, an immunohistochemical diagnosis of myocarditis was established during the 1990s. Here, intramyocardial quantification and qualification of interstitial leukocytes, T-lymphocytes, and macrophages are performed in association with the immunohistochemical detection of proinflammatory molecules.

This immunohistochemical myocarditis diagnosis was first applied in stillborn infants, early death in newborns, and in cases of suspected SIDS in the 1990s and later (Dettmeyer et al. 2006b, c, d; Dettmeyer et al. 1999a, b, 2001a, b, 2002; Lazda et al. 2000; Ino et al. 1997). Analogous to the procedure used for diagnosing adult myocarditis, the procedure for suspected SIDS cases entails taking a minimum of eight myocardial samples from defined areas (Table 17.3).

Other investigations ($n = 39$) of SIDS cases at the age of 3–9 months increased the number of myocardial specimens taken at autopsy to 15 from defined sites. Of these, nine specimens were used for histological and immunohistochemical tests, and six were frozen at −80 °C for later investigation for viruses. This study found nine cases of, in part, significantly elevated numbers of lymphocytes in the myocardium and molecular genetic evidence of enteroviruses (coxsackieviruses), corresponding to 23%. Neither increased numbers of lymphocytes nor enteroviruses were found in the age-matched control group of non-natural deaths using identical specimens (Gaaloul et al. 2016a, b). Based on these results, it should be made a requirement in the future that the number of myocardial specimens investigated histologically, immunohistochemically, as well as molecular genetically should be as high as possible. At the same time, and with regard to the acuteness of death, acute arrhythmogenic cardiac death should be considered and the cardiac conduction system, as well as its surrounding tissue, investigated for inflammatory infiltrates and the presence of viruses (Dettmeyer et al. 2016). Lymphocytic infiltration of perineural nerve sheaths near the cardiac conduction system is detected in some cases (Fig. 17.31).

Table 17.3 Areas for taking myocardium samples from suspected SIDS victims, chosen to prevent "sampling errors" (Dettmeyer et al. 1999a)

Sample	Localization of tissue samples
A	Right ventricle, anterior wall
B	Right ventricle, posterior wall
C	Septum interventricular, cranial
D	Septum interventricular, caudal
E	Left ventricle, anterior wall, cranial
F	Left ventricle, anterior wall, caudal
G	Left ventricle, posterior wall, cranial
H	Left ventricle, posterior wall, caudal

Heart valves, coronary arteries, cardiac conduction system, epicardium, and endocardium should be examined separately

Immunohistochemical methods that characterize and quantify inflammatory cells in the myocardial interstitium demonstrate proinflammatory molecules in the myocardium, and use molecular pathological techniques to detect viral genomes in myocardial samples, among others, have improved diagnosis significantly (Chap. 13; Fig. 17.32, 17.33, 17.34, 17.35, 17.36, 17.37, 17.38, and 17.39).

Information on the recommended methodological approach to potential SIDS cases can be found in Table 17.4. Immunohistochemical diagnosis is suitable when myocarditis is undiagnosable using conventional histological methods or, according to own experience, suspected cases can be chosen in an attempt to more probably demonstrate the existence of a virus.

Important: When qualifying single leukocytes, T-lymphocytes, and macrophages, the otherwise standard positive control of lymphatic tissue (e.g., tonsil tissue) is not reliable since there is always summary staining. Thus, an identically processed myocardial sample with definite loose, cellular infiltration throughout the indicated cells should be chosen for the positive control. Furthermore, the quality of immunohistochemical staining needs to be checked critically in order to avoid diagnostic errors (see Chap. 2, Dettmeyer 2016).

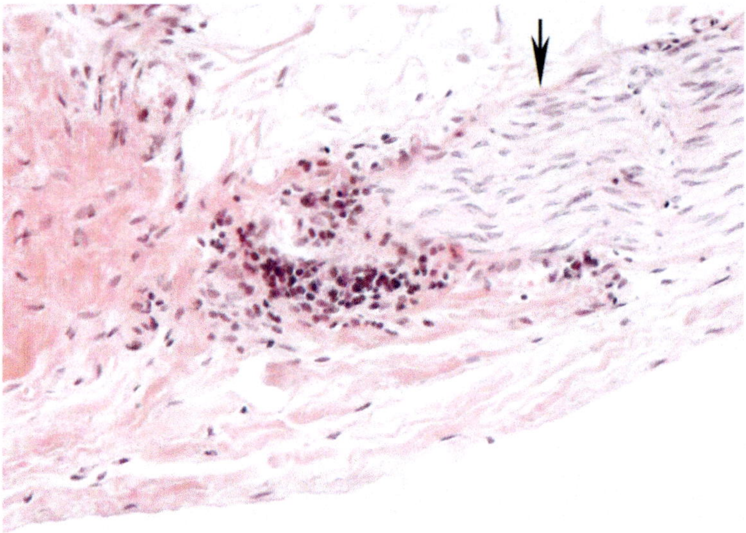

Fig. 17.31 Nerve fibers (arrow) with lymphomonocytic infiltration of the perineural nerve sheaths near the cardiac conduction system in a case of suspected sudden infant death syndrome (H&E ×200)

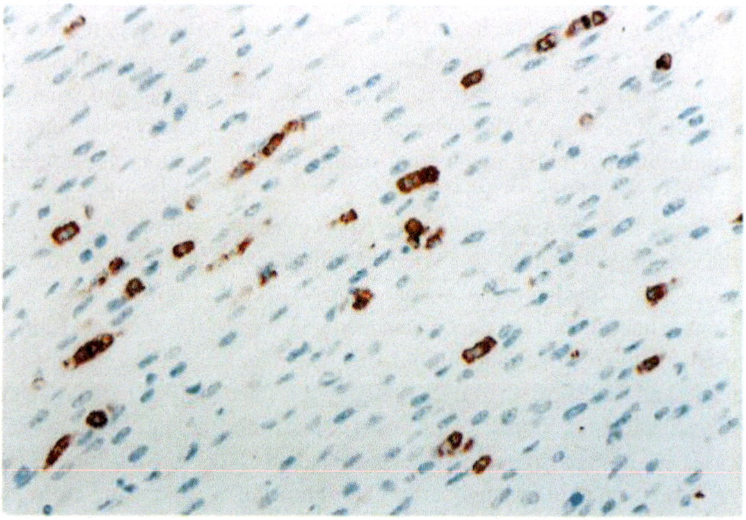

Fig. 17.32 Increased focal infiltration with LCA+-leukocytes in the myocardium of an infant left ventricle, posterior wall (×400)

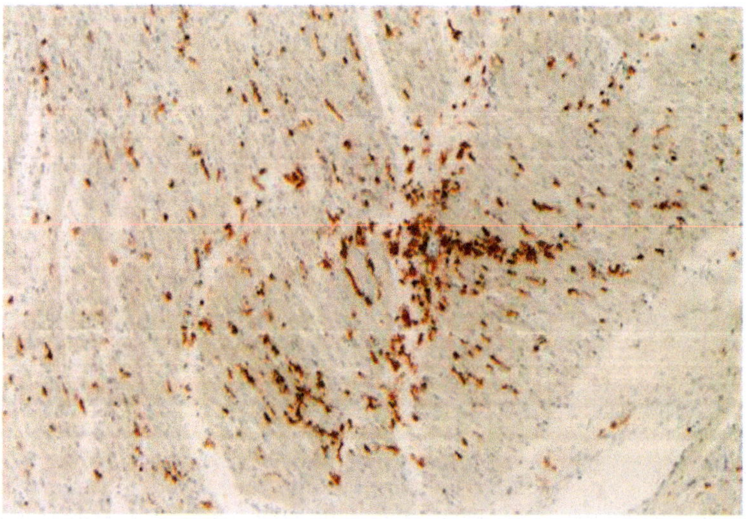

Fig. 17.33 Strong focal and weak diffuse infiltration with LCA+-leucocytes in the myocardium (×100)

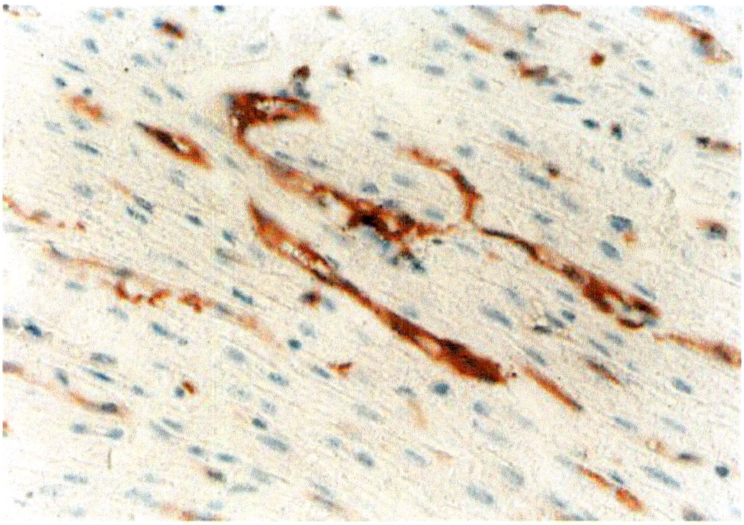

Fig. 17.34 Significantly marked endothelial and cellular expression of the MHC class II molecules in the left ventricle, posterior wall, close to the base (×400)

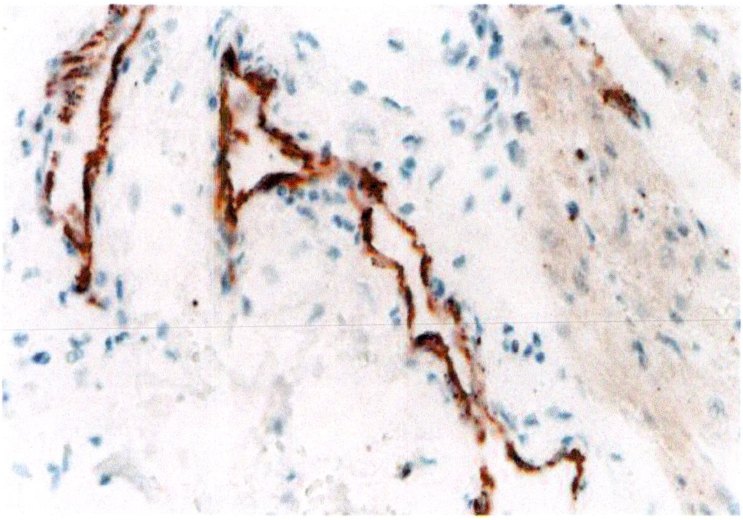

Fig. 17.35 Strong endothelial expression of proinflammatory E-selectin in peripheral coronary artery branches (×400)

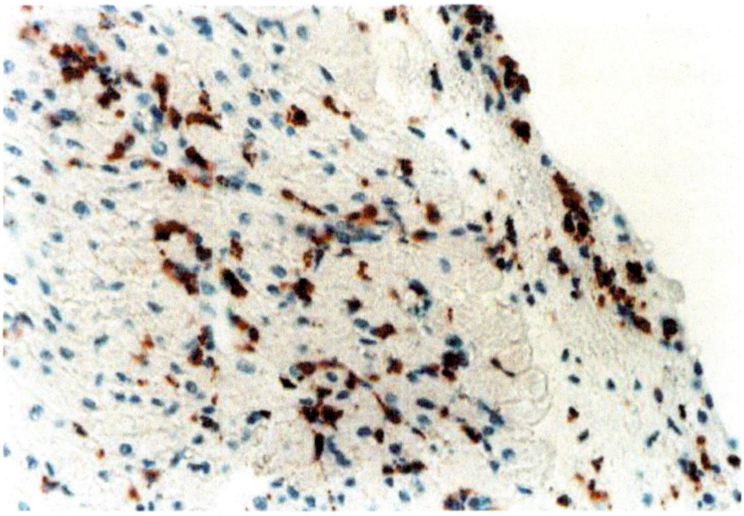

Fig. 17.36 Increased focal cellular infiltration of the myocardium by CD68-positive macrophages with epicardial involvement (×400)

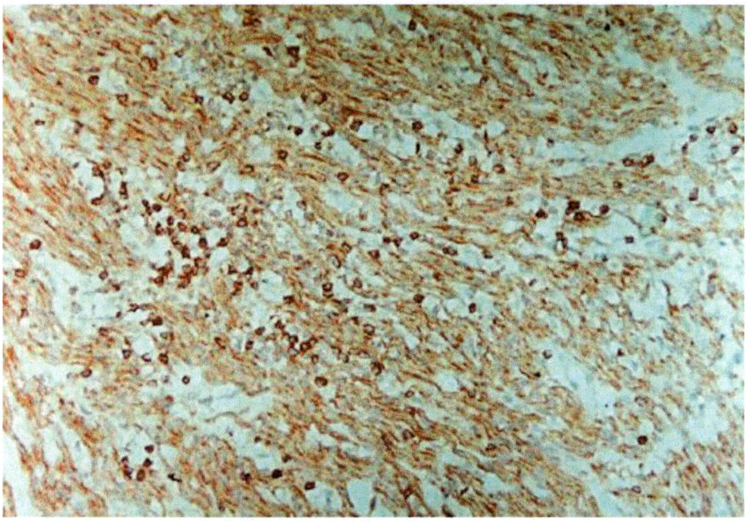

Fig. 17.37 Multiple CD3+-T-lymphocytes demonstrating myocarditis in a 7-month-old male (×200)

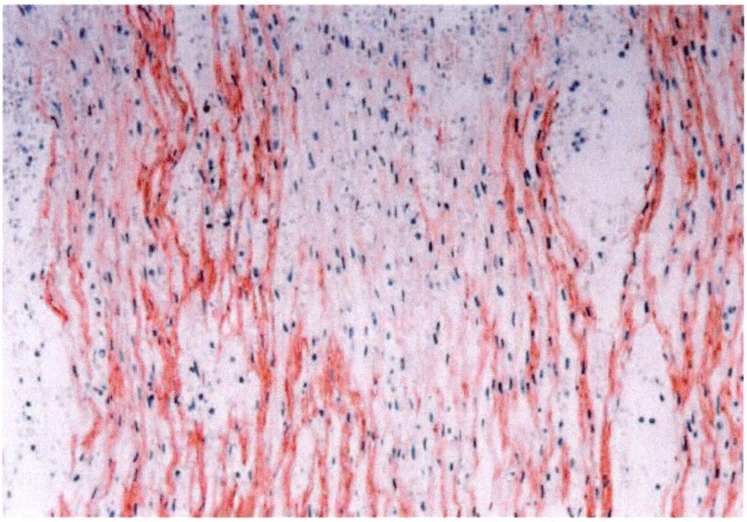

Fig. 17.38 Myocarditis with expression of troponin C in a 7-month-old male (×200)

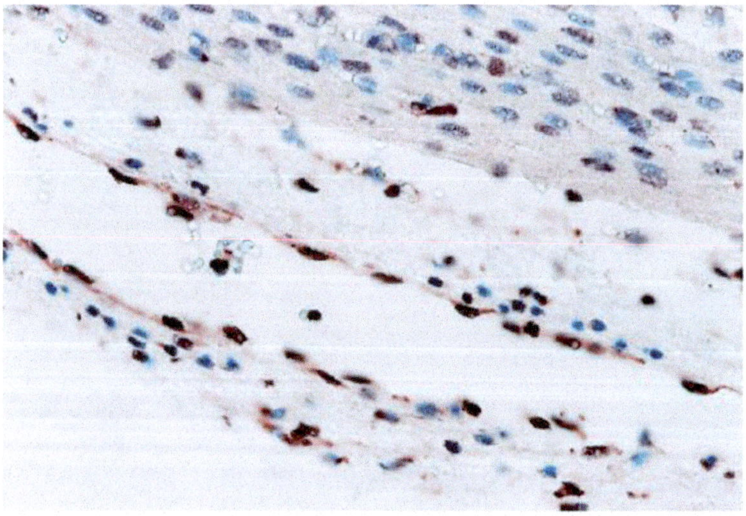

Fig. 17.39 Endothelial expression of ubiquitin in subepicardial coronary branches (×400)

Table 17.4 Suggested procedure when selecting myocardial samples for immunohistochemical myocarditis diagnosis in suspected SIDS cases (Dettmeyer et al. 1999a; Dettmeyer 2004)

Procedure	Important
Death scene investigation	Aged 8 days up to 365 days, no signs of natural or unnatural death. Room temperature too high? Co-sleeping with parents?
Storage of corpse	If possible, prompt cooling at +4 °C, early autopsy
Anamnesis	Family anamnesis, preexisting illnesses, position at death, immunizations, number of siblings, earlier SIDS cases in the family, breastfeeding period, etc.
Autopsy	Exclusion of excessive violence, typical macroscopic findings (petechiae: subpleural, subepicardial, under the capsule, and inside the thymus) but no cause of death
Sample taking	Taking of a minimum of eight myocardial samples from defined areas (Table 17.3)
Fixative	Neutral phosphate-buffered formaldehyde (pH 7.0); there is currently insufficient experience with alternative fixatives in association with tissue removed at autopsy
Fixation time	Maximum 48 h
Additional processing	Bath <60 °C (58 °C)
Section thickness	4–6 μm
Pretreatment	Differs depending on selection of primary antibodies (autopsy tissue), e.g., cooking in citrate buffer, pronase digestion
A selection of established immunohistochemical markers for myocarditis diagnosis	LCA, CD3, CD45R0, CD68, MHC class I, and MHC class II, cytokines, selectins (see Chap. 13)
Microscopic quality control	Evaluation of the suitability of the tissue sections: section thickness, staining, artifacts; obligatory review of simultaneous positive and negative controls
Quantification of LCA^+-leukocytes, e.g., $CD45R0^+$- or $CD3^+$-T-lymphocytes, $CD68^+$ macrophages, evidence of early necrosis marker $C5b\text{-}9_{(m)}$-complement complex	Previously: Quantification per visual field = high power field (hpf) = ×400 Currently: quantification per mm^2
Proinflammatory molecules	Semiquantitative evaluation per level of expression: –, +, ++, +++
Sample selection for the molecular pathological identification of a viral genome	Selection of tissue samples with the immunohistochemically strongest inflammatory and in particular cellular reaction (Dettmeyer 2004)
Molecular pathological evidence of a viral genome	Tissue probes from the paraffin block. Evidence of DNA and RNA viruses: PCR or RT-PCR, positive control, housekeeping gene, sequencing of PCR products, matching with NCBI database
Interpretation of findings	Cautious and specific to the individual case; requirements concerning the level of expression of the immunohistochemical finding must be clarified; the interpretation of evidence of PVB19 in particular is sometimes controversial; interpretation of findings must also consider further results (e.g., cytomegalovirus-induced pneumonia and sialoadenitis)

In comparison to the collective myocardial samples in controls, SIDS cases showed a more marked infiltration of the myocardial interstitium with $CD45R0^+$-T-lymphocytes, LCA^+-leukocytes, and $CD68^+$ macrophages. Rarely, there are cases with microfocal expression of the necrosis marker $C5b\text{-}9_{(m)}$-complement complex. The expression of the proinflammatory MHC class II molecules can be displayed with various intensities; this is also true for the endothelial proinflammatory marker E-selectin. Immunohistochemical characterization and quantification of interstitial myocardial leukocytes permit diagnostic limit values to also be suggested for infants on the basis of completed examinations (Table 17.5) (Dettmeyer et al. 2004a).

Table 17.5 Suggested preliminary criteria for cellular immunohistochemical diagnosis of viral myocarditis in cases of suspected SIDS (Dettmeyer et al. 2004a, 2006b, c, d)

Number of cells	Interpretation
LCA$^+$-leukocytes >15/hpf	Myocarditis
CD45R0$^+$-T-lymphocytes >10/hpf	Myocarditis
CD45R0$^+$-T-lymphocytes 5–9/hpf	Suspicion of myocarditis
CD68$^+$ macrophages >10/hpf	Suspicion of myocarditis

Hpf high power field; average of 20 hpf (×400)

Knowledge of immunologic reactions, not only of the myocardium to viruses, is still incomplete. One may imagine that, despite the presence of a viral infection, the early immune reaction may be rapid and mild. This is supported by the fact that viruses causing viral myocarditis are ubiquitously distributed, but only rarely do patients develop a manifest myocarditis. Thus, one should consider the potential of rapid viral elimination with limited conventional, histological, and immunohistochemical findings. The chronology of acute viral myocarditis described in the literature is presented in Table 17.6.

Currently, myocarditis is typically seen as the cause of death only when marked inflammatory infiltrates are present, or when the cardiac conduction system is inflamed. Less significant histopathological findings are not accepted as valid causes of death. However, a different evaluation may result when myocardial samples are shown with detectable viruses. In general, evidence of viruses in the myocardium is alone a pathological finding. In regard to parvovirus B19, the relevance of evidence of viral presence in the myocardium is under discussion. The most common agents of viral myocarditis enteroviruses, particularly coxsackieviruses, are regarded as cardiotropic. Detection of a viral genome is regarded as evidence of viral myocarditis, even when the morphological findings are less significant. Abnormal clinical development occurs (Heusch et al. 1996; Hebert et al. 1995; Henson and Mufson 1971); thus it is possible that a viral PVB19 myocarditis as well as myocardial infection with Epstein–Barr virus (EBV) may simulate myocardial infarction (Bültmann et al. 2003b; Kühl et al. 2003; Tyson et al. 1989; Miller et al. 1973). It is also possible that cytomegaloviruses (CMV) may trigger myocarditis much more often than previously thought (Kytö et al. 2005).

Table 17.6 Diagnostic phases of an acute viral myocarditis: findings postinfection (Feldman and McNamara 2000; Mall 1995)

Phase	Findings
Early phase (hours postinfection)	Ultrastructural and molecular pathological diagnosis: evidence of ultrastructural changes (electron microscopy), molecular pathological evidence of a virus
Approximately 24–48 h	Immunohistochemical diagnosis: increasingly immunohistochemically detectable findings (expression of non-cellular, proinflammatory molecules adhesion molecules, cytokines), leukocytic infiltration, expression of non-cellular, proinflammatory molecules
After 24–48 h	Conventional histological diagnosis: gradually increasing cellular infiltration, originating focally at the site of myocarditis development according to the Dallas criteria (Aretz et al. 1987)

Molecular Genetic Virus Identification in Myocardial Samples

By following the specifications listed in Table 17.3, viral genomes may be proven using molecular pathology with the help of PCR or RT-PCR on EV, adenovirus (Towbin et al. 1993), parvovirus B19 (PVB19; Cherry 1999; Cassinotti et al. 1993), EBV (Byard 2002), and CMV (Dettmeyer et al. 2004a, b, 2006a, 2008; Baasner et al. 2003a, b; Shimizu et al. 1995; Martin et al. 1994). In some cases, evidence of the viral genome of human herpes simplex virus type 1 (HHSV1) and *Toxoplasma gondii* was successful in the myocardium of suspected SIDS cases. PVB19 in the myocardium was shown in SIDS cases; the pathophysiological significance of PVB19 in the myocardium is debatable, even when more recent evaluations have shown endothelial dysfunction due to PVB19 and the cause of death attributable to PVB19-induced myocarditis (Klingel and Kandolf 2008; Bültmann et al. 2003a, b; Dettmeyer et al. 2003). Therefore, it should be highlighted that a PVB19 variant also caused myocarditises with sudden death in young dogs (Lenghaus et al. 1980; Hayes et al. 1979). Further investigations in cases of sudden unexpected death in infancy (SUDI) and sudden infant death syndrome (SIDS) also result in the detection of numerous viruses: enterovirus (EV), adenovirus (AV), Epstein–Barr virus (EBV), parvovirus B19 (PVB19), human herpes simplex virus (HHSV), cytomegalovirus (CMV), human rhinovirus (HRV), influenza virus, rotavirus, as well as other types of virus isolated in samples from the myocardium, lungs, intestine, and liver (la Grange et al. 2014; Burger et al. 2014). Coxsackievirus A16 infection has been demonstrated in infants following sudden unexplained death in extremely rare cases (Astrup et al. 2016).

Nevertheless, analysis of the individual case is needed to show whether the virus was significantly related to the cause of death, not least because a strict correlation to histological and histochemical findings is unproven (Dettmeyer et al. 2004a, 2009a, b). Other studies for which the conditions described in Table 17.3 were not met have not resulted in the demonstration of enteroviral genomes in myocardial samples of SIDS cases (Krous et al. 2009; Dettmeyer et al. 2009a). The different regional and seasonal distribution of enteroviruses might be important, as well as the fact that some viruses are endemic (Mounts et al. 2001). Meanwhile, a molecular foundation was identified for increased cardiotropy, particularly for enteroviruses (Badorff et al. 1999, 2000a, b; Bergelson et al. 1997). After respective preliminary evaluations, enteroviral myocarditis is regarded as the most thoroughly researched myocarditis (Klingel et al. 1992a, b, 1994, 2000; Kandolf 1995; Moral et al. 1993; McManus et al. 1993; Kandolf et al. 1993; Klump et al. 1990; Seko et al. 1990; Morens 1978), whereby smaller epidemics were already described decades ago (Mertens et al. 1982; Philipps et al. 1980). It is apparent that stool samples and spleen tissue are currently not systematically examined to prove enteroviral genomes in cases of assumed SIDS (Bendig et al. 2001).

17.4.3 Cardiomyopathies and SIDS

Cardiomyopathies frequently remain undetected in infants, children, teenagers, and young adults and can lead to sudden death (Schmaltz 2004; Schmaltz and Kreuder 1999; Bryant 1999; Arola et al. 1997; Friedman et al. 1991; Harris et al. 1968). Nevertheless, cardiomyopathies currently do not play an important role in the differential diagnosis of SIDS cases (Bajanowski and Brinkmann 2006), and there are relatively few relevant publications (Dettmeyer and Kandolf 2010), especially in regard to histological and immunohistochemical findings (overall relevant to children: Lewis et al. 1985). Genetic clarification should be considered in individual cases (Schwartz et al. 1996). If, in the case of dilative cardiomyopathies, a virus has been identified during childhood, enteroviruses seem to dominate as triggering agents (Arola et al. 1998).

Macroscopic autopsy findings of an infant heart involving cardiomyopathies frequently do not show the expression levels necessary for diagnosis. It is possible that dilative and hypertrophic forms of cardiomyopathy are more common (Kanter et al. 1997; Muller et al. 1995; Jacob et al. 1989), while the histiocytoid form of cardiomyopathy is extremely rare in infants (Saffitz et al. 1980; Witzleben and Pinto 1978; Reid et al. 1968). From the histopathological perspective, multiple findings may point to cardiomyopathy.

Primary Cardiomyopathy

Attention should be paid to the irregular arrangement or storiform pattern of myocardial fibers in infant hearts (myocardial disarray; Chap. 13). If these changes are found outside the interventricular septum, primary cardiomyopathy should be considered as the underlying disease, and genetic clarification is recommended.

Inflammatory Cardiomyopathy

An inflammatory cardiomyopathy should be considered when, relative to age, abnormally marked interstitial and/or perivascular fibrosis is found. Inflammatory cardiomyopathy is characterized by a moderately increased number of infiltrating lymphocytes and macrophages, together with interstitial and perivascular fibrosis findings which are unusual in infants. In such cases, an increased number of inflammatory cells in the myocardium can be immunohistochemically shown via qualification and quantification of interstitial cells. For adults, the cause is a chronic inflammatory process with possible immunological progressive myocarditis with no potential of successfully determining a causal agent. In one case, it was possible to show molecular pathological enteroviruses (coxsackievirus type B3; CVB3) in the myocardium (Dettmeyer and Kandolf 2010); relevant reports can be found in the literature (Archard et al. 1987).

Left Ventricular Noncompaction Cardiomyopathy (LVNC) (Also Called Spongy Myocardium, Spongiform Cardiomyopathy, Left Ventricular Hypertrabeculation)

LVNC is a cardiomyopathy characterized anatomically by deep trabeculations in the ventricular wall with defined recesses communicating with the main ventricular chamber. Major clinical correlates include systolic and diastolic dysfunction, sometimes associated with arrhythmias and systemic embolic events. The frequency of LVNC is not well known. The annual incidence of unclassified cardiomyopathies among children 0–10 years of age is 0.17 per 100,000 children. A genetic cause is generally suggested and there is evidence that mutations in several genes play a role: G4.5 is located on Xq28 and was initially described in patients with Barth syndrome. Alpha dystrobrevin is an autosomal gene first identified in a Japanese family with six members affected by LVNC. FRKBP12 is a gene that modulates the release of calcium from the sarcoplasmatic reticulum via the ryanodine receptor 2. FRKBP12 deletions in mice lead to a feature of nonompaction and congenital heart defects. Mutations in lamin A/C (LMNA) have been reported in patients with dilated cardiomyopathy; one was reported to have features of LVNC. The 11p15 locus was suggested by genome-wide linkage analysis in one family with autosomal dominant LVNC (Kenton et al. 2004; Sasse-Klaassen et al. 2004; Bleyl et al. 1997).

17.4.4 Hypoxia-Related Changes

Reports of hypoxia-induced histopathological findings in the myocardium describe structural changes which were found to occur after already 10 min (Janssen 1997). Investigators found that periocular localized vacuoles were involved in connection with hydropic swelling of the cardiomyocytes in cases of dehydration and acidophile cytoplasm. Prolonged hypoxia causes fatty degeneration and cardiomyolysis originating from homogenization and reduction of the cristae mitochondriales, only seen by electron microscopy (Büchner and Onishi 1968). An additional indicator of hypoxia-induced myocardial damage is a histochemically detectable reduction of ATPase activity with reduced color intensity and a slightly increased accumulation of fibronectin seen immunohistochemically (Bajanowski et al. 2003a). Proposals that recurring hypoxia caused by sleep apnea would lead to right ventricular hypoxia could not be confirmed. In addition, there was no increase in the number of mast cells (Risse and Weiler 1997; Valdes-Dapena et al. 1980; Williams et al. 1979). Also, myocardial necrosis caused by hypoxia could not be proven (Thomsen and Saternus 1994). Alternately, immunohistochemical antibodies against troponin C and fibronectin were shown to be suitable to demonstrate previous hypoxic myocardial damage and have also proved to be useful in the differential diagnosis of asphyxia versus SIDS (Ortmann et al. 2000; Brinkmann et al. 1993). Contraction band necrosis (CBN) is diagnostically less meaningful. Various types of CBN have been described as supposedly originating from adrenogenous stress rather than previous hypoxia. However, the causes and appearance of CBN are rather speculative. A Luxol fast blue stain is preferred for the detection of CBN. The histopathological differentiation between other causes and autolytic changes can be very difficult if not impossible, such that hypoxia-related findings in the myocardium are not suitable to prove, for example, lethal asphyxia. Further examinations of myocardial samples of SIDS victims are lacking in the literature. Only in individual cases is it possible to demonstrate pronounced intracellular vacuolar degeneration of cardiomyocytes in the setting of a proven impairment to pulmonary oxygen uptake due to chronic hypoxia, or hypoxia lasting at least several days. As a result of large-scale intracytoplasmic vacuole formation, one sees a honeycomb-like pattern of apparently empty sarcolemmal tubes when looking at the myocardial fibers in cross section (Fig. 17.40). One also sees vacuolar degeneration in the hepatocyte cytoplasm in such cases.

In addition the concept of position-dependent cerebral hypoxemia as a mechanical cause of sudden death in infants was presented, based on the possibility of flow impairment in the large neck vessels, carotid, and vertebral arteries (Saternus and Adam 1985). Otherwise, in cases of suspected sudden infant death (SID), sequelae of any past traumata including lesions of the vertebral artery due to birth trauma could not be detected (Saternus and Hebold 1986; Hebold et al. 1986).

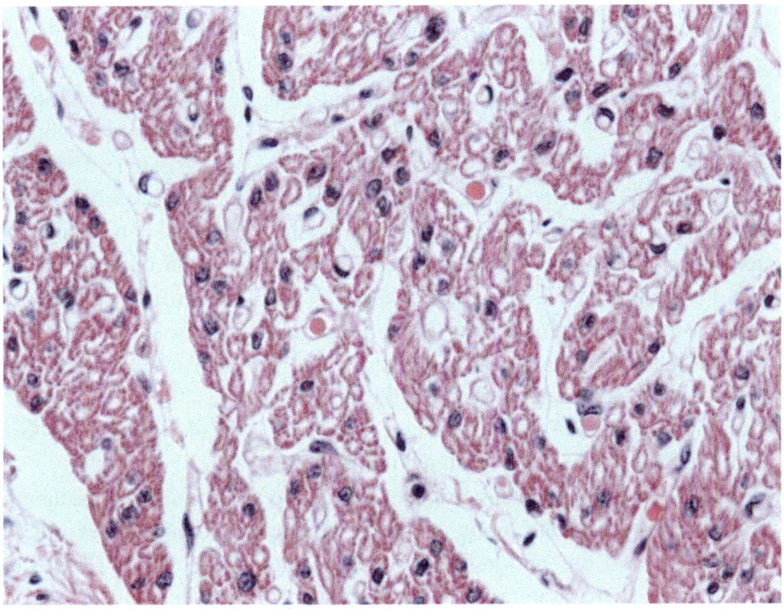

Fig. 17.40 Vacuolar degeneration in the cardiomyocyte cytoplasm due to chronic hypoxia in an infant that lived to 7 days with virtually empty sarcolemmal tubes that are striking for their partially ring-like configuration in cross section (H&E ×100; image kindly provided by Prof. J. Preuß-Wössner, Kiel/Lübeck, Germany)

17.4.5 Histopathological Findings in the Cardiac Conduction System

Since ventricular fibrillation or other arrhythmias have been suggested as a cause of unexplained sudden infant death, many authors focused their studies on the cardiac conduction system (Fineschi et al. 2006; Dudorkinowa and Bouska 1993; Fu et al. 1994; Kozakewich et al. 1982; Anderson and Hill 1982; Jankus 1976; Lie et al. 1976; Suarez-Mier and Aguilera 1998; Ferris 1973). Histological examinations of the cardiac conduction system require regular serial sections after tissue removal (Zack and Wegener 1994; Valdes-Dapena et al. 1973). The defined findings were descriptive (resorptive degeneration, necrotic fibers, fibroblasts) and did not thoroughly examine inflammatory processes, clear necrosis, or histopathologically diagnosed standard variants in increased numbers. A larger study (Matturri et al. 2000) did not show significant differences in comparison to a group of non-SIDS cases, with the exception of resorptive degenerative changes, which were visually evident in 97% of SIDS victims and in only 75% of the control group. The authors considered the frequency of His bundle hypoplasia, atrioventricular node dispersion, left-sided His bundle, intramural right bundle, His bundle dispersion, resorptive degeneration, Mahaim fibers, cartilaginous metahyperplasia, and anatomical abnormalities (Matturri et al. 2000). Immunocytochemical demonstration of a relative lack of nerve fibers in the atrioventricular node and His bundle was possible using the S100 antibody. S100 selectively marks Schwann cells associated with both myelinated and nonmyelinated nerves. While examining immunocytochemically the age difference of the nerve fiber content of the cardiac conduction system (CCS), it became evident that in certain SIDS cases, there was a lack of S100 positive nerve fibers in the atrioventricular node and His bundle. The authors concluded that, when taken in conjunction with the epidemiology of SIDS, results suggested that the lack of atrioventricular node and His bundle innervation most probably reflects a delay in the development or maturation of the nerve elements of the CCS, similar to that noted for other parts of the central and peripheral nervous systems in SIDS (Fu et al. 1994).

In own examinations of approximately 40 SIDS cases, the cardiac conduction system was processed using serial sections, followed by an immunohistochemical examination of CD45R0^{+}-T-lymphocyte, LCA^{+}-leukocyte, and CD68^{+}-macrophage infiltration. In addition, expression of MHC class II molecules was determined semiquantitatively, together with expression of the endothelial proinflammatory marker E-selectin. The immunohistochemical findings were compared across samples from eight defined areas of the same myocardium; however, there were no findings of more frequent or more intense inflammatory activities within the periphery of the cardiac conduction system (Dettmeyer, not published). Findings such as fetal dispersion of the AV node and/or His bundle were described, in addition to other findings. Mahaim tracts, especially of the fasciculoventricular type, were not found in controls and thus may be the cause of death. Fibromuscular hyperplasia of the AV node artery was very rarely found but may be the cause of death when the lumen is extremely narrowed (Paz Suárez-Mier and Aguilera 1998). Nevertheless, studies of the cardiac conduction system can explain some cases of sudden infant death; thus it must be investigated in all cases of SIDS. A simplified method for studying the cardiac conduction system must be extensive enough to identify the most important abnormalities (Paz Suárez-Mier and Aguilera 1998; see also Zack and Wegener 1994). Indeed, histological examinations of the cardiac conduction system are carried out too seldom in cases of sudden cardiac death caused by cardiac conduction disturbances as well as in cases of suspected SIDS.

17.4.6 Salivary Glands

The submandibular and parotid glands may show evidence of an infection in cases of suspected SIDS (Fig. 17.41; Püschel et al. 1988; Variend and Pearse 1986; Molz et al. 1985). Information

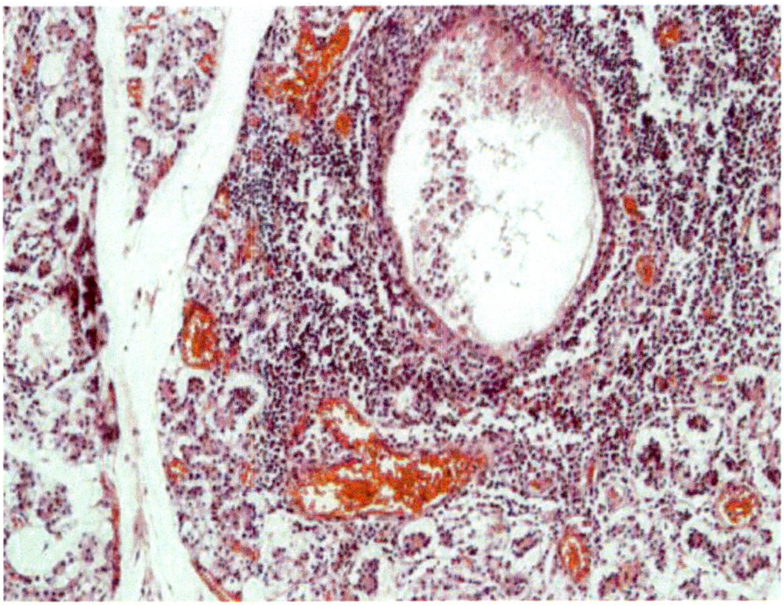

Fig. 17.41 Chronic sialoadenitis of the parotid gland with lymphomonocytic infiltration in a 5-month-old girl (H&E ×200)

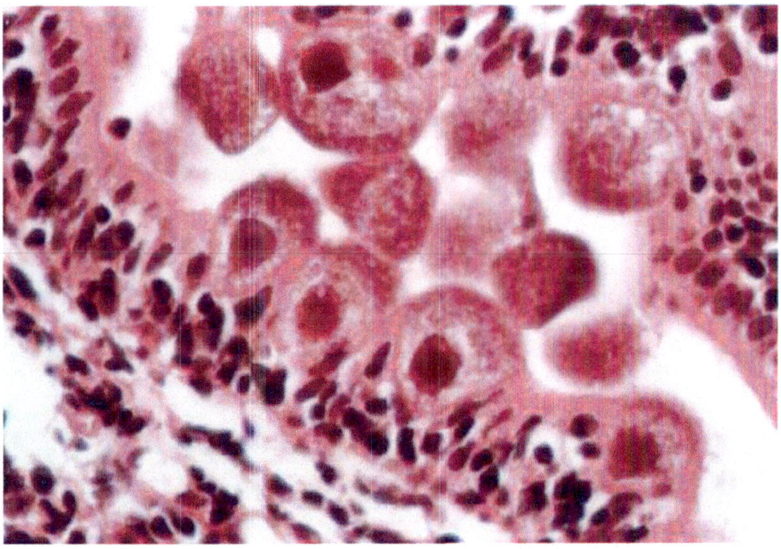

Fig. 17.42 Inclusions typical for cytomegaly in the epithelium of the parotid gland (H&E ×400) (Photo courtesy of Prof. M. Risse, Gießen, Germany)

regarding the frequency of sialadenitises in SIDS cases varies across studies. Involvement of the glandular epithelium with CMV can typically be seen in the parotid gland. These findings can already be seen with conventional H&E staining in approximately 10–30% of cases (Püschel et al. 1988): the enlarged glandular epithelia showed a similarly enlarged cell nucleus surrounded by an optically brightened margin (Fig. 17.42). There is marked accompanying unspecified lymphomonocytic sialoadenitis (Figs. 17.43 and 17.44). Such results must be interpreted within the context of all findings, particularly in lung tissue and the myocardium. Immunohistochemical markers and samples for in situ hybridization are available to show the presence of CMV (Bajanowski et al. 1994; Löning et al. 1986). Using immunohistochemical analysis and in situ hybridization, viral substances were detected in CMV-infected cells as well as in morphologically healthy cells. The literature on the clinical and epidemiological aspects of cytomegaly indicates that a localized

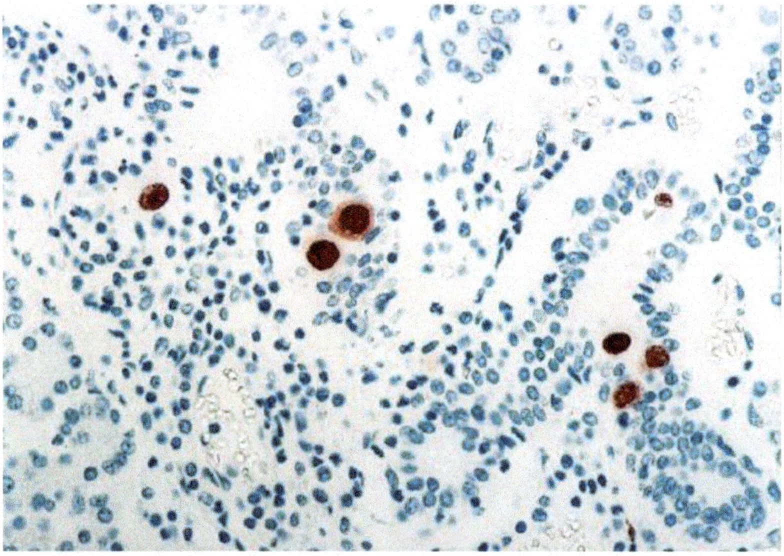

Fig. 17.43 Immunohistochemical detection of cytomegalovirus-positive epithelial cells and lymphomonocytic sialoadenitis of the parotid gland (CMV ×200)

Fig. 17.44 Partially dense infiltrate with LCA+-leukocytes in the parotid gland with chronic parotitis and no evidence of cytomegalovirus-positive cells (×200)

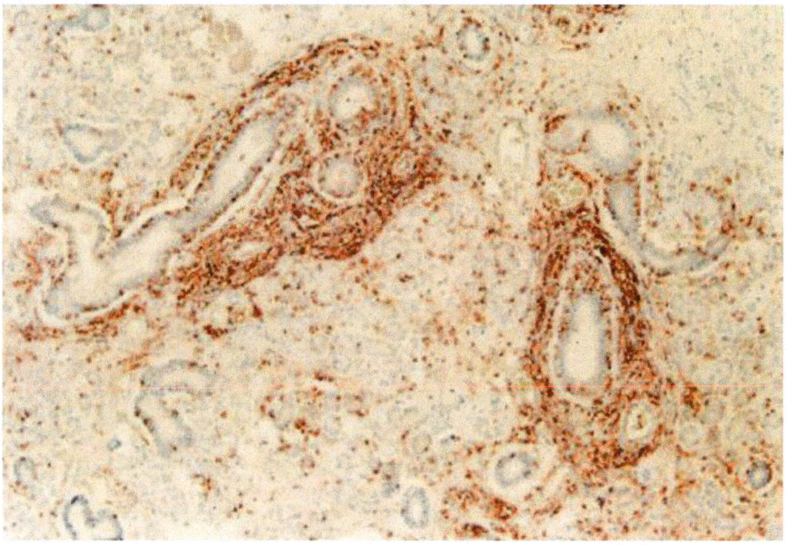

CMV infection of the salivary glands does not sufficiently explain the SIDS. While it should be emphasized that the presence of cytomegaly alone can influence the immunological status of the organism, a CMV-induced pneumonia and myocarditis should also be taken into account. However, other internal organs may also exhibit CMV infection (Yagmur et al. 2016; Ludwig 1969). It is estimated that the prospective mother sustains a human cytomegalovirus infection in 0.5–4% of pregnancies (Buxmann et al. 2017). Past investigations indicate that the frequency of CMV infection is not age dependent within the first 12 months of life (Püschel et al. 1988).

17.4.7 The Liver

Hemosiderin may sometimes be found in the liver of infants, predominantly localized in the periphery of the lobules (Risse and Weiler 1987a). No significant differences were found in cases of SIDS compared to controls. Earlier studies discussed metabolism or electrolyte disorders as the causes of sudden infant death (Vawter et al. 1986; Steele et al. 1984; Raie and Smith 1981; Lapin et al. 1976). When diffuse microvesicular steatosis of the liver can be shown, a mitochondriopathy-type illness should be considered, for example, medium-chain acyl-coenzyme A dehydrogenase (MCAD) deficiency (Stanley and Hale 1994). Sudden death due to MCAD can be referred to the coroner's physician as sudden unexplained infant death. Detailed death investigation including autopsy findings and biochemical and molecular studies can reveal the cause and natural manner of death (Manoukian et al. 2009).

Liver-cell hydrops seems to represent a frequent morphological equivalent to acute oxygen deficiency in asphyxia in childhood and is a common finding in SIDS cases. One may observe balloon-shaped hepatocytes with brightened cytoplasm and centrally located cell nuclei (Fig. 17.45). Frequently, the liver sinusoids are no longer visible or increasingly constricted. Evidence of liver-cell hydrops is not suitable for the differential diagnosis of asphyxia due to external violence in infants and toddlers, as well as asphyxia linked to SIDS. Partially focal liver-cell hydrops was found after cases of fatal violent compression to the neck, death by drowning, and following amniotic fluid and chyme aspiration (Weiler and Ritter 1988). The number of diffuse extramedullary hematopoietic cells was found higher in SIDS cases compared to non-SIDS (Törő et al. 2007).

17.4.8 The Thymus

It is well known that there may be numerous petechiae both under the thymus capsule and inside the parenchyma in SIDS cases (Kleemann 1997; Beckwith 1988; Krous 1984). Previously, systematic histological investigations were carried out on the thymus in cases of suspected SIDS. Cases with unsuccessful attempts at resuscitation were compared with cases with no resuscitation attempts; the histological distribution pattern of petechial thymus hemorrhage did not notably differ between the two groups (Risse and Weiler 1989b, 1990b). The pattern of findings indicated that the hemorrhages had developed during the agonal period prior to death and that the typical histological distribution pattern with an increased occurrence of petechiae in the cortical zone was altered by massive attempts at resuscitation in individual cases (Hood et al. 1988).

The literature describes acute exposure reaction, adjustment reaction, and inversion stages I and II as a thymus tissue reaction (Entrup and Brinkmann 1990a, b). However, such differentiations depend on the examiner's experience, as

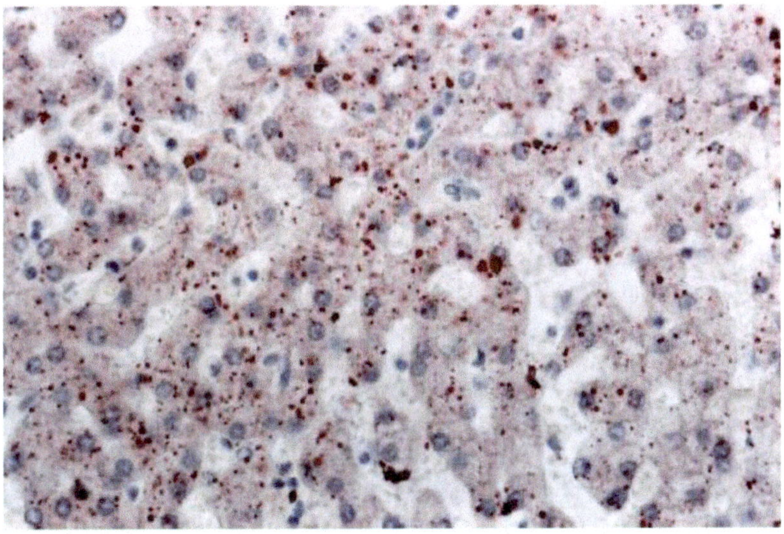

Fig. 17.45 Diffuse microvesicular steatosis of the liver, suspicious for mitochondriopathy, in a case attributed to SIDS (Sudan III ×400)

well as his subjective evaluation, and on the number of samples examined. In certain cases, histological findings in the thymus may point to systemic processes. No connection between the number and size of the Hassall bodies inside the thymus tissue and SIDS has been assumed.

17.4.9 Endocrine Organs (Pancreas, Thyroid, Pituitary)

Histological examinations of the endocrine organs in SIDS victims include the pancreas, thyroid, pituitary, pituitary gland, and adrenal gland (Pérez-Platz et al. 1994).

Pancreas

Examinations of the pancreas and pancreatic islets in cases of suspected SIDS yielded no serious histopathological findings. A higher number of enlarged islet cells were morphometrically described, as well as "cytoplasm shrinking" in SIDS victims (Klensang et al. 1997). In one case, it was possible to immunohistochemically show a mild, isolated leukocytic infiltration of pancreatic islet cells with simultaneously proven enteroviral myocarditis (Dettmeyer et al. 2006b). This finding supports the idea that viral insulitis may cause juvenile diabetes (Roivainen et al. 1995; Foulis et al. 1990).

Thyroid

The morphological picture of the thyroid gland, the only endocrine organ with a follicle structure, allows a limited conclusion to be drawn with respect to its functional state, despite any physiological variability. The thyroid of newborns shows total colloid release and collapse of the follicles. The typical structure of the thyroid gland will be formed within several weeks after birth (Müller and Rämsch 1966). Total colloid absorption can be found in cases of stress-activated thyroids as well as in cases of death due to freezing. Many SIDS cases present findings which may be interpreted as morphological correlates of a premortal chronic or recurrent stress reaction (Byard and Bellis 2016; Risse and Weiler 1984).

In comparison to a control group, histological, immunohistochemical, and morphometric examinations of the thyroids of SIDS victims more frequently showed fibrotic zones and "depleted follicles"; inflammatory processes and criteria for increased functional activity did not occur at significantly higher frequency (Risse and Weiler 1984, 1990a; Risse et al. 1986; Rothfuchs et al. 1995). The interpretation of the findings was that in some cases, there had been previous "near-death episodes" and repeated hypoxia. No further interpretation was possible in regard to acute congestive hypoxia being added to the diagnosis, including clearing of the follicles and squamous epithelium (Werne and Garrow 1953; Sagreiya and Emery 1970). An increased incidence of thyroid activation was seen only from the second month of life in SIDS cases (Risse and Weiler 1990a, b). Conclusions involving the histomorphological findings and the respective functional state of the thyroid should be made with great care.

Pituitary Glands

A more expansive series of examinations shows necrosis and hemorrhage only in rare cases, while hypoxia was present in approximately 50% of cases. With no deviation from control groups, there were cysts in the intermediate zone (14%), persistence of Rathke's pouch (44%), Erdheim's squamous epithelium (8%), or heterotopic salivary glands (3%). The semiquantitative immunohistochemical evaluation of the different cell types also showed no significant variations from the control group. Additionally, the pattern of distribution of the intracytoplasmic vacuolizations of the ACTH and gonadotropic cells showed no significant differences (Reuss et al. 1994).

Adrenal Glands

In 146 SIDS cases, normal maturation of the adrenal glands was found with no necrosis or extensive hemorrhage. There were no signs of inflammation, but a focal lipid depletion of the fasciculate zone was seen in 92% of the adrenal glands in SIDS and control cases. Additionally, calcium deposits were found (13%) due to hyperemic involution of the fetal zone. No pathological findings were seen in the S100 protein-positive sustentacular cells of the medulla; additionally, chromogranin A-positive cells were unchanged.

17.4.10 Lymph Nodes and Spleen

Lymph Nodes

Histological findings in lymphatic tissue (lymph node, spleen, thymus) revealed a substantial increase in evidence of acute infections in SIDS cases when compared to control cases (Entrup and Brinkmann 1990b).

The spectrum of histological findings in lymphatic tissue includes well-developed germinal centers, which may represent diffuse, follicular, or frequently paracortical hyperplasia. In addition, there are reports of colored pulpa hyperplasia with an increased number of immunoblasts and sinus histiocytosis. However, follicular lymphatic hyperplasia in infancy may be regarded as a physiological reaction. In individual cases, attention should be paid to epithelioid cells that may be evaluated as an indication of toxoplasmosis or an infectious mononucleosis, especially when they appear in the lymph nodes of the neck (so-called Piringer's lymphadenitis). Some authors conclude that changes in the reaction pattern of the lymphoid tissue could be a more sensitive detection method of early stages of inflammation than local histology (Bajanowski et al. 1997). Not all studies in the literature were able to demonstrate a substantial lack of reactivity in the immune system of SIDS victims. Also, immunohistochemical investigations of the B- and T-cell antigens showed normal reactivity. In some SIDS cases, it was possible to observe reaction patterns that are normally associated with acute inflammation, but the findings were not regarded as compatible with a rapidly overwhelming infection leading to death.

Spleen

In the case of systemic infection, the lymphatic tissue of the spleen may react by developing periarterial germinal centers. In most cases, the sinuses of the spleen are completely filled with erythrocytes following acute blood congestion, and the border to the lymphatic tissue of the white spleen pulp is relatively sharp. The spleen in newborns and infants may show diffuse siderosis of the red pulp (Risse and Weiler 1987a, b).

17.4.11 Additional Histopathological Findings

Gastroesophageal Reflux

Gastroesophageal reflux has been discussed in the context of findings in cases of suspected SIDS (Risse and Weiler 1989a; Walsh et al. 1981; Herbst et al. 1978; Leape et al. 1977; Ismail-Beigi et al. 1970). Systematic histological investigations were carried out on the esophagus of SIDS and control cases. The results consisted of focal epithelial defects (14%) and fresh inflammatory wall changes (7%) in SIDS cases without preferential localization. There were also lymphocytic reactions of varying extent, but mainly in the upper third of the esophagus (Risse and Weiler 1989a). It appears doubtful that the inflammatory changes are the result of gastroesophageal reflux.

Phrenic nerves and Diaphragms

Disturbances of the respiratory system may be an important factor in the series of events leading to sudden infant death (Weis et al. 1994; Silver and Smith 1992). As stated by Weis et al. (1998), the diaphragm is the major respiratory muscle in infants, but little is known about alterations to this muscle and the phrenic nerve in SIDS cases. Morphologic analysis revealed only slightly larger cross-sectional areas of phrenic nerve axons, but no increase in myelin sheath thickness in SIDS cases. Using electron microscopy, several nerve fibers of SIDS cases showed focal accumulations of neurofilaments. Muscle fiber diameters in SIDS diaphragms were significantly larger compared to controls ($p < 0.0001$). In most SIDS and control cases, axons and myelin sheaths were artificially swollen, and acute segmental muscle fiber ruptures and contracture bands were found (Weis et al. 1998; Weber et al. 1994). However, all these findings are nonspecific. Nevertheless, it was postulated that decreased density of phrenic nerve myelinated axons may contribute to sudden infant death.

Allergen Hypersensitivity Reaction

Individual investigations discuss an acute allergic reaction as an accompanying cause of sudden infant death (Hagan et al. 1998; Raven et al. 1978). An anaphylactic reaction shortly after multiple immunizations is occasionally considered, particularly if an elevated concentration of ß-tryptase together with an increase in degranulated mast cells is detected, e.g., immunohistochemically in lung tissue (D'Errico et al. 2008).

References

Adelson I, Kinney ER (1956) Sudden and unexpected death in infancy and childhood. Pediatrics 17:663–697

Aherne W, Bird T, Court SDM, Garnder PS, McQulillen J (1970) Pathological changes in virus infection of the lower respiratory tract in children. J Clin Pathol 23:7–18

Aita K, Doi M, Tanno K, Oikawa H, Oo MT, Ohashi N, Misawa S (2000) Pulmonary neuroendocrine cell distribution in sudden infant death syndrome. Legal Med 2:134–142

Al Senaidi K, Lacson A, Rebeyka IM, Mackie AS (2009) Echocardiographic detection of early myocardial calcification in acute neonatal myocarditis due to Coxsackie virus type B. Pediatr Cardiol 30:862–863

Althoff H (1968) Der forensische Beweiswert histopathologischer Bronchien- und Lungenveränderungen beim plötzlichen Kindstod. Beitr Gerichtl Med 25:253–262

Feldman AM, McNamara D (2000) Myocarditis. N Engl J Med 343:1388–1398

Amann G (2000) Spezielle Pathologie des Frühgeborenen. Pathologe 21:339–348

An SF, Gould S, Keeling JW (1993) The role of viral infection in SIDS: detection of viral nucleic acid by in situ hybridisation. J Pathol 171:271–278

Andersen FW, Hogan JG, Ansbacher R (2004) Sudden death: ectopic pregnancy mortality. Obstet Gynecol 103:1218–1223

Anderson KR, Hill RW (1982) Occlusive lesions of cardiac conducting tissue arteries in sudden infant death syndrome. Pediatrics 69:50–52

Aoki Y (1994) Histopathological findings in the lung and trachea in sudden infant death syndrome: review of 105 cases autopsied at Dade County Medical Examiner Department. Jpn J Leg Med 48:141–149

Archard CC, Bowles EG, Olsen EGJ, Richardson PJ (1987) Detection of persistent coxsackie-B-virus RNA in dilated cardiomyopathy and myocarditis. Eur Heart J 8:437–440

Aretz HT, Billingham ME, Edwards W, Factor SM, Fallon JT, Fenoglio JJ, Olsen EGJ, Schoen FJ (1987) Myocarditis: a histopathologic definition and classification. Am J Cardiovasc Pathol 1:5–14

Arola A, Jokinen E, Ruuskanen O, Saraste M, Pesonen E, Kuusela AL, Tikanojja T, Paavilainen T, Simell O (1997) Epidemiology of idiopathic cardiomyopathies in children and adolescents. A nationwide study in Finland. Am J Epidemiol 146:385–393

Arola A, Kallajoki M, Ruuskanen O, Hyypia T (1998) Detection of enteroviral RNA in end-stage dilated cardiomyopathy in children and adolescents. J Med Virol 56:364–371

Astrup BS, Johnsen IBG, Engsbro AL (2016) The role of Coxsackievirus A16 in a case of sudden unexplained death in an infant – a SUDI case. Forensic Sci Int 259:e9–e13

Baasner A, Dettmeyer R, Graebe M, Madea B (2003a) PCR-based diagnosis of enterovirus and parvovirus B19 in paraffin-embedded heart tissue. In: Brinkmann B, Carracedo A (eds) Progress in forensic fgenetics 9, 19th international ISFG congress, Münster, August 28–September 1 2001. International congress series, vol 1239, p 715–717

Baasner A, Dettmeyer R, Graebe M, Rissland J, Madeda B (2003b) PCR-based diagnosis of enterovirus and parvovirus B19 in paraffin-embedded heart tissue of children with suspected sudden infant death syndrome. Lab Investig 83:1451–1452

Badorff C, Lee GH, Lamphear BJ, Martone ME, Campbell KP, Rhoads RE, Knowlton KU (1999) Enteroviral protease 2A cleaves dystrophin: evidence of cytoskeletal disruption in an acquired cardiomyopathy. Nat Med 5:320–326

Badorff C, Berkely N, Mehrotra S, Talhouk JW, Rhoads RE, Knowlton KU (2000a) Enteroviral protease 2A directly cleaves dystrophin and is inhibited by a dystrophin-based substrate analogue. J Biol Chem 275:1191–1197

Badorff C, Lee GH, Knowlton KU (2000b) Enteroviral cardiomyopathy: bad news for the dystrophin-glycoprotein-complex. Herz 25:227–232

Bajanowski T (2008) Significance of respiratory infections for fatalities of infants and children. Rechtsmedizin 18:377–382

Bajanowski T, Brinkmann B (1995) Pulmonary viral infection in SIDS. In: Rognum TO (ed) Sudden infant death syndrome. New trends in the nineties. Scandinavian University Press, Oslo, pp 199–202

Bajanowski T, Brinkmann B (2000) Thickness of the air-blood tissue barrier in infants. Int J Legal Med 113:332–337

Bajanowski T, Brinkmann B (2006) Cardiac alterations in sudden infant death (SID). In: Fineschi V, Baroldi G, Silver MA (eds) Pathology of the heart and sudden death in forensic medicine. CRC Press, Boca Raton

Bajanowski T, Verhoff MA (2008) Obduktionen der Leichen von Neugeborenen. Säuglingen und Kleinkindern. Empfehlungen für die Praxis. Rechtsmedizin 18:91–98

Bajanowski T, Wiegand P, Brinkmann B (1994) Comparison of different methods for CMV detection. Int J Legal Med 106:219–222

Bajanowski T, Wiegand P, Cecchi R, Pring-Akerblom P, Adian T, Jorch G, Brinkmann B (1996) Detection and significance of adenoviruses in cases of sudden infant death. Virchows Arch 428:113–118

Bajanowski T, Ortmann C, Hernandez M, Freislederer A, Brinkmann B (1997) Reaction patterns in selected lymphatic tissues associated with sudden infant death (SID). Int J Legal Med 110:63–68

Bajanowski T, Rossi D, Biondo B, Ortmann C, Haverkamp W, Wedekind H, Jorch G, Brinkmann B (2001) Prolonged QT interval and sudden infant death – report of two cases. Forensic Sci Int 115:147–153

Bajanowski T, Ortmann C, Teige K, Wedekind H, Zack F, Röse I, Brinkmann B (2003a) Pathological changes of the heart in sudden infant death. Int J Legal Med 177:193–302

Bajanowski T, Rolf B, Jorch G, Brinkmann B (2003b) Detection of RNA viruses in sudden infant death (SID). Int J Legal Med 117:237–240

Bajanowski T, Brinkmann B, Vennemann M (2006) The San Diego definition of SIDS: practical application and comparison with the GeSID classification. Int J Legal Med 120:331–336

Bajanowski T, Vege Å, Byard RW, Krous HF, Arnestad M, Bachs L, Banner J, Blair PS, Borthne A, Dettmeyer R, Fleming P, Gaustad P, Gregersen M, Grøgaard J, Holter E, Isaksen CV, Jorgensen JV, de Lange C, Madea B, Moore I, Morland J, Opdal SH, Råsten-Almqvist P, Schlaud M, Sidebotham P, Skullerud K, Stoltenburg-Didinger G, Stra-Pedersen A, Sveum L, Rognum TO (2007) Sudden infant death syndrome (SIDS) – standardised investigations and classification: recommendations. Forensic Sci Int 165:129–143

Baker AM, Morey MK, Berg KK, Crosson J (2000) Trophoblastic microemboli as a marker for preeclampsia-eclampsia in sudden unexpected maternal death. A case report and review of the literature. Am J Forensic Med Pathol 21:354–358

Banaschak S, Janßen K, Becker K, Friedrich K, Rothschild MA (2014) Fatal postpartum air embolism due to uterine inversion and atonic hemorrhage. Int J Legal Med 128:147–150

Barbesier M, Duncanson ER, Mackey-Bojack SM, Roe SJ, Thomas LC (2013) Sudden death due to spontaneous acute dissection of the left subclavian artery with rupture during postpartum period: a case report. Int J Legal Med 127:453–457

Baxendine J, Moore I (1995) Pulmonary eosinophilia in sudden infant death syndrome. J Pathol 177:415–421

Beckwith JB (1970) Observations on the pathological anatomy of the sudden infant death syndrome. In: Bergmann AB, Beckwith JB, Ray CG (eds) International conference on causes of sudden death in infants. University of Washington Press, Seattle, pp 83–139

Beckwith JB (1988) Intrathoracic petechial hemorhages: a clue to the mechanism of death in sudden infant death syndrome? Ann N Y Sci 533:37–47

Beckwith JB (1989) The mechanism of death in sudden infant death syndrome. In: Culbertson JL, Krous HK, Bendell RD (eds) Sudden infant death syndrome. Medical aspects and physiological management. Arnold, London, pp 48–61

Beckwith JB, Bergman AB, Beckwith JB, Ray CG (eds) (1970) Discussion of terminology and definition of the sudden infant death syndrome. In: Proceedings of the second international conference on the causes of sudden death in infants, Seattle, 1970. University of Washington Press, p 14

Becroft DM, Thompson JM, Mitchell EA (1998) Epidemiology of intrathoracic petechial hemorrhages in sudden infant death syndrome. Pediatr Dev Pathol 1:200–209

Beech DJ, Sibbons PD, Howard CV, van Velzen D (2000) Renal development delay expressed by reduced glomerular number and is associated with growth retardation in victims of sudden infant death syndrome and in "normal" infants. Pediatr Dev Pathol 3:450–454

Bendig JWA, O'Brien PS, Muir P, Porter HJ, Caul EO (2001) Enterovirus sequences resembling coxsackievirus A2 detected in stool and spleen from a girl with fatal myocarditis. J Med Virol 64:482–486

Berg S, Kijewski S (1978) Histologische Befunde an 224 Fällen von plötzlichem Säuglingstod im norddeutschen Raum. Beitr Gerichtl Med 36:153–160

Bergelson JM, Cunningham JA, Droguett G, Kurt-Jones EA, Krithivas A, Hong JS, Horwitz MS, Crowell RL, Finberg RW (1997) Isolation of a common receptor for coxsackie B viruses and adenoviruses 2 and 5. Science 275:1320–1323

Berkovich S, Rodriguez-Torres R, Lin JS (1968) Virologic studies in children with acute myocarditis. Am J Dis Child 115:207–212

Berry PJ (1992) Pathological findings in SIDS. J Clin Pathol 45:11–16

Bickell NA, Bodian C, Anderson RM, Kase N (2004) Time and risk of ruptured tubal pregnancy. Obstet Gynecol 104:789–794

Blackwell CC, Weir DM (1999) The role of infection in sudden infant death syndrome. FEMS Immunol Med Microbiol 25:1–6

Blackwell CC, Weir DM, Busuttil A (1995) Infectious agents, the inflammatory responses of infants and sudden infant death syndrome. Mol Med Today 1(2):72–78

Blackwell CC, Weir DM, Busuttil A (1999) Infection, inflammation and sleep: more pieces to the puzzle of sudden infant death syndrome (SIDS). APMIS 107:455–473

Bleyl SB, Mumford BR, Brown-Harrison MC, Pagotto LT, Carey JC, Pysher TJ, Ward K, Chin TK (1997) Xq28-linked noncompaction of the left ventricular myocardium: prenatal diagnosis and pathologic analysis of affected individuals. Am J Med Genet 72:257–265

Brinkmann B, Sepulchre MA, Fechner G (1993) The application of selected histochemical and immunohistochemical markers and procedures to the diagnosis of early myocardial damage. Int J Legal Med 106:135–141

Bryant RM (1999) Hypertrophic cardiomyopathy in children. Cardiol Rev 7:92–100

Büchner F, Onishi S (1968) Der Herzmuskel bei acuter Coronarinsuffizienz im elektronenmikroskopischen Bild. Urban & Schwarzenberg, München

Bültmann B (1992) Virusnachweis im Gewebe. Verh Dtsch Ges Pathol 76:400

Bültmann BD, Klingel K, Sotlar K, Bock CT, Kandolf R (2003a) Parvovirus B19: a pathogen responsible for more than hematologic disorders. Virchows Arch 442:8–17

Bültmann BD, Klingel K, Sotlar K, Bock T, Baba HA, Sauer M, Kandolf R (2003b) Fatal parvovirus B19-associated myocarditis clinically mimicking ischemic heart disease: an endothelial cell-mediated disease. Hum Pathol 34:92–95

Burger MC, Dempers JJ, de Beer C (2014) Profiling the approach to the investigation of viral infections in cases of sudden unexpected death in infancy in the Western Cape Province, South Africa. Forensic Sci Int 239:27–30

Burgmeister G (1963) Infektiöse Myokarditis im Kindesalter. Dtsch Gesundheit 18:26

Burkhardt S, Padosch SA, Schmidt PH, Dettmeyer R, La Harpe R, Harding TW, Madea B (2005) Suspicion de syndrome de mort subite du nourisson: pathologie cardiaque congenitale meconnue avec congestion pulmonaire severe bilaterale. J Med Leg Droit Med 48:7–10

Busuttil A, Burchell A (1992) The SIDS phenomene: an update. J Clin Pathol 45:1–2

Bux R, Bratzke H, Rothschild MA, Lutz FU (2002) Plötzlicher Tod einer 12-Jährigen mit klinisch inapparenter Myokarditis unter psychischer und physischer Belastung. Rechtsmedizin 12:229–232

Buxmann H, Hamprecht K, Meyer-Wittkopf M, Friese K (2017) Primary human cytomegalovirus (HCMV) infection in pregnancy. Dtsch Ärztbl Int 114:45–52

Byard RW (2002) Unexpected death due to infectious mononucleosis. J Forensic Sci 47:202–204

Byard R, Krous H (1995) Minor inflammatory lesions and sudden infant death: cause, coincidence or epiphenomena? Pediatr Pathol Lab Med 15:649–654

Byard RW, Krous H (2001) Sudden infant death syndrome. Oxford University Press, New York

Byard RW, Bellis M (2016) Histological changes in the thyroid gland in cases of infant and early childhood asphyxia – a preliminary study. J Forensic Sci 61:674–675

Carter N, Rutty GN (2004) The maternal death. In: Rutty GN (ed) Essentials of autopsy practice: recent advances, topics and developments. Springer, London, pp 73–92

Cassinotti P, Weitz M, Siegl G (1993) Human parvovirus B19: routine diagnosis by a new nested polymerase chain reaction assay. J Med Virol 40:228–234

Castro EC, Peres LC (1999) Vocal cord basement membrane in non-sudden infant death syndrome cases. Pediatr Dev Pathol 2(5):440–445

Cecchi R, Bajanowski T, Kahl B, Wiegand P (1995) CMV-DNA detection in parenchymatous organs in cases of SIDS. Int J Legal Med 107:291–295

Cherry JD (1999) Parvovirus infections in children and adults. Adv Pediatr Infect Dis 46:245–269

Christiansen LR, Collins KA (2006) Pregnancy-associated deaths: a 15-year retrospective study and overall review of maternal pathophysiology. Am J Forensic Med Pathol 27:11–19

Cittadini F, Loyola G, Caradonna L, Minelli N, Rossi R (2014) A case of toxic shock due to clandestine abortion by misoprostol self-administration. J Forensic Sci 59:1662–1664

Cremer U, Althoff H (1991) Nachweis und Inzidenz von Zytomegalievirusinfektionen bei plötzlichen Kindstodesfällen (SIDS). Rechtsmedizin 1:25–28

Cubie HA, Duncan LA, Marshall LA (1997) Detection of respiratory syncytial virus nucleic acid in archival post mortem tissue from infants. Pediatr Pathol Lab Med 17:927–938

Cutz E, Perrin DG, Hackman R, Czegledy-Nagy EN (1996) Maternal smoking and pulmonary neuroendocrine cells in sudden infant death syndrome. Pediatrics 98:668–672

Daley AJ, Isaacs D, Dwyer DE, Gilbert GL (1998) A cluster of cases of neonatal Coxsackievirus B meningitis and myocarditis. J Paediatr Child Health 34:196–198

de la Grandmaison GL, Dorandeu A, Carton M, Patey A, Durigon M (1999) Increase of pulmonary density of macrophages in sudden infant death syndrome. Forensic Sci Int 104:179–187

De Mello DE, Heyman S, Phelps DS, Floros J (1993) Immunogold localization of SP-A in lungs of infants dying from respiratory distress syndrome. Am J Pathol 142:1631–1640

Debertin AS, Tschernig T, Schürmann A, Bajanowski T, Brinkmann B, Pabst R (2006) Coincidence of different structures of mucosa-associated lymphoid tissue (MALT) in the respiratory tract of children: no indications for enhanced mucosal immunostimulation in sudden infant death syndrome (SIDS). Clin Exp Immunol 146:54–59

deSa DJ (1986) Isolated myocarditis as a cause of sudden death in the first year of live. Forensic Sci Int 30:113–117

Dettmeyer R (2004) Plötzlicher Kindstod (sudden infant death syndrome; SIDS) – Neue Aspekte zur Bedeutung der virusbedingten Herzmuskelentzündung. Shaker-Verlag, Aachen

Dettmeyer R (2008) Virus-induced myocarditis in suspected sudden infant death syndrome. New knowledge from immunohistochemical and molecular pathological investigations. Rechtsmedizin 18:365–376

Dettmeyer RB, Kandolf R (2010) Cardiomyopathies – misdiagnosed as sudden infant death syndrome (SIDS). Forensic Sci Int 194:e21–e24

Dettmeyer R, Madea B (2002) Myokarditis durch Enteroviren in Griechenland – und bei uns? Leserbrief zum Beitrag aus Dtsch Med Wochenschr 127:1364 (2002a). Dtsch Med Wochenschr 27:2467–2468

Dettmeyer R, Madea B (2003) Commentary to the letter of Arya SC and Agarval N to our report "Fatal parvovirus B19 myocarditis in an 8-year-old boy", J Forensic Sci 2003; 48:183–186 – authors response. J Forensic Sci 48:1205

Dettmeyer R, Madea B (2004) Sudden, unexpected death related to viral myocarditis. A survey of histological, immunohistochemical, and molecularpathological methods for the postmortem diagnosis. In: Tsokos M (ed) Forensic pathology reviews, 2nd edn. Humana Press, Tatowa, pp 169–186

Dettmeyer R, Schlamann M, Madea B (1999a) Immunohistochemical techniques improve the diagnosis of myocarditis in cases of suspected sudden infant death syndrome (SIDS). Forensic Sci Int 105:83–94

Dettmeyer R, Schlamman M, Madea B (1999b) Myokarditisdiagnostik bei SIDS-Verdacht. Klin Padiatr 211:456–458

Dettmeyer R, Baasner A, Winkelmann S, Greabe M, Madea B (2001a) Myocarditis and sudden death in infancy – immunohistochemical and moelcularpathological investigations. J Perinat Med 29(Suppl II):25

Dettmeyer R, Kandolf R, Schmidt P, Schlamann M, Madea B (2001b) Lympho-monocytic enteroviral myocarditis: traditional, immunohistological and molecularpathological methods for diagnosis in a case of suspected sudden infant death syndrome (SIDS). Forensic Sci Int 119:141–144

Dettmeyer R, Baasner A, Schlamann M, Haag C, Madea B (2002) Coxsackie B3 myocarditis in 4 cases of suspected sudden infant death syndrome: diagnosis by immunohistochemical and molecular-pathologic investigations. Pathol Res Pract 198:689–696

Dettmeyer R, Kandolf R, Baasner A, Banaschak S, Eis-Hübinger AM, Madea B (2003) Fatal parvovirus B19 myocarditis in an 8-year-old boy. J Forensic Sci 48:183–186

Dettmeyer R, Baasner A, Schlamann M, Padosch SA, Haag C, Kandolf R, Madea B (2004a) Role of virus-induced myocardial affections in sudden infant death syndrome (SIDS): a prospective postmortem study. Pediatr Res 55:947–952

Dettmeyer R, Padosch SA, Baasner A, Madea B (2004b) PCR-based diagnosis of adenovirus and Epstein-Barr virus in paraffin-embedded heart tissue. In: Doutremépuich C, Morling N (eds) Progress in forensic genetics 10. Proceedings of the 20th international ISFG congress, Arcachon, 9–13 September 2003. International congress series 1261, pp 605–607

Dettmeyer R, Müller J, Letzner J, Madea B (2005) Histologische und immunhistochemische Untersuchungen zur Inzidenz interstitieller Pneumonien bei mutmaßlichem Plötzlichen Kindstod – Sudden Infant Death Syndrome (SIDS). In: 14th spring meeting, German Society of Forensic Medicine – Northern Region, Bremen, 20–21 May 2005

Dettmeyer R, Müller J, Poster S, Madea B (2006a) PCR-based diagnosis of cytomegaloviruses in paraffin-embedded heart tissues in cases of suspected sudden infant death syndrome (SIDS). In: Progress in forensic genetics 11. Proceedings of the 21st international ISFG congress, Ponta Delgada, 2006. International congress series, vol 1288, pp 771–773

Dettmeyer R, Padosch SA, Madea B (2006b) Lethal enterovirus-induced myocarditis and pancreatitis in a 4-month-old boy. Forensic Sci Int 156:51–54

Dettmeyer R, Strehler M, Winkelmann S, Madea B (2006c) Myokarditis. Rechtsmedizin 16:138–142

Dettmeyer R, Winkelmann S, Letzner J, Müller J, Madea B (2006d) Immunohistochemical and molecular pathological diagnosis of myocarditis and pneumonia – investigations of 121 cases of suspected sudden infant death syndrome (SIDS). In: 20th congress of international academy of legal medicine, Budapest, 23–26 Aug 2006

Dettmeyer R, Sperhake JP, Müller J, Madea B (2008) Cytomegalovirus-induced pneumonia and myocarditis in three cases of suspected sudden infant death syndrome (SIDS): Diagnosis by immunohistochemical techniques and molecularpathologic methods. Forensic Sci Int 174:229–233

Dettmeyer R, Baasner A, Haag C, Bruch S, Schlamann M (2009a) Immunohistochemical and molecular-pathological diagnosis of myocarditis in cases of suspected sudden infant death syndrome (SIDS) – a multicenter study. Legal Med 11:S124–S127

Dettmeyer R, Bruch S, Haag C (2009b) Letter to the. Pediatr Res 66:714

Dettmeyer R, Baasner A, Haag C, Schlamann M (2016) Letter to the editor: Gaaloul et al., Postmortem diagnosis of infectious heart diseases: a mystifying cause of Sudden Infant Death. Forensic Sci Int 267:e18

Dettmeyer R (2016) Postmortem diagnostics of a (post-) viral myocarditis in putative sudden infant death syndrome. Case report for avoidance of errors in the diagnostics. Rechtsmedizin 26:514–519

D'Errico S, Neri M, Riezzo I, Rossi G, Pomara C, Turillazzi E, Fineschi V (2008) ß-Tryptase and quantitative mast-cell increase in a sudden infant death following hexavalent immunization. Forensic Sci Int 179:e25–e29

Doi M, Tanno K, Obashi N, Aita K, Oikawa MS (2000) The lung pathology of the sudden infant death syndrome. J Pediatr Pract 63:361–365. (in Japanese)

Douglas AS, Gupta R, Helms PJ, Jolliffe IT (1997) Months of birth as an independent variable in sudden infant death syndrome. Paediatr Perinat Epidemiol 11:57–66

Douglas AS, Helm PJ, Jolliffe IT (1998a) Seasonality of sudden infant death syndrome in mainland Britain und Ireland 1985–95. Arch Dis Child 79:269–270

Douglas AS, Helms PJ, Jolliffe IT (1998b) Seasonality of sudden infant death syndrome (SIDS) by age at death. Acta Paediatr 87:1033–1038

Druyts-Voets E, Van Renterghem L, Gerniers S (1993) Epidemiology. Coxsackie B virus epidemiology and neonatal infection in Belgium. J Infect Dis 27:311–316

Dudorkinowa D, Bouska I (1993) Histochemistry of the atrioventricular conducting system during postnatal development. Pediatr Pathol 13:191–201

Entrup M, Brinkmann B (1990a) Histologische Lungenbefunde beim plötzlichen Kindstod. Z Rechtsmed 103:425–433

Entrup M, Brinkmann B (1990b) Histologische Untersuchungen des lymphatischen Gewebes beim plötzlichen Kindstod. Z Rechtsmed 103:415–424

Fairley CK, Ryan M, Wall PG, Weinberg J (1996) The organisms reported to cause infective myocarditis and pericarditis in England and Wales. J Infect 32:223–225

Ferris JAJ (1973) Hypoxic changes in conducting tissue of the heart in sudden infant death syndrome. Br Med J 2:23–25

Ferris JAJ, Aherne WA, Locke WS, McQuillan J, Gardner PS (1973) Sudden and unexpected death in infancy: histology and virology. Br Med J 2:439–442

Fineschi V, Baroldi G, Silver MD (2006) Pathology of the heart and sudden death in forensic medicine. CRC Taylor & Francis, Boca Raton, pp 248–251

Fitzgerald K (2001) The "reduced risk" campaign, SIDS international. The Global Strategy Task Force and the European Society of the study and prevention of infant death. In: Byard RW, Krous HF (eds) Sudden infant death syndrome. Arnold, London, pp 310–318

Forcada P, Beigelman J, Milei J (1996) Inapparent myocarditis and sudden death in pediatrics. Diagnosis by immunohistochemical staining. Int J Cardiol 56:93–97

Forsyth KD (1999) Immune and inflammatory responses in sudden infant death syndrome. FEMS Immunol Med Microbiol 25:79–83

Forsyth KD, Weeks SC, Kohl HL, Skinner J, Bradley J (1989) Lung immunoglobulins in the sudden infant death syndrome. Br Med J 298:23–26

Foulis AK, Farquharson MA, Cameron SO, McGill M, Schonke H, Kandolf R (1990) A search for the presence of the enteroviral capsid protein VP1 in pancreases of patients wih type 1 (insulin-dependent) diabetes and pancreases and hearts of infants who died of coxsackieviral myocarditis. Diabetologia 33:290–298

Fracasso T, Karger B, Vennemann M, Bajanowski T, Golla-Schindler UM, Pfeiffer H (2010) Amniotic fluid aspiration in cases of SIDS. Int J Legal Med 124:113–117

Freitag L, von Kaisenberg C, Kreipe HH, Hussein K (2014) Evaluation of intrauterine death. Importance of examination of fetal, placental and maternal factors. Pathologe 35:77–82

Freund MW, Kleinveld G, Krediet TG, von Loon AM, Verboon-Maciolek MA (2010) Prognosis for neonates with enterovirus myocarditis. Arch Dis Child Fetal Neonatal Ed 95:F206–F212

Fried K, Beer S, Vure E, Algom M, Shapira Y (1979) Autosomal recessive sudden unexpected death in children probably caused by a cardiomyopathy associated with myopathy. J Med Genet 16:341–346

Friedman RA, Moak JP, Garson A Jr (1991) Clinical course of idiopathic dilated cardiomyopathy in children. J Am Coll Cardiol 18:157–158

Fu C, Jasani B, Vujanic GM, Leadbatter S, Berry PJ, Knight BH (1994) The immunocytochemical demonstration of a relative lack of nerve fibres in the atrioventricular node and bundle of His in the sudden infant death syndrome (SIDS). Forensic Sci Int 66:175–185

Funayama M, Kageyama N, Ohtani S, Tokudome S, Tabata N, Morita M (1994) An immunohistochemical study on pulmonary surfactant of infants diagnosed as sudden infant death syndrome. Jpn J Legal Med 48:225–230

Gaaloul I, Riabi S, Evans M, Hunter T, Huber S, Aouni M (2016a) Postmortem diagnosis of infectious heart

diseases: a mystifying cause of sudden infant death. Forensic Sci Int 262:166–172
Gaaloul I, Riabi S, Evans M, Hunter T, Huber S, Aouni M (2016b) Coxsackievirus B heart infections and their putative contribution to sudden unexpected death: an 8-year review of patients and victims in the coastal region of Tunisia. Forensic Sci Int 268:73–80
Garstang J, Ellis C, Sidebotham P (2015) An evidence-based guide to the investigation of sudden unexpected death in infancy. Forensic Sci Med Pathol 11:345–357
Gold E, Carver DH, Heineberg H, Adelson L, Robbins FC (1961) Viral infection. A possible cause of sudden unexpected death in infants. N Engl J Med 264:53–60
Gould SJ, Isaacson PG (1993) Bronchus-associated lymphoid tissue (BALT) in human fetal and infant lung. J Pathol 169:229–234
Gray ES, Hauptmann S, Dietel M, Sobrinho-Simoes M (eds) (2001) Surgical pathology. update 2001. In: 18th European congress of pathology. Acquired myocardial disease as a cause of death in neonates and infants, Berlin, 2001. ABW Wissenschaftsverlag GmbH, pp 529–530
Guilleminault C (1988) SIDS, near miss SIDS and cardiac arrythmia. Ann N Y Acad Sci 533:358–367
Guntheroth WG, Spiers PS, Naeye R (1994) Redefinition of the sudden infant death syndrome: the disadvantages. Pediatr Pathol 14:127–132
Gurudut KS, Gouda HS, Aramani SC, Patil RH (2011) Spontaneous rupture of unscarred gravid uterus. J Forensic Sci 56:S263–S265
Haddad J, Gut J, Wendling M, Struc D, Jernite M, Obert G, Messer J (1993) Enterovirus infections in neonates. A retrospective study of 21 cases. Eur J Med 2:209–214
Hagan LL, Goetz DW, Revercomb CH, Garriott J (1998) Sudden infant death syndrome: a search for allergen hypersensitivity. Ann Allergy Asthma Immunol 80:227–231
Harris LC, Rodin AE, Nghiem QX (1968) Idiopathic, nonobstructive cardiomyopathy in children. Am J Cardiol 21:153–165
Harrison LM, Morris A, Telford DR, Brown SM, Jones K (1999) The nasopharyngeal bacterial flora in infancy: effects of age, gender, season, viral upper respiratory tract infection and sleeping position. FEMS Immunol Med Microbiol 25:19–28
Hayes MA, Russell RG, Babiuk LA (1979) Sudden death in young dogs with myocarditis caused by parvovirus. J Am Vet Med Assoc 174:1197–1203
Hebert MM, Yu C, Towbin JA, Rogers BB (1995) Fatal Epstein-Barr virus myocarditis in a child with repetitive myocarditis. Pediatr Pathol Lab Med 15:805–812
Henson D, Mufson MA (1971) Myocarditis and pneumonitis with type 21 adenovirus infection. Association with fatal myocarditis and pneumonitis. Am J Dis Child 121:334–336
Hebold K, Saternus KS, Schleicher A (1986) Morphometric studies on the vertebral arteries in infants. Z Rechtsmed 97:41–48
Herbst JJ, Book LS, Bray PF (1978) Gastroesophageal reflux in the "near-miss" sudden infant death syndrome. J Pediatr 92:73–75
Herbst J, Winskog C, Byard RW (2010) Cardiovascular conditions and the evaluation of the heart in pregnancy-associated autopsies. J Forensic Sci 55: 1528–1533
Heusch A, Kühl U, Rammos S, Krogmann ON, Schultheiss HP, Bourgeois M (1996) Complete AV-block in two children with immunohistological proven myocarditis. Eur J Pediatr 155:633–636
Hiller AS, Kracke A, Tschernig T, Kasper M, Kleemann WJ, Tröger HD (1997) Comparison of the immunohistology of mucosa-associated lymphoid tissue in the larynx and lungs in cases of sudden infant death and controls. Int J Legal Med 110:316–322
Hood I, Ryan D, Spitz WU (1988) Resuscitation and petechiae. Am J Forensic Med Pathol 9:35–37
Hoppenbrouwers T, Calub M, Arakawa K, Hodgman JE (1981) Seasonal relationship of sudden infant death syndrome and environmental pollutants. Am J Epidemiol 113:623–635
Ino T, Kishiro M, Okubo M, Akimoto K, Nishimoto K, Yabuta K, Okada R (1997) Late, persistent expressions of ICAM-1 and VCAM-1 on myocardial tissue in children with lymphocytic myocarditis. Cardiovasc Res 34:323–328
Ismail-Beigi F, Horton PF, Pope CE (1970) Histological consequences of gastroesophageal reflux in man. Gastroenterology 58:163–174
Jacob B, Haarhoff K, Neuen-Jacob E, Burring KF, Frenzel H, Rammos S, Bonte W (1989) Unexpected infant death attributed to cardiac tumor or cardiomyopathy. Z Rechtsmed 103:335–343
Jänisch S, Germerott T, Bange FC, Schmidt A, Debertin AS (2009) Postnatal sepsis due to group A Streptococcus in a mother and her newborn. Arch Kriminol 224:93–100
Jänisch S, Schmidt A, Günther D, Fieguth A, Debertin AS (2010) Plazentabefunde bei perinatalen Todesfällen. Arch Kriminol 225:159–166
Jankus A (1976) The cardiac conduction system in sudden infant death syndrome: a report of three cases. Pathology 8:275–280
Janssen W (1997) Forensische histopathologie. Schmidt-Römhild, Lübeck
Jensen LL, Rohde MC, Banner J, Byard RW (2012) Reclassification of SIDS cases – a need for adjustment of the San Diego classification? Int J Legal Med 126:271–277
Johnstone JM, Lawy HS (1966) Role of infection in cot deaths. Br Med J 1:706–709
Jones AM, Weston JT (1976) The examination of the sudden infant death syndrome infant: investigative and autopsy protocols. J Forensic Sci 21:833–841
Jordán I, Esteva C, Esteban E, Noguera A, Garcia JJ, Muñoz-Almagro C (2009) Severe enterovirus disease in febrile neonates. Enferm Infecc Microbiol Clin 27:399–402

Kandolf R (1995) Molekulare Pathogenese der Enterovirusmyokarditis. Viruspersistenz und chronische Entzündung. Internist 36:438
Kandolf R, Klingel K, Zell R, Canu A, Fortmuller U, Hohenadl C et al (1993) Molecular mechanisms in the pathogenesis of enteroviral heart disease: acute and persistent infections. Clin Immunol Immunopathol 68:153–158
Kanter RJ, Gravatt A, Bharati S (1997) Pathological findings following sudden death in an infant with hypertrophic cardiomyopathy and supraventricular tachycardia. J Cardiovasc Electrophysiol 8:222–225
Kaplan M (1983) Coxsackie virus infections in infants younger than three months. Rev Infect Dis 5(6):1019–1032
Karger B, Fracasso T, Brinkmann B, Bajanowski T (2004) Evaluation of the Reid index in infants and cases of SIDS. Int J Legal Med 118:221–223
Kariks J (1988) Cardiac lesions in sudden infant death syndrome. Forensic Sci Int 39:211–225
Kariks J (1992) Myocardial lesions in SIDS. Med J Aust 156:741
Kenton AB, Sanchez X, Coveler KJ, Kavar KA, Jiminez S, Ichida F, Murphy RT, Elliott PM, McKenna W, Bowles KR et al (2004) Isolated left ventricular noncompaction is rarely caused by mutations in G4.5, alpha-dystrobrevin and FK Binding Protein-12. Mol Genet Metab 82(2):162–166
Kinney HC, Rognum TO, Nattie EE, Haddad GG, Hyma B, McEntire B, Paterson DS, Crandall L, Byard RW (2012) Sudden and unexpected death in early life: proceedings of a symposium in honor of Dr. Henry F. Krous. Forensic Sci Med Pathol 8:414–425
Kleemann WJ (1997) Intrathorakale und subkonjunktivale Petechien bei Säuglingstodesfällen. Z Rechtsmed 7:139–146
Kleemann WJ, Schuk M, Verhagen W, Burutha U, Tröger HD (1988) Influenza-Todesfälle beim plötzlichen Kindstod. Zentralbl Rechtsmed 31:882–883
Kleemann WJ, Schlaud M, Poets C, Rothämel T, Tröger HD (1996) Hyperthermia in sudden infant death. Int J Legal Med 109:139–142
Klein RM, Vester EG, Perings C, Strauer BE (1995) Arrhythmien bei myokarditis. Internist 36:458–468
Klensang U, Hagemann S, Saeger W, Bajanowski T, Freislederer A (1997) Morphology, immunohistochemistry and morphometry of pancreatic islets in cases of sudden infant death syndrome. Int J Legal Med 110:199–203
Klingel K, Kandolf R (2008) Virale Myokarditis im Kindesalter. Stellenwert der modernen kardiopathologischen Diagnostik. Rechtsmedizin 18:349–358
Klingel K, Albrecht M, Canu A, Hofschneider PH, Kandolf R (1992a) Molekulare Pathogenese der Myokarditis: Viruspersistenz und chronische Herzmuskelentzündung. Verh Dtsch Ges Pathol 76:394
Klingel K, Hohenadl C, Canu A, Albrecht M, Seemann M, Mall G et al (1992b) Ongoing enterovirus-induced myocarditis is associated with persistent heart muscle infection: quantitative analysis of virus replication, tissue damage, and inflammation. Proc Natl Acad Sci U S A 89:314–318
Klingel K, Rieger P, Selinka HC, Zell R, Kandolf R (1994) Nachweis virusinduzierter zytopathogener Effekte bei der enteroviralen Myokarditis durch elektronenmikroskopische in situ Hybridisierung. Verh Dtsch Ges Pathol 78:469
Klingel K, Selinka HC, Huber M, Sauer M, Leube M, Kandolf R (2000) Molecular pathology and structural features of enteroviral replication. Towards understanding the pathogenesis of viral heart disease. Heart 25:216–220
Klump WM, Bergmann I, Muller BC, Ameis D, Kandolf R (1990) Complete nucleotide sequence of infectious Coxsackievirus B3 cDNA: two initial 5`uridine residues are regained during plus-strand RNA syntheses. J Virol 64:1573–1583
Kopp N, Chigr F, Denoroy L, Gilly R, Jordan D (1993) Absence of adrenergic neurons in nucleus tractus solitarius in sudden infant death syndrome. Neuropediatrics 24:25–59
Kozakewich HPW, McManus BM, Vawter GF (1982) The sinus node in sudden infant death syndrome. Circulation 65:1242–1246
Krous HF (1984) The microscopic distribution of intrathoracic petechiae in sudden infant death syndrome. Arch Pathol Lab Med 108:77–79
Krous HF, Beckwith JB, Byard RW, Rognum TO, Bajanowski T, Corey T, Cutz E, Hanzlick R, Keens TG, Mitchell EA (2004) Sudden infant death syndrome and unclassified sudden infant deaths: a definitonal and diagnostic approach. Pediatrics 114:234–238
Krous HF, Ferandos C, Masoumi H, Arnold J, Haas EA, Stanley C, Crossfeld PD (2009) Myocardial inflammation, cellular death, and viral detection in sudden infant death, caused by SIDS, suffocation, or myocarditis. Pediatr Res 66:17–21
Kühl U, Pauschinger M, Bock T, Klingel K, Schwimmbeck CPL, Seeberg B, Krautwurm L, Poller W, Schultheiss HP, Kandolf R (2003) Parvovirus B19 infection mimicking acute myocardial infarction. Circulation 108:945–950
Kuroki Y, Dempo K, Akino T (1986) Immunohistochemical study of human pulmonary surfactant apoproteins with monoclonal antibodies. Pathologic application for hyaline membrane disease. Am J Pathol 124:25–33
Kytö V, Vuorinen T, Saukko P, Lautenschlager I, Lignitz E, Saraste A, Voipio-Pulkki LM (2005) Cytomegalovirus infection of the heart is common in patients with fatal myocarditis. Clin Infect Dis 40:683–688
la Grange H, Verster J, Dempers JJ, de Beer C (2014) Review of immunological and virological aspects as contributory factors in sudden unexpected death in infancy (SUDI). Forensic Sci Int 245:12–16
Lapin CA, Morrow G, Chvapil M, Belke DP, Fisher RS (1976) Heptic trace elements in the sudden infant death syndrome. J Pediatr 89:607–608
Lau G (1994) Amniotic fluid embolism as a cause of sudden maternal death. Med Sci Law 34:213–220

Lavezzi WA, McKenna BJ, Wolf BC (2004) The significance of pulmonary interstitial emphysema in live birth determination. J Forensic Sci 49:546–552
Lazda EJ, Batchelor WH, Cox PM (2000) Immunohistochemical detection of myocardial necrosis in stillbirth and neonatal death. Pediatr Dev Pathol 3(1):40–47
Leape LL, Holder TM, Franklin JD, Amoury RA, Ashcraft KW (1977) Respiratory arrest in infants secondary to gastroesophageal reflux. Pediatrics 60:924–928
Lemke R, Schäfer AT (1992) Histochemischer Immunglobulinnachweis bei plötzlichen Säuglingstodesfällen (SIDS). Pathologe 13:252–254
Lenghaus C, Studdert MJ, Finnie JW (1980) Acute and chronic canine parvovirus myocarditis following intrauterine innoculation. Vet J 56:465–468
Lewis AB, Neustein HB, Takahashi M, Lurie PR (1985) Findings on endomyocardial biopsy in infants and children with dilated cardiomyopathy. Am J Cardiol 55:143–145
Lie JT, Rosenberg HS, Erickson EE (1976) Histopathology of the conduction system in the sudden infant death syndrome. Circulation 53:3–8
Loewe C, Dragovic LJ (1998) Acute coronary artery thrombosis in a postpartum woman receiving bromocriptine. Applicatin of biotinylated CMV-DNA probes on paraffin-embedded specimens. Am J Forensic Med Pathol 19:258–260
Löning T, Milde K, Foss HD (1986) In situ hybridization for the detection of cytomegalovirus (CMV) infection. Virch Arch A Pathol Anat Histopathol 409:777–790
Ludwig J (1969) Sudden unexpected unexplained death in infants. Virch Arch A Path Anat 346:287–301
Lunetta P, Penttilä A (1996) Immunohistochemical identification of syncytiotrophoblastic cells and megakaryocytes in pulmonary vessels in a fatal case of amniotic fluid embolism. Int J Legal Med 108:210–214
Mall G (1995) Morphologie der Myocarditis. Internist 36:426–429
Manoukian AA, Ha CE, Seaver LH, Bhagavan NV (2009) A neonatal death due to medium-chain acyl-CoA dehydrogenase deficieny. Am J For Med Pathol 30:284–286
Maron BJ, Fisher RS (1977) Sudden infant death syndrome (SIDS): cardiac pathologic observations in infants with SIDS. Am Heart J 93:762–766
Martin AB, Webber S, Fricker FJ, Jaffe R, Demmler G, Kearney D et al (1994) Acute myocarditis: rapid diagnosis by PCR in children. Circulation 90:330–339
Matturri L, Ottaviani G, Ramos SG, Rossi L (2000) Sudden infant death syndrome (SIDS): a study of cardiac conduction system. Cardiovasc Pathol 9:147–148
McManus BM, Chow LH, Wilson JE, Anderson DR, Gulizia JM, Gauntt CJ, Klingel KE, Beisel KW, Kandolf R (1993) Direct myocardial injury by enterovirus: a central role in the evolution of murine myocarditis. Clin Immunol Immunopathol 68:159–169
Melinte PR, Dragoi GS, Dinca I, Patrascu E (2015) Placenta – the "black box" for the evolution of gestation and evidence in forensic expertise of pregnancy. Rom J Leg Med 23:269–274
Mertens T, Hager H, Eggers HJ (1982) Epidemiology of an outbreak in a maternity unit of infections with an antigenic variant of Echovirus 11. J Med Virol 9:81–91
Miller R, Ward C, Amsterdam E (1973) Focal mononucleosis myocarditis simulating myocardial infarction. Chest 63:102–105
Mirchandani HG, Michandani IH, Parikh SR (1988) Hypernatremia due to amniotic fluid embolism during a saline-induced abortion. Am J Forensic Med Pathol 9:48–50
Missliwetz J, Reiter CH, Zoder G (1986) Periventrikuläre fettige Metamorphose der Neuroglia – Ein morphologisches Substrat beim SIDS. Z Rechtsmed 96:173–182
Modlin JF (1988) Perinatal echovirus and group B coxsackievirus infections. Clin Perinatol 15:233–246
Molz G, Hartmann HP, Michels L (1985) Plötzlicher Kindstod: Histologische Befunde in den Kopfspeicheldrüsen. Pathologe 6:8–12
Moon RY, Horne RSC, Hauck FR (2007) Sudden infant death syndrome. Lancet 370:1578–1587
Moral GL, Rubio-Calduch EM, Broto-Escapa P, Caballero-Requero E, Calico-Bosch I, Bertran-Sangues JM (1993) Enteroviral infections in children: clinical and epidemiological findings in 530 patients (1984–1991). An Esp Pediatr 39:521–527
Morens DM (1978) Enteroviral disease in early infancy. J Pediatr 92:374–377
Morey AL, Keeling JW, Porter HJ et al (1992) Clinical and histopathological features of parvovirus B 19 infection in the human fetus. Br J Obstet Gynaecol 99:566–574
Morita M, Tabata N, Maya A (1985) Studies on asphyxia: on the changes of the alveolar walls of rats in the hypoxic state. Forensic Sci Int 27:81–92
Mounts AW, Amr S, Jamshidi R, Graves C, Dwyer D, Guarner J, Dawson JE, Oberstse MS, Parashar U, Spevak P, Alexander J (2001) A cluster of fulminant myocarditis cases in children, Baltimore, Maryland, 1997. Pediatr Cardiol 22:34–39
Müller G (1963) Der plötzliche Kindstod. Thieme, Stuttgart
Müller E, Rämsch R (1966) Schilddrüsenbefunde bei Tot- und Neugeborenen. Frankf Z Pathol 75:425–431
Muller G, Ulmer HE, Hagel KJ, Wolf D (1995) Cardiac dysrhythmias in children with idiopathic dilated or hypertrophic cardiomyopathy. Pediatr Cardiol 16:56–60
Nathan M, Walsh R, Hardin JT, Einzig S, Connor BO, Balaguru D, Verma R, Starr JP (2008) Enteroviral sepsis and ischemic cardiomyopathy in a neonate: case report and review of literature. ASAIO J 54:554–555
Noren GR, Stanley NA, Bandt CM, Kaplan EL (1975) Occurrence of myocarditis in sudden death in children. J Forensic Sci 22:188–196
Oehmichen M, Linke P, Zilles K, Saternus KS (1989) Reactive astrocytes and macrophages in the brain stem of SIDS victims? Eleven age- and sex-matched SIDS and control cases. Clin Neuropathol 8:276–283
Oehmichen M, Theuerkauf I, Bajanowski T, Merz H, Meissner C (1998) Enhanced reactivity of Alz-50 antibody in brains of sudden infant death syndrome victims versus brains with lethal hypoxic/ischemic

injury. Diagnostic significance after applications of the ImmunoMax technique on routine paraffin material. Acta Neuropathol 95:280–286
Ogbuihi S, Zink P (1987) Lungengerüstveränderungen beim plötzlichen Kindestod. Z Rechtsmed 98:191–205
Ogbuihi S, Zink P (1988) Über Veränderungen des Mengenverhältnisses von Kollagen Typ I und III im interlobulären Lungeninterstitium beim plötzlichen Kindstod – eine Pilotstudie. Z Rechtsmed 101:247–254
Ogbuihi S, Zink P (1989) Zelluläre Komponenten im Lungeninterstitium beim plötzlichen Kindstod immunhistochemische Charakterisierung. Z Rechtsmed 102:133–142
Opdal SH, Rognum TO (2011) Gene variants predisposing to SIDS: current knowledge. Forensic Sci Med Pathol 7:26–36
Ortmann C, Pfeiffer H, Brinkmann B (2000) A comparative study on the immunohistochemical detection of early myocardial damage. Int J Legal Med 113:215–220
Oyer CE, Ongeapin EH, Ni J, Bowles NE, Towbin JA (2000) Fatal intrauterine adenoviral endomyocarditis with aortic and pulmonary valve stenosis: diagnosis by polymerase chain reaction. Hum Pathol 31:1433–1435
Parham DM, Cheng R, Schutze GE, Dilday B, Nelson R, Erickson S, Kokes C, Peretti F, Sturner WQ (1998) Enzyme-linked immunoassay for respiratory syncytial virus is not predictive of bronchiolitis in sudden infant death syndrome. Pediatr Dev Pathol 1:375–379
Pattison CP, Marshall BJ (1997) Proposed link between *Helicobacter pylori* and sudden infant death syndrome. Med Hypotheses 49:365–369
Paz Suárez-Mier M, Aguilera B (1998) Histopathology of the conduction system in sudden infant death. Forensic Sci Int 93:143–154
Pérez-Platz U, Saeger W, Dhom G, Bajanowski T (1994) The pathology of the adrenal glands in sudden infant death syndrome. Int J Legal Med 106:244–248
Philipps CA, Aronson MD, Tomkow J, Philipps ME (1980) Enteroviruses in Vermont 1969–1978: an important cause of illness throughout the year. J Infect Dis 141:162–164
Püschel K, Hashimoto Y, Löning T, Lignitz E (1988) Cytomegalie der Kopfspeicheldrüsen bei SIDS. Z Rechtsmed 99:281–289
Pucci A, Zanini C, Ferreo F, Arisio R, Valori A, Abbruzzese P, Forni M (2003) Misalignment of lung vessels: diagnostic role of conventional histology and immunohistochemistry. Virchows Arch 442: 597–600
Quan L, Zhu BL, Ishida K, Taniguchi M, Oritani S, Kamikodai Y, Fujita MQ, Maeda H (2000) Sudden infant death attributed to peracute pulmonary infection: two autopsy cases. Legal Med 2:79–83
Raie RM, Smith H (1981) Trace elements deficiency and cot deaths. Med Sci Law 21:41–46
Rajs J, Hammarquist F (1988) Sudden infant death in Stockholm. Acta Paediatr Scand 77:812–820
Rambaud C, Cieuta C, Canioni D, Rouzioux C, Lavaud J, Hubert P, Brousse N, Rudle M, Chéron G (1992) Cot death and myocarditis. Cardiol Young 2:266–271
Randall B, Donelan K, Koponen M, Sens MA, Krous HF (2012) Application of a classification system focusing on potential asphyxia for cases of sudden unexpected infant death. Forensic Sci Med Pathol 8:34–39
Rasten-Almqvist P, Eksborg S, Rajs J (2000) Heart weight in infants – a comparison between sudden death syndrome and other causes of death. Acta Paediatr 89(9):1062–1067
Rasten-Almqvist P, Eksborg S, Rajs J (2002) Myocarditis and sudden infant death syndrome. APMIS 110:469–480
Raven C, Maverakis NH, Eveland WC, Ackermann WW (1978) The sudden infant death syndrome made possible hypersensitivity reaction determined by distribution of IgG in lungs. J Forensic Sci 23:116–128
Ray C, Beckwith JB, Hebestreit NM, Bergham AB (1970) Studies of the sudden infant death syndrome in King County. Washington. I. The role of viruses. JAMA 211:619–623
Reid JD, Hajdu SI, Attah E (1968) Infantile cardiomyopathy: a previously unrecognized type with histiocytoid reaction. J Pediatr 73:335–339
Reuss W, Saeger W, Bajanowski T (1994) Morphological and immunohistochemical studies of the pituitary in sudden infant death syndrome. Int J Legal Med 106:249–253
Risse M, Weiler G (1984) Histologische Schilddrüsenbefunde beim Neugeborenen und Säugling unter besonderer Berücksichtigung des plötzlichen Säuglingstodes. Z Rechtsmed 92:205–213
Risse M, Weiler G (1987a) Hämosiderinbefunde in Leber, Milz und Lunge bei Neugeborenen und Säuglingen. Z Rechtsmed 98:181–190
Risse M, Weiler G (1987b) Spontaneous dissecting coronary arterial aneurysm as a rare cause of postpartum maternal death. Z Rechtsmed 99:143–150
Risse M, Weiler G (1989a) Histologische Befunde der Speiseröhre im Säuglingsalter. Ein Beitrag zur Frage des gastro-oesophagealen Refluxes beim plötzlichen Kindstod. Z Rechtsmed 102:521–530
Risse M, Weiler G (1989b) Vergleichende histologische Untersuchungen zur Genese petechialer Thymusblutungen. Z Rechtsmed 102:33–40
Risse M, Weiler G (1990a) Altersabhängige morphologische Schilddrüsenbefunde beim plötzlichen Kindstod. Z Rechtsmed 103:507–512
Risse M, Weiler G (1990b) Reanimationsmaßnahmen und petechiale Thymus-Blutungen beim plötzlichen Kindstod. Z Rechtsmed 103:207–212
Risse M, Weiler G (1997) Quantitative myokardiale Mastzellbefunde bei Säuglingen und Kleinkindern zur Ermittlung altersabhängiger Normwerte und als Grundlage differentialdiagnostischer Überlegungen. Rechtsmedizin 7:49–72
Risse M, Weiler G, Benker G (1986) Vergleichende histologische und hormonelle Untersuchungen der Schilddrüse unter besonderer Berücksichtigung

des plötzlichen Kindstodes (SIDS). Z Rechtsmed 96:31–38
Risse M, Weiler G, Glanz H, Dreyer TH (1997) Histomorphologic studies of the glottic region to elucidate the pathogenesis and functional significance of fibrinoid vocal cord lesions in infants and young children. Int J Pediatr Otorhinolaryngol 42:125–134
Rognum TO (2004) New SIDS definition presented at the conference. Scand J Forensic Sci 2:25–56
Rognum TO, Arnestad M, Bajanowski T et al (2003) Consensus on diagnostic criteria for the exclusion of SIDS. Scand J Forensic Sci 9:62–73
Roivainen M, Rasilainen S, Ylipaasto P, Nissinen R, Ustinov J, Bouwens L, Eizirik D, Hovi T, Otonkoski T (1995) Mechanisms of coxsackievirus-induced damage to human pancreatic-cells. J Clin Endocrinol Metab 85:432–440
Rothfuchs D, Saeger W, Bajanowski T, Freislederer A (1995) Morphology, immunohistochemistry and morphometry of the thyroid gland in cases of sudden infant death syndrome (SIDS). Int J Legal Med 107:187–192
Saffitz JE, Ferrans VJ, Rodriguez ER, Lewis FR, Roberts WC (1980) Histiocytoid cardiomyopathy: a cause of sudden death in apparently healthy infants. Am J Cardiol 52:215–217
Sagreiya K, Emery JL (1970) Perinatal thyroid discharge. A histological study of 1225 infant thyroids. Arch Dis Child 45:746–754
Sarioglu N, Turowski G (2015) Obduktion von Kindern, Neonaten, Feten und Embryonen. Vorbereitung, Präparation und Berichterstellung. Pathologe 36:343–354
Sasse-Klaassen S, Probst S, Gerull B, Oechslin E, Nurnberg P, Heuser A, Jenni R, Hennies HC, Thierfelder L (2004) Novel gene locus for autosomal dominant left ventricular noncompaction maps to chromosome 11p15. Circulation 109:2720–2723
Saternus KS, Adam G (1985) Sudden death in children: post-mortem flow measurements in the large neck vessels to demonstrate position-dependent hypoxaemia. Dtsch Med Wschr 110:297–303
Saternus KS, Hebold K (1986) Zum Stellenwert geburtstraumatischer Schädigungen der Arteria vertebralis beim plötzlichen Kindstod. Beitr Gerichtl Med XLIV:569–571
Sawaguchi T, Kato I, Franco P, Sottiaux M, Kadhim H, Shimizu S, Groswasser J, Togari H, Kobayashi M, Nishida H, Sawaguchi A, Kahn A (2005) Apnea, glial apoptosis and neuronal plasticity in the arousal pathway of victims of SIDS. Forensic Sci Int 149:205–217
Schmaltz AA (2004) Inflammatorische Kardiomyopathie – chronische Myokarditis. Monatsschr Kinderheilkd 152:632–638
Schmaltz AA, Kreuder J (1999) Kardiomyopathien im Kindesalter. Pädiat Prax 56:601–611
Schwartz ML, Cox GF, Lin AE, Korson MS, Perez-Atayde A, Lacro RV, Lishultz SE (1996) Clinical approach to genetic cardiomyopathy in children. Circulation 94:2021–2038
Seifert G (1961) Zur Pathologie der Virusmyokarditis (insbes. durch Coxsackie-Viren) im Säuglings- und Kindesalter. Zentralbl Allg Pathol Anat 102:274
Seko Y, Tsuchimochi H, Nakamura T, Okumura K, Naito S, Imatako K (1990) Expression of major histocompatibility complex class I antigen in murine ventricular myocytes infected with Coxsackievirus B3. Circ Res 67:360–367
Shanes JG, Ghali J, Billingham ME, Ferrans VJ, Fenoglio JJ, Edwards WD, Tsai CC, Saffitz JE, Isner J, Furner S (1987) Interobserver variability in the pathologic interpretation of endomyocardial biopsy results. Circulation 75:401–405
Shatz A, Hiss J, Arensburg B (1991) Basement-membrane thickening of the vocal cords in sudden infant death syndrome. Laryngoscope 101:484–486
Shatz A, Hiss Y, Hammel I, Arensburg B, Varend S (1994) Age related basement membrane thickening of the vocal cords in sudden infant death syndrome (SIDS). Laryngoscope 104:865–868
Shatz A, Hiss J, Arensburg B (1997) Myocarditis misdiagnosed as sudden infant death syndrome (SIDS). Med Sci Law 37:16–18
Shimizu H, Rambaud C, Cheron G, Rouzioux C, Anuradha R, Stanway G et al (1995) Molecular identification of viruses in sudden infant death associated with myocarditis and pericarditis. Pediatr Infect Dis J 14:584–588
Shinagawa S, Katagari S, Noro S, Nishihira M (1983) An autopsy study of 306 cases of maternal death in Japan. Nippon Sanka Fujinka Gakkai Zasshi 35:194–200
Silver MM, Smith CR (1992) Diaphragmatic contraction band necrosis in a perinatal and infantile autopsypopulation. Hum Pathol 23:817–827
Srettabunjong S (2013) Spontaneous rupture of acute ascending aortic dissection in a young pregnant woman: a sudden unexpected death. Forensic Sci Int 232:e5–e8
Stallmach T, Hebisch G (2004) Placental pathology: its impact on explaining prenatal and perinatal death. Virchows Arch 445:9–16
Stanley CA, Hale DE (1994) Genetic disorders of mitochondrial fatty acid oxidation. Curr Opin Pediatr 6:476–481
Steele RJ, Fogerty AC, Willcox ME, Clancy SL (1984) Metal content of the liver in sudden infant death syndrome. Aust Paediatr J 20:141–142
Stewart S, Fawcett J, Jacobsen W (1985) Interstitial haemosiderin in the lungs of sudden infant death syndrome: a histological hallmark of "near-miss" episodes? J Clin Pathol 145:53–58
Stojanovic I, Milić M, Ilić G, Antović A, Todorović S, Trandafilović M (2013) Ruptured splenic artery aneurysm in the 35th week of pregnancy. Medical error or bad luck? Rom J Leg Med 21:5–8
Stoltenberg L, Saugstad OD, Rognum TO (1992) Sudden infant death syndrome victims show local immunoglobulin M response in tracheal wall and immunoglobulin A response in duodenal mucosa. Pediatr Res 31:372–375

Stramba-Badiale M, Grancini F, Porta N, Schwartz P (1992) Pathophysiological mechanisms of sudden infant death syndrome. Cardiol Young 2:272–276

Strehler M, Dettmeyer R, Madea B (2006) Plötzlicher Tod bei unerkannter rupturierter Eileiterschwangerschaft mit intraperitonealer Blutung. Rechtsmedizin 16:219–222

Suarez-Mier MP, Aguilera B (1998) Histopathology of the conduction system in sudden infant death. Forensic Sci Int 93:143–154

Sudnerland REJ (1981) Febrile convulsions and cot death. Lancet 2(8239):176–178

Takahashi O, Kamiya T, Echigo S, Yutani C, Manabe H (1983) Myocarditis in children – clinical findings and myocardial biopsy findings. Jpn Circ J 47:1298–1303

Thomsen H, Saternus KS (1994) Myocardnekrosen beim plötzlichen und unerwarteten Säuglingstod (SIDS)? – eine Untersuchung mit polyclonalen Antikörpern gegen C5b-9(m)-Komplement-Komplex. Z Rechtsmed 5:6–9

Törő K, Hubay M, Keller E (2007) Extramedullary haematopoiesis in liver of sudden infant death cases. Forensic Sci Int 170:15–19

Towbin J, Ni J, Demmler G, Martin A, Kearney D, Bricker JT (1993) Evidence for adenovirus as common cause of myocarditis in children using polymerase chain reaction (PCR). Pediatr Res 33:27A

Tschernig T, Kleemann WJ, Pabst R (1995) Bronchus-associated lymphoid tissue (BALT) in the lungs of children who had died from sudden infant death syndrome and other causes. Thorax 50:658–660

Tsokos M (2004) Pathological features of maternal death from HELPP syndrome. In: Tsokos M (ed) Forensic pathology reviews, vol 1. Humana Press Inc., Totowa, pp 275–290

Tsokos M, Longauer F, Kardosova V, Gavel A, Anders S, Schulz F (2002) Maternal death in pregnancy from HELLP syndrome. A report of three medico-legal autopsy cases with special reference to distinctive histopathological alterations. Int J Legal Med 116:50–53

Tyson AA, Hackshaw BT, Kutcher MA (1989) Acute Epstein-Barr virus myocarditis simulating myocardial infarction with cardiogenic shock. South Med J 82:1184–1187

Uren EC, Williams AL, Jack I, Rees JW (1980) Association of respiratory virus infection with sudden infant death syndrome. Med J Aust 1:417–419

Valdes-Dapena MA (1982) The pathologist and the sudden infant death syndrome. Am J Pathol 106:118–131

Valdes-Dapena MA (1986) Sudden infant death syndrome. Morphology update for forensic pathologists – 1985. Forensic Sci Int 30:177–186

Valdes-Dapena M, Greene M, Basavanand N, Catherman R, Truex RC (1973) The myocardial conduction system in sudden death in infancy. N Engl J Med 289:1179–1180

Valdes-Dapena M, Gillane MM, Catherman R (1980) The question of right ventricular hypertrophy in sudden infant death syndrome. Arch Pathol Lab Med 104:184–186

Van Landeghem FK, Brinkmann B, Bajanowski T (1999) Basement membrane thickness of the vocal cord in cases of sudden infant death. Int J Legal Med 112:31–34

Variend S, Pearse RG (1986) Sudden infant death and cytomegalovirus inclusion disease. J Clin Pathol 39:383–386

Vawter GF, McGraw CA, Hug G, Kozakewich HPW, McNaulty J, Mandell F (1986) An hepatic metabolic profile in sudden infant death (SIDS). Forensic Sci Int 30:93–98

Vege Å, Rognum TO (1999) Inflammatory responses in sudden infant death syndrome – past and present views. FEMS Immunol Med Microbiol 25:67–78

Vege A, Rognum TO, Scott H, Aasen AO, Saugstad OD (1995) SIDS cases have increased levels of interleukin-6 in cerebrospinal fluid. Acta Paediatr 84:193–196

Vege A, Rognum TO, Aasen AO, Saugstad OD (1998) Are elevated cerebrospinal fluid levels of IL-6 in sudden unexplained deaths, infectious deaths and deaths due to heart/lung disease in infants and children due to hypoxia? Acta Paediatr 87:819–824

Vege A, Rognum TO, Anestad G (1999) IL-6 cerebrospinal fluid levels are related to laryngeal IgA and epithelial HLA-DR response in sudden infant death syndrome. Pediatr Res 45:803–809

Vennemann MM, Butterfass-Bahloul T, Jorch G, Brinkmann B, Findeisen M, Sauerland C, Bajanowski T, Mitchell EA, GeSID Group (2007) Sudden infant death syndrome: no increased risk after immunisation. Vaccine 25:336–340

Ventura F, Rutigliani M, Bellini C, Bonsignore A, Fulcheri E (2013) Clinical difficulties and forensic diagnosis: histopathological pitfalls of villus mesenchymal dysplasia in the third trimester causing foetal death. Forens Sci Int 229:e35–e41

Ventura F, Landolfa MC, Portunato F, Stefano FD (2011) Sudden death due to aortic dissection in pregnancy: case report. Rom J Leg Med 19:17–22

Verboon-Maciolek MA, Krediet TG, Gerards LJ, de Vries LS, Groenendaal F, van Loon AM (2008) Severe neonatal parechovirus infection and similarity with enterovirus infection. Pediatr Infect Dis J 27:241–245

Vogel M (1986) Histologische Entwicklungsstadien der Chorionzotten in der Embryonal- und der frühen Fetalperiode (5. bis 20. SSW). Pathologe 7:59–61

Walsh JK, Farrell MK, Keenan WJ, Lucas M, Kramer M (1981) Gastroesophageal reflux in infants: relation to apnea. J Pediatr 99:197–201

Weber U, Lemke R, Althoff H, Schröder JM, Weis J (1994) Alterations of diaphragmatic muscle fibres in sudden infant death. Clin Neuropathol 13:276

Weber MA, Ashworth MT, Risdon RA, Malone M, Sebire NJ (2009) The frequency and significance of alveolar haemosiderin-laden macrophages in sudden infant death. Forensic Sci Int 187:51–57

Weiler G, Ritter C (1988) Häufigkeit und Beweiswert eines Leberzellhydrops bei äußerer Erstickung und bei plötzlichem Kindstod. Z Rechtsmed 100:113–121

Weis J, Weber U, Schröder JM, Lemke R, Althoff H (1994) Neuro- und myopathologische Veränderungen beim plötzlichen Kindstod. Zentralbl Rechtsmed 42:454–455

Weis J, Weber U, Schröder JM, Lemke R, Althoff H (1998) Phrenic nerves and diaphragms in sudden infant death syndrome. Forensic Sci Int 91:133–146

Werne J, Garrow I (1953) Sudden apparently unexplained death during infancy. I. Pathologic findings in infants found dead. Am J Pathol 29:633–675

Wigglesworth JS, Keeling JW, Rushton D (1987) Pathological investigations in cases of sudden infant death. J Clin Pathol 40:1481–1483

Williams RB, Emery JL (1987) Endocardial fibrosis in apparently normal infant hearts. Histopathology 2:283–288

Williams A, Vawter G, Reid L (1979) Increased muscularity of the pulmonary circulation in victims of the sudden infant death syndrome. Pediatrics 63:18–23

Williams AL, Uren EC, Brotherton L (1984) Respiratory viruses and sudden infant death. Br Med J 288:1491–1493

Willinger M, James LS, Catz C (1991) Defining the sudden infant death syndrome (SIDS): deliberations of an expert panel convened by the National Institute of Child Health and Human Development. Pediatr Pathol 11:677–684

Wilske J (1984) Der plötzliche Säuglingstod (SIDS). Morphologische Abgrenzung, Pathomechanismus und Folgerung für die Praxis. Springer, Berlin

Windorfer A, Sitzmann FC (1971) Acute virus myocarditis in infants and children. Dtsch Med Wschr 96:1177

Witzleben CL, Pinto M (1978) Foamy myocardial transformation of infancy. Arch Pathol Lab Med 102:306–311

Wu JH, Parsons S (2017) Fatal disseminated neonatal herpes simplex virus type 1 infection in neonates in a forensic setting. Forensic Sci Med Pathol 13:99–101

Yagmur G, Ziyade N, Elgormus N, Das T, Sahin MF, Yildirim M, Ozgun A, Akcay A, Karayel F, Koc S (2016) Postmortem diagnosis of cytomegalovirus and accompanying other infection agents by real-time PCR in cases of sudden unexpected death in infancy (SUDI). J Forensic Legal Med 38:18–23

Zack F, Wegener R (1994) Zur Problematik der Diagnose "rhythmogener Herztod" durch histologische Untersuchungen des Erregungsbildungs- und -leitungssystems. Rechtsmedizin 5:1–5

Zhu BL, Maeda H, Fukita K, Sakurai M, Kobayashi Y (1996) Immunohistochemical investigation of pulmonary surfactant in perinatal fatalities. Forensic Sci Int 83:219–227

Zink P (1986) Pathologisch-anatomische Befunde bei plötzlichen, unerwartetem Tod von Kindern und Erwachsenen mit Influenza-A-Infektion. Z Rechtsmed 97:165–184

Zink P, Drescher J, Verhagen W, Flik J, Milbrandt H (1987) Serological evidence of recent influenza virus A infections in forensic cases of sudden infant death syndrome. Arch Virol 93:223–232

Forensic Cytology 18

Cytological investigation can, in individual cases, aid significantly in the clarification of forensic questions (Lee et al. 2016; Weitzig et al. 2015; Mittal et al. 2010; Murphy 1981; Oehmichen 1984). Locating and identifying cells, assigning cells to particular organs or anatomic locations, as well as isolating cell groups or single cells for further molecular genetic examinations must be considered as an option in certain cases. This includes the cytological determination of foreign bodies, e.g., *Lycopodium* spores after condom use or diatoms following freshwater drowning.

Forensic practice deals with the following in particular:

- Determination of cells at a crime scene, on crime instruments, or on other materials
- Isolation, identification, preparation, and work-up of cells
- Immunohistochemical species identification: human or nonhuman cells or tissue
- Cytological diagnosis of sexual offenses with evidence of sperm in smears or in sperm-containing substances on the victim's body, clothing, or other materials
- Evidence of condom use
- Evidence of epithelial cells and localization (vaginal, oral or buccal, anal, penile)
- Evidence of diatoms following freshwater drowning (Pachar and Cameron 1992)
- Cytological diagnosis in cases of potential mix-up of cytological and other specimens (contamination)
- Immunohistochemical diagnosis of blood groups, e.g., in the case of transfusion incidents

Cytological diagnosis is possible in samples of organs and body surfaces extracted during autopsy. The literature mentions, for example, changes to alveolar cells in cases of protracted asphyxia (Janssen and Bärtschi 1964), drowning (Brinkmann et al. 1983), or strangulation. The absence of lectin receptors on bronchial epithelia is considered an indication of viral pneumonia (Schaefer 1981). Cytological diagnosis performed on intact tissue and organs, rather than single cells or small cell groups, is not considered cytological diagnosis in the strictest sense of the term.

18.1 Detection, Isolation, and Species Identification of Cells

Smears can be taken from material where tissue and cells are found or suspected; alternatively, cells can be mounted on microscope slides by other means. For example, biological substances on projectiles and crime instruments may be considered (Karger et al. 1996; Knudsen 1993;

R. B. Dettmeyer, *Forensic Histopathology*, https://doi.org/10.1007/978-3-319-77997-3_18

Nichols and Sens 1990; Maresch 1961). Thus, it was possible, for example, to detect respiratory epithelial cells on the crime instrument following suffocation using a soft cover (Luke 1969).

The condition of cells is first assessed microscopically, as well as by means of immunocytochemical methods if available (Wehner et al. 2007, 2008). Based on these results, type and origin of cells are assigned. The following substances can be found:

- Epithelial cells with nuclei, sometimes as epithelial cell groups
- Keratinized, nucleated, shed skin cells (keratinocytes)
- Intact spermatozoa or sperm heads
- Cells that can be assigned to an organ or tissue (e.g., adipose cells, blood cells, nerve cells, muscle cells, liver cells)
- Squamous epithelial cells of nonkeratinized squamous epithelium (anal, vaginal, buccal, or penile)
- Blood components with red and white blood cells, to be characterized in greater detail
- Sometimes only cellular debris, the utility of which remains undetermined in differential studies

Species Diagnostics

Cell groups and single cells for immunocytochemical and genetic investigations can be extracted from tissue or organs by means of laser dissection microscopy. This applies in particular to the extraction of spermatozoa following sexual offenses (Vandewoestyne et al. 2009; Anoruo et al. 2007; Anslinger et al. 2007; Di Martino et al. 2004; Murray et al. 2007; Sanders et al. 2006a; Elliot et al. 2003).

Immunocytochemical species identification plays a limited role in forensic practice. However, in principle, it is possible to label tissue with anti-human immunoglobulin as a primary antibody, while this is not possible with primary antibodies against immunoglobulins of different animal species in human tissue (Pedal 1995).

Cell Extraction

If only single cells of trace material are available, DNA analysis, including amplification of short tandem repeats (STR) of complementary DNA (cDNA), should be performed (Brinkmann 2004). In 1997, successful amplification of six STR systems on single epithelial cells of the buccal mucosa was reported but without detailing the method of cell extraction and isolation used (Findlay et al. 1997). A method of cellular uptake ("picking") under microscopic control with the aid of a glass pipette has been described, in which the amplification and sequencing of the HV1 region and HV2 region in mitochondrial DNA was possible (success rate 80%) (Brück et al. 2010). In the case of mixed traces, cell selection may be problematic. In this context, it has been suggested that at least ten cells are examined using molecular genetics. If no consistent pattern can be determined, further cells may be examined (Brück et al. 2010).

18.2 Cytological Diagnosis in Sexual Offenses

In sexual offenses, cytological diagnosis concentrates initially on the detection of sperm in smear samples (vaginal, anal, oral, penile, and other skin areas) and on textiles (Evers et al. 2009). If condom use is suspected, investigation is needed to establish whether condom residues can be determined microscopically. In the case of an offender with azoospermia and evidence of squamous epithelial cells, one should question whether these cells originated as vaginal epithelial cells from the victim or as penile epithelial cells from the offender. However, if a penile smear from a suspect is taken early enough, some cells on the penis could have originated from the female victim as a result of sexual intercourse. In addition, the examination of textiles and other materials for condom residues or cells of the suspect and victim must be considered. After a smear has been taken, a cytological examination may follow.

18.2.1 Sperm Detection

Even if different staining methods can be applied (Oppitz 1969), the characteristic morphology of sperm with a round- or oval-shaped head with or without tail is decisive for microscopic detection. If a sperm tail is present, trichomonads must be considered in the differential diagnosis. Staining is performed after air-drying according to Stiasny-H&E, Baecchi, or Papanicolaou methods.

The microscopic detection of sperm is carried out using smear samples. In the first step, vaginal smear samples from three different localizations should be examined:

- Rear side of the labia
- Vaginal vestibule
- Posterior third of the vagina

The vaginal epithelium in adolescent girls and premenopausal women is typically thickened to varying degrees. However, superficial cells with small central nuclei and broad cytoplasm predominate. Additional inflammatory cells, in particular granulocytes, are frequently seen. Depending on cell plication, a cytological determination of cycle phase can be made, which requires specialized experience, but is rarely of interest in forensic practice. The focus lies on the detection of intact sperm or sperm heads (Table 18.1; Fig. 18.1). Other cells, which may be transmitted during sexual intercourse from the offender to the victim, are difficult to differentiate in conventional smear specimens, regardless of the staining method chosen.

Ejaculate substances on items of clothing or objects, for example, can be examined cytologically using various staining methods (Albrecht et al. 2004; Allery et al. 2001). Frequently, sperm or sperm heads attached to textile fibers (Fig. 18.2) can only be seen sporadically (Fig. 18.3). When only a few spermatozoa are present in an overwhelming number of epithelial cells, automatic detection of spermatozoa for laser capture microdissection allows precise identification (Vandewoestyne et al. 2009).

The loss of sperm tails is used to approximate the age of the sperm; however, storage conditions play a substantial role in this regard.

Table 18.1 Microscopic detection of sperm in smear samples

Staining or detection	Findings
Stiasny-H&E staining	Blue spermatozoa
Native sample	Motile spermatozoa for 5–8 h
Regular detection	Up to 12 h
Longest detection	24–48 h, only occasional spermatozoa or sperm heads (possibly much longer on the corpse)
Additional findings	Vaginal epithelial cells with blue nucleolus, signs of inflammation (granulocytes), basophilic bacterial colonies (likely cocci), potentially foreign material
Condom use	Detection of starch granules, possibly *Lycopodium* spores

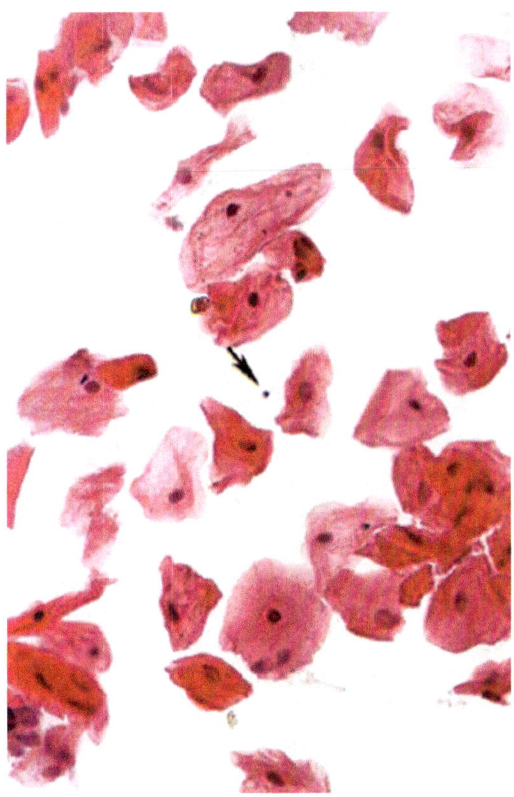

Fig. 18.1 Typical smear sample with vaginal epithelial cells (superficial cells) and single spermatozoon with intact sperm tail (*arrow*) (Papanicolaou ×200)

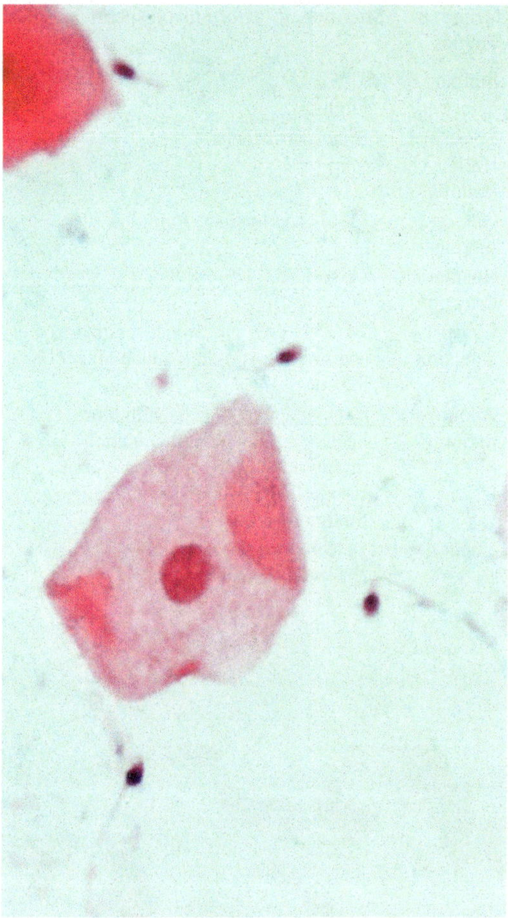

Fig. 18.2 Vaginal smear: epithelial cell with individual spermatozoa demonstrating preserved sperm tails (Baecchi ×400)

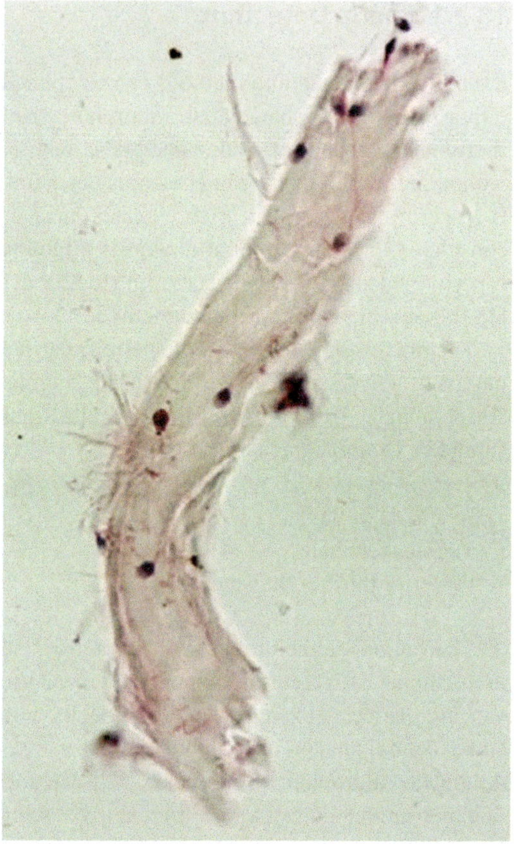

Fig. 18.3 Substances of single sperm heads without detection of sperm tails on textile fibers following a sexual offense (Baecchi ×400)

Single sperm can also be taken directly from specimen slides by means of laser microdissection for further molecular genetic diagnosis or DNA analysis of the offender (Sanders et al. 2006b; Martino et al. 2004; Elliott et al. 2003). Nevertheless, archived slides of cell smears with histological stains are often the only source of DNA available when cold cases are reopened. The negative effects of particular histological stains on DNA recovery and quality from human cells are discussed in the literature (Simons and Vintiner 2011).

18.2.2 Detection of Condom Residues

The detection of condom residues is carried out by determining the substances that have been applied to the condom surface during manufacturing to prevent the condom from rolling up (Maynard et al. 2001). These substances include starch granules, primarily corn starch and *Lycopodium clavatum* spores (club moss) (Cremer 1994; Berkefeld 1993; Balick 1988, 1989). Silicone polymers, such as dimethicone, are used as lubricants. Some manufacturers add spermicides, as well as scents or flavoring agents.

The starch granules are polyhedral to round with a diameter of 2–32 μm and show a typical cross detectable with polarization effects. The starch granules appear deep blue when stained with Lugol's solution (Fig. 18.4).

Lycopodium spores have a diameter of 25–40 μm, a characteristic tetrahedral form, and a reticular surface. In cell-rich specimens containing blood, it is sometimes challenging and time-consuming to determine single *Lycopodium* spores and starch granules (Fig. 18.5).

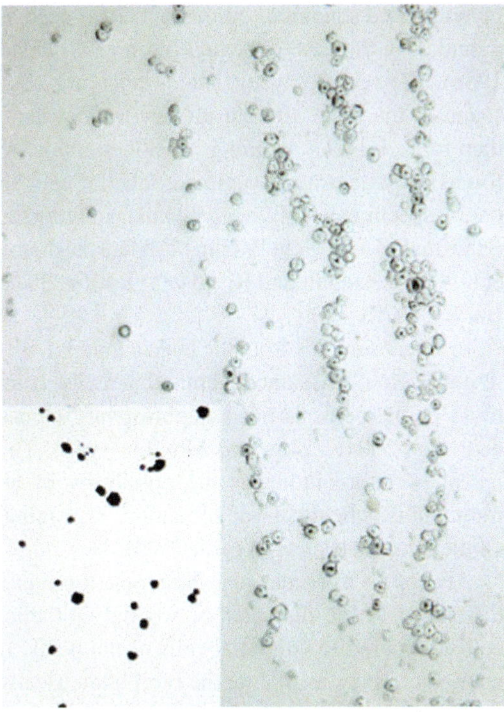

Fig. 18.4 Abundant starch granules (native sample ×100) and starch granules stained deep blue with Lugol's solution (×200)

In addition, evidence of lubricants and spermicides in vaginal wet mounts is possible by means of infrared or mass spectrometry (Blackledge and Vincenti 1994). Due to their high oil concentration, *Lycopodium* spores stain yellow in Sudan III staining, while corn starch granules stain blue with Lugol's solution (Keil et al. 1997). Both *Lycopodium* spores and corn starch granules are relatively storage stable and can be detected in swab specimens up to 72 h post coitum, in Sudan III staining up to 48 h post coitum, and in penis specimens up to at least 24 h post coitum (Keil et al. 1997). However, the determination of starch granules is nonspecific, since starch granules are also present in numerous foodstuffs, suppositories, and cosmetics. Powdered gloves also contain starch, which is why contamination unrelated to the crime must also be considered when determining starch granules. *Lycopodium* spores are mainly derived from the club moss plant, however, and are almost exclusively used in condom manufacturing. For this reason, the detection of *Lycopodium* spores is a significant indication of condom use.

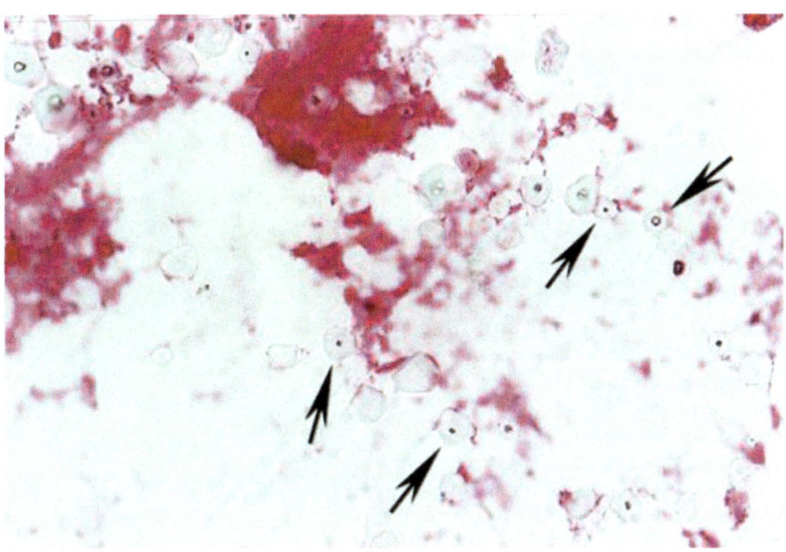

Fig. 18.5 Vaginal smear with starch granules after condom use, autolytically changed cells and agglutinated erythrocytes (Papanicolaou ×200)

18.2.3 Detection of Vaginal Epithelial Cells

In general, epithelial cells can be differentiated cytologically, e.g., keratinous epithelial cells in keratinized squamous epithelium, ciliated epithelial cells from the respiratory tract, epithelial cells from the transitional epithelium of the genitourinary tract, cells from nonkeratinized squamous epithelium of the buccal mucosa, as well as epithelial cells of the penis and in anal and vaginal smears (French et al. 2008). Specimen preparations after a sex crime are also partly stained according to Baecchi, sometimes with Lugol's solution. Other smear samples are frequently stained according to the Papanicolaou method. The potassium iodide-containing Lugol's solution is suitable for demonstrating glycogen-containing vaginal epithelium cells, which can be obtained, for instance, from the surface of a condom following condom use during vaginal sexual intercourse (Fig. 18.6).

Vaginal epithelial cells have a relatively high glycogen concentration and can be shown with Lugol's staining method. Therefore, evidence of glycogenated squamous epithelial cells is used as a marker in the case of sexual offenses (Randall 1988). However, glycogenated cells are also found in the male efferent urinary tract system; therefore, Lugol's staining is not suitable to forensically determine vaginal epithelial cells in penis specimens following sexual intercourse (Hausmann and Schellmann 1994; Hausmann et al. 1994; Randall and Riss 1985; Rothwell and Harvey 1978).

In smear samples from the buccal mucosa, differentiation of squamous epithelial cells from those of the penis is not straightforward (Jones and Leon 2004; Ziskin and Moulton 1948). The recent literature indicates the possibility of an immunohistochemical identification of vaginal epithelial cells (Paterson et al. 2006).

According to recent investigations, there is a difference in the diameter of vaginal epithelial cells compared to epithelial cells of the penis. If enough cells are available, the morphometrically measured diameter of epithelial cells in the stereomicroscope can be an important indication of whether specific cells are of vaginal or penile origin (Fig. 18.7). A diameter of more than 60 μm suggests vaginal epithelial cells.

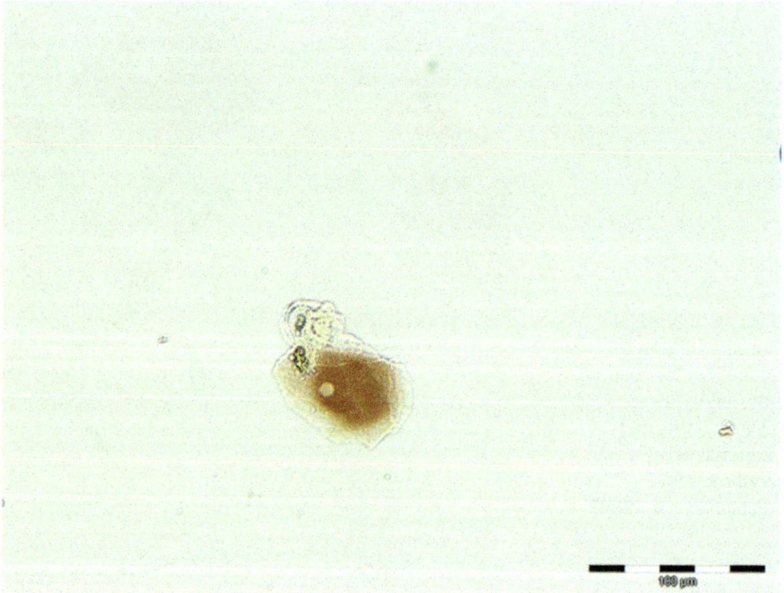

Fig. 18.6 Large glycogen-positive vaginal epithelial cell and nucleus taken from the surface of a condom following sexual intercourse (Lugol's solution; ×400; image kindly provided by Dr. G. Lasczkowski, Gießen, Germany)

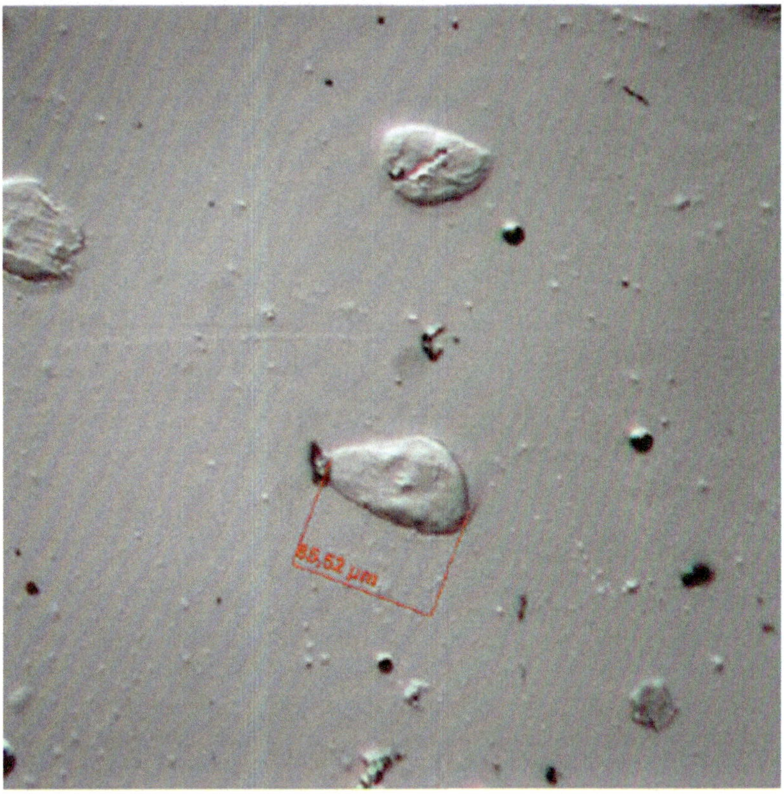

Fig. 18.7 Morphometric measurement of cell size using a stereomicroscope; detection of a vaginal epithelial cell (Photo courtesy of Prof. M.A. Verhoff, Gießen, Germany; ×1000)

18.3 Identification of Cells and Tissues in the Case of Suspected Material Contamination or Mix-Up

Occasionally, intentional or unintentional contamination or mix-up of tissue or cytological samples is suspected (Banaschak et al. 1997). In such cases, histological or cytological diagnosis is able to precisely localize and select those tissues or cells that should be examined for further diagnosis. Cells from medical treatments may have been mistakenly mounted on neighboring microscope slides and subsequently may lead to a suspected disease which does correspond to the anamnesis and clinical diagnosis, for example, cells from an ascites puncture in an elderly female tumor patient with papillary adenocarcinoma of the ovary finding their way onto the vaginal smear specimen of a young woman with an inconspicuous anamnesis. The arrangement of cells on the microscope slides as well as the composition of the remaining cell image may already give cause to suspect contamination or mix-up (Junge et al. 2008). If analysis of the different cell types shows different DNA profiles, the material originates from two different individuals, and the question arises, whether the puncture of one patient took place in the same room where the cytological slide preparation was taken from another patient (Fig. 18.8).

18.4 Transfusion Reactions

The erroneous transfusion of ABO-incompatible red blood cells can lead to life-threatening and complement-induced shock, resulting in death in less than 10% of cases with an acute hemolytic transfusion reaction (Leo and Pedal 2010).

In transfusion incidents, e.g., following a mix-up of units of stored blood and administration of incompatible blood, recipient blood reacts with hemolysis and phagocytosis. Foreign erythrocytes and the resulting decomposition products

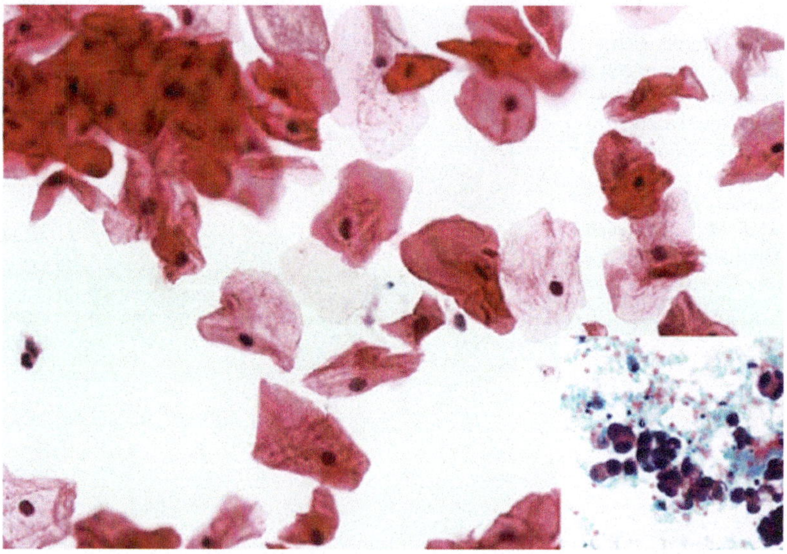

Fig. 18.8 Typical superficial squamous epithelium with small cell nuclei in the vaginal smear of a young woman with a singular sperm and tumor cells in one area. These tumor cells (inlet) originate from the fluid of pleural aspirate taken from an older female patient with a metastasized adenocarcinoma, who has been treated in the same room before (Papanicolaou ×400)

can be determined immunocytochemically in the case of short survival times. Here, immunocytochemically marked erythrocyte agglutination must be considered, particularly in larger vessels and also later in terminal vasculatures.

Following a survival time of more than 24 h, intravascular foreign erythrocytes can typically no longer be determined. After only a few hours, macrophages in the liver, spleen, and adrenals with pronounced phagocytosis of foreign erythrocytes (erythrophagia) are described. After a survival time of more than 48 h, evidence of foreign erythrocytes is very difficult to obtain, unless these erythrocytes have not undergone phagocytosis in older hematomas or necrosis after shock, in which case, immunocytochemical marking may still be possible.

Thus, in the case of the processing procedure for foreign erythrocytes described, immunocytochemical diagnosis after transfusion incidents always enables determination of an approximate survival time (Pedal 1987, 1995; Mukoyama and Seta 1986; Pedal et al. 1990). Human antigens of the ABO system can also be detected immunocytochemically in biological traces, such as hair medulla. However, due to irregular expression, these antigens cannot always be detected in the epidermis. For this reason, only a positive detection is meaningful here (Pedal 1995).

Immunohistochemically, blood group antigens with monoclonal antibodies against A, B, and, for example, the two antigens of the Lewis system, Le-a and Le-b, can also be determined in tissue sections. When interpreting the results, it should be borne in mind that some people excrete their group-specific antigens with the secretions, termed secretors (approximately 75%). Depending on the investigated matrix, it must be considered that secretors, for example, in the tracheal glands, show an intense marking of the mucous but not the serous glands for the group-specific antigens of the ABH system (Pedal 1995).

The differential diagnosis should rule out transfusion-related acute lung injury and other immunologically triggered causes such as febrile nonhemolytic transfusion reaction or allergic reactions, as well as nonimmunological causes (e.g., bacterial contamination, transfusion-associated circulatory overload, and rare events such as air or debris embolism).

18.5 Additional Methods of Forensic Cytological Diagnosis

Other cytological diagnostic techniques are described in the literature:

- The determination of blood group antigens by means of immunohistochemical diagnosis in squamous epithelial cells of the buccal mucosa (Ito and Hirota 1992; Noda et al. 2002)

- Cytological examinations of dried blood stains (Undritz and Hegg 1959, 1960)
- Cytological evidence of amniotic fluid embolism (Lee et al. 1986; Giampalo et al. 1987; Marcus et al. 2005)
- Microvascular cytological findings in cases of pulmonary fat embolism (Castella et al. 1992)
- Cytological techniques can be used to detect particulate matter on bullets (Knudsen 1993)

In addition, cytological diagnosis of specific cells or cell types forms an integral part of any histological examination.

References

Albrecht K, Schultheiss D, Rothämel T, Breitmeier D, Tröger HD (2004) Der Nachweis von Spermaspuren in der forensischen Medizin. Kriminalistik 8:552–558

Allery JP, Telmon N, Mieusset R, Rouge BD (2001) Cytological detection of spermatozoa: comparison of three staining methods. J Forensic Sci 46:349–351

Anoruo B, van Oorschot R, Mitchell J, Howells D (2007) Isolating cells from non-sperm cellular mixtures using the PALM microlaser micro dissection system. Forensic Sci Int 173:93–96

Anslinger K, Bayer B, Mack B, Eisenmenger W (2007) Sex-specific fluorescent labelling of cells for laser microdissection and DNA profiling. Int J Legal Med 121:54–56

Balick MJ (1988) *Lycopodium* spores found in condom dusting agent. Nature 332:591

Balick MJ (1989) *Lycopodium* spores used in condom manufacture: associated health hazards. Econ Bot 43:373–377

Banaschak S, Sibbing U, Brinkmann B (1997) Identifizierung von Gewebeproben bei Verdacht auf Materialvertauschung. Pathologe 18:385–389

Berkefeld K (1993) Einc Nachweismöglichkeit füı Kondombenutzung bei Sexualdelikten. Arch Kriminol 192:37–42

Blackledge RD, Vincenti M (1994) Identification of polydimethylsiloxane lubricant traces from latex condoms in cases of sexual assault. J Forensic Sci Soc 34:245–256

Brinkmann B (2004) Forensische DNA-Analytik. Dtsch Ärztebl 101:A2329–A2335

Brinkmann B, Fechner G, Püschel K (1983) Zur Lungenhistologie bei experimentellem Ertrinken. Z Rechtsmed 89:267–277

Brück S, Thias V, Heidorn F, Gruber C, Kramer N, Evers H, Verhoff MA (2010) Sequenzierung aus einzelnen Epithelzellen. HV1 und HV2-Region der mitochondrialen DNA. Rechtsmedizin 20:25–33

Castella X, Valles J, Cabezuelo MA, Fernandez R, Artigas A (1992) Fat embolism syndrome and pulmonary microvascular cytology. Chest 101:1710–1711

Cremer U (1994) Zum Nachweis von Präservativrückständen in Vaginalabstrichen. Zbl Rechtsmed 42:425

Di Martino D, Giuffrè G, Staiti N et al (2004) Single sperm cell isolation by laser dissection. Forensic Sci Int 146:S151–S153

Elliot K, Hill DS, Lambert C et al (2003) Use of laser microdissection greatly improves the recovery of DNA from sperm on microscope slides. Forensic Sci Int 137:28–36

Elliott K, Hill DS, Lambert C, Burroughes TR, Gill P (2003) Use of laser microdissection greatly improves the recovery of DNA from sperm on microscopic slides. Forensic Sci Int 137:28–36

Evers H, Heidorn F, Gruber C, Lasczkowski G, Risse M, Dettmeyer R, Verhoff MA (2009) Investigative strategy for the forensic detection of sperm traces. Forensic Sci Med Pathol 5:182–188

Findlay I, Taylor A, Quirke P et al (1997) DNA-fingerprinting from single cells. Nature 389:555–556

French CEV, Jensen CG, Vintiner SK, Elliot DA, McGlashan SR (2008) A novel histological technique for distinguishing between epithelial cells in forensic casework. Forensic Sci Int 178:1–6

Giampalo C, Schneider V, Kowalski BH, Bellaver LA (1987) The cytologic diagnosis of amniotic fluid embolism: a critical reappraisal. Diagn Cytopathol 3:126–128

Hausmann R, Schellmann B (1994) Forensic value of the Lugol's staining method: further studies on glycogenated epithelium in the male urinary tract. Int J Legal Med 107:147–151

Hausmann R, Pregler C, Schellmann B (1994) The value of the Lugol's iodine staining technique for the identification of vaginal epithelial cells. Int J Legal Med 106:298–301

Ito N, Hirota T (1992) Histochemical and cytochemical localisation of blood group antigens. Prog Histochem Cytochem 25:1–85

Janssen W, Bärtschi G (1964) Vitale und supravitale Reaktionen der Alveolarzellen nach protrahiertem Sauerstoffmangel. Dtsch Z Gesamt Gerichtl Med 55:47–60

Jones EL, Leon JA (2004) Lugol's tcst rc-cxamincd again: buccal cells. J Forensic Sci 49:64–67

Junge A, Dettmeyer R, Madea B (2008) Identification of biological samples in a case of contamination of a cytological slide preparation. J Forensic Sci 53:739–741

Karger B, Meyer E, Knudsen PJT, Brinkmann B (1996) DNA typing of cellular material on perforating bullets. Int J Legal Med 10:177–179

Keil W, Kutschka G, Sachs H (1997) Spuren bei sexualstraftaten: zum nachweis von kondomrückständen in vaginal- und penisabstrichen. Kriminalistik 51:439–440

Knudsen PJT (1993) Cytology in ballistics – an experimental investigation of tissue fragments on full metal jacketed bullets using routine cytological techniques. Int J Legal Med 106:15–18

Lee KR, Catalano PM, Ortiz-Giroux S (1986) Cytologic diagnosis of amniotic fluid embolism. Report of a case with a unique cytologic feature and emphasis on the difficulty of eliminating squamous contamination. Acta Cytol 30:177–182

Lee WC, Khoo BE, Abdullah AFL (2016) Enhancement of seminal stains using background correction algorithm with colour filters. Forensic Sci Int 263:1–9

Leo A, Pedal I (2010) Diagnostic approaches to acute transfusion reactions. Forensic Sci Med Pathol 6:135–145

Luke JL (1969) Recovery of intact respiratory epithelium from a cloth pillowcase four days following its utilization as a smothering instrument. J Forensic Sci 14:398–401

Marcus BJ, Collins KA, Harley RA (2005) Ancillary studies in amniotic fluid embolism: a case report and review of the literature. Am J Forensic Med Pathol 26:92–95

Maresch W (1961) Zum Nachweis von Gewebsteilchen an Tatwerkzeugen. Dtsch Z Gesamte Gerichtl Med 51:560–562

Martino D, Giuffre G, Staiti N, Simone A, Le Donne M, Saravo L (2004) Single sperm cell isolation by laser microdissection. Forensic Sci Int 146(Suppl):S151–S153

Maynard P, Allwell K, Roux C, Dawson M, Royds D (2001) A protocol for the forensic analysis of condom and personal lubricants found in sexual assault cases. Forensic Sci Int 124:140–156

Mittal T, Muralidhar Saralaya K, Kuruvilla A, Achary C (2010) Sex determination from buccal mucosa scrapes. Int J Legal Med 123:437–440

Mukoyama H, Seta S (1986) The determination of blood groups in tissue samples. In: Forensic science progress, vol 1. Springer, Berlin

Murphy GK (1981) Applications of cytology to forensic pathology. Acta Cytol 25:153–156

Murray C, McAlister C, Elliot K (2007) Identification and isolation of male cells using fluorescence in situ hybridisation and laser dissection, for use in the investigation of sexual assault. Forensic Sci Int Genet 1:247252

Nichols CA, Sens MA (1990) Recovery and evaluation by cytologic techniques of trace material retained on bullets. Am J Forensic Med Pathol 11:17–34

Noda H, Yokota M, Tatsumi S, Sugiyama S (2002) Determination of ABO blood grouping from human oral squamous epithelium by the highly sensitive immunohistochemical staining method EnVision+. J Forensic Sci 47:341–344

Oehmichen M (1984) Fortschritte zytologischer Methoden in der forensischen Pathologie. Pathologe 5:200–203

Oppitz E (1969) A new colouring method for the determination of sperm cells in sexual assault cases. Arch Kriminol 144:145–148

Pachar JV, Cameron JM (1992) Scanning electron microscopy: application in the identification of diatoms in cases of drowning. J Forensic Sci 37:860–866

Paterson SK, Jensen CG, Vintiner SK, McGlashan SR (2006) Immunhistochemical staining as a potential method for the identification of vaginal epithelial cells in forensic casework. J Forensic Sci 51:1138–1143

Pedal I (1987) Blutgruppen-immunhistochemie. Thieme-Verlag, Stuttgart

Pedal I (1995) Immunhistochemische Blutgruppendiagnostik (ABH, Lewis) in der Rechtsmedizin. In: Bratzke HJ, Schröter A (eds) Immunhistochemie in der Rechtsmedizin. Deutsche Hochschulschriften, Egelsbach, pp 14–21

Pedal I, Freislederer A, Reiter C, Depastas G (1990) Zur Immunhistochemie tödlicher Transfusionszwischenfälle. Pathologe 11:143–147

Randall B (1988) Gylcogenated squamous epithelia cells as a marker of foreign body penetration in sexual assault. J Forensic Sci 33:511–514

Randall B, Riss RE (1985) Penile glycogenated epithelial cells as an indicator of recent vaginal intercourse. Am J Clin Pathol 84:524–526

Rothwell TJ, Harvey KJ (1978) The limitations of the Lugol's iodine staining technique for the identification of vaginal epithelial cells. J Forensic Sci Soc 18:181–184

Sanders CT, Sanchez N, Ballantyne J, Petersen DA (2006a) Laser microdissection separation of pure spermatozoa. J Forensic Sci 51:748–757

Sanders CT, Sanchez N, Ballantyne J, Peterson DA (2006b) Laser microdissection separation of pure spermatozoa from epithelial cells for short tandem repeat analysis. J Forensic Sci 51:748–757

Schaefer HE (1981) Virus und Respirationstrakt – morphogenetische Aspekte pulmonaler Veränderungen. Verh Dtsch Ges Pathol 65:107–127

Simons JL, Vintiner SK (2011) Effects of histological staining on the analysis of human DANN from archived slides. J Forensic Sci 56. https://doi.org/10.1111/j.1556-4029.2010.01595.x

Undritz E, Hegg P (1959) Die morphologisch-hämatologische und cytologische Untersuchung eingetrockneter Blutflecken. Schweiz Med Wschr 89:1088–1091

Undritz E, Hegg P (1960) Die morphologische Untersuchung eingetrockneter Blutflecken. II. Teil: Anwendung an einem Beispiel. Schweiz Med Wschr 90:1223–1230

Vandewoestyne M, van Hoofstat D, van Nieuwerburgh F, Deforce D (2009) Automatic detection of spermatozoa for laser capture microdissection. Int J Legal Med 123:169–175

Wehner F, Stiegler A, Schulz MM, Wehner HD, Martin D (2007) Immunzytochemische Untersuchungen biologischer Spuren an Tatklingen. Arch Kriminol 219:180–190

Wehner F, Moos NRM, Wehner HD, Martin D, Schulz MM (2008) Immunocytochemical examinations of biological traces on expanding bullets (QD-PEP). Forensic Sci Int 182:66–70

Weitzig L, Schroeder AS, Augustin C, Raupach T, Sehner S, Anders S (2015) Diagnostic value of PSA and AP tests for the detection of spermatozoa in postmortem swabs from the genital and anal region in males. J Forensic Sci 60:41–44

Ziskin D, Moulton R (1948) A comparison of oral and vaginal epithelial smears. J Clin Endocrinol Metab 8:146–165

19 Histothanatology: Autolysis, Putrefaction, and Mummification

Histological and histopathological findings following prolonged postmortem intervals have been subject of several investigations in the past (Galloway 1997; Emson 1991; Weimann 1958; Walcher 1928, 1938). The detection of usable microscopic findings in relation to the postmortem interval, especially in the context of exhumation, is by nature temporary and dependent on many factors. Thus, forensic–histological diagnostics are limited due to autolysis and putrefaction (Vock et al. 1989; Janssen 1977). These techniques are of limited utility, for example, in autopsies on bodies from mass graves (Ubelaker 2008). In the case of mummification, tissue and organoid structures, as well as potential pathological findings, can be shown microscopically for a significantly longer period of time in contrast to autolysis and putrefaction in non-mummified bodies (Schulz et al. 1999). However, microscopically, there are numerous demarcation problems, for example, when differentiating tubular necrosis in the kidney from solely autolytic changes (Kocovski and Duflou 2009). Detecting acute myocardial infarction can also be challenging and is only possible for a limited time period. Finally, structures are prone to various autolytic processes in the postmortem period. Leukocytes and nuclei of granulocytes are seen as exceedingly resistant to autolysis and putrefaction (Walcher 1928). Evidence of bronchopneumonia was shown even after 392 days following exhumation (Naeve and Bandmann 1981). Others have diagnosed confluent bronchopneumonia after a postmortem interval of 95 days (Althoff 1974). However, there is no specific sequence and timeline for changes in internal tissues and organs due to autolysis and putrefaction, nor can a fixed time or period of time be determined for single organs. In general, the uterus is considered to be an organ relatively resistant to putrefaction.

Microscope diagnostics are influenced by several factors, including:

- Physical status at the time of death (age, constitution, and preexisting diseases, such as fever, sepsis, or injuries)
- Type and duration of the position or storage of the body after death, especially weather conditions (temperature, humidity, etc.)
- Type of burial (with or without coffin, type of wood used to make the coffin, prior embalming, or surface disinfection)
- Location of cemetery, depth of grave, soil temperature, and soil properties
- Length of time since burial, cadaver fauna, and cadaver flora

Many of the above factors are unknown prior to exhumation, and in most cases, it is impossible to safely determine them retroactively. In order to clarify death and determine identity, exhumations are classically performed in cases of intoxication, suspected homicide, medical malpractice, or accidents, including traffic accidents. The authorities concerned are often interested in those

R. B. Dettmeyer, *Forensic Histopathology*, https://doi.org/10.1007/978-3-319-77997-3_19

findings which can be reasonably expected from exhumation, depending on both the nature of the diagnostic question being asked and the specific length of time since burial.

Histological findings in organs and tissues following prolonged postmortem periods have previously been described (Evans 1961; Schmidt 1951; Weimann 1928; Schmeißer 1926; Schwarz 1926; Geill 1924). Recognizability of histopathological findings can be significantly extended due to changes in preserved bodies, such as mummification or formation of lipids. In principle, chronic diseases with post-inflammatory fibrosis and calcifications can often be proven for a longer period of time than acute, pathological processes (Breitmeier et al. 2003, 2005; Althoff 1974). Thus, while acute myocardial infarction may no longer be detectable histologically after a very short burial period (Naeve and Bandmann 1981), it may be possible to prove myocardial infarction with the help of the necrosis marker C5b-$9_{(m)}$ after 12 months (Karger et al. 2004) or longer (Ortmann et al. 2000). Depending on environmental conditions, some organs can show marked resistance to autolysis (Cotton et al. 1987). Organotypic structures and particularly connective tissue structures, such as portal fields of the liver, are often present for a prolonged period of time and therefore enable the identification of organs (Schulz et al. 1999).

In some cases, it is difficult to differentiate certain findings from autolytic changes, for example, the demarcation of acute ischemic tubular necrosis; however, combined examinations using immunohistochemical markers should permit a reliable diagnosis (Kocovski and Duflou 2009).

19.1 Time Frame for the Reliable Detection of Microscopic Findings

There are currently insufficient data on human brain tissue preservation following prolonged postmortem periods; however, neuropathological examinations of human brain tissue extracted from the skull and fixed after prolonged body storage in a cool environment can feasibly diagnose neurological disorders, even several months after death. Histomorphology of the cerebral and cerebellar cortex can be well preserved, and many histological and immunohistochemical stainings can be performed with positive results (Gelpi et al. 2007; Fechner and Sivaloganathan 1987). Nevertheless, the significance of negative immunohistochemical staining results must be interpreted with caution in all cases of exhumation.

Thanatological changes in cells are mostly of the autolytically destructive kind, often with subsequent bacterial decomposition. Two questions need to be addressed:

1. How does one differentiate between vital and avital findings?
2. What is the time frame for the detection of biochemical traces or for performing histological and immunohistochemical staining for the purposes of determining postmortem intervals, among others?

In occasional cases, immunohistochemical determination of blood type antigens may be considered. In particular, erythrocytes, their precursors, and endothelial cells of the blood vessels show relatively constant marking of the ABH secretor status of an individual. After storage in 15 °C water for 1 month, it was still possible to show ABH antigens of the skeletal muscles; marked blood vessels were still visible after 3 months. Only the destruction of vascular antigens by bacteria, fungi, amoeba, etc. with extensive degradation of the antigens prevents marking of ABH antigens (Pedal 1995). Epithelial cell antigens are more resistant to putrefaction. Attempts to immunohistochemically diagnose blood type are seen as promising, as long as parts of the tissue structure remain macroscopically recognizable; this applies to skeletal and heart muscles; the laryngeal, tracheal, and bronchial wall; as well as kidney tissue (Pedal 1995).

Evidence of acute myocardial infarction remains immunohistochemically possible with the markers C5b-$9_{(m)}$ and NP57 when conventional H&E staining no longer shows results (Ortmann et al. 2000). C5b-$9_{(m)}$, a marker of early myocardial necrosis, gave positive results even after prolonged periods of artificial and natural putrefaction. NP57 stains neutrophilic leukocytes, which could be demonstrated considerably longer after humid putrefaction than after dry putrefaction (Ortmann et al. 2000). These two markers—C5b-$9_{(m)}$ and NP57—should be regarded as the markers of choice for the detection of early myocardial infarction and leukocyte infiltration in advanced stages of putrefaction.

It is also important in forensic practice to diagnose whether a discolored area of a corpse has been caused by postmortem hypostasis or bruises. Therefore, the usefulness of glycophorin A (GPA) as a marker of bleeding was investigated in decomposed bodies by immunohistochemistry using an antihuman GPA monoclonal antibody. The authors concluded that the detection of GPA by immunohistochemistry can help to differentiate between bleeding and hemoglobin diffusion from blood vessels in a decomposed body (Tabata and Morita 1997).

For information on the detectability of histological and immunohistochemical findings after postmortem intervals of varying duration, please refer to the data selected in Table 19.1.

Typically, epithelial cells die earlier than connective tissue, cartilage tissue, and bones. Nevertheless, macroscopic and histological investigations, in particular of the heart and lung, are valuable even several years postmortem. Exhumations are an adequate and frequently successful tool to recover evidence which should have been collected immediately after the death of a person. Additionally, exhumations can be seen as an instrument to evaluate the quality of death investigations. The various conditions found long after burial justify optimism for successful results from an exhumation. In many cases, decomposing lungs characterized by gas bubbles caused by decomposition, pyknosis, hyperchromatosis with partial chromatolysis, interstitial eosinophilic opacity, and hemolysis could be found (Zhu et al. 1996).

Finally, it should be pointed out that—as with the detection of histological findings in relation to postmortem intervals—there are numerous investigations into the use of chemical–toxiclogical examinations after prolonged postmortem periods (Høiseth et al. 2008; Politi et al. 2008; Spiller and Pfiefer 2007; Lech 2006; Below and Lignitz 2003; Grellner 1998; Arnold et al. 1984; Käferstein 1981; Sticht et al. 1981; Sierra-Callejas and Pribilla 1978; Weinig 1958). Moreover, exhumations have proven to be useful for clarifying insurance-related medical questions (Stachetzki et al. 2001; Seibel et al. 1997).

Depending on the selected antibody, immunohistochemical examinations can provide evidence of the detected antigen for various lengths of time (Hilbig et al. 2004; Wehner et al. 1999, 2000, 2001a, b; Betz et al. 1993; Lorente et al. 1992).

The expression of glucagon in pancreatic cells was immunohistochemically examined with regard to varying postmortem intervals. Results showed that pancreatic α-cells from up to 6-day-old corpses produce a positive immunoreaction toward glucagon, whereas none of the corpses older than 14 days showed such a reaction (Wehner et al. 2001a).

The expression of calcitonin in thyroid C-cells was examined to determine the postmortem interval of a cadaver. Results showed that thyroid C-cells from up to 4-day-old corpses produce a positive immunoreaction toward calcitonin, whereas none of the corpses older than 13 days showed a positive reaction (Wehner et al. 2001b).

Autolysis and Putrefaction

Autolysis and bacterial decomposition with spread of gas-producing agents are findings that can typically be seen relatively early at autopsy conducted shortly after death (within 1–3 days). In most cases, autolysis with partial digestion of cells and tissue can first be seen in pancreatic tissue with a relatively early loss of dyeability of the nuclei. In addition, there are increasingly depleted erythrocytes (Pentillä and Laiho 1981), which initially results in a canalicular spread of microorganisms, in particular, bacteria. Gas-producing bacteria lead to the development of intraparenchymal gas bubbles; organs appear foamy or honeycomb-like (e.g., comb-like liver). In the case of such changes due to putrefaction, the organoid structure is often microscopically incomplete or can no longer be traced (Padosch et al. 2005). Thus hepatocytes, for example, not only lose dyeability of the nuclei, but in addition, the trabecular arrangement of the cells is lost and cell disintegration begins. Typically, fiber structures as well as embedded pigments (gall pigment, iron pigment, lipofuscin, anthracotic pigment, etc.) are more resistant. Calcification can also be shown for a prolonged period of time. Prior to the loss of dyeability of the nuclei, extensive spread of microorganisms is already possible. With marked gas production, detection of an air embolism becomes more difficult (Bajanowski et al. 1998). In differential diagnostic terms, it may also be difficult to differentiate between shock-related changes in the liver and focal autolytic changes (see Figs. 19.1, 19.2, 19.3, 19.4, and 19.5).

Table 19.1 Detectability of histological findings subject to postmortem periods according to data in the literature (selection)

Finding	Approximate postmortem period	Author(s)
Electrical burn	3 weeks	Walcher (1937)
Peritonitis, sepsis, septicopyemia	17 days/42 days	Althoff (1974)
Polynuclear alveolar cells	15 days	Althoff (1974)
Early cell infiltration	65 days	Althoff (1974)
Subserous hemorrhage	65 days	Althoff (1974)
Chronic meningitis	52 days	Althoff (1974)
Coronary thrombosis and myocardial fibrosis	90 days	Althoff (1974)
Chronic bronchitis	27 days	Althoff (1974)
Bronchopneumonia	133 days/95 days	Althoff (1974)
	392 days	Naeve and Bandmann (1981)
Immunohistochemical finding with myeloperoxidase	19 months	Schulz et al. (1999)
Brain metastasis of lung cancer	44 days	Althoff (1974)
Liver metastasis of a hemangiosarcoma	27 days	Althoff (1974)
Bronchial anthracofibrosis	80 days	Althoff (1974)
Stenosing coronary sclerosis	133 days	Althoff (1974)
Intimal sclerosis of the coronary arteries	19 months	Schulz et al. (1999)
Ganglion and glial cells	114 days	Walcher (1937)
	1212 days	Althoff (1974)
Positive evidence of iron in the tissue	1–2 years	Walcher (1937)
Fat embolism	8–10 days (experimental data)	Lubarsch (1900)
	4–8 weeks	Walcher (1925, 1928)
	4.5 months	Strassmann (1921, 1924, 1931)
Coronary thrombosis	8 months	Banaschak et al. (1998)
	3.5 months	Grellner and Glenewinkel (1997)
	3.9 months	Althoff (1974)
	96 days	Stachetzki et al. (2001)
Acute myocardial infarction	11 days	Thomsen and Held (1994)
Detected immunohistochemically with necrosis marker C5b-9(m)	6 weeks	Breitmeier et al. (2003)
	12 months	Karger et al. (2004)

Table 19.1 (continued)

Finding	Approximate postmortem period	Author(s)
NP57 (indicates neutrophilic leukocytes)	63 days, 487 days	Ortmann et al. (2000)
	128 days	Ortmann et al. (2000)
Detection of hemosiderin in the dura	8.5 months	Breitmeier et al. (2005)
Liver fibrosis	4.5 months	Breitmeier et al. (2005)
Shock liver	6 months	Breitmeier et al. (2005)
Glomerulonephritis	3.2 months	Breitmeier et al. (2005)
Cervical artery dissection	20 months	DeGiorgio et al. (2007)
Alzheimer's disease	2 months	Gelpi et al. (2007)
	20 months	Omalu et al. (2005)
Former cerebral contusion	3.5 weeks	Grellner and Glenewinkel (1997)
Cerebral edema	13 weeks	Grellner and Glenewinkel (1997)
Thyroiditis	3.75 months	Grellner and Glenewinkel (1997)
Nodular goiter	7 weeks	Grellner and Glenewinkel (1997)
	13.5 weeks	Althoff (1974)
Thyroid adenoma	3 months	Grellner and Glenewinkel (1997)
Tracheitis	2 weeks	Grellner and Glenewinkel (1997)
Epicarditis	3.75 months	Grellner and Glenewinkel (1997)
Lipomatosis cordis	2.5 years	Grellner and Glenewinkel (1997)
Myocardial hypertrophy	3.5 months	Grellner and Glenewinkel (1997)
	4.25 months	Naeve and Bandmann (1981)
Myocardial granulation tissue	3.5 months	Grellner and Glenewinkel (1997)
Myocardial fibrosis or scarring	2.5 years	Grellner and Glenewinkel (1997)
	2 years	Nordmann (1939)
Acute pulmonary trauma	5 weeks	Grellner and Glenewinkel (1997)
Pulmonary edema	3 months	Grellner and Glenewinkel (1997)
	2.5 years	Thomas et al. (1979)
Chronic pulmonary congestion	2.1 months	Grellner and Glenewinkel (1997)
	3.5 months	Naeve and Bandmann (1981)
Pulmonary amyloid bodies	3.5 years	Grellner and Glenewinkel (1997)
Shock lung	2 weeks	Grellner and Glenewinkel (1997)
Pneumonia	3.75 months	Grellner and Glenewinkel (1997)
	1.1 years	Naeve and Bandmann (1981)
Immunohistochemical detection of neutrophilic granulocytes with NP57	24 months	Karger et al. (2004)
Lung emphysema	2.5 years	Grellner and Glenewinkel (1997)
	2 years	Nordmann (1939)
	26 days	Raestrop (1926)
Anthracosis	7.5 years	Grellner and Glenewinkel (1997)
Tuberculosis	1.5 months	Grellner and Glenewinkel (1997)
	10 months	Nordmann (1939)
Pulmonary artery sclerosis	2.5 years	Grellner and Glenewinkel (1997)
Pulmonary thromboembolism	1.5 months	Grellner and Glenewinkel (1997)
Pulmonary fat embolism	4.5 months	Strassmann (1921, 1924, 1931)
	1–2 months	Walcher (1925–1928)
	1.2 months	Naeve and Bandmann (1981)
Hepatic capsular fibrosis	2.5 years	Grellner and Glenewinkel (1997)
Hepatocellular necrosis	6 days	Grellner and Glenewinkel (1997)
Fatty degeneration of the liver	3 months	Grellner and Glenewinkel (1997)
	10 years	Siegel et al. (1985)
Fatty liver hepatitis	2 weeks	Grellner and Glenewinkel (1997)

(continued)

Table 19.1 (continued)

Finding	Approximate postmortem period	Author(s)
Periportal infiltration	16 days	Althoff (1974)
Splenic artery hyalinosis	3.75 months	Grellner and Glenewinkel (1997)
Septic spleen	8 days	Grellner and Glenewinkel (1997)
	16 days	Althoff (1974)
Scarring of the renal cortex	3 months	Grellner and Glenewinkel (1997)
	4.8 months	Naeve and Bandmann (1981)
Renal shrinkage	6 weeks	Grellner and Glenewinkel (1997)
	3 years	Walcher (1937)
(Chronic) pyelonephritis	6 months	Grellner and Glenewinkel (1997)
	5 weeks	Althoff (1974)
Prostatic hypertrophy	2.5 years	Grellner and Glenewinkel (1997)
	2.5 months	Riepert et al. (1993)
Corticoadrenal hyperplasia	3.5 weeks	Grellner and Glenewinkel (1997)
Adipose tissue	2 years	Grellner and Glenewinkel (1997)
Alveolar structure and epithelium	4.8 years	Grellner and Glenewinkel (1997)
	1.25 years	Walcher (1937)
	2 weeks	Althoff (1974)
Amniotic fluid components	4.5 months	Strassmann (1921, 1924, 1931)
Bone marrow	3 months	Grellner and Glenewinkel (1997)
Brain tissue remains in adipoceratous cadavers	73 years	Erman (1882)
Brain structures	3 months	Grellner and Glenewinkel (1997)
Myocardium	2.5 years	Grellner and Glenewinkel (1997)
Hepatic cells	2.5 years	Grellner and Glenewinkel (1997)
Neuronal and glial cells	17 years	Grellner and Glenewinkel (1997)
	3.3 years	Althoff (1974)
Pancreas	4.8 years	Grellner and Glenewinkel (1997)
	4 weeks	Walcher (1937)
Renal structures and cells	2.5 years	Grellner and Glenewinkel (1997)
	3 years	Walcher (1928)
Skeletal muscle, including transverse striation	4.8 years	Grellner and Glenewinkel (1997)
Thyroid structure	2.5 years	Grellner and Glenewinkel (1997)
Infectious arteritis of the hepatic artery	9 days	Dedouit et al. (2010)
Reticulum cell sarcoma	16 months	Sierra-Callejas and Pribilla (1978)
Expanded lung tissue in a newborn caused by breathing	4.5 months	Strassmann (1921)
Displaced textile fibers at the site of bullet entry	7 months	Strassmann (1921)
	1 year	Strassmann (1921)
Interstitial lung fibrosis	223 days	Stachetzki et al. (2001)
Keratinizing squamous cell lung cancer	43 days	Stachetzki et al. (2001)
Brain metastasis of small-cell bronchial cancer	73 days	Stachetzki et al. (2001)
Immunohistochemical evidence of glucagon	Negative from 14 days postmortem	Wehner et al. (2001b)
Immunohistochemical evidence of calcitonin	Negative from 13 days postmortem	Wehner et al. (2001a)

Sometimes only the postmortem interval is stated in the literature but not if mummification or autolysis and putrefaction can be assumed

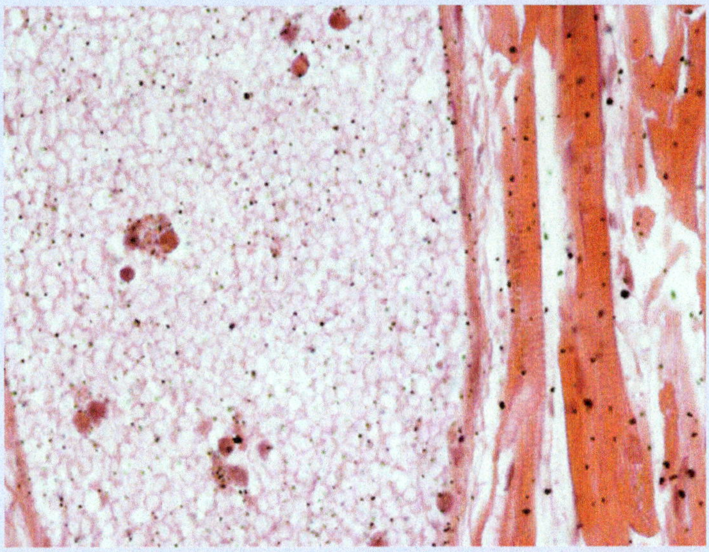

Fig. 19.1 Acute blood congestion with depleted and barely recognizable erythrocytes within the vascular lumen (H&E ×40)

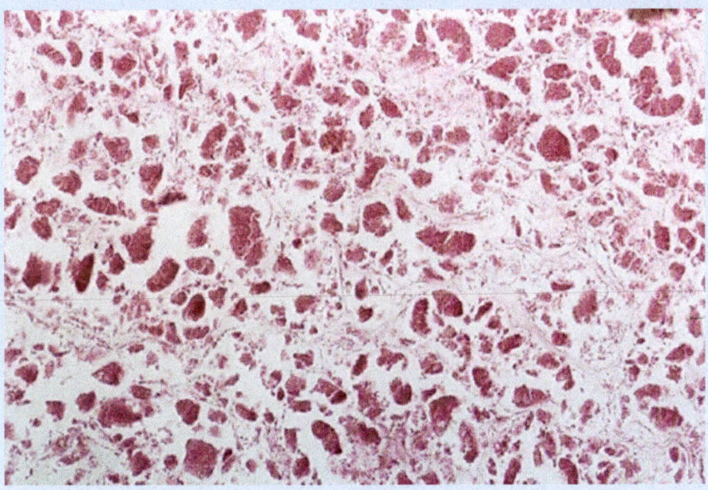

Fig. 19.2 Myocardial changes due to putrefaction with expired nuclear dyeability and irregular cardiomyocyte disintegration (H&E ×400)

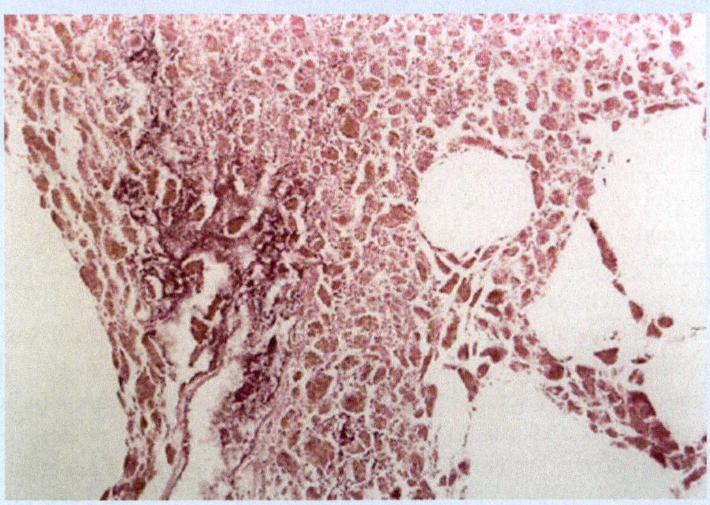

Fig. 19.3 Gas bubbles from putrefaction in the liver with elimination of the preexisting organic structure—macroscopically termed comb-like liver; simultaneous spread of bacteria in the liver sinusoids (H&E ×200)

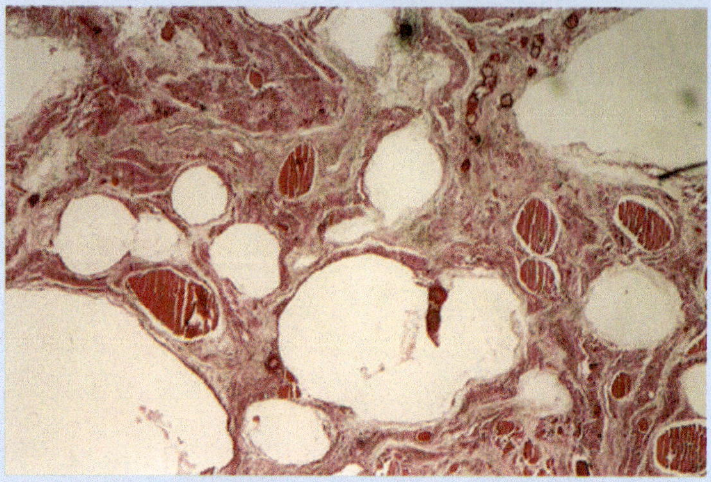

Fig. 19.4 Thyroid tissue changes due to putrefaction with barely recognizable organic structures and gas bubbles from putrefaction (H&E ×40)

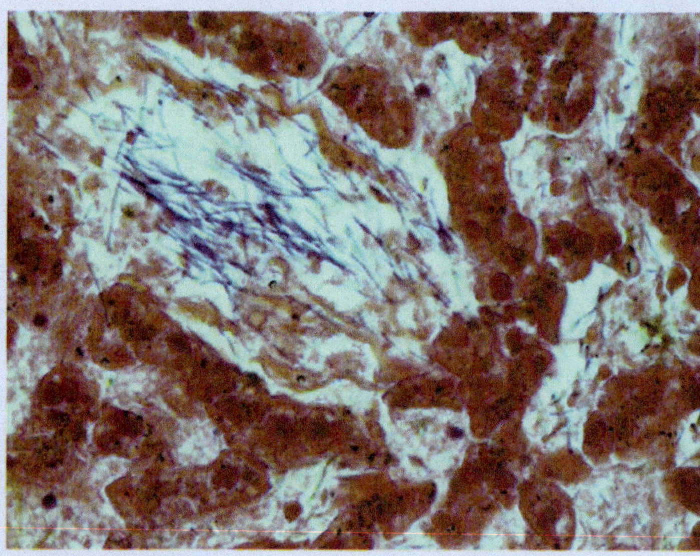

Fig. 19.5 Canalicular spread of microorganisms in the blood vessels (within the lumen of a central vein of the liver) and in liver sinusoids (H&E ×400)

Adipocere (Grave Wax)

Adipocere, which can be observed in particular in drowned bodies immersed in water for prolonged periods of time, can be useful to determine postmortem intervals (Fründ and Schoenen 2009; O'Brien and Kuehner 2007; Mellen et al. 1993). The formation of grave wax is the transformation of subcutaneous fatty tissue into a whitish-gray granular mass with an initially waxy and somewhat greasy consistency (Takatori and Yamaoka 1977; Takatori 2001; Yan et al. 2001).

The consistency becomes more solid over time due to drying out. Histologically, the developing structures may appear radially crystalline (Fig. 19.6). In fact, the term "grave wax" is incorrect since it is actually comprised of long-chain fatty acids and calcium salt. Adipocere develops when a corpse is stored in a wet environment with a lack of oxygen. Excess water causes hydrolytic cleavage of body fat into glycerine and fatty acids followed by saponification. The saponification of human adipose tissue is a preservation process resulting in a tissue called adipocere. Formation of adipocere develops in the water after several weeks and in the grave after several months. In most cases, however, it takes several years until the formation of adipocere in the corpse is complete. The formation of adipocere in the muscles begins after 3–4 months at the earliest.

In some cases, autolysis and putrefaction can develop quickly under certain environmental conditions, e.g., when the body is stored in a warm and humid environment or in the digestion tower of a sewage plant. In addition, putrefactive changes may occur more rapidly when the body is electrocuted, as could be the case if a hairdryer continued to operate in a water-filled bathtub (Fig. 19.7). However, added bath salts may have a certain preserving effect if they form a thick film that clings to the body (Fig. 19.8).

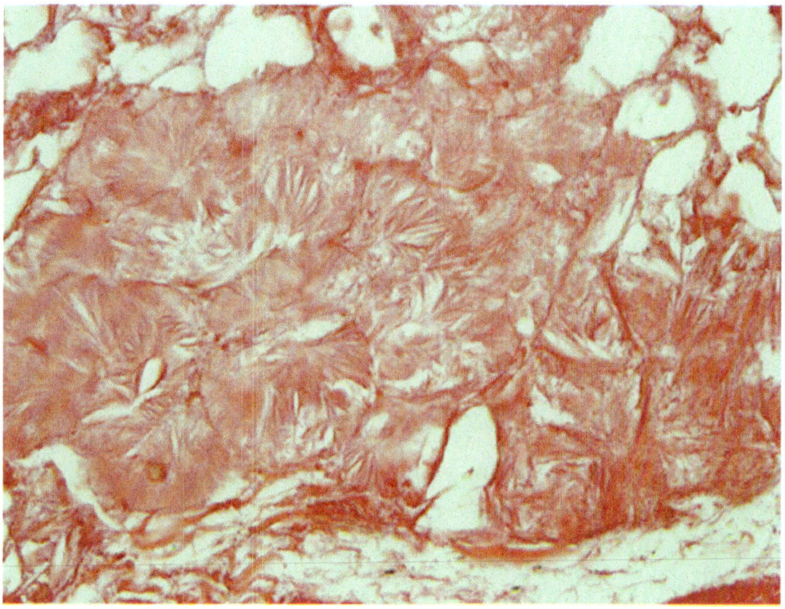

Fig. 19.6 Histological findings in the case of formation of adipocere with radial structures with a somewhat crystalline appearance (H&E ×200)

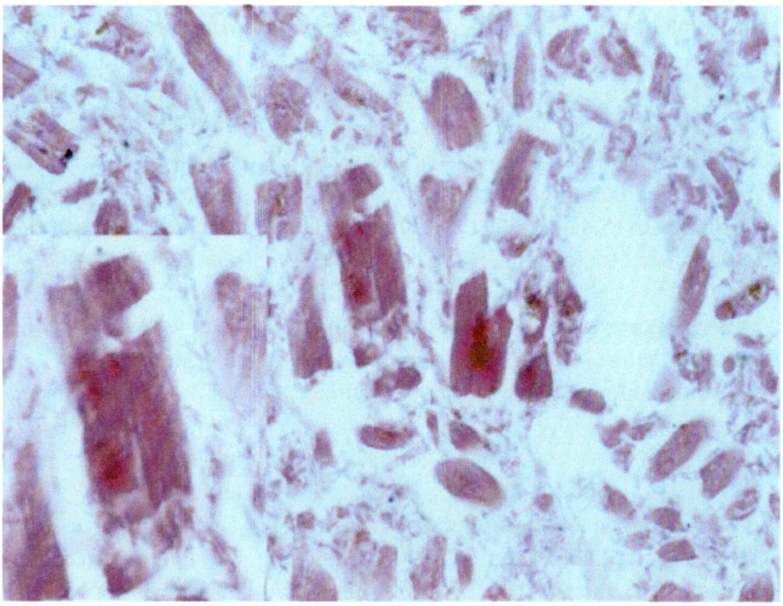

Fig. 19.7 A body electrocuted while a hairdryer continued to operate: dissolved structures in the myocardium, remaining lipofuscin pigment (H&E ×40), and partial horizontal striping of cardiomyocytes (H&E ×400)

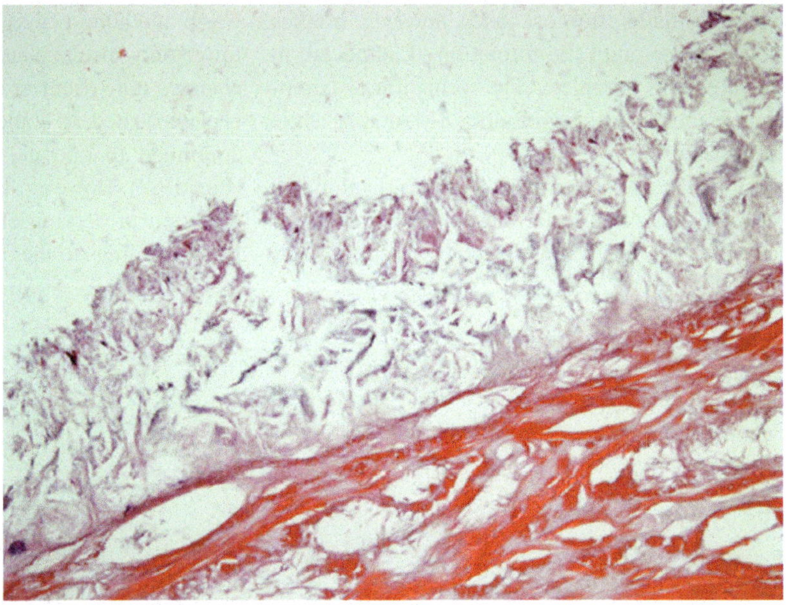

Fig. 19.8 After 7-week emersion in a water-filled bathtub: a film of bath salt covers the body surface and has a preserving effect (H&E ×100)

Mummification

In the case of mummification of a body, microscopic structures can be seen for a significantly longer period of time (Schulz et al. 1999), and the tissue can be rehydrated for histological investigation (Katzgraber et al. 1997). Confluent bronchopneumonia could be detected, for example, in a mummified body after 19 months with the aid of immunohistochemical methods. Conventional staining also permits the detection of connective tissue (Elastica van Gieson) for prolonged periods of time. In comparison, fibrin can no longer be differentiated at relatively early stages (Schulz et al. 1999; Olivecrona 1920). For exhumations, it can be assumed that microscope diagnosis is rarely possible after a postmortem period of more than 2 years. However, organic diagnoses may be possible for up to 5 years and sometimes even longer.

Microscopy evaluation becomes easier if already mummified structures that have undergone significant autolytic and putrefaction-related changes can be pretreated, thereby permitting better microscopic evaluation. Postmortem changes to human skin have been described when using immunohistochemical markers to, e.g., lysozyme and fibronectin (Fieguth et al. 1997). This could be shown for skin samples taken after a long postmortem interval using Sandison's rehydrating solution. As part of this process, the skin samples were treated with the rehydrating solution prior to fixation in formalin (Collini et al. 2014). Micromorphologically detectable changes to bone depending on the postmortem interval have been demonstrated in animal models, while histological changes in the bone matrix due to high temperatures have also been seen (Zangarini et al. 2016; Castillo et al. 2013). At the same time, one must expect to find fungal colonization and a wide variety of fungal species at autopsy (Hawksworth and Wiltshire 2011). Some fungal species possibly harbor an allergic potential, e.g., *Aspergillus fumigatus* and *Candida albicans* (Fig. 19.9; Schwarz et al. 2015). Unusual patterned skin lesions can be caused by postmortem fungal activity (Byard 2014).

In addition to fungi on the corpse, it is also possible to detect fly eggs deposited by various fly species depending on the postmortem interval and environmental conditions (Fig. 19.10).

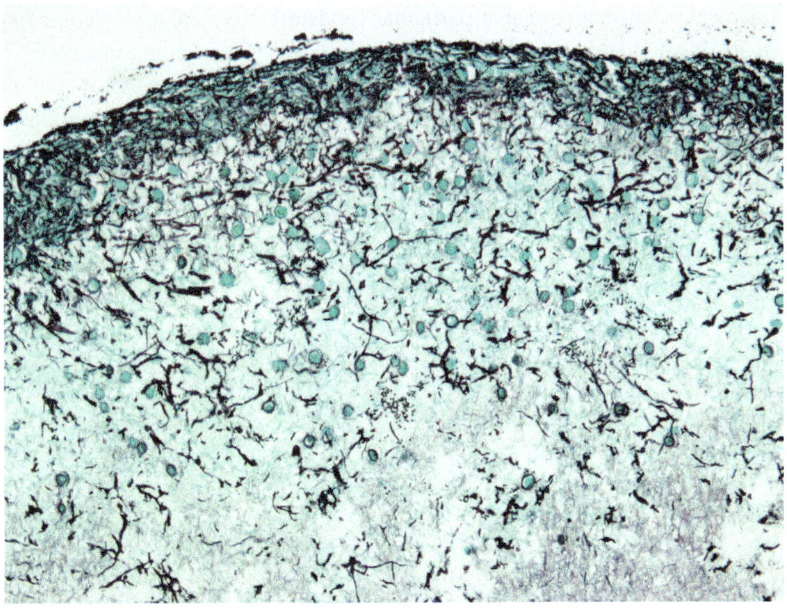

Fig. 19.9 Fungal colonization visible in the subepidermal soft tissue following a postmortem interval of several weeks (Grocott ×20)

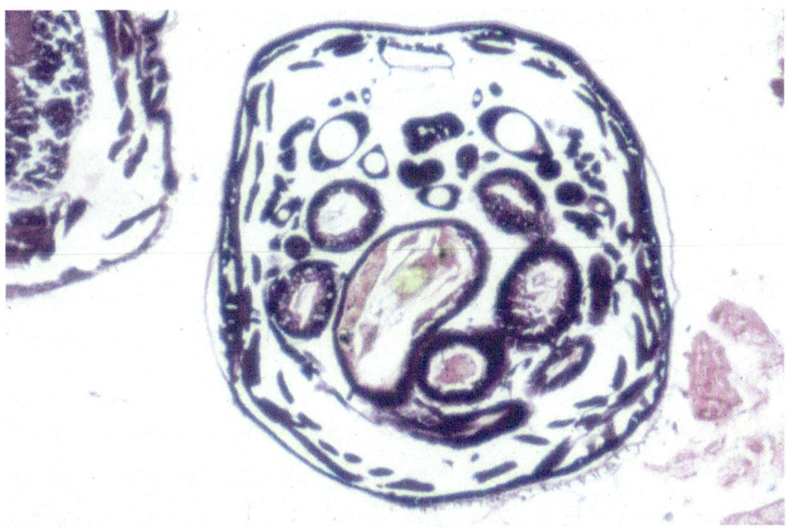

Fig. 19.10 Histological demonstration of a fly egg (HE ×100)

19.2 Microscopic Examination of Stomach Contents

The microscopic examination of stomach contents serves more to demonstrate specific nutritional components for criminological purposes than to clarify cause of death. The quantity of stomach contents, how quickly the contents passed through the stomach, as well as the type of food may be interesting in certain cases for the verification of other information by the investigating authorities (Tröger et al. 1987).

A number of foodstuffs show relatively characteristic findings (Gottschaldt 1934; Volger 1934; Drude 1933), and often only an approximate classification is possible (herbal components, meat).

However, in practice, any microscopic structure that can be identified as a certain food component should always be compared with the microscopic structure of that particular foodstuff in its fresh, undigested state. This applies, for instance, to microscopic structures in peanut in the case of known peanut allergy (see Chap. 15, Fig. 15.29), as well as to other relatively typical food components. Attention should also be paid during histological analysis of stomach contents to foreign material such as components of tablets. Figures 19.11 and 19.12 show examples of some typical microscopic findings for undigested, fresh food components.

When analyzing chyme particles histologically, it is important to bear in mind that even undigested food components can exhibit great similarity under microscopy, e.g., cucumber, eggplant, and olives. Differentiation can be extremely challenging in the undigested state. There are only scant investigations on defined

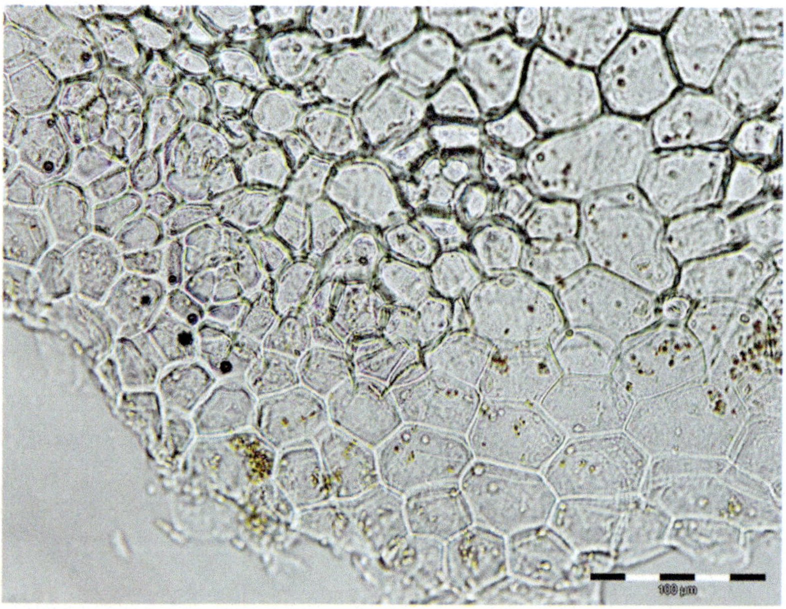

Fig. 19.11 Cucumber (×100)

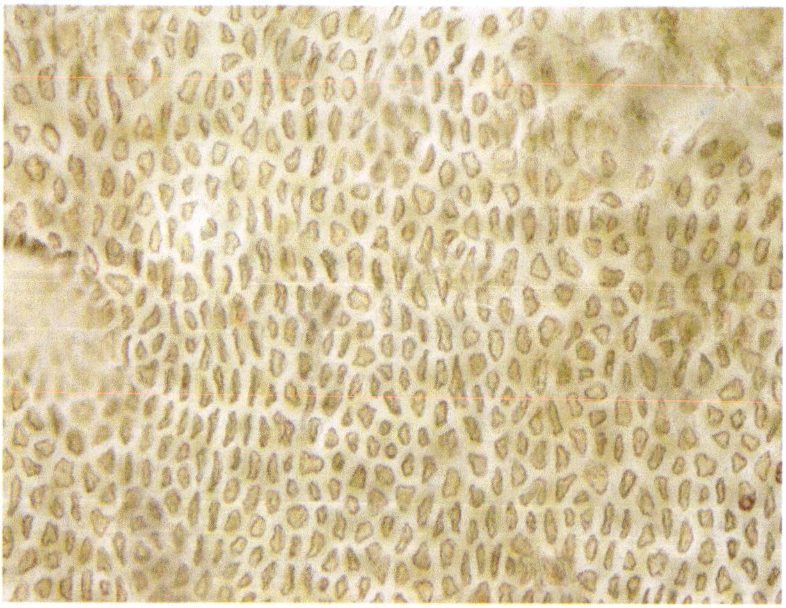

Fig. 19.12 Cherry (×100)

Fig. 19.13 Microscopic detection of tobacco fibers in the stomach in a case of oral tobacco ingestion with suicidal intent (H&E ×40; H&E ×400)

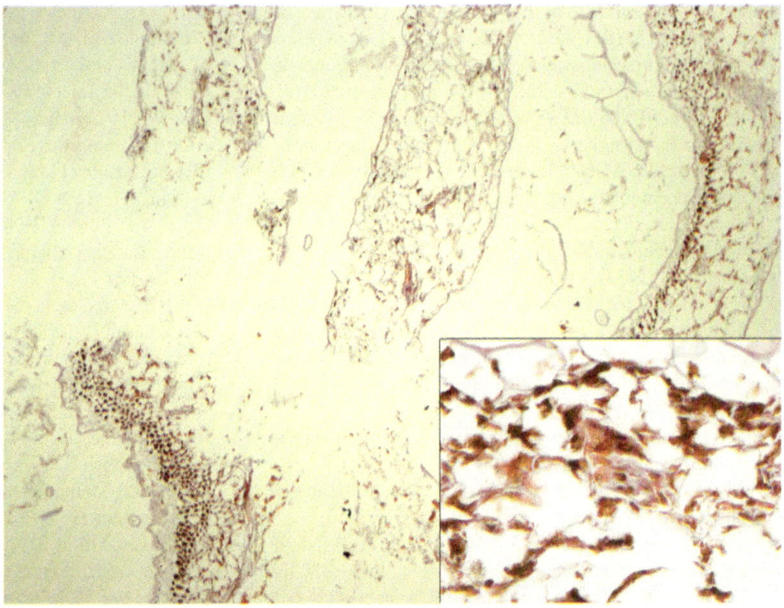

food components that can be systematically induced to undergo acidic and enzymatic digestion at body temperature and that can be analyzed by microscopy at defined time intervals.

In practice, the microscopic examination of gastric contents may well be decisive, for example, if it is able to provide evidence that peanuts were consumed despite a known peanut allergy (see Chap. 15, Figs. 15.34 and 15.35). Similarly, in the case of high levels of nicotine and cotinine detected in postmortem blood, microscopic examination of gastric contents can enable the detection of tobacco ingestion (Fig. 19.13).

References

Althoff H (1974) Bei welchen Fragestellungen kann man aussagefähige pathomorphologische Befunde nach Exhumierung erwarten. Z Rechtsmedizin 75:1–20

Arnold D, Naeve W, Arnold W (1984) Toxikologische Befunderhebungen an Fäulnisleichen – Leichenfäulnis an der Luft. Z Rechtsmedizin 93:151–164

Bajanowski T, Köhler H, DuChesne A, Koops E, Brinkmann B (1998) Proof of air embolism after exhumation. Int J Legal Med 112:2–7

Banaschak S, Eisenmenger W, Kuznik J, Brinkmann B (1998) Exhumierungen und kein Ende. Arch Kriminol 202:39–43

Below E, Lignitz E (2003) Cases of fatal poisoning in post-mortem examinations at the Institute of Forensic Medicine in Greifswald – analysis of five decades of post-mortems. Forensic Sci Int 133:125–131

Betz P, Nerlich A, Wilske J, Tubel J, Penning R, Eisenmenger W (1993) The immunohistochemical analysis of fibronectin, collagen type III, laminin, and cytokeratin 5 in putrified skin. Forensic Sci Int 61:35–42

Breitmeier D, Graefe-Kirci U, Albrecht K, Günther D, Kleeman WJ, Tröger HD (2003) Exhumierungen – Aussagekraft in Abhängigkeit von der Grabliegezeit. Kriminalistik 10:611–615

Breitmeier D, Graefe-Kirci U, Albrecht K, Weber M, Träger HD, Kleemann WJ (2005) Evaluation of the correlation between time corpses spent in in-ground graves and findings at exhumation. Forensic Sci Int 154:218–233

Byard RW (2014) Unusual patterned skin lesions caused by postmortem fungal activity. Forensic Sci Med Pathol 10:651–653

Castillo RF, Ubelaker DH, Acosta JAL, Cañadas de la Fuente GA (2013) Effects of temperature on bone tissue. Histological study of the changes in the bone matrix. Forensic Sci Int 226:33–37

Collini F, Adreola SA, Gentile G, Marchesi M, Muccino E, Zoja R (2014) Preservation of histological structure of cells in human skin presenting mummification and corification processes by Sandison's rehydrating solution. Forensic Sci Int 244:207–212

Cotton GE, Aufderheide AC, Goldschmidt VG (1987) Preservation of human tissue immersed for five years in fresh water of known temperature. J Forensic Sci 32:1125–1130

Dedouit F, Piercecchi-Marti MD, Leonetti G, Rougé D, Telmon N (2010) Cause of internal hemorrhage determined after exhumation: report of one case. Forensic Sci Int 204:e20–e23. https://doi.org/10.1016/j.forsciint.2010.05.028

DeGiorgio F, Vetrugno G, Fucci N, Rainio J, Tartaglions T, DiLazzaro V, Carbone A (2007) Fatal stroke in a young cocaine drug addict: chemical hair analysis and cervical artery examination twenty months after death. Folia Neuropathol 45:149–152

Drude W (1933) Beiträge zur mikroskopischen Diagnostik der Gemüse. I. Zwiebeln, Kohlarten, Tomate, Aubergine, Okra, Finocchio-Fenchel, Cardy und Artischocke. Z Unters Lebensm 65:497–540

Emson HE (1991) The case of the empty body. Am J Forensic Med Pathol 12:332–333

Erman P (1882) Beitrag zur Kenntnis der Fettwachsbildung. Vjschr Gerichtl Med 37:51

Evans WE (1961) Some histological findings in spontaneously preserved bodies. Med Sci Law 2:155

Fechner G, Sivaloganathan S (1987) Demonstration of myocardial infarction in putrefying bodies. J Clin Pathol 40:922–929

Fieguth A, Kleemann WJ, von Wasielewski R, Werner M, tröger HD (1997) Influence of postmortem changes on immunohistochemical reactions in skin. Int J Legal Med 110:18–21

Fründ HC, Schoenen D (2009) Quantification of adipocere degradation with and without access to oxygen and to the living soil. Forensic Sci Int 18:18–22

Galloway A (1997) The process of decomposition: a model from the Arizona-Sonoran desert. In: Hagland WD, Sorg MH (eds) Forensic taphonomy: the post-mortem fate of human remains. CRC Press, Boca Raton, pp 139–150

Geill T (1924) Mikroskopische Untersuchung von Organen einer exhumierten Leiche. Beitr Gerichtl Med 6:10

Gelpi E, Preusser M, Bauer G, Budka H (2007) Autopsy at 2 months after death: brain is satisfactorily preserved for neuropathology. Forensic Sci Int 168:177–182

Gottschaldt H (1934) Beiträge zur mikroskopischen Diagnostik der Gemüse. III. Salate und Spinate. Z Unters Lebensm 67:465–510

Grellner W (1998) Toxikologische Nachweismöglichkeiten bei Fettwachsumwandlung und mehrjähriger Liegezeit. Arch Kriminol 202:81–84

Grellner W, Glenewinkel F (1997) Exhumations: synopsis of morphological and toxicological findings in relation to the post-mortem interval. Survey on a 20-year period and review of the literature. Forensic Sci Int 90:139–159

Hawksworth DL, Wiltshire PEJ (2011) Forensic mycology: the use of fungi in criminal investigations. Forensic Sci Int 206:1–11

Hilbig H, Bidmon HJ, Oppermann OT, Remmerbach T (2004) Influence of post-mortem delay and storage temperature on the immunohistochemical detection of antigens in the CNS of mice. Exp Toxicol Pathol 56:159–171

Høiseth G, Karinen R, Johnsen L, Normann PT, Christophersen AS, Mørland J (2008) Disappearance of ethyl glucuronide during heavy putrefaction. Forensic Sci Int 176:147–151

Janssen W (1977) Histologische Untersuchung exhumierter Leichen. In: Forensische histologie. Schmidt-Römhild, Lübeck, pp 54–72

Käferstein H (1981) Schwer flüchtige organische Gifte in Fäulnisleichen – Nachweisbarkeit und Beurteilungsmöglichkeit. Beitr Gerichtl Med 39:119–124

Karger B, Lorin de la Grandmaison G, Bajanoswki T, Brinkmann B (2004) Analysis of 155 consecutive forensic exhumations with emphasis on undetected homicides. Int J Legal Med 118:90–94

Katzgraber F, Rabl W, Steinlechner M (1997) Histologische Ergebnisse nach Rehydrierung mumifizierten Gewebes: experimentelle Überprüfung verschiedener Methoden. In: 76th Annual meeting of the German Society of Forensic Medicine, Jena, 1997

Kocovski L, Duflou J (2009) Can renal acute tubular necrosis be differentiated from autolysis at autopsy? J Forensic Sci 54:439–442

Lech T (2006) Exhumation examination to confirm suspicion of fatal lead poisoning. Forensic Sci Int 158:219–223

Lorente JA, Lorente M, Villanueva E (1992) Postmortem stability of lung surfactant phospholipids. J Forensic Sci 37:1341–1345

Lubarsch O (1900) Über die Veränderungen vergrabener Leichentheile. Kriminalistik 57:611–615

Mellen PF, Lowry MA, Micozzi MS (1993) Experimental observations on adipocere formation. J Forensic Sci 38:91–93

Naeve W, Bandmann H (1981) Über Fragestellungen, Ergebnisse und Aussagewert versicherungsmedizinischer Obduktionen nach Exhumation. Lebensversicher Med 33:37–42

Nordmann M (1939) Erfahrungen bei Exhumierungen. Zbl Allg Path Anat 73:81–86

O'Brien T, Kuehner AC (2007) Waxing grave about adipocere: soft tissue change in an aquatic context. J Forensic Sci 52:294–301

Olivecrona H (1920) Untersuchungen über die Fäulnisveränderungen der menschlichen Lunge. Vjschr Gerichtl Med Öffentl Sanitätswesen 60:102–120

Omalu BI, Mancuso JA, Cho P, Wecht CH (2005) Diagnosis of Alzheimer's disease in an exhumed decomposed brain after twenty months of burial in a deep grave. J Forensic Sci 50:1453–1458

Ortmann C, Pfeiffer H, Brinkmann B (2000) Demonstration of myocardial necrosis in the presence of advanced putrefaction. Int J Legal Med 114:50–55

Padosch SA, Dettmeyer R, Kröner LU, Preuss J, Madea B (2005) An unusual occupational accident: fall into a sewage plant tank with lethal outcome. Forensic Sci Int 149:39–45

Pedal I (1995) Immunhistochemische Blutgruppendiagnostik (ABH, Lewis) in der Rechtsmedizin. In:

Bratzke HJ, Schröter A (eds) Immunhistochemie in der Rechtsmedizin. Deutsche Hochschulschriften, Egelsbach, pp 14–21
Pentillä A, Laiho K (1981) Autolytic changes in blood cells of human cadavers. II. Morphological studies. Forensic Sci Int 17:121–132
Politi L, Morini L, Mari F, Groppi A, Bertol E (2008) Ethyl glucuronide and ethyl sulfate in autopsy samples 27 years after death. Int J Legal Med 122:507–509
Raestrop G (1926) Über Exhumierungen. Dtsch Z Gerichtl Med 6:34–48
Riepert T, Lasczkowski G, Rittner C (1993) Zusammenhang zwischen Arbeitsunfall und Todeseintritt 55 Jahre später. Versicherungsmedizin 45:91–93
Schmeißer H (1926) Beitrag zur Frage der Zweckmäßigkeit gerichtlicher Exhumierungen unter besonderer Berücksichtigung histologischer Organbefunde bei exhumierten Leichen. Dtsch Z Gerichtl Med 8:162
Schmidt W (1951) Histologische Befunde an Felsenbeinen exhumierter Leichen. Dtsch Z Gerichtl Med 40:400
Schulz F, Tsokos M, Püschel K (1999) Natürliche Mumifikation im häuslichen Milieu. Rechtsmedizin 10:32–38
Schwarz F (1926) Über histologisch-bakteriologische Befunde an Organen einer exhumierten Leiche. Schweiz Med Wschr 56:996
Schwarz P, Dannaoui E, Gehl A, Felske-Zech H, Birngruber CG, Dettmeyer RB, Verhoff MA (2015) Molecular identification of fungi found on decomposed human bodies in forensic autopsy cases. Int J Legal Med 129:785–791
Seibel O, Heinemann A, Hildebrand E, Püschel K (1997) 131 cases of exhumination in Hamburg and their significance for legal medicine and medical insurance (1971–1995). Versicherungsmedizin 49:209–215
Siegel H, Rieders F, Holmstedt B (1985) The medical and scientific evidence in alleged tubocurarine poisonings. A review of the so-called Dr. X case. Forensic Sci Int 29:29–76
Sierra-Callejas JL, Pribilla O (1978) Exhumierung bei Verdacht auf Vergiftung – Retikulumzellsarkom. Z Rechtsmed 81:335–340
Spiller HA, Pfiefer E (2007) Two fatal cases of selenium toxicity. Forensic Sci Int 171:67–72
Stachetzki U, Verhoff MA, Ulm K, Müller KM (2001) Morphologische Befunde und versicherungsmedizinische Aspekte bei 371 Exhumierungen. Pathologe 22:252–258
Sticht G, Ramme H, Dotzauer G (1981) Morphologische und toxikologische Befunde nach 17jähriger Liegezeit einer Leiche. Beitr. Ger Med 39:177–183
Strassmann G (1921) Mikroskopische Untersuchungen an exhumierten und verwesten Organen. Vjschr Gerichtl Med 62:131
Strassmann G (1924) Beobachtungen bei Exhumierungen. Ärztl Sachverst Ztg 34:241
Strassmann G (1931) Lehrbuch der Gerichtlichen Medizin. Enke-Verlag, Stuttgart
Tabata N, Morita M (1997) Immunohistochemical demonstration of bleeding in decomposed bodies by using anti-glycophorin A monoclonal antibody. Forensic Sci Int 87:1–8
Takatori T (2001) The mechanism of human adipocere formation. Legal Med 3:193–204
Takatori T, Yamaoka A (1977) The mechanism of adipocere formation. I. Identification and chemical properties of hydroxy fatty acids in adipocere. Forensic Sci 9:63–73
Thomas F, La Barre J, Renaux J, Draux E (1979) A therapeutic catastrophe, entailing 16 exhumations, following the administration of digitoxin instead of oestradiol benzoate to prostate cancer patients: identification of the poison. Med Sci Law 19:8–18
Thomsen H, Held H (1994) Susceptibility of $C5b\text{-}9_{(m)}$ to postmortem changes. Int J Legal Med 106:291–293
Tröger HD, Baur C, Spann KW (1987) Mageninhalt und Todeszeitbestimmung. Methodik und gerichtsmedizinische Bedeutung. Schmidt-Römhild, Lübeck
Ubelaker DH (2008) Review of: the scientific investigation of mass graves: towards protocols and standard operating procedures. J Forensic Sci 53:1014
Vock R, Wünsch PH, Müller-Wallraf R (1989) Exhumierung – eine sinnvolle diagnostische Maßnahme. Dt Ärztebl 86:352–353
Volger H (1934) Beiträge zur mikroskopischen Diagnostik der Gemüse. II. Leguminosenhülsen, Wurzel- und Knollengemüse, Blatt- und Stengelgemüse. Z Unters Lebensm 67:1–41
Walcher K (1925) Beitrag zur praktischen Bedeutung der Exhumierungen für die Erkennung der Todesursache. Ärztl Sachverst Ztg 31:255
Walcher K (1928) Studien über die Leichenfäulnis mit besonderer Berücksichtigung der Histologie derselben. Virchows Arch A Pathol Anat Histopathol 268:17–180
Walcher K (1937) Die späten Leichenveränderungen. Ergebni Path 33:55
Walcher K (1938) Studien über die Leichenfäulnis mit besonderer Berücksichtigung der Histologie derselben. Virch Arch Path Anat 268:17
Wehner F, Wehner HD, Schieffer MC, Subke J (1999) Delimination of the time of death by immunohistochemical detection of insulin in pancreatic beta-cells. Forensic Sci Int 105:161–169
Wehner F, Wehner HD, Schieffer MC, Subke J (2000) Delimination of the time of death by immunohistochemical detection of thyreoglobulin. Forensic Sci Int 110:199–206
Wehner F, Wehner HD, Subke J (2001a) Delimitation of the time of death by immunohistochemical detection of calcitonin. Forensic Sci Int 122:89–94
Wehner F, Wehner HD, Subke J (2001b) Delimitation of the time of death by immunohistochemical detection of glucagons in pancreatic alpha-cells. Forensic Sci Int 124:192–199
Weimann W (1928) Histologische Hirnbefunde bei Exhumierungen. Dtsch Z Gerichtl Med 11:388

Weimann W (1958) Histologische Hirnbefunde bei Exhumierungen. Dtsch Z Gerichtl Med 47:397–416

Weinig E (1958) Die Nachweisbarkeit von Giften in exhumierten Leichen. Dtsch Z Gerichtl Med 47:397–416

Yan F, McNally R, Kontanis EJ, Sadik OA (2001) Preliminary quantitative investigation of post-mortem adipocere formation. J Forensic Sci 46:609–614

Zangarini S, Trombino L, Cattaneo C (2016) Micromorphological and ultramicroscopic aspects of buried remains: time-dependent markers of decomposition and permanence in soil in experimental burial. Forensic Sci Int 263:74–82

Zhu BL, Maeda H, Fukita K, Sakurai M, Kobayashi Y (1996) Immunohistochemical investigation of pulmonary surfactant in perinatal fatalities. Forensic Sci Int 83:219–227

20 Forensic Neuropathology

Forensic neuropathology has established itself as an independent discipline within forensic science. More specific information can be found by referring to the relevant literature (e.g., Leestma 2009; Oehmichen et al. 2006; Itabashi et al. 2007; Chan and Lowe 2002; Oehmichen and König 1997; Bratzke and Krauland 1988; Bratzke et al. 1986; Krauland 1973, 1981, 1982). For some investigations, there are more differentiated proposals on the neuropathological diagnostic work-up, e.g., in sudden infant death syndrome (SIDS) (Matturri et al. 2008).

However, the most significant neuropathological findings in forensic practice will be described here in more detail. These include traumatic injuries, such as intracranial bleeding, inflammation (e.g., meningitis or meningoencephalitis), aneurysms of the basilar arteries, intracerebral arteriovenous malformations, and rare diseases that may explain sudden and unexpected death in some cases.

Although histopathological findings in the hypophysis have rarely been examined (Ishikawa et al. 2006a, b, 2009), findings relevant to cause of death have been observed (Bauer et al. 2001). Axonal damage in drug-related deaths could be determined immunohistochemically (Büttner et al. 2006). The central nervous system (CNS) also plays a role in systemic diseases, such as amyloidosis (Büttner et al. 2001). Incidental findings sometimes occur, e.g., intracranial plasma cell granuloma (Dettmeyer et al. 1998a, b) or subarachnoid hemorrhage originating from ecchordosis physaliphora (Fracasso et al. 2008). *Hippocampal malformations* are believed to be associated with sudden death in childhood; however, the evidence here is scant, and conceivable pathophysiological links remain unelucidated (Rutecki und Sutula 2016; Ackerman et al. 2016; Smith 2016; Noebels 2016; Hefti et al. 2016; Rodriguez et al. 2012).

Neuropathological findings may help to explain accidents (e.g., motor vehicle accidents) (Kibayashi and Shojo 2002; Ng'walali et al. 2002; Viitanen et al. 1998). Some immunohistochemical markers have been used to help explain cause of death or determine intravital damage to nervous tissue, such as ubiquitin (Piette et al. 2010; Quan et al. 2001, 2005a, b, c), S-100 (Li et al. 2006), or β-amyloid precursor protein (ß-APP) as a marker for early damage to brain tissue (Dolinak and Reichard 2006; Reichard et al. 2003; Gleckman et al. 1999; Sherriff et al. 1994).

20.1 Forensic Neurotraumatology

By definition, there are no morphological correlates for clinical and neurological symptoms in the case of cerebral concussion. However, cerebral concussion may sometimes have lethal effects if the trauma induces lethal thrombosis of the basilar arteries (Kind 1991). Traumatic changes in the CNS also include macroscopically undetectable results of trauma, such as diffuse

R. B. Dettmeyer, *Forensic Histopathology*, https://doi.org/10.1007/978-3-319-77997-3_20

axonal injury (DAI) (Oehmichen et al. 2009; Orihara et al. 2003; Geddes et al. 2000; Hausmann et al. 1999; Nogami et al. 1999a, b; Ogata and Tsuganezawa 1999; Herczeg et al. 1995; Kitamura 1994; Vowles et al. 1987). Sudden cerebral swelling and death secondary to cranio-cerebral trauma have also been observed in children and young adults. Although the etiology is unknown, the basic pathophysiology includes vasodilatation and initial hyperemia with redistribution of blood from the subarachnoid and pial vessels into the parenchyma of the brain (McQuillen et al. 1988).

Some authors have looked for morphological parameters to grade brain swelling (cerebral edema), which is a common finding after traumatic brain injury due to a dysfunction of the blood–brain barrier, microcirculation failure, or reactions of the local glial cells. Cerebral edema is characterized by abnormally large amounts of fluid in the extracellular compartment of brain tissue, preferentially in the white matter. Nevertheless, histological findings are of minimal significance when grading brain swelling (Hausmann et al. 2006).

20.1.1 Intracranial Hematomas or Hemorrhages

In forensic science, intracranial hemorrhages are of special interest in everyday practice, i.e., epidural and subdural hematomas, subarachnoid hemorrhages, and hemorrhages within the CNS.

Epidural Hematomas

Acute epidural hematomas are relatively infrequent, usually unilateral, and often seen as a result of a fall or motor vehicle accident. The majority of cases present with a fracture at the site of impact (Padosch et al. 2006). Lacerated meningeal vessels lead to hemorrhage, typically with involvement of the middle meningeal artery. Epidural hematomas due to venous bleeding are rare and usually due to the laceration of meningeal veins, diploic veins, or dural sinuses. Chronic epidural hematomas, which, by definition, present or are identified 48–72 h after injury, are also rare and may or may not be associated with skull fracture.

Subdural Hematomas

Subdural hematomas can be acute (symptoms present within 72 h), subacute (symptoms present between 3 days and 2–3 weeks), or chronic (more than 3 weeks after injury). Subdural hemorrhage is caused by shear force acting upon the parasagittal bridging veins during acceleration–deceleration injuries (DiMaio and Dana 2007). It may occur on either the ipsilateral or contralateral side of impact or bilaterally and must not be associated with skull fractures. Otherwise, although it is said *that* traumatic subdural hemorrhage results from rupture of bridging veins, new insights into the anatomy of infant dura suggest a dural origin for the thin-film subdural bleeding seen in young infants (Squier and Mack 2009). In cases of subdural hematoma in children, glutaric aciduria type 1 (GA1) may represent a differential diagnosis from child abuse in rare cases (Vester et al. 2015). In association with an underlying disease, fatal subdural hematoma in infancy that is initially suggestive of shaken baby syndrome may occur. If bridging veins are intact and there is no hemorrhage at the level of the optic nerve sheath, a nontraumatic cause of subdural hematoma should be considered (Ceauşu et al. 2015; Guddat et al. 2011); the same is true for forms of von Willebrand disease (Stray-Pedersen et al. 2011). A chronic subdural hematoma can rebleed spontaneously or as a result of a relatively minor trauma. Ruptures of bridging veins as a cause of subdural bleeding are not easy to verify. It appears that these blood vessels do not rupture completely, even in cases of serious accidents (Gumpert and Maxeiner 2008).

The organization of a subdural hematoma can be divided microscopically into different stages such that an approximate age determination of a subdural hematoma may be possible if the tissue samples to be investigated have been carefully selected (Table 20.1).

Once organization is complete, only a thin yellow-gold-colored membrane adherent to the dura may remain.

Organization of a subdural hematoma typically begins with fibrinogen and fibrin deposits, the build-up of fibroblasts, collagen fiber formation, the migration of leukocytes and macrophages, and capillary blood vessel sprouting. If, in addition to the findings listed in Table 20.1, linear lipophage deposits (Fig. 20.1) are found histologically at the brain tissue border, one should consider the possibility of additional damage to the immediately adjacent cerebral cortex.

Subarachnoid Hemorrhage

Subarachnoid hemorrhage is the most common intracranial bleeding due to blunt head trauma (Thornstedt and Voigt 1960). Blunt head trauma can cause lethal basal subarachnoid hemorrhage (Bratzke and Eisenmenger 1989) due to overstretching ruptures and/or bursting ruptures. The vast majority of traumas appear to result from fights under the influence of alcohol and can be classified as minor traumata (Simonsen 1963, 1984). A case of subarachnoid hemorrhage due to whiplash trauma involving dissection of the internal carotid artery, as conceivable in the context of a traffic accident, has been described (Uhrenholt et al. 2015). Histological evidence of the origin of a subarachnoid hemorrhage can be helpful for a precise answer to legal questions (Krauland 1981). In the case of fatal basal subarachnoid hemorrhage due to rupture of the normal intracranial vertebral artery, rupture can be caused by overstretching of the vertebral artery from traumatic hyperextension of the neck (Miyazaki et al. 1990).

Organization of subarachnoid hemorrhages yields the same microscopic picture on the side between the clot and arachnoid, as described for subdural hematomas in Table 20.1 (Fig. 20.2). Intracerebral hemorrhages resulting from blunt force injury are organized in a similar manner to hemorrhages due to cortical contusions with bleeding.

Table 20.1 Stages in the organization of subdural hematomas

Time period following injury	Possible microscopic findings
Up to 24 h	Erythrocytes, a thin layer of fibrin between the dura and clot
48–72 h	Erythrocytes, rare fibroblasts at the interface on the side of the membrane facing the dura
4–5 days	Breakdown of erythrocytes, two- to five-cell-thick layer of fibroblasts on the side of the membrane facing the dura
5–10 days	Early capillary formation/granulation tissue of clot, some siderophages, thicker layer of fibroblasts, and, occasionally, small capillaries may be present on the side of the membrane facing the dura
10–20 days	Granulation tissue with capillary formation within the clot, fibroblast layer 1/3–1/2 as thick as the dura; siderophages; early fibroblastic membrane evident on the side of the membrane between the clot and arachnoid
3–4 weeks	Clot nearly liquefied, membrane equal to the dura in thickness on the side of the membrane facing the dura; siderophages
1–3 months	Large capillaries, possibility of rebleeding, hyalinized membranes on the side facing the dura and on the side between the clot and arachnoid

According to DiMaio and Dana (2007) and Squier and Mack (2009)

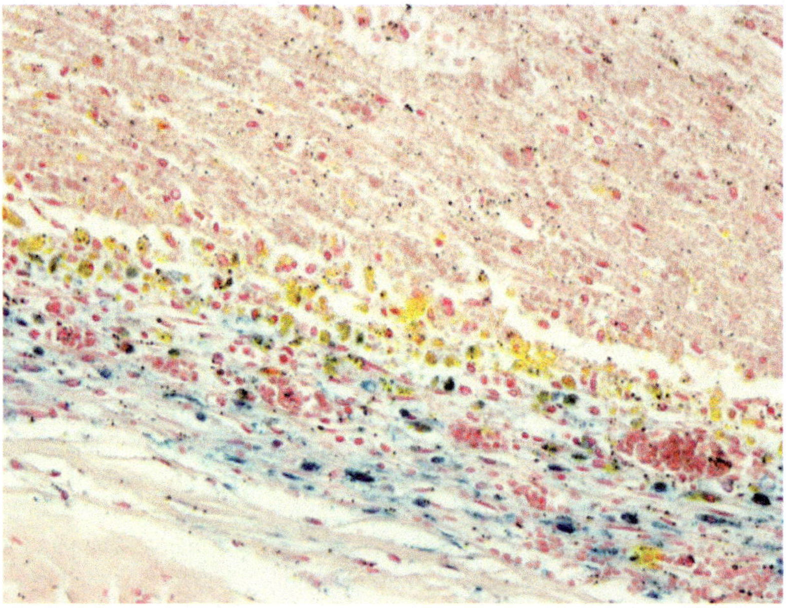

Fig. 20.1 An old subdural hematoma with linear deposits of hemosiderin-containing macrophages (siderophages) in the Prussian blue reaction, as well as a linear, parallel accumulation of yellow lipophages at the border to brain tissue in a case of evident traumatic injury also affecting adjacent cerebral cortex tissue (Prussian blue, ×200)

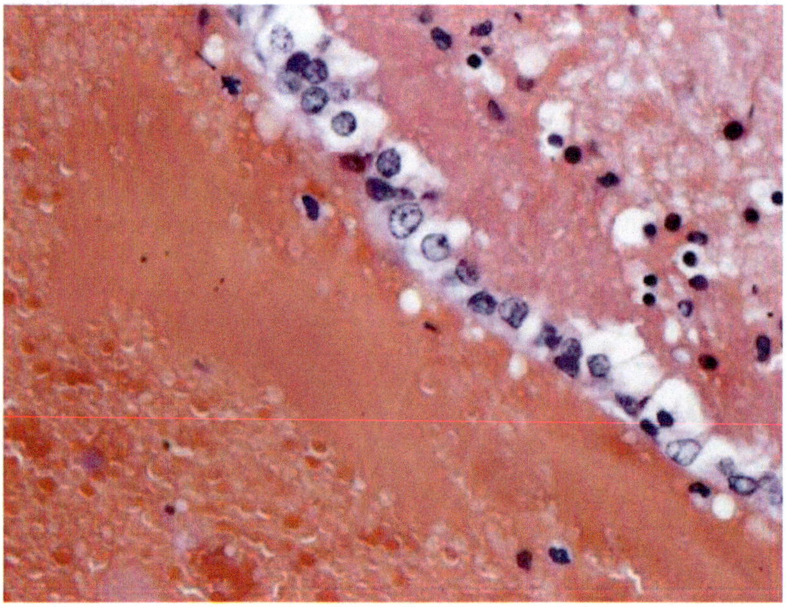

Fig. 20.2 Acute arachnoid hemorrhage: early signs of organization with rare fibroblasts on the side of the membrane between the clot and arachnoid 36 h post-blunt head trauma (H&E ×400)

20.1.2 Wound Age Estimation of Cortical Contusions

Cerebral contusions are bruises to the cortical surface of the brain, which can extend to the white matter. Several studies have examined the temporal course of the wound-healing process in the CNS by using conventional histological and enzyme-histochemical or immunohistochemical techniques. Cortical contusions are characterized by early morphological changes, such as hemorrhage or microscopically visible signs of neuronal degeneration, followed by local cellular reactions (Figs. 20.3, 20.4, 20.5, and 20.6) (Hausmann 2004).

DAI of the brain describes immediate prolonged coma (>6 h) after head trauma not associated with intracranial hemorrhage or macroscopically visible lesions (DiMaio and Dana 2007; Iino et al. 2003; Oehmichen et al. 1998; Sheriff et al. 1994;

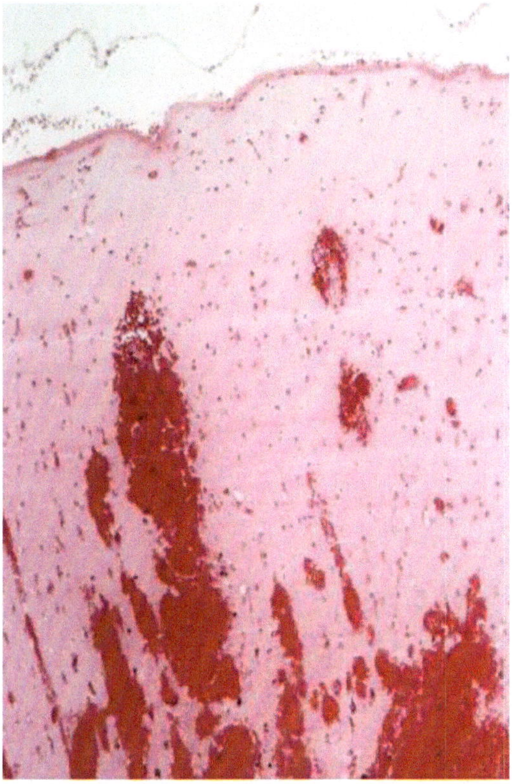

Fig. 20.3 Cerebral contusion with acute intracerebral hemorrhage of the cortical surface of the brain (contrecoup contusion) accompanied by a skull fracture at the point of impact (coup contusion) and without any signs of organization (H&E ×100)

Gentleman et al. 1993). Axonal injuries in cases of DAI are not visible by light microscopy using H&E staining until about 12 h after head trauma (DiMaio and Dana 2007), but they may be seen 2–3 h after injury by means of immunohistochemical techniques showing ß-amyloid precursor protein (ß-APP). However, DAI is not specific for trauma.

In cases of traumatic brain injury (TBI), using routine histology as well as immunohistochemical techniques, the earliest appearance and observation period of various parameters are of interest (Wang et al. 2011, 2012; Tao et al. 2006; Cervós-Navarro and Lafuente 1991; Oehmichen and Raff 1980):

- Cellular response
- Neuronal changes
- Glial changes
- Mesenchymal changes
- Vascular reactions

An overview including some important histological and immunohistochemical parameters for approximate age determination of brain tissue injury is shown in Table 20.2. In addition to the immunohistochemical markers listed in Table 20.2, the following are also mentioned: LCA, UCHL-1, MIB-1, vimentin, tenascin, alpha-1-antichymotrypsin, laminin, type IV collagen, thrombomodulin, and factor VIII (Hausmann et al. 2006).

Nevertheless, it should be noted that the majority of the parameters mentioned in the literature are not specific for brain trauma and may also occur under pathological conditions, such as ischemia, toxic lesions, encephalomyelitis, or brain tumors. It is also important to bear in mind that the results of relevant expression studies in the literature are presented differently: some studies present the results for the earliest expression of a marker, while others give the time point at which a marker disappears. Yet other studies report time-dependent changes in expression, differentiated according to acute, subacute, and delayed. In none of these cases is it possible to speak of high accuracy in terms of the statements made, not least since effects such as postmortem interval, fixation time of the tissue analyzed, and the postmortem stability of individual markers were frequently not taken into consideration. A macroscopic grading system for cerebral contusions depending on the number and localization of the contusions has been proposed (Omalu et al. 2005).

When determining the age of a cerebral contusion, a separate consideration of immunohistochemical reactions according to their microscopic localization is recommended, i.e., distinguishing between vascular findings (tenascin, MIB-1) and reactive gliosis (tenascin, MIB-1, GFAP, vimentin) and cellular infiltration (CD15, LCA, CD3, UCHL-1). Only by considering several parameters is it possible to make an approximate wound age determination in terms of hours, days, or weeks according to wound age specification as fresh, no longer fresh, and older. ß-APP can be demonstrated immunohistochemically in marginal zones of injured brain tissue relatively early (<35 min; see Fig. 20.23), whereas using Bodian's silver impregnation, changes are not visible until

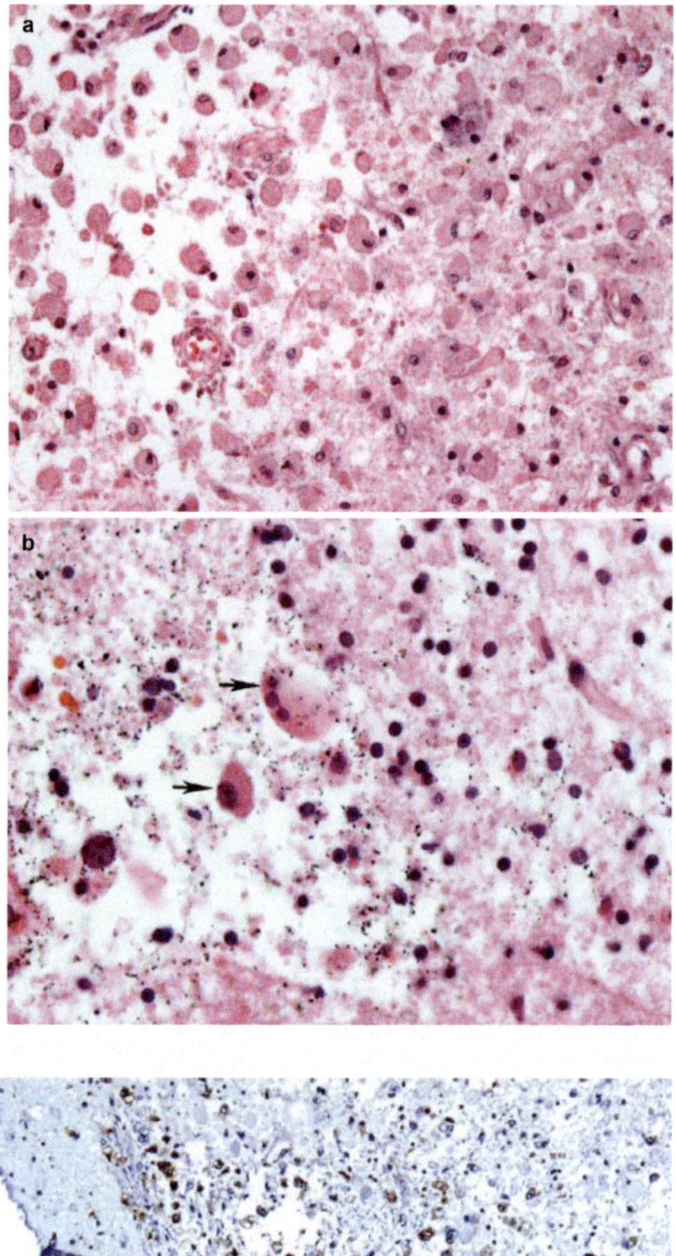

Fig. 20.4 (**a**) Nonfresh craniocerebral trauma with resorbing histiocytic reaction (H&E x200) and (**b**) lipophage involvement (*arrows*) at the edge of brain tissue necrosis (H&E ×500)

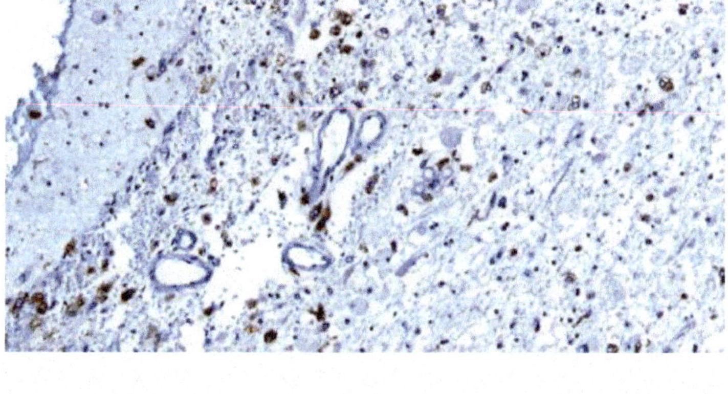

Fig. 20.5 Small contusion with immunohistochemically phagocytosing CD68+ macrophages (CD68 ×400)

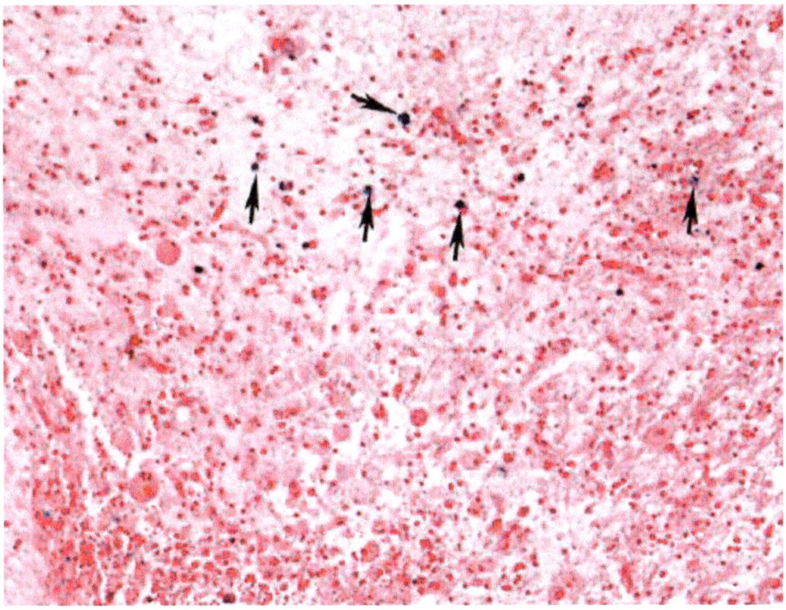

Fig. 20.6 Contusion with single siderophages (*arrows*) (Prussian blue ×250)

Table 20.2 Selected parameters for age estimation of *cortical lesions* using routine histology and immunohistochemistry

Parameter	Earliest appearance
Edematous swelling	Immediately
Neuronal degeneration, shrinkage	Immediately
Neuronal vacuolization	Immediately
CD15	10 min
DAI, demonstrated with ß-APP	2–3 h
Apolipoprotein E (ipsilateral hemisphere)	>3–4 h
Axonal swelling	10–20 h
Nuclear swelling	12–24 h
GFAP – loss of astrocyte marking (Fig. 20.7)	3 h
GFAP – in the peri-contusion zone	*From 4/5 days*
Neutrophils	>2 h
Leukocyte common antigen	>1 day
$CD3^+$ T lymphocytes	>2–4 days
$CD68^+$ macrophages (Fig. 20.4)	Several hours
Erythrophages	8 h–4 days
Apoptosis	>45–120 min
Siderophages (Fig. 20.5)	>2–5 days
Lipophages	24–72 h
NSE (neuron-specific enolase) in the peri-contusion zone	*>2 h*
Hematoidin	>6 days
Vascular proliferation	>12–24 h
Ceroid (lipopigment)	>100 h
Tenascin	7 days

According to Goede et al. (2015), DiMaio and Dana (2007), Dressler et al. (2007), Hausmann et al. (2006), Hausmann (2004), Orihara and Nakasono (2002), Hausmann and Betz (2000, 2001), Hausmann et al. (2000), Ng et al. (2000), Oehmichen et al. (1986), Eisenmenger (1977), Lindenberg and Freytag (1957), and Strassmann (1949)

DAI diffuse axonal injury. For detailed information on further histological and immunohistochemical parameters, please refer to the relevant literature

approximately 15–18 h following trauma. Likewise, reactive astrogliosis can only be identified immunohistochemically 4–5 days after trauma using anti-GFAP antibodies. Reactive microglia are reported to be detectable after 36–48 h using anti-CD68 antibodies (Woischneck et al. 2014).

20.1.3 Apoptosis in Human Traumatic Brain Injury

The loss of neuronal and glial cells as a result of traumatic head injury has generally been regarded as a consequence of necrosis combined with the appearance of inflammatory cells. Additionally, research has increasingly demonstrated the significance of programmed cell death or apoptosis (Dressler et al. 2007). Apoptosis is a genetically determined active death program without any accompanying inflammatory reaction (Padosch et al. 2001; Ng'walali et al. 2002). Effector mechanisms of apoptotic cell death include the activation of cysteine proteinases termed caspases 1–9 (Suzuki and Shiraki 2001). Using the TUNEL technique (TdT-mediated dUTP nick end labeling), apoptotic neurons have been observed after a posttraumatic interval of about 2 h and frequently up to 12 days (Dressler et al. 2007). *Neuronal apoptosis* was found localized in and adjacent to the damaged area in cortical lesions older than 3 days (Dressler et al. 2005; Hausmann et al. 2004); the majority of these cells showed MIB-1 expression, as described for cerebral macrophages following human brain injury (Hausmann and Betz 2002). Summarizing the detection of neuronal and glial apoptosis can be of utility in forensic wound age estimation. However, results showed a significant interindividual variability (Hausmann et al. 2004). The detection of neuronal cells seems most promising for the timing of cortical contusions, particularly in the early stage of wound healing (Dressler et al. 2005; Hausmann et al. 2004; Hausmann 2002), but other disorders of the CNS that could act as possible triggers of apoptosis should be absent. Additionally, apoptosis may also play an important role in forensic autopsy cases to detect cardiomyocyte apoptosis (Nakatome et al. 2002), apoptotic cell death in HIV encephalitis (Petito and Roberts 1995), apoptosis in human skin injuries (Suárez-Peñanranda et al. 2002), or apoptotic and necrotic brain lesions in cases of carbon monoxide poisoning (Uemura et al. 2001).

Another marker of apoptosis and programmed cell death is single-stranded DNA (ssDNA), which has been examined with regard to cause of death (Michiue et al. 2008). Neuronal immunopositivity of ssDNA was globally detected in the brain, independent of age, gender, and postmortem interval but dependent on cause of death. Higher positivity was typically found in the pallidum for delayed brain injury death and fatal carbon monoxide intoxication and in the cerebral cortex, pallidum, and substantia nigra for drug intoxication. For mechanical asphyxiation, high positivity was detected in the cerebral cortex and pallidum, while positivity was low in the substantia nigra (Michiue et al. 2008).

20.1.4 Boxing

Cerebral concussions ("knockouts") are the most relevant acute consequences of boxing. There are reports on cases of death in the boxing ring (Strassmann and Helpern 1968). Epidural hemorrhages are rare (Kreft 1952). A ruptured tentorium at the connection of the falx and rupture of the longitudinal sinus in an amateur boxer were caused by a punch to the point of the chin that was apparently strong enough to produce considerable skull deformation and therefore overstraining of the dural duplicature (Unterharnscheidt 1970, 1975). Subdural hemorrhage is a frequent finding after blows to the head. Numerous observations of fatal subdural hemorrhages, mostly involving amateur boxers, have been published (Krauland 1961). Traumatic dissection of extracranial vertebral artery can lead to a subtentorial infarction (Saito et al. 2009).

Neuronal and glial injuries correlate with the number and severity of blows to the head, including altered total tau, β-amyloid, neurofilament light protein, glial fibrillary acidic protein, and neuron-specific enolase, leading to chronic traumatic encephalopathy (CTE). One of the most important findings is increased phosphorylation of tau and deposits of neurofibrils in the upper parts of the frontal and temporal lobes (Förstl et al. 2010). Initially described as "punch drunk" (Martland 1928), CTE in boxers was later termed "dementia pugilistica" by Millspaugh (1937). The now commonly used term CTE refers to clinical neurological deficits and morphological changes: generalized brain atrophy that is more pronounced in frontal and temporal regions, an enlarged ventricular system, as well as marked neurofibrillary and astrocytic tangles primarily in the frontotemporal region around small blood vessels and deep in the sulci. Pathological deposits of hyperphosphorylated tau proteins (tangles) in the limbic system, the interbrain, and the brainstem nuclei have also been reported. No increase in ß-amyloid deposits, as in Alzheimer's disease, was seen. The detection of hyperphosphorylated tau protein AT8 combined with the demonstration of glial fibrillary acidic protein (GFAP) and a macrophage/microglia marker, e.g., KiM1P, is paramount in histomorphological and immunohistochemical diagnostics (Günther et al. 2017). A neuropathological staging system for CTE has been proposed in the literature (Table 20.3).

Table 20.3 Neuropathological findings in correlation to clinical findings as a staging system for chronic traumatic encephalopathy (according to McKee et al. 2013, 2016)

Stage	Neuropathological findings	Clinical symptoms
1	Discrete perivascular foci Tau-positive deposits in the frontal region	Headache, attention and concentration difficulties
2	Multiple foci of tau-positive deposits deep in the sulci and localized spread to superficial parts of the cortex	Additionally depression, mood swings, irritability, impaired short-term memory
3	Mild cerebral atrophy, widespread tau-positive deposits (with sparing of the medial temporal lobe)	Additionally, cognitive deficits
4	Moderately pronounced cerebral atrophy, marked tau-positive deposits in most cortical regions	Additionally, dementia with marked loss of short-term memory, aggressive behavior

20.1.5 Agonal Stress and Survival Time

Working on the assumption that cerebral tissue damage can be detected histologically and immunohistochemically depending on survival time following trauma, Piette and coworkers performed investigations. For example, the expression and distribution of ubiquitin, a heat shock protein, in the locus coeruleus is reported to be more readily demonstrated the longer the survival time. Additional agonal stress was assumed as part of these investigations (Piette et al. 2010).

20.2 Ischemic and Hypoxic Changes

The morphological manifestation of hypoxia and ischemia in brain tissue is relatively homogeneous. The morphological demonstration of hypoxic brain injury is of considerable interest in forensic pathology for determining cause of death (Oehmichen and Meissner 2006; Oehmichen et al. 2003; Krauland 1973). The most important general microscopic criteria include (Hausmann et al. 2007):

- Plasmolysis
- Cellular degeneration with shrinkage
- Acidophilic behavior
- Loss of Nissl substance

Additionally, morphological studies revealed considerable polymorphism of ganglion cell lesions, predominantly determined by the severity, duration, and form of hypoxia; survival interval after the onset of oxygen deficiency also plays an important role (Hausmann et al. 2007). A selective vulnerability to hypoxic and ischemic damage is well known for definite regions of the CNS, such as layers 3, 5, and 6 in the cerebral cortex, the CA1 area (Sommer sector), the end plate in the hippocampus, and the Purkinje neurons of the cerebellum (Hausmann et al. 2007; Horn and Schote 1992; Sato et al. 1990).

Ischemia

Ischemia is a temporary or permanent reduction of cerebral blood flow with cerebral function failure. Complete irreversible ischemia is differentiated from global and regional ischemia (Oehmichen 2001). Regional ischemia leads to a cerebral stroke (Figs. 20.7 and 20.8). Another cause of traumatic cerebral stroke may be intermittent dissection of extracranial cervical arteries (Maxeiner and Finck 1989) as well as posttraumatic thrombosis following vascular wall injury (Bratzke and Krauland 1988; Hartman and Lindlar 1987).

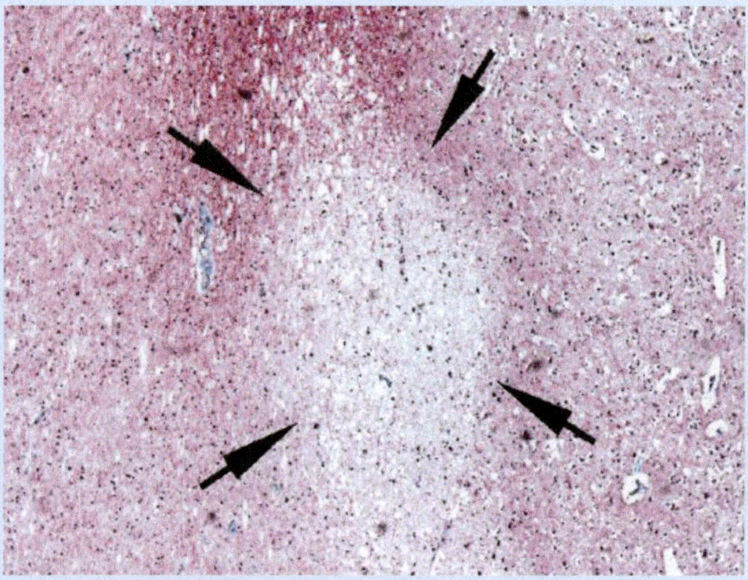

Fig. 20.7 Fresh cerebral stroke in the parietal cortex: pallid area in Masson trichrome staining, no recognizable cellular reaction at the margin (Masson trichrome ×100)

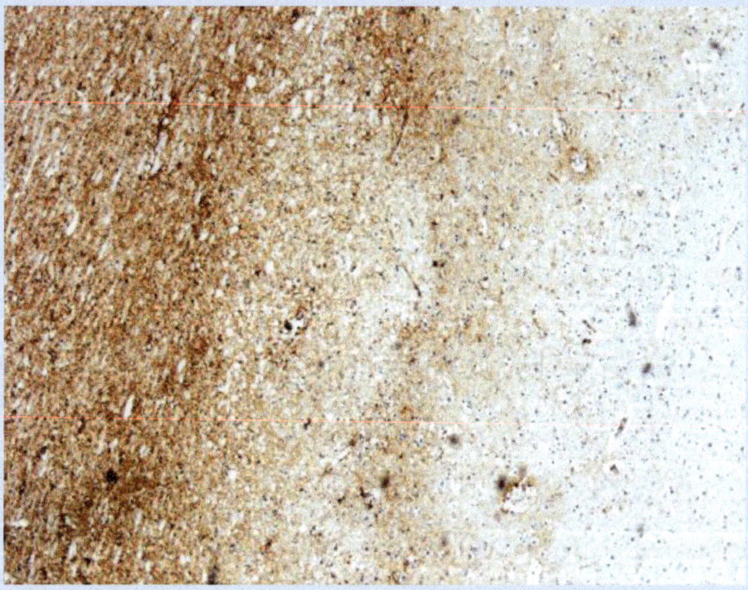

Fig. 20.8 Fresh cerebral stroke in the parietal cortex: immunohistochemical physiological marking of astrocytes with glial fibrillary acidic protein (*GFAP*) and pallor in the infarct area (×100)

Hypoxia or anoxia of tissue describes a lack of oxygen in a cell. Reduced oxygen content is called hypoxemia.

Asphyxia

Asphyxia, on the other hand, is shortness of breath or a metabolic disorder within the organism, which may lead to reduced oxygen content in the blood with increased carbon dioxide levels and lactic acidosis.

Frequently, only small lesions can be found in the brain tissue due to local hypoxia or ischemia. The histological changes mentioned in Table 20.4 allow for a rough age estimation of such lesions. Purkinje cells of the cerebellum have been found to be most vulnerable to oxygen demand. Currently, only a limited number of systematic studies on ischemic damage in human Purkinje cells are described in the literature, many of which were performed on animals (Hausmann et al. 2007; Sato et al. 1990). It was reported that hypoxic Purkinje cells had a smaller somata than those of normal cells by 15% and that the density was decreased by 10% compared to normal cells. In addition, in contrast to healthy Purkinje cells, hypoxically altered Purkinje cells exhibited a more rounded, shrunken appearance with less average diameter compared to controls (Lee et al. 2001).

20.3 Meningitis

A first manifestation of bacterial or viral meningitis in the case of acute death is very rare, but does occur. Fungal meningitides and tuberculous meningitis are both extremely rare (Fig. 20.9).

Purulent meningitides are predominant (frequent pathogens: *Neisseria meningitidis*, *Streptococcus pneumoniae*, *Listeria monocytogenes*, *Escherichia coli*, *Haemophilus influenzae*). Nevertheless, meningococcemia without meningitis can result in rapid, fulminant death in fewer 12 h from onset of symptoms. Autopsy findings in such cases include petechiae and typically bilateral adrenal hemorrhage (Waterhouse–Friderichsen syndrome). Viral meningitides are typically less fulminant but also show a wider range of possible viral pathogens (Ishigami et al. 2004).

Table 20.4 Morphological changes with ischemic and hypoxic brain damage

Findings	Occurrence
Chromatin agglutination in nerve cells	Ultrastructural changes after a few minutes
Loosening of Nissl bodies	After approximately 20 min
Decay of Nissl bodies	After approximately 2 h
Homogenization of karyoplasm with shrinkage of nucleus and cytoplasmic eosinophilia:	After approximately 7 h, typically visible after 12–18 h
H&E staining: pink cytoplasm	
Klüver–Barrera staining: turquoise cytoplasm	
Cresyl violet staining: discolored cytoplasm	
Swelling of endothelial cells, pericytes, and astrocytic appendages	Visible after 12 h
Axonal swelling at the margin of the swelling	After approximately 24 h
First occurrence of macrophages at the border of the source	After 30 h
Macrophages clearly increased; after microhemorrhages, siderophages are also visible	After approximately 48 h
So-called fat-granule cells (Sudan III staining) or lipophages	After approximately 48 h
Capillary sprouts beginning at the periphery	2–3 weeks
Macrophages, as well as lipophages, remain at the periphery; after microhemorrhages, siderophages are also visible	Still detectable after many weeks to years
After completed resorption and organization, a pseudocystic area may remain with peripheral lipophages	Visible for years; lipophages have still been found after 4 years (Wojahn 1970)

If a softening lesion is present close to the surface, the molecular layer can be preserved, which is an indication of ischemic necrosis with a nontraumatic origin

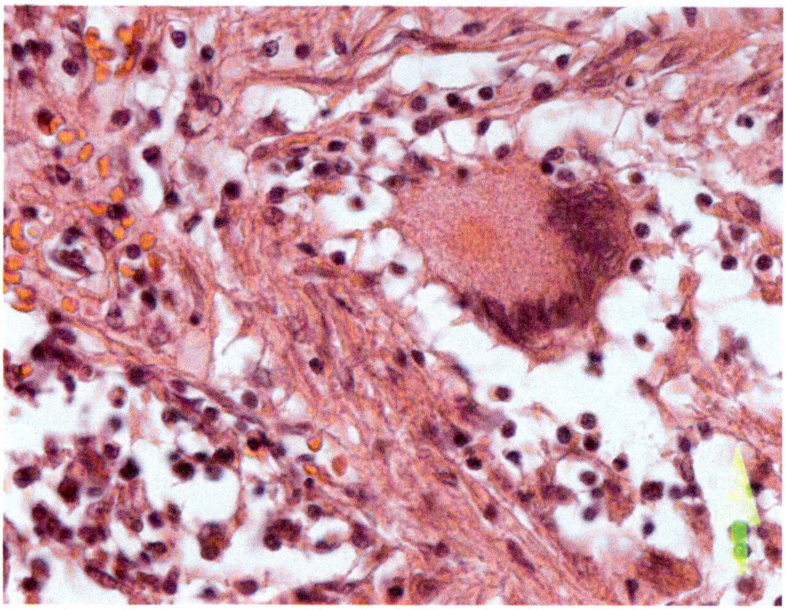

Fig. 20.9 Tuberculous meningitis with evidence of a Langerhans giant cell and marked pulmonary tuberculosis (HE ×400)

20.3.1 Waterhouse–Friderichsen Syndrome

Waterhouse–Friderichsen syndrome (WFS), the most severe form of peracute meningococcal sepsis, typically presents with bilateral adrenal hemorrhage, disseminated skin purpura, and multiple petechiae as manifestations of systemic sepsis. Fatal courses of WFS in immunocompetent healthy adults are regarded as very rare events (Varchmin-Schultheiß et al. 1990; Althoff 1982; Böhm 1982). The diagnosis of WFS as the cause of death is established postmortem based on autopsy findings, microscopic examination, measurement of serum procalcitonin concentration, and outcome of postmortem bacteriologic cultures from heart and spleen blood samples (Sperhake and Tsokos 2004; Tsokos 2003; Tsokos and Püschel 2001). Apoplexy of the adrenals was first described by Waterhouse in 1911 and Friderichsen in 1918 (Waterhouse 1911; Friderichsen 1918). WFS also occurs in infancy and childhood (Ryan et al. 1993). Diagnosis is additionally based on morphological criteria: fulminant sepsis, patchy purpura of the skin as a result of disseminated intravascular coagulation (DIC), and bilateral hemorrhagic necroses of the adrenals (Sperhake and Tsokos 2004). Usually, all cases have a very rapid clinical course of at most 1 day. Postmortem microbiological examinations yield different infective agents, mainly meningococci (Mirza et al. 2000; Ip et al. 1995; Jacobs et al. 1983; Böhm 1982). Meningococcemia can lead to lethal complete heart block (Riordan et al. 1995; Detesky and Salit 1983). Negative postmortem microbiological results are possible due to antibiotics given prior to death or a postmortem interval of 2 days or more. Therefore, the postmortem interval prior to microbiological examinations should be as short as possible (Sperhake and Tsokos 2004). There is potential for the postmortem detection of infective agents in the leptomeninges. Cases of WFS may present with myocarditis involving the cardiac conduction system as well as the potential for a clinically undiagnosed interstitial myocarditis with vasculitis. Therefore, myocarditis and endotoxinic vascular damage could be the leading cause of death in many cases of WFS (Böhm 1982). Myocardial infiltrates in myocardial lesions include granulocytes, lymphocytes, and mast cells. Sometimes, gram-negative diplococci can be visible by light microscopy (Sperhake and Tsokos 2004).

In cases of WFS, a transmission of pathogens during autopsy is in principle possible. For this reason, forensic scientists are recommended to wear appropriate protective clothing, including eye and face protection. As postexposure prophylaxis, antibiotic administration is recommended, e.g., one dose of 500-mg ciprofloxacin (Centers for Disease Control and Prevention (CDC) 1997).

A macroscopically suspected diagnosis can be confirmed microscopically by detection of a granulocytic inflammatory infiltrate in the meninges, with alternating density. At the time of death, this inflammatory infiltrate may have already spread to the brain parenchyma (meningoencephalitis; Fig. 20.10). Early phases, which cannot be reliably detected macroscopically, show less dense and loosely spread polymorphonuclear neutrophil granulocytes, the detection of which is facilitated by means of ASD staining.

In very rare cases, a fungal meningitis or fungal encephalitis is present (Fig. 20.11). Cases of lethal subarachnoid hemorrhage as a complication of actinomycosis meningitis have been reported in which the pathogens were detected primarily in lung tissue. In addition, polyarteritis nodosa-like vascular changes were detectable due to actinomyces as pathogenic agents (Koda et al. 2003).

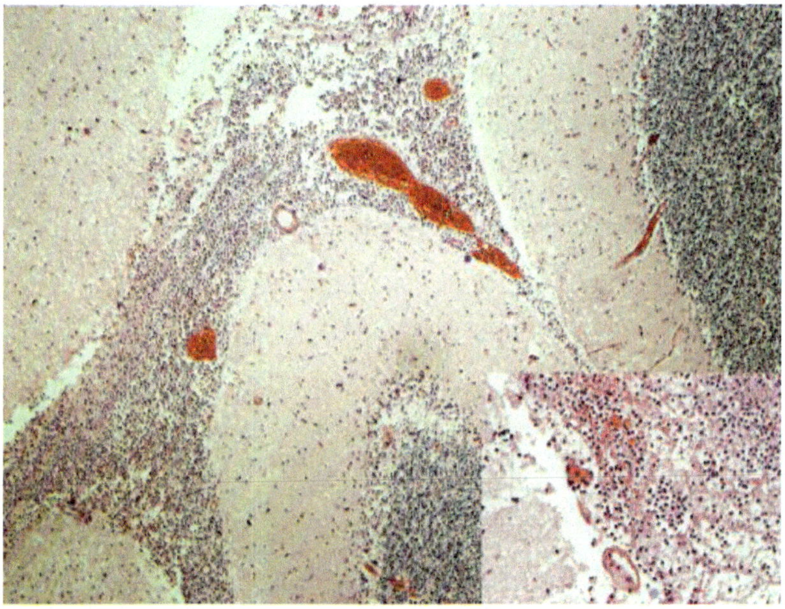

Fig. 20.10 Granulocytic inflammatory infiltrate above the cerebellar cortex in a case of acute purulent meningitis (H&E ×40) with numerous polymorphonuclear granulocytes, spread of inflammation to the adjacent tissue of the cortex (meningoencephalitis), and signs of early organization (H&E ×200)

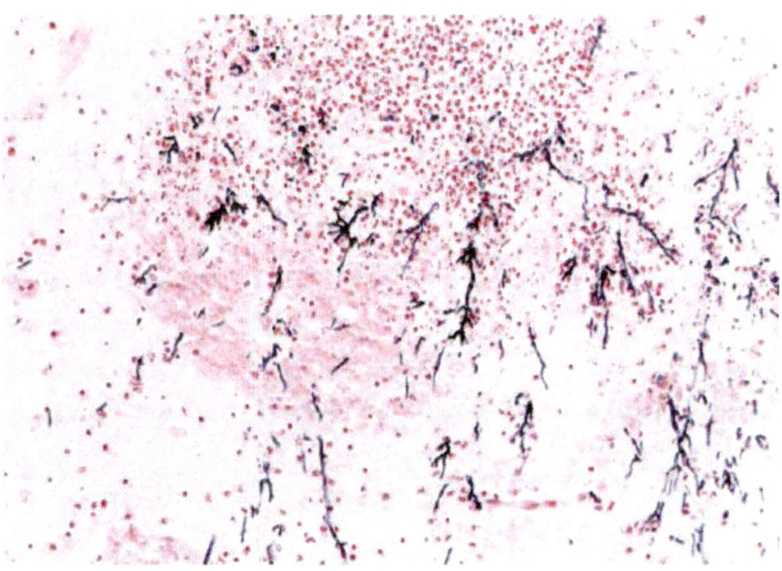

Fig. 20.11 Fungal meningitis and fungal encephalitis with numerous fungal fibers in the barely recognizable cerebellar matter and in the cortex (Grocott ×200)

20.3.2 Posttraumatic Meningitis

Infections of the leptomeninges in which the infectious agent gains access to the intracranial compartment via traumatic means are termed posttraumatic. Meningeal swabs often yielded *Streptococcus pneumoniae* (Matschke and Tsokos 2001).

In addition to trauma-related hemorrhage and necrosis, as well as early organization (depending on survival time), bacterial and granulocytic meningitis can also be seen histologically. Craniocerebral trauma does not necessarily have to be the point of origin of the infection.

20.4 Unknown Brain Tumors and Malignant Diseases of the Central Nervous System as Cause of Death

In rare cases, sudden unexpected death may occur if CNS diseases remained previously undetected, including glioblastomas (Fig. 20.12), neurocytomas, and ependymal or subependymal brain tumors remained previously undetected (Sakai et al. 2007; Matschke and Tsokos 2005; Black and Graham 2002; Matschke et al. 2000), Matschke et al. 1999; Balko and Schultz 1999; Lindboe et al. 1997; Matsumoto and Yamamoto 1994; Zappi et al. 1993; Byard et al. 1991; Schwarz et al. 1987; Nelson et al. 1987; Abu et al. 1986; Mork et al. 1986; Poon and Solis 1985; DiMaio et al. 1980; Huntington et al. 1965). A fatal case of Lhermitte–Duclos syndrome due to an unknown dysplastic ganglioma of the cerebellum (synonyma Purkinjeoma) as a benign (grade 1) tumor according to the WHO classification was described. Histopathologically, impressive dysplastic Purkinje cells were present, which were hypertrophic and swollen with vacuolization (Buschmann et al. 2008). In some cases, preceding epilepsy was known (Büttner et al. 1999; Prahlow et al. 1995). In very rare cases, intracranial cysts or pseudocystic changes, such as colloid cysts of the third ventricle (Demirci et al. 2009; Büttner et al. 1997), epidermoid cysts (Matschke et al. 2002), other cysts (Igari et al. 2014), intracranial chordoma (Li et al. 2010), and von Recklinghausen neurofibromatosis (Unger et al. 1984), can cause sudden. The mortality rate for neurosarcoidosis is approximately 10%, and histological and immunohistochemical findings have been described (D'Errico et al. 2011).

Occasionally, a clinical and radiological diagnosis of meningitis is later proven to be

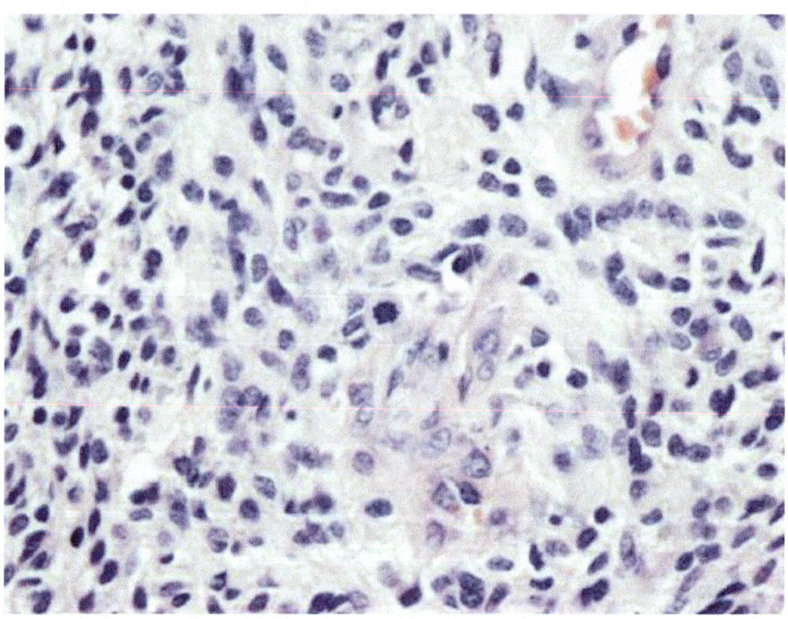

Fig. 20.12 Sudden and unexpected death of a 43-year-old woman: multiform glioblastoma with a single mitose – undetected prior to death (H&E ×400)

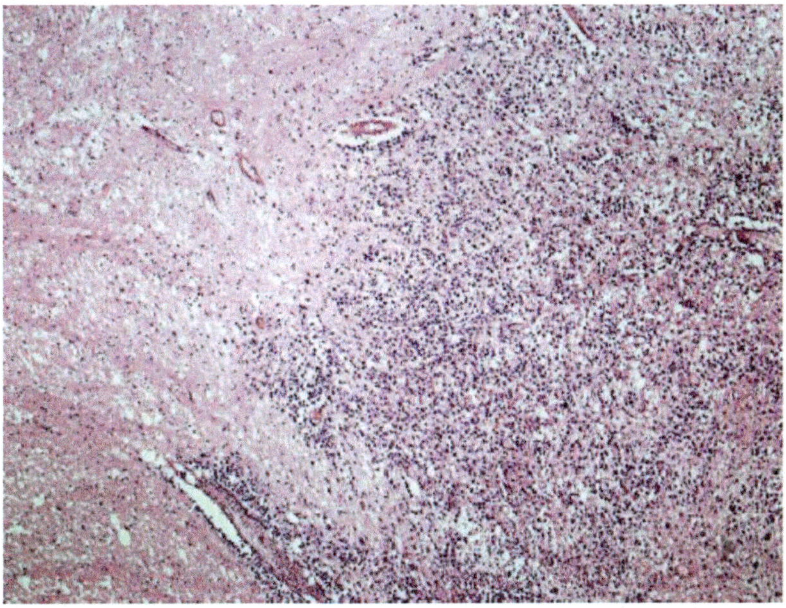

Fig. 20.13 Widespread lymphomatous meningeosis with lymphomatous infiltration of the adjacent brain tissue by a malignant non-Hodgkin lymphoma, misdiagnosed as meningitis (H&E ×40)

meningeosis lymphomatosa (Fig. 20.13). In this case, the exact cause of death can only be clarified microscopically. A review of the literature demonstrated that the incidence of sudden death as a result of primary intracranial neoplasms has declined in recent decades (Matsche 2005; Eberhart et al. 2001).

20.5 Nontraumatic Subarachnoid and Intracerebral Hemorrhages

Common causes of spontaneous nontraumatic intracerebral and/or subarachnoid hemorrhages (Klages 1970) include:

- Hypertension
- Ischemic stroke with secondary hemorrhage
- Ruptured congenital cerebral aneurysms, mainly within the circle of Willis
- Arteriovenous malformations
- Amyloid angiopathy
- Cerebral vasculitis
- Tumors: primary brain tumors or metastases
- Bleeding diatheses due to thrombocytopenia, DIC, leukemia, and anticoagulant therapy
- Drug-induced bleeding, particularly associated with cocaine or amphetamine use
- Sturge–Weber syndrome (encephalofacial angiomatosis)

Intracerebral hemorrhage, which can also rapidly lead to sudden death, occurs in cases of stroke and—most commonly—hypertension. Typical sites include the basal ganglia, thalamus, pons, cerebellum, and subcortical white matter, demonstrating macroscopically as lobar hemorrhages. Brain sections from the areas adjacent to hemorrhage may show sclerosed and hyalinized walls of arteries and arterioles.

20.5.1 Ruptured Congenital Cerebral Aneurysms Within the Circle of Willis

The most common cause of nontraumatic subarachnoid hemorrhage is a ruptured congenital intracranial aneurysm (berry aneurysm; Fig. 20.14) (Bratzke et al. 1986). Of these, 90% are silent until rupture; approximately 2–4% of adults present an intracranial aneurysm at autopsy. About two thirds of patients become

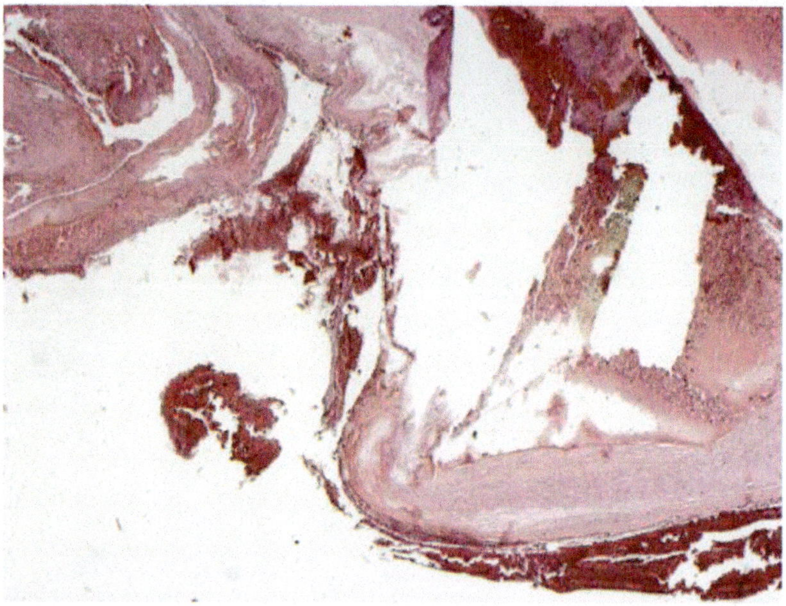

Fig. 20.14 Ruptured aneurysm of the anterior cerebral artery (H&E ×20)

symptomatic between the ages of 40 and 65 years (Bowen 1984). Aneurysms of large cerebral arteries can be divided into:

- Saccular aneurysms
- Atherosclerotic aneurysms
- Inflammatory aneurysms
- Dissecting aneurysms

Approximately 85% of berry aneurysms are found on the anterior region of the circle of Willis. Rupture is uncommon in aneurysms less than 5 mm in diameter. Rupture into the brain and ventricles, as well as the subarachnoid space, is possible. At autopsy, the ruptured aneurysm must be examined fresh after carefully excising the arachnoid membrane and flushing the coagulated blood from the area of greatest concentration (DiMaio and Dana 2007). Intramural hemorrhages in the wall of ruptured aneurysms can be found (Fig. 20.15).

If neurological surgery was performed following aneurysm rupture, remains of surgical suture material may be visible microscopically (Fig. 20.16).

So-called pseudoaneurysms as acute traumatic lesions of arteries with periarterial hematoma must be differentiated from true aneurysms not only by radiological and clinical findings but also by histological investigation (Weiler et al. 1980).

20.5.2 Intracerebral Arteriovenous Malformations

Cerebral cavernous or arteriovenous malformations are common sporadic or autosomal dominantly inherited vascular lesions predisposing to recurrent headaches, seizures, and hemorrhagic stroke. An arteriovenous malformation (AVM) (Fig. 20.17), such as a localized congenital malformation of the vascular system, can lead to acute intracerebral and/or subarachnoid hemorrhage (Tomcik et al. 2011; Kominato et al. 2004; Racette and Sauvageau 2007). The majority of AVM involves the central parietal cortex. Histologically, a conglomeration of arteries and veins without a capillary bed can be found, located in the cerebral cortex and usually extending into the contiguous white matter (DiMaio and Dana 2007). If previous microhemorrhages were present, it may be possible to detect accumulations of hemosiderin-laden macrophages in the vicinity of the AV malformation (Fig. 20.18).

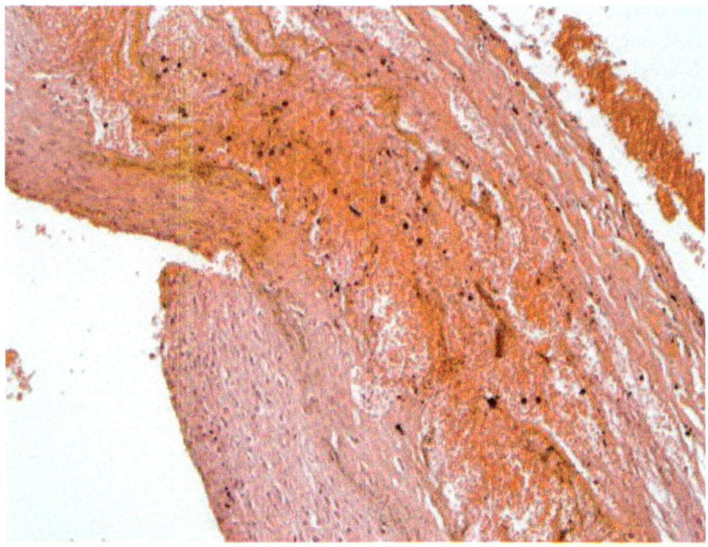

Fig. 20.15 Intramural hemorrhages in the wall of the ruptured aneurysm of the anterior cerebral artery (H&E ×100)

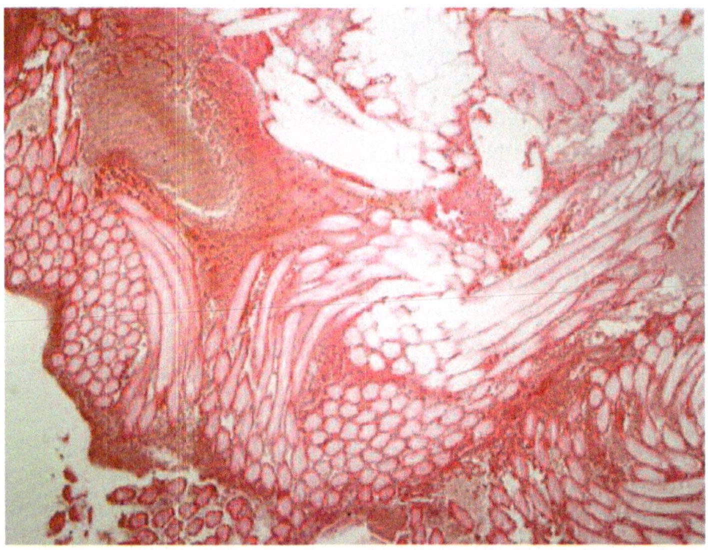

Fig. 20.16 Microscopically detected surgical suture material at the base of an aneurysm of the anterior cerebral artery due to failed neurosurgical intervention (H&E ×40)

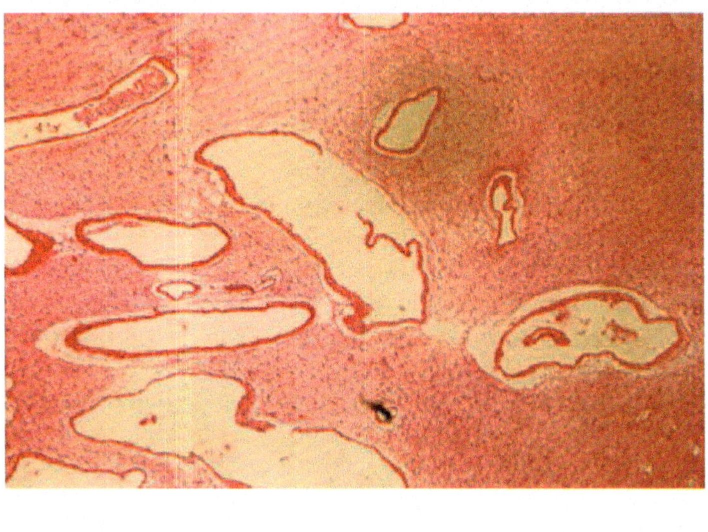

Fig. 20.17 Intracerebral vascular malformation (H&E ×40)

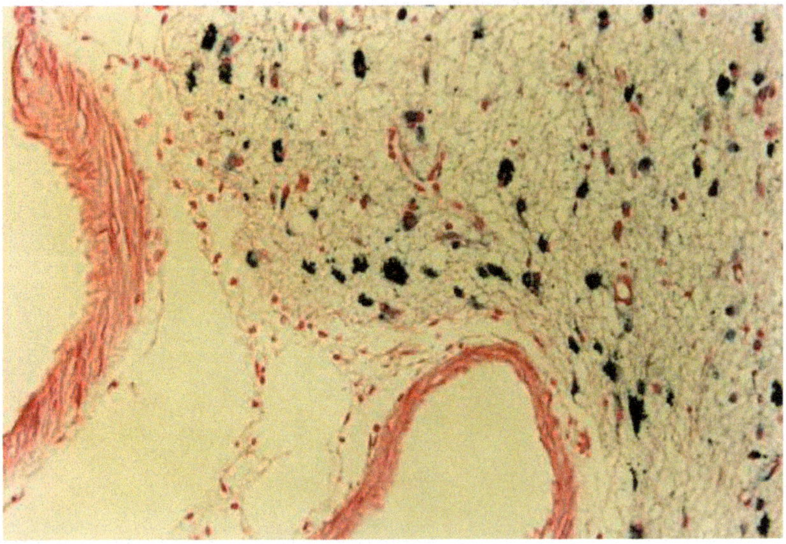

Fig. 20.18 Hemosiderin-laden macrophages in the vicinity of a vascular malformation (Prussian blue ×200)

Not all intracranial vascular malformations are necessarily detectable macroscopically, and the actual rupture in a vessel wall as the source of bleeding may require complex histological evaluation in order to be identified (Tomcik et al. 2011).

20.5.3 Amyloid Angiopathy

Amyloid angiopathy (Fig. 20.19), a rare cause of intracranial hemorrhage, may be found multifocally but is most frequently localized in the occipital cortex. Victims of amyloid angiopathy are usually older patients; intracerebral or subarachnoid hemorrhage can occur suddenly and unexpectedly with a fatal course.

20.6 Shaken Baby Syndrome (SBS)

Shaken baby syndrome (SBS) is the most common variant of inflicted neurotrauma in infants. The first description of subdural hemorrhage in association with child abuse was documented in the late nineteenth century (Matschke 2008; Tardieu 1860). Later, Henry Kempe et al. published their seminal paper on "battered child syndrome" (Kempe et al. 1962), and John Caffey described SBS (Caffey 1972). Nevertheless, some authors have reported on shaken adult syndrome, which is also possible (Pounder 1997). Meanwhile, SBS is accepted as a form of child abuse (American Academy of Pediatrics 2001) combining:

- Subdural hemorrhage
- Acute encephalopathy
- Retinal hemorrhage
- Optic nerve sheath hemorrhage
- Sparse or absent signs of external injury

SBS occurs nearly exclusively in children under 2 years of age and can be considered a common component of "non-accidental head injury" (NAHI) (Duhaime et al. 1992). Retinal hemorrhage and optic nerve sheath hemorrhage in SBS (NAHI) are typically bilateral, symmetrical, preretinal, subretinal, or intraretinal, as well as subhyaloid or submembranous; they are mostly located at the posterior pole and/or the midperiphery near the ora serrata (Matschke et al. 2009) (Figs. 20.20, 20.21, 20.22, and 20.23).

Retinal hemorrhage, either bilateral or unilateral (Arlotti et al. 2007; Tyagi et al. 1997), can occur in more than 30% of newborns, but its incidence declines substantially within the first days of life (Emerson et al. 2001; Sezen 1971; Baum and Bulpitt 1970).

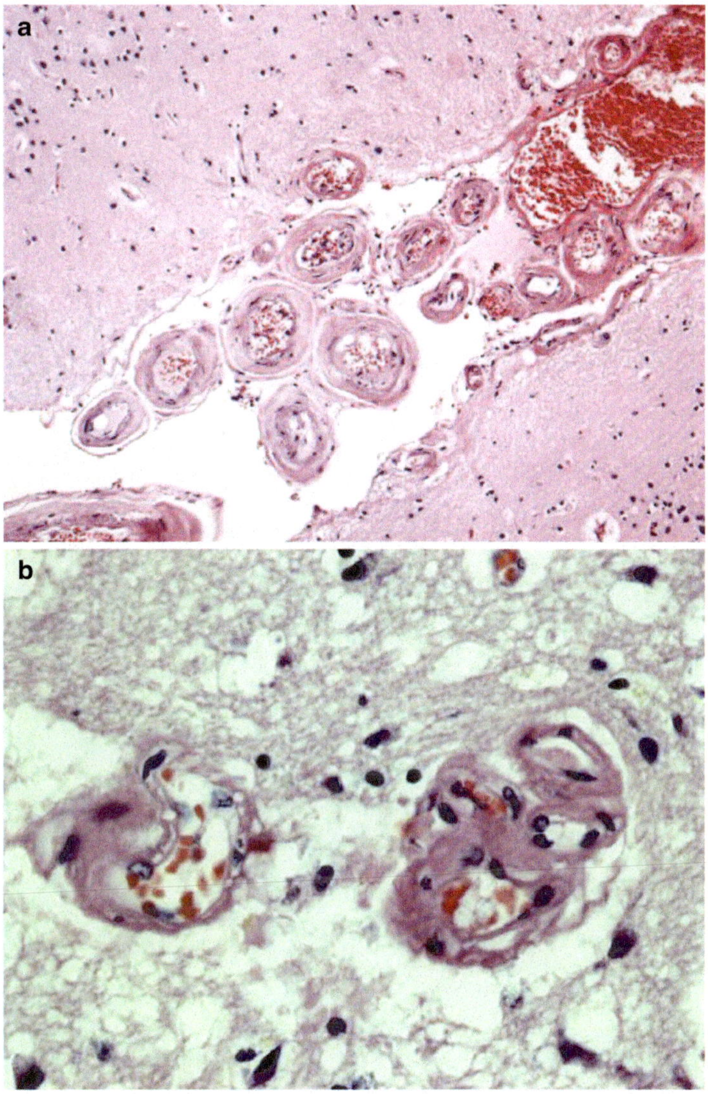

Fig. 20.19 (**a**) Amyloid angiopathy (already suspected on the basis of H&E staining; H&E ×100) with (**b**) widened, seemingly homogenous vascular walls as the cause of an intracerebral and subarachnoid hemorrhage in a 76-year-old man who died suddenly (H&E ×400)

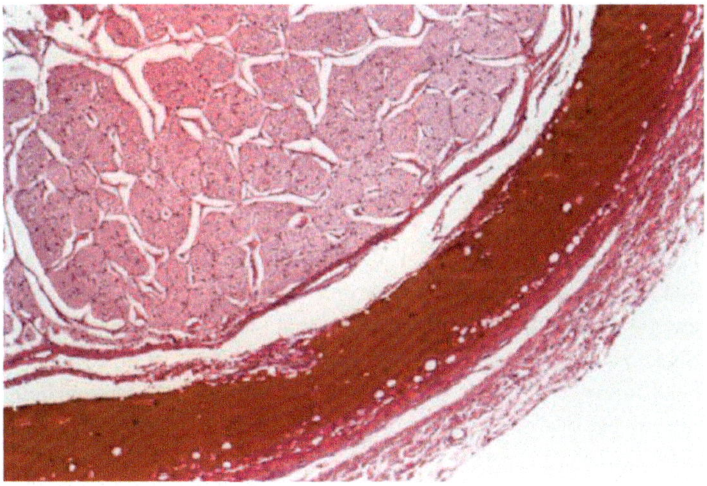

Fig. 20.20 Optic nerve sheath hemorrhages in a case of SBS in a 4-month-old female infant (H&E ×40)

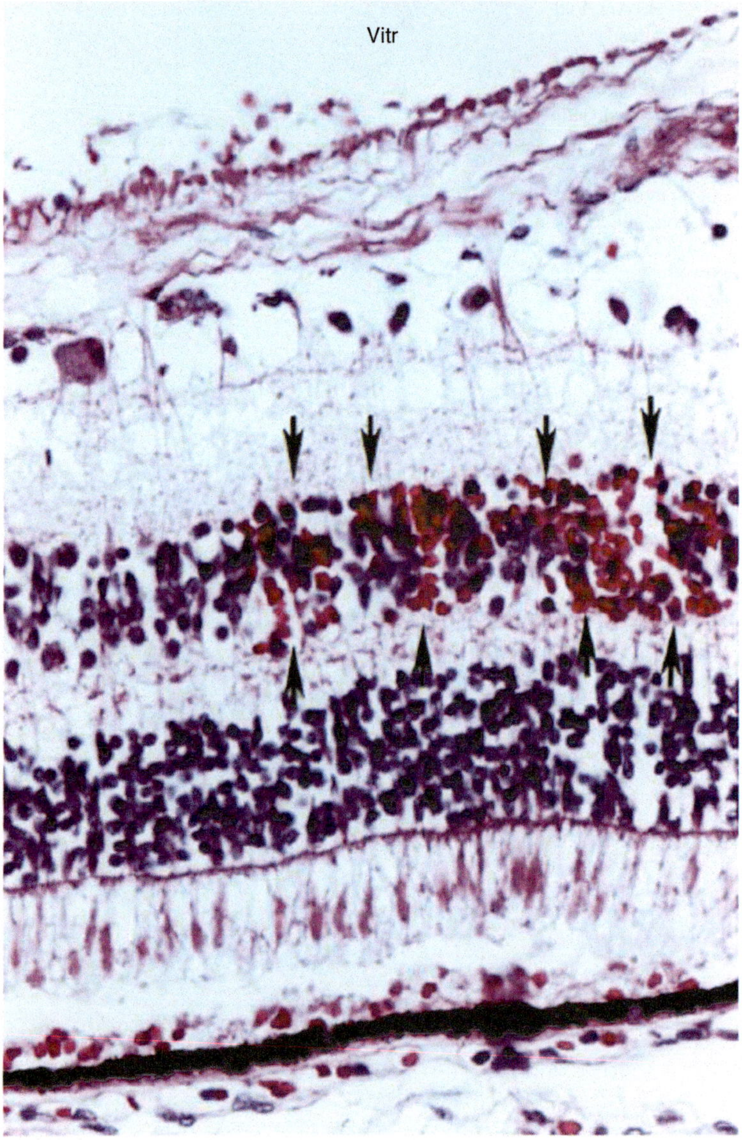

Fig. 20.21 Section through the retina with intraretinal hemorrhage (*between arrows*) in a case of SBS diagnosed in a 4-month-old female infant (H&E ×400) and with anatomical designations: vitreous (*vitr*), nerve fiber layer (*nfl*), ganglion cell layer (*gcl*), inner plexiform layer (*ipl*), inner nuclear layer (*inl*), outer plexiform layer (*opl*), outer nuclear layer (*onl*), photoreceptors (*pc*)

Alternative explanations for detected retinal bleeding include: severe vomiting, possibly due to pyloric stenosis (Herr et al. 2004), an accident (Johnston et al. 1993), cramps or epileptic seizures (Tyagi et al. 1998), previous resuscitation measures (Gilliland et al. 1994; Gilliland and Luckenbach 1993; Weedn et al. 1990; Goetting and Sowa 1990; Kanter 1986), or preexisting disease, such as glutaric aciduria (Gago et al. 2003). Shaken baby syndrome (or rather: non-accidental head injury, NAHI), on the other hand, remains the subject of discussion despite the fact that, in principle, the macroscopic and microscopic findings are reliable (Sperhake and Matschke 2014; Byard 2014; Scheimberg and Mack 2014). In individual cases, microscopic retinal hemorrhage is also seen in adults following traffic accidents involving severe whiplash head and neck injury (Parsons et al. 2005). Retinal hemorrhage may also occur in isolated cases in the setting of meningitis or a congenital metabolic disorder (Ong et al. 2009).

Retinal hemorrhage cannot always be detected macroscopically. For this reason, microscopic

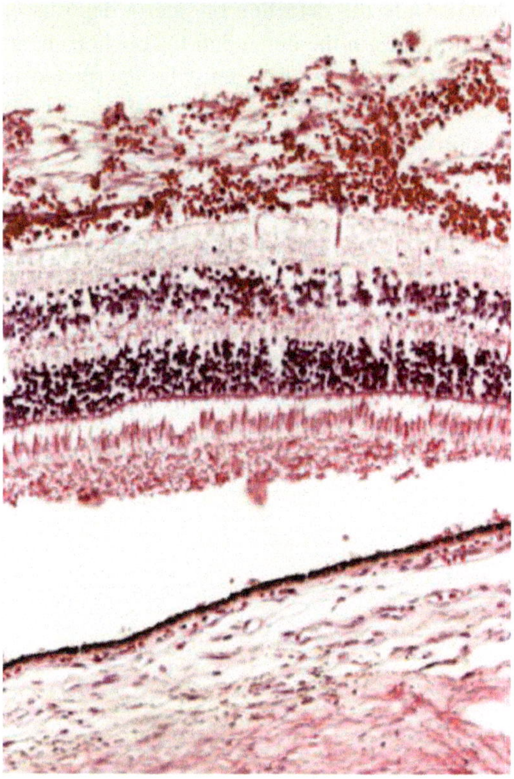

Fig. 20.22 Subhyaloid hemorrhage, not covered by the internal membrane limitans, in a case of SBS (H&E ×200)

investigations may help clarify an equivocal diagnosis (Matschke and Glatzel 2008; Gilliland et al. 2007; Gilliland and Luthert 2003). In addition to retinal hemorrhage and subdural hematomas (Ommaya and Yarnell 1969), further findings based on SBS or other child abuse offenses can be determined (Raul et al. 2008; Roth et al. 2007; Munger et al. 1993; Riffenburgh and Sathyavagiswaran 1991).

Massive transretinal hemorrhage cannot easily be explained by a single trauma, such as a trivial fall. In combination with other typical signs of SBS, e.g., subdural hematoma, bleeding in the dorsal neck muscles, or periadventitial extracranial vertebral artery hemorrhage (Gleckman et al. 2000), the detection of extensive bleeding almost certainly indicates violent shaking. Since considerable asymmetry between the eyes of an individual can occur, it must be emphasized that both eyes should be removed and investigated (Gilliland et al. 2007; Betz et al. 1996). Morphometric analysis of retinal hemorrhages can help to differentiate between SBS and severe head injury, intravital brain death, nontraumatic intracranial hemorrhage, or SIDS, including cardiopulmonary resuscitation (Betz et al. 1996).

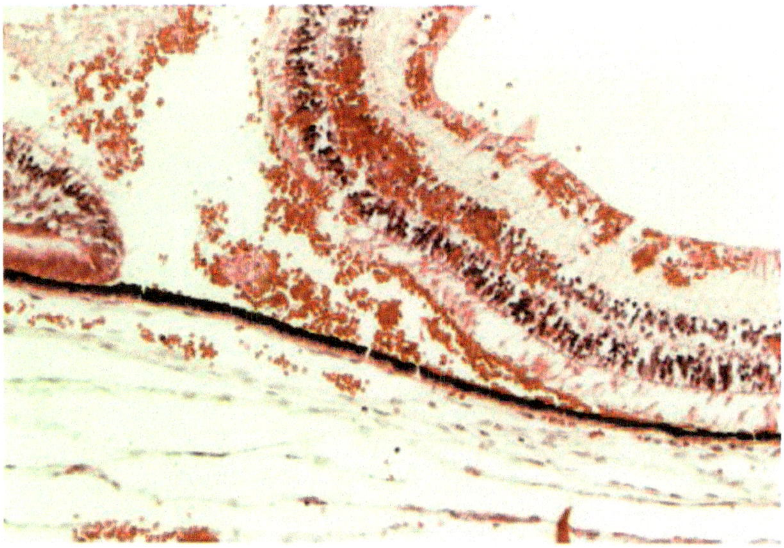

Fig. 20.23 Subretinal, intraretinal, and subhyaloid hemorrhage in a case of SBS together with artificial tearing of the retina from the underlying pigmented epithelium as a common phenomenon and inevitable artifact of tissue processing. This phenomenon should not be confused with retinal folds due to shaking (H&E ×200)

While retinal hemorrhage is usually indicative of preceding SBS, isolated fresh intradural hemorrhage cannot be considered sufficient evidence of acute SBS (Fig. 20.24). Cohen et al. observed the highest incidence of an association among intradural hemorrhage, subdural hemorrhage, and hypoxia during the perinatal period (Cohen et al. 2010). Others found intradural hemorrhage at autopsy unrelated to trauma in 72% of children younger than 5 months of age (Geddes et al. 2003). Only the detection of siderin deposits or siderophages in the dura confirms previous hemorrhage, which however, must be interpreted in the context of additional findings. In particular, hemorrhage as the result of an asphyctic processes must be considered (Hauser et al. 2001). Deposits of ß-APP due to DAI and depending on survival time have been reported; such deposits can occur following traumatic and nontraumatic axonal injury (Fig. 20.25; Hayashi et al. 2009, 2015).

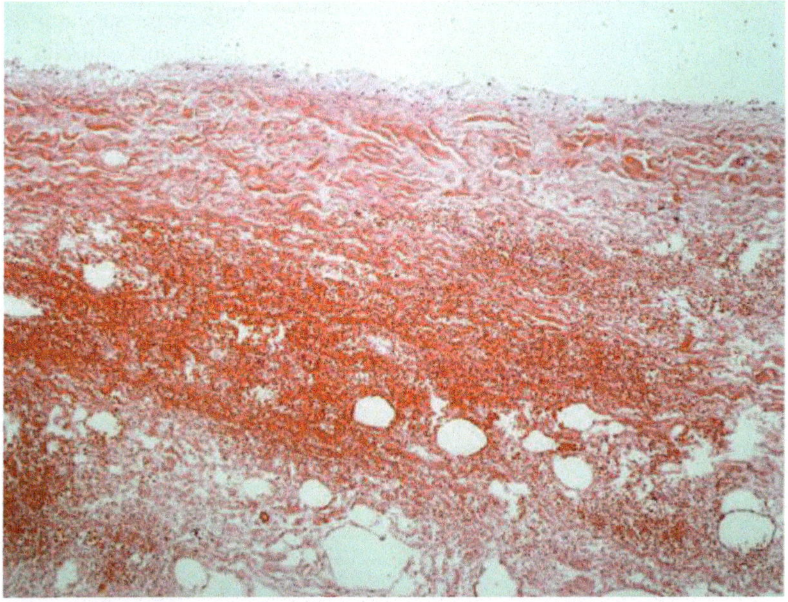

Fig. 20.24 A 17-month-old female infant: isolated fresh intradural hemorrhages, not suggestive of SBS (H&E ×40)

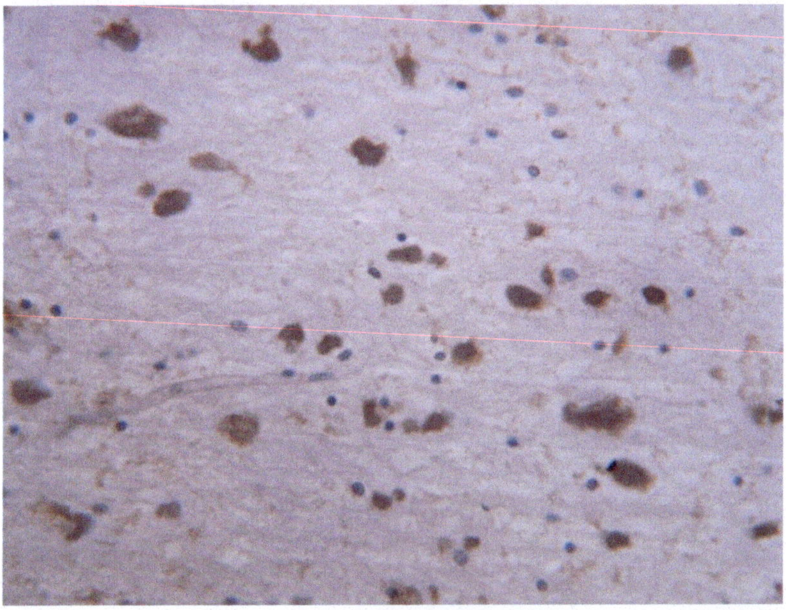

Fig. 20.25 ß-amyloid precursor protein deposits following axonal injury (image kindly provided by Dr. D. Farkaš, Kosice, Slovakia)

Depending on survival time again, the immunohistochemical detection of interleukin 8 (IL-8) in injured axons and surrounding oligodendrocytes following TBI may be helpful (Hayashi et al. 2016). Particularly in shaken baby syndrome, an investigation of the brainstem region can potentially lead to the identification of trauma-related ischemic hypoxic injury (Matschke et al. 2015). However, the demonstration of ß-APP in spinal nerves alone has in itself little validity (Squier et al. 2011). For detailed information, please refer to the relevant neuropathological literature.

20.7 Neuropathology of Drug Abuse

A broad spectrum of neuropathologic changes are encountered in the brain of drug abusers, particularly heroin, cocaine, and amphetamine abusers, but also following the intake of other drugs (Mu et al. 2017; Ishikawa et al. 2007; Quan et al. 2005a; De Letter et al. 2003). Heroin-associated cerebral arteritis, as well as neurosurgical complications in cases of heroin addiction, has been described, as well as neurosurgical complications in cases of heroin addiction (Amine 1997; King et al. 1978; Halpern and Citron 1971).

Nevertheless, while the main findings are due to infection, other complications may include hypoxic-ischemic changes with cerebral edema, ischemic neuronal damage, and neuronal loss. These are assumed to occur under conditions of prolonged heroin-induced respiratory depression, stroke due to thromboembolism, vasculitis, septic emboli, hypotension, and positional vascular compression (Büttner et al. 2000). Other than these, there are no specific lesions of the CNS hallmarking heroin abuse. Thus, the exact etiology of various neuropathological alterations is still unclear in many cases. However, bilateral, symmetrical ischemic necrosis of the globus pallidus has been reported to occur in 5–10% of heroin addicts after intravenous or intranasal abuse (Fig. 20.24; Andersen and Skullerud 1999; Riße and Weiler 1984). Bipallidal hemorrhage following ethylene glycol intoxication is also described (Caparros-Lefebvre et al. 2005). After cocaine, amphetamines are the second most common cause of ischemic or hemorrhagic stroke. Besides stroke, subarachnoid and intracerebral hemorrhages have been described after acute amphetamine and methamphetamine abuse (Büttner and Weis 2004), and immunohistochemical investigations include dopaminergic terminal markers and caspase-3 activation in the striatum of human methamphetamine users (Kitamura et al. 2007). Additionally, animal experiments have been undertaken to investigate drug-induced neuropathologic changes, including the induction of apoptotic cell death in rat thymus and spleen after a bolus injection of methamphetamine (Iwasa et al. 1996). Neuronal loss, a reduction in the number of GFAP-positive astrocytes, vascular hyalinosis, and ß-APP deposits, as well as endothelial proliferation and reduced immunoreactivity for type IV collagen in the vascular basal lamina, have been described in the setting of drug abuse (Büttner and Weis 2006). Drug abusers with bacterial endocarditis may develop nontraumatic subdural hematoma secondary to septic brain embolism (Geisenberger et al. 2015).

There are only scant investigations based on the immunohistochemical demonstration of drugs in tissue samples. In principle, however, 3,4-methylenedioxymethamphetamine (MDMA) and 3,4-methylenedioxyamphetamine (MDA), for instance, can also be demonstrated immunohistochemically in brain tissue or the pituitary gland when using the appropriate antibodies (de Letter et al. 2003). The same applies to the demonstration of morphine in hippocampal ganglion cells (Wehner et al. 2000). On the other hand, evident changes in preexisting physiological processes are seen, at least following methamphetamine use, e.g., in relation to tyrosine hydroxylase (TH), the dopamine transporter (DAT), and the vesicular monoamine transporter 2 (VMAT2) (Kitamura 2009).

20.8 Central Pontine Myelinolysis

Central pontine myelinolysis (CPM) is a demyelinating disease of the central part of the base

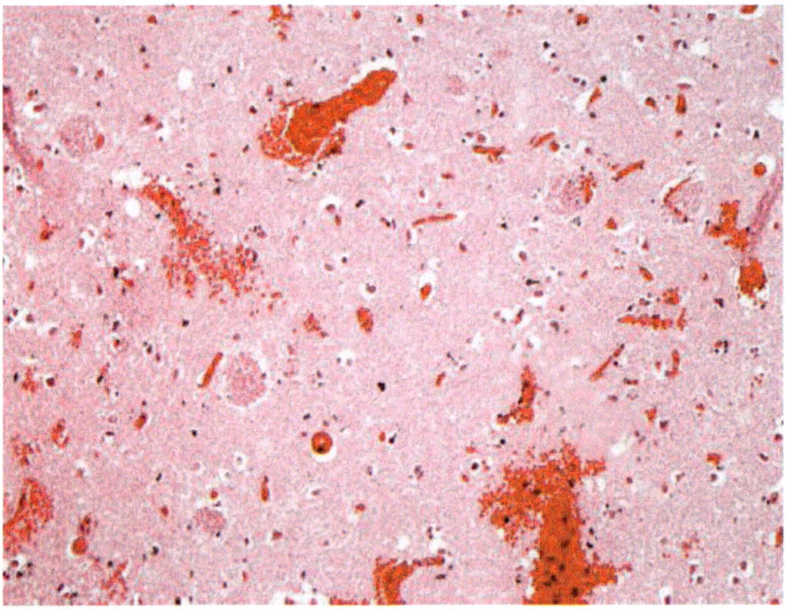

Fig. 20.26 Histology in a case of acute, symmetrical bilateral ischemic necrosis of the globus pallidus following heroin abuse: neuronal and glial necrosis and microhemorrhages (H&E ×400)

of the pons and was first described in patients with long-term alcoholism and malnutrition (Adams et al. 1959; Büttner and Weis 2008; Fersini et al. 2015). Besides alcohol and drugs in the narrower sense, other toxic substances can cause immunohistochemically detectable neuropathological findings consistent with CPM (Fig. 20.26; Unuma et al. 2010), as well as necrosis of the basal ganglia with and without carbon monoxide poisoning (Yarid and Harruff 2015). Although Wernicke encephalopathy has been described in alcoholics in particular, it refers in the stricter sense to a neurological disorder caused by thiamine (vitamin B-1) deficiency (Sechi and Serra 2007).

20.9 Fahr Disease

Clinical studies and reviews have described a wide range of symptoms to be associated with Fahr disease. Widespread calcifications combined with movement disorders, e.g., Parkinson disease, ataxia, psychological disorders, and dementia, have been observed. Macroscopically, the brain does not present any pathological findings. Routine histology with H&E staining reveals thickening of intracerebral arterial walls caused by poorly structured eosinophilic material not reacting to Congo red staining (Fig. 20.27). Iron (Prussian blue reaction) is not detectable. Since these changes are only present in the CNS, von Kossa staining unmasks the material associated with calcium (Fig. 20.28). Intracerebral small vessel mineralization primarily of cerebellar structures, of white brain matter, along the border between gray and white matter, and of the basal ganglia can be detected (Preusser et al. 2007; König and Haller 1985). Characteristically, symmetrical intracerebral calcinosis is predominantly present in capillaries and arterioles. Mandani et al. reported on an association between basal ganglia calcification and spontaneous bleeding (Mandani et al. 2007). Currently, Fahr disease is not considered to be associated with sudden death, but calcium metabolism disturbances may have potentially lethal courses (e.g., cardiac arrhythmia, hypocalcemia, tetanic fit, laryngospasm) (Unkrig et al. 2010).

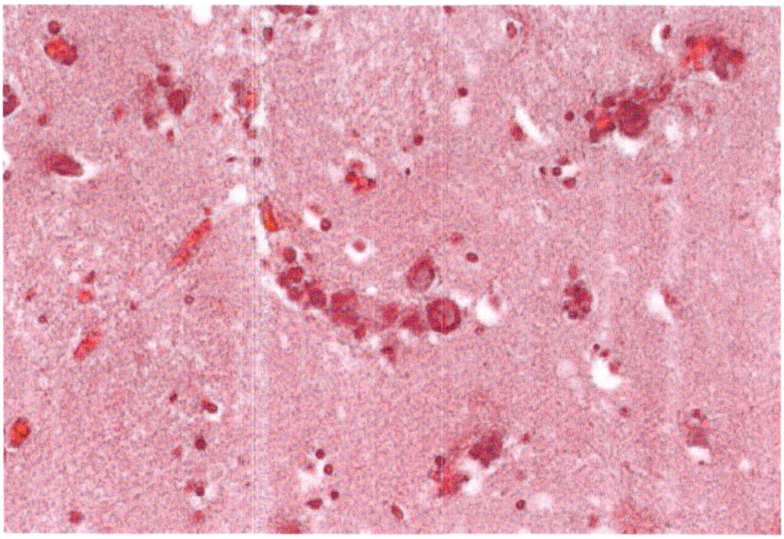

Fig. 20.27 Thickening of small intracerebral blood vessels (detectable using H&E staining) in a case of Fahr disease (H&E ×400)

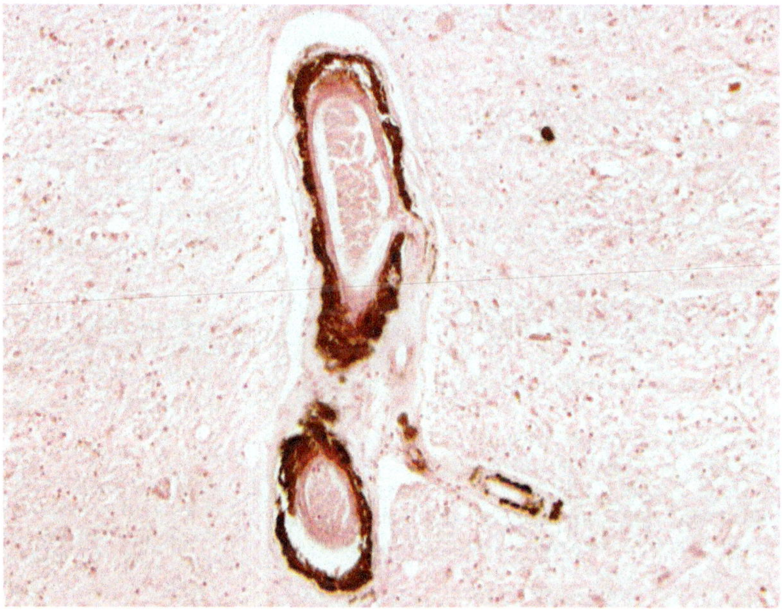

Fig. 20.28 Vessel wall thickening in intracerebral peripheral branches and detectable mineralization in Fahr disease (von Kossa ×100)

20.10 Epilepsy

Sudden death in epileptics occurs in the acute status epilepticus on the one hand or independent of an acute seizure, termed sudden unexpected death in epilepsy (SUDEP), on the other. SUDEP has been defined as

> sudden, unexpected, witnessed or unwitnessed, non-traumatic, and non-drowning death in patients with epilepsy, with or without evidence of a seizure and excluding documented status epilepticus where necropsy examination does not reveal a toxicological or anatomical cause of death. (Milroy 2011; Matschke et al. 2010; Oehmichen et al. 2006; Lear-Kaul et al. 2005; Byard 2004; Sperling 2001)

Alternatively, forms of epilepsy exist for which histomorphological diagnoses are possible, such as in the case of Lafora disease, which is a rare form of autosomal recessive progressive myoclonic epilepsy characterized by grand mal seizures, myoclonic jerking, difficulties in voluntary movements, ataxia, and progressive dementia (Wick and Byard 2006; Andrade et al. 2003). Causes of sudden death in cases of epilepsy include status epilepticus, SUDEP, trauma, cardiac arrhythmia, choking/aspiration of gastric contents, positional asphyxia, or miscellaneous, including suicide and homicide (Wick and Byard 2006). Only a handful of studies report histological or immunohistochemical findings in sudden unexpected death in epilepsy (SUDEP). For example, the expression of HSP 70 and c-Jun is presumed to indicate acute neuronal injury (Thom et al. 2003).

References

Abu AL, Ragheb SY, Koussous KJ, Amr SS (1986) Intracranial neoplasms associated with sudden death: a report of seven cases and a review of the literature. Med Sci Law 26:270–272

Ackerman MJ, Andrew TA, Baker AM, Devinsky O, Upshaw Downs JC, Keens T, Kuntz J, Lin P, Lear-Kaul KC, Reichard R, Robinson DA (2016) An association of hippocampal malformations and sudden death? We need mor data. Forensic Sci Med Pathol 12:229–231

Adams R, Victor M, Mancall E (1959) Central pontine myelinolysis. A hitherto undescribed disease occurring in alcoholic and malnourished patients. Arch Neurol Psychiatr 81:154–172

Althoff H (1982) Zur Ätiologie und Pathogenese des Waterhouse-Friderichsen-Syndroms. Z Rechtsmed 88:173–184

American Academy of Pediatrics (2001) Shaken baby syndrome: rotational cranial injuries – technical report. Pediatrics 108:206–210

Amine ARC (1997) Neurosurgical complications of heroin addiction: brain abscess and mycotic aneurysm. Surg Neurol 7:385–386

Andersen SN, Skullerud K (1999) Hypoxic/ischaemic brain damage, especially pallidal lesions, in heroin addicts. Forensic Sci Int 102:51–59

Andrade DM, Ackerley CA, Minett TS, Teive HA, Bohlega S, Scherer SW, Minassian BA (2003) Skin biopsy in Lafora disease: genotype-phenotype correlations and diagnostic pitfalls. Neurology 61:1611–1614

Arlotti SA, Forbes BJ, Dias MS, Bonsall DJ (2007) Unilateral retinal hemorrhages in shaken baby syndrome. J AAPOS 11:175–178

Balko MG, Schultz DL (1999) Sudden death due to a central neurocytoma. Am J Forensic Med Pathol 20:180–183

Bauer M, Lang C, Patzelt D (2001) Sudden death due to pituitary apoplexy. Legal Med 3:183–186

Baum JD, Bulpitt CJ (1970) Retinal and conjunctival haemorrhage in the newborn. Arch Dis Child 45:344–349

Betz P, Püschel K, Miltner E, Lignitz E, Eisenmenger W (1996) Morphometrical analysis of retinal hemorrhages in the shaken baby syndrome. Forensic Sci Int 78:71–80

Black M, Graham DI (2002) Sudden unexplained death in adults caused by intracranial pathology. J Clin Pathol 55:44–50

Böhm N (1982) Adrenal, cutaneous and myocardial lesions in fulminating endotoxinemia (Waterhouse-Friderichsen syndrome). Pathol Res Pract 174:92–105

Bowen DA (1984) Ruptured berry aneurysms: a clinical, pathological and forensic review. Forensic Sci Int 26:227–234

Bratzke H, Eisenmenger W (1989) Traumatische Ruptur der Arteria communicans anterior. Beitr Gerichtl Med 47:437–440

Bratzke H, Krauland W (1988) Zur Genese und Morphologie des traumatischen Mediainfarktes (Fallbericht). In: Bauer G (ed) Gerichtsmedizin – Festschrift für Wilhelm Holczabek. Deutike-Verlag, Wien

Bratzke H, Püschel K, Colmant HJ (1986) The phenomena and morphology for fatal aneurysms causing brain hemorrhage. Z Rechtsmed 96:245–273

Buschmann CT, Matejic D, Semm K, Tsokos M (2008) Lhermitte-Duclos syndrome as the cause of sudden death. Rechtsmedizin 19:34–36

Büttner A, Weis S (2004) Central nervous system alterations in drug abuse. In: Tsokos M (ed) Forensic pathology reviews, vol 1. Humana Press, Totowa, pp 79–136

Büttner A, Weis S (2006) Neuropathological alterations in drug abusers. Forensic Sci Med Pathol 2:115–126

Büttner A, Weis S (2008) Central nervous system alterations in alcohol abuse. In: Tsokos M (ed) Forensic pathology reviews, vol 5. Humana Press, Totowa, pp 69–89

Büttner A, Winkler PA, Eisenmenger W, Weis S (1997) Colloid cysts of the third ventricle with fatal outcome: a report of two cases and review of the literature. Int J Legal Med 110:260–266

Büttner A, Gall C, Mall C, Weis S (1999) Unexpected death in persons with symptomatic epilepsy due to glial brain tumors: a report of two cases and review of the literature. Forensic Sci Int 100:127–136

Büttner A, Mall G, Penning R, Weis S (2000) The neuropathology of heroin abuse. Forensic Sci Int 113:435–442

Büttner A, Weis S, Mall G, Gall C, Eisenmenger W (2001) The diagnostic relevance of cerebral amyloid angiopathy in the setting of forensic pathology – a report of two cases and review of the literature. Legal Med 3:141–148

Büttner A, Rohrmoser K, Mall G, Penning R, Weis S (2006) Widespread axonal damage in the brain of drug abusers as evidenced by accumulation of beta-amyloid precursor protein (beta-APP): an immunohistochemical investigation. Addiction 101:1339–1346

Byard RW (2004) Neurologic conditions. In: Sudden death in infancy, childhood and adolescence, 2nd edn. Cambridge University Press, Cambridge, pp 366–372. Chapter 8

Byard RW (2014) "Shaken baby syndrome" and forensic pathology: an uneasy interface. Forensic Sci Med Pathol 10:239–241

Byard RW, Bourne AJ, Hanieh A (1991) Sudden and unexpected death due to hemorrhage from occult central nervous system lesions. A pediatric autopsy study. Pediatr Neurosurg 17:88–94

Caffey J (1972) On the theory and practice of shaking infants. Its potential residual effects of permanent brain damage and mental retardation. Am J Dis Child 124:161–169

Caparros-Lefebvre D, Policard J, Sengler C, Benabdallah E, Colombani S, Rigal M (2005) Bipallidal haemorrhage after ethylene glycol intoxication. Neuroradiology 47:105–107

Ceauşu M, Dragoteanu C, Hostiuc S, Negoi I (2015) Sudden death due to non-traumatic subdural hematoma in a patient with a myeloproliferative disorder. Rom J Leg Med 23:251–256

Centers for Disease Controal – CDC (1997) Control and prevention of meningococcal disease: recommendations of the Advisory Committee on Immunization Practices (ACIP). MMWR Recomm Rep 46(5):1–10

Cervós-Navarro J, Lafuente JV (1991) Traumatic brain injuries: structural changes. J Neurol Sci 103:3–14

Chan KK, Lowe J (2002) Techniques in neuropathology. In: Bancroft JD, Gamble M (eds) Theory and practice of histological techniques, 5th edn. Churchill Livingstone, London, pp 371–414

Cohen MA, Sprigg A, Whitby EH (2010) Subdural hemorrhage, intradural hemorrhage and hypoxia in the pediatric and perinatal post mortem: are they related? An observational study combining the use of post mortem pathology and magnetic resonance imaging. Forensic Sci Int 200:100–107

D'Errico S, Bello S, Cantatore S, Neri M, Riezzo I, Turillazzi E, Fineschi V (2011) Immunohistochemical characterization and TNF-α expression of the granulomatous infiltration of the brainstem in a case of sudden death due to neurosarcoidosis. Forensic Sci Int 208:e1–e5

De Letter EA, Espeel MF, Craeymeersch ME et al (2003) Immunohistochemical demonstration of the amphetamine derivatives 3,4-methylenedioxymethamphetam ine (MDMA) and 3,4-methylenedioxyamphetamine (MDA) in human post-mortem brain tissues and the pituitary gland. Int J Legal Med 117:2–9

Demirci S, Dogan KH, Erkol Z, Gulmen MK (2009) Sudden death due to a colloid cyst of the third venricle: report of three cases with a special sign at autopsy. Forensic Sci Int 189:e33–e36

Detesky AS, Salit IE (1983) Complete heart block in meningococcemia. Ann Emerg Med 12:391–393

Dettmeyer R, Varchmin-Schultheiß K, Madea B (1998a) Intracranial plasma cell granuloma and homocystinuria. Pathol Res Pract 194:205–208

Dettmeyer R, Varchmin-Schultheiß K, Madea B (1998b) Sudden death of an 18-year-old man with homocystinuria and intracranial inflammatory pseudotumor (IPT). Forensic Sci Int 94:19–24

DiMaio VJM, Dana SE (2007) Handbook of forensic pathology, 2nd edn. Taylor & Francis, Boca Raton

DiMaio SM, DiMaio VJ, Kirkpatrick JB (1980) Sudden unexpected death due to primary intracranial neoplasms. Am J Forensic Med Pathol 1:29–45

Dolinak D, Reichard R (2006) An overview of inflicted head injury in infants and young children, with a review of beta-amyloid precursor protein immunohistochemistry. Arch Pathol Lab Med 130:712–717

Dressler J, Hanisch U, Busuttil A (2005) Comments on Hausmann et al.: neuronal apoptosis following human brain injury. Int J Legal Med 119:177–178

Dressler J, Hanisch U, Kuhlisch E, Geiger KD (2007) Neuronal and glial apoptosis in human traumatic brain injury. Int J Legal Med 121:365–375

Duhaime AC, Alario AJ, Lewander WJ et al (1992) Head injury in very young children: mechanisms, injury types, and ophthalmologic findings in 100 hospitalized patients younger than 2 years of age. Pediatrics 90:179–185

Eberhart CG, Morrison A, Gyure KA, Frazier J, Smialek JE, Troncoso JC (2001) Decreasing incidence of sudden death due to undiagnosed primary intracranial tumors. Arch Pathol Lab Med 125:1024–1030

Eisenmenger W (1977) Zur histologischen und histochemischen Altersbestimmung gedeckter Hirnverletzungen. Med Habil, München

Emerson MV, Pieramici DJ, Stoessel KM, Berreen JP, Gariano RF (2001) Incidence and rate of disappearance of retinal hemorrhage in newborns. Ophthalmology 108:36–39

Fersini F, Govi A, Tsokos M (2015) Central pontine myelinolysis. Forensic Sci Med Pathol 11:130–132

Förstl H, Haass C, Hemmer B, Meyer B, Halle M (2010) Boxing-acute complications and late sequelae: from concussion to dementia. Dtsch Arztebl Int 107:835–839

Fracasso T, Brinkmann B, Paulus W (2008) Sudden death due to subarachnoid bleeding from ecchordosis physaliphora. Int J Legal Med 122:225–227

Friderichsen C (1918) Nebennierenapoplexie bei kleinen Kindern. Jahrb Kinderheilk 87:109

Gago LC, Wegner RK, Capone A Jr, Williams GA (2003) Intraretinal hemorrhages and chronic subdural effusions: glutaric aciduria type 1 can be mistaken for shaken baby syndrome. Retina 23:724–726

Geddes JF, Whitwell HL, Graham DI (2000) Traumatic axonal injury: practical issues for diagnosis in medicolegal cases. Neuropathol Appl Neurobiol 26:105–116

Geddes JF, Tasker RC, Hackshaw AK, Nickols CD, Adams CGW, Whitwell HL, Scheimberg I (2003) Dural hemorrhage in non-traumatic infant deaths: does it explain the bleeding in "shaken baby syndrome"? Neuropathol Appl Neurobiol 29:14–22

Geisenberger D, Huppertz LM, Büchsel M, Kramer L, Pollak S, Große Perdekamp M (2015) Non-traumatic subdural hematoma secondary to septic brain embolism: a rare cause of unexpected death in a drug addict suffering from undiagnosed bacterial endocarditis. Forensic Sci Int 257:e1–e5

Gentleman SM, Nash AJ, Sweeting CJ, Graham DI, Roberts GW (1993) ß-Amyloid precursor protein (ß-APP) as a marker of axonal injury in traumatic brain injury. Neurosci Lett 160:139–144

Gilliland MG, Luckenbach MW (1993) Are retinal hemorrhages found after resuscitation attempts? A study of the eyes of 169 children. Am J Forensic Med Pathol 14:187–192

Gilliland MG, Luthert P (2003) Why do histology on retinal haemorrhages in suspected non-accidental injury? Histopathology 43:592–602

Gilliland MG, Luckenbach MW, Chenier TC (1994) Systemic and ocular findings in 169 prospectively studied child deaths: retinal hemorrhages usually mean child abuse. Forensic Sci Int 68:117–132

Gilliland MG, Levin AV, Enzenauer RW et al (2007) Guidelines for postmortem protocol for ocular investigation of sudden unexplained infant death and suspected physical child abuse. Am J Forensic Med Pathol 28:323–329

Gleckman AM, Bell MD, Evans RJ, Smith TW (1999) Diffuse axonal injury in infants with nonaccidental craniocerebral trauma: enhanced detection by beta-amyloid precursor protein immunohistochemical staining. Arch Pathol Lab Med 123:146–151

Gleckman AM, Kessler SC, Smith TW (2000) Periadventitial extracranial vertebral artery hemorrhage in a case of shaken baby syndrome. J Forensic Sci 45:1151–1153

Goede A, Dreßler J, Sommer G, Schober K, Franke H, Ondruschka B (2015) Wound age diagnostics after fatal brain injury. Expression of neuron-specific enolase and glial fibrillary acidic protein in brain tissue. Rechtsmedizin 25:261–267

Goetting MG, Sowa B (1990) Retinal hemorrhage after cardiopulmonary resuscitation in children: an etiologic reevaluation. Pediatrics 85:585–588

Guddat SS, Ehrlich E, Martin H, Tsokos M (2011) Fatal spontaneous subdural bleeding due to neonatal giant cell hepatitis: a rare differential diagnosis of shaken baby syndrome. Forensic Sci Med Pathol 7:294–297

Gumpert S, Maxeiner H (2008) Sturzbedingte tödliche Schädel-Hirn-Traumen. Rechtsmedizin 18:247–250

Günther M, Becker J, Wegner C, Brück W, Pauli R (2017) Death of a boxer. An example of chronic traumatic encephalopathy. Rechtsmedizin 27:33–36

Halpern M, Citron BP (1971) Necrotizing angiitis associated with drug abuse. Am J Roentgenol 111:663–671

Hartman CA, Lindlar F (1987) Hirninfarkt nach traumatischer Karotisthrombose. Z Rechtsmed 99:219

Hauser R, Jankowski Z, Gos T, Krzyżanowski M (2001) Hemorrhages in head tissues during the asphyxiation process. Forensic Sci Int 124:235–236

Hausmann R (2002) Die Altersbestimmung von Hirnkontusionen bei gedecktem Schädel-Hirn-Trauma des Menschen. In: Arbeitsmethoden der Medizinischen und Naturwissenschaftlichen Kriminalistik, vol 25. Schmidt-Römhild, Lübeck

Hausmann R (2004) Timing of cortical contusions in human brain injury: morphological parameters for a forensic wound-age estimation. In: Tsokos M (ed) Forensic pathology reviews, vol 1. Humana Press Inc, Totowa, pp 53–75

Hausmann R, Betz P (2000) The time course of the vascular response to human brain injury – an immunohistochemical study. Int J Legal Med 113:288–292

Hausmann R, Betz P (2001) Course of glial immunoreactivity for vimentin, tenascin and alpha1-antichymotrypsin after traumatic injury to human brain. Int J Legal Med 114:338–342

Hausmann R, Betz P (2002) The course of MIB-1 expression by cerebral macrophages following human brain injury. Legal Med 4:79–83

Hausmann R, Kaiser A, Lang C, Bohnert M, Betz P (1999) A quantitative immunohistochemical study on the time-dependent course of acute inflammatory cellular response to human brain injury. Int J Legal Med 112:227–232

Hausmann R, Rieß R, Fieguth A, Betz P (2000) Immunohistochemical investigations on the course of astroglial GFAP expression following human brain injury. Int J Legal Med 113:70–75

Hausmann R, Biermann T, Wiest I, Tübel J, Betz P (2004) Neuronal apoptosis following human brain injury. Int J Legal Med 118:32–36

Hausmann R, Vogel C, Seidl S, Betz P (2006) Value of morphological parameters for grading of brain swelling. Int J Legal Med 120:219–225

Hausmann R, Seidl S, Betz P (2007) Hypoxic changes in Purkinje cells of the human cerebellum. Int J Legal Med 121:175–183

Hayashi T, Ago K, Ago M, Ogata M (2009) Two patterns of beta-amyloid precursor protein (APP) immunoreactivity in cases of blunt head injury. Legal Med 11(Suppl. 1):S171–S173

Hayashi T, Ago K, Nakamae T, Higo E, Ogata M (2015) Two different immunostaining patterns of beta-amyloid precursor protein (APP) may distinguish traumatic from non-traumatic axonal injury. Int J Legal Med 129:1085–1090

Hayashi T, Ago K, Nakamae T, Higo E, Ogata M (2016) Interleukin (IL)-8 immunoreactivity of injured axons and surrounding oligodendrocytes in traumatic head injury. Forensic Sci Int 263:48–54

Hefti MM, Cryan JB, Haas EA, Chadwick AE, Crandall LA, Trachtenberg FL, Armstrong DD, Grafe M, Krous HF, Kinney HC (2016) Hippocampal malformation associated with sudden death in early childhood: a neuropathologic study. Forensic Sci Med Pathol 12:14–25

Herczeg L, Gorombey S, Vaszily M (1995) Morphological damage to the central nervous system (CNS) following open heart surgery. Forensic Sci Int 79:103–111

Herr S, Pierce MC, Berger RP, Ford H, Pitetti RD (2004) Does Valsalva retinopathy occur in infants? An initial investigation in infants with vomiting caused by pyloric stenosis. Pediatrics 113:1658–1661

Horn M, Schote W (1992) Delayed neuronal death and delayed neuronal recovery in the human brain following global ischemia. Acta Neuropathol 85:79–87

Huntington RW, Cummings KL, Moe TI, O'Connell HV, Wybel R (1965) Discovery of fatal primary intracranial neoplasms at medicolegal autopsies. Cancer 18:117–127

Igari Y, Hosoya T, Hayashizaki Y, Usui A, Kawasumi Y, Usui K, Funayama M (2014) Sudden death due to a cystic lesion in the cerebellum. Forensic Sci Int 245:e25–e28

Iino M, Nakatome M, Ogura Y, Fujimura H, Kuroki H, Inoue H et al (2003) Real-time PCR quantification of FE65 a ß-amyloid precursor protein-binding protein after traumatic brain injury in rats. Int J Legal Med 117:153–159

Ip M, Teo JG, Cheng AF (1995) Waterhouse-Friderichsen syndrome complicating primary biliary sepsis due to *Pasteurella multocida* in a patient with cirrhosis. J Clin Pathol 48:775–777

Ishigami A, Kubo S, Ikematsu K, Kitamura O, Tokunaga I, Gotohda T, Nakasono I (2004) An adult autopsy case of acute encephalopathy associated with influenza A virus. Legal Med 6:252–255

Ishikawa T, Zhu BL, Li DR, Zhao D, Michiue T, Maeda H (2006a) Postmortem stability of pituitary hormones in the human adenohypophysis. Legal Med 8:34–38

Ishikawa T, Zhu BL, Li DR, Michiue T, Maeda H (2006b) Age-dependent increase of clusterin in the human pituitary gland. Legal Med 8:28–33

Ishikawa T, Zhu BL, Miyaishi S, Ishizu H, Maeda H (2007) Increase of clusterin-containing follicles in the adenohypophysis of drug abusers. Int J Legal Med 121:395–402

Ishikawa T, Michiue T, Quan L, Zhao D, Komatsu A, Bessho Y, Maeda H (2009) Morphological and functional alterations in the adenohypophysis in cases of brain death. Legal Med 11:S234–S237

Itabashi HH, Andrews JM, Tomiyasu U et al (2007) Forensic neuropathology. A practical review of the fundamentals. Elsevier, Amsterdam

Iwasa M, Maeno Y, Inoue H, Koyama H, Matoba R (1996) Induction of apoptotic cell death in rat thymus and spleen after a bolus injection of methamphetamine. Int J Legal Med 109:23–28

Jacobs RF, His S, Wilson CB, Benjamin D, Smith AL, Morrow R (1983) Apparent meningococcemia: clinical features of disease due to *Haemophilus influenzae* and *Neisseria meningitides*. Pediatrics 7:469–472

Johnston DL, Braun D, Friendly D (1993) Accidental head trauma and retinal hemorrhage. Neurosurgery 33:231–234

Kanter RK (1986) Retinal hemorrhage after cardiopulmonary resuscitation or child abuse. J Pediatr 108:430–432

Kempe H, Silverman FN, Steele BF, Droegemueller W, Silver HK (1962) The battered child syndrome. JAMA 181:17–24

Kibayashi K, Shojo H (2002) Incipient Alzheimer's disease as the underlying cause of a motor vehicle crash. Med Sci Law 42:233–236

Kind M (1991) Tödliche basilaris-thrombose nach commotio cerebri. Verh Dtsch Ges Pathol 75:518

King J, Richards M, Tress B (1978) Cerebral arteritis associated with heroin abuse. Med J Aust 2:444–445

Kitamura O (1994) Immunohistochemical investigations of hypoxic/ischemic brain damage in forensic autopsy cases. Int J Legal Med 107:69–76

Kitamura O (2009) Detection of methamphetamine neurotoxicity in forensic autopsy cases. Legal Med 11:S63–S65

Kitamura O, Tokunaga I, Gotohda T, Kubo S (2007) Immunohistochemical investigation of dopaminergic terminal markers and caspaser-3 activation in the striatum of human methamphetamine users. Int J Legal Med 121:163–168

Klages U (1970) Spontaneous versus traumatic lethal subarachnoid hemorrhage. J Leg Med 67:67–86

Koda Y, Seto Y, Takeichi S, Kimura H (2003) Fatal subarachnoid hemorrhage complicating actinomycotic meningitis. Forensic Sci Int 134:169–171

Kominato Y, Matsui K, Hata Y, Matsui K, Kuwayama N, Ishizawa S, Takizawa H (2004) Acute subdural hematoma due to arteriovenous malformation primarily in dura mater: a case report. Legal Med 6:256–260

König P, Haller R (1985) Results of a study of a family with aggregated occurrence of bilateral symmetrical basal ganglia calcinosis. Eur Arch Psychiatry Neurol Sci 234:325–334

Krauland W (1961) Über die Quellen des akuten und chronischen subduralen Hämatoms. Thieme-Verlag, Stuttgart

Krauland W (1973) Über die Zeitbestimmung von Schädelhirnverletzungen. Beitr Gerichtl Med 30:226–251

Krauland W (1981) Die traumatische subarachnoidale Blutung. Z Rechtsmed 87:1–18

Krauland W (1982) Verletzungen der intrakraniellen Schlagadern. Springer, Berlin

Kreft F (1952) Über Todesfälle beim Boxen. Dtsch Gesundheit 7:1559–1564

Lear-Kaul KC, Coughlin L, Dobersen MJ (2005) Sudden unexpected death in epilepsy: a retrospective study. Am J Forensic Med Pathol 26:11–17

Lee CH, Kim DW, Jeon GS, Roh EJ, Seo JH, Wang KC, Cho SS (2001) Cerebellar alterations induced by chronic hypoxia: an immunohistochemical study using a chick embryonic model. Brain Res 901:271–276

Leestma JE (2009) Forensic neuropathology, 2nd edn. CRC Press/Taylor & Francis Group, Boca Raton

Li DR, Zhu BL, Ishikawa T, Zhao D, Michiue T, Maeda H (2006) Immunohistochemical distribution of S-100 protein in the cerebral cortex with regard to the cause of death in forensic autopsy. Legal Med 8:78–85

Li DR, Ishikawa T, Zhao D, Michiue T, Quan L, Zhu BL, Maeda H (2010) Unexpected sudden death due to intracranial chordoma: an autopsy case. Forensic Sci Int 200:e15–e18

Lindboe CF, Svenes KB, Slordal L (1997) Sudden unexpected death in subjects with undiagnosed gliomas. Am J Forensic Med Pathol 18:271–275

Lindenberg R, Freytag E (1957) Morphology of cortical contusions. Arch Pathol 63:23–42

Mandani N, Repp AL, Seyoum B, Berhanu P (2007) Idiopathic hypoparathyroidism presenting with severe hypocalcemia and asymptomatic basal ganglia calcification followed by acute intracerebral bleed. Endocr Pract 13:487–492

Martland HS (1928) Punch drunk. JAMA 91:1103–1107

Matsche J (2005) Primary cerebral neoplasms as a cause of sudden, unexpected death. In: Tsokos M (ed) Forensic pathology reviews, vol 2. Humana Press, Totowa, pp 45–58

Matschke J (2008) Historical overview of non-accidental head injury in toddlers and infants. Rechtsmedizin 18:7–8

Matschke J, Glatzel M (2008) Neuropathologische Begutachtung des nichtakzidentellen Schädel-Hirn-Traumas bei Säuglingen und Kleinkindern. Rechtsmedizin 18:29–35

Matschke J, Tsokos M (2001) Post-traumatic meningitis: histomorphological findings, post-mortem microbiology and forensic implications. Forensic Sci Int 115:199–205

Matschke J, Tsokos M (2005) Sudden unexpected death due to undiagnosed glioblastoma: report of three cases and review of the literature. Int J Legal Med 119:280–284

Matschke J, Tsokos M, Schulz F, Lockemann U (1999) Differential diagnostic aspects of forensically relevant findings in the brain stem. Arch Kriminol 203:108–116

Matschke J, Tsokos M, Püschel K (2000) Pilocytic astrocytoma of the brainstem as the cause of death in a 29-year-old man. Rechtsmedizin 10:221–225

Matschke J, Stavrou D, Püschel K (2002) Sudden unexpected death due to epidermoid cyst of the brain. Am J Forensic Med Pathol 23:368–370

Matschke J, Püschel K, Glatzel M (2009) Ocular pathology in shaken baby syndrome and other forms of infantile non-accidental head injury. Int J Legal Med 123:189–197

Matschke J, Glatzel M, Püschel K, Andresen H (2010) Fatalities in patients with epilepsy. Rechtsmedizin 20:437–446

Matschke J, Büttner A, Bergmann M, Hagel C, Püschel K, Glatzel M (2015) Encephalopathy and death in infants with abuse head trauma is due to hypoxic-ischemic injury following local brain stem trauma to vital brainstem centers. Int J Legal Med 129:105–114

Matsumoto H, Yamamoto K (1994) A case of sudden death by undiagnosed glioblastoma multiforme. Jpn J Legal Med 47:336–339

Matturri L, Ottaviani G, Lavezzi AM (2008) Guidelines for neuropathologic diagnostics of perinatal unexpected loss and sudden infant death syndrome (SIDS) – a technical protocol. Virchows Arch 452:19–25

Maxeiner H, Finck GA (1989) Traumatischer Hirninfarkt bei mehrzeitig verlaufender Dissektion der extrakraniellen Arteria carotis interna. Unfallchirurg 92:321–327

McKee AC, Stern RA, Nowinski CJ, Stein TD, Alvarez VE, Daneshvar DH, Lee HS, Wojtowicz SM, Hall G, Baugh CM, Riley DO, Kubilus CA, Cormier KA, Jacobs MA, Martin BR, Abraham CR, Ikezu T, Reichard RR, Wolozin BL, Budson AE, Goldstein LE, Kowall NW, Cantu RC (2013) The spectrum of disease in chronic traumatic encephalopathy. Brain 136:43–64

McKee AC, Cairns NJ, Dickson DW, Folkerth RD, Keene CD, Litvan I, Perl DP, Stein TD, Vonsattel JP, Stewart W, Tripodis Y, Crary JF, Bieniek KF, Dams-O'Connor K, Alvarez VE, Gordon WA (2016) The first NINDS/NIBIB consensus meeting to define neuropathological criteria for the diagnosis of chronic traumatic encephalopathy. Acta Neuropathol 131:75–86

McQuillen JB, McQuillen E, Morrow P (1988) Trauma, sport and malignant cerebral edema. Am J Forensic Med Pathol 9:12–15

Michiue T, Ishikawa T, Quan L, Li DR, Zhao D, Komatsu A, Zhu BL, Maeda H (2008) Single-stranded DNA as an immunohistochemical marker of neuronal damage in human brain: an analysis of autopsy material with regard to the cause of death. Forensic Sci Int 178:185–191

Millspaugh J (1937) Dementia pugilistica. US Nav Med Bull 35:297–303

Milroy CM (2011) Sudden unexpected death in epilepsy in childhood. Forensic Sci Med Pathol 7:336–340

Mirza I, Wolk J, Toth L, Rostenberg P, Kranwinkel R, Sieber SC (2000) Waterhouse-Friderichsen syndrome secondary to Capnocytophaga canimorsus septicaemia and demonstration of bacteremia by peripheral blood smear. Arch Pathol Lab Med 124:859–863

Miyazaki T, Kojima T, Chikasue F, Yashiki M, Ito H (1990) Traumatic rupture of intracranial vertebral artery due to hyperextension of the head: reports on three cases. Forensic Sci Int 47:91–98

Mork SJ, Morild I, Giertsen JC (1986) Subependymoma and unexpected death. Forensic Sci Int 30:275–280

Mu J, Li M, Lv B, Qiu M, Dong H (2017) Methamphetamine-induced toxic leukoencephalopathy: clinical, radiological and autopsy findings. Forensic Sci Med Pathol 13:362–366

Munger CE, Peiffer RL, Bouldin TW, Kylstra JA, Thompson RL (1993) Ocular and associated neuropathologic observations in suspected whiplash shaken infant syndrome. A retrospective study of 12 cases. Am J Forensic Med Pathol 14:193–200

Nakatome M, Matoba R, Ogura Y et al (2002) Detection of cardiomyocyte apoptosis in forensic autopsy cases. Int J Legal Med 116:17–21

Nelson J, Frost JL, Schochet SS (1987) Sudden unexpected death in a 5-year-old boy with an unusual primary intracranial neoplasm. Am J Forensic Med Pathol 8:148–152

Ng I, Yeo TT, Tang WY, Soong R, Ng PY, Smith DR (2000) Apoptosis occurs after cerebral contusions in humans. Neurosurgery 46:949–956

Ng'walali PM, Yonemitsu K, Kibayashi K, Tsunenari S (2002) Neuropathological diagnosis of Alzheimer's disease in forensic autopsy of elderly persons with fatal accident. Legal Med 4:223–231
Noebels J (2016) Hippocampal abnormalities and sudden childhood death. Forensic Sci Med Pathol 12:198–199
Nogami M, Takatsu A, Endo N, Ishiyama I (1999a) IgG immunohistochemistry for the assessment of brain injuries in forensic autopsies. Legal Med 1:76–79
Nogami M, Takatsu A, Endo N, Ishiyama I (1999b) Immunohistochemical localization of heat shock protein 70 in the human medulla oblongata in forensic autopsies. Legal Med 1:198–203
Oehmichen M (2001) Brain hypoxia and ischemia. Schmidt-Römhild, Lübeck
Oehmichen M, König HG (1997) Neurotraumatology: biomechanic aspects, cytologic and molecular mechanisms. In: Research in legal medicine, vol 17. Schmidt-Römhild, Lübeck, pp 239–259
Oehmichen M, Meissner C (2006) Cerebral hypoxia and ischemia: the forensic point of view: a review. J Forensic Sci 51:880–887
Oehmichen M, Raff G (1980) Timing of cortical contusion. Correlation between histomorphological alterations and post-traumatic interval. Z Rechtsmed 84:79–94
Oehmichen M, Eisenmenger W, Raff G, Berghaus G (1986) Brain macrophages in human cortical contusions as an indicator of survival period. Forensic Sci Int 30:281–301
Oehmichen M, Meißner C, Schmidt V, Pedal I, König HG, Saternus KS (1998) Axonal injury – a diagnostic tool in forensic neuropathology? A review. Forensic Sci Int 95:67–83
Oehmichen M, Meissner C, von Wurmb-Schwank N, Schwank T (2003) Methodological approach to brain hypoxia/ischemia as a fundamental problem in forensic neuropathology. Legal Med 5:190–201
Oehmichen M, Auer RN, König HG (2006) Forensic neuropathology and associated neuropathology. Springer, Berlin
Oehmichen M, Jakob S, Mann S, Saternus KS, Pedal I, Meissner C (2009) Macrophage subsets in mechanical brain injury (MBI) – a contribution to timing of MBI based on immunohistochemical methods: a pilot study. Legal Med 11:118–124
Ogata M, Tsuganezawa O (1999) Neuron-specific enolase as an effective immunohistochemical marker for injured axons after fatal brain injury. Int J Legal Med 113:19–25
Omalu BI, Nnebe-Agumadu UH, Shakir AM, Rozin L, Wecht CH (2005) Postmortem grading of cerebral contusions. A proposed modification of the Adam`s Contusion Index with re-definition of anatomic markers. Forensic Sci Med Pathol 1:105–112
Ommaya AK, Yarnell P (1969) Subdural hematoma after whiplash injury. Lancet 2:237–239
Ong BB, Gole GA, Robertson T, McGill J, de Lore D, Crawford M (2009) Retinal hemorrhages associated with meningitis in a child with a congenital disorder of glycosylation. Forensic Sci Med Pathol 5:307–312
Orihara Y, Nakasono I (2002) Induction of apolipoprotein E after traumatic brain injury in forensic autopsy cases. Int J Legal Med 116:92–98
Orihara Y, Tsuda R, Ikematsu K, Nakasono I, Ogata M (2003) Immunohistochemical study on the induction of heme oxygenase-1 by traumatic brain injury. Legal Med 5:S278–S279
Padosch SH, Vogel P, Böttiger BW (2001) Neuronale apoptose nach zerebraler Ischämie. Anaesthesist 50:905–920
Padosch SA, Dettmeyer RB, Schmidt PH, Musshoff F, Madea B (2006) Spinal epidural haematoma after blunt trauma to the neck and hyperflection of the cervical spine. Forensic Sci Int 159:230–234
Parsons MA, Talbot JF, Mudhar HS, Rutty GN (2005) The pathology of whiplash maculopathy and retinopathy. Forensic Sci Med Pathol 1:19–25
Petito CK, Roberts B (1995) Evidence of apoptotic cell death in HIV encephalitis. Am J Pathol 146:1121–1130
Piette MHA, Pieters SEP, de Letter EA (2010) Evaluation of the agonal stress: can immunohistochemical detection of ubiquitin in the locus coeruleus be useful? Int J Legal Med 125(3):333–340
Poon TP, Solis OG (1985) Sudden death due to massive intraventricular hemorrhage into an unsuspected ependymoma. Surg Neurol 24:63–66
Pounder DJ (1997) Shaken adult syndrome. Am J Forensic Med Pathol 18:321–324
Prahlow JA, Teot LA, Lantz PE, Stanton CA (1995) Sudden death in epilepsy due to an isolated subependymal giant cell astrocytoma of the septum pellucidum. Am J Forensic Med Pathol 16:30–37
Preusser M, Kitzwoegener M, Budka H, Brugger S (2007) Bilateral striopallidodentate calcification (Fahr's syndrome) and multiple system atrophy in a patient with longstanding hypoparathyroidism. Neuropathology 27:453–456
Quan L, Zhu BL, Ishida K, Oritani S, Taniguchi M, Fujita MQ, Maeda H (2001) Intranuclear ubiquitin immunoreactivity of the pigmented neurons of the substantia nigra in fatal acute mechanical asphyxiation and drowning. Int J Legal Med 115:6–11
Quan L, Ishikawa T, Michique T et al (2005a) Ubiquitin-immunoreactive structures in the midbrain of methamphetamine abusers. Legal Med 7:144–150
Quan L, Ishikawa T, Michiue T, Li DR, Zhao D, Zhu BL, Maeda H (2005b) Quantitative analysis of ubiquitin-immunoreactivity in the midbrain periaqueductal gray matter with regard to the causes of death in forensic autopsy. Legal Med 7:151–156
Quan L, Ishikawa T, Michiue T, Li DR, Zhao D, Zhu BL, Maeda H (2005c) Ubiquitin immunoreactivity in the midbrain as a marker of stress to motor nervous systems in fatal injury. Legal Med 7:157–163
Racette S, Sauvageau A (2007) Brain arteriovenous malformation and its implication in forensic pathology. J Forensic Sci 52:189–191

Raul JS, Roth S, Ludes B, Willinger R (2008) Influence of the benign enlargement of the subarachnoid space on the bridging veins strain during a shaking event: a finite element study. Int J Legal Med 12:337–340

Reichard RR, White CL 3rd, Hladik CL, Dolinak D (2003) Beta-amyloid precursor protein staining in nonhomicidal pediatric medicolegal autopsies. J Neuropathol Exp Neurol 62:237–247

Riffenburgh RS, Sathyavagiswaran L (1991) The eyes of child abuse victims: autopsy findings. J Forensic Sci 36:741–747

Riordan FAI, Marzouk O, Thomson APJ, Sills JA, Hart CA (1995) The changing presentations of meningococcal disease. Eur J Pediatr 154:472–474

Riße M, Weiler G (1984) Heroinsucht als seltene Ursache einer symmetrischen Pallidumnekrose. Z Rechtsmed 93:227–235

Rodriguez ML, McMillan K, Crandall LA, Minter ME, Grafe MR, Poduri A, Kinney HC (2012) Hippocampal asymmetry and sudden unexpected death in infancy: a case report. Forensic Sci Med Pathol 8:441–446

Roth S, Raul JS, Ludes B, Willinger R (2007) Finite element analysis of impact and shaking inflicted to a child. Int J Legal Med 121:223–228

Rutecki PA, Sutula TP (2016) Hippocampal abnormalities and sudden childhood death. Forensic Sci Med Pathol 12:200–201

Ryan CA, Wenman W, Hennigsen C, Tse S (1993) Fatal childhood pneumococcal Waterhouse-Friderichsen syndrome. Pediatr Infect Dis J 12:250–251

Saito K, Takda A, Kuroda N, Hara M, Arai M, Ro A (2009) Traumatic dissection of extracranial vertebral artery with massive subtentorial cerebral infarction: report of an autopsy case. Legal Med 11:S520–S522

Sakai K, Takatsu A, Shigeta A, Abe S, Ikegami M, Takagi K (2007) Sudden death due to undiagnosed acute promyelocytic leukaemia: a case report. Int J Legal Med 121:311–314

Sato M, Hashimoto H, Kosaka F (1990) Histological changes of neuronal damage in vegetative dogs induced by 18 minutes of complete global brain ischemia: two phase damage of Purkinje cells and hippocampal CA1 pyramidal cells. Acta Neuropathol 80:527–534

Scheimberg I, Mack J (2014) "Shaken baby syndrome" and forensic pathology. Forensic Sci Med Pathol 10:242–243

Schwarz KO, Perper JA, Rozin I (1987) Sudden, unexpected death due to fourth ventricular subependymoma. Am J Forensic Med Pathol 8:153–157

Sechi G, Serra A (2007) Wernicke`s encephalopathy: new clinical settings and recent advances in diagnosis and management. Lancet Neurol 6:442–455

Sezen F (1971) Retinal haemorrhages in newborn infants. Br J Ophthalmol 55:248–253

Sheriff FE, Bridges LR, Sivaloganatham S (1994) Early detection of axonal injury after human head trauma using immunocytochemistry for ß-amyloid protein. Acta Neuropathol 87:55–62

Simonsen J (1963) Traumatic subarachnoid hemorrhage in alcohol intoxication. J Forensic Sci 8:97–116

Simonsen J (1984) Fatal subarachnoid haemorrhages in relation to minor injuries in Denmark from 1967 to 1981. Forensic Sci Int 24:57–63

Smith C (2016) Hippocampal abnormalities and sudden childhood death. Forenic Sci Med Pathol 12:202–203

Sperhake J, Matschke J (2014) "Shaken baby syndrome" and forensic pathology. Forensic Sci Med Pathol 10:251–252

Sperhake JP, Tsokos M (2004) Pathological features of Waterhouse-Friderichsen syndrome in infancy and childhood. In: Toskos M (ed) Forensic pathology reviews, vol 1. Humana Press Inc, Totowa, pp 219–231

Sperling MR (2001) Sudden unexplained death in epilepsy. Epilepsy Curr 1:21–23

Squier W, Mack J (2009) The neuropathology of infant subdural haemorrhage. Forensic Sci Int 187:6–13

Squier W, Scheimberg I, Smith C (2011) Spinal nverve root ß-APP staining in infants is not a reliable indicator of trauma. Forensic Sci Int 212:e31–e35

Strassmann G (1949) Formation of hemosiderin after traumatic and spontaneous cerebral hemorrhages. Arch Pathol 47:205–210

Strassmann G, Helpern M (1968) Tödliche Hirnverletzungen im Boxkampf. Dtsch Zschr Gerichtl Med 63:70–83

Stray-Pedersen A, Omland S, Nedregaard B, Klevberg S, Rognum TO (2011) An infant with subdural hematoma and retinal hemorrhages: does von Willebrand disease explain the findings? Forensic Sci Med Pathol 7:37–41

Suárez-Peñanranda JM, Rodríguez-Calvo MS, Ortiz-REy JA et al (2002) Demonstration of apoptosis in human skin injuries as an indicator of vital reaction. Int J Legal Med 116:109–112

Suzuki A, Shiraki K (2001) Tumor cell "dead or alive": caspase and surviving regulate cell death, cell cycle and cell survival. Histol Histopathol 16:583–593

Tao L, Chen X, Qin Z, Bian S (2006) Could NF-kB and caspase-3 be markers for estimation of post-interval of human traumatic brain injury? Forensic Sci Int 162:174–177

Tardieu A (1860) Étude medico-légale sur les sévices et mauvais traitements exercés sur des enfants. Ann d'Hygiène Publ Med Lég 13:361–398

Thom M, Seetah S, Sisodiya S, Koepp M, Scaravilli F (2003) Sudden and unexpected death in epilepsy (SUDEP): evidence of acute neuronal injury using HSP-70 and c-Jun immunohistochemistry. Neuropathol Appl Neurobiol 29:132–143

Thornstedt H, Voigt GE (1960) Tödliche, basale Subarachnoidalblutung nach Trauma. Dtsch Zschr Gerichtl Med 50:254–277

Tomcik MA, Gerig NR, Prahlow JA (2011) Sudden death from ruptured intracranial vascular malformation. Forensic Sci Med Pathol 7:185–191

Tsokos M (2003) Fatal Waterhouse-Friderichsen syndrome due to Ewingella americana infection. Am J Forensic Med Pathol 24:41–44

Tsokos M, Püschel K (2001) Postmortem bacteriology in forensic pathology: diagnostic value and interpretation. Legal Med 3:15–22

Tyagi AK, Willshaw HE, Ainsworth JR (1997) Unilateral retinal haemorrhages in non-accidental injury. Lancet 349:1224

Tyagi AK, Scotcher S, Kozeis N, Willshaw HE (1998) Can convulsions alone cause retinal haemorrhages in infants? Br J Ophthalmol 82:659–660

Uemura K, Harada K, Sadmitsu D, Tsuruta R, Takahashi M, Aki T, Yasuhara M, Maekawa T, Yoshida K (2001) Apoptotic and necrotic brain lesions in a fatal case of carbon monoxide poisoning. Forensic Sci Int 116:213–219

Uhrenholt L, Freeman MD, Webb AL, Pedersen M, Boel LWT (2015) Fatal subarachnoid hemorrhage associated with internal carotid artery dissection from whiplash trauma. Forensic Sci Med Pathol 11:564–569

Unger PD, Song S, Taff ML, Schwarz IS (1984) Sudden death in a patient with von Recklinghausen's neurofibromatosis. Am J Forensic Med Pathol 5:175–179

Unkrig S, Gulotta F, Madea B (2010) Morbus Fahr – considerations on a case of sudden death. Forensic Sci Int 204:e12–e15

Unterharnscheidt F (1970) About boxing: review of historical and medical aspects. Tex Rep Biol Med 28:421–495

Unterharnscheidt F (1975) Injuries due to boxing and other sports. In: Winken PJ, Bruyn GW (eds) Handbook of clinical neurology, vol 23, pp 527–593

Unuma K, Harada K, Nakajima M, Eguchi H, Tsushima K, Ito T, Shintani-Ishida K, Kojima H, Yoshida K (2010) Autopsy report on central pontine myelinolysis triggered by vomiting associated with digoxin intoxicaton. Forensic Sci Int 194:e5–e8

Varchmin-Schultheiß K, Holtz J, Horn M (1990) Waterhouse-Friderichsen-Syndrom im Erwachsenenalter. Beitr Gerichtl Med 48:229–231

Vester MEM, Bilo RAC, Karst WA, Daams JG, Duijst WLJM, van Rijn RR (2015) Subdural hematomas: glutaric aciduria type 1 or abuse head trauma? A systematic review. Forenic Sci Med Pathol 11:405–415

Viitanen M, Johansson K, Bogdanovic N et al (1998) Alzheimer changes are common in aged drivers killed in single car crashes and at intersections. Forensic Sci Int 96:115–127

Vowles GH, Cl S, Cameron JM (1987) Diffuse axonal injury in early infancy. J Clin Pathol 40:185–189

Wang Q, Ishikawa T, Michiue T, Zhu BL, Maeda H (2011) Evaluation of human brain damage in fire fatality by quantification of basic fibroblast growth factor (bFGF), glial fibrillary acidic protein (GFAP) and single-stranded DNA (ssDNA) immunoreactivities. Forensic Sci Int 211:19–26

Wang Q, Ishikawa T, Michiue T, Zhu BL, Guan DW, Maeda H (2012) Quantitative immunohistochemical analysis of human brain basic fibroblast growth factor, glial fibrillary acidic protein and single-stranded DNA expressions following traumatic brain injury. Forensic Sci Int 221:142–151

Waterhouse R (1911) A case of suprarenal apoplexy. Lancet 1:577

Weedn VW, Mansour AM, Nichols MM (1990) Retinal hemorrhage in an infant after cardiopulmonary resuscitation. Am J Forensic Med Pathol 11:79–82

Wehner F, Wehner HD, Subke J, Meyermann R, Fritz P (2000) Demonstration of morphine in ganglion cells of the hippocampus of heroin overdose by means of anti-morphine antiserum. Int J Legal Med 113:117–120

Weiler G, Reinhardt V, Nau HE, Gerhard L (1980) Contribution to intracranial traumatic aneurysm. Z Rechtsmed 85:225–233

Wick R, Byard RW (2006) Mechanisms of unexpected and/or sudden death in Lafora disease. Forensic Sci Int 163:144–147

Woischneck D, Kapapa T, Scheuerle A, Schütze M, Pauli S (2014) Der histologische Nachweis des diffusen axonalen Hirnschadens bei Überlebenden schwerer Schädel-Hirntraumen. Versicherungsmedizin 66:188–192

Wojahn H (1970) Klärung einer Abtreibung mit zentraler Luftembolie nach 4 Jahren. Beitr Gerichtl Med 27:97–100

Yarid NA, Harruff RC (2015) Globus pallidus necrosis unrelated to carbon monoxide poisoning: retrospective analysis of 27 cases of basal ganglia necrosis. J Forensic Sci 60:1484–1487

Zappi E, Zappi M, Breithaupt M, Zugibe FT (1993) Cerebral intraventricular lipoma and sudden death. J Forensic Sci 38:489–492

Index

R. B. Dettmeyer, *Forensic Histopathology*, https://doi.org/10.1007/978-3-319-77997-3

I

The manufacturer's authorised representative in the EU is Springer Nature Customer Service Centre GmbH, Europaplatz 3, 69115 Heidelberg, Germany. If you have any concerns regarding our products, please contact ProductSafety@springernature.com

Printed and bound by CPI Group (UK) Ltd, Croydon, CR0 4YY
15/05/2026
02111380-0006